The Female Athlete

The Female Athlete

Mary Lloyd Ireland, M.D.
Orthopaedic Surgeon and President
Kentucky Sports Medicine Clinic
Lexington, Kentucky
Team Physician for Eastern Kentucky University, Richmond, Kentucky
Team Consultant for Georgetown College, Georgetown, Kentucky
Medical Director for the Women's United Soccer Association (WUSA)
Consultant in Orthopaedic Surgery for
Shriner's Hospitals for Children, Lexington, Kentucky

Aurelia Nattiv, M.D.
Associate Professor
UCLA Department of Family Medicine, Division of Sports Medicine and
Department of Orthopaedic Surgery
Director, UCLA Osteoporosis Center
UCLA School of Medicine
Los Angeles, California
Team Physician, UCLA Department of Intercollegiate Athletics, Los Angeles, California
Volunteer Team Physician, USA Track and Field, USA Gymnastics, and
the United States Olympic Committee [USOC]

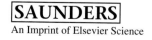
An Imprint of Elsevier Science

SAUNDERS
An Imprint of Elsevier Science

The Curtis Center
Independence Square West
Philadelphia, Pennsylvania 19106

THE FEMALE ATHLETE
Copyright 2002, Elsevier Science (USA). All rights reserved.

ISBN 0–7216–8029–1

Notice

Medicine is an ever-changing field. Standard safety precautions must be followed but as new research and clinical experience broaden our knowledge, changes in treatment and drug therapy may become necessary or appropriate. Readers are advised to check the most current product information provided by the manufacturer of each drug to be administered to verify the recommended dose, the method and duration of administration, and contraindications. It is the responsibility of the treating physician relying on experience and knowledge of the patient, to determine dosages and the best treatment for each individual patient. Neither the publisher nor the author assume any liability for any injury and/or damage to persons or property arising from this publication.

The Publisher

Library of Congress Cataloging in Publication Data

The female athlete / [edited by] Mary Lloyd Ireland and Aurelia Nattiv.
    p. ; cm.
  ISBN 0-7216-8029-1
    1. Sports medicine. 2. Sports injuries. 3. Women–Health and hygiene. I. Ireland, Mary Lloyd II. Nattiv, Aurelia.
    [DNLM: 1. Athletic Injuries. 2. Sports Medicine. 3. Women's Health. QT 261 F3291 2003]
  RC1210 .F365 2003
  617.1′027′082–dc21

2002075772

KI/MBY

Printed in the United States of America.

Last digit is the print number: 9 8 7 6 5 4 3 2 1

Dedication

A book is like a patient. She arrives on crutches. She complains loudly for frequent attention, but responds well to team intervention. So now that this patient has completed its course of treatment and is raring to get back in the race, we can only sit back and watch from the stands. When we hear the starter's pistol, we probably won't say very much, but you know what we'll be thinking: "You go, girl! Run like the wind." We hope the crowd will encourage the athlete and that she remains forever healthy and active. We are happy to get this text out to you. We are listening for your cheers.

We dedicate this book to the future female athlete and exercising female. May she have the opportunities, resources, knowledge, and tools to participate in sport and exercise to enhance her well-being, spirit, and health and may she do so with enjoyment and vitality.

Mary Lloyd Ireland, M.D.
Aurelia Nattiv, M.D.

To my parents who encouraged me to do my very best and to do the right thing. To my husband Wood, for his love and for his counsel. To those mentors, friends, family, and patients who allowed me to learn so much from them. I am truly blessed.

Mary Lloyd Ireland, M.D.

I would like to thank my mentor for many years, James C. Puffer, M.D., for the opportunities, support and friendship he has brought forth to me throughout my career, and Barbara Drinkwater, Ph.D., for her mentorship and example. Many thanks to my husband Joel, my parents, sister, and friends for their encouragement, love, and support that helped make this book a reality.

Aurelia Nattiv, M.D.

Many thanks to Tom Adler, Mark DeMars, Carolyn Large, and Cathy Truda for their technical support.

Contributors

James W. Akin, Jr., M.D.
Assistant Professor
Division of Reproduction Endocrinology
and Infertility
Department of Obstetrics and Gynecology
University of Kentucky College of Medicine
Lexington, Kentucky
Contraception
Hormonal Disorders

James R. Andrews, M.D.
Medical Director
American Sports Medicine Institute
Birmingham, Alabama
Clinical Professor
Orthopaedic and Sports Medicine
University of Virginia
Charlottesville, Virginia
Clinical Professor
Department of Orthopaedics
University of Kentucky Medical School
Lexington, Kentucky
Clinical Professor
Division of Orthopaedic Surgery
University of Alabama Medical School
Birmingham, Alabama
Elbow Injuries

William R. Barfield, Ph.D.
Associate Professor
College of Charleston
Associate Research Professor
Orthopaedic Surgery
Medical University of South Carolina
Charleston, South Carolina
Stress Fractures

Robert R. Bell, M.D.
El Paso Orthopaedic Surgery Group
El Paso, Texas
Hand and Wrist Injuries

Holly J. Benjamin, M.D.
Assistant Professor
Clinical Pediatrics and Surgery
Director, Primary Care Sports Medicine
University of Chicago
Chicago, Illinois
Volleyball

Joseph S. Bird, Jr. M.D.
Associate Professor
Obstetrics and Gynecology, Reproductive
Endocrinology
University of Tennessee at Chattanooga
Chattanooga, Tennessee
Menstrual Dysfunction

Christine M. Bonci, M.S., A.T.,C.
Co-Director
Division of Athletic Training/Sports
Medicine
Intercollegiate Athletics
The University of Texas at Austin
Austin, Texas
Development of Studies and Wellness:
The Texas Experience

William W. Briner, Jr., M.D.
Assistant Professor
Family Practice
University of Illinois at Chicago
Sports Medicine Fellowship Director
Lutheran General Hospital
Park Ridge, Illinois
Volleyball

William H. Brooks, M.D.
Chief of Neurosurgery
Cental Baptist Hospital
Lexington, Kentucky
Head and Neck Injuries

Douglas W. Brown, M.D.
Orthopaedic Association of Portland
Portland, Maine
Head Team Physician
US Women's National Soccer Team
Soccer

J. W. Thomas Byrd, M.D.
Assistant Clinical Professor
Department of Orthopaedics and
Rehabilitation
Vanderbilt University School of Medicine
Nashville Sports Medicine and Orthopaedic
Center
Nashville, Tennessee
Equestrian

Lisa R. Callahan, M.D.
Assistant Professor of Medicine
Cornell University Medical College
Medical Director
Women's Sports Medicine Center
Hospital for Special Surgery
New York, New York
  The Female Athlete Triad

T. Jeff Chandler, Ed.D., C.S.C.S., FACSM
Associate Professor and Chairman
Division of Exercise Science, Sports, and
Recreation
Marshall University
Huntington, West Virginia
  Racquet Sports

Cindy J. Chang, M.D.
Head Team Physician
Departments of Intercollegiate Athletics and
University Health Services
University of California, Berkeley
Berkeley, California
Assistant Clinical Professor
Department of Family and Community Medicine
University of California, San Francisco (UCSF)
San Francisco, California
Assistant Clinical Professor
Department of Family and Community
Medicine
University of California, Davis (UC Davis)
Davis, California
  The Physically Challenged Athlete

Jeffrey S. Christian, M.D.
Lakewood Obstetrics and Gynecology Inc.
Lakewood, Ohio
  Pregnancy: Physiology and Exercise
  Return to Activity Postpartum

Stefanie Schupp Christian, M.D.
Lakewood Obstetrics and Gynecology Inc.
Lakewood, Ohio
  Pregnancy: Physiology and Exercise
  Return to Activity Postpartum

Ellen J. Coleman, M.A., M.P.H., R.D.
Nutrition Consultant
The Sport Clinic
Riverside, California
  Sports Supplements and Ergogenic Aids

Scott Crook, P.T., C.S.C.S.
Director of Physical Therapy
Perimeter Physical Therapy Associates
Certified Strength and Conditioning Specialist
National Strength and Conditioning
Association
Lexington, Kentucky
  Rehabilitation Concerns–Lower Extremity
  Upper and Lower Extremity Strength
  Training

Leigh Ann Curl, M.D.
Assistant Professor
Department of Orthopaedic Surgery
Johns Hopkins Bayview Medical Center
Team Physician
Baltimore Ravens
Baltimore, Maryland
  Basketball

Carolyn Newton Curry, Ph.D.
Former Instructor in Women's Studies
University of Kentucky
Lexington, Kentucky
  The Impact of the Female Athlete: From
  Sojourner to Tegla

**George J. Davies, M.Ed., P.T., S.C.S.,
A.T.C., C.S.C.S.**
Professor
Physical Therapy
University of Wisconsin–Lacrosse
Graduate Physical Therapy Program
Director
Clinical and Research Services
Gundersen Lutheran Sports Medicine
Lacrosse, Wisconsin
  Evaluation of Strength

Lauren Bari Davis, B.A.
Research Assistant
Department of Obstetrics and Gynecology
Columbia College of Physicians and
Surgeons
New York, New York
  Updates in Exercise-Associated Amenorrhea
  and Leptin

Kathleen J. DeBoer, B.A., M.B.A.
Senior Associate Athletics Director
University of Kentucky
Lexington, Kentucky
  Optimizing Performance in Team Sports for
  Female Athlete

Katherine L. Dec, M.D.
Medical Director
Mind/Body Medical Institute Bon Secour
Richmond
An affiliate of Beth Israel Deaconess and
Harvard Medical University
Private Practice
Richmond, Virginia
  The Physically Challenged Athlete

John P. DiFiori, M.D.
Associate Professor and Chief
Division of Sports Medicine
UCLA Department of Family Medicine
UCLA School of Medicine
Team Physician, UCLA Department of
Intercollegiate Athletics
Los Angeles, California
Softball

Sandra A. Eisele, M.D.
Consultant
Cincinnati Bengals
Miami University of Ohio
Director
Dance Medicine
Cincinnati Ballet
Past President
Wellington Orthopaedic and Sports Medicine
Cincinnati, Ohio
Foot and Ankle Injuries

Wade F. Exum, M.D., M.B.A.
Former Director of Drug Control
Administration
US Olympic Committee
Colorado Springs, Colorado
Substance Abuse

Gerald A. M. Finerman, M.D.
Professor and Chair
UCLA Department of Orthopaedic Surgery
UCLA School of Medicine
Head Team Physician
UCLA Department of Intercollegiate Athletics
Los Angeles, California
Pelvis and Hip Injuries

Renata J. Frankovich, M.D.
University of Ottawa
Sport Medicine and Physiotherapy Centre
Ottawa, Ontario, Canada
Cycling and In-Line Skating

Peter G. Gerbino, II, M.D.
Instructor in Orthopaedic Surgery
Harvard Medical School
Assistant in Orthopaedic Surgery
Division of Sports Medicine
Children's Hospital
Boston, Massachusetts
Thoracic and Lumbar Injuries

Diane L. Gill, Ph.D.
Professor
Department of Exercise and Sport Science
Area–Social Psychology of Sport and Exercise
University of North Carolina at Greensboro

Greensboro, North Carolina
*Social and Psychological Aspects of Athletic
Participation*

Ann C. Grandjean, Ed.D., R.D.
Executive Director
The Center for Human Nutrition
Omaha, Nebraska
Nutrition

W. David Hager, M.D., FACOG
Professor
Department of Obstetrics and Gynecology
University of Kentucky
Director
Affiliated University of Kentucky Residency
Training Program
Central Baptist Hospital
Athletic Consultant
University of Kentucky
Women's Teams
Private practice
Women's Care Center
Lexington, Kentucky
Gynecologic Problems
Sexually Transmitted Diseases

Sharon L. Hame, M.D.
Assistant Professor
UCLA Department of Orthopaedic Surgery
UCLA School of Medicine
Attending Physician, UCLA Medical Center
Attending Physician, Santa Monica–UCLA
Medical Center
Attending Physician, West Los Angeles Veterans
Administration Hospital
Team Physician, UCLA Department of
Intercollegiate Athletics
Los Angeles, California
Pelvis and Hip Injuries

Jo A. Hannafin, M.D., Ph.D.
Associate Professor of Orthopaedic Surgery
Weill Medical College of Cornell University
Orthopaedic Director
Women's Sports Medicine Center
Hospital for Special Surgery
Team Physician, US Rowing
Team Physician, WUSA New York Power
New York, New York
Rowing

Suzanne S. Hecht, M.D.
Assistant Professor
UCLA Department of Family Medicine
Division of Sports Medicine and Department
of Orthopaedic Surgery
UCLA School of Medicine

Team Physician, UCLA Department of
Intercollegiate Athletics
Los Angeles, California
Anemia

Susan K. Hillman, M.S., M.A.
Director
Human Anatomy
Associate Professor
Physical Therapy
Arizona School of Health Sciences
Mesa, Arizona
Sport-Specific Rehabilitation Program

William H. Hindle, M.D.
Professor Emeritus
Department of Obstetrics and Gynecology
University of Southern California
Keck School of Medicine
Los Angeles, California
The Breast: Disorders and Injury

Robert J. Homm, M.D., FACOG
Clinical Faculty
Department of Obstetrics and Gynecology
University of Kentucky School of Medicine
Chairperson
Department of Obstetrics and Gynecology
Central Baptist Hospital
Lexington, Kentucky
Director
Fertility and Endocrine Associates
Lexington/Louisville, Kentucky
Fertility

Timothy M. Hosea, M.D.
Clinical Associate Professor
Department of Orthopaedic Surgery
UMDNJ Robert Wood Johnson Medical School
New Brunswick, New Jersey
Chair–Sports Medicine and Research
Committee
US Rowing
Indianapolis, Indiana
Rowing

Robert G. Hosey, M.D.
Assistant Professor
Family Medicine
Associate Director
Primary Care Sports Medicine Fellowship
University of Kentucky
Lexington, Kentucky
Softball

Mark R. Hutchinson, M.D.
University of Illinois at Chicago
Director

Sports Medicine Services
Associate Professor
Orthopaedics and Sports Medicine
University of Illinois at Chicago
Chicago, Illinois
Cheerleading
Knee Injuries
Rehabilitation Concerns–Lower Extremity

Mary Lloyd Ireland, M.D.
President, Kentucky Sports Medicine
Lexington, Kentucky
Team Physician
Eastern Kentucky University
Richmond, Kentucky
Consultant in Orthopaedic Surgery
Shriner's Hospitals for Children
Lexington, Kentucky
Medical Director
Women's United Soccer Association (WUSA)
Epidemiology of Injuries—Section 2 High
School and Collegiate
Knee Injuries
Participation and Historical Perspective—
Section 2 High School and Collegiate
Rehabilitation Concerns–Lower Extremity
Shoulder Injuries

Elizabeth Joy, M.D.
Clinical Associate Professor
Department of Family and Preventive Medicine
Director
University of Utah/TOSH Primary Care
Sports Medicine Fellowship
University of Utah
Team Physician
University of Utah
Salt Lake City, Utah
Cardiac Concerns

David M. Joyner, M.D.
Former Vice-Chairperson
Orthopaedic Surgical Department
Harrisburg Hospital
Harrisburg, Pennsylvania
Former Chairman
USOC (US Olympic Committee)
Sports Medicine Committee
Colorado Springs, Colorado
Present member
USOC Sports Medicine Advisory
Committee
US Olympic Committee
Colorado Springs, Colorado
Olympic Sports
Winter Sports: Skiing, Speed Skating, Ice
Hockey

Ariella Kelman-Sherstinsky, M.D.
Fellow, Division of Immunology and
Rheumatology
Stanford University Hospital
Palo Alto, California
The Female Athlete Triad

W. Ben Kibler, M.D.
Medical Director
Lexington Clinic Sports Medicine Center
Lexington, Kentucky
Racquet Sports
Soft Tissue Injuries

Mandy Kimball, M.S., P.T., A.T.C.
American Sports Medicine Institute
Birmingham, Alabama
Rehabilitation Concerns–Upper Extremity

Joseph M. Lane, M.D.
Professor of Orthopaedic Surgery
Weill Medical College of Cornell University
Chief, Metabolic Bone Disease Service
Hospital for Special Surgery
New York, New York
Osteoporosis

John A. LeBlanc, D.O.
Orthopaedic Surgeon
Grand River Hospital District
Rifle, Colorado
Shoulder Injuries

Scott M. Lephart, Ph.D., A.T.C.
Associate Professor and Chairperson
Department of Sports Medicine and
Nutrition
University of Pittsburgh
Director
Neuromuscular Research Laboratory
UPMC Center for Sports Medicine
Pittsburgh, Pennsylvania
Upper and Lower Extremity
Proprioception Testing and Practical Use

Barney F. LeVeau, Ph.D., P.T.
Professor
Department of Physical Therapy
Alabama State University
Montgomery, Alabama
Biomechanical Considerations

Beven P. Livingston, M.S., P.T., A.T.C.
Ph.D. candidate: Neuroscience
Emory University
Atlanta, Georgia
Racquet Sports

Robert M. Malina, Ph.D.
Director, Institute for the Study of Youth Sports
Professor of Physical Education and Exercise
Science
Department of Kinesiology
Michigan State University
East Lansing, Michigan
*Performance in the Context of Growth and
Maturation*

Terry R. Malone, Ed.D., P.T., A.T.C.
Director
Department of Physical Therapy
University of Kentucky
Chandler Medical Center
Professor of Physical Therapy
University of Kentucky
Lexington, Kentucky
Evaluation of Strength

Bert R. Mandelbaum, M.D.
Fellowship Director
Santa Monica Orthopaedic Research and
Education Foundation
Team Physician
US Soccer
Team Physician Pepperdine University
Santa Monica, California
Soccer

David A. Mattingly, M.D.
New England Baptist Bone and Joint Institute
Chestnut Hill, Massachusetts
*Total Hip and Knee Arthroplasty in Active
Women*

Angus M. McBryde, Jr., M.D.
Professor
Sports Medicine and Orthopaedic Surgery
Clinical Professor
Orthopaedic Surgery
University of South Carolina School of
Medicine
Columbia, South Carolina
Stress Fractures

John R. McCarroll, M.D.
Clinical Assistant Professor
Department of Orthopaedics
Indiana University School of Medicine
Indianapolis, Indiana
Golf

Frank C. McCue, III, M.D.
Alfred R. Shands Professor of Orthopaedic
Surgery and Plastic Surgery of the Hand
Director

Division of Sports Medicine and Hand Surgery
Team Physician
Department of Athletics
University of Virginia School of Medicine
Department of Orthopaedics
Charlottesville, Virginia
Hand and Wrist Injuries

James A. McGregor, M.D., C.M.
Visiting Professor
Cedars Sinai Medical Center
Obstetrics and Gynecology
University of California, Los Angeles
Los Angeles, California
Practitioner, Obstetrics
Tucson, Arizona
Pregnancy: Physiology and Exercise
Return to Activity Postpartum

William C. McMaster, M.D.
Attending, St. Joseph Hospital
Clinical Professor
Department of Orthopaedic Surgery
University of California Irvine
Irvine, California
Swimming and Diving

Jordan D. Metzl, M.D.
Medical Director
The Sports Medicine Institute for Young Athletes
Assistant Professor, Department of Pediatrics
Cornell Medical College
New York, New York
Growth and Development

Lyle J. Micheli, M.D.
Director, Division of Sports Medicine
Associate in Orthopaedic Surgery
Department of Orthopaedic Surgery
Division of Sports Medicine
Boston Children's Hospital
Associate Clinical Professor
Orthopaedic Surgery
Harvard Medical School
Boston, Massachusetts
Thoracic and Lumbar Injuries

Jean A. Miles P.T., A.T.C., C.S.C.S
Skaneateles, New York
Women's Field Hockey and Lacrosse

Julie Moyer-Knowles, Ed.D., A.T.C., P.T.
University of Delaware
Lecturer
Newark, Delaware
Thomas Jefferson University
Philadelphia, Pennsylvania
Partner, HealthSouth Sports Medicine and
Rehabilitation Center

Wilmington, Delaware
Founding Member
Delaware Women's Alliance for Sports Fitness
Fencing

Aurelia Nattiv, M.D.
Associate Professor
UCLA Department of Family Medicine
Division of Sports Medicine and
Department of Orthopaedic Surgery
UCLA School of Medicine
Director
UCLA Osteoporosis Center
Team Physician
UCLA Department of Intercollegiate Athletics
Los Angeles, California
The Female Athlete Triad

Duc T. Nguyen, M.D.
Private Practice
Cleveland, Tennessee
Hand and Wrist Injuries

Susan M. Ott, D.O.
Orthopedic Surgeon
Co-Director Sports Medicine
Guthrie Clinic
Sayre, Pennsylvania
Gymnastics

John D. Perrine, M.D.
Associate Clinical Professor of Medicine
University of Kentucky
Past President of Staff
Central Baptist Hospital
Lexington, Kentucky
Preparticipation Physical Examination

Joan M. Price, B.A., B.S.N., R.N.
Senior Manager and Acting Director
National Anti-Doping Program
US Olympic Committee
Colorado Springs, Colorado
Substance Abuse

Margot Putukian, M.D.
Director
Primary Care Sports Medicine
Penn State University
University Park, Pennsylvania
Associate Professor
Hershey Medical Center
Department of Orthopaedics and
Rehabilitation
Hershey, Pennsylvania
Second Vice President
American Medical Society for Sports Medicine
Soccer

Russalind Ramos, M.D.
Associate Researcher
Department of Obstetrics and Gynecology
Columbia University
New York, New York
*Updates in Exercise-Associated Amenorrhea
and Leptin*

Kristin J. Reimers, M.S., R.D.
Associate Director
The Center for Human Nutrition
Omaha, Nebraska
Nutrition

Cheryl Riegger-Krugh, Sc.D., P.T.
Associate Professor
Physical Therapy Program
University of Colorado
Health Sciences Center
Denver, Colorado
Biomechanical Considerations

Susan L. Rozzi, Ph.D., A.T.,C.
Assistant Professor
Department of Physical Education and Health
Director
Athletic Training Education Program
College of Charleston
Charleston, South Carolina
*Upper and Lower Extremity
Proprioception Testing and Practical Use*

Jaime Ruud, M.S., R.D.
Nutrition Link Consulting, Inc.
Lincoln, Nebraska
Nutrition

Jack B. Ryan, M.D.
Private Practice
St. John Macomb Hospital
Orthopaedic and Sports Medicine
Warren, Michigan
Epidemiology of Injuries—Section 1 West Point

Randa Ryan, Ph.D.
Associate Athletics Director
University of Texas at Austin
Austin, Texas
*Development of Studies and Wellness: The
Texas Experience*

Marc R. Safran, M.D.
Associate Professor
Department of Orthopaedic Surgery
Co-Director Sports Medicine
University of California, San Francisco
San Francisco, California
Racquet Sports

Joseph S. Sanfilippo, M.D.
Professor
Obstetrics, Gynecology, and Reproductive
Sciences
The University of Pittsburgh School of
Medicine
Vice Chairman, Reproductive Sciences
Magee-Women's Hospital
Pittsburgh, Pennsylvania
Menstrual Dysfunction

Cynthia A. Slater, M.A.
Manager
Department of Information Resources
US Olympic Committee
Colorado Springs, Colorado
*Participation and Historical
Perspective–Section 1 Olympic*

Angela D. Smith, M.D.
Associate Professor, Clinical Faculty
Department of Orthopaedics
University of Pennsylvania
Attending faculty
The Sports Medicine and Performance
Center
Children's Hospital of Philadelphia
Philadelphia, Pennsylvania
Figure Skating

Susan L. Snouse, A.T.C.
Professional Staff
Peachtree Orthopaedic Clinic
Atlanta, Georgia
USOC Sports Medicine
Colorado Springs, Colorado
*Track and Field
Winter Sports: Skiing, Speed Skating, Ice
Hockey*

Dennis B. Sprague, Ph.D.
Adjunct Professor
University of Kentucky
Lexington, Kentucky
*Psychology and Motivation of the Female
Athlete*

Carol A. Stamm, M.D.
Assistant Professor
Department of Obstetrics and Gynecology
University of Colorado Health Sciences Center
Staff Physician
Denver Health Medical Center
Denver, Colorado
*Pregnancy: Physiology and Exercise
Return to Activity Postpartum*

Jennifer A. Stone, M.S., A.T.C.
Monument, Colorado
  Participation and Historical Perspective—
  Section 1 Olympic
  Judo and Taekwondo

Sabrina M. Strickland, M.D.
Sports Medicine and Shoulder Fellow
Hospital for Special Surgery
New York, New York
  Growth and Development

Jorunn Sundgot-Borgen, Ph.D.
Professor
Department of Physical Activity and Health
The Norwegian University of Sport and the
Olympic Training Centre
Oslo, Norway
  Disordered Eating

Carol C. Teitz, M.D.
Professor
Department of Orthopaedics and Sports
Medicine
University of Washington
Team Physician
University of Washington Huskies
Seattle, Washington
  Dance

Kenneth B. Tepper, M.D.
Orthopaedic Surgeon
Advanced Centers for Orthopaedic Surgery
and Sports Medicine
Owings Mills, Maryland
  Shoulder Injuries

Geoffrey J. Van Flandern, M.D.
Assistant Professor
Tufts University Medical School Staff Surgeon,
New England Baptist Bone and Joint Institute
New England Baptist Hospital
Boston, Massachusetts
  Total Hip and Knee Arthroplasty in Active
  Women

Michelle P. Warren, M.D.
Professor

Department of Medicine and Obstetrics and
Gynecology
Columbia College of Physicians and Surgeons
Medical Director
Columbia-Presbyterian Medical Center
Center for Menopause, Hormonal Disorders,
and Women's Health
New York, New York
  Updates in Exercise-Associated Amenorrhea
  and Leptin

James A. Whiteside, M.D.
Professor of College Health and Human
Services
HealthSouth Scholar in Sports Medicine
Athletic Team Physician
Troy State University
Emeritus Director of Medical Aspects of Sports
Medicine
HealthSouth
Birmingham, Alabama
  Elbow Injuries

Kevin E. Wilk, P.T.
National Director, Research and Clinical
Education
HealthSouth Rehabilitation and Sports
Medicine
Birmingham, Alabama
Adjunct Assistant Professor
Physical Therapy Program
Marquette University
Milwaukee, Wisconsin
  Rehabilitation Concerns–Upper Extremity

Richard I. Williams, M.D.
Head Team Physician
Tennessee Technical University
Cookeville, Tennessee
Member, American Orthopaedic Society for
Sports Medicine
  Knee Injuries

Leisure Yu, M.D., Ph.D.
Associate Professor
Department of Orthopaedics
Loma Linda University Medical Center
Loma Linda, California
  Figure Staking

Foreword

The year of the publication of *The Female Athlete* represents 30 years since Congress passed Title IX of the Education Amendments Act, ensuring equal opportunity for females to participate in organized sports. Over these last three decades, sports participation for females has grown exponentially. Today, women in sport symbolize health, strength, and endurance. They are considered great role models, are respected by society, and are even able to pursue professional opportunities and endorsements. Young girls often aspire to be great female athletes.

With this increasing participation of women in sport and exercise, a heightened level of knowledge regarding medical and orthopaedic concerns of the female athlete has emerged. Sports medicine research specific to the female athlete has become an *in vogue* area of study and interest among orthopaedic and primary care sports medicine circles.

Differences that exist between boys and girls, men and women socially, psychologically, and physiologically need to be understood and stud-

ied by sports medicine physicians and health care providers who work with the active and athletic female. We must continue to emphasize the important benefits of exercise, fitness, and sport for females of all ages, and educate parents, athletes, administrators, and health care providers to these important messages. The potential risks of participation need to be further explored and educational efforts to prevent these risks implemented.

This comprehensive book on the female athlete addresses the latest in research and clinical practice relating to the multifaceted medical, psychological, social, nutritional, orthopaedic, and rehabilitative concerns of the female athlete. I challenge all of you to educate yourselves and others in these areas and to continue to expand the field of women's sports medicine through sound research and clinical application.

Donna Lopiano, Ph.D.
Executive Director
Women's Sports Foundation
East Meadow, New York

Contents

The Female Athlete

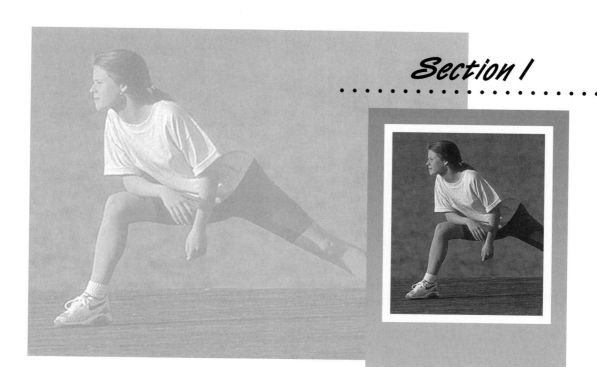

History of Female Athletic Participation

Chapter 1

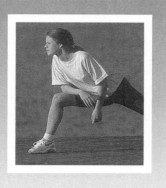

The Impact of the Female Athlete
FROM SOJOURNER TO TEGLA

Carolyn Newton Curry, Ph.D.

As we enter the 21st century, it is the best time in history to be born female. In the last 100 years, more progress has been made in the lives of women than was achieved in all the years prior to 1900. Women now have political, social, educational, and economic opportunities that were denied them for centuries. However, these rights are not enjoyed equally around the world, but slowly—far too slowly in some nations—change for women is beginning to be felt. Even in those countries where freedom is restricted, women are seeing examples of strong women who have taken advantage of opportunities and who serve as role models to their nation. Very often these pioneers are female athletes. One such woman is a Kenyan, only 4 feet 11 inches tall and weighing 82 pounds, named Tegla Laroupe. She can run the marathon, the longest and most grueling event in international track, at a speed once undreamed of for a woman.

On April 19, 1998, Laroupe astounded the world of athletics by running the Rotterdam Marathon in 2 hours 20 minutes and 47 seconds, smashing the world record that had stood for 13 years. When she was interviewed, she said she had begun running at the age of 6 when she ran 6 miles to and from school with books strapped on her back. Naturally gifted, but very hard working as well, she soon began entering competitions and winning. Her many victories have inspired great pride in her countrymen. They were especially proud of the marathon record since she was the first African woman to hold the record. But when she won at Rotterdam, she pointed out, "For me it was a long struggle, especially since women from my country have a difficult time breaking through. When I was racing for the record, I focused on what I'd gone through. It was such hard work."[1]

Tegla's victory, televised on TV in Kenya, has made her a national heroine. But she has also had an impact on my life and me. Being an his-torian of women, I have followed Laroupe's career with great interest. But there has been the added dimension that I saw her attempt her first marathon on the same day my 27-year-old daughter, Kristin, attempted her first marathon—the New York Marathon in 1994. Tegla Laroupe, an internationally renowned, world-class runner, and Kristin Curry, an amateur from Atlanta, Georgia, came from two vastly different worlds and had almost nothing in common, but that day they were both beneficiaries of the changes that have occurred in this century to open opportunities for female athletes to compete.

The events of that marathon weekend came to symbolize much more than they might have normally. They afforded me the opportunity to reflect on the history of women in general; but more specifically, I reflected on my life and my daughter's life. My husband, Bill Curry, played professional football for 10 years and was a professional or college coach for 22 years. Our son, Billy, played almost every competitive sport growing up and finished his playing years in football at the University of Virginia. Season after season I have shouted my encouragement to them through more exciting games than I can remember, but the New York Marathon was the first big athletic event I had attended to cheer for my daughter, Kristin. After all, she is a female athlete and sports have traditionally provided far fewer opportunities for women than men.

I grew up in the late 1940s and 1950s and never knew what it was like to be a member of a team, or play a competitive sport. My high school had one women's sport, basketball, which provided places for only a few. I was a cheerleader. Girls watched and cheered while boys played. I regret never learning to compete or knowing the joy of challenging my mind and body as an athlete.

In my adult life my interest in running was stirred quite accidentally. When my husband, Bill, was in training for football I would go to the track with him and sit in the stands and watch as he ran round and round the field. When I grew bored one day, I decided I would see if I could run around the track without stopping. When I learned that was one fourth of a mile, I tried another lap and then another. A few years later, in my thirties, a mother of 2 young children, I ran a 13.1-mile half marathon and finally felt the joy of athletic achievement.

Running, especially for women, was just catching on in the United States. In those days, I can recall hearing the debate about whether women had the ability to run the marathon in the Olympic games. There was a strong argument against it. Skeptics argued women's bodies were not suited to run 26 miles. The distance was simply too difficult for women's weaker bodies. Some argued the marathon could kill women. I remember how thrilled I was in 1984 when the petite Joan Benoit won the first Women's Olympic Marathon in the heat of Los Angeles. She was anything but weak and fragile. After Benoit's exciting victory my interest in the marathon, the ultimate physical challenge, continued and it was the one event in the Olympic games I never missed watching.

Why have women not been encouraged to join teams and compete the same way men have? Furthermore, why have we historically had fixed attitudes about what males and females can and cannot do? I have spent the last 25 years trying to understand the history of women and their dilemma in the modern world. What can we learn from the past and how can that knowledge help us understand the status of women in our present society? What has been myth and folklore? What has been reality?

Our country was founded in the late 17th and early 18th centuries by hard-working, devout people who believed very strongly in a hierarchy of beings. God was at the top of the chain. Men were subservient to God, and women subservient to men. This chain of being was not questioned by the vast majority of people. When a literal interpretation of the Bible was combined with English Common Law, the resulting system negated the legal existence of women. Because a woman was one with her husband, she was supposedly protected by his legal rights and required none of her own. A married woman could not make a contract, nor could she sue or be sued. She could not own property and she could not own her own wages in the rare incidence that she had any sort of wage. Since most professions were closed to women, she did not very often earn wages independent of her husband. She did not even have legal guardianship of her children, who could be willed away from her at her husband's death. She was a jural minor along with children and slaves. In the colonial period there were some rare occasions when single female property owners voted, but it was assumed to be a male privilege.

Women's primary role in life was to have children and remain in the private, domestic sphere. She did not participate in politics or business, because her mind was not suited for such activity. Education was considered dangerous and could hurt her reproductive powers. In 1645 the governor of Massachusetts Bay, John Winthrop, wrote of the madness of one Mistress Hopkins, a godly woman,

who was fallen into a sad infirmity, the loss of her understanding and reason . . . by occasion of her giving herself wholly to reading and writing, and had written many books . . . . For if she had attended her household affairs, and such things as belong to women, and not gone out of her way and calling to meddle in such things as are proper for men whose minds are stronger etc. she had kept her wits, and might have improved them usefully and honorably in the place God had set her.[2]

ANATOMY DETERMINED DESTINY

The female was the weaker sex and Puritan girls were given names to remind them of their limitations: Silence, Patience, Prudence, Mindwell, and even Fear. Women were to be submissive, pious, and obedient.

When the constitution of the United States was written, there was no mention of women. Despite the admonition of Abigail Adams to her husband, John, to "Remember the Ladies, and be more generous and favourable to them than your ancestors," women were given no rights whatsoever.[3] Women were not citizens of the New Republic. Only white male property owners had the vote.

The great debate of the 19th century centered on the rights of white women and African-American slaves, both male and female. Early in the struggle, women's issues became enmeshed with the abolitionist movement. Working in the background of the antislavery movement, white women in the northern United States began to identify with African-American slaves. Along with male and female slaves, white women began to see that they were chattel, too.

In 1848 the first women's rights convention was held in Seneca Falls, New York. Led by Lucretia Mott, Elizabeth Cady Stanton, and Lucy Stone, the women wrote a "Declaration of Sentiments" using the Declaration of Independence as a model. They simply inserted "women" in the Declaration so that it read, "We hold these truths to be self-evident: that all men and women are created equal; that they are endowed by their creator with certain inalienable rights; that among these are life, liberty and the pursuit of happiness."[4] After much debate, the ex-slave, Frederick Douglass, persuaded the women to include the "first right of a citizen, the elective franchise" in their document. It was a radical idea because it would take women from the private sphere and thrust them into the public world of politics.

One of the most famous women of the 19th century, Sojourner Truth, spoke out about the injustices to women and particularly the injustices of slavery against African-American women. A former slave and a Quaker, she was in attendance at a women's rights convention in 1851 in Akron, Ohio. A large meeting of theologians, abolitionists, and interested women debated whether women should have the same rights as men. One theologian voiced the sentiments of the 19th century that women were weak and needed to be cared for by men. His remarks did not ring true for Sojourner and she was moved to speak. Frances Gage, a woman in attendance at this meeting, left the only account of this famous speech: A "profound hush" fell over the audience as Sojourner, 6 feet tall, with "head erect and eyes piercing" began,

But what's all this talking about? That man over there says that women need to be helped into carriages, and lifted over ditches and to have the best place everywhere. Nobody ever helps me into carriages or over mud puddles or gives me any best place! (And raising herself to her full height, and her voice to a pitch like rolling thunder she asked) And ain't I a woman?

Look at me! Look at my arm! (and she bared her right arm to the shoulder, showing her tremendous muscular power). I have ploughed and planted, and gathered into barns, and no man could help me! And ain't I a woman? I could work as much and eat as much as man—when I could get it—and bear the lash as well! And ain't I a woman? I have born thirteen children and seen them most all sold off to slavery and when I cried out with my mother's grief, none but Jesus heard me! And ain't I a woman?[5]

Sojourner's colorful, blistering attack on the thinking of the day ended with thunderous applause. Her life personified what some women already knew: women had always done hard physical work. Despite the fact women gave birth, their bodies were not weak, but physically strong.

Sojourner and other men and women of like mind traveled all over the country trying to convince people of the need for change. Progress was slow, but gradually state legislatures passed laws guaranteeing property rights for married women and guardianship of children, and in 1920 the Susan B. Anthony Amendment was passed, giving women the right to vote.

In the 20th century great strides have been made by women. Life expectancy was only 49 years at the turn of the century. Between 1910 and 1925, 350,000 women died in childbirth—a number equal to that of men who died in battle from the Revolution to World War I. But because of birth control and progress in medicine, women rarely die in childbirth today and life expectancy has risen to 79 years.

Likewise, women have gained full access to education. Today women earn more professional degrees than ever before, and virtually all professions are open to women. The Equal Rights Amendment, which guaranteed "equality of rights under the law" for women, was passed by Congress in 1972, but it fell short of ratification by 3 states. The rights that women have today are protected primarily by Title VII of the Civil Rights Act of 1964 and legal victories based on the "due process" clause of the Fourteenth Amendment. Despite the problems of unequal pay, inadequate childcare and the ever-present glass ceiling, women are making progress toward equality in the work place.

In the field of athletics, we are just now beginning to see what women can do. Science is now telling us that perhaps women's bodies are better suited than men's for some athletic events requiring flexibility and endurance, such as gymnastics and long-distance running. Today the best female athletes can run, swim, and skate faster that the top male athletes of a few decades ago. Studies have shown that since 1964, women's marathon times have dropped 32% while men's have dropped only 4.2%. If this progress continues, some have even suggested that world-class female runners could possibly catch up with male runners in the 21st century.[6] More time and research are needed to discover just how far and fast women can go.

CONCLUDING REMARKS

As I stood and watched as thousands of women finished the 1994 New York Marathon, I was excited about what the women had accomplished. A total of 29,535 men and women ran the marathon. Of the 7728 first-time marathoners that day, over 50% were women. But the most amazing thing about the race was that the female winner was a first-time marathoner, Tegla Laroupe. She was 21 years old at the time and won the women's race in 2 hours 27 minutes and 37 seconds. On that day she was also the first black-African female to win a major marathon. I was so happy for the many women, my daughter included, who were doing something they had once been told women could not do—and they were doing it well!

Kenya, an African country famous for the marathon success of its men, heaps lavish resources on them, but actively discourages women from running. Despite these obstacles, Tegla was determined to run. As Tegla accepted her award for winning, she said, "I was not expecting to win. It was my first time."[7] But win she did.

What will happen when countries give women the resources, the encouragement, and the expectation of winning? Only time will tell what female athletes will accomplish in the years ahead. No longer referred to as the weaker sex, women are getting stronger and faster every day. I look forward to seeing what strong, confident women will be able to achieve in the future.

Around the world more young women are flocking to soccer fields, softball diamonds, basketball courts, swimming pools, and running tracks in numbers far greater than ever before in history. Televised events give young women role models in formerly male-dominated sports. Professional leagues have formed that finally give women a way to make a living and still play their sport. The vast majority of women will continue to play just for the exhilaration and sense of well-being athletics gives them.

In 1998 when Tegla Laroupe set the new world record for the marathon, one reporter asked her if, since she had become such a heroine to Kenyans, would she someday consider going into politics. She replied, "Maybe, if I can do something to help the women."[8] But like her forerunner, Sojourner Truth, she does not have to go into politics to help women. Her example of hard work and dedication has already spoken to women around the world and told them that maybe they can do something special, too.

As this book goes into print, it is fitting to note that a new world record in the women's marathon has been set by another woman from Kenya. On October 7, 2001 Catherine Ndereba ran the Chicago Marathon in 2 hours 18 minutes and 47 seconds exactly 2 minutes faster than Tegla's record. No doubt this young woman was inspired to follow in the footsteps of Tegla and prove that we have only begun to discover what the female athlete can accomplish.

References

1. Gambaccini P: Simply smashing. Runner's World, July 1998, Vol. 33, No. 7, p 78.
2. Norton MB (ed): Major Problems in American Women's History: Documents and Essays. Lexington, Mass, D.C. Heath, 1989, p 21.
3. Levin PL: Abigail Adams. New York, St. Martin's Press, 1987, p. 82.
4. Norton, p 203.
5. Ibid, p 205. [Original dialect and spelling have been changed to modern usage.]
6. Ehrenreich B: The real truth about the female body. Time, March 8, 1999, Vol. 153, No. 9, p 58.
7. Thomas Robert McG Jr: Kenyan runs far away from doubts. The New York Times, November 7, 1994, p D1.
8. Gambaccini, p 78.

Chapter 2

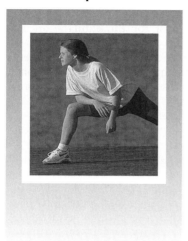

Participation and Historical Perspective
Section 1   OLYMPIC

Cynthia A. Slater, M.A.
Jennifer A. Stone, M.S., A.T.,C.

April 6, 1896: The opening ceremony of the Games of the I Olympiad. Over 200 athletes from 14 countries participated in the opening of the first Olympic Games of the modern era. None were female.

September 15, 2000: The opening ceremony of the Games of the XXVII Olympiad in Sydney, Australia. Australian Cathy Freeman bears the Olympic torch, celebrating the Olympic spirit and marking 100 years of women's participation at the Olympic Games.

Women have participated in all but the first of the modern Olympic Games. They don't participate in the same numbers as their male peers and they don't compete in the same number of events as the men. But, as the steady growth of female competitors and events indicates, women are as driven and as fiercely competitive as male athletes. Their desire to excel and win is not diminished by their gender.

The inclusion of women's events on the Olympic program has been a long but rewarding struggle (Tables 2-1 and 2-2). The founder of the modern Olympic Games, Pierre de Fredy, Baron de Coubertin, like many of his contemporaries, believed that " . . . the Olympic Games must be reserved for men . . . ".[3] As vital as de Coubertin's ideals are to the Olympic movement, this one could not withstand the growing need of women to compete in the Games. Each successive International Olympic Committee (IOC) Executive Board has labored to review and add events that would increase women's presence in the Games. The program for the 1996 Olympic Games, held in Atlanta, included 26 sports, and women competed in 21 of those sports. Women's weightlifting and modern pentathlon, as well as trampoline,

Table 2-1. Participants in the Olympic Games, 1896–2000

YEAR	WOMEN	MEN
1896	0	245
1900	15	1206
1904	6	681
1908	36	1999
1912	57	2490
1920	77	2591
1924	136	2956
1928	290	2724
1932	127	1281
1936	328	3738
1948	385	3417
1952	518	4407
1956	384	2958
1960	610	4738
1964	683	4457
1968	781	4750
1972	1058	6065
1976	1247	4781
1980	1125	4092
1984	1567	5230
1988	2186	6279
1992	2708	6659
1996	3684	7060
2000	4254	6862

water polo, hammer, pole vault, tae kwon do, triathlon, sailing 49er class, trap and skeet shooting, and synchronized swimming duet were included in the 2000 Olympic Games in Sydney, Australia.

ANCIENT OLYMPIC GAMES

Archaeological evidence tells us that women were present at the ancient Olympic Games, but they did not participate in the events.[16]

Table 2-2. Participants in the Olympic Winter Games, 1924–2002

YEAR	WOMEN	MEN
1924	13	281
1928	26	468
1932	21	274
1936	80	675
1948	77	636
1952	109	623
1956	132	686
1960	143	521
1964	200	986
1968	211	1081
1972	206	1015
1976	231	900
1980	233	837
1984	274	1000
1988	313	1110
1992	488	1318
1994	523	1313
1998	815	1489
2002	886	1513

Sculptures, paintings, and documents recovered from ancient Greece suggest that young virgins could watch the competitors, as could the woman designated the priestess of the goddess Demeter. The priestess was actually a honorary position periodically awarded to a "noble and moneyed" woman, who then took her place on a small white marble altar located on one side of the stadium. There is also the often-repeated story of Kallipateira, a woman who dressed herself as a male trainer in order to watch her son compete. She accidentally revealed herself while rejoicing at his success. She was spared the decreed punishment, a death sentence, because she was the daughter, wife, and mother of Olympic champions.[5]

But neither Kallipateira, the priestess of Demeter, nor the young virgins actually participated in the Olympic Games. When women wanted to demonstrate their athletic prowess, they had to go elsewhere. The festival best recorded among the women's competitions was the Heran Games.[16] Instituted in honor of the goddess Hera, the Heraia were held every 4 years and consisted of a foot race for the competitors. Accounts of the race indicate that the Heraia was structured on an age-group principle, with participants separated into 3 age groups. Winners' names were inscribed on commemorative tablets that would later be mounted on the columns of the Heraion.[6]

Records from 3 other pan-Hellenic festivals reveal women victors. A trio of sisters, Trifose, Hedea, and Dionysia, were listed among the individual winners in the Isthmian, Pythian, Nemean, Sicyonian, and Asclepian Games.[6] However, information is scant regarding whether or not these women competed against men or if they competed in a separately held event.

As difficult as information about the ancient Olympic Games is to find, it is that much more difficult to uncover specifics about women's participation in these, and other, athletic events. However, it is clear, even from the minimal records, that women included sports and athletic activities in their daily lives.

MODERN OLYMPIC GAMES

Commitment to the revival of the Olympic Games came from the delegates of the "Paris International Athletic Congress" held at the Sorbonne in June 1894.[10] Called together to discuss problems inherent in amateur athletics, these delegates unanimously agreed to support de Coubertin's dream—to re-establish an international competition for the best of the amateur sportsmen. De Coubertin's dream did not include women. He was opposed to women participating in the Games from the very beginning, through his long tenure as president of the International Olympic Committee, and long after his retirement. In one way or another, he used then-popular theories to support nonparticipation: the female body is controlled by nerves rather than muscles, children run the risk of being left motherless, order and decorum at events would be completely destroyed, and, of course, it's not "natural."[8]

Fortunately, not all of de Coubertin's peers agreed with him. The support of some IOC members, combined with a growing women's reform movement, convinced the French Organizing Committee to include 2 women's events—tennis and golf—on the program for the 1900 Olympic Games.[15]

Eleven women, from the United States, France, and Great Britain, registered to compete in the 2 events, with Charlotte Cooper, of Great Britain, becoming the first woman medallist by winning both the singles and mixed-doubles titles in tennis. Margaret Abbott, of the United States, followed a few months later with a win in the golf championship. Abbott's mother, Mary, finished seventh in the same competition.[14]

The Olympic Games of 1904 produced another woman champion; Lida Howell won 3 gold medals in the archery event, the only event open to women in 1904. She and 7 other women competed as members of the Cincinnati and Washington, DC, archery clubs.[15]

Both the 1900 and 1904 Olympic Games were held in conjunction with the Paris and St Louis World's Fairs, respectively. The events of the Olympic Games were staged over several months, and, at times, were not clearly distinguished from the events of the World's Fair. Scholars continue to debate just which events were "official" Olympic events and which were not. Hence, the important step taken by the organizers of the 1908 Olympic Games.

After a tenuous and worrisome start, the Olympic Games were on the verge of becoming the powerful separate entity of which de Coubertin dreamed. The organizing committee of the 1908 Games declared 3 "official" events for women: tennis, archery, and figure skating. In addition to the official sports, 4 new events were demonstrated to the audience: swimming, diving, fencing, and team gymnastics. Thirty-six women from 4 countries competed in London. Unfortunately, the United States was not among the 4, the American Olympic Committee having decided to not send any women competitors.

They still had not changed their minds in 1912, the first year women's swimming was added to the program (for an excellent review of the machinations involved in this decision, see the 1974 dissertation by Leigh[8]). In addition to the swimming events, women also competed in tennis and diving. Team gymnastics was again a crowd-pleasing demonstration sport. One other sport, the 3-day equestrian event, was open to women, though none registered. In all, 57 women vied for the gold in Stockholm.

The Olympic Games held between the 2 World Wars included more women athletes competing in more events. But this slow increase did not occur without a struggle. One of the key players in the struggle was the Federation Sportive Feminine Internationale (FSFI). The FSFI was formed in Paris, in 1921, to counteract the International Amateur Athletic Federation's (IAAF) decision to not support women's track and field. FSFI, headed by Frenchwoman Alice Milliat, organized the First Women's Olympic Games in 1922. The Women's Games, undergoing various name changes, continued for 3 more quadrenniums. The success of these games, combined with savvy negotiations by Madame Milliat, forced the IAAF and the IOC to review their lackadaisical approach to women's participation in the Olympic Games.[11] The FSFI's dedication to women's sports helped to ensure a permanent and growing Olympic program for women.

The Olympic Games of 1920, held in Antwerp, Belgium, saw the hoisting of a new Olympic flag, the taking of a new athlete's oath, and 64 female competitors.[13] Finally, this contingent included an "official" women's team from the United States. In 1914, the Amateur Athletic Union (AAU) reversed its previous decision and became a champion of women's athletics.[8] With their support, the American Olympic Committee fielded a women's team to the 1920 Games. The 1936 Olympic Games were privileged to host 328 women, competing in 5 sports. Introduced during this era were fencing, team gymnastics, and various events on the swimming and track and field program. Tennis was dropped from the program after the 1924 Olympic Games.

The Games of 1924 also marked the first separately competed Olympic Winter Games. Women did participate in these Games and in each Olympic Winter Games held since. The pattern of slow growth established in the Summer Games is mirrored by the women's program for the Winter Games. Until the 1936 Winter Games in Garmish-Partenkirsch, Germany, when alpine skiing was added, only figure skating was open to women.

This era produced legendary athletes like Mildred "Babe" Didrikson, who stunned the athletic community with her versatility and her commitment to excellence; Gertrude Ederle, winner of 3 swimming medals in 1924 and, in 1926, the first woman to swim the English Channel; Lira Radke, holder of the world record in the 800-meter run for 16 years; and Sonja Henie, winner of 3 consecutive gold medals in women's figure skating.

However, even the legendary stars had to struggle to participate. Women's teams were assigned chaperons, regardless of their age, housed hours away from the competition venues, and patronized in press reports. Erroneous reports of collapsing competitors spurred the IOC to ban women from races longer than 200 meters, a ban that lasted almost 32 years.[15] By IOC rules, Didrikson was limited to 3 events, even though she qualified in 5; and, Eleanor Holm, a 1932 gold medallist, was forced to watch the 1936 swimming events after being removed from the team for behavior considered unfit for a female competitor.[1] Great steps forward had been made during this era, but, clearly, there were still great steps left to be made.

The next 20 years witnessed the addition of only one women's sport, volleyball, to the Summer Games program, although several events in swimming, track and field, and gymnastics were included. Women's cross-country skiing, speed skating, and luge were added to the Olympic Winter Games program. Women's athletics benefited from the politics of the Cold War, which brought a strong sense of nationalism to the Olympic Games. In the drive to increase medal counts, the United States Olympic Committee (USOC), the AAU, and the National Amateur Athletic Federation (NAAF) combined forces to promote and support women's sports programs in both the academic and community setting.[15]

The Olympic Games of 1948 were held in London and marked the return, amazing at that time, of Fanny Blankers-Koen. Amazing because, since her first appearance in the 1936 Olympic Games, Blankers-Koen had married and given birth to 2 children. In 1948, she entered 4 of the 9 women's track and field events and won gold in each.[2] Of the 385 women competing in London, Blankers-Koen emerged as the best proof of women's dedication and commitment to athletic excellence. Two new alpine events—downhill and slalom—were introduced at the Olympic Winter Games held in St Moritz, Switzerland. An American, Gretchen Fraser, won the downhill and a Swiss, Heidy Schlunegger, won the slalom. Seventy-seven women participated in the alpine skiing and figure skating events that year.

1952 heralded the entrance of the Soviet athletes to both the Summer and Winter Games. Of the 109 women entered in the Olympic Winter Games, 20 competed in the inaugural 10-kilometer cross-country race. A record 518 women competed in the Summer Games, which were marked by Soviet dominance in gymnastics, track and field, and swimming. These Summer Games marked the first female equestrian athletes; 4 women entered the individual dressage, competing directly against men. Lis Hartel, of Denmark, won the silver medal. She repeated this victory in 1956, the same year that Patricia McCormack successfully defended her 1952 victories in platform and springboard diving. The decreased turnout of only 384 women athletes at the 1956 Games probably reflected the difficult travel arrangements necessary to attend the Games in Melbourne, Australia.[7]

However, an increased number of women, 109, participated in the 1952 Olympic Winter Games, held in Oslo, Norway. Spectators watched the first American skier to win 2 medals in an Olympic Winter Games, Andrea Mead Lawrence. Another first took place in 1956; Cuilana Minuzzo, of Italy, was the first woman to take the athletes' oath on behalf of all competitors.

Little expansion of the women's program took place in 1960 and 1964. Fencing, kayaking, and volleyball were new sports added, while events such as the 800-meter (track and field) and the 4×100-meter medley relay (swimming) were included on the Summer Games program.

Winter athletes could add luge and speed skating to their selections. There were 610 women athletes in Rome in 1960 and 683 women in Tokyo in 1964. The number of women athletes participating in the Winter Games also grew from 144 in Squaw Valley, Idaho, in 1960 to 200 in Innsbruck, Austria, in 1964.

The program may not have expanded much, but performances were setting records. Wilma Rudolf won 3 gold medals in 1960, while Lairs Latynina won 6 medals in gymnastics, a performance she repeated in 1964. Lydia Skobilkova won all 4 women's speed skating events in Innsbruck.

If the 20 years between 1948 and 1968 were slow-growth years, then the next 20 years could be considered explosive. In 1968, the IOC Executive Board reached a consensus of opinion that favored the expansion of the women's program.[9] This agreement marked the beginning of a sincere effort by the IOC to convince sports federations to expand opportunities for women within their respective sports. Beginning in 1976, several new sports were added to the program, including rowing, team handball, basketball, field hockey, cycling, table tennis, tennis, and judo. Also added during this time were new events within the sport disciplines, including the marathon, the soloing class in sailing, the 20-kilometer cross-country skiing race, and the 5000-meter speed-skating event. The return of archery and the addition of several mixed competitions (in shooting, equestrian, and sailing) expanded opportunities to new levels. Women immediately took advantage of the new opportunities: 781 women competed in the 1968 Olympic Games; 2186 competed in 1988.

The Olympic Games of 1968, held in Mexico City, marked the first time a woman was selected to light the Olympic flame and the first time a woman lead the United States contingent, carrying the American flag. Americans dominated the swimming events, winning 11 of 14 possible gold medals. For the first time, women competed against men in shooting events.

One athlete of the 1299 women competing in 1972 emerged as a crowd favorite: Olga Korbut. Her winning combination of athleticism, flexibility, and determination spurred a world-wide renewed interest in gymnastics. Korbut was succeeded by Nadia Comaneci in 1976, raising women's gymnastics to a new pinnacle of performance and popularity.[2] The East German women's team dominated track and field, swimming, and rowing, setting a precedent they would continue for many years. In the 1976 Summer Games, 1251 women competed, setting yet another record for attendance.

By 1980, *boycott* was not a new word within the Olympic movement. For a variety of political and nationalistic reasons, individual countries had boycotted the Olympic Summer Games of 1976, 1964, and 1956.[7] But the withdrawal of the United States from the 1980 Olympic Games in Moscow created the largest void of participants to date. In all, over 60 nations boycotted the 1980 Games, hurting the level of competition. In turn, 14 Eastern bloc countries boycotted the Games of the 23rd Olympiad, held in Los Angeles in 1984. Although the playing field was much more level, the lack of Soviet, Cuban, or East German athletes was felt by all competitors.

On the positive side, these 2 Olympic Games offered more events for women athletes than any previous Games. Field hockey was added in 1980 and 13 new events were added in 1984. Years of lobbying for long-distance races finally paid off with the inclusion of the women's marathon in 1984. Also included in these Olympic Games was cycling, one of the first sports in which women participated at the turn of the century. Over 1500 women participated in the 75 events held during the 1984 Games, a record that was broken at the very next Olympic Games in Seoul, Korea, in 1988. More than 2100 women athletes converged in Seoul, many to compete in 5 new women's events. The standout performer of these Games was Florence Griffith Joyner, who took home 4 medals, 3 gold and 1 silver. Her sister-in-law, Jackie Joyner-Kersee, set a world record in the heptathlon, establishing her as one of the world's best all-around athletes.

The 20 years from 1968 to 1988 saw limited growth opportunities for women wishing to compete at the Olympic Winter Games. The number of competitors rose each year, but only slightly—211 women participated in the 1968 Winter Games in Grenoble, France, and 313 in the 1988 Winter Games in Calgary, British Columbia, Canada. New events were added in 1976, 1984, and 1988, bringing the total to 17 events in 5 sports. Nevertheless, there were some outstanding performances. Peggy Fleming invigorated the figure-skating world with a dynamic and graceful gold-medal performance. Diane Holum tied for the silver in the 500-meter speed-skating event in 1968, then won the gold in the 1500-meter in 1972. Sheila Young joined an elite club of athletes by winning 3 medals in speed skating, after winning a world championship in cycling. Sonja Henie's long-standing record of figure-skating titles was tied by Irina Rodnina, when she won the gold in the pairs competition.[15] Jane Torvill, with partner Christopher Dean, electrified the audience with a perfect score for their ice dance interpretation of Ravel's Bolero. A Finnish cross-country skier, Marja-Liisa Haemaelaeinen, won 3 individual gold medals and a team bronze. Bonnie Blair began her domination of women's speed skating with a gold and a bronze in 1988.

The Olympic Games of the closing decade of this century have featured, and will continue to feature, more sports and events for women athletes. New events on the Olympic Winter Games program for 1992 and 1994 included biathlon, short-track speed skating, mogul skiing, and aerial skiing. The 1992 Olympic Winter Games were hosted by Albertville, France; 488 women competed. The number increased to 521 in Lillehammer, Norway, 2 years later. 1994 was the inaugural year of a separate cycle for the Olympic Winter Games, which will be held every 4 years, alternating every 2 years with the Olympic Summer Games.

Bonnie Blair continued her winning streak in 1992, bringing home 2 more medals, and, in 1994, became the leading US women's gold medalist. Raissa Smetanina, a Russian cross-country skier, became the most decorated Winter Games athlete with a total of 10 Olympic medals.[4] Lillehammer audiences witnessed the outstanding performance of Manuela Di Centa, an Italian cross-country skier, as she won a medal in each of the 5 cross-country events.

The Olympic Games of 1992 were held in Barcelona, Spain, and were the first Olympic Games, for decades, not marred by boycotts. A record number of athletes participated: 9367, of whom 2708 were women. Although no single athlete dominated these Games, performances by Krisztina Egerzegi, Shannon Miller, Tatyana Gutsu, and Summer Sanders will be remembered by all who watched.

The Atlanta Olympic Games in 1996 featured 21 sports available to over 3700 female athletes. The 2000 Olympic Games in Sydney marked the 100th anniversary of women's participation in the Olympics. More women than ever before competed in the Sydney 2000 Olympics, which included 8 new women's events. At the 2002 Olympic Winter Games in Salt Lake City, women's bobsled, skeleton, and cross-country ski sprints were added to the Games, thus leaving only 2 sports—nordic combined and ski jumping—without female events. One hundred years of struggle have brought triumph.

In addition, at the initiative of the IOC Executive Board, all National Olympic Committees and national and international governing bodies filled at least 10% of their decision-making bodies with women. This percentage should increase to at least 20% by 2005.[12]

Section 2 HIGH SCHOOL AND COLLEGIATE

Mary Lloyd Ireland, M.D.

Participation in high school sports continues to increase. Growth in female sports exceeds that in male sports. According to the National Federation of State High School Associations, for the 1999–2000 season, 3,861,749 males and 2,675,874 females participated in high school athletics, and coed participation totaled 19,289 (Table 2-3). The top 10 high school sports for males and females are listed in Table 2-4. For sports in which both males and females compete, the numbers of participants are as follows: basketball, 541,130 males and 451,600 females; track, 480,791 males and 405,305 females; and soccer, 330,044 males and 270,273 females. The athletics participation survey summary shows that the numbers have consistently grown since recording began in 1971 (Table 2-5). The number of boys participating in 1971 was 3,666,917 and the number of girls, 294,015. The most recent (1999–2000) survey of participants found 3,861,749 boys and 2,675,874 girls.

Growth also may be expressed as a ratio; in 1970, the male:female ratio was 12.5:1, in

Table 2-5. National Federation of State High School Associations 1999–2000 Athletics Participation Summary Survey Totals

YEAR	BOY PARTICIPANTS	GIRL PARTICIPANTS
1971	3,666,917	294,015
1972–73	3,770,621	817,073
1973–74	4,070,125	1,300,169
1975–76	4,109,021	1,645,039
1977–78	4,367,442	2,083,040
1978–79	3,709,512	1,854,400
1979–80	3,517,829	1,750,264
1980–81	3,503,124	1,853,189
1981–82	3,409,081	1,810,671
1982–83	3,355,558	1,779,972
1983–84	3,303,599	1,747,346
1984–85	3,354,284	1,157,884
1985–86	3,344,215	1,807,121
1986–87	3,354,082	1,836,356
1987–88	3,425,777	1,849,684
1988–89	3,416,844	1,839,352
1989–90	3,398,192	1,858,659
1990–91	3,406,355	1,892,316
1991–92	3,429,853	1,940,801
1992–93	3,416,389	1,997,489
1993–94	3,472,967	2,130,315
1994–95	3,536,359	2,240,461
1995–96	3,634,052	2,367,936
1996–97	3,706,225	2,474,043
1997–98	3,763,120	2,570,333
1998–99	3,832,352	2,652,726
99–2000	3,861,749[a]	2,675,874[a]

[a]Total does not include a portion of 19,289 participants in combined sports.

Table 2-3. Total Participation by High School Athletes, 1999–2000

MALES	3,861,749	(59%)
FEMALES	2,675,874	(41%)
COED	19,289[a]	
	6,537,623	

[a]Combined sports.

Data compiled by the National Federation of State High School Associations.

1985–1986, 1.9:1, and in 1999–2000, 1.4:1 (Fig. 2-1). Further information regarding a particular state is available from the National Federation of State High School Associations (NFHS, PO Box 20626, Kansas City, Mo 64195; www.nfhs.org). Summaries of athletic participa-

Table 2-4. Top 10 High School Sports, 1998–1999

MALES		FEMALES	
Football	1,002,734	Basketball	451,600
Basketball	541,130	Track & field	405,305
Track & field	480,791	Volleyball	382,755
Baseball	451,701	Fast-pitch softball	343,001
Soccer	330,044	Soccer	270,273
Wrestling	239,105	Tennis	159,740
Cross-country	183,139	Cross-country	154,021
Golf	165,857	Swimming & diving	138,475
Tennis	139,507	Competitive spirit squads	64,319
Swimming & diving	86,640	Field hockey	58,372
	3,620,648 (94%)		2,427,861 (91%)

Data compiled by the National Federation of State High School Associations.

Table 2-6. 1999–2000 Collegiate Participants (NCAA) by Division, All Sports

MALES		FEMALES	
Division I	85,812	Division I	62,802
Division II	45,288	Division II	29,519
Division III	79,889	Division III	57,865
TOTAL	210,989	TOTAL	150,186

Total numbers include "emerging sports," ie, rowing and squash for men and ice hockey, squash, synchronized, swimming, and water polo for women.

tion by state and numbers of schools and participants for each sport are available from the National Collegiate Athletic Association (NCAA, PO Box 6222, Indianapolis, Ind 46207; www.ncaa.org). The number of athletes in each state is also available from the NCAA. Information regarding a particular state can also be obtained through the state high school athletic association.

At the collegiate level, the NCAA keeps statistics on the number of competitors in each of 3 divisions. In 1999–2000, the total numbers of participants for all sports were 210,989 males and 150,186 females (Table 2-6).[17] Figure 2-2 presents graphically the growth of participation by males and females since 1989. One can see from this graph that, excluding male partici-

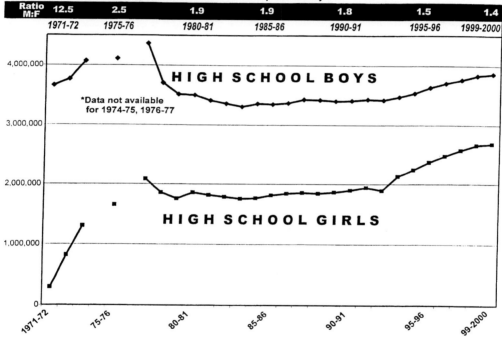

Figure 2-1. High school athletic participation, 1971–2000. (From the National Federation of State High School Associations Participation Survey. Kansas City, Mo.)

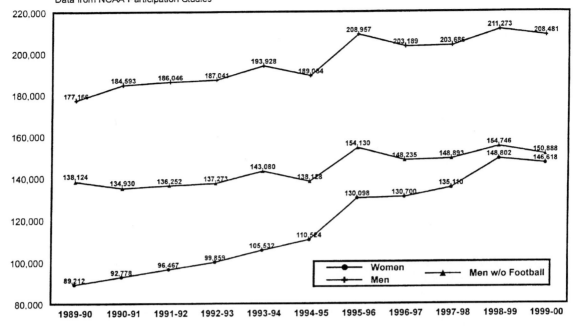

Figure 2-2. Total number of college athletes, 1989–2000. (Data from NCAA Participation Studies. NCAA, Indianapolis, Ind.)

pation in football, equality of participation was achieved in 1998.

References

1. Associated Press and Grolier: Pursuit of Excellence: The Olympic Story. Danbury, Conn, Grolier Enterprises, 1979, p 160.
2. Blue A: Faster, higher, further: Women's triumphs and disasters at the Olympics. London, Virago, 1988, pp 47–54.
3. Davenport J: Women's sports—the Olympics. Olympian 5:16, 1979.
4. Davies L: The results of the XVII Olympic Winter Games in Lillehammer. Olympic Rev 317:153,178, 1994.
5. Durantz C: Women at Olympia II. The cursed judgement. Olympic Rev 103/104:296–300, 1976.
6. Durantz C: Women at Olympia. 1. The Heran Games. Olympic Rev 101/102:171–5, 1976.
7. Kamper E, Mallon B: The golden book of the Olympic Games. Milan, Vallardi & Associati, 1992, p 627.
8. Leigh MH: The evolution of women's participation in the Summer Olympic Games, 1900–1948 [Dissertation]. Columbus, Ohio, Ohio State University, 1974, pp 55–90.
9. Lekarska N: The entry marathon of the second sex. Olympic Rev 275/276:457, 1990.
10. MacAloon JJ: This Great Symbol. Chicago, University of Chicago Press, 1981, p 166.
11. Segrave J, Chu D: Olympism. Champaign, Ill, Human Kinetics, 1981, p 77.
12. Sotelo J (ed): Highlights of the week's Olympic news. Lausanne, International Olympic Committee, 179:1, 1995.
13. United States Olympic Committee: Legacy of Gold. Clearwater, Fla, Rococo International, 1992, pp 86–89,117.
14. Welch P: Shrouded Olympic achievements. In Fitzgerald A (ed): Olympic education: breaking ground for the 21st century. Proceedings of the USOA XIII, Evergreen State College, Colorado Springs, Colo. US Olympic Committee, 1990, pp 47–53.
15. Wollum J: Outstanding women athletes, who they are and how they influenced sports in America. Phoenix, Oryx Press, 1992, pp 32–65.
16. Yalouris N: The Olympic Games in Ancient Greece. Athens, Greece, Ekdotike Athenon SA, 1976, p 108.
17. National Collegiate Athletic Association: NCAA Injury Surveillance System. NCAA, Indianapolis, Ind, 1999–2000.

Chapter 3

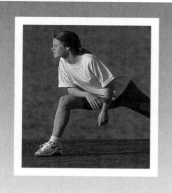

Epidemiology of Injuries
Section 1   WEST POINT

Jack B. Ryan, M.D.
(Colonel [retired], Medical Corps, US Army)

Following the creation of the all-volunteer military force in 1972, women interested in joining noncombat military specialties as officers were admitted to Reserve Officer Training Corps (ROTC) and Officer Candidate School (OCS) programs. Military physical training programs were modified to make women's training programs as challenging as those required for men. Initially, training was segregated by gender. However, by 1975 women soldiers were integrated with their male counterparts in training and barracks living. In 1975 women in the Armed Services totaled 75,000, the highest number of any nation in the world.

On October 8, 1975, President Gerald Ford signed into law a modification of Chapters 403, 603, and 903 of the United States Code, Title 10. This law directed the Secretaries of the Army, Navy, and Air Force to appoint, train, educate, and commission in the noncombat arms women at the nation's military academies. The Secretary of the Army, Bo Calloway, indicated that female cadets would be admitted to the United States Military Academy with no change in the present admissions standards except those minimum essential adjustments demanded by physiologic differences. This "single-track" program in military duties, leadership, and education ensured that the mission of the United States Military Academy would remain "the preparation of each graduate for progressive and continued development through a career as an officer of the Regular Army."

The physical requirements and training standards at West Point exceed those of the active Army. The standards were refined over the first 175 years of this all-male military college. "Project 60," performed early in 1976 as reported by Tomasi and coworkers, attempted to answer questions about training injuries associated with rigorous physical activities performed by female volunteer high school seniors.[12] After having 3 participants fail the medical examination, and 2 drop out early secondary to leg pain during initial fitness testing, the 58 remaining women completed the training. Reported injuries were related primarily to overuse (shin splints, anterior knee pain, muscle strains, tendinosis, and blisters). Participants scoring highest on the initial fitness test had no or fewer injuries compared to less-fit individuals. Since the project utilized training techniques similar to those for cadet basic training, the leadership at West Point felt confident that women could safely participate in training beginning in 1976.

In July 1976, 119 women and 1366 men entered West Point as freshman candidates for the Class of 1980. The initial summer training program included daily running, calisthenics, military parade training, individual military skills training, organized daily athletics, and progressively lengthening road marching. By the end of the training, 102 women and 1228 men completed the mandatory 10-mile march with full combat gear, becoming full members of the Corp of Cadets. Protzman reviewed the medical records and fitness scores from this initial class.[9] Women had lower scores on the physical aptitude examination, although the difference was thought to be physiologic since the test measured upper-body strength, leg strength, and power endurance. Hospital records indicated an incidence of stress fractures of 1% (12 of 1220) in men and 10% (10 of 102) in women. Twenty-five percent of women were withheld from training by the eighth week of summer training because of physical limitation as compared to 5% of men. Hospital records demonstrated 25% of female cadets were admitted for illness as compared to 7% of male cadets. Injury admissions were only slightly higher for women at 3.9% as compared to those for men, which were 2.5%. During the ensuing academic year, however, data from intramural, club and intercollegiate teams indicated that men and women showed an equal loss of practice or game time when identical sports were compared.

Over the next few summer training cycles modifications were made to the program. Running shoes were substituted for combat boots during daily distance and conditioning runs. A regimented prearrival training program was mailed to each new cadet candidate 3 months prior to summer training. Following an initial fitness test, cadets were placed in 3 different groups according to run times. Over the course of summer training the pace of each of these groups was gradually increased. Shorter cadets (men and women) were assigned to the front ranks during marching, thus setting the stride. A review of the Class of 1990 during summer training in 1986 indicated an incidence of stress fracture of 0.5% for men and 5.1% for women.[14]

During the mid 1980s a computerized medical surveillance system was developed at the United Stated Military Academy. Any West Point cadet unable to participate fully in activities (military formations and training, physical education, and varsity club or intramural athletics) must obtain a cadet excusal form that lists the diagnosis and duration of limited activities. Data from each excusal are entered into a computerized injury record using a predetermined injury vocabulary agreed upon by all physicians, physicians' assistants, and therapists. Orthopaedic sick call is held Monday through Friday at 6:30 AM in the cadet health center and 5:00 PM at the intramural and varsity training rooms. Injured cadets must attend physical therapy in lieu of extracurricular activities. Return to full activities requires a change or termination of profile by the orthopaedic surgeon or physical therapist. Although not impossible, it is difficult for injured cadets to avoid diagnosis and treatment.

McBride and coworkers performed a retrospective analysis of illness and injury data in randomly selected cadets of the Class of 1992 (74 women and 74 men) from July 1988 until June of 1991.[7] The results indicated that women had a higher incidence of overuse injuries (stress fracture, 0 males, 11 females; shin splints, 3 males, 10 females; patellofemoral pain syndrome, 5 males, 18 females). The lack of any stress fractures in the selected male group was attributed to selection bias. From this review the investigators found that men and women were excused on average an equal amount of time for similar diagnoses. One exception was low back pain, where men were excused for an average of 4 weeks as opposed to 2 weeks for women. More men (4) than women (1) sustained anterior cruciate injuries during the study period, although men had a greater exposure to contact sports.

Table 3-2. Required and Elective Athletic Activities

ACTIVITY	MEN	WOMEN	COED
DPE classes (required)			
Boxing	x		
Swimming			x
Gymnastics			x
Wrestling	x		
Self-defense		x	
Combatives			x
Intramurals (required)			
Basketball			x
Football	x		
Team handball			x
Racquetball			x
Wrestling/boxing	x		
Area hockey			x
Wallyball			x
Swimming			x
Flickerball			x
Cross-country			x
Softball	x		
Lacrosse	x		
Corps squad (varsity)			
Baseball	x		
Basketball	x	x	
Cross-country	x	x	
Football	x		
150-lb football	x		
Gymnastics	x	x	
Hockey	x		
Lacrosse	x		
Soccer	x	x	
Softball		x	
Swimming	x	x	
Tennis	x	x	
Track	x	x	
Wrestling	x		
Volleyball		x	
Powerlifting	x	x	
Club sports			
Crew	x	x	
Cycling	x	x	
Fencing	x	x	
Judo	x	x	
Karate	x	x	
Lacrosse		x	
Marathon	x	x	
Rugby	x		
Skiing			
Nordic	x	x	
Alpine	x	x	
Volleyball	x		
Team handball	x	x	

Table 3-1. Distribution of the Study Population

	WOMEN	MEN
Volunteered	133	136
Withdrew from study	7 (5%)	14 (10%)
Withdrew from Academy	42 (31%)	28 (21%)
Available for study	84 (63%)	94 (69%)

Between June 1989 and May 1993 a prospective study was approved and performed to document traumatic and overuse injuries.[13] Of 144 female cadet candidates at the military academy in July 1989, 133 volunteered for participation in this study. Of 150 male cadet candidates selected randomly, 136 volunteered and signed informed consent. Table 3-1 documents the composition of the final study group. The cadets were interviewed on a regular basis (approximately every 6 months) by the study team. Medical records were reviewed for accuracy and correlated with entries into the computerized medical data records during these review periods. Withdrawal from the study was defined as no data provided for 24 months.

During summer training women and men trained together in a "single-track" program involving basic military skills, endurance activities, and strength training (road marches, unit runs, and calisthenics). During the academic year women are expected to meet Army Fitness Standards and the traditional standards of the Academy in all physical education training except boxing, wrestling, and contact sports.

Table 3-2 demonstrates the similarities and exceptions by gender of activities at West Point during the academic year.

Table 3-3 presents average physical parameters of the study population. Aerobic fitness is indicated by the run times in the 2-mile fitness test over the course of the study. As these data indicate, this is a select population of highly fit, college-age students who met preadmission physical fitness and medical standards required by the Academy.

There were 664 injuries over 47 months involving the extremities and back (316 occurred in males and 328 in females). Table 3-4 demonstrates the frequency of injury by gender and location.

During the study there were 421 traumatic injuries (254 in men and 167 in women). Shoulder injuries were 3 times more frequent in men (Table 3-5). Knee, ankle, and foot traumatic injuries were more frequent in men and consistent with greater participation in contact sports, more aggressive free-time activities, and perhaps more risk taking. There were four anterior cruciate ligament injuries in both men and

Table 3-3. Average Physical Parameters

DATE	AUG 1989	AUG 1990	AUG 1991	AUG 1992
Height (cm)				
Women	167±0.7	167±0.7	167±0.7	168±0.7
Men	179±0.7	180±0.7	180±0.7	180±0.7
Body weight (kg)				
Women	60±0.9	63±0.9	62±0.9	62±0.9
Men	74±0.8	76±0.8	77±0.8	79±0.8
Body fat (%)				
Women	24.8±0.41	25.7±0.40	25.4±0.41	24.8±0.41
Men	13.6±0.38	14.5±0.38	15.2±0.38	16.1±0.40
2-mile run (min)				
Women	16.5±0.17	15.2±0.17	15.3±0.17	15.1±0.17
Men	13.3±0.16	13.2±0.16	13.1±0.16	13.0±0.16

Table 3-4. Injuries by Location and Gender

	MEN	WOMEN
Shoulder	53	16
Arm	2	3
Elbow, forearm	5	9
Wrist	12	7
Hand	25	22
Pelvis/hip	10	20
Thigh	14	15
Knee	61	69
Leg	21	37
Ankle	41	47
Foot	50	68
Back	22	25

Table 3-5. Traumatic Injuries by Gender

	MEN	WOMEN
Shoulder	51	14
Arm	2	2
Elbow, forearm	4	6
Wrist	12	5
Hand	25	19
Pelvis/hip	9	11
Thigh	12	13
Knee	50	28
Leg	8	8
Ankle	39	24
Foot	21	12
Back	21	25

Table 3-6. Most Common Traumatic Injuries in Men

	NUMBER	AVERAGE DAYS EXCUSAL
Sprain	89	32
Strain	46	15
Contusion	32	10
Fracture	24	45
Subluxation/instability	25	50
Spider bite	10	10
Torn meniscus/labrum	10	65
Dislocation	8	11
Closed head injury/concussion	7	12
Back pain	7	27
Abrasion	7	4
Bursitis traumatic	7	20

Table 3-7. Most Common Traumatic Injuries in Women

	NUMBER	AVERAGE DAYS EXCUSAL
Sprain	57	22
Strain	51	16
Contusion	32	13
Fracture	16	50
Instability/subluxation	10	30
Back pain	9	15
Abrasion	7	4
Spider bite	5	4
Traumatic bursitis	3	18
Closed head injury	3	8

women, representing an injury rate in men of 4.3% and an injury rate in women of 4.8%. The incident and excusal times for the most common traumatic injuries are presented in Tables 3-6 and 3-7.

There were 223 overuse injuries in this study (62 in men and 167 in women) (Table 3-8). The vast majority involved the lower extremities (Table 3-9). Women had significantly more overuse injuries. The most common overuse injuries are presented in Tables 3-10 and 3-11. There were 8 stress fractures in women (10%) and 2 in men (2%).

Table 3-8. Overuse Injuries by Gender

	MEN	WOMEN
Shoulder	2	2
Arm	0	1
Elbow, forearm	1	3
Wrist	0	2
Hand	0	3
Pelvis/hip	1	9
Thigh	2	2
Knee	11	41
Leg	13	29
Ankle	2	13
Foot	29	56
Back	1	0

During the study men and women performed together in a "single-track" military training program for 6 weeks during 4 consecutive summers (1989–1992). The first and second summers are extremely demanding physically. During the third summer most cadets are assigned to military units for training in the United States and overseas. During the fourth year cadets are placed in leadership roles training the first- and second-year cadets. The fourth-year cadets are expected to lead by example, performing all activities, including daily rigorous fitness training. Summer traumatic injuries are listed in Table 3-12. Over the 4 summers the average summer traumatic injury rate was 9 injuries per 100 cadets per month training. The rates were similar for men and women and were highest during the second summer (26 injuries/100 cadets/month training). The average summer overuse injury rate was 6.0/100 male cadets/month training and 14.1/100 female cadets/month training. The summer overuse injury rate changed over the course of the study (Tables 3-13 and 3-14).

During the course of this study the number of days required for adequate rehabilitation of either overuse or traumatic injuries (excusal time—number of days of limited activity) was similar for both genders for traumatic and overuse injuries.

Table 3-9. Most Common Overuse Injuries in Men

	NUMBER	AVERAGE DAYS EXCUSAL
Tendinitis	12	10
Ingrown toenails	10	16
Blisters	11	7
Shin splints	8	28
Patella femoral pain syndrome	8	11
Iliotibial band friction syndrome	3	24
Compartment syndrome	3	11
Plantar fasciitis	2	6
Fracture stress	2	75
Bursitis	2	27

Table 3-10. Most Common Overuse Injuries in Women

	NUMBER	AVERAGE DAYS EXCUSAL
Tendinitis	49	14
Blisters	38	9
Shin splints	26	19
Patella femoral pain syndrome	25	19
Ingrown toenails	13	16
Iliotibial band friction syndrome	12	19
Plantar fasciitis	12	25
Synovitis	9	19
Stress fracture	8	66
Stress reaction	10	27

Table 3-11. Summer Trauma by Gender

	MEN	WOMEN
Shoulder	7	2
Arm	0	0
Elbow, forearm	1	2
Wrist	2	0
Hand	2	3
Pelvis/hip	5	4
Thigh	2	7
Knee	6	5
Leg	0	2
Ankle	10	12
Foot	5	3
Back	7	7

Table 3-12. Summer Overuse by Gender

	MEN	WOMEN
Shoulder	0	1
Arm	0	0
Elbow, forearm	0	1
Wrist	0	1
Hand	0	0
Pelvis/hip	1	3
Thigh	0	1
Knee	7	15
Leg	4	14
Ankle	1	6
Foot	11	29
Back	0	0

Table 3-13. Summer Traumatic Injury Rate (Injuries /100 Cadets / Month Training)

	AVERAGE	1989	1990	1991	1992
Women	9.33	15.5	29.8	1.2	8.33
Men	8.33	18.1	23.4	1.0	4.26

Table 3-14. Summer Overuse Injury Rates (Injuries / 100 Cadets / Month Training)

	AVERAGE	1989	1990	1991	1992
Women	14.1	34.1	13.49	3.17	5.35
Men	6.0	8.51	4.97	1.42	2.13

Men had more traumatic shoulder problems, probably associated with the strong emphasis on contact sports (football, boxing, and wrestling). There were no differences in the incidences of anterior cruciate ligament injuries in this group of young adults. In this select population women have more overuse injuries than men, but the rate can be decreased in both genders by progressive and sustained training. The ratio of stress fractures between women and men in this study population was 5:1. These findings are consistent with those of Jones and coworkers, who found the risk of stress fracture during soldier basic training to be 12.3% in women and 2.4% in men.[5] In the past researchers have found a cadet stress fracture ratio of 10:1 for women and men.[9,12] The decrease in this ratio may indicate changes in the cadet selection pool, improved monitoring of prestress fracture injuries with an open door policy of early intervention, and perhaps better training techniques.

Since 1976 women have made a positive impact on the Corp of Cadets in the United States Military Academy at West Point by being pioneers, athletes, scholars, and leaders. There are well-recognized physiologic differences in age-matched men and women.[2,4-6,10,11] Experience has demonstrated that women can be successful in a career in the active military. More and more women are participating in rigorous physical activities during childhood and adolescence. This increased activity level is reflected in the improved fitness of female cadet candidates entering our military academies.[1-3,8,13] During the course of training at West Point women respond to increased physical demands and demonstrate a lower incidence of overuse injuries.

Acknowledgments

The author wishes to thank his co-investigators—Charles E. Wade, Ph.D., John Copley, M.D., Virginia L. Gildengorin, Ph.D., Marjorie M. Hunt, M.B.A., James H. Swain, M.P.T., Daniel E. Brooks, M.T.(A.S.C.P.), Charles R. Scoville, M.Ed., M.P.T., and Jill Lindberg, M.D.; the US Army Joint and Soft Tissue Trauma Fellows—Jack F. McBride, M.D., Richard Gardner, M.D., Dean C. Taylor, M.D., and John M. Uhorchuk, M.D.; fellow orthopaedists—Robert A. Arciero, M.D., Bruce Wheeler, M.D., Robert Stanton, M.D., William Meade, M.D., and James McComb, M.D.; the administrative staff—Jane Reddington, Ruth Travers, Jung Soon Napoli, and Trudy Sharpe; the staff and faculty of the United States Military Academy, Keller Army Hospital, Letterman Army Institute of Research, and the US Army Institute of Surgical Research; and the West Point Class of 1993 study participants. This research was funded by the US Army Medical Research and Development Command under grant #91MM-1502. The views expressed in this chapter are those of the author and do not reflect the official policy or position of the Department of the Army, Department of Defense, or the United States Government.

Section 2   HIGH SCHOOL AND COLLEGIATE

Mary Lloyd Ireland, M.D.

Research institutes provide injury rates at the collegiate and high school level. The injury must be defined and reported rates—numerator and denominator made clear. The National Collegiate Athletic Association (NCAA, P. O. Box 6222, Indian apolis, IN 64207, www.ncaa.org) has an injury surveillance system that follows the types and body parts of athletes sustaining injuries in 16 sports. Sixteen percent of member institutions of all 3 divisions are surveyed. Data are compiled from injury reports completed by athletic trainers from participating institutions. The reports indicate the number of injuries per 1000 exposure hours. Injury rates by the type of injury and whether the injury occurred in practice or during a game are shown in Table 3-15. The 2 sports that can be compared by gender are basketball and soccer. There are gender-based differences in the college lacrosse rules, as well as in the apparati used in gymnastics. The NCAA injury rates by body part are shown in Table 3-16.

Comparison of injuries in different sports and between genders is an important aspect of planning for coverage of events and prevention strategies. One must compare the rates of injury and not the absolute numbers. The information should be assessed carefully to determine the common denominator. The National Center for Catastrophic Sports Injury Research, Chapel Hill, NC, has been recording fatalities and catastrophic and serious injuries in US high schools and colleges. Data on fall sports fatalities and catastrophic and serious injuries in US high school and colleges reported from 1982 to 1996 are listed in Table 3-17.[14] Similar tracking was done for winter sports from 1982 to 1997 (Table 3-18).[14] Spring sports were also followed from 1983 to 1997 (Table 3-19).[14]

The numbers of deaths from catastrophic injury in high school and college football are depicted in Figure 3-1. Cheerleading incidents resulted in the highest number of catastrophic injuries in female athletes. With the new injury-reporting and computer packages now available, better documentation of injury types and severity is possible.

Table 3-15. NCAA Injury Rate by Type of Injury, 1999–2000[a]

	CONTUSION		TENDINITIS		LIGAMENT SPRAIN (INCOMPLETE TEAR)		LIGAMENT SPRAIN (COMPLETE TEAR)		MUSCLE-TENDON STRAIN (INCOMPLETE TEAR)		MUSCLE-TENDON STRAIN (COMPLETE TEAR)		FRACTURE		STRESS FRACTURE		CONCUSSION		HEAT EXHAUSTION		INFLAMMATION	
	Practices	Games	P	G	P	G	P	G	P	G	P	G	P	G	P	G	P	G	P	G	P	G
Gymnastics-W	0.55	0.96	0.30	0.48	1.66	2.40	0.30	1.44	1.36	1.92	0.05	0.48	0.40	1.44	0.35	0.00	0.10	0.00	0.00	0.00	0.15	0.48
Gymnastics-M	0.41	0.85	1.22	0.00	1.01	1.70	0.20	0.85	1.22	0.85	0.00	0.00	0.20	0.85	0.20	0.00	0.00	0.00	0.00	0.00	0.71	0.00
Basketball-W	0.26	1.03	0.22	0.14	1.54	3.10	0.18	0.62	0.88	0.45	0.02	0.07	0.16	0.79	0.21	0.07	0.22	0.86	0.00	0.00	0.13	0.03
Basketball-M	0.33	1.43	0.14	0.06	1.58	3.26	0.08	0.18	0.55	1.22	0.01	0.03	0.28	0.97	0.11	0.18	0.14	0.58	0.01	0.00	0.09	0.06
Soccer-W	0.34	2.65	0.30	0.26	1.01	4.64	0.16	1.62	1.97	2.72	0.05	0.04	0.13	1.10	0.07	0.07	0.13	1.95	0.07	0.22	0.24	0.18
Soccer-M	0.53	4.80	0.17	0.08	1.15	6.09	0.06	0.31	1.37	3.74	0.01	0.00	0.16	1.09	0.02	0.08	0.03	1.37	0.06	0.00	0.08	0.12
Lacrosse-W	0.37	1.05	0.45	0.23	0.87	1.29	0.08	0.70	1.11	1.64	0.03	0.00	0.13	0.47	0.40	0.00	0.16	0.59	0.03	0.00	0.00	0.23
Lacrosse-M	0.59	2.38	0.07	0.00	0.84	2.22	0.09	0.33	0.72	2.71	0.00	0.00	0.05	0.57	0.01	0.00	0.18	1.64	0.00	0.00	0.05	0.08
Field Hockey-W	0.14	1.51	0.24	0.18	0.60	0.71	0.02	0.09	1.33	0.71	0.02	0.09	0.17	0.80	0.10	0.00	0.05	0.44	0.07	0.00	0.14	0.09
Volleyball-W	0.16	0.17	0.38	0.17	1.06	1.87	0.07	0.26	1.33	0.99	0.02	0.00	0.07	0.09	0.17	0.06	0.09	0.14	0.00	0.00	0.15	0.06
Softball-W	0.43	1.22	0.23	0.16	0.43	0.97	0.05	0.11	0.70	0.77	0.02	0.01	0.14	0.49	0.03	0.00	0.15	0.33	0.02	0.00	0.07	0.07
Spring Football-M	0.86	0.00	0.03	0.00	3.20	0.00	0.48	0.00	2.19	0.00	0.04	0.00	0.59	0.00	0.02	0.00	0.67	0.00	0.02	0.00	0.04	0.00
Wrestling-M	0.44	1.84	0.04	0.10	1.50	9.79	0.13	1.53	1.14	4.49	0.05	0.10	0.18	1.02	0.00	0.00	0.30	1.73	0.00	0.00	0.13	0.31
Football-M	0.44	6.66	0.09	0.16	1.16	14.81	0.14	2.39	1.19	5.59	0.04	0.21	0.21	2.64	0.02	0.07	0.34	4.20	0.16	0.09	0.06	0.25
Ice Hockey-M	0.41	3.21	0.01	0.05	0.32	4.38	0.09	0.51	0.61	1.96	0.03	0.09	0.19	1.58	0.01	0.00	0.11	1.63	0.00	0.00	0.03	0.00
Baseball-M	0.15	1.15	0.24	0.27	0.40	0.96	0.04	0.14	0.57	1.33	0.01	0.04	0.11	0.61	0.02	0.02	0.03	0.29	0.00	0.00	0.06	0.11

[a] All data are shown as rate per 1000 athletic exposures for 1999–2000.

From the NCAA Injury Surveillance System, 1999–2000. NCAA, Indianapolis, Ind.

Table 3-16. NCAA Injury Rate by Body Part, 1999–2000[a]

	NECK		SHOULDER		WRIST		HAND		LOWER BACK		PELVIS, HIPS, GROIN		UPPER LEG		KNEE		PATELLA		LOWER LEG		ANKLE		FOOT	
	Practices	*Games*	P	G	P	G	P	G	P	G	P	G	P	G	P	G	P	G	P	G	P	G	P	G
Gymnastics-W	0.35	0.48	0.30	0.48	0.15	0.00	0.05	0.00	0.71	0.48	0.30	0.00	0.15	0.96	1.01	4.32	0.15	0.00	0.55	0.48	1.01	2.40	0.25	0.48
Gymnastics-M	0.41	0.00	1.82	0.85	0.20	0.00	0.00	0.00	0.61	0.85	0.00	0.00	0.00	0.85	0.41	1.70	0.00	0.00	0.20	0.00	0.91	1.70	0.20	0.85
Basketball-W	0.03	0.03	0.14	0.41	0.01	0.10	0.01	0.17	0.23	0.21	0.18	0.28	0.43	0.21	0.68	1.97	0.11	0.17	0.25	0.14	1.32	2.14	0.29	0.59
Basketball-M	0.01	0.09	0.09	0.33	0.05	0.30	0.05	0.12	0.24	0.37	0.16	0.46	0.21	0.55	0.48	1.13	0.08	0.15	0.17	0.21	1.28	2.62	0.22	0.64
Soccer-W	0.02	0.29	0.09	0.40	0.02	0.26	0.01	0.11	0.15	0.44	0.53	0.52	1.20	1.77	0.68	3.98	0.06	0.15	0.34	1.33	0.98	3.57	0.19	0.77
Soccer-M	0.01	0.12	0.09	0.66	0.04	0.20	0.02	0.04	0.08	0.43	0.47	1.21	0.72	2.77	0.55	3.24	0.07	0.16	0.32	1.21	0.92	4.37	0.28	1.05
Lacrosse-W	0.05	0.12	0.16	0.47	0.00	0.00	0.03	0.00	0.05	0.35	0.21	0.23	0.50	1.05	0.37	1.88	0.05	0.00	0.53	0.23	0.74	0.35	0.50	0.47
Lacrosse-M	0.04	0.25	0.23	2.22	0.03	0.16	0.03	0.25	0.19	0.41	0.15	0.49	0.46	2.14	0.42	1.23	0.00	0.08	0.11	0.57	0.76	0.82	0.04	0.33
Field Hockey-W	0.02	0.00	0.02	0.00	0.00	0.09	0.07	0.09	0.21	0.18	0.33	0.18	0.67	0.53	0.45	0.98	0.07	0.09	0.29	0.27	0.33	0.62	0.10	0.18
Volleyball-W	0.01	0.06	0.55	0.51	0.05	0.06	0.03	0.00	0.37	0.26	0.20	0.17	0.27	0.09	0.44	0.54	0.10	0.06	0.30	0.09	0.75	1.56	0.16	0.17
Softball-W	0.03	0.07	0.29	0.44	0.07	0.11	0.04	0.21	0.19	0.12	0.09	0.17	0.23	0.38	0.18	0.68	0.09	0.08	0.10	0.32	0.36	0.62	0.10	0.04
Spring Football-M	0.32	0.00	1.13	0.00	0.14	0.00	0.19	0.00	0.35	0.00	0.43	0.00	1.36	0.00	1.85	0.00	0.12	0.00	0.23	0.00	1.50	0.00	0.23	0.00
Wrestling-M	0.43	1.63	0.85	5.51	0.06	0.20	0.05	0.10	0.28	0.71	0.07	0.20	0.11	0.61	1.29	8.06	0.07	0.20	0.07	0.20	0.59	2.04	0.11	0.31
Football-M	0.17	1.63	0.50	5.85	0.05	0.47	0.07	0.68	0.15	0.96	0.29	1.69	0.66	3.10	0.69	9.41	0.05	0.36	0.16	1.71	0.60	8.09	0.16	0.96
Ice Hockey-M	0.04	0.05	0.22	2.28	0.10	0.56	0.00	0.42	0.22	0.42	0.30	1.12	0.14	0.93	0.29	2.75	0.01	0.09	0.05	0.19	0.10	1.07	0.09	0.33
Baseball-M	0.00	0.02	0.39	0.81	0.03	0.20	0.06	0.35	0.10	0.14	0.06	0.15	0.14	0.69	0.11	0.47	0.03	0.07	0.06	0.21	0.25	0.47	0.06	0.16

[a]All data are shown as rate per 1000 athletic exposures for 1999–2000

From the NCAA Injury Surveillance System, 1999–2000. NCAA, Indianapolis, Ind.

Table 3-17. Fall Sports Fatalities and Catastrophic and Serious Injuries in US High Schools and Colleges, 1982–1996

SPORT	TOTAL NUMBER OF PARTICIPANTS (PERCENT MALE/FEMALE)	(100,000 PARTICIPANTS)		TOTAL DIRECT INJURIES (AND RATE PER 100,000 PARTICIPANTS)		TOTAL DIRECT FATALITIES AND INJURIES (AND RATE PER 100,000 PARTICIPANTS)
		DIRECT[a]	INDIRECT[b]	NONFATAL[c]	SERIOUS[d]	
High School						
Cross-country	4,063,203 (59/41)	0	10 (0.25)	1 (0.02)	0	1 (0.02)
Football	21,302,466 (99/1)	61 (0.29)	89 (0.42)	147 (0.69)	166 (0.78)	374 (1.76)
Soccer	5,263,083 (64/36)	4 (0.08)	16 (0.30)	2 (0.04)	6 (0.11)	12 (0.23)
Total	30,628,752 (88/12)	65 (0.21)	115 (0.38)	150 (0.49)	172 (0.56)	387 (1.26)
College						
Cross-country	262,050 (56/44)	0	1 (0.38)	0	0	0
Football	1,250,000 (100/0)	5 (0.40)	24 (1.92)	21 (1.68)	62 (4.88)	88 (6.96)
Soccer	331,212 (67/33)	0	2 (0.60)	0	1 (0.30)	1 (0.30)
Total	1,843,262 (88/12)	5 (0.27)	27 (1.47)	21 (1.14)	63 (3.42)	89 (4.84)
Overall	32,472,014	70 (0.22)	142 (0.43)	171 (0.53)	235 (0.72)	476 (1.47)

[a]Caused by performing the activities of a sport.
[b]Caused by systemic failure as a result of exertion while participating in a sport.
[c]Resulting in permanent severe functional spinal cord disability.
[d]Resulting in transient functional spinal cord disability.

From Cantu RC, Mueller FO: Fatalities and catastrophic injuries in high school and college sports, 1982–1997: Lessons in improving safety. Physician Sports Med 27(8): 35–49, 1999, with permission.

Table 3-18. Winter Sports Fatalities and Catastrophic and Serious Injuries, US High Schools and Colleges, 1982–1997

SPORT	TOTAL NUMBER OF PARTICIPANTS (PERCENT MALE/FEMALE)	TOTAL FATALITIES (AND RATE PER 100,000 PARTICIPANTS)		TOTAL DIRECT INJURIES (AND RATE PER 100,000 PARTICIPANTS)		TOTAL DIRECT FATALITIES AND INJURIES (AND RATE PER 100,000 PARTICIPANTS)
		DIRECT[a]	INDIRECT[a]	NONFATAL[a]	SERIOUS[a]	
High School						
Basketball	13,878,343 (56/44)	0	54 (0.39)	2 (0.01)	5 (0.04)	7 (0.05)
Gymnastics	486,597 (14/86)	1 (0.21)	0	7 (1.44)	4 (0.82)	12 (2.46)
Ice hockey	354,135 (98/2)	2 (0.56)	2 (0.56)	4 (1.13)	5 (1.41)	11 (3.11)
Swimming	2,556,181 (46/54)	0	4 (0.16)	4 (0.16)	3 (0.12)	7 (0.27)
Wrestling	3,556,640 (99/1)	2 (0.06)	13 (0.37)	20 (0.56)	11 (0.31)	33 (0.93)
Total	20,831,896 (62/38)	5 (0.02)	73 (0.35)	37 (0.18)	28 (0.13)	70 (0.34)
College						
Basketball	367,225 (54/46)	0	12 (3.27)	1 (0.27)	2 (0.54)	3 (0.81)
Gymnastics	34,543 (33/67)	0	0	5 (14.49)	1 (2.90)	6 (17.39)
Ice hockey	60,603 (96/4)	0	1 (1.65)	4 (6.60)	3 (4.95)	7 (11.55)
Swimming	234,566 (50/50)	0	4 (1.70)	1 (0.43)	0	1 (0.43)
Wrestling	108,673 (100/0)	0	0	1 (0.92)	0	1 (0.92)
Total	805,610 (61/39)	0	17 (2.11)	12 (1.49)	6 (0.74)	18 (2.23)
Overall	21,637,506	5 (0.02)	90 (0.42)	49 (0.23)	34 (0.16)	88 (0.41)

[a]See Table 3-17 footnotes for definitions.

From Cantu RC, Mueller FO: Fatalities and catastrophic injuries in high school and college sports, 1982–1997: Lessons in improving safety. Physician Sports Med 27(8): 35–49, 1999, with permission.

Table 3-19. Spring Sports Fatalities and Catastrophic and Serious Injuries, US High Schools and Colleges, 1983–1997

SPORT	TOTAL NUMBER OF PARTICIPANTS (PERCENT MALE/FEMALE)	TOTAL FATALITIEs (AND RATE PER 100,000 PARTICIPANTS)		TOTAL DIRECT INJURIES (AND RATE PER 100,000 PARTICIPANTS)		TOTAL DIRECT FATALITIES AND INJURIES (AND RATE PER 100,000 PARTICIPANTS)
		DIRECT[a]	INDIRECT[a]	NONFATAL[a]	SERIOUS[a]	
High School						
Baseball	6,279,333 (99/1)	6 (0.10)	7 (0.11)	11 (0.18)	11 (0.18)	28 (0.45)
Lacrosse	442,785 (66/34)	1 (0.23)	2 (0.45)	0	0	1 (0.23)
Track and field	12,684,649 (56/44)	16 (0.13)	19 (0.15)	10 (0.08)	13 (0.10)	39 (0.31)
Tennis	3,951,505 (51/49)	0	1 (0.03)	0	0	0
Total	23,358,272 (67/33)	23 (0.10)	29 (0.12)	21 (0.09)	24 (0.10)	68 (0.29)
College						
Baseball	319,679 (100/0)	2 (0.63)	2 (0.63)	1 (0.31)	1 (0.31)	4 (1.25)
Lacrosse	121,114 (61/39)	0	1 (0.83)	2 (1.65)	2 (1.65)	4 (3.30)
Track and field	836,624 (60/40)	2 (0.24)	1 (0.12)	2 (0.24)	3 (0.36)	7 (0.84)
Tennis	227,035 (51/49)	0	2 (0.88)	0	0	0
Total	1,504,452 (67/33)	4 (0.27)	6 (0.40)	5 (0.33)	6 (0.40)	15 (1.0)
Overall	24,862,724	27 (0.11)	35 (0.14)	26 (0.10)	30 (0.12)	83 (0.33)

[a]See Table 3–17 footnotes for definitions.

From Cantu RC, Mueller FO: Fatalities and catastrophic injuries in high school and college sports, 1982–1977: Lessons in improving safety. Physician Sports Med. 27(8): 35–49, 1999, with permission.

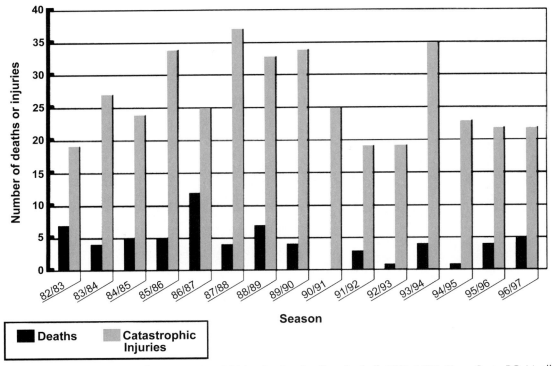

Figure 3-1. Deaths and catastrophic injuries in US high school and college football, 1982–1997. (From Cantu RC, Mueller FO: Fatalities and catastrophic injuries in high school and college sports, 1982–1997: Lessons in improving safety. Physician Sportsmed 27 (8): 35–49, 1999, with permission.)

References

1. Amoroso PJ, Bell NS, Jones BH: Injury among female and male army parachutists. Aviat Space Environ Med 68(11):1006–11, 1997.
2. Baldi KA: An overview of physical fitness of female cadets at the military academies. Milit Med 156(10):537–9, 1991.
3. Bielenda CC, Knapik J, Wright DA: Physical fitness and cardiovascular disease risk factors of female senior U.S. military officers and federal employees. Milit Med 158(3):177–81, 1993.
4. Bishop GD: Gender, role, and illness behavior in a military population. Health Psychol 3(6):519–34, 1984.
5. Jones BH, et al: Intrinsic risk factors for exercise-related injuries among male and female army trainees. Am J Sports Med 21(5):705–10, 1993.
6. Jones BH, Cowan DN, Knapik JJ: Exercise, training and injuries. Sports Med 18(3):202–14, 1994.
7. McBride J, Meade WC III, Ryan JB: Incidence and pattern of injury in female cadets at West Point Military Academy. In Pearl A (ed): The Athletic Female. Champaign, Ill, Human Kinetics, 1993, pp 219–33.
8. Petosa S: Women in the military academies: US Air Force Academy (Part 2 of 3). Physician Sports Med 17(3):133–42, 1989.
9. Protzman R: Women in Sports: can women be overextended in physical conditioning programs? Am J Sports Med 7(2):145–6, 1979.
10. Stauffer R: A Follow-Up Study to: The Comparison of USMA Men and Women on Selected Physical Performance Measures—"Project Summertime." West Point, NY, United States Military Academy, 1977.
11. Stauffer RW, et al: Comparison of metabolic responses of United States Military Academy men and women in acute military load bearing. Aviat Space Environ Med 58(11):1047–56, 1987.
12. Tomasi L, Peterson JA, Pettit GP, et al: Women's response to army training. Physician Sports Med, 1977.
13. Wade CE, Ryan JB, copley JB, et al: Longitudinal monitoring of healthy young adults: gender differences of exercise on gonadal steroid levels, bone mineral density, and stress fractures. Institution Report 91MM1502, US Army Medical Research and material command, Fort Detrick, Frederick, MD21702–5012, 1996.
14. Welch M: Women in the military academies: US Army (Part 3 of 3). Physician Sports Med 17(4):89–96, 1989.
15. Cantu RC, Mueller FO: Fatalities and catastrophic injuries in high school and college sports, 1982–1997: Lessons in improving safety. Physician Sportsmed 27(8):35–49, 1999.

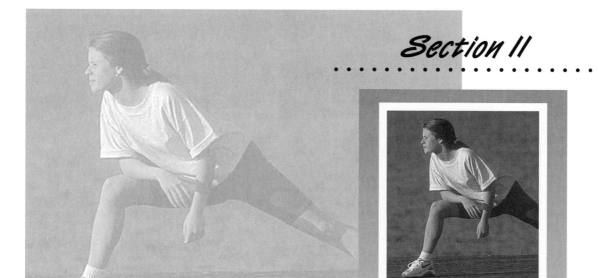

Section II

Psychology and Motivation

Chapter 4

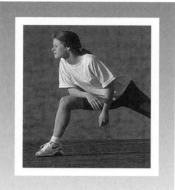

Social and Psychological Aspects of Athletic Participation

Diane L. Gill, Ph.D.

Recently I watched a television commercial in which several young women argued that they would be better physically (e.g., have a lower risk of cancer and heart disease), mentally (have less depression), and socially (have better grades, less teenage pregnancy, greater career success) "if you let [us] play sports." The athletic company that developed the commercial drew upon the literature that documents these claims and supports the many benefits of athletic participation for women. The business world sees females as athletes (and athletic consumers), and indeed, female athletic participation has exploded in the last generation. Still, the numbers of female and male participants are not equal. More important, even if the numbers were equal, female athletes are not the same as male athletes. The main point of this chapter is that we must look beyond numbers, biologic sex characteristics, and simple dichotomous sex differences to the powerful, gendered psychosocial context of athletics to understand the female athlete.

In this chapter I will consider sports psychology research and practice related to the female athlete as I advocate a feminist, social dynamics approach. Gender is a key feature of social context and social processes in athletics. Gender varies with culture, and in fact, culture defines gender. Although biologic sex is innate, all meanings, social roles, expectations, standards of appropriate behavior and beauty, power, and status are created by culture. We are not born to wear high heels or high-top sneakers. In addition, gender varies with other cultural categories. For example, in the United States field hockey is almost entirely a women's sport, whereas in India field hockey is largely a men's sport, and in Australia and New Zealand both women and men play.

Before considering the research and practice literature on gender, consider how gender affects your interpretations, responses, and possible approaches to the following athletes:

- A soccer player who lacks control and is prone to angry outbursts.
- A 16-year-old figure skater who may have an eating disorder, but is working to keep that "line," make it to nationals, and get endorsements.

Did gender influence your responses? Did you identify these athletes as male or female? Do you think coaches, sports psychologists, trainers, and parents would behave the same with female and male athletes? If you try to be nonsexist, treat everyone the same, and assume that gender does not matter, you will probably have difficulty. Gender does matter. Imagine each case with a female athlete, then go back and imagine the same scenario with a male athlete. Trying to treat everyone the same does a disservice to the athletes.

From the time we are born our world is shaped by gender. Our parents, teachers, peers, and coaches reacted to us as girls or boys. The influence of gender is seen in every aspect of our lives, and athletics is no exception. Anyone who works with female or male athletes should be aware of gender influences in the sports world as well as in the larger society.

THE GENDERED CONTEXT OF SPORTS

To understand the psychology of the female athlete, we must first understand the social and historical context of female athletes. In the United States, the civil rights and women's movements of 1970s helped women gain a place in sports, and women now constitute about one third of U.S. high school, college, and Olympic athletes. But one third is not one half, and in other ways women have lost ground. Women have not become coaches, administrators, sports writers, or sports medicine personnel in significant numbers. Before Title IX of the Educational Amendments of 1972, nearly all (over 90%) women's athletic teams were coached by women and had a woman athletic director. Today less than half of the women's teams are coached by women, and only 16% have a woman director.[7,16,17,28,35] While women have moved into previously all-male competitive athletics, other programs with more emphasis on participation, skill development, and recreation have been lost to both men and women. Even a cursory review of sports psychology conferences, journals, and organizations reveals that males dominate sports psychology research and practice as well as competitive athletics. Thus, sport is male dominated with a clear hierarchical structure that is widely accepted and communicated in so many ways that we seldom notice.

GENDER SCHOLARSHIP IN SPORTS PSYCHOLOGY

Given the social and historical context of women's sports, it is not surprising that our limited gender scholarship did not develop within sports science. Instead, gender scholarship in sports psychology largely follows gender scholarship within psychology. Generally, that scholarship has progressed from sex differences to an emphasis on gender role as personality, to more current social psychology models that emphasize social context and processes.

Sex Differences

The early sex difference work, exemplified by Maccoby and Jacklin's review,[24] assumed dichotomous biology-based psychological differences—that male and female are opposites. In practice, dichotomous sex differences are typically interpreted as meaning that we should treat males one way and females the other way. Today, consensus holds that psychological characteristics associated with females and males are neither dichotomous nor biology based.[4,9,14,16,17,20] Even most biologic factors are not dichotomously divided, but are normally distributed within both females and males. For example, the average male basketball center is taller than the average female center, but the average female center is taller than most men. For social psychological characteristics such as aggressiveness or confidence, even average differences are elusive, and the evidence does not support biologic dichotomous sex-linked connections. With criticisms of the sex differences approach, and its failure to shed light on gender-related behavior, psychologists turned to personality.

Personality and Gender Role Orientation

Psychologists, particularly Sandra L. Bem,[3,5] have focused on gender role orientation as the relevant personality construct. Personality is *not* a function of biology. Instead, both males and females can have masculine or feminine personalities, and androgyny is best. Advocates of androgyny argue that practitioners should treat everyone the same and encourage both masculine and feminine personalities. Masculine and feminine categories and measures such as, Bem's Sex Role Inventory, a widely used instrument in psychology that measures masculine and feminine gender role perceptions, have been widely criticized, and even Bem[4] has progressed to a more encompassing gender perspective, but most sports psychology gender research is based on her early work. Overall, this research suggests that female athletes possess more masculine personality characteristics than do female nonathletes.[16,17] This is not particularly enlightening. Athletics, especially competitive athletics, demands instrumental, assertive behaviors, and the higher masculine scores of female athletes probably reflect an overlap with competitiveness. Today, most psychologists recognize the limits of earlier sex differences and gender role approaches, and look beyond the male–female and masculine–feminine dichotomies to socialization and social cognitive models for explanations.

Gender and Social Processes

In the 1980s, gender research moved away from the sex differences and personality approaches to a more social approach, emphasizing gender beliefs and stereotypes. How people *think* males and females differ is more important than how they actually differ. Although actual differences between females and males with respect to such characteristics as independence or competitiveness are small and inconsistent, we maintain our stereotypes.[2,9–12,33] These gender stereotypes are pervasive. We exaggerate minimal differences into larger perceived differences through social processes. These perceptions exert a strong influence that may elicit further gender differences. This cycle reflects the feminist position that gender is socially constructed.

Similar gender beliefs seem alive and well in the sports world. Metheny[27] identified gender stereotypes in her classic analysis. Acceptable sports for women (e.g., gymnastics, swimming, tennis) emphasize aesthetic qualities and tend to be individual activities rather than direct competitive and team sports. Recently, Kane and Snyder[22] confirmed gender stereotyping and identified the emphasis on the male's physical muscularity, strength, and power as the key feature.

These persistent gender beliefs and stereotypes are found everywhere. Socialization pressures are pervasive, and strong, and begin early. Parents, teachers, peers, and societal institutions treat girls and boys differently from birth.[1,15,31,36] Overall, differential treatment is consistent with producing independence and efficacy in boys, and emotional sensitivity, nurturance, and helplessness in girls.

One prominent source of differential treatment in athletics is the media.[21,26] First, females receive little coverage. Women receive less than 10% of the coverage whether we consider television air time, newspaper space, feature articles, or photographs. Moreover, female and male athletes receive *different* coverage that reflects gender hierarchy. Generally, athletic ability and accomplishments are emphasized for males, but femininity and physical attractiveness are emphasized for females.

The social aspect of gender is more than perceptions and stereotypes; it's the whole context. In *The Female World*, Jesse Bernard[6] proposed that the social worlds of females and males are different, even when they appear similar. In earlier times we created actual separate sport worlds for females and males with segregated physical education and athletic programs. Although we now have coed activities, the separate worlds have not disappeared. The social world differs for female and male university basketball players, for male and female joggers, and for the girl and boy in a youth soccer game.

Stereotypes are of concern because we act on them; we exaggerate minimal gender differences and restrict opportunities for both females and males. Gender beliefs keep many women out of sports, and gender beliefs restrict the behaviors of both men and women in sports. Both girls and boys can participate in youth gymnastics or baseball, and at early ages physical capabilities are similar. Yet, children see female gymnasts and male baseball players as role models, peers gravitate to sex-segregated activities, and most parents, teachers, and coaches support gender-appropriate activities of children.

To illustrate the role of social context, consider athletic confidence. Considerable earlier research suggested gender differences, with females displaying lower confidence than males across varied settings.[16] Lenney[23] concluded that the social situation was the primary source of gender differences. Specifically, gender differences emerged with masculine tasks, in competitive settings, when clear, unambiguous feedback was missing. Several studies confirmed Lenney's propositions.[8] However, these studies were experimental studies involving novel motor tasks rather than athletic skills, conducted in controlled lab settings that purposely stripped away social context. We cannot ignore social context in the real world of sport. Sport tasks typically are seen as masculine, competition is the norm, and males and females develop their confidence along with their athletic skills through radically different experiences and opportunities.

Although sport is stereotypically masculine, feminist scholars recognize that gender stereotypes and beliefs affect men. For example, Messner[25] describes sports as a powerful force that socializes boys and men into a restricted masculine identity. Messner notes that sport bonds men together as superior to women. And, sport is not only male, but white, middle-class, heterosexual male. Gender stereotypes and their influence likely vary across other social categories such as race, class, sexuality, and age. Duda and Allison[13] cited the need for sports psychology research on race and ethnicity. Pat Griffin[18] has contributed important work on sexual orientation and homophobia. However, as Yevonne Smith[32] concluded in her review of the scholarship on women of color, we have a deafening silence on the experiences of diverse women in sports. Overall, we lack scholarship on diversity, and have little information to guide our work with diverse female athletes.

So, the literature does not support dichotomous sex differences; males and females are not opposites. But, women and men are not the same and we can not ignore gender. Gender is part of a complex, dynamic social network, and a particularly salient, powerful part of sport. Clearly, recognition of gender and diversity is critical to effective sports psychology practice.

FROM GENDER SCHOLARSHIP TO FEMINIST PRACTICE

To translate gender scholarship into feminist practice we must first avoid sexist assumptions, standards, and practices. Then, we might follow the lead of psychologists who have moved beyond nonsexist practices to more actively feminist approaches. Feminist practice[37] incorporates gender scholarship, emphasizes neglected women's experiences (e.g., sexual harassment), and takes a more nonhierarchical, empowering, process-oriented approach that shifts emphasis from personal change to social change.

First, sports psychology consultants and others who work with female athletes might consider how gender influences interactions and communication. Although we stereotype females as more talkative, research[19] indicates that men talk more, interrupt more, and take more space and dominant postures. Training in communication and interpersonal skills, as well as familiarity with gender scholarship, may help professionals adjust. Still, the larger world is different for female and male athletes, and we can go beyond the immediate consultant-athlete setting to more social, egalitarian practice.

To take a more active feminist approach, we might consider going beyond gender awareness in the scenarios presented earlier. In the first scenario the aggressive soccer player could be male or female, but a male soccer player is more likely to grow up in a world that reinforces aggressive behavior, and a male athlete is more likely to continue to have such behaviors reinforced. The less aggressive, more tentative approach is more typical of female athletes. Even talented, competitive female athletes are socialized to keep quiet, be good, and let others take the lead. Moreover, most female athletes have a male coach, trainer, athletic director, and professors, and deal with males in most other power positions.

Overly aggressive, uncontrolled behavior is not exclusively male, nor all tentative styles exclusively female. Still, we will work more effectively if we recognize gender influences in the athlete's background and situation. Anger control and confidence-building have different contexts, and likely require different strategies for female and male athletes. For example, a consultant might examine the media and public relations for the women's team as well as the status of women's sports in general. How does sport fit into the player's life? How do others (coach, teammates, family, spectators, friends) react to the player? Behavior is not just within the athlete, but is within a particular sport context, and within a larger social context, and both the immediate situation and larger context are gender related.

The figure skater's scenario (potential eating disorder) could involve clinical psychologists, as well as other professionals (e.g., physicians, nutrition specialists), but we will focus on the social psychological aspects here. Gender influences psychological disorders and diagnoses.[30,34] For example, women are more likely to present with major depression and simple phobias, whereas men are more likely to present with antisocial personality disorder or alcohol abuse. In the United States the largest gender gap, by far, is in the context of eating disorders. Although the overall incidence is lower than for other psychological disorders, females are nine times as likely as males to exhibit anorexia or bulimia. Moreover, the incidence is increasing, the disorders are prominent in adolescence and early adulthood, and participants in certain activities, including dance and sports, may be at higher risk. The figure skater is much more likely to be female than male (as well as white, middle-upper class, and adolescent). But personality and gender are not the only considerations; eating disorders are social phenomena and body image plays a major role.[29] Females in certain sports may have exaggerated body image concerns related to appearance and performance. Judges do look for a "line," and appearance does affect endorsements. For such cases an educational approach stressing proper nutrition, without discounting the athlete's understandable concern for body image, might be effective. Feminist practitioners might move to social action—to educate others and try to change the system that leads athletes to pursue an unhealthy body image.

CONCLUDING REMARKS

Gender is so ingrained in our athletic structure and practice that we must be aware of the many overt and subtle ways that gender affects everyone in the athletic setting to practice effectively. First, valuing the female perspective and familiarity with the scholarship on women and gender contributes to a thorough understanding of the female athlete. Then, we can further enrich our practice by moving beyond awareness of gender scholarship to feminist practice. The key to feminist practice, a focus on women and women's experiences, is essential for a consultant working with female athletes. Moreover, the guiding principles of feminist practice are relevant to all practitioners. Sports psychologists who contextualize their practice by considering both the immediate athletic situation and larger social context can help athletes recognize constraints and options, and incorporate that social context into their psychological skills training and performance.

Finally, we can move beyond the immediate situation. In feminist practice, education and empowerment extend to social and political action. Sports psychologists can work with coaches, other sports participants, and the general public to empower women and to incorporate diversity on our campuses, in our communities, and in the larger society. Such a feminist approach to research and practice ensures that the social world of athletics is empowering and enriching for the female athlete and for all who participate.

References

1. American Association of University Women: The AAUW Report: How Schools Shortchange Girls. Executive Summary. Washington, DC, American Association of University Women Educational Foundation, 1992.
2. Bem SL: Androgyny and gender schema theory: A conceptual and empirical integration. In Sonderegger TB (ed): Psychology and Gender: Nebraska Symposium on Motivation, 1984, Vol 32. Lincoln, Neb, University of Nebraska Press, 1985, pp 179–226.
3. Bem SL: Beyond androgyny: Some presumptuous prescriptions for a liberated sexual identity. In Sherman J, Denmark F (eds): Psychology of Women: Future Directions for Research. New York, Psychological Dimensions, 1978, pp 1–23.
4. Bem SL: The Lenses of Gender. New Haven, Conn, Yale University Press, 1993.
5. Bem SL: The measurement of psychological androgyny. J Consult Clin Psychol 42:155–62, 1974.
6. Bernard J: The Female World. New York, The Free Press, 1981.
7. Carpenter LJ, Acosta RV: Back to the future: Reform with a woman's voice. In Eitzen DS (ed): Sport in Contemporary Society: An Anthology (4th edition). New York, St. Martin's Press, 1993, pp 398–9.
8. Corbin CB, Nix C: Sex-typing of physical activities and success predictions of children before and after cross-sex competition. J Sport Psychol 3:30–4, 1979.
9. Deaux K: From individual differences to social categories: Analysis of a decade's research on gender. Am Psychol 39:105–16, 1984.
10. Deaux K, Kite ME: Gender stereotypes. In Denmark FL, Paludi MA (eds): Psychology of Women: A Handbook of Issues and Theories. Westport, Conn, Greenwood Press, 1993, pp 107–39.
11. Deaux K, Kite ME: Thinking about gender. In Hess BB, Ferree MM (eds): Analyzing Gender. Beverly Hills, Calif, Sage, 1987, pp 92–117.
12. Deaux K, Major B: Putting gender into context: An interactive model of gender-related behavior. Psychol Rev 94:369–89, 1987.
13. Duda JL, Allison MT: Cross-cultural analysis in exercise and sport psychology: A void in the field. J Sport Exerc Psychol 12:114–31, 1990.
14. Eagley AH: Sex Differences in Social Behavior: A Social-Role Interpretation. Hillsdale, NJ, Lawrence Erlbaum, 1987.
15. Geis FL: Self-fulfilling prophecies: A social psychological view of gender. In Beall AE, Sternberg RJ (eds): The Psychology of Gender. New York, Guilford, 1993, pp 9–54.
16. Gill DL: Gender and sport behavior. In Horn TS (ed): Advances in Sport Psychology. Champaign, Ill, Human Kinetics, 1992, pp 143–60.
17. Gill DL: Gender issues: A social-educational perspective. In Murphy SM (ed): Sport Psychology Interventions. Champaign, Ill, Human Kinetics, 1995, pp 205–34.
18. Griffin P: Changing the game: Homophobia, sexism, and lesbians in sport. Quest 44:251–65, 1992.
19. Hall JA: On explaining sex differences: The case of nonverbal communication. In Shaver P, Hendrick C (eds): Sex and Gender. Newbury Park, Calif, Sage, 1987, 177–200.
20. Hyde JS, Linn MC (eds): The Psychology of Gender: Advances Through the Meta-Analysis. Baltimore, Johns Hopkins University Press, 1986.
21. Kane MJ, Parks JB: The social construction of gender difference and hierarchy in sport journalism—few new twists on very old themes. Women Sport Phys Activity J 1:49–83, 1992.
22. Kane MJ, Snyder E: Sport typing: The social "containment" of women. Arena Rev 13:77–96, 1989.
23. Lenney E: Women's self-confidence in achievement settings. Psychol Bull 84:1–13, 1977.
24. Maccoby E, Jacklin C: The Psychology of Sex Differences. Stanford, Calif, Stanford University Press, 1974.
25. Messner MA: Power at Play: Sports and the Problem of Masculinity. Boston, Beacon Press, 1992.
26. Messner MA, Duncan MC, Jensen K: Separating the men from the girls: The gendered language of televised sports. In Eitzen DS (ed): Sport in Contemporary Society: An Anthology (4th edition). New York, St. Martin's Press, 1993, pp 219–33.
27. Metheny E: Symbolic forms of movement: The feminine image in sports. In Metheny E (ed): Connotations of Movement in Sport and Dance. Dubuque, Iowa, WC Brown, 1965, pp 43–56.
28. Nelson MB. Are We Winning Yet: How Women Are Changing Sports and Sports Are Changing Women. New York, Random House, 1991.
29. Rodin J, Siberstein L, Striegel-Moore R: Women and weight: A normative discontent. In Sonderegger TB (ed): Psychology and Gender: Nebraska Symposium on Motivation, 1984, (Vol 32). Lincoln, Neb, University of Nebraska Press, 1985, pp 267–307.
30. Russo NF, Green BL: Women and mental health. In Denmark FL, Paludi MA (eds): Psychology of women: A Handbook of Issues and Theories. Westport, Conn, Greenwood Press, 1993, pp 379–436.
31. Sadker M, Sadker D, Klein S: The issue of gender in elementary and secondary education. Review of Research in Education. Washington, DC, American Educational Research Association, 1991, pp 269–334.
32. Smith YR: Women of color in society and sport. Quest 44:228–50, 1992.
33. Spence JT, Helmreich RL: Masculinity and Femininity. Austin, Texas, University of Texas Press, 1978.
34. Travis CB: Women and Health Psychology: Mental Health Issues. Hillsdale, NJ, Lawrence Erlbaum, 1988.
35. Uhlir GA: Athletics and the university: The post-women's era. Academe 73:25–9, 1987.
36. Unger R, Crawford M: Women and Gender: A Feminist Psychology. New York, McGraw-Hill, 1992.
37. Worell J, Remer P: Feminist Perspectives in Therapy: An Empowerment Model for Women. Chichester, UK, John Wiley, 1992.

Chapter 5

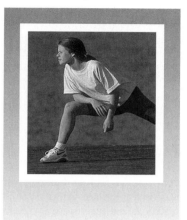

Psychology and Motivation of the Female Athlete

Dennis B. Sprague, Ph.D.

OVERVIEW

In the contemporary sports arena, athletes are constantly trying to find the competitive edge. In spite of social constraints, women have not been excluded from this pursuit of excellence. In the early 1960s, under the leadership of younger faculty members, many colleges and universities began to institute women's sports. In most settings, no budget was allotted for expenses, so faculty members volunteered their time to coach, advise, and officiate events and each team raised its own money for travel, equipment, and uniforms. Winning was important, but the programs' primary emphasis was to provide an enjoyable and competitive experience for women.[10]

With the advent of Title IX of the Education Amendments Act of 1972, which bans sex discrimination in academics and athletics, the number of women participating in sports at the collegiate level has increased dramatically. Search committees now attempt to seek out the most qualified coaches for female sports and monies have been channeled through university administrative networks to pay the coaches adequate salaries. Media coverage has also created a phenomenon of sorts, influencing the younger generation to place more emphasis on the value of the sports experience. As a result, more young women aspire to play high school and college sports than ever before. In this process of evolution, athletes and coaches have described crucial psychological, biologic, and motivational factors that have had a great impact on women's sports and how women approach and deal with competition.

GENDER ISSUES

Initially, the emphasis on women and gender involved a sex difference approach. This emphasis progressed to one of gender role as a personality orientation, and more recently to a sociopsychological model that emphasizes social factors and processes within the social structure of the athletic experience.[17] Traditionally, researchers have looked specifically at male behavior as the norm. Horner focused her attention on gender issues and gender roles.[9] She found that athletic successes often have negative consequences for women because success requires competitive achievement behaviors that conflict with the traditional feminine image. Oftentimes, a conflict develops between the desire for success through competitive achievement behavior and the traditional feminine role, which creates confusion and other forms of abberant behavior. Critics[2,21] noted that men as well as women have behavioral symptoms such as confusion that are consistent with competitive achievement behavior rather than gender issues alone. Supporting these findings, McElroy and Willis[14] concluded that there was no evidence to support the theory that achievement and stereotyped attitudes in females are different from those in males.

Weinburg and Gould[22] reviewed gender differences and levels of confidence. They infer that expectations, as well as social environment, gender roles, and individual differences, are determinants of achievement choices and behavior. Females appear to have lower expectations when they view the task as masculine, feedback is ambiguous, and social comparisons are high.

Similarly, when the task is gender neutral and social comparison is at a minimum, females did not show lower levels of confidence in competition.[20] Coaching feedback regarding performance can also improve self-confidence.

SOCIOLOGICAL FACTORS

More recent research has focused on a sociopsychological model that emphasizes social factors and social behaviors. Results indicate that behaviors consistent with men and women are neither dichotomous nor biologically based and that psychosociological factors play a more dominant role than originally anticipated.[17]

DeBoer[5] cites that appropriate behaviors for female athletes are situation specific and sociologically influenced and not separated into neat, gender-bound packages. Women are taught to be externally focused and may have some difficulty with an all-consuming need to win. Women may choose to follow their socialized instincts and be "nice people" regardless of whether or not it results in winning. Parents, schools, churches, media, and peers have often influenced expectations for girls and women. Girls and women, according to DeBoer, are taught to be placating, caring, and maternal. Their focus is often on the well-being of others. Nurturing behavior might be a motivator for the female team athlete, but it may not be appropriate for the female athlete in an individual sport. There is some evidence to suggest that females are more susceptible to social influence than males,[3] although the results of the social facilitation research have been inconsistent.[1] Women also appear more prone to internalize criticism and take perceived failures personally. This may affect the level of play during competition as well as consistency in performance.

SEX DIFFERENCES

In reviewing sex differences between males and females, recent studies[6,11] suggest that specific sex differences in terms of abilities are minimal and not biologically based. There appears to be more similarity and overlap than originally assumed.[12,13] More recent research[7] measured different types of motivation in sports and found differences between men and women, reflecting some interesting trends. Men scored higher on competitiveness and win orientation than did women and appear more oriented to social comparison. Women, on the other hand, scored higher on goal orientation, or achievement orientation, than did men, appearing more interested in personal improvement. Women appear highly motivated to achieve in the athletic realm, but conflicts sometimes arise when achievement-related behaviors of men are generalized to females.

MOTIVATION

As we review psychological factors bearing on the level of motivation of female athletes, it is apparent that research is rather limited. Some research has been done in the area of attribution theory. From a cognitive perspective, attribution relates to task outcomes being a function of ability, effort, task difficulty, and luck.[23] Deaux and Farris[4] found that males tend to attribute success internally (i.e., to ability), whereas females attribute success more to situational factors and luck.

Horner[9] formulated "fear of success" as a primary concept in motivation, the premise being the motive to avoid success as a stable personality characteristic acquired early in life in conjunction with one's sex role. She believed that this motive is more common in women than men and is strongly aroused in competitive achievement circumstances. It is presumed that the fear of success should be more strongly aroused in women highly motivated to achieve or highly capable of success. Thus, the fear of success was proposed by Horner as a highly feminine characteristic. This hypothesis was not, however, confirmed by other researchers. The work of Silva,[19] Zuckerman and Allison,[24] and McElroy and Willis[14] did not find women to be motivated by a "fear of success."

McHugh, Duquin, and Frieze[15] indicated that highly motivated women were found to be generally self-confident, autonomous, and achievement oriented. Women were found to be more intrinsically motivated than men and reported playing more for the fun of the game than for winning. They were also more likely to attribute winning to luck.

In the achievement motivation literature, Henchen, Edwards, and Mathinos[8] found virtually no differences between males and females on masculinity or femininity dimensions. They did find that females had significantly higher achievement motivation.

Today, women at all organizational levels and in the sports arena continue to create opportunities for themselves, often under adverse conditions.[18] In this process of continued evolution, psychological and sociological factors have had an effect on motivation. Research on the psychological preparation of women athletes indicates that it is essential for coaches to understand that they cannot prepare all female athletes nor all male athletes in the same way, neither androgynously nor based on gender–sex role expectations. Some female athletes may be comfortable with an androgynous approach, but many prefer a traditional approach owing to social and traditional feminine role expectations.[16] Therein lies the continued challenge for coaches and others who work directly with the female athlete.

References

1. Carron AV: Social Psychology of Sport: An Experimental Approach. Ithaca, NY, Mouvement, 1980.
2. Condry J, Dyer S: Fear of success: attribution of cause to the victim. J Soc Issues 32:63–8, 1976.
3. Crowne D, Marlowe D: The Approval Motive: Studies in Evaluative Dependence. New York, Harper & Rowe, 1964.
4. Deaux K, Farris E: Attributing causes for one's own performance: the effects of sex, norms, and outcomes. J Res Pers 11:59–72, 1977.
5. DeBoer K: Growing up female and athlete. Coaching Womens Basketball 3:9–30, 1993.
6. Eagly AH: Sex differences in social behavior: A Social–Role Interpretation. Hillsdale, NJ Lawrence Erlbaum, 1987.
7. Gill DL, Deeter TE: Development of the sport orientation questionnaire. Res Q Exerc Sport 59:191–202, 1988.
8. Henchen K, Edwards S, Mathinos C: Achievement motivation and sex-role orientation of high school female track and field vs. nonathletes. Percept Mot Skills 55:183–7, 1982.
9. Horner M: Toward an understanding of achievement–related conflicts in women. J Soc Issues 28(2):157–76, 1972.
10. Hulstrand B: The growth of collegiate women's sports: the 1960's. Women in sport leadership: The legacy and the challenge. Phys Educ Recreat Dance. (3), 41–4, 1993.
11. Hyde JS: Linn MC (eds): The Psychology of Gender. Advances Through the Meta-Analysis. Baltimore, Johns Hopkins University Press, 1986.
12. Jacklin CN: Female and male: issues of gender. Am Psychol 44:128–33, 1989.
13. Maccoby E, Jacklin C: The Psychology of Sex Differences. Stanford, Calif, Stanford University Press, 1974.
14. McElroy MA, Willis JD: Women and the achievement conflict in sport: a preliminary study. J Sport Psychol 1: 241–7, 1979.
15. McHugh MC, Duquin ME, Frieze IH: Beliefs about success and failure: attributes and female athletes. In Oglesby CA (ed): Women & Sport: From Myth to Reality. Philadelphia, Lea & Febiger, 1978, pp 172–91.
16. Mechikoff RA, Evans V: Sport Psychology for Women. New York, Harper & Rowe, 1987.
17. Murphy S: Sport Psychology Interventions. Champaign, Ill, Human Kinetics, 1995.
18. Park J, Hult J: Women as leaders in physical education and school-based sports, 1865 to the 1930's. (Women in Sport Leadership: The Legacy and the Challenge). J Phys Educ Recreat & Dance 3:33–8, 1993.
19. Silva JM: An evaluation of fear of success in female and male athletes and nonathletes. J Sport Psychol 4:92–6, 1982.
20. Stewart MJ, Corbin CB: Feedback dependence among low confidence preadolescent boys and girls. Res Q Exerc Sport 59:160–4, 1988.
21. Tresemer DW: Fear of Success. New York, Plenum, 1977.
22. Weinberg RS, Gould D: Foundations of Sport & Exercise Psychology. Champaign, Ill, Human Kinetics, 1995.
23. Weiner B: An attribution theory of achievement, motivation and emotion. Psychol Rev 92:548–73, 1985.
24. Zuckerman M, Allison SN: An objective measure of fear of success: construction and validation. J Pers Assess 40: 422–30, 1976.

Chapter 6

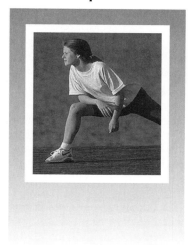

Optimizing Performance in Team Sports for Female Athletes
AN EXPLORATION OF GENDER-SPECIFIC PSYCHOLOGICAL DIFFERENCES AND THEIR EFFECT ON ATHLETIC PERFORMANCE IN TEAM SPORTS

Kathleen J. DeBoer, B.A., M.B.A.

This is a chapter about coaching. My intent is to improve our coaching of female athletes by examining our assumptions about motivation, competition, and reinforcement. My hypothesis is that psychosocial differences influencing males and females produce disparate worldviews. These worldviews affect competitive behavior, achievement motivation, and team dynamics. By becoming aware of these differences we will choose different approaches to coaching females that will yield better results.

INTRODUCTION

Until about 20 years ago, athletics was synonymous with maleness in this country. With few exceptions, males were the participants. Men coached the teams, and men or boys played the games. Participation at some level was encouraged for all boys. Sport was a training ground for manhood.

Theories about competition, techniques of motivation, and methods of discipline were well established by the late 1960s when females started entering the athletic scene in large numbers. Coaches of female teams mimicked what coaches had done before them. The profession had been male, so the models were masculine.

Even though many of the early coaches of girls' and women's teams were female, few people questioned the efficacy of this model. The logic seemed sound: if females were going to participate in an activity that formerly only males had participated in, the best way to succeed would be to emulate successful male models.

In the area of technical training, this assumption was and is correct. Shooting a basketball, serving a volleyball, and throwing a softball are all technical skills in which males and females are trained similarly. Coaches must be aware of differences in strength that may influence the number of repetitions appropriate for training a female versus a male athlete, but the mechanics taught are identical.

Successful women athletes continue to be those who execute skills similarly to their male counterparts. The reason for this is simply biomechanical proficiency. This proficiency has nothing to do with gender. Nevertheless, our history of putting greater emphasis on athletic participation for males at a young age has resulted in a cultural perception that males are inherently more adept than females in sports skills. Hence, on playing fields you will hear the taunt that a boy throws "like a girl"; in a game you will hear a male berate his athletic performance by saying he is playing "like his sister"; on a golf course you will hear male golfers tease each other on short putts by saying "bring your purse, Alice." Each of these comments is meant to insult the male by comparing his skills or performance to that of a female.

Actually, the development of a specific athletic skill in both males and females is closely linked to three things: the number of hours of repetition of that skill; the athlete's ability to model the correct technique; and, to a great extent, the quality of feedback and type of reinforcement the athlete has received.

PSYCHOLOGICAL DIFFERENCES

Technical expertise, while important, is only one element of successful coaching. The ability to motivate, teach, and discipline athletes is equally important. My hypothesis is that, in this area of coaching, use of male models may not be the most effective route to success with female athletes because of the psychological differences between men and women.

A friend of mine had been the assistant coach with the men's national volleyball team for several years, and was now coaching his own women's college team. He shared this story with me.

During his tenure with the men, he recalled a match that was critically important to the team's advancement internationally. The head coach called a timeout. After a few technical instructions, he turned to the team's best player and shouted, "It is time for you to step it up. You're our best player; you're supposed to be one of the world's best. Show me that now! Make a difference!" The star player looked the coach straight in the eye and nodded.

He played the rest of the match aggressively and with great self-confidence. His attitude stimulated the rest of the team; they raised their level of play, and the team won the match.

Several years later my friend was in a similar situation with his women's collegiate team. He approached his best player in the timeout and repeated to her the words of his mentor. Her reaction was markedly different. She looked away from him nervously, and a slight paleness came over her face. In response, he increased the intensity of his praise for her skills and finished by saying, "You are the only one on this team who can win this for us. Do you understand? You're the best; now prove it!"

After he finished, she thrust her hand out for the final cheer and said abruptly to her teammates, "We're all in this together, now let's go." Her play after the timeout was hesitant and tentative. She seemed unsure of herself and made a critical error on a routine play. Her indecisiveness confused her teammates: they lost all sense of rhythm, and the team lost the match.

The same situation and the same words solicited a radically different response from the two athletes. This could be an isolated example, attributable to personality differences between the two stars. However, my experience in working with male and female athletes, and my discussions with male and female coaches of both genders, leads me to believe this is not an isolated incident. I have observed exceptions, but on the whole, there is a pattern of differences in the way male and female athletes respond to coaching.

THE DISCUSSION OF DIFFERENCES IN TODAY'S POLITICAL CONTEXT

The discussion of gender differences is one I approach with great trepidation. This is a time of concern with "political correctness." We are cautious when speaking or writing about people based on historic biases and generalized stereotypes.

I hesitate to write a chapter about general patterns in male/female behavior lest it discourage you from evaluating athletes as individuals. Of course, behaviors range within each gender. Some females will demonstrate more masculine traits; some males, more feminine traits.

Nevertheless, I believe there are observable patterns of similarities within each gender. In fact, blindness to these patterns in behavior causes much frustration and misunderstanding in both female athletes and their coaches.

Another reason for my hesitation is that the perception that females lack interest in participating in athletics has been the basis for discrimination in access to athletic opportunities. I anticipate objections to this chapter from those who posit that, if there really is an alternate motivation in females for the desire to compete, then we will reinforce negative stereotypes about female athletes, and thereby undermine the progress that has been made.

We will go backward only if we presume the male agenda for competition is the ideal and the female agenda is an inferior imitation. Historically, this has been a tacit assumption. In other words, if a motivational technique works well with male athletes but does not work well with female athletes, we have criticized the female athletes rather than questioned the efficacy of the method. Overcoming the bias in athletics to view the male model as the prototype is a major challenge. Nevertheless, we must realize that ignoring gender differences rather than legitimizing them only exaggerates the disenfranchisement of female athletes.

AN EXPLORATION OF WORLDVIEWS

One of my premises is that males and females have different worldviews. The paradigms that shape values, the situations that cause fear, and the circumstances that define success are distinct.

The question of whether these disparate world-views are a function of biology, socialization, or a combination of the two is a worthwhile and intriguing debate, but is well beyond the scope of this chapter.

The literature on the subject credits early childhood as the time of worldview development.[11] There seems to be little debate that boys and girls, from birth, face different challenges in the struggle to define themselves as individuals.

The source of the difference, according to Nancy Chodorow, is that historically the primary caregiver for children has been the mother; therefore, the source of identity for girls is attachment; the source of identity for boys is separation.[1]

Carol Gilligan, in her 1982 book entitled *In a Different Voice: Psychological Theory and Women's Development* says, ". . . girls, in identifying themselves as female, experience themselves as like their mothers, thus fusing the experience of attachment with the process of identity formation. In contrast, . . . boys, in defining themselves as masculine, separate their mothers from themselves. . . . Consequently, male development entails a 'more emphatic individuation and a more defensive firming of experienced ego boundaries'."[2]

Sam Keen, in his book, *Fire in the Belly: On Being a Man*, reinforces Gilligan's premise about male development when he says, ". . . the first major crisis in a boy's life [is] severing his attachment to his mother and identifying with his father. . . . This successful resolution of the Oedipus complex, like ancient initiation rites, involves identification with power, authority, and the values of the father and the male establishment."[8]

The male worldview that boys learn is that of a hierarchical social order. Self-esteem and self-definition are closely linked to one's position in the order. Independence, learned painfully during differentiation from the mother, is highly valued. Status is rewarded and is achieved by moving up the ranks. Differentiating oneself from others through accomplishment is closely linked to self-esteem.

By contrast, the female worldview, shaped by imitating the same-sex parent, is that of a web of relationships. Views of self are linked to one's place in the web. The interconnectedness of the attachments is closely linked to self-esteem. Status is ascribed by linkage to those, usually males, who have achieved it.

These different worldviews shape what males and females value and fear most. Males value independence, freedom, and success or status; they fear dependency, suffocation, and failure. Females value connectedness, intimacy, and belonging; they fear isolation, separation, and loneliness.

The operative word in the preceding paragraph is "most." Obviously, at some level, men value connectedness, and women value independence; at some level, men fear isolation, and women fear failure. By generalizing, we identify patterns of behavior in each sex, granting that neither sex demonstrates these characteristics to the total exclusion of those prominent in the other sex.

Gilligan explains the result of these disparate worldviews when she says, ". . . The images of hierarchy and web . . . convey different ways of structuring relationships and are associated with different views of morality and self. . . . [The male has] . . . the wish to be alone at the top and the consequent fear that others will get too close; [the female has] . . . the wish to be at the center of connection and the consequent fear of being too far out on the edge. These images create a problem in understanding because each distorts the other's presentation . . . each image marks as dangerous the place which the other defines as safe."[3]

Given these concepts, let's return to the responses of the male and female volleyball players in the previous stories. The male player felt singled out as the best, a position he craved, a position of high status in the team's hierarchy. The coach's motivational words matched his mindset, and he responded positively.

The female player, on the other hand, felt separated from the team, a position she feared, a position at the perimeter of the web. The same words inappropriately motivated her, and she responded negatively.

Both athletes were capable volleyball players, clearly able to lead their teams to victory and desiring to do so. However, they needed to be motivated in different ways to respond to that challenge.

CONVERSATION AS A WINDOW ON WORLDVIEW

Sociolinguist Deborah Tannen reinforces Gilligan's principles about male and female mindset differences in her research on conversations. In *You Just Don't Understand: Men and Women in Conversation*, she describes the male worldview as ". . . an individual in a hierarchical social order in which he [is] either one-up or one-down. In this world, conversations are negotiations in which people try to achieve and maintain the upper hand if they can, and protect themselves from others' attempts to put them down and push them around. Life, then, is a contest, a struggle to preserve independence and avoid failure."

Her description of the female worldview is ". . . an individual in a network of connections. In this world, conversations are negotiations for closeness in which people try to seek and give confirmation and support, and to reach consensus. They try to protect themselves from others' attempts to push them away. Life, then, is a community, a struggle to preserve intimacy and avoid isolation."[12]

I remember an exchange I had with an athlete during a match. I was irritated because she was not following my instructions. In a scolding tone, I said to her, "You're not following the game plan. I told you to establish the middle attack, do you understand?" Without waiting for her answer, I snapped, "Do you want our outside hitters to get blocked off the court? Now, set the middle!" Instead of acknowledging my request, or defending her delinquency, she said to me, "You hate me, don't you?"

The disgust in my voice had hurt her feelings. There was a breach in our relationship that, to her, was more important than my instructions. When she returned to the court, she performed poorly. She mechanically followed my instructions, looking at me after every unsuccessful play. I had made a coaching mistake. My harsh words and sarcastic tone had taken her mind off winning the match and focused her attention on our relationship.

I have seen this happen with female teams on many occasions. The importance of relationships is a factor that coaches must consider when managing and motivating a female team. When relationships rupture, the team will be easily distracted from playing to win. Coaches of female teams ignore this fact at their own peril.

WORLDVIEW AS A WINDOW ON BEHAVIOR

A colleague of mine used to coach both male and female cross-country teams. In his observation, the groups responded differently to a time breakthrough by a particular runner.

On the men's team, when one of the runners dramatically reduced his time, several others were likely to experience a similar surge after a period of training. The breakthrough provided motivation to the athlete's teammates. It showed them possibilities; it made them fear falling behind; it challenged them to push harder.

With his women's teams, when one runner excelled, the other runners reacted differently. They teased her by calling her the coach's pet; they said she was trying to make the rest of them look bad, and that she wanted to be the star. They often expressed discouragement with their own running and performances.

In other words, the breakthrough caused a tear in the comfortableness of the relationship web on the team. By taunting her, the group isolated the offending runner. Instead of gaining status for achievement, she was punished.

Fearing this isolation, the breakthrough runner often worked hard to win back the favor of her teammates. She encouraged her teammates' efforts. She slowed herself slightly in training, running just at the head of the group, as if pulling them along by not putting too much distance between herself and the group.

This behavior may not have helped the individual runner excel, but it helped improve the performance of the team. My colleague observed that when his female runners ran as a pack, the individuals put tremendous pressure on themselves to stay with the group. The women drove themselves to personal bests on a regular basis in their attempt to stay with the group and not disappoint the team.

This example demonstrates the differences between the sexes in the source of self-esteem. Men achieve their sense of self from their position in the hierarchy, women from their position in the web. For men, their place in the hierarchy is determined by what they do and how well they do it; it is only peripherally associated with their ability to connect and maintain relationships. For women, their place in the web is determined by their ability to connect and maintain relationships; it is only peripherally associated with what they do and how well they do it. Hence, male runners will punish themselves to catch a colleague who has outdistanced them; female runners will punish themselves to fulfill their commitment to the group. In both cases, the performance of the group is improved, the motivations for the individual runners, however, may be quite different.

ACHIEVEMENT MOTIVATION

While both sexes are driven to succeed, and both fear the embarrassment of failure, the rewards and punishments for particular successes and failures often differ by gender.

Matina Horner did research in this area in the late 1960s, developing the "fear of success" theory. Horner reports that ". . . Women appeared to have a problem with competitive achievement, and that problem seemed to emanate from a perceived conflict between femininity and success. . . ."[6] Her theory provided insight into the observed under-achievement of women in competitive situations where their skills would predict that they would succeed.

Horner continues, ". . . when success is likely or possible, threatened by negative consequences they expect to follow success, young women become anxious and their positive achievement strivings become thwarted."[6] In a related paper, she posits that this fear of achieving "exists because for most women, the anticipation of success in competitive achievement activity, especially against men, produces anticipation of certain negative consequences, for example, threat of social rejection and loss of femininity."[7]

When I was in my mid-twenties, I was coaching volleyball at a Midwestern university. I had played a lot of tennis as an adolescent and retained a certain degree of proficiency in that sport. I was single at the time and was asked to substitute for a sick wife at a mixed doubles tennis outing.

Although competition was involved, the outing was intended to be social. The hours of tennis were matched with hours of eating and drinking. Men and women were paired at random; the only stipulation being that spouses could not play on the same team. I drew a man named Jack as my partner. He was a college administrator with average tennis skills but above-average competitiveness.

Jack and I made a good team, defeating all of our opponents. He was especially thrilled when we defeated the athletics director, a man who prided himself on his tennis ability, and who was just as competitive as Jack was. In fact, when I aced the athletics director to win the set, Jack could barely contain his glee. He threw his racket in the air, gave me a bear hug, and said, "What a serve! God, who is ever going to marry you?"

The not-so-hidden message in his comment was that, in his mind, my success as an athlete was diminishing my chances of finding a mate. Barbara A. Kerr, in her book *Smart Girls, Gifted Women*, reinforces this thought when she says, "It is likely that society's emphasis on the impossibility of combining love and achievement forces many gifted girls to become preoccupied with their relationships rather than personal achievement."[9]

I remember feeling both hurt and disappointed when one of my best friends and our star forward told me before her junior year in high school that she was not going to try out for the basketball team because her parents had told her she needed to get a job. I asked her why her brother, a senior and average performer on our high school swim team, did not have to quit to get a job. She said her brother might be swimming in college and therefore had a reason to continue athletics. I argued that, with her skills, she had a better chance than her brother did of participating in college. She said there was no reason for her to continue, and she had made up her mind.

At the time neither of us realized we were in a common struggle for adolescent girls, one dealing with what Barbara Kerr calls "issues of conformity versus achievement." She found in her research on gifted children that at about age 14, girls become more concerned with relationships than self-actualization.[10]

This shift from "what I can be" to "where I fit" is one coaches of female teams must deal with. Adolescent girls are very sensitive to peers' evaluations of their activities. The negative taunts of tomboy, Amazon, and lesbian, while never reinforcing to female athletes, are most frightening to athletic girls in adolescence.

SANCTIONS FOR SUCCESS/FAILURE

Not only does athletic success carry with it certain penalties for females, but also failure is acceptable, often expected, and routinely encouraged, especially in competitions with males. John Gray, in his book, *Men Are from Mars, Women Are from Venus*, goes so far as to say that women have a lose/win philosophy, meaning, "I lose so that you can win." Men, on the other hand, have a win/lose philosophy, meaning: "I want to win, and I don't care if you lose."[5] He characterizes both of these extremes as dysfunctional for building lasting interpersonal relationships. Nevertheless, these differences may provide insight into the different types of competitiveness displayed by male and female athletes.

Athletic success is not viewed as a defining element of female development. In other words, it's not an integral part of "becoming a woman." Therefore, females may be greatly embarrassed by athletic failure, but they will not feel as if they are failures as women. No one views a failed female athlete as less feminine than her conqueror; in fact, just the opposite may be true. For female athletes, losing can be devastating, but winning is more likely to be associated with questioned gender identity than losing.

This is different for males. The personal embarrassment of failure is combined with gender diminishment. Recently a football-coaching friend was describing the effect a very convincing loss had on his team. He said the team's sports psychologist had likened the feelings of the players after the loss with those experienced by a woman who had been raped. He said that the margin of defeat not only embarrassed his players, but also made them feel shamed, powerless, and afraid. The loss made them doubt their masculinity.

I have observed many motivational speeches by coaches of men's teams that are full of references to a contest as a test of manhood, that abound with challenges to the participants to prove their manliness, and that are peppered with adjectives associated with masculinity. The message is clear: to succeed is to succeed in "being a man"; to fail is to fail in that regard.

I have never heard a motivational speech to female athletes that makes reference to womanhood, womanliness, or femininity. In fact, most locker room speeches to female teams are just as full of adjectives associated with masculinity as the speeches given to male teams. Female athletes are encouraged to be aggressive, powerful, strong, assertive and competitive. When the ball is in play, a "lose/win" philosophy is a major liability.

When a male succeeds athletically, he is rewarded with high reinforcement of his gender identity. The successful male athlete is a highly sought-after date and mate. He is regarded as the prototype of his sex, particularly during the critical identity-forming adolescent years. For males, then, the rewards of athletic success and the penalties for failure are greater than those for females.

These distinct patterns of social reinforcement have a direct impact on the achievement motivation of male and female athletes. For male teams the social rewards of success and penalties for failure are such that winning, simply for the sake of winning, is usually sufficient motivation to produce maximum commitment.

Female teams, on the other hand, may experience social censure if they are too successful, and our culture readily forgives them for failure. Therefore, female teams may need additional incentives, beyond winning for the sake of being the best, to produce maximum commitment.

MESHING WORLDVIEW WITH TEAM MANAGEMENT

One of these incentives that coaches of female teams can facilitate is the development of team chemistry. As mentioned earlier, females generally are extremely committed to a group they feel connected to, so winning for the team can be an important motivator. The group whose members are dedicated to each other and to the legitimacy of their cause will experience the synergy necessary to overachieve.

I had an experience with one of my teams several years ago that made me painfully aware of the importance of interpersonal relationships on a women's team. I was taking time during practice to explain to one of my best players a new formation for receiving the opponent's serve. She looked at my diagrams, then told me there was no way those formations would work because I had positioned her receiving the serve next to a player she did not like. When I questioned her dedication to our success, she calmly explained that she and this other player would not communicate on line calls and had no investment in making each other look good; therefore, if I were dedicated to our success, I would not have them play next to each other.

Arguing that the rotation I was proposing would be our strongest pattern, I started the season that way. Very quickly I observed a tense, icy atmosphere on the court. I swallowed my pride, switching the line-up to separate the rivals. Our team chemistry improved immediately. We went on, with a theoretically weaker rotation, to a very successful season.

Once I began to examine coaching in the context of worldview, I realized how often my colleagues and I were using "challenges to manliness" motivational statements with our females.

I played professional basketball for a man who had spent his entire coaching career coaching men's teams. During a particularly close game, he screamed at me from the sideline, "You chased that ball just like a woman." He was obviously displeased with the intensity of my effort, and he associated lack of effort with my sex. He also was trying to chastise me in the harshest manner he could. I was angered by his rebuke and shot back a retort that earned me a seat on the bench for the rest of the game.

This experience as an athlete obviously taught me little about effective coaching because I frequently used "challenges to manliness" techniques with my own teams. I assumed the validity of the hierarchical model for motivating athletes. I pitted one player against another in a drill and, in my feedback, I appealed to their desire for one-upmanship. I ranted about the loss of status that accompanied failure.

One day one of my athletes shouted at me, "I don't care if she beats me; she is my friend." At first I chalked up her remark to a lack of competitiveness. Then I came to realize that my feedback was inappropriate for her mindset. She had no need to feel superior to her friend or to win the drill for winning's sake. In fact, protecting her place in the interconnectedness of the group was much more important to her than winning the drill, and potentially singling herself out.

From that realization forward, my feedback centered on challenging each player to make her teammate better. I convinced them that the harder they made the exercise for their counterpart, the better each of them would become. I equated effort in the drill with commitment to the team. The motivational task was to convince them that to retain their position in the web, they had to raise their level of effort or play. This type of motivation had a much more powerful effect on my athletes because it appealed to the things they valued.

Instead of chastising a player when she failed to execute a support task (such as covering a hitter in volleyball, calling out a pick in basketball, or backing up a throw in softball), I challenged her commitment to her teammate. I scolded her for making her counterpart look bad, telling her that her play indicated to me that she did not care about her teammate. Because keeping the web intact is important to females, this type of censure was painful, and much more powerful than appealing to her desire to be great.

I also learned to avoid the "star" label with my female teams. An elevation of status may push a player out of the web. Isolation from the group is an uncomfortable place for females, even if the cause is self-actualization.

When I was in my junior year of high school, I won the Most Valuable Player Award in every sport that our school offered for girls. I had high achievement motivation so I craved those awards, and I was the best athlete in those sports, so I deserved the awards. In spite of those factors, however, I remember feeling embarrassed, and somewhat angry, that no one else had won. I feared being alone at the top.

I encountered this same discomfort when I was recruiting high school stars to my college program. Parents frequently expressed dismay at the vindictiveness directed toward their daughters by teammates and other parents. The young women I was recruiting could not wait for college volleyball, where, they perceived, all the players were dedicated and highly skilled, and their dedication and superior skills would not single them out. They desperately wanted to succeed, but they also craved conformity and acceptance.

Another coaching tactic that I changed after repeated mistakes was that of chastising a player in front of her teammates. I found it had the opposite effect from the one I sought. I was using negative feedback to change a player's behavior, but she often received positive feedback from her teammates when she returned to the court. Her teammates would rally around her, assuring her that she was an important part of the group, and that I was the ogre. My criticism usually went unheeded.

Once I became aware of this dynamic, I separated the player I was disciplining from the group. Not only did I avoid the sympathy backlash, but also the player realized she needed to heed my instructions to be allowed to return to the group. For most players, this was a strong incentive to cooperate.

One of the advantages of coaching female athletes is that, in keeping with their concern for attachment, they are very sensitive to their relationship with the coach. The result is that female athletes are generally eager to please. They attempt to follow instructions, change bad habits, and focus on a practice task more readily than their male counterparts, who are not as obsessed with approval.

The drawback to this preoccupation with attachment is that female athletes tend to take criticism very personally. Corrective feedback is often taken as criticism, especially if a raised voice or sarcastic tone accompanies it. A breach in the coach—player relationship may distract a female athlete from her focus on competition. A key element in her self-esteem is her relationship with her coach. If that is damaged, she may lose confidence in her ability to perform, or may lose one of her prime incentives to succeed.

In my observation, the result of this factor is that frequently coaches train male and female teams differently. Female teams spend most of their practice time in drills of specific fundamentals; male teams spend most of their practice time in modified game situations. Generally, female participants seem to have a higher tolerance for the banality of task repetition; and male participants, a greater addiction to the thrill of competition. In reality, the great athlete, of either gender, combines intensity and focus on skill development in practice with tenacity and single-mindedness to win in competition.

CONCLUDING REMARKS

During my coaching years, I remember many male colleagues lamenting that their female players were not as competitive as males. The most fervent complainers were those who had been athletes themselves. They followed the hierarchical model automatically in their coaching. They had lived it; it had worked for them.

These coaches were frustrated and mystified by their lack of effectiveness when leading a female group that valued team chemistry more than winning, that refused "the star" label as much as they craved success, that practiced intensely but, at times, struggled with competition, and that disabled themselves by personalizing corrective feedback.

My female colleagues who, like me, had made liberal use of the hierarchical model in their coaching did not attribute their frustration to a lack of competitiveness among their athletes. Forgetting the memories of our own experiences and reactions, we said that athletes had changed, that they were not as tough as we used to be.

All of us were missing the point. The issue was not lack of competitiveness among female athletes or of a significant change in female character, but rather that our methods of motivating and reinforcing our athletes did not match their worldview. We were trying to get them to respond to things that did not matter to them, and we were ignoring things that mattered deeply to them. We were, in essence, talking in a foreign language to them. Their feelings of being misunderstood were as profound as our own.

I would love to conclude this chapter by claiming that, after examining my coaching in the context of male/female worldview differences, I never lost another match. I know it would be the best motivation I could give you to examine your own methods. Unfortunately, this was not the case.

I continued to have a moderately high level of success in terms of wins and losses because I had a moderately high level of skill among the players in my program. I also continued to succeed in motivating some players and to fail in motivating others.

My understanding of these matters did, however, make me a better coach. I did not rant and rave more or less; I simply ranted and raved about different things. I did not ask any less of my athletes; I simply asked it in a different way. I understood myself better and I understood them better. These factors made me, and will make you, a better coach.

References

1. Chodorow N: Family structure and feminine personality. In Rosaldo MZ, Lamphere L (eds): Woman, Culture and Society. Stanford, Calif, Stanford University Press, 1974, pp 43–4.
2. Gilligan C: In a Different Voice: Psychological Theory and Women's Development. Cambridge, Mass, Harvard University Press, 1982, pp 7–8.
3. Ibid, p 62.
4. Ibid, p 14.
5. Gray J: Men Are from Mars, Women Are from Venus. New York, HarperCollins, 1992, pp 44–8.
6. Horner MS: Sex Differences in Achievement Motivation and Performance in Competitive and Noncompetitive Situations. Ph.D. Thesis, University of Michigan, 1968, University Microfilms #6912135:125.
7. Horner MS: Toward an understanding of achievement-related conflicts in women. J Soc Issues 28:157–75, 1972.
8. Keen S: Fire in the Belly: On Being a Man. New York, Bantam Books, 1991, pp 19–20.
9. Kerr BA: Smart Girls, Gifted Women. Dayton, Ohio, Psychology Press, 1985, p 101.
10. Ibid, p 100.
11. Stoller RJ: A contribution to the study of gender identity. Int J Psychoanal 45:220–6, 1964.
12. Tannen D: You Just Don't Understand: Women and Men in Conversation. New York, William Morrow, 1990, pp 24–5.

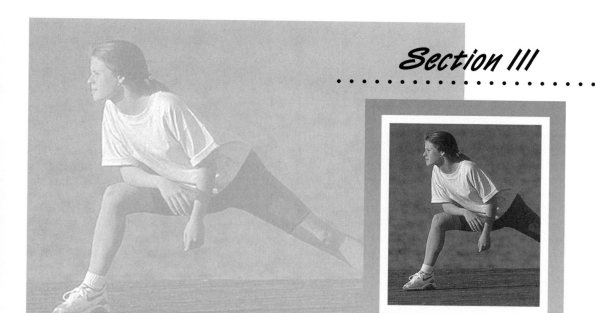

Performance
Issues

Chapter 7

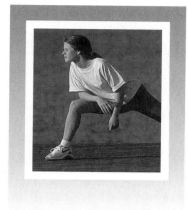

Performance in the Context of Growth and Maturation

Robert M. Malina, Ph.D.

Athletes by definition are skilled in the performance demands of their respective sports. It is reasonable to assume that athletes as a group are proficient in motor skills and perhaps in a variety of physiologic indicators of performance, such as aerobic power and muscular strength and endurance.

The performance and training demands of a sport tend to be specific. As such, it is difficult to compare athletes in different sports, or athletes and nonathletes. Nevertheless, the outcomes of tasks performed under specified conditions can be quantified and compared between athletes and nonathletes, athletes in several sports, and male and female athletes within the same sport. Such tasks include, for example, the vertical jump and long jump (power), medicine ball throw (power and coordination), dashes (speed) and shuttle runs (speed and agility), sit-ups per unit time (abdominal strength and endurance), the force expressed against a fixed resistance (strength), and maximal aerobic power (VO_2 max).

The performances of young athletes must be viewed in the context of normal growth and maturation; performances ordinarily change in concert with progress in these 2 biologic processes that dominate the first 2 decades of life. Size, physique, and body composition, outcomes of growth processes, all influence performance. Individual differences in the timing and tempo of biologic maturation are additional factors to consider.

This chapter addresses the performances of females in general, and female athletes in particular, in the context of growth and maturation. Several factors that influence performance are also considered. The performances of females are compared with those of males as needed to illustrate specific points. Concepts

of growth and maturation, and the growth and maturation of female athletes in particular, are initially considered. With this information as background, age-, sex-, and maturity-associated variation in motor performances, strength, and aerobic power are then discussed. Finally, the influence of physique and body composition on performance is considered.

OVERVIEW OF GROWTH AND MATURATION

Children, both athletes and nonathletes, grow, mature, and develop as they progress from childhood to adulthood. Although the 3 processes are often treated interchangeably, each has a specific meaning.[47]

Growth refers to the increase in the size of the body as a whole and of its parts. Thus, as children grow, they become taller and heavier, they increase in lean and fat tissues, their organs increase in size, and so on. Heart volume and mass, for example, follow a growth pattern like that for body weight, while the lungs and lung functions grow proportionally to height. Different parts of the body grow at different rates and different times, resulting in changes in body proportions.

Maturation refers to progress toward the biologically mature state. It is an operational concept because the mature state varies with the body system. All tissues, organs, and systems of the body mature. Studies of children and adolescents focus on sexual, skeletal, and somatic maturation. Maturation can be viewed in 2 contexts, timing and tempo. The former refers to when specific maturational events occur (eg, age at the beginning of breast development in girls, the age at the appearance of pubic hair in boys and girls, or the age at maximum growth during the adolescent growth spurt). *Tempo* refers to the rate at which maturation progresses (eg, how quickly or slowly the youngster passes from initial stages of sexual maturation to the mature state). Timing and tempo vary considerably among individuals.

In healthy, adequately nourished children and adolescents, growth and maturation are largely genetically regulated.[9] Development, on the other hand, is largely culturally mediated. It refers to the acquisition of behavioral competence, that is, the learning of appropriate behaviors and skills expected by society. Nevertheless, it is important to recognize that the 3 processes—growth, maturation, and development—occur simultaneously and interact. These biocultural interactions influence the youngster's self-concept, self-esteem, body image, and perceived competence. Individuals working with young athletes should be aware of these interactions. How an adolescent is coping with her sexual maturation or adolescent growth spurt may influence her behaviors, including sport-related behaviors and performance. Further, the demands of specific sports are superimposed upon those associated with normal growth, maturation, and development, and a mismatch between the demands of a sport and those of normal growth and maturation may be a source of stress among elite young athletes.

GROWTH AND MATURITY STATUS OF FEMALE ATHLETES

Athletes are variably defined during childhood and adolescence. The majority of studies of young athletes include youth who can be classified as select, elite, or junior national caliber.[37] The growth and maturity characteristics of young athletes are selective factors in many sports. It is often size, physique, and maturity that bring young athletes to the attention of adults involved in youth sports. In some sports, young children are selected for their physical characteristics. Growth and maturity status, in turn, influence performances on a variety of tasks. Thus, an understanding of the growth and maturation of youngsters active in sport, and of young athletes in specific sports, is essential.

Height and Weight

Young female athletes in a variety of sports have, on average, heights that equal or exceed reference medians from childhood through adolescence (Table 7-1). Gymnastics and figure

Table 7-1. Stature and Weight of Young Female Athletes Relative to Percentiles (P) of United States Reference Data

SPORT	STATURE	WEIGHT
Basketball	P 75– >P90	P 50–P 75
Volleyball	P 75	P 50–P 75
Soccer	P 50	P 50
Track		
Distance runs	≥P 50	<P 50
Sprints	≥P 50	≤P 50
Swimming	P 50–P 90	P 50–P 75
Diving	≤P 50	P 50
Gymnastics	≤P 10–<P 50	P 10–<P 50[a]
Tennis	>P 50	±P 50
Figure skating	P 10–<P 50	P 10–<P 50
Ballet	≤P 50	P 10–<P 50

[a]More recent samples of gymnasts are closer to P 10.
Adapted from Malina RM: Physical growth and biological maturation of young athletes. Exerc Sport Sci Rev 22:389–433, 1994 and Malina RM: Growth and maturation of young athletes: Is training for sport a factor? In Chan K-M, Micheli LJ (eds): Sports and Children. Hong Kong, Williams & Wilkins Asia-Pacific, 1998, p 133.

skating are the only sports that consistently present a profile of short stature. More recent samples of elite female gymnasts are, on average, shorter than those of 20 years ago.[40] Female ballet dancers tend to have shorter statures during childhood and early adolescence, but catch up to nondancers in late adolescence.[37] Stature is a selective factor in some sports, for example, shortness in gymnastics and tallness in the high jump and basketball.

Body mass presents a similar pattern. Female athletes in a variety of sports tend to have body masses that, on average, equal or exceed the reference medians. Gymnasts, figure skaters, and ballet dancers consistently show lighter body masses. However, body mass is appropriate for height in gymnasts and figure skaters, while it is low for height in ballet dancers. A similar trend is demonstrated in female distance runners.[37]

Maturity Status and Progress

Information on the maturity status and progress of young female athletes is not extensive (Table 7-2), with the exception of data for the age at menarche (see below). Maturity differences are most apparent during the transition into adolescence and the adolescent growth spurt, and reflect the individuality in timing and tempo of maturation. Skeletal maturation is the only maturity indicator that spans childhood through adolescence. Data for skeletal age are available for female gymnasts and swimmers, with less data for ballet dancers and track athletes. The data for track and field are to some extent confounded by event.

Table 7-2. Maturity Status Based on Skeletal Age and Secondary Sex Characteristics (Excluding Menarche) in Female Athletes During Middle Childhood and Adolescence, and in Late Adolescence

FEMALES	CHILDHOOD (< 10.0 YRS)[a]	ADOLESCENCE (10.0–14.9 YRS)[a]	LATE ADOLESCENCE (>15.0 YRS)[a]
Distance runs	[b]	Later/average	Later/average
Track and field	[b]	Average	Average
Swimming	Average/advanced	Average/advanced	Average
Gymnastics	Average	Later/average	Later
Ballet	[b]	Later/average	Later

Characterizing maturity status in late adolescence is influenced by the early attainment of maturity in advanced maturers and catch-up of average and later maturers, that is, all youth eventually reach skeletal and sexual maturity. The upper limit of one skeletal maturity assessment system is 16.0 years (maturity).
[a]Indicated ages are approximate.
[b]Satisfactory data are not available.
Adapted from Malina RM: Physical growth and biological maturation of young athletes. Exerc Sport Sci Rev 22:389–433, 1994, and Malina RM: Growth and maturation of young athletes: Is training for sport a factor? In Chan K-M, Micheli LJ (eds): Sports and Children. Hong Kong, Williams & Wilkins Asia-Pacific, 1998, p 133.

During childhood, gymnasts have skeletal ages that can be classified as "average" or "on time" for chronologic age. A skeletal age within plus or minus 1 year of chronologic age is considered average.[44] Most gymnasts are classified as average and late (skeletal age lags behind chronologic age by more than 1 year), and few early-maturing girls (skeletal age is in advance of chronologic age by more than 1 year) are in the samples. In later adolescence, most gymnasts are late maturing.[37] The data suggest that early- and average-maturing girls are systematically less represented among gymnasts as girls pass from childhood through adolescence. This trend probably reflects the selection criteria of the sport, and perhaps the performance advantage of later-maturing girls in gymnastics activities. Corresponding data for secondary sex characteristics are less extensive, but are consistent with the trends in skeletal age. Although data are not as extensive as for gymnasts, female ballet dancers and distance runners show a similar maturity gradient in adolescence. In contrast, young female swimmers tend to have skeletal ages that are average or advanced in childhood and adolescence.[37,41] The data for later adolescence are difficult to evaluate because maturity status at this time is influenced by the early attainment of maturity by youth advanced in maturation and the catch-up of average and later maturing youth (ie, all youth eventually reach skeletal and sexual maturity).

Pubertal progress refers to the tempo of change from one stage of a secondary sex characteristic to another, or from initial appearance to the mature state. Such data for female athletes are not extensive. Limited data for girls active in sport (track and rowing) suggest no differences in tempo compared to nonathletes. Mean intervals for progression from one stage to the next or across 2 stages of breast and pubic hair development are similar to those for nonactive youth, and are well within the range of normal variation in longitudinal studies of nonathletes.[52] The interval between ages at peak height velocity (PHV) and menarche for girls active in sport and nonactive girls also does not differ, and is similar to those for several samples of nonathletic girls, mean intervals of 1.2 to 1.5 years.[24]

Menarche

Most discussions of biologic maturation of female athletes focus on the age at menarche, which is a late-pubertal event. Later mean ages at menarche are reported in athletes in many, but not all, sports.[36,39,42,57] There is confusion about later ages at menarche in athletes, which is related in part to the methods of estimating age at which this indicator of maturity occurs.[44] Age at menarche can be estimated in 3 ways. In longitudinal studies, girls are ordinarily examined at 3-month intervals so that interviewing the girl or her mother on each occasion can usually provide a reasonably accurate estimate of when menarche occurs. This is the prospective method based on longitudinal data. Sample sizes in prospective studies are generally small. Longitudinal studies of athletes followed from prepuberty through puberty are ordinarily short term and limited to small, select samples; a potentially confounding issue is selective drop-out.

The status quo method provides a sample or population estimate for the age at menarche. It is a statistical method (based on probits) that requires a sample that spans approximately 9 to 17 years of age. Two pieces of information are needed, the exact age of each girl, and whether or not she has attained menarche. Status quo data for young athletes actively involved in systematic training provide estimates for the sample, but these samples often include athletes of different skill levels and training histories. Only prospective and status quo data deal with maturing athletes.

The vast majority of data on the age at menarche of athletes are retrospective and are based on samples of postmenarcheal late-adolescent and adult athletes. Retrospective data, of course, include potential error associated with accuracy of recall.

Prospective and status quo data for adolescent athletes and retrospective data for a sample of university athletes are summarized in Table 7-3. Other retrospective data for athletes in a variety of sports are summarized elsewhere.[4,36,39,57] Retrospective mean ages at menarche in athletes vary among athletes in different sports, tend to be later than average, and tend to be later in athletes within a sport who are at a higher competitive level. Prospective and status quo data for gymnasts and ballet dancers, and status quo data for Junior Olympic divers and soccer players are generally consistent with the retrospective data. The limited prospective and status quo data for tennis players, rowers, track athletes, and more available data for age group swimmers indicate earlier mean ages at menarche than retrospective estimates for each sport respectively, that is, late-adolescent and young adult athletes (retrospective data) in these sports tend to attain menarche later than those involved in the respective sports during the pubertal years (prospective and/or status quo data). The differences probably represent the interaction of several factors, including the longer growth period associated with later maturation, selective success of late-maturing girls in some sports, selective drop-out of early-maturing girls, and increased opportunity in sport at the collegiate level or older ages.

Does Regular Training for Sport Influence the Growth and Maturation?

Training refers to systematic, specialized practice for a specific sport or sport discipline for most of the year or to specific short-term experimental programs. Training programs are ordinarily specific (eg, endurance running, strength training, sport skill training), and vary in intensity and duration. Some have suggested that sport training has a stimulatory or accelerating influence on growth and maturation, while others have suggested potentially negative influences. Discussions of potentially negative effects of training almost exclusively concern female athletes.

Table 7-3. Ages at Menarche (Years) in Adolescent and University Athletes

	M/Md	SD
Adolescent Athletes—Prospective		
Gymnasts, Polish	15.1	0.9
Gymnasts, Swiss	14.5	1.2
Gymnasts, Swedish	14.5	1.4
Gymnasts, British[a]	14.3	1.4
Swimmers, British	13.3	1.1
Tennis players, British	13.2	1.4
Track, Polish	12.3	1.1
Rowers, Polish	12.7	0.9
Elite ballet dancers, U.S.	15.4	1.9
Adolescent Athletes—Status Quo		
Gymnasts, world[b]	15.6	2.1
Gymnasts, Hungarian	15.0	0.6
Swimmers, age group, U.S.	13.1	1.1
Swimmers, age group, U.S.	12.7	1.1
Divers, Junior Olympic, U.S.	13.6	1.1
Ballet dancers, Yugoslavia	13.6	
Ballet dancers, Yugoslavia	14.1	
Track, Hungarian	12.6	
Soccer players, age group, U.S.	12.9	1.1
Team sports, Hungarian	12.7	
Adolescent Nonathletes[c]		
Range of medians	12.1–13.5	
University Athletes		
Swimming	14.2	1.5
Diving	14.0	1.7
Tennis	13.9	1.5
Golf	13.4	1.1
Volleyball	13.8	1.5
White	13.8	1.5
Black	13.6	1.4
Basketball	13.3	1.4
White	13.6	1.3
Black	13.0	1.4
Track and field	13.7	1.6
Distance: White	14.0	1.4
Middle Distance:		
White	15.2	0.9
Black	14.3	1.5
Sprints:		
White	14.5	1.7
Black	13.1	1.5
Jumps:		
White	13.9	1.0
Black	13.2	2.0
Throws:		
White	13.0	1.5
Black	12.9	1.1
University Nonathletes		
1970	13.0	1.2
1987–1994	12.9	1.3

Adapted from Malina RM: Growth and maturation of young athletes: Is training for sport a factor? In Chan K-M, Micheli LJ (eds): Sports and Children. Hong Kong, Williams & Wilkins Asia-Pacific, 1998, p 133, which includes the specific references. The data for university athletes and nonathletes were collected between 1985 and 1994; the nonathletes were students at the same university as the athletes (Malina, unpublished). Prospective data report means, while status quo data report medians based on probit analysis.
[a]Among the British athletes, 13% had not yet attained menarche, therefore the estimated mean ages will be somewhat later. Small numbers of Swiss and Swedish gymnasts and ballet dancers also had not reached menarche at the time the results were reported.
[b]This sample is from the 1987 world championships in Rotterdam. It did not include girls under 13 years of age so that the estimate may be biased towards an older age.
[c]Status quo estimates for European girls from the mid-1960s through the 1980s. All except 2 of the 39 ages were between 12.5 and 13.5 years. There is a geographic gradient in the distribution of menarcheal ages within Europe, median ages decline from the north to south. The status quo estimate for United States girls is 12.8 years.

Growth in Height and Weight

Sport participation and training for sport have no apparent effect on growth in height and the rate of growth in height in healthy, adequately nourished children and adolescents. With few exceptions, athletes of both sexes in a variety of sports have, on average, heights that equal or exceed reference values for nonathletes (see above). Exceptions among athletes are gymnasts and figure skaters, who present shorter heights than average. This trend probably reflects the selection criteria of the sports. The smaller size of elite gymnasts is evident long before any systematic training started,[54] and is part familial, that is, gymnasts have parents who are shorter than average.[43] There is also a size difference between those who persist in the sport and those who drop out.[43,62,65]

Short-term longitudinal studies of athletes in several sports (volleyball, diving, distance running, basketball) indicate rates of growth in height that, on average, closely approximate rates observed in the nonathletes. The growth rates are well within the range of normally expected variation among youth.[37,52]

In contrast to height, body weight can be influenced by regular training for sport, resulting in changes in body composition. Training is associated with a decrease in fatness in both sexes and occasionally with an increase in fat-free mass. Changes in fatness depend on continued, regular activity or training (or caloric restriction, which often occurs in sports like gymnastics, ballet, figure skating, and diving in girls) for their maintenance. When training is significantly reduced, fatness tends to accumulate. It is difficult to partition specific effects of training on fat-free mass from changes that occur with normal growth and sexual maturation during adolescence.[47]

Biologic Maturation

Does regular training for and participation in sport influence the timing and tempo of biologic maturation? Variation is the rule in the timing and tempo of biologic maturation, especially during adolescence. The timing and tempo of maturation are highly individual characteristics that often show a tendency to run in families, that is, mothers and their daughters may both be early or late maturers. The following summarizes the general trends in the literature for young female athletes.[37,41]

Skeletal Maturation

Although regular activity functions to increase bone mineralization, it does not influence the rate of maturation of the skeleton. Short-term longitudinal studies of girls in several sports indicate similar gains in skeletal maturation in athletes and nonathletes. In other words, skeletal age proceeds in concert with the child's chronolgic age. It should be noted that in later adolescence, differences in maturity status among participants at younger ages are reduced and are eventually eliminated as skeletal maturity is attained by all individuals.

Somatic Maturation

Age at PHV is the primary indicator of somatic maturation. Estimates of the age at PHV and peak velocity for individuals require longitudinal data that span adolescence, approximately 9 to 10 to 16 to 17 years. Based upon observations that spanned only 2.0 to 3.7 years in individual athletes with a mean span of 2.3 years,[60] it has been cautioned that " . . . gymnasts advance through puberty without a normal pubertal growth spurt."[61] The data are not sufficiently longitudinal to warrant such a conclusion, let alone provide an accurate estimate of the age at PHV and peak velocity of growth. Other data for gymnasts that span 6 years across adolescence indicate a clearly defined growth spurt that reaches its peak about 1 year later than average.[65] Many potentially confounding factors are not considered in these studies, especially the rigorous selection/exclusion criteria for female gymnastics, marginal diets, parental size, and so on. Closer examination of the available data suggests that female gymnasts as a group show the growth and maturation characteristics of short normal, slow-maturing children with short parents.[43]

Sexual Maturation

Longitudinal data on the sexual maturation of girls who are regularly active or training for sport are not extensive. The available data are largely cross-sectional so that it is difficult to make clear statements on potential effects of training for sport. The limited longitudinal data indicate no effect of activity or training on the timing and progress of breast and pubic hair development.[37,40,52]

Most discussions of the potential influence of training on sexual maturation focus on later mean ages at menarche that are often observed in females athletes. Training for sport is often indicated as the factor that is responsible for the later mean ages at menarche, with the inference that training "delays" the onset of this maturational event. Unfortunately, studies of athletes ordinarily do not consider other factors that are

Table 7-4. Familial Correlations for Age at Menarche in Athletes

Mother–Daughter	Ballet	0.32
	Athletes in seven sports	0.25
Sister–Sister	Swimmers	0.37
	Athletes in seven sports	0.44

Adapted from Malina RM, Ryan RC, Bonci CM: Age at menarche in athletes and their mothers and sisters. Ann Hum Biol 21:417–22, 1994, which includes the primary references for the ballet dancers and swimmers. Corresponding mother–daughter interclass correlations for samples of nonathletes range from 0.15 to 0.40; corresponding sister–sister intraclass correlations for samples of nonathletes range are 0.25 to 0.30. Assuming no dominance, the expected correlation between first-degree relatives is 0.50.[51]

known to influence menarche. For example, there is a familial tendency for later maturation in athletes (Table 7-4). Mothers of athletes in several sports attain menarche later than mothers of nonathletes, and sisters of elite swimmers and university athletes attain menarche later than average.[51] Although the data are limited, the familial correlations for athletes are similar to those for families of nonathletes. In addition, age at menarche in athletes varies with number of children in the family (Table 7-5). Athletes from larger families attain menarche later than those from smaller families, and the estimated family size effect is similar in athletes and nonathletes.

Allowing for the many factors that are known to influence menarche, it is exceedingly difficult to implicate training per se as the causative factor.[48] The conclusions of 2 comprehensive discussions of exercise and reproductive health of women summarize the situation as follows:

Table 7-5. Estimated Effects of Family Size (Number of Children in the Family) on the Age at Menarche in Samples of Athletes and Nonathletes

	ESTIMATED YEARS PER ADDITIONAL SIBLING IN THE FAMILY
Athletes	
High school varsity	0.15
Olympic (Montreal Games)	0.22
University	
White	0.22
Black	0.20
Nonathletes	
High school students	0.12
University students, 1970	0.08
University students, 1987	0.19

[1]Adapted from Malina RM, Katzmarzyk PT, Bonci CM, et al: Family size and age at menarche in athletes. Med Sci Sports Exerc 29:99–106, 1997. The reported values are partial regression coefficients controlling for birth order. Corresponding estimates for samples of European girls, not controlling for birth order, range from 0.11 to 0.18 years per additional sibling in the family.[48]

"although menarche occurs later in athletes than in nonathletes, it has yet to be shown that exercise delays menarche in anyone"[34]

and

"the general consensus is that while menarche occurs later in athletes than in nonathletes, the relationship is not causal and is confounded by other factors"[15]

AGE- AND SEX-ASSOCIATED VARIATION IN PERFORMANCE

Characteristics of the adolescent growth spurt and sexual maturation, and of interrelationships among indices of sexual, skeletal, and somatic maturity, are reasonably well documented.[47] Changes in physical performance during childhood and adolescence are less well documented. The data are largely cross-sectional, with but few longitudinal observations spanning the immediate prepubertal and pubertal years.

Motor Performance and Strength

Average performances of girls in a variety of motor tasks (dash, standing long jump, vertical jump, shuttle run, and others) improve more or less linearly from childhood through about 14 to 15 years of age, followed by a slight increase in some tasks or a plateau in others.[8,25] There is much overlap between the sexes during childhood. In early adolescence, the average performances of girls fall within 1 standard deviation of the averages for boys; subsequently, the average performances of girls are often outside the limits defined by 1 standard deviation below the boys' mean performance. Overhand throwing performance and the sit and reach are exceptions. Few girls approximate the throwing performances of boys at all ages from late childhood, while girls are more flexible than boys at all ages.

Motor performance is in part related to muscular strength. Strength improves linearly with age from early childhood through about 15 years of age in girls, followed by slower improvement. This pattern is in contrast to the marked acceleration of strength development during male adolescence, so that sex differences in muscular strength are considerable at this time.[3,6,28]

A question that merits more detailed study is the relative flatness of the performance curves of girls during adolescence, that is, their level of performance shows little improvement in many tasks after 14 to 15 years of age. Is this trend related to the biologic changes associated with female adolescence (eg, sexual maturation, fat accumulation, changes in physique), or is it related to cultural factors (eg, changing social interests and expectations, pressure from peers, lack of motivation, limited opportunities to participate in performance-related physical activities)? It probably reflects an interaction of biologic and cultural factors. With recent emphasis on and opportunity for athletic competition for young girls and wider acceptability of women in the role of an athlete, the overall age-related pattern of physical performance during female adolescence may change.

Motor Performance and Strength during the Adolescent Growth Spurt

Longitudinal data relating the motor performances of girls to the timing of the adolescent growth spurt, and specifically PHV, are not extensive. Trends for girls based on mixed-longitudinal data show peak velocities of growth in the standing long jump and medicine ball throw (power) after PHV, and in the dash (speed) and shuttle run (speed and agility) before PHV.[26] Corresponding trends are similar in boys. Maximal gains in the flexed arm hang (functional strength) and vertical jump (power) occur, on average, after PHV, while maximal gains in the shuttle run (speed and agility), speed of hand movement (limb speed), and the sit and reach (hamstring and lower back flexibility) occur before PHV.[3]

The relationship between strength development and the growth spurt and sexual maturation in girls is also not as clear as in boys. Maximum strength gains occur, on the average, after PHV in boys.[3,6] The available longitudinal data for girls are variable. In an early study of California girls, the time of maximum strength (composite score of right and left grip and pushing and pulling tests) gain does not correspond closely to PHV, and a significant percentage of girls experience peak strength gains prior to PHV.[19] On the other hand, in a study of Dutch girls, peak gain in strength (arm pull) occurs, on average, one-half year after PHV (the same time as it occurs in Dutch and Belgian boys on the same task). Maximum gain in strength at this time, however, is about 6.0 kg/year in girls, which contrasts to the maximum gain of 12.0 kg/year in boys.[3,6]

Motor Performances of Female Athletes

Although the performances of girls tend to level off or improve only slightly after 14 to 15 years of age, some girls do, in fact, improve in their performances through adolescence. Measures of flexibility increase with age during female adolescence. The sit and reach, a measure of hamstring/lower-back flexibility, for example, is often included in motor performance and physical fitness test batteries. Hence, generalization across difference performance items needs to be done with caution.

How do young female athletes compare to nonathletes in motor performance? A priori, it might be assumed that athletes will perform better given the premium placed on skill and practice, and sport-related motor skills. However, data comparing the performances of female athletes and nonathletes on standard tasks are limited. This is due in part to the lack of comparable test items; in addition, even though the same items are used, test protocols may vary so that comparisons may have limitations.

Comparisons of females athletes in several sports and nonathletes on two tasks commonly used in assessment batteries are shown in Figures 7-1 and 7-2. For the vertical jump (Fig. 7-1), divers consistently exceed the reference values at all ages, while alpine skiers approximate the reference value. Distance runners are near the reference to about 13 years of age and then lag behind. The trends for athletes in these 3 sports probably reflect the specific training demands of the respective sports. Diving places a premium on vertical jumping ability, while the other sports do not. Skiing places more emphasis on side-to-side jumping, while distance running often focuses on endurance training to the neglect of explosive power. In contrast to the vertical jump, both divers and distance runners have greater flexibility of the hamstrings/lower back (Fig. 7-2). This trend probably reflects the emphasis on stretching as a preliminary to more specific training activities in a sport.

A comparison of elite female distance runners with nonathletes on 2 other motor items is shown in Figures 7-3 and 7-4. The flexed arm hang is a measure of functional strength/muscular endurance. Young distance runners show better functional strength in late childhood and early adolescence and then decline linearly with age in this task so that by 16 to 17 years of age they are similar to nonathletes (Fig. 7-3). One might expect this given the lack of concern for upper-body muscular strength and endurance in training for distance running. In contrast to the flexed arm hang, distance runners do not differ from nonathletes in the standing long jump from late childhood to about 15 years of age; then they do not perform as well as nonathletes (Fig. 7-4). The pattern is similar to that for the vertical jump (Fig. 7-1).

The limited data emphasize the need for further comparative research with young female athletes.

Text Continued on Page 58

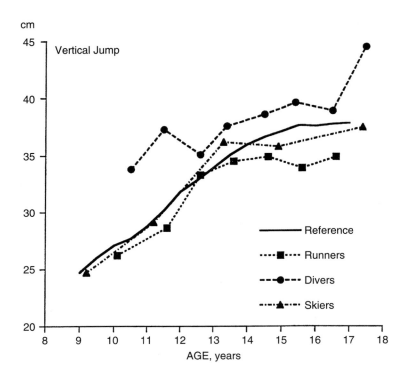

Figure 7-1. Vertical jumping performances of elite distance runners,[17] Junior Olympic divers,[23] and alpine skiers[29] compared to reference values for nonathletes.[25]

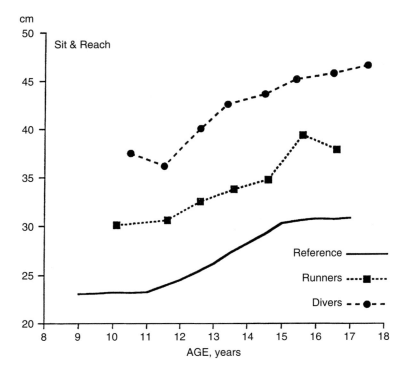

Figure 7-2. Sit and reach performances of elite distance runners[17] and Junior Olympic divers[23] compared to reference values for nonathletes.[25]

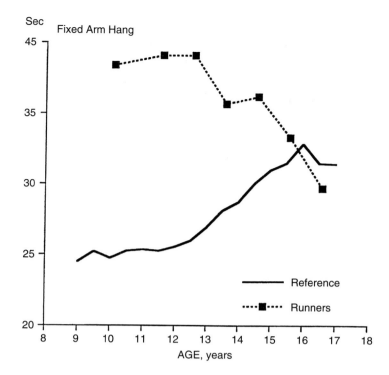

Figure 7-3. Flexed arm hang performances of elite distance runners[17] compared to reference values for nonathletes.[25]

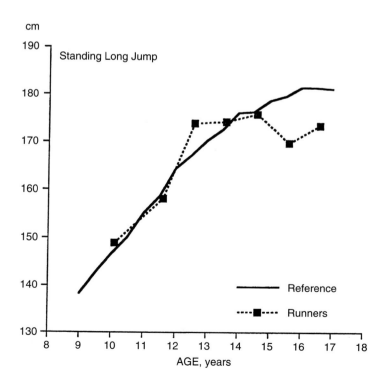

Figure 7-4. Standing long jump performances of elite distance runners [17] compared to reference values for nonathletes. [25]

They also emphasize the specificity of training. Training programs emphasize the specific skills or demands of a sport. Other basic skills are perhaps taken for granted, or perhaps neglected. Early specialization and exclusive training in a specific sport may be an additional contributing factor.

Motor Performances of Female and Male Athletes in the Same Sports

Sex differences in motor performance are well described for the general population of youth, but not for young female and male athletes within the same sport. Such comparisons may shed some light on the issue of sex differences. What is the magnitude of sex differences in the performances of elite young athletes within the same sport? Such data are not extensive, but suggest several interesting contrasts. Comparative data are available for elite female and male athletes in 3 sports: diving, downhill skiing, and distance running.

Divers

Performances of 121 male and 151 female Junior Olympic divers, 11 to 18 years of age, were assessed on 5 tests: timed sit-ups (trunk flexion power), a quadrant jump (agility), vertical jump (explosive power of the legs), the sit and reach (flexibility of the hamstrings and lower back), and an overhead, backward 1-kg medicine ball throw (explosive power of the upper body). Consistent with nonathletes, female divers have a better sit and reach at all ages. There are no consistent sex differences in timed sit-ups. In the quadrant jump, female divers perform, on average, better from 11 to 14 years, and there are no consistent differences subsequently. The vertical jump does not differ at 11 to 12 years; male divers then perform better from 14 to 18 years. The medicine ball throw does not differ between males and females from 11 to 14 years; subsequently, males perform better. Thus, in contrast to the general population, sex differences in the motor performances of elite divers are not marked, with the exception of greater upper- and lower-body power in males later in adolescence.[23]

Skiers

The motor performances of 300 competitive alpine skiers, 8 to 18 years of age, were compared on 5 motor tasks deemed specific to downhill skiing: explosive power (vertical jump), agility (hexagonal jump, and single leg lateral jump), muscular endurance (high box),

and dynamic balance (Bass test). For explosive power and muscular endurance, there are no sex differences from 8 to 13 years; subsequently, males perform significantly better. Results for the agility tests indicate no significant differences for any age-group comparisons, while boys are significantly faster than girls on the single-leg lateral vault only in the older age groups, 14 to 18 years. Mean balance scores are relatively similar for all age groups, but females perform better in the oldest age group, 16 to 18 years. The results thus suggest that sex differences in the motor performances of elite young skiers 8 to 13 years are minor. During the adolescent growth spurt, sex differences emerge in power and muscular endurance. On the other hand, trends for the agility tests and balance indicate small sex differences in most age groups.[29]

Distance Runners

The performances of a mixed-longitudinal sample of 27 male and 27 female elite young distance runners were compared on 7 tasks: side leap, quadrant jump, figure 8 run, standing long jump, vertical jump, flexed arm hang, and sit and reach. Female and male runners do not differ significantly in the side leap or quadrant jump across all age groups. They likewise do not differ in the figure 8 run, long jump and vertical jump before 14 years of age; subsequently male runners have better performances. Male runners perform consistently better on the flexed arm hang, while female runners perform consistently better on the sit and reach. Between 13 and 18 years of age, the magnitude of the sex difference for the long jump and vertical jump increases with age. The results suggest that sex differences in neuromuscular agility and explosiveness (quadrant jump, long jump, vertical jump) are attenuated prior to 13 years of age in elite young runners. However, during the adolescent growth spurt, sex differences emerge as a result of continued increase in the motor performance of males and a plateau in the motor performance of females. Sex differences for upper-body neuromuscular endurance (flexed arm hang) favoring males and low back/hamstring flexibility (sit and reach) favoring females persist through the age range.[17]

The comparisons suggest that sex differences in the performances of elite young athletes in the same sport are relatively minor until the male adolescent spurt. The male adolescent growth spurt in muscle mass, specifically upper-body musculature, and in strength and power contributes to the sex difference in

combination of the two factors. Endomorphy is based on the sum of 3 skinfolds adjusted for stature in the Heath-Carter anthropometric protocol.[11] Mean endomorphy in this international sample of elite gymnasts is uniformly low and homogeneous across 13 to 20 years of age, ranging from 1.4 to 1.9,[14] which markedly contrasts the trend toward increasing endomorphy with age across adolescence in nonathlete females. Among a national sample of Flemish girls, mean endomorphy increases from 2.9 at 10 years of age to 4.1 at 18 years of age (A.L. Claessens, personal communication). Thus, it may be difficult to detect a negative influence of such low endomorphy on competition scores. The issue of the perception of fatness or endomorphy by gymnastics judges, or the aesthetic demands of the sport that place an emphasis on petiteness and leanness, should perhaps be systematically addressed. This, of course, has relevance for the health of young gymnasts, many of whom are in negative energy balance in an attempt to limit weight gain and fat accumulation when the normal course of growth and especially sexual maturation is to gain in both.

A similar trend is suggested for elite young divers. In a sample of 121 male and 151 female Junior Olympic divers 11 to 18 years of age observed in 1991 and 1992, 12 males and 17 females were identified as eventually successful in national and international competitions. As youth, the successful female divers were more muscular (greater estimated arm and calf muscle circumferences), and had less relative fatness and lower endomorphy than those who were not successful. Female divers as a group are higher in endomorphy than gymnasts, mean values ranging from 2.5 to 3.5 among divers 11 to 18 years of age.[21] In contrast, the successful male divers were shorter and lighter, lower in ectomorphy, and higher in mesomorphy, and had relatively broad shoulders compared to those who were not successful.[22]

The results of these 2 analyses suggest a need for further study of the influence of the selective criteria of specific sports and perhaps the judging criteria on the physique and body composition of young competitors. Undue emphasis on leanness can potentially have a negative influence on the health of the young athletes, in particular females. The same applies to other sports in which coaches and/or the sport system place undue emphasis on fatness in female athletes, such as distance running, ballet, swimming, and so on.

A Period in Need of Study: The Transition from Adolescence to Adulthood

This chapter has focused on the growth and motor performance of female athletes during childhood and primarily in adolescence. There is a gap in the data for the important transitional years from adolescence into adulthood, or from interscholastic to intercollegiate athletic competition. Changes in size, physique, body composition, and performance of female athletes in the transition from adolescence into young adulthood, or from high school into college, need study. Many freshman collegiate athletes will continue to grow, especially in muscle mass, and many will gain weight. The demands of collegiate sport are different from those of high school sport, the major demand perhaps being year-round training. In addition, many collegiate sports require off-season aerobic and strength training, which is not characteristic of high school programs. Lifestyle changes associated with the move from home to campus place additional demands on the young athlete.

References

1. Armstrong N, Welsman JR: Assessment and interpretation of aerobic fitness in children and adolescents. Exerc Sport Sci Rev 22:435–76, 1994.
2. Beunen G, Claessens A, Ostyn M, et al: Motor performance as related to somatotype in adolescent boys. In Binkhorst RA, Kemper HCG, Saris WHM (eds): Children and Exercise XI. Champaign, Ill, Human Kinetics, 1985, p 279.
3. Beunen G, Malina RM: Growth and physical performance relative to the timing of the adolescent spurt. Exerc Sport Sci Rev 16:503–40, 1988.
4. Beunen G, Malina RM: Growth and biological maturation: Relevance to athletic performance. In Bar-Or O (ed): The Child and Adolescent Athlete. Oxford: Blackwell Science, 1996, p 3.
5. Beunen G, Malina RM, Ostyn M, et al: Fatness, growth and motor fitness of Belgian boys 12 through 20 years of age. Hum Biol 55:599–613, 1983.
6. Beunen G, Malina RM, Van't Hof MA, et al: Adolescent Growth and Motor Performance: A Longitudinal Study of Belgian Boys. Champaign, Ill, Human Kinetics, 1988.
7. Beunen G, Rogers DM, Woynarowska B, Malina RM: Longitudinal study of ontogenetic allometry of oxygen uptake in boys and girls grouped by maturity status. Ann Hum Biol 24:33–43, 1997.
8. Beunen G, Simons J: Physical growth, maturation, and performance. In Simons J, Beunen G, Renson R, et al (eds): Growth and Fitness of Flemish Girls: The Leuven Growth Study. Champaign, Ill, Human Kinetics, 1990, p 69.
9. Bouchard C, Malina RM, Perusse L: Genetics of Fitness and Physical Performance. Champaign, Ill, Human Kinetics, 1997.

10. Carter JEL: Somatotypes of children in sports. In Malina RM (ed): Young Athletes: Biological, Psychological, and Educational Perspectives. Champaign, Ill, Human Kinetics, 1988, p 153.

11. Carter JEL, Heath BH: Somatotyping—Development and Applications. Cambridge, Cambridge University Press, 1990.

12. Claessens AL, Beunen G, Lefevre J, et al: Relation between physique and performance in outstanding female gymnasts. In Hermans GPH, Mosterd WL (eds): Sports, Medicine and Health. Amsterdam, Elsevier Science, 1990, p 725.

13. Claessens AL, Lefevre J, Beunen G, Malina RM: The contribution of anthropometric characteristics to performance scores in elite female gymnasts. J Sports Med Phys Fit 39:355–60, 1999.

14. Claessens AL, Malina RM, Lefevre J, et al: Growth and menarcheal status of elite female gymnasts. Med Sci Sports Exerc 24:755–63, 1992.

15. Clapp JF, Little KD: The interaction between regular exercise and selected aspects of women's health. Am J Obstet Gynecol 173:2–9, 1995.

16. Eisenmann JC, Malina RM: Body size and endurance performance. In Shephard RJ (ed): Endurance in Sport, 2nd edition. Oxford, Blackwell Science, 2000, p 37.

17. Eisenmann JC, Malina RM: Sex differences in selected motor performances of elite young distance runners. Submitted for publication.

18. Falls HB, Humphrey LD: Body type and composition differences between placers and nonplacers in an AIAW gymnastics meet. Res Q 49:38–43, 1978.

19. Faust MS: Somatic development of adolescent girls. Mon Soc Res Child Develop 42 (serial no 169), 1977.

20. Geithner CA: Somatic growth, maturation, and submaximal power output of Polish adolescents: A longitudinal study. Doctoral dissertation, University of Texas at Austin, 1995.

21. Geithner CA, Malina RM: Somatotypes of Junior Olympic divers. In Malina RM, Gabriel JL (eds): U.S. Diving Sport Science Seminar 1993: Proceedings. Indianapolis, United States Diving, 1993, p 36.

22. Malina RM, Geithner CA: Successful divers: Characteristics as Junior Olympic participants. Inside USA Diving 9:3, 6-7 (Fall), 2001.

23. Geithner CA, O'Brien RO, Gabriel JL, Malina RM: Sex differences in the motor performances of elite young divers. Med Sci Sports Exerc 31 (suppl):S170, 1999.

24. Geithner CA, Woynarowska B, Malina RM: The adolescent spurt and sexual maturation in girls active and not active in sport. Ann Hum Biol 25:415–23, 1998.

25. Haubenstricker JL, Wisner DM, Seefeldt V, Branta CF: Gender differences and mixed-longitudinal reference values for selected motor skills for children and youth. Unpublished data, Department of Kinesiology, Michigan State University.

26. Heras Yague P, de la Fuente JM: Changes in height and motor performance relative to peak height velocity: A mixed-longitudinal study of Spanish boys and girls. Am J Hum Biol 10:647–60, 1998.

27. Ismail AH, Christian JE, Kessler WV: Body composition relative to motor aptitude for preadolescent boys. Res Q 34:463–70, 1963.

28. Jones HE: Motor Performance and Growth: A Developmental Study of Static Dynamometric Strength. Berkeley, University of California Press, 1949.

29. Klika RJ, Malina RM: Sex differences in motor performance in elite young alpine skiers. Med Sci Sports Exerc 31 (suppl):S319, 1999.

30. Krahenbuhl GS, Skinner JS, Kohrt WM: Developmental aspects of maximal aerobic power in children. Exerc Sport Sci Rev 13:503–38, 1985.

31. Leedy HE, Ismail AH, Kessler WV, Christian JE: Relationships between physical performance items and body composition. Res Q 36:158–63, 1965.

32. Lefevre J, Beunen G, Steens G, et al: Motor performance during adolescence and age thirty as related to age at peak height velocity. Ann Hum Biol 17:423–35, 1990.

33. Little NG, Day JAP, Steinke L: Relationship of physical performance to maturation in perimenarcheal girls. Am J Hum Biol 9:163–71, 1997.

34. Loucks AB, Vaitukaitis J, Cameron JL, et al: The reproductive system and exercise in women. Med Sci Sports Exerc 24:S288–93, 1992.

35. Malina RM: Anthropometric correlates of strength and motor performance. Exerc Sport Sci Rev 3:249–74, 1975.

36. Malina RM: Menarche in athletes: A synthesis and hypothesis. Ann Hum Biol 10:1–24, 1983.

37. Malina RM: Physical growth and biological maturation of young athletes. Exerc Sport Sci Rev 22:389–433, 1994.

38. Malina RM: Anthropometry, strength and motor fitness. In Ulijaszek SJ, Mascie-Taylor CGN (eds): Anthropometry: The Individual and the Population. Cambridge, Cambridge University Press, 1994, p 160.

39. Malina RM: The young athlete: Biological growth and maturation in a biocultural context. In Smoll FL, Smith RE (eds): Children and Youth in Sport: A Biopsychosocial Perspective. Dubuque, Ia, Brown and Benchmark, 1996, p 161.

40. Malina RM: Growth and maturation of female gymnasts. Spotlight on Youth Sports (Institute for the Study of Youth Sports, Michigan State University) 19(3):1–3, 1997.

41. Malina RM: Growth and maturation of young athletes: Is training for sport a factor? In Chan K-M, Micheli LJ (eds): Sports and Children. Hong Kong, Williams & Wilkins Asia-Pacific, 1998, p 133.

42. Malina RM: Physical activity, sport, social status and Darwinian fitness. In Strickland SS, Shetty PS (eds): Human Biology and Social Inequality. Cambridge, Cambridge University Press, 1998, p 165.

43. Malina RM: Growth and maturation of elite female gymnasts: Is training a factor? In Johnston FE, Zemel B, Eveleth PB (eds): Human Growth in Context. London, Smith-Gordon, 1999, p 291.

44. Malina RM, Beunen G: Monitoring growth and maturation. In Bar-Or O (ed): The Child and Adolescent Athlete. Oxford: Blackwell Science, 1996, p 647.

45. Malina RM, Beunen G, Claessens AL, et al: Fatness and physical fitness of girls 7 to 17 years. Obes Res 3:221–232, 1995.

46. Malina RM, Beunen G, Lefevre J, Woynarowska B: Maturity-associated variation in peak oxygen uptake in active adolescent boys and girls. Ann Hum Biol 24:19–31, 1997.

47. Malina RM, Bouchard C: Growth, Maturation, and Physical Activity. Champaign, Ill, Human Kinetics, 1991.

48. Malina RM, Katzmarzyk PT, Bonci CM, et al: Family size and age at menarche in athletes. Med Sci Sports Exerc 29:99–106, 1997.
49. Malina RM, Meleski BW, Shoup RF: Anthropometric, body composition, and maturity characteristics of selected school-age athletes. Pediatr Clin North Am 29:1305–23, 1982.
50. Malina RM, Rarick GL: Growth, physique, and motor performance. In Rarick GL (ed): Physical Activity: Human Growth and Development. New York, Academic Press, 1973, p 125.
51. Malina RM, Ryan RC, Bonci CM: Age at menarche in athletes and their mothers and sisters. Ann Hum Biol 21:417–22, 1994.
52. Malina RM, Woynarowska B, Bielicki T, et al: Prospective and retrospective longitudinal studies of the growth, maturation, and fitness of Polish youth active in sport. Int J Sports Med 18 (suppl 3):S179–85, 1997.
53. Mirwald RL, Bailey DA: Maximal Aerobic Power. London, Ontario, Sports Dynamics, 1986.
54. Peltenburg AL, Erich WBM, Zonderland ML, et al: A retrospective growth study of female gymnasts and girl swimmers. Int J Sports Med 5:262–7, 1984.
55. Pool J, Binkhorst RA, Vos JA: Some anthropometric and physiological data in relation to performance in top female gymnasts. Int Z Angew Physiol 27:329–38, 1969.
56. Rowland TW: Developmental Exercise Physiology. Champaign, Ill, Human Kinetics, 1996.
57. Skierska E: Age at menarche and prevalence of oligo/amenorrhea in top Polish athletes. Am J Hum Biol 10:511–7, 1998.
58. Slaughter MH, Lohman TG, Misner JE: Relationship of somatotype and body composition to physical performance in 7- to 12-year old boys. Res Q 48:159–68, 1977.
59. Slaughter MH, Lohman TG, Misner JE: Association of somatotype and body composition to physical performance in 7–12-year-old girls. J Sports Med Phys Fit 20:189–98, 1980.
60. Theintz GE, Howald H, Weiss U, Sizonenko PC: Evidence for a reduction of growth potential in adolescent female gymnasts. J Pediatr 122:306–13, 1993.
61. Tofler IR, Stryer BK, Micheli LJ, Herman LR: Physical and emotional problems of elite female gymnasts. New Engl J Med 335:281–3, 1996.
62. Tönz O, Stronski SM, Gmeiner CYK: Wachstum und Pubertät bei 7-bis 16 jährigen Kunstturneirinnen: eine prospektive Studie. Schweiz med Wschr 120:10–20, 1990.
63. Welsman JR, Armstrong N, Nevill AM, et al: Scaling peak VO2 for differences in body size. Med Sci Sports Exerc 28:259–65, 1996.
64. Wilmore JH: Advances in body composition applied to children and adolescents in sport. In Malina RM (ed): Young Athletes: Biological, Psychological, and Educational Perspectives. Champaign, Ill, Human Kinetics, 1988, p 141.
65. Ziemilska A: Wplyw intensywnego treningu gimnastycznego na rozwoj somatyczny i dojrzewanie dzieci. Warsaw, Akademia Wychowania Fizycznego, 1981.

Chapter 8

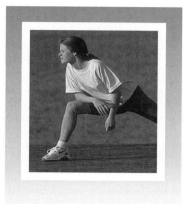

Development of Studies and Wellness

THE TEXAS EXPERIENCE

Christine M. Bonci, M.S., A.T.,C.
Randa Ryan, Ph.D.

"More equals better."
"The more variables I can control, the better my athlete's performance will be."
"Champions work through pain and fatigue, the ultimate tests."

These philosophical positions guide coaches' approach to the design of training programs, the establishment of team rules, decisions related to injuries, and how players are treated on and off the playing fields. Under such a system of popularized beliefs, players are at risk. "More" is not necessarily better. "More" can produce chronic fatigue, lack of recovery from the previous training bout, injuries, over-training, and deterioration in performance. Coaches, trying to control every variable in their players' lives, from diet to sleep and study habits, are not contributing to student-athletes learning how to make good decisions or to take charge of their own lives.

Yet, these are common refrains among coaches at all levels. They are saying what has been said to them and what they have experienced. They are repeating popular clichés. They want to win. They are committed to making their athletes perform to their potential. They know the game—all about skills and X's and O's. They care about their players.

Unfortunately, there are many coaches who are lacking expertise in one or more crucial areas—motor learning, skill analysis, game theory, conditioning techniques, and the psycho-physiological responses to stress. Few have been formally trained as physical educators or have had courses in exercise physiology, coaching methodology, or sports medicine. And, even fewer have good knowledge of the major stu-

dent-athlete issues in educational or open amateur sport. The United States is one of the few countries in the world without coach certification programs. This is incomprehensible considering that coaches play an important role in safeguarding the athlete's physical and mental health.

Can athletes protect themselves? Probably not. In most athletics environments, the student-athlete is in the least advantageous position to prevent physiological or psychological injury to self. Athletes know that to question the coach may mean being misperceived as a "wise guy" or "complainer" at best and disrespectful or deserving of being benched at worse. Student-athletes look up to coaches as experts. The coach knows best. Blind obedience is the rule rather than the exception.

Where does this situation leave the responsible athletics administrator and coach? How do we protect our student-athletes and deliver the right information and right expert advice to coaches so they can be better at what they do? The establishment of certification standards for coaches is a good start, but a politically difficult path that may take years to accomplish. The best immediate course is to restructure support programs to include: (1) an interdisciplinary approach to health care vested in the pursuit of holistic solutions to problems unique to the athlete; (2) ongoing health service and support programs that treat problems earlier rather than later; (3) in-service coach training programs and regular dissemination of information that helps coaches examine their training and communication practices and recognize their role in preventing injuries and other health problems; (4) student-athlete educational programs that give them the tools to balance the competing forces in their lives and to recognize bad health and nutrition habits; and, (5) administrative oversight mechanisms that deal with specific situations that affect the health and well-being of student-athletes.

This chapter is the end result of such an effort. It is the product of more than 15 years of experience in trying to design health care systems and educational support programs that protect athletes and coaches, make student-athletes more responsible for their lives and more informed about their rights, and provide coaches with the most up-to-date information and best advice. It is about recognizing the extraordinary talent, expertise and interest that resides in a University—expertise that can solve almost any problem reaching out to acquire this knowledge.

It is about dedicated health care professionals, athletics coaches, academicians, and athletics administrators learning how to best work together to address these problems because they care about their student-athletes.

It is about good people learning to be better with each other's help.

Donna Lopiano, Ph.D.
Director, Women's Sports Foundation
Former Athletics Director,
Intercollegiate Athletics for Women
The University of Texas at Austin

Substantial and measurable improvement in the health and performance status of female student-athletes at The University of Texas at Austin can be directly attributed to an interdisciplinary model of health care that was established in 1985. This prototypical model, coined *the performance team,* demonstrates how intercollegiate sports systems, university academicians and researchers, and medical practitioners can be integrated within the framework of higher education to positively influence the health and well-being of student-athletes.[8] Highlighted by a non-hierarchical group of experts representing a cross section of disciplines, the team encourages, supports, and participates in the pursuit of improved health care strategies that have preventive, therapeutic, and performance-enhancing potential. To fully relate how this model has enhanced our ability to respond to the health needs of women and intercollegiate sport simultaneously requires a review of the past with special reference to the key players responsible for the model's inception.

HISTORICAL SKETCH

The Department of Intercollegiate Athletics for Women at The University of Texas at Austin was established in 1975. By the end of the decade, a competitive framework and governance structure, separate from the Department of Intercollegiate Athletics for Men, was firmly in place. From this reference point, the athletics environment for women changed dramatically as reflected in the increased availability of scholarships, expanded media coverage, demanding competitive schedule and travel obligations, higher performance expectations, and a budget allocation that ballooned from $57,000 at the time of the department's inception to over $2 million by the late 1980s and over $9 million by the year 2000. At the outset, women were afforded opportunities for athletics participation in 8 sports: basketball, cross-country, golf, swimming and diving, tennis, track and field, and volleyball. Soccer, softball, and rowing were added in the mid-1990s.

In 27 years of intercollegiate athletics participation, the women's teams have claimed 24 national championship titles. A total of 121 individual National Champions have been crowned and 33 have been singled out for National Player of the Year honors. Forty-nine have participated in the Olympic Games over a cross section of 6 sports with 30 winning medals—14 gold—in the sports of basketball, diving, softball, swimming, and track and field. Additionally, the department's student-athletes have received 1557 individual National All-America honors, 21 National Academic All-America honors, and 11 NCAA post-graduate scholarships. For those participants who have exhausted their athletics eligibility, there is a 95% graduation rate.

Student-athletes became associated with a sports system that was committed to performance excellence. It was also a system that placed great demands on their physical and emotional well-being and many facets of their college life, most notably, personal development, social life, and academics. Whether our support programs were keeping pace with the needs and interests of student-athletes in light of these demands was a pressing issue requiring objective evaluation.

In evaluating the effectiveness of our health care delivery and support programs, we found that student-athletes were being shortchanged when studied in the context of the availability and procurement of untapped resources. This was best exemplified in the limitations of a clinical practice agenda that operated primarily from the traditional model of reaction-based medicine oriented toward diagnosis and treatment. The department was well equipped to handle the immediate health care needs of student-athletes who presented with injuries and illnesses that are known to routinely occur with participation in elite competitive sports. However, prevention, health maintenance/protection, and health promotion activities were slighted, especially in circumstances unrelated to physical impairment or those necessitating the sound implementation of applied research. Balancing our clinical practice agenda to include these activities required a more proactive stance.

From a certified athletic trainer's perspective, the "big picture" was often lost in the reality of working "in the trenches." Efforts in coordinating and implementing services beyond physical restoration, particularly in the area of prevention, were handcuffed by time constraints, understaffing, and in some instances, managerial inexperience. Because health status is known to be influenced by physical, environmental, behavioral, psychological, and social factors, in addition to medical care, frustrations were further heightened when operating within the confines of a health care delivery system that failed to appreciate the interaction of all these factors.

From a performance-enhancement perspective, a similar level of frustration was manifesting itself in the coaching ranks. With competition becoming keener and the physique and athleticism of female athletes changing, new advances in training methodology were required. There was a need for the application of knowledge based on proven scientific principles rather than on anecdotal reports or "this is how I do-it-isms." Even though the department's coaches were master teachers and had a good working knowledge of basic exercise science, their coaching commitments left very little time to keep abreast of all scientific breakthroughs related to conditioning/training, technique, and equipment considerations. Moreover, when pertinent research findings stimulated their interest, the availability of resources that enabled a systematic translation of the findings into procedures that could potentially enhance the performance capabilities of athletes were limited.

The University's internationally recognized exercise scientists who were engaged in cutting-edge research on performance issues could have readily dealt with this logistical problem. However, it was disconcerting to note there was no mechanism in place to access the expertise of these scientists or to disseminate information regarding their ongoing research projects.

There was no link to our Human Performance Laboratory. Establishing this link was imperative if our athletes were to realize their performance potential.

The goal was to move toward a more complete, integrated health care delivery and support system encompassing an interdisciplinary team of sports medicine specialists, exercise scientists, coaches, administrators, and academicians. The key to success of the team would rest in its ability to share academic and practical knowledge to a level compatible with the needs and interests of our student-athletes. Accomplishing this goal would require the support and direction of a progressive administration. At the time, the department was fortunate to have had one of the most dynamic woman athletics administrators in the business, Dr. Donna Lopiano, presently Director of the Women's Sports Foundation. Through her guidance and creativity, a better understanding was developed on how an interdisciplinary team works, how goals are generated, and how those goals could be supported by different disciplines in the context of health care delivery and the collegiate female athlete. Dr. Lopiano had a gift for bringing diverse groups of people together and facilitating mutually interactive pathways to problem solving that prevented too much comfort in the theoretical and technical practice associated with individual disciplines. To her credit, she believed that everything was doable and more positively enhanced with a collaborative team effort rather than the sum of individual contributions. This management style had its strength in developing a shared direction that proved vital to the early success of *The Performance Team.*

With the administration's support, *The Performance Team* was prepared to develop and implement a broad-based strategy for restructuring health care delivery and support programs with emphasis on clinical practice, research, and educational initiatives (Fig. 8-1). Specific objectives[8] encompassed: (1) establishing protocols related to the prevention of athletics injury or deficiencies induced by training which may negatively affect the health and safety of student-athletes; (2) recommending the initiation of research or collection of data related to improving health and performance status; (3) advising the Athletics Director regarding policies or procedures related to the administration of testing or prevention programs; (4) advising coaches on performance and health issues in which they have limited expertise; (5) initiating and progressing health promotion activities that provide student-athletes with

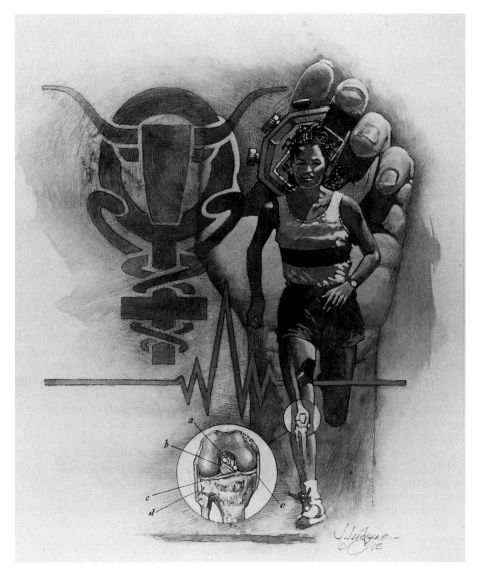

Figure 8-1. The *Performance Team* demonstrates how medical practitioners, athletics administrators, coaches, and university academicians and researchers, share their expertise to favorably impact the health and well-being of student-athletes. The team encourages, supports, and participates in the design and implementation of health care strategies and support programs that have preventive, therapeutic, and performance-enhancing potential.

resources to heighten personal responsibility for their own health; and, (6) raising ethical, health, safety, and procedural questions related to the adoption of new supplementation, treatment, or training protocols.

To realize the model's potential in these areas required facilitators—individuals who could marshal and allocate resources necessary to get the job done. The authors of this chapter assumed the role of the facilitators. Besides directing, coordinating, and monitoring the team's activities in these areas, their role leaned heavily toward fostering productive working relationships among team members.

Strong people-management skills were required to overcome barriers known to hinder effective functioning of interdisciplinary teams, in particular, turf issues and self-serving attitudes that weaken relationships among team members and disrupt the continuity and comprehensiveness of health care services.[4] The facilitators' ability to blend the talents, temperaments, and experience of team members to the particular problem at hand was the key to developing clinical practice, research, and educational initiatives that greatly impacted the type and quality of services provided to student-athletes.

PERFORMANCE TEAM INITIATIVES

The following list of initiatives reflects the views held by a fast-growing number of experts in the medical community with respect to women's health issues and their response to physical activity—that biology does matter, that girls and women have been neglected by researchers in the biomedical sciences, education, physical education, and the social sciences, and moreover, that they exhibit unique physiological, emotional, and social outcomes that merit special consideration and investigation.[13] The following initiatives relative to clinical practice, research, and education influenced a number of important program changes that had major significance for health care delivery, policy, and planning.

Clinical Practice Initiatives

Expanded physician and allied health support and leadership to address the needs of female athletes presenting with conditions beyond the traditional orthopaedic and primary care practice arenas to include a range of medical disciplines. Specialty-physician consultants were recruited to share their expertise in the disciplines of gynecology, endocrinology, neurology, radiology, cardiology, allergy and immunology, ophthalmology, psychiatry, and dentistry. Similarly, allied health care professionals were recruited in the fields of exercise physiology, pharmacology, psychology, physical therapy, nutrition, massage therapy, chiropractic/applied kinesiology, and orthotics and prosthetics. Engaging practitioners who were sincerely committed to restructuring health care services for our student-athletes and who were receptive to working with relevant disciplines in the pursuit of multifaceted solutions to treating the whole person rather than individual body systems was a priority. An important consideration was the practitioner's willingness to develop collaborative relationships and to become more familiar with another's language, ideas, and perspectives. This was essential to heightening our understanding of the role that physical, social, emotional, and cultural environments play in the overall health of the student-athlete.

Defined an alternative organizational structure for the provision of services complete with policies and procedures that reflected internal operating standards and performance outcomes that were integral to establishing a coordinated approach to health care delivery and support programs. A broad range of support personnel directly involved in maintaining and promoting the student-athlete's health and well-being characterizes an interdisciplinary team approach. Ensuring continuity and comprehensiveness of services with such an approach is highly dependent on a model that educates and reeducates practitioners about the programs' scope, articulates optimal standards of practice, and delegates responsibilities based on professional training, experience, and competence. In addition, the model must be driven by in-house facilitators who possess the following qualities: (1) the administrative savvy to incorporate a managerial style that is collegial rather than hierarchical in nature; (2) the people-oriented skills to influence a higher level of communication artistry and teamwork among colleagues and affiliates; and (3) the creativity to employ a strategic plan that acknowledges the roles and positions of affiliates, encourages a sharing of roles and tasks according to skills and services, and promotes a broad and integrative view of relevant health and sports performance disciplines through the association of all providers in planned actions. The importance of and the necessity for mutual support, shared learning experiences, professional courtesies, and joint accountability cannot be overemphasized.

Developed and implemented a woman-centered multiphasic screening approach with special reference to tailoring medical history questionnaires and evaluations to health care concerns unique to the female athlete. The screening process, characterized by a methodical collection and interpretation of information based on the use of algorithms, leads practitioners through the evaluation process and simplifies decision-making in circumstances where further work-ups and/or remedial programs are indicated.[3] *Performance Team* sub-group clinicians representing the fields of internal medicine, gynecology, orthopaedics, allergy and immunology, dentistry, ophthalmology, athletic training, and nutrition participate in the screening process. Particular attention is paid to addressing orthopaedic, biomechanical, physiological, gynecological, psychological, and training considerations that place female athletes at risk for developing a host of limiting conditions, particularly joint ligamentous injury, degenerative joint disease, exercise-induced bone stress injury, premature osteoporosis, disordered eating, allergy/asthma symptomology, and stress-anxiety disorders. An ongoing medical surveillance system, characterized by periodic check-ups and serial health testing, helps practitioners monitor the progress of at-risk athletes

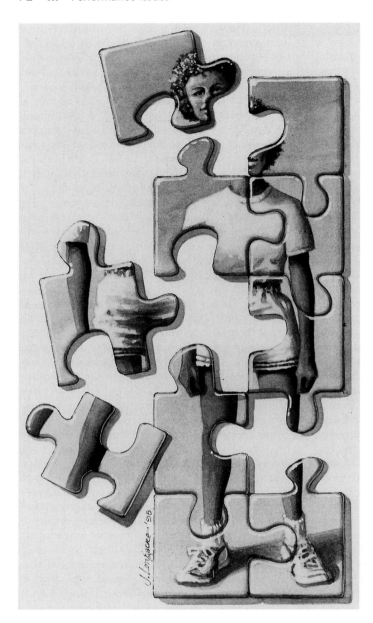

Figure 8-2. An interdisciplinary model heightens understanding of the role that physical, environmental, behavioral, psychological, and social factors, in addition to medical care, play in the overall health and well-being of student-athletes. Inherent to the model's success is the pursuit of holistic solutions to meeting the needs and interests of student-athletes through emphasis on clinical practice, research, and educational initiatives.

and determine if treatment plans are in line with meeting their special health care needs. Even though the major purpose of the screening is to identify athletes with high risk factors and initiate early intervention strategies to decrease the morbidity associated with these factors, efforts are not restricted solely to this at-risk group. The "well" population is attended to with education and counseling activities designed to improve their current health status by orienting them to positive health behaviors.

Established a program for the prevention of eating disorders. The Athletics Department recognized the constant source of stress created for female athletes in the area of body weight and performance and the relationship of those perceived stressors to the manifestation of eating disorders. Environmental and cultural issues provided the impetus for the development and implementation of "The Eating Disorders Prevention and Education Model."[11,14] The model is based on changing the athletes' environment as well as changing the athletes' perceptions about their environment. It contains 4 components: (1) an educational component for the student-athlete that focuses on nutrition, body composition, and eating disorders; (2) an educational component for the coach that facilitates a better understanding of eating disorders and personality characteristics that increase susceptibility; (3) a counseling and referral component that specializes in eating disorders, developmental issues, and nutrition; and, (4) a programming component that helps both coaches and athletes become aware of their differences in perception about body weight issues. Since its inception, the program is considered to be a model for colleges and universities across the country and has been featured by the NCAA, American College of Sports Medicine, several sport national governing bodies, and numerous high school and club sport programs.

Capitalized on the expertise of exercise scientists working in the University of Texas Human Performance Laboratory to help initiate and progress a battery of physical performance tests aimed at identifying an athlete's strengths and weaknesses relative to her sport. The composition of the test battery, mutually agreed upon by the coach, athletic trainer, and exercise scientist, includes the following routine evaluation components: body composition and anthropometry; aerobic capacity (VO_2 max); hematology with special reference to hemoglobin, hematocrit, and serum ferritin values; musculoskeletal strength and endurance; joint range of motion/flexibility; and, sport-specific functional performance tests.

Data collected from these tests, highly technical in its raw form, is only as good as its interpretation. If it is not handled from a practical standpoint, it will be of little clinical or performance significance. Care is taken to exchange information from this premise and in a manner in which athletes and coaches become students of the process.

Established a comprehensive record keeping system for short and long term medical, legal, and research reference. Computerized databases were developed and implemented in collaboration with *Performance Team* subgroup members specializing in preventive medicine and biostatistics to enhance decision making options related to health and performance issues. Two file sources, in particular, characterized our efforts in this area. One file source, a continuous injury/illness surveillance system, was developed to maintain documentation of the nature and extent of care provided to injured or ill athletes throughout their playing careers. Pertinent biographical, medical, and training variables are recorded and accumulated specific to the diagnosis, treatment, and progress of injuries or illnesses significant enough to warrant physician intervention, activity restrictions, and return-to-play guidelines. In addition, a physiological testing file was developed to maintain data specific to the aforementioned physical performance test battery.

As data are accumulated, analyzed, and consolidated into a composite picture, the coach, clinician, and exercise scientist can develop a more comprehensive understanding of an individual athlete's response to physically demanding training regimens. The databases have proven invaluable in providing ongoing feedback as to the immediate health status of the athlete and in evaluating progress resulting from the implementation of a particular training methodology or a particular course of remedial action (eg, dietary modifications, iron supplementation, biofeedback, plyometrics). Visual formatting of the data for prompt athlete and coach reference is essential to an ongoing educational process that reinforces the positive influences of healthy training and lifestyle practices.

Research Initiatives

Despite changes in the clinical practice agenda, there were health problems that our program strategies were not immediately affecting. Our student-athletes were sustaining a high incidence of exercise-induced bone stress injuries and noncontact anterior cruciate ligament injuries, demonstrating unsafe body-weight regulation practices and presenting with mental health concerns. In order to address these issues with systematic plans of action, active involvement in research endeavors was required.

Initiated and furthered the progress of research for the development of intervention strategies to decrease the incidence of exercise-induced bone stress injuries.[7] A prospective study was initiated in 1985 to document all cases of bone stress injuries and to follow their progress through recovery. Subjects were 105 yearly program participants representing a cross section of 8 intercollegiate sports: basketball, cross-country, diving, golf, swimming, tennis, track and field, and volleyball. A comprehensive database was established for injury tracking. Data were compiled from August 1985 through August 1992. Special emphasis was placed on the collection of relevant biographical, medical, and training variables that, when analyzed and interpreted, provided injury information regarding: (1) the rates of occurrence; (2) the distribution by skeletal site, sport, race, and class of athletic eligibility; (3) the prognostic value of a classification system that differentiates grades of stress reaction by correlating the athlete's clinical and training history with bone imaging findings[5]; and (4) the degree of disability as measured by treatment intervention strategies (eg, rest only or cast immobilization plus rest), treatment results, time to recovery, and final competitive status.

Bone radiography and scintigraphy were the main diagnostic tools used by the sports medicine team to contrast the differences in bone stress manifested by abnormal remodeling (stress reaction) and stress fracture. Scintigrams or bone scans were considered diagnostic of stress reaction when a well-marginated area of increased uptake was found. Athletes with diffuse uptake of technetium 99m were excluded from the study. The interpretations of the bone scans were then correlated with the athlete's clinical and training history, physical examination findings, and radiographic findings to differentiate four grades of symptomatic stress reactions along a scale from grade I through IV. Stress reactions were subdivided into those injuries which represented local efforts of remodeling of appropriate degree to adapt to a new physical loading exposure; those that were clinically significant in that they represented a significant weakening of the bone; and those that resulted in complete structural failure, that is stress fracture.[5] For the purposes of this study, the term *stress fracture* was operationally defined as a break in the continuity of bone with associated healing that was verified on radiographs. Using this classification scheme, 40 cases of bone stress injuries were recorded with a final diagnosis of stress reaction or stress fracture.

It is beyond the scope and purpose of this section to present a comprehensive description of the data from these cases or to discuss the prognostic value of classifying the grade of bone stress injury. However, a discussion limited to the distribution of bone stress injuries by sport, skeletal site, and class of athletic eligibility is appropriate.

In analyzing the distribution of bone stress injuries by sport, 19 track and field/cross-country athletes sustained 27 of the 40 injuries. This accounted for 67.5% of the injuries documented over the 7 years of data collection. The 27 injuries incurred by the track and field athletes were further subdivided into their specialty events. The injury rate was highest among long-distance runners ($N=17$), followed by mid-distance runners ($N=3$), hurdlers ($N=3$), sprinters ($N=2$), vertical jumpers ($N=1$), and throwers ($N=1$). An appreciable decline in the number of injuries was noted with respect to athletes participating in other sports. Only 6 bone stress injuries were diagnosed in 4 basketball players and 5 in 5 volleyball players accounting for 16% and 12.5% of the injuries, respectively. The sports of tennis and swimming accounted for the lowest percentage of injuries at 2.5% with only 1 injury diagnosed in 1 tennis player and 1 in 1 swimmer. No bone stress injuries were diagnosed in golfers/divers.

Distribution of injuries by skeletal site revealed that the tibia was implicated in the majority of the injuries. In descending order of frequency, there were 12 (30%) tibial injuries followed by 7 (17.5%) in the fibula, 5 (12.5%) in the tarsal navicular, 5 (12.5%) in the metatarsals, 3 (7.5%) in the calcaneus, 3 (7.5) in the pars interarticularis, 2 (5.0%) in the femoral neck, 2 (5.0%) in the femoral shaft, and 1 (2.5%) in the sacrum.

Data on the distribution of bone stress lesions by class of athletic eligibility revealed that athletes in transition (high school to college) were prone to bone stress injuries with over 52% occurring in freshman and 32% in sophomores. As the participants became more experienced and seasoned as competitors, a decrease in the overall number of injuries was noted. Third-year participants sustained only 15% ($N=6$) of the injuries while no injuries were diagnosed in athletes partaking in their final year of eligibility.

These findings provided the impetus for validating our current intervention strategies and developing new plans of action for injury reduction. The procedures established for prevention and treatment of bone stress injuries were highly dependent on information collected during preseason screenings. Athletes presenting with menstrual irregularities, static postural malalignments, nutritional deficiencies, and low fitness markers were targeted. Those with a history of menstrual dysfunction, specifically amenorrhea and oligomenorrhea, were referred for further work-ups, and, when indicated, estrogen replacement therapy was encouraged. Athletes presenting with multiple risk factors and a history of previous injury were referred for bone density studies to assess the status of bone health. Correcting pelvic assymetries, restoring muscle balance with appropriate stretching and strengthening exercises, and controlling abnormal foot mechanics with fabrication of orthotic devices were essential from a biomechanical standpoint. Addressing nutritional deficiencies was facilitated through the implementation of a computerized program for analysis of dietary recall. The information collected and analyzed served as a baseline for assessing adequate calcium, protein, and caloric intake. Body composition measurements were of importance in determining healthy weight control practices. From a training perspective, careful surveillance of freshman training practices was indicated relative to the magnitude of the loading and/or frequency with which the load was applied. Since most freshman reported with low fitness markers and were unaccustomed to particular training techniques (eg, intervals, weight training, plyometrics), individualized programs were required at the outset. Also, educating athletes about bone stress injury recognition and early presentation of symptoms was paramount to preventing complete structural failure of bone especially at high risk anatomical sites involving the femoral neck, pars interarticularis, tarsal navicular, and anterior mid-tibia. In summary, these intervention strategies proved successful in decreasing the number of injuries and/or reducing the morbidity associated with them.

Initiated and furthered the progress of research for the design and implementation of screening and training protocols for the prevention of anterior cruciate ligament (ACL) injuries. Over an 8-year period, from 1984 to 1992, a high incidence of noncontact ACL injuries were sustained by our basketball players. Our first step towards prevention was standardization of a screening protocol designed to investigate possible risk factors that may increase an athlete's susceptibility to noncontact ACL injuries.[2] As early as 1990, screening evaluations were routinely employed by our clinicians as part of pre-season clinical work-ups to establish musculoskeletal profiles when our athletes are healthy and in top form. This approach gives us an opportunity to maximize both structural and functional outcome strategies when deficiencies in test results are observed in subgroups of athletes matched for age, sex, and training and performance expectations.

The screening components for the assessment of predisposing factors to ACL injury are threefold and include variables thought to be measurable and easily obtainable by clinicians and researchers. The first part focuses on static postural malalignments that contribute to abnormal pre-loading stress on the ACL, along with lower extremity musculoskeletal strength and neuromuscular control considerations. The second part, an assessment tool designed primarily for physicians, includes manual tests of knee pathology for documentation of ligamentous integrity and other pertinent anatomical considerations. The last part consists of a questionnaire that solicits important information about the athlete's prior injury history, present knee status, conditioning and training experiences, and equipment considerations.

The variables included in the screening protocol and their various interactions have provided us with a range of intervention strategies that have been instrumental in decreasing injury incidence. These strategies range from maximizing structural outcomes through orthotic and footwear interventions to maximizing functional outcomes through postural and training interventions.

Initiated research designed to evaluate body weight regulation practices with respect to the coach's role in monitoring body weight as a performance factor.[11] The impetus for this study came from athlete inquiries into how goal weights were determined by coaches. Through training, female athletes were increasing their muscle mass and decreasing their fat mass. They felt leaner and stronger, yet the scale frequently reflected an increase in their body weight. However, few athletes understood the relationship of body composition and body weight in accounting for the increase. The sole use of body weight as measured by a scale to determine goal weights and guide decisions about performance was confusing at best.

In an attempt to change the weighing in procedure and its related problems, 120 athletes from 7 sports complied with a different policy for 1 year. Body composition was measured and body weight recorded 4 to 6 times during the year by a body composition and anthropometric expert accessed through the Department of Kinesiology and Health Education. Coaches received feedback on this information from the sports medicine staff. However, coaches were not permitted to weigh in athletes, to set goal weights, or to initiate interaction with them in any manner about body composition or body weight. Athletes were given educational assistance in all relevant areas and access to professionals in support areas such as nutrition and exercise physiology if they desired. At the end of the year, the athletes' mean body weight and body composition indices were compared to corresponding values from the previous year to determine the extent of changes, if any, that occurred under the new policy. During the period when coaches were restricted from regulating body weight, data showed that the athletes' body composition values were lower and the documented incidence of eating disorders declined. In other words, the athletes were healthier, leaner, and fitter.

Removing the potential pressure imposed by coaches in the area of weight control and using an educational approach to help athletes understand the relationships between body weight, body composition, and performance produced a significantly healthier, happier, and more responsible group of individuals. The athletes were self-motivated to optimize their body composition and to do so in healthy ways. Moreover, the policy restricting coaches from weighing in athletes, setting weight goals, and conferring with them about their body weight or body composition was permanently adopted by the administration. *Performance Team* subgroup members representing the disciplines of internal medicine, athletic training, nutrition, and psychology are the only core support personnel authorized to address any concerns regarding body composition or weight control issues.

Initiated and progressed research to explore mental health problems from the perceptions and experiences of female student-athletes.[9,15] The commitment on the part of female student-athletes to achieve success in the academic and athletics arena is characterized by immense pressure. Central to academic and athletic success is the student-athlete's mental health status. There is no strong research evidence to suggest that female student-athletes suffer from more mental health problems than their nonathletic peers. However, there is evidence indicating that the combination of particular personality characteristics common to female athletes, coupled with the stressors inherent in achieving at competitive academic and athletic levels, can lead to serious developmental crises and mental disorders.[1,6,12,16]

The Performance Team recognized these issues early and sought grant money to initiate and further the progress of research in this area. The project's major goal was to explore mental health issues from the point of view of the female athlete and to identify both stressors and mediators for women in competitive academic and athletics environments.

Research methods combined ethnographic interviews and a battery of psychological tests. The interview data highlighted the following issues: extensive male influences in sport from the early years through college, different perceptions about early coaches as compared to college coaches, difficulty in transition to and out of the university environment, and high levels of stress due to the combined issues of limited time, extensive structure, confused body image, low self-esteem, stereotypes, injury, and difficulty in balancing a multitude of roles and demands. The psychological data identified these issues: rejection of the traditional female gender role, some symptoms of depression, developmental issues, reluctance to discuss emotional needs and utilize traditional mental health supports, somatic manifestation of psychologically generated problems, high levels of stress, difficulty in decision-making, perfectionism, and negative health behaviors.

In addition to these points, the most important observation from the data was the difference in perception between the athletes, parents, coaches, and support staff. For example, experienced coaches, who had spent years in sports, framed situations and concepts in one way, while female athletes endorsed different perceptions regarding their environment.

These observations became critical in planning interventions for this population. Intervention strategies, piloted and modified based on the sociological and psychological data in addition to feedback from coaches, athletes and support staff, were implemented as full programming during the last year of the study. Observations on the effectiveness of the intervention strategies highlighted the need for the following:

1. Counseling services that are readily accessible to the student-athletes. The athletes' vulnerability to a number of psychological factors relating to their multiple involvement and roles in the university setting emphasized the necessity for increased availability, accessibility, and utilization of counseling services. Counseling supports were deemed critical in helping to minimize emotional distress and to aid the student-athletes in achieving both scholastic and athletic goals. On-campus counseling and mental health services were an important resource in assisting student-athletes in addressing psychological concerns. However, on-campus services should not be their only accessible resource. Consideration should be given to the availability of resources off-campus due to issues of anonymity, scheduling conflicts, patient overload at on-campus facilities and, in some situations, lack of on-campus expertise in the specific needs of this population.

2. Ongoing supports for seniors, fifth-year athletes, or athletes no longer competing due to injury or retirement. Student-athletes representing these groups were often surprised with how little time they had devoted to future planning, how their friendships were limited to teammates and how much of their identity was attached to their sport. Also, when the highly demanding days and structured activities associated with sports participation were no longer a part of their lifestyle, they were left to make a series of daily decisions about time use and activity choices that they had no experience in making.

3. Academic program supports. The data suggested a need for student-athletes to increase their interactions with faculty and

teaching assistants, to join study groups with students who were not athletes, to seek assistance from resources and opportunities across campus, and to better maximize study and academic counseling times.

4. Opportunities for team building and team decision-making. Often coaches would set rules or establish protocols that athletes perceived as too structured. Yet, when the athletes were questioned about how they would handle a situation, often they would identify with the same rules and procedures the coaches had established. In working with the coaches, it was agreed they could get the athletes to more willingly support team rules and exhibit appropriate behavior if the athletes were invested in the decision-making process. By having team meetings to decide issues, coaches could often direct the athletes to arrive at what they felt were good team policies without the coach feeling the athletes were in charge of the team. This approach to team decision-making also provided opportunities for both coaches and athletes to identify issues which may unfavorably impact the overall functioning and success of the team. Ongoing attention to team-related group process concerns are critical to achieving successful working interrelationships among team members and between the coaching staff and teams. Examples of issues or types of concerns which can be addressed at team discussions include: identifying and working through potentially destructive team dynamics, extreme competitiveness of teammates, strained working relationships, generating team confidence and sportsmanship, and miscommunication between team members and coaches.

5. Coach and staff education in addition to athlete education. When the coaches and staff learned what the athletes were perceiving and made changes to bring those perceptions more in line with their own perceptions as they related to the department's philosophical goals and values, the mental health issues of the athletes and the athletics department's environment improved. Creating a shared perception that had investment by all groups was critical to the overall changes. The Athletics Director played a key role in disseminating the study information to coaches and staff. Through group awareness, sharing, problem solving, and brainstorming, a greater understanding has been created about this group of young women. In turn, the coaches and staff who work daily to help the athletes grow, learn,

and achieve are now focusing on this shared perception—how to help athletes identify their perceptions and draw conclusions that are similar with what the environment is saying and how their values and beliefs affect daily choices and behaviors.

The rich and complex set of data, collected and interpreted on elite female student-athletes, indicates that their mental health issues are connected to a wide range of factors. The stressors in the lives of these athletes, specifically, transition into and out of sport, transition into and out of college, injury, performance failure, academic difficulty, and social issues provide the backdrop for intervention strategies. Providing educational support and environmental changes to minimize the influence of stressors are important contributions to improving the athletes' mental health status and underscores the necessity for a biosocial and interactive approach to addressing their needs.

Education Initiatives

The research findings generated by the mental health project provided the impetus for educational initiatives designed to inform, teach, and motivate student-athletes to take better care of themselves. Some of the health promotional programs already in existence were revised to take advantage of the project's findings.

Developed and implemented health promotion curricula for dissemination to freshmen athletes in an organized classroom setting. The purpose of the noncredit class, piloted during the fall of 1991, was to provide freshmen athletes with a variety of information and strategies on health promotion topics that had the potential to effect positive health behaviors. The curriculum developed and taught by athletics department personnel, covers the following topics: Transition to College, Managing Stress, Performance Issues, Public Relations Skills, The Utilization of Health Services, Academic Survival Skills, Substance Abuse, Multiculturalism, The Careers Program, Mental Health Issues, Social Issues, and Putting It All Together (a former athlete's panel). In an effort not to impose additional time constraints on student-athletes, the class was held weekly throughout the fall semester during an hour of mandatory freshman study hall.

Over the past 8 years, the NCAA devised a similar program called *"Champs Life Skills."* It was piloted at 50 institutions across the country during the 1994–1995 academic year. The University of Texas at Austin was one of these pilot institutions. Since initial feedback on this program was so promising in terms of its value to student-athletes, it has become a featured educational component of the NCAA.

Revised "The Student-Athlete Orientation Program," which acquaints freshmen with the resources to help them succeed and thrive in their new academic and athletics environments.[10] The transition period to a university is characterized by a range of differences and adjustments. This program focuses on the dissemination of information to new student-athletes to help prepare them for this transition. The "how to" of accessing and utilizing resources in the areas of health care delivery, psychological support, academic support, and public relations is a priority. The orientation program is a time to allay freshmen athletes' fears, to minimize homesickness tendencies, and to address feelings of being overwhelmed. Presenting the university as a friendly environment is essential to this process. Even though most orientation activities center on freshmen, all other student-athletes are required to participate in selected parts of the program.

Developed and implemented a "mentoring program" with special reference to minority and/or academically gifted student-athletes. The focus of the program is to enrich the academic and personal development of student-athletes by connecting them with professors, mentors, and programs available across campus. This enhances the student's ability to capitalize on the resources of higher education and cultivate relationships outside self-selected peer groups associated with athletic participation such as teammates, coaches, and departmental support staff.

Demonstrated and disseminated information about program developments or procedures which emerge from the efforts of the *Performance Team*. These activities include publishing of *The Performance Team* newsletters,[7-11] conducting athlete and/or coach workshops, participating in national symposia and conferences, and developing self-help/guide booklets (eg, Stress in Female College Student-Athletes—What Parents Should Know; Eating Disorders—What Coaches, Athletes, and Parents Should Know; Guidelines for "Right" Actions by Athletes, Coaches, and Other Sport Leaders Regarding the Use of Drugs).

FUTURE PERSPECTIVES

With increasing opportunities for women's participation in sports comes the need to provide them with answers to questions regarding their health, safety, and performance capabilities. Those of us who govern, coach, and assist student-athletes in the pursuit of performance excellence are challenged with optimizing the care, support, direction and information they need and must have to excel athletically with minimal dysfunctional consequences on their minds and bodies. Reflecting on the past from the perspective of Jody Conradt, former Director of Intercollegiate Athletics for Women at The University of Texas at Austin and Hall of Fame Basketball Coach, underscores the magnitude of this challenge.

As women's athletics began to gain a foothold with increased participation and commitment on the part of colleges across the country, we had more and more students seeking opportunity in sports. Their skill levels were notably improved. They had received better coaching during their formative years. They were more committed to high-level performance.

The pressures associated with performance changed as well. There was competition for collegiate scholarships, a result of intense scouting and recruiting by head coaches. On the academic side, eligibility standards increased, resulting in a need for excellence and discipline in study habits. And socially, we were seeing a myriad of changes which affect the lives of young people: the family structure may be unconventional, with one-parent or no-parent homes; public education endures funding cuts, which negatively impact learning environments and limit some extra-curricular activities; and, daily, young people are subjected to temptations of drugs, alcohol and other harmful elements.

In short, the typical student-athlete of this decade is likely the product of a different environment than one we previously governed and coached. What occurs outside the practice arena indeed may affect the athlete's performance more so than what is derived from practice sessions.

As administrators and coaches, we feel responsible for the development of a well-rounded individual, a challenge that we enjoy and want to fulfill as best we can. And so, restructuring support programs in the spirit of mutual support, shared learning and collaborative problem-solving can do more for improving the health status and quality of life of our student-athletes than perhaps any other program endeavor.

Acknowledgments

The authors wish to thank the following founding members of the *Performance Team* who provided invaluable assistance and expertise in improving the type and quality of health services and support programs for student-athletes at The University of Texas at Austin:

Dr. Bob Dodd, Internal Medicine; Dr. Laura Flawn, Orthopaedic Surgery; Dr. John Pearce, Orthopaedic Surgery; Dr. Jesse DeLee, Orthopaedic Surgery; Dr. Margaret Thompson, Gynecology; Dr. Tom Blevins, Endocrinology; Dr. Rogene Tesar, Bone Densitometry; Dr. Sue Ellen Young, Ophthalmology; Dr. Robert Morrow, Dentistry; Dr. James B. Carter, Allergy and Immunology; Dr. Alice Lawler, Psychology; Dr. Eddie Coyle, Exercise Physiology; Dr. John Ivy, Exercise Physiology; Dr. Jack Wilmore, Exercise Physiology; Dr. Bob Malina, Body Composition and Anthropometry; Dr. Larry Abraham, Biomechanics; Dr. Marcus Pandy, Biomechanics; Lisa Kessler, Nutrition; Dr. Roseann Kutschke, Nutrition; Laurie McDonald, Nutrition; Dr. Steve Leslie, Pharmacology; Neil Walsdorf, Pharmacology; Julie Cain, Athletic Training; Spanky Stephens, Athletic Training; Joy Davenport, Physical Therapy; Dr. Terry Todd, Strength Training.

The authors gratefully acknowledge Dr. Donna Lopiano, Jody Conradt, Chris Plonsky, and Dr. Sheila Rice for their administrative support and guidance, in addition to the following head coaches, past and present, who provided the impetus for formation of The Performance Team—Mike Brown (Diving), Terry Crawford (Track and Field), Mick Haley (Volleyball); Jeff Moore (Tennis); Richard Quick (Swimming); and Pat Weis (Golf). We are also indebted to the Hogg Foundation and RGK Foundation for their funding and support of our programming endeavors. A special thanks is extended to our physician consults, allied health care professionals, coaches, and athletics staff affiliated with our department over the years for their contributions in maintaining, enhancing, and promoting the health and performance of our student-athletes. And lastly, thanks to Jimmy Longacre for his exceptionally fine art work.

Acknowledgments

The authors wish to thank the following *Performance Team* members who have provided invaluable assistance and expertise in improving the type and quality of health services and support programs for student-athletes at The University of Texas at Austin: Dr. Mark Chassay, Primary Care; Dr. Bob Dodd, Internal Medicine; Dr. Jerry Julian, Orthopaedics; Dr. Laura Flawn, Orthopaedics; Drs. John and Stephen Pearce, Orthopaedics; Dr. Jesse DeLee, Orthopaedics; Dr. J. Christopher Reynolds, Orthopaedics; Dr. Margaret Thompson, Gynecology; Dr. Tom Blevins, Endocrinology; Dr. Rogene Tesar, Bone Densitometry; Dr. Sue Ellen Young, Ophthalmology; Dr. Robert Morrow, Dentistry; Dr. Ivy Schwartz, Dentistry; Dr. James B. Carter, Allergy and Immunology; Dr. Bernard Crosby, Allergy and Immunology; Dr. Alice Lawler, Psychology; Dr. Madonna Constantine, Psychology; Dr. Eddie Coyle, Exercise Physiology; Dr. John Ivy, Exercise Physiology; Dr. Jack Wilmore, Exercise Physiology; Dr. Bob Malina, Body Composition and Anthropometry; Dr. Larry Abraham, Biomechanics; Dr. Marcus Pandy, Biomechanics; Drs. John and Mike Bandy, Chiropractic/Applied Kinesiology; Dr. Roy Mullins, Chiropractic/Applied Kinesiology; Marsha Beckerman, Nutrition; Michelle Cross, Nutrition; Laurie McDonald, Nutrition; Leslie Bonci, Nutrition; Becky Marshall, Athletic Training; Julie Cain, Athletic Training; Kim Minger, Athletic Training; Connie Grauer; Athletic Training; LaGwyn Durden, Athletic Training; Jenny Posey, Athletic Training; Angela Rich, Athletic Training/Physical Therapy; Laurie King, Massage Therapy; Dana LeDue, Strength Training; Angel Spassov, Strength Training; and, Ed Nordenschild, Strength Training. The authors gratefully acknowledge the support and encouragement of Dr. Donna Lopiano, Jody Conradt, Chris Plonsky, and Dr. Sheila Rice. Special appreciation is also extended to teh coaches and staff of the Department of Intercollegiate Atheletics for Women.

References

1. Allison MT: Role conflict and the female athlete. J Appl Sport Psychol 3:49–60, 1991.
2. Bonci CM: Assessment and evaluation of predisposing factors to anterior cruciate ligament injury. J Athl Train 34:15–25, 1999.
3. Bonci CM, Ryan R: Pre-participation screening in intercollegiate athletics. Postgraduate Advances in Sports Medicine. Forum Medicum, 1988.
4. Given B, Simmons S: The interdisciplinary healthcare team: fact or fiction. *Nurs Forum* 15:165–84, 1977.
5. Jones, BH, Harris, JM, Vinh, TN, Rubin, C: Exercise induced stress fractures and stress reactions of bone: epidemiology, etiology and classification. Exerc Sports Sci 17:379–422, 1989.
6. Ogilvie BC, Tutko TA: Security. In Larson L (ed): Encyclopedia of Sport Sciences and Medicine: The American College of Sports Medicine. New York, Macmillan, 1971, pp 910–3.

7. The Performance Team Newsletter. Bone stress injury project. The University of Texas at Austin, Department of Intercollegiate Athletics for Women, 1990, 2(3).

8. The Performance Team Newsletter. Establishment of the interdisciplinary model for health care. The University of Texas at Austin, Department of Intercollegiate Athletics for Women, 1987, 1(1).

9. The Performance Team Newsletter. Mental health services for elite female athletes. The University of Texas at Austin, Department of Intercollegiate Athletics for Women, 1989, 2(2).

10. The Performance Team Newsletter. Student athlete orientation program. The University of Texas at Austin, Department of Intercollegiate Athletics for Women, 1988, 1(3).

11. The Performance Team Newsletter. Weight regulation practices/disordered eating. The University of Texas at Austin, Department of Intercollegiate Athletics for Women, 1988, 1(2).

12. Pinkerton RS, Hinz LD, Barrow JC. The college student-athlete: psychological considerations and interventions. *J Am Coll Health* 1989; 37:218–226.

13. The President's Council on Physical Fitness and Sports—Executive Summary. Bunker LK (ed): Physical activity and sport in the lives of girls: physical and mental health dimensions from an interdisciplinary approach. May 1977.

14. Ryan R (ed): The mental health of female college student-athletes: research and interventions on a university campus. Final report to The Hogg Foundation, The RGK Foundation. The University of Texas at Austin, June 1994.

15. Ryan R: Management of eating problems in athletic settings. In Brownell KD, Roden J, Wilmore JH (eds): Eating, Body Weight and Performance in Athletes: Disorders of a Modern Society. Philadelphia, Lea & Febiger, 1992, pp 344–62.

16. West C: The female athlete-who will direct her destiny? Rethinking services for college athletes. London, Jossey-Bass, 1984, pp 21–30.

Chapter 9

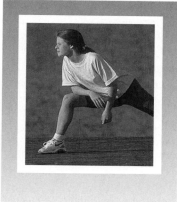

Nutrition

Ann C. Grandjean, Ed.D., R.D.
Kristin J. Reimers, M.S., R.D.
Jaime Ruud, M.S., R.D.

As we enter the 21st century, few can disagree that nutrition has ceased being the poor stepchild in the world of athletic performance, and has reached a level of prominence. Concurrently, nutrition has received a great deal of attention in the public health arena as a preventive weapon against chronic diseases. An interesting phenomenon that has resulted is the blending—and often confusion—of these areas of nutrition. Certainly, nutritional principles for enhancing performance and nutritional principles for disease prevention do intersect, but the distinct differences often are not acknowledged. Not surprisingly, many athletes and coaches do not recognize the difference between nutrition for enhancing performance and nutrition for general health and disease prevention. The inherent danger therein is, at best, the adoption of an oversimplified or "cookie-cutter" approach to nutrition, and at worst, the development of eating habits that are helpful for neither sport performance nor disease prevention.

Quite naturally, health professionals typically counsel athletes with an emphasis placed on health implications—acute illness or chronic disease. The athlete, however, rarely is motivated (beyond lip service) by health implications. Instead, motivation lies in such factors as decreasing body fat for appearance, speed, agility, or jumping; increasing lean body mass for increased strength and performance; or taking supplements for faster recovery following injury. The following discussion will examine, and attempt to clarify, nutritional issues encountered primarily within the female athletic population from the standpoints of both health and performance. A sound working knowledge and pragmatic approach to nutrition and performance will increase the likelihood that nutritional recommendations will be implemented.

WEIGHT ISSUES

The emphasis on performance and appearance at the expense of health is evident in some athlete's effort to manipulate body composition. Short of being pathologically driven to lose weight, as is seen in anorexia nervosa, many female athletes attempt to achieve and maintain body weight or body fat at levels significantly lower than what is genetically determined or would be defined as normal. The motivating forces usually include the need to be thin for sports in which scores are influenced by appearance; to increase jumping ability, speed, or agility; to improve appearance in the suit or uniform; or to achieve a body type consistent with societal ideals. The challenge when working with such an athlete is to facilitate achieving the goal to the extent possible without "crossing the line" to where dietary practices and training practices become detrimental to health and performance.

Assessment

When an athlete seeks to lose body fat, the first step is to assess current body composition and set realistic goals. Body weight is a poor measure of body composition because increased lean body mass cannot be distinguished from fat mass. Many female athletes will weigh more but have less body fat than sedentary counterparts. Several methods exist to measure body composition indirectly. None are without error. Valid, reliable methods include underwater weighing, bioelectrical impedance, and, the most readily available and inexpensive, skinfold thickness measurement. Skinfold testing, when using population-specific equations, reliable calipers, and a trained measurer, yields percent body fat estimations with an accuracy of ±3%.[25] The "ideal" percent body fat for each individual is elusive.

Some data exist on average percent body fat levels of female athletic groups, but these group averages cannot be extrapolated to the individual. Secondly, specific numbers tend to be helpful clinically as a monitoring tool, but have little relevance to performance. The athlete and coach should focus on strength, speed and general performance abilities to determine the level of body fat appropriate for each individual, and avoid using arbitrary numbers or guidelines. Some athletes will feel tired and weak at body fat levels well above the expected body fat minimum, and others will thrive at body fat levels less than the theoretic minimum.

Initial body composition assessment usually places the female athlete into either of 2 categories: relatively lean wanting to be leaner, or moderately to significantly overfat. Of the 2 types, the relatively lean athlete often presents more dilemmas for the clinician: "Should this athlete be dissuaded from weight loss?" "How low is too low?" "If I dissuade weight loss attempts, will she proceed anyway, and perhaps use extreme measures?" The decision as to whether the weight loss has the potential to improve performance and not negatively impact health is a decision involving the coach, athlete, and physician. Indications that weight loss should be avoided or discontinued from a health standpoint include a change from eumenorrhea to amenorrhea or oligomenorrhea (barring other causes), fat loss cessation despite continued calorie restriction, recurrent illness or injury, incidence of extreme behaviors such as fasting, or adoption of dietary habits too restrictive to meet nutrient needs.

Guidelines for Fat Loss

If the assessment indicates that the athlete is a candidate for weight loss, the basis for achieving weight loss in either the relatively lean athlete or the overly fat athlete is the same—create a caloric deficit—however, the rate of weight loss, the ability to maintain the weight loss, and the effect of weight loss on performance will vary with each situation. The following are practical considerations for the female athlete attempting to decrease body fat:

TIMING

It is usually best to achieve fat loss during the off-season or early pre-season.

RATE

Expected rate of fat loss for the lean athlete is less than 0.5 pound per week. For the athlete with excessive adipose tissue the rate can safely be 1% body weight per week initially, slowing to 0.5 to 1 pound per week thereafter.

FOOD INTAKE

Some athletes prefer a regimented meal plan. Referral to a dietitian or sports nutritionist for a customized plan is appropriate in these cases. For those athletes who prefer more general guidelines, the following can help in achieving a negative calorie balance: reducing fat intake, establishing a set meal schedule, substituting lower-calorie snacks, decreasing use of caloric beverages, and other reasonable modifications as indicated by usual intake. It is often helpful for the athlete to record all food and beverage intake to become aware of quality and quantity of her diet: for example, to identify eating patterns, to recognize where, if at all, calories can be reduced, and to monitor the nutrient content of foods consumed. It is not uncommon to observe an athlete who is omitting entire groups of food or consuming snack foods as the majority of caloric intake. Without written records, these qualitative issues often go unnoticed.

SUPPLEMENTS

When caloric intake declines to less than 1200 to 1500 kcal/day, it is difficult to meet vitamin and mineral requirements without a vitamin and/or mineral supplement.

TRAINING

Based on current training, determine whether aerobic activity can be increased. If the athlete is already at a maximum level of daily training, the caloric deficit has to be accomplished primarily by reducing food intake.

The Fat Phobia Phenomenon

The importance placed on thinness coupled with a pervasive public health message about the dangers of eating a high-fat diet have resulted in a trend observed in many Americans: the fear of eating fat. For many female athletes this fat phobia encompasses fear of fat on the plate and fear of fat on the body.

Many athletes perceive avoidance of fat as a nutrition truth and cure-all. They attempt to avoid foods containing even a few grams of fat. Parents, peers, and coaches often accept this behavior because of the prevalent negative attitude about fat. However, when pressed, the athlete will usually not cite fear of dying from a heart attack as her primary motivation for this extreme dietary practice. In most cases, she believes that if fat is consumed, her body fat will increase. In nonobese, active athletes who are not consuming excess calories, there is no correlation between fat content of the diet and fat content of the body. Actually, some of the leanest athletes have the highest dietary fat intake. The amount of body fat an athlete carries remains an issue of calorie balance and genetics.

The fat-free eating that the athlete perceives as being extremely healthy *and* performance enhancing is neither. Excessively low fat intake often leads to exclusion of entire food groups, such as meats and dairy foods. For many female athletes, the exclusion of these foods means nutrients important for health and performance are lacking. Two key nutrients often affected by restricting food intake are iron and calcium.

Female athletes who significantly restrict calorie intake are the group at highest risk for nutrient shortfalls in their diets, however, other groups are also at risk. This group includes those athletes with naturally low calorie intakes, those who exclude food groups, and those who simply make poor food choices because of a lack of food availability, time, or resources.

IRON

Iron is present in all cells of the body and plays a key role in numerous biochemical reactions. It performs a vital role in the transport of oxygen and the synthesis of hemoglobin and myoglobin. It is also present in a number of enzymes responsible for electron transport. Thus, a deficiency of iron can affect several metabolic functions related to energy production.

Iron deficiency has long been a health and performance issue for female athletes. Studies assessing the diets of female athletes show that they frequently consume less than the recommended amount of iron.[26,28,36,42] Biochemical analyses reveal suboptimal hemoglobin and serum ferritin levels, particularly among female distance runners.[2,18,23,33] It has been speculated that these suboptimal levels represent hemodilution, which is a normal adaptation to endurance training. There are, however, a number of other factors that can contribute to poor iron status of female athletes, including increased iron losses (ie, menstruation, pregnancy, gastrointestinal bleeding), decreased iron absorption, and inadequate dietary intake.[2,11,35]

Regardless of the cause, low iron stores can lead to iron-deficiency anemia, which can impair athletic performance by decreasing physical work capacity.[10] Awareness, early detection, and adequate knowledge are important steps in preventing iron deficiency.

For those readers interested in a more comprehensive review, several have been written describing the prevalence of iron deficiency and anemia in female athletes, the effects of training on iron status, and the effects of iron status on performance.[7,17,19,27,30,43] The focus here will be on effective intervention strategies: screening, treatment, and prevention of iron deficiency.

Screening for Deficiency

Ideally, all female athletes should be screened for symptoms of iron-deficiency anemia, including fatigue and decreased performance. The yearly pre-participation examination is an opportune time for such a screen. A comprehensive screen includes obtaining a brief medical history; information on diet, weight-control practices, menstrual history, and drug usage (eg, aspirin, alcohol, and inflammatory agents); and laboratory values if history and symptoms are suggestive of anemia or iron deficiency.

A complete battery of tests to determine iron status will include serum iron, total iron-binding capacity (TIBC), transferrin saturation, and serum ferritin concentration, in addition to hemoglobin, hematocrit, and mean corpuscular volume (MCV). The serum ferritin level is the most sensitive screen for iron deficiency. Normal serum ferritin levels for females range from 12 to 150 ng/mL, with 30 ng/mL being average.[17] However, there is disagreement as to what values represent "depletion." In classic iron-deficiency anemia, serum ferritin values are generally less than 12 ng/mL; however, some clinicians prefer to use a cutoff of 20 ng/mL in the high-performance athlete.

Low hemoglobin levels do not always indicate anemia or the need for iron therapy. To determine if a borderline hemoglobin level in an athlete is indicative of anemia necessitates comparison to the individual's normal baseline hemoglobin level[17] and further workup as indicated.

Treatment of Deficiency

If an athlete has been diagnosed with iron deficiency, dietary counseling and iron supplementation are the most efficient methods of treatment. Ferrous sulfate (325 mg/day) is the preparation most often recommended, but if not well tolerated, ferrous fumarate or ferrous gluconate can be prescribed.

Gastrointestinal side effects such as epigastric discomfort, nausea, and vomiting make iron therapy troublesome for many. A slow-release iron supplement, with or without a stool softener, is an option that may decrease gastrointestinal symptoms. Recent data have shown that in some populations, iron supplementation less than once daily (eg, 30 mg elemental iron 2 times per week) is as effective as, though not superior to, daily administration of iron in improving the iron status of individuals with low iron stores.[38] These preliminary data suggest that if an athlete is experiencing negative side effects while on daily iron supplements, the physician may consider prescribing less frequent iron supplementation to improve compliance while not significantly affecting therapeutic benefit.

Supplementation

Many nonanemic female athletes take iron supplements to increase energy and enhance performance. Although iron supplementation increases blood iron levels, it has not been shown to have a positive effect on performance.[22,31,41] One concern with taking iron supplements prophylactically is interaction with other nutrients. Studies have reported that iron supplementation decreases absorption of zinc and copper.[37,40,45] Thus, prophylactic iron supplementation, above that which might be contained in a multivitamin pill, is not recommended.

Prevention of Deficiency

In most cases, iron deficiency can be prevented with an adequate diet. At-risk athletes should be aware of good sources of dietary iron (Table 9-1). Bioavailability (the total amount of iron available for absorption) depends on several factors, including the individual's iron status, the form of iron (heme vs nonheme), the presence of inhibitors (ie, phytates, bran, polyphenols in tea, antacids) and the presence of enhancers.

Meat consumption is a key dietary determinant of iron status.[9] Meat contains heme iron, which is absorbed at a much higher rate (23%) than nonheme iron (3% to 8%).[29] In addition, heme iron promotes absorption of nonheme iron, and the effect increases as the amount of meat increases.[15] Vitamin C has been shown to enhance nonheme iron absorption, although the effects may be less significant than once thought.[20]

The Recommended Dietary Allowances state that a daily intake of 15 mg iron from a typical diet is adequate to replace iron losses of most women.[13] Based on calculations by Hallberg and Rossander-Hulten,[16] the amount of iron needed to be absorbed to cover the iron requirements of adult menstruating women is 2.84 mg/day. For this amount to be absorbed, the diet should contain about 18 mg/day of iron, or approximately 9 mg/1000 kcal/day.

Female athletes who restrict calories or consume monotonous diets will have difficulty meeting iron requirements. This is especially true for athletes who consume vegetarian diets. In female runners consuming a modified vegetarian diet (less than 100 g red meat/week), Snyder et al[39] reported the bioavailability of iron was significantly lower ($p < 0.05$) than in female runners consuming red meat, 0.66 mg/day and 0.91 mg/day, respectively. There were no significant differences in total caloric intake, and both groups consumed approximately 14 mg/day of dietary iron. However, athletes who ate red meat consumed greater amounts of heme iron (1.2 mg/day vs 0.2 mg/day, respectively) and had higher serum ferritin levels than athletes consuming a modified vegetarian diet (19.8 μg/L and 7.4 μg/L, respectively). Yokoi et al[46] also reported a positive influence on iron status in women consuming red meat.

CALCIUM

Optimal calcium intake during childhood and adolescence is important for attainment of peak bone mass and for the prevention of osteoporosis. Calcium is especially important for amenorrheic women, who are already at risk for low bone mineral density because of decreased estrogen levels.

The role of calcium in bone metabolism, amenorrhea, and osteoporosis is covered elsewhere in this book. This section reviews current calcium requirements and calcium contribution of foods.

Recommendations

The current recommended dietary allowance for calcium is 1200 mg/day for females ages 11 to 24 and 800 mg/day for those over age 25.[13] However, participants at a National Institutes of Health (NIH) conference recommended higher calcium intakes to achieve maximum bone mass and minimize bone loss.[32] Table 9-2 lists the recommendations of the NIH expert panel on calcium.

There exists a wide gap between the recommendations for increasing calcium intake and the actual intake of many Americans, particularly females. The National Health and Nutrition Examination Survey (NHANES III)[1] reported mean calcium intakes less than the RDA for almost all female ethnic race groups over age 12.[1] Low calcium intakes are also prevalent

Text continued on Page 83

Table 9-1. Dietary Sources of Iron

Heme Sources of Iron

FOOD (3 OZ, COOKED, LEAN ONLY)	TOTAL IRON (MG)	AVAILABLE IRON (MG)
Beef		
Liver, pan fried	5.34	.60
Chuck, arm pot roast, braised	3.22	.48
Tenderloin, roasted	3.05	.46
Sirloin, broiled	2.85	.42
Roundtip, roasted	2.50	.38
Top round, broiled	2.45	.37
Top loin, broiled	2.10	.31
Ground, lean, broiled	1.79	.27
Eye round, roasted	1.65	.25
Pork		
Shoulder, blade, Boston, roasted	1.36	.15
Tenderloin, roasted	1.31	.15
Ham, boneless, 5–11% fat	1.19	.14
Loin chop broiled	.78	.09
Lamb		
Loin, roasted	2.07	.31
Leg, shank half, roasted	1.75	.26
Veal		
Loin, roasted	.93	.14
Cutlet, pan fried	.74	.11
Chicken		
Liver, simmered	7.2	.81
Leg, roasted	1.11	.17
Breast, roasted	.88	.13

Nonheme Sources of Iron

FOOD	TOTAL IRON (MG)	AVAILABLE IRON (MG)
Cereals		
Raisin bran (enrich), dry, 1/2 c	4.5	.23
Corn flakes (enrich), dry, 1 oz	1.8	.09
Shredded wheat, dry, 1 oz	1.20	.06
Oatmeal, cooked, 1/2 c	.80	.04
Whole wheat hot cereal, 1/2 c	.75	.04
Grains		
Bagel, 1	1.8	.09
Bran muffin, home recipe, 1	1.4	.07
Whole wheat bread, 1 sl	1.0	.05
White rice (enrich), cooked, 1/2 c	.9	.05
White Bread (enrich), 1 sl	.7	.04
Brown rice, cooked, 1/2 c	.5	.03
Fruits		
Apricots, dried, 7 halves	1.16	.06
Prunes, dried, 3 medium	.84	.04
Raisins, 2 Tbsp	.38	.02
Banana, 1 medium	.35	.02
Apple, 1 medium	.25	.01
Orange, 1 medium	.13	.01
Vegetables		
Potato, baked w/skin, 1 medium	2.75	.14
Peas, cooked, 1/2 c	1.26	.06
Spinach, raw, 1/2 c	.76	.04
Broccoli, raw, 1/2 c	.39	.02
Carrots, 1 medium	.36	.02
Lettuce, iceberg, 1/8 head	.34	.02
Corn, cooked, 1/2 c	.25	.01
Beans/Legumes		
Kidney beans, boiled, 1/2 c	2.58	.13
canned, 1/2 c	1.57	.08
Chickpeas, boiled, 1/2 c	2.37	.12
canned, 1/2 c	1.62	.08
Baked beans, canned, plain, 1/2 c	.37	.02

Table continued on following Page

Table 9-1. Dietary Sources of Iron (*Continued*)

FOOD (3 OZ, COOKED, LEAN ONLY)	TOTAL IRON (MG)	AVAILABLE IRON (MG)
Turkey		
Leg, roasted	2.26	.34
Breast, roasted	.99	.14
Fish		
Tuna, light meat, canned	2.72	.31
white meat, canned	.51	.06
Halibut, dry heat	.91	.10
Salmon, sockeye, dry heat	.47	.06
Flounder/sole, dry heat	.23	.03
Shellfish		
Oysters, 6 medium, raw	5.63	.63
Shrimp, moist heat	2.63	.30
Crab, Alaskan king, moist heat	.65	.07

FOOD	TOTAL IRON (MG)	AVAILABLE IRON (MG)
Meat Substitutes		
Tofu, 2 1/2 × 2 3/4 × 1 in	2.3	.12
Egg, whole	1.0	.05
yolk	.95	.05
white	tr	–
Peanut Butter, 2 Tbsp	.6	.03
Dairy		
Milk, lowfat, 1 c	.12	.01
Yogurt, plain lowfat, 1 c	.18	.01
Cheese, cheddar, 1 oz	.19	.01
Molasses		
Cane, blackstrap, 1 Tbsp	5.05	.25

From Iron in Human Nutrition. Chicago, Ill, National Live Stock and Meat Board, 1990.

Table 9-2. Comparison of NIH Expert Panel Recommendation to the Recommended Dietary Allowance of Calcium

AGES	NIH EXPERT PANEL	RDA
11–24 years	1200–1500 mg	1200 mg
Women:		
25–49 years	1000 mg	800 mg
50–65 years (taking estrogen)	1000 mg	800 mg
50–65 years (not taking estrogen)	1500 mg	800 mg
65+ years	1500 mg	800 mg
Men:		
25–64 years	1000 mg	800 mg
65+ years	1500 mg	800 mg

From Optimal calcium intake. NIH Consensus Statement, 1994, June 6–8, vol 12(4), pp 1–31.

among female athletes, specifically those who restrict calories to maintain thinness.[3,8,28,34] Many calcium-deficient women are unaware of the problem, and thus are not overly concerned about increasing their calcium intake.[6] The per-

ception may be that a few servings of dairy products a day is adequate, while the reality is that many women need to consume 5 servings a day. Another explanation for inadequate calcium consumption is the fact that many women, including female athletes, believe that milk and dairy products are high in fat and calories.[6] However, data show that it is possible to increase calcium intake without increasing fat intake.[21] Adolescent girls who consumed higher-calcium diets, achieved primarily by adding 2% milk, skim milk, and American cheese, did not have higher fat and caloric intakes than those who had lower-calcium diets with fewer dairy products.[5] Increasing the athlete's knowledge and awareness about calcium is the first step the physician can take to promote increased calcium intake. One excellent means of increasing awareness is to ask the athlete to review her calcium intake. While this might be as simple as providing a verbal history, completing a brief screening tool (Table 9-3) is also effective.

Table 9-3. Screening Tool for Assessing Calcium Intake

FOODS WITH CALCIUM	SERVING SIZE	NO. SERVINGS	CALCIUM (MG)	CALCIUM SUBTOTAL
Yogurt (plain or with fruit)	1 cup	☐		
Evaporated skim milk	1/2 cup	☐		
Nonfat dry milk powder	1/2 cup	+ ☐		
	Total servings	☐	× 400 =	☐ mg
Milk (nonfat, lowfat, lactose reduced, whole, chocolate, buttermilk)	1 c	☐		
Parmesan cheese (grated)	1/4 c	☐		
Ricotta cheese (part skim, nonfat)	1/2 c	☐		
Swiss and Gruyere cheese	1 oz	☐		
Tofu (calcium set)	1/2 c	+ ☐		
	Total servings	☐	× 300 =	☐ mg
Hard cheeses (most others)	1 oz	☐		
	Total servings	☐	× 200 =	☐ mg
Instant oatmeal	1 packet	☐		
Pudding, custard, flan	1/2 c	+ ☐		
	Total servings	☐	× 150 =	☐ mg
Beans (white)	1/2 c	☐		
Cream cheese (nonfat)	1 oz	☐		
Turnip greens, bok choy	1/2 c	☐		
Almonds (shelled)	1 oz	☐		
Ice cream, ice milk, frozen yogurt	1/2 c	+ ☐		
	Total servings	☐	× 100 =	☐ mg
Broccoli	1/2 c	☐		
Kale, mustard greens	1/2 c	☐		
Beans (most dried)	1/2 c	☐		
Cottage cheese	1/2 c	☐		
Corn tortilla	1 medium	☐		
Orange	1 medium	+ ☐		
	Total servings	☐	× 50 =	☐ mg
Dates, raisins	1/4 c	☐		
Whole wheat bread	1 sl	☐		
Soy milk	1 c	+ ☐		
	Total servings	☐	× 25 =	☐ mg

- Your calcium score:
- Your calcium needs:
- The difference is:

☐ mg
☐ mg
☐ mg
☐ mg

From Nutrition Education Services. Oregon Dairy Council, Portland, Or.

Table 9-4. Food Sources of Calcium

FOODS*	SERVING SIZE (G)	CALCIUM CONTENT (MG)	ESTIMATED ABSORBABLE CALCIUM/SERVING (MG)
Milk	240	300	96.3
Almonds, dry roasted	28	80	17.0
Beans, pinto	86	44.7	7.6
Beans, red	172	40.5	6.9
Beans, white	110	113	19.2
Broccoli	71	35	18.4
Brussel sprouts	78	19	12.1
Cabbage, Chinese	85	79	42.5
Cabbage, green	75	25	16.2
Cauliflower	62	17	11.7
Citrus punch with CCM	240	300	150
Fruit punch with CCM	240	300	156
Kale	65	47	27.6
Kohlrabi	82	20	13.4
Mustard greens	72	64	37.0
Radish	50	14	10.4
Rutabaga	85	36	22.1
Sesame seeds, no hulls	28	37	7.7
Soy milk	120	5	1.6
Spinach	90	122	6.2
Tofu, calcium set	126	258	80.0
Turnip greens	72	99	51.1
Watercress	17	20	13.4

*Based on 1/2-c CCM, calcium serving size except for milk, citrus punch, and fruit punch (1 cup) and almonds and sesame seeds (1 oz).

Adapted from Weaver CM, Plawecki KL: Dietary calcium: adequacy of a vegetarian diet. *Am J Clin Nutr* 59: 1238S–41S, 1994.

Dairy products are the richest source of calcium, providing more than 50% of the calcium in a typical diet.[12] Other calcium-rich foods include sardines (with bones), turnip greens, kale, calcium-fortified fruit drinks, and calcium-fortified soy milk. Calcium from soybeans and green leafy vegetables such as broccoli contain less calcium per serving than milk but are absorbed as well. Table 9-4 lists calcium-rich foods.

Supplementation

A diet void of dairy products typically contains about 300 mg calcium. Considering this as a baseline, the female patient who cannot or will not increase dairy product consumption will need an additional 600 to 1200 mg of calcium daily. This amount can be achieved through a combination of consumption of other calcium-rich foods and use of supplements. For example, an 8-oz glass of calcium-fortified orange juice provides about 300 mg, as much as many calcium supplements.

Calcium carbonate is the most widely available preparation for supplements. Other supplements with good bioavailability include calcium citrate, calcium lactate, calcium gluconate, and calcium citrate maleate.[24] Bone meal dolomite and fossilized oyster shell preparations are not recommended because they may be contaminated with heavy metals.[4,44] Patients should be advised that calcium in supplements is best absorbed when doses of less than 500 mg are taken between meals, and that calcium supplements taken with meals or with iron supplements significantly decrease iron absorption.[14]

CONCLUDING REMARKS

The unique nutritional needs of the female athlete pose many questions; however, by remaining mindful of the relationship between good health and the occasionally questionable messages of performance nutrition, the credibility and efficacy of the physician will be enhanced.

References

1. Alaimo K, McDowell MA, Briefel RR, et al. Dietary Intake of Vitamins, Minerals, and Fiber of Persons Ages 2 Months and Over in the United States: Third National Health and Nutrition Examination Survey, Phase 1, 1988–91. Advanced data from Vital and Health Statistics. Hyattsville, Md, National Center for Health Statistics, 1994.
2. Balaban EP, Cox JV, Snell P, et al: The frequency of anemia and iron deficiency in the runner. Med Sci Sports Exerc 21:643–8, 1989.

3. Benson JE, Geiger CJ, Eiserman PA, Wardlaw GM: Relationship between nutrient intake, body mass index, menstrual function, and ballet injury. J Am Diet Assoc 89:58–63, 1989.

4. Bourgoin BP, Evans DR, Cornett JR, et al: Lead content in 70 brands of dietary calcium supplements. Am J Public Health 83:1155–60, 1993.

5. Chan GM, Hoffman K, McMurry M: Effects of dairy products on bone and body composition in pubertal girls. J Pediatr 126:551–6, 1995.

6. Chapman KM, Chan MW, Clark CD: Factors influencing dairy calcium intake in women. J Am College Nutr 14:336–40, 1995.

7. Clarkson PM, Haymes EM. Exercise and mineral status of athletes: calcium, magnesium, phosphorus, and iron. Med Sci Sports Exerc 27:831–43, 1995.

8. Cohen JL, Potosnak L, Frank O, Baker H: A nutritional and hematologic assessment of elite ballet dancers. Phys Sportsmed 13:43–54, 1985.

9. Cook JD, Dassenko SA, Lynch SR: Assessment of the role of nonheme-iron availability in iron balance. Am J Clin Nutr 54:717–22, 1991.

10. Davies KJA, Maguire JJ, Brooks GA, et al: Muscle mitochondrial bioenergetics, oxygen supply, and work capacity during dietary iron deficiency and repletion. Am J Physiol 242:E418–27, 1982.

11. Eichner ER: Runner's macrocytosis: a clue to footsrike hemolysis. Am J Med 78:321–5, 1985.

12. Fleming KH, Heimbach JT: Consumption of calcium in the U.S.: food sources and intake levels. J Nutr 124:1426S–30S, 1994.

13. Food Nutrition Board. Recommended Dietary Allowances (10th edition). Washington, DC, National Academy of Sciences, 1994.

14. Gleerup A, Rossander-Hulten L, Gramatkovski E, Hallberg L: Iron absorption from the whole diet: comparison of the effect of two different distributions of daily calcium intake. Am J Clin Nutr 61:97–104, 1995.

15. Hallberg L: Bioavailability of dietary iron in man. In Darby WJ (ed): Annual Review of Nutrition. Palo Alto, Calif, Annual Reviews, 1981.

16. Hallberg L, Rossander-Hulten L: Iron requirements in menstruating women. Am J Clin Nutr 54:1047–58, 1991.

17. Harris SS: Helping active women avoid anemia. Phys Sportsmed 23:35–48, 1995.

18. Haymes EM, Spillman DM: Iron status of women distance runners, sprinters, and control women. Int J Sports Med 10:430–3, 1989.

19. Haymes EM: Dietary iron needs in exercising women: A rational plan to follow in evaluating iron status. Med Exerc Nutr Health 2:203–12, 1993.

20. Hunt JR, Gallagher SK, Johnson LK: Effect of ascorbic acid on apparent iron absorption by women with low iron stores. Am J Clin Nutr 59:1381–5, 1994.

21. Karanja N, Morris CD, Rufolo P, et al: Impact of increasing calcium in the diet on nutrient consumption, plasma lipids, and lipoproteins in humans. Am J Clin Nutr 59:900–7, 1994.

22. Klingshirn LA, Pate RR, Bourque SP, et al: Effect of iron supplementation on endurance capacity in iron-depleted female runners. Med Sci Sports Exerc 24:819–24, 1992.

23. Lampe JW, Slavin JL, Apple FS: Poor iron status of women runners training for a marathon. Int J Sports Med 7:111–4, 1986.

24. Levenson DI, Bockman RS: A review of calcium preparations. Nutr Rev 52:221–32, 1994.

25. Lohman TG: Skinfolds and body density and their relation to body fatness: A review. Hum Biol 53:181–225, 1981.

26. Loosli AR, Benson J, Gillien DM, Bourdet K: Nutrition habits and knowledge in competitive adolescent female gymnasts. Phys Sportsmed 14:118–30, 1986.

27. Loosli AR: Reversing sports-related iron and zinc deficiencies. Phys Sportsmed 21:70–8, 1993.

28. Moffatt RJ: Dietary status of elite female high school gymnasts: inadequacy of vitamin and mineral intake. J Am Diet Assoc 84:1361–3, 1984.

29. Monsen ER, Hallberg L, Layrisse M, et al: Estimation of available dietary iron. Am J Clin Nutr 31:134–41, 1978.

30. Newhouse IJ, Clement DB: Iron status in athletes: An update. Sports Med 5:337–52, 1988.

31. Newhouse IJ, Clement DB, Taunton JE, McKenzie DC: The effects of prelatent/latent iron deficiency on physical work capacity. Med Sci Sports Exerc 21:263–8, 1989.

32. Optimal calcium intake. NIH Consensus Statement, 1994, June 6–8, Vol 12(4):1–31.

33. Pate RR, Sargent RG, Baldwin C, Burgess ML: Dietary intake of women runners. Int J Sports Med 11:461–6, 1990.

34. Perron M, Endres J: Knowledge, attitudes, and dietary practices of female athletes. J Am Diet Assoc 85:573–6, 1985.

35. Raunikar RA, Sabio H: Anemia in the adolescent athlete. Am J Dis Child 146:1201–5, 1992.

36. Reggiani E, Arras GB, Trabacca S: Nutritional status and body composition of adolescent female gymnasts. J Sports Med 29:285–8, 1989.

37. Sandstrom B, Davidsson L, Cederblad A, Lonnerdal B: Oral iron, dietary ligands and zinc absorption. J Nutr 115:411–4, 1985.

38. Schultink W, Gross R, Gliwitzki M, et al: Effect of daily vs twice weekly iron supplementation in Indonesian preschool children with low iron status. Am J Clin Nutr 61:111–5, 1995.

39. Snyder AC, Dvorak LL, Roepke JB: Influence of dietary iron source on measures of iron status among female runners. Med Sci Sports Exerc 21:7–10, 1989.

40. Solomons NW: Competitive interaction of iron and zinc in the diet: consequences for human nutrition. J Nutr 116:927–35, 1986.

41. Telford RD, Bunney CJ, Catchpole EA, et al: Plasma ferritin concentration and physical work capacity in athletes. Int J Sport Nutr 2:335–42, 1992.

42. van Erp-Baart AMJ, Saris WHM, Binkhorst RA, et al: Nationwide survey on nutritional habits in elite athletes. II. Mineral and vitamin intake. Int J Sports Med 10:S11–6, 1989.

43. Weaver CM, Rajaram S: Exercise and iron status. J Nutr 122:782–7, 1992.

44. Whiting SJ: Safety of some calcium supplements questioned. Nutr Rev 52:95–7, 1994.

45. Yadrick MK, Kenney MA, Winterfeldt EA: Iron, copper, and zinc status: response to supplementation with zinc or zinc and iron in adult females. Am J Clin Nutr 49:145–50, 1989.

46. Yokoi K, Alcock NW, Sandstead HH: Iron and zinc nutriture of premenopausal women: Associations of diet with serum ferritin and plasma zinc disappearance and of serum ferritin with plasma zinc and plasma zinc disappearance. J Lab Clin Med 124:852–61, 1994.

Chapter 10

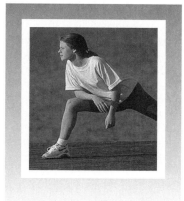

Sports Supplements and Ergogenic Aids

Ellen Coleman, M.A., M.P.H., R.D.

According to the advertisements in many fitness magazines, there is no shortage of products that claim to increase speed, enhance endurance, improve strength, increase muscle mass or reduce body fat. Some advertisements even claim that their product does all of the above.

Fitness-oriented women (and men) want to believe in some product that will improve their performance beyond what they can achieve by following a sound diet and training program. In many events, the difference between winning and losing is measured in fractions of seconds, so it is not surprising that athletes are vulnerable to miraculous claims for supplements.

Nutritional ergogenic aids are dietary supplements that supposedly enhance performance above levels anticipated under normal conditions. The term *ergogenic* means "work producing."

Sarah Short, PhD, RD, an ardent crusader against sports nutrition fraud, suggests several factors that may contribute to the increased use of ergogenic aids and dietary supplements among athletes.[31] Athletes, coaches, and the public have an inadequate knowledge of sports nutrition and nutrition in general. A poor understanding of nutrition, combined with locker room talk and the influence of slick ads in sports magazines, help to perpetuate myths regarding nutrition. Although coaches believe they should be the ones to provide nutritional advice to their athletes, few coaches have any formal nutritional training. Some misinformed but well-intentioned coaches suggest that their athletes consume specific foods or dietary supplements, such as protein, amino acids, or vitamins.

Melvin Williams, PhD, an expert on ergogenic aids, notes three other factors in the athletic environment that contribute to the use of supplements.[48] There is an abundance of advertisements of nutritional products marketed specifically to athletes in leading sports magazines. These publications also have a substantial amount of nutritional misinformation in their articles. Furthermore, athletes often follow the dietary habits or recommendations of successful athletes who have no formal nutrition training.

THE 1994 DIETARY SUPPLEMENT HEALTH AND EDUCATION ACT

The 1994 Dietary Supplement Health and Education Act (DSHEA) was passed by Congress after the health food industry and its allies urged Congress to "preserve the consumer's freedom to choose dietary supplements." The result was a law that greatly weakened the ability of the US Food and Drug Administration (FDA) to protect consumers.[2]

The DSHEA prohibits the FDA from regulating dietary supplements as food additives and expanded the types of products that could be marketed. "Dietary supplements" now include vitamins, minerals, herbs or other botanicals, amino acids, other dietary substances, and any concentrate, metabolite, constituent, extract, or combination of such ingredients.[2]

Although many of these products are marketed for their alleged preventive and therapeutic (ie, drug) effects, the DSHEA has made it difficult or impossible for the FDA to regulate them as drugs. Even hormones, such as DHEA, melatonin, and androstenedione, are being hawked as supplements.[2]

Thanks to the DSHEA, dietary supplements and ergogenic aids do not have to be proven safe or effective to be sold. There is also no guarantee that the products are what they say they are on their labels.[2]

While prescription and over-the-counter drugs and food additives must meet FDA safety and effectiveness requirements, supplements that are marketed with medical claims bypass these regulations. These products can go to market with no testing for efficacy, thus skipping the years-long process that drugs must undergo. The FDA is also prohibited from taking a product off the market unless the agency can prove that using the supplement will create a medical problem. Unfortunately, this law places the burden of proof of a supplement's safety on the overtaxed FDA rather than on the companies profiting from the sale of the supplement. Furthermore, supplements that are worthless but harmless are protected.[2]

FDA approval is not required for package or marketing claims, so supplement manufacturers can put unsupported health claims, called "nutritional support" statements, on their labels; however, the DSHEA stipulates that labeling must be truthful and not misleading, and that "nutritional support" statements must be followed by the phrase, "This statement has not been evaluated by the FDA. This product is not intended to diagnose, treat or prevent disease." This disclaimer (usually in very small print) should raise a red flag of suspicion about the accuracy of the supplement manufacturer's information.[2]

Lastly, supplements do not have to be manufactured according to any standards. Since supplements such as herbs are not regulated as drugs, no legal standard exists for their processing, harvesting, or packaging. In many cases contents and potency are not accurately listed on the label.[2]

THE MARKETING OF ERGOGENIC AIDS

More than a hundred companies are marketing worthless (but profitable) ergogenic aids. It is estimated that the total sales of these products through health food stores exceeded $204 million in 1996.[1] They are also sold in pharmacies and supermarkets. Ads for such products often display trim, muscular individuals and/or endorsements from respected professional athletes and National Collegiate Athletic Association or Olympic champions. Locker room conversations also perpetuate nutritional myths and misinformation.

In 1991, researchers from the US Centers for Disease Control and Prevention surveyed 12 popular health and body building magazines (one issue each) and found ads for 89 brands and 311 products, with a total of 235 single ingredients. The most frequent ingredients were amino acids and herbs. Among the 221 products for which an effect was claimed, 59 were said to produce muscle growth, 27 were said to increase testosterone levels, 17 were said to enhance energy, 15 were said to reduce fat, and 12 were said to increase strength.[28]

The National Council Against Health Fraud's Task Force on Ergogenic Aids has outlined a number of deceptive tactics used in selling these products.[20] The Task Force reviewed the claims made by 45 companies, most of which advertise in popular athletic and body building magazines. A number of deceptive marketing tactics for ergogenic aids were identified by the Task Force:

- Taking published research out of context, claiming products are "university tested" when no research has been done
- Using unauthorized endorsements by professional organizations
- Making false statements that research is currently being performed
- Using testimonials, referencing research inappropriately, patenting products (which is proof of uniqueness, not effectiveness)
- Engaging in mass media publicity.[20]

The Task Force suggests two reasons athletes believe that various products have helped them: first, the use of the product often coincides with natural improvement due to training; second, increased self-confidence or a placebo effect inspires greater performance. This psychological benefit should be weighed against the dangers of misinformation, wasted money, misplaced faith, and adverse side effects that can result from some of these products.[3]

In a 1992 report titled "Magic Muscle Pills! Health and Fitness Quackery in Nutrition Supplements,"[22] the New York Department of Consumer Affairs (DCA) reported that the manufacturers they contacted were unable to provide a single study from a scientific journal to support claims made for their products.

The DCA warned consumers to beware of such terms as "fat burner," "fat fighter," "fat metabolizer," "energy enhancer," "performance booster," "strength booster," "ergogenic aid," "anabolic optimizer," and "genetic optimizer." DCA officials urged the FDA and the US Federal Trade Commission (FTC) to stop the "blatantly drug-like claims" and fraudulent advertising used to promote these products.[22]

SPECIFIC ERGOGENIC AIDS

In this section, the currently popular dietary supplements and ergogenic aids used by active women are described.

Amino Acids: Arginine, Ornithine, and Lysine

CLAIM

Stimulate release of human growth hormone, promote muscle growth, increase strength.

FACT

These supplements do not increase growth hormone levels or muscle mass in men. Weight lifting and endurance training both increase growth hormone levels significantly. Combining these supplements with exercise has not been found to increase growth hormone levels in men above those seen with exercise. Although there is a lack of information on amino acid supplementation in women, it is unlikely that the supplements would be anabolic for female athletes.[7,19]

Androstenedione

Androstenedione is an adrenal hormone that functions as a metabolic precursor of testosterone.

CLAIM

Increases testosterone levels, increases muscle mass and strength.

FACT

Little is known about the safety and effectiveness of androstenedione. It may be converted to testosterone in the body and produce muscle growth like other anabolic steroids. The known side effects of anabolic steroid use include liver problems, unfavorable changes in blood lipids (decreased high-density lipoprotein [HDL] and increased low-density lipoprotein [LDL] levels), blood-clotting disorders, uncontrolled aggressive behavior ("roid rage"), increased acne, extra growth of body hair, reduction of testicle size and breast growth in men, and increased size of the clitoris and lowering of the voice in women. Anabolic steroids can also shut off bone growth in adolescents, stunting height. Pregnant women should avoid androstenedione altogether. Androstenedione is banned by the National Football League, the National Collegiate Athletic Association, and the US Olympic Committee.[26]

Antioxidant Vitamins: C, E, and Beta-Carotene

CLAIM

Protect against exercise-induced oxidative tissue damage due to free-radical production.

FACT

These vitamins may protect against oxidative damage following prolonged endurance exercise, but they do not improve performance. In the small quantities found in food, antioxidants help to stop the production and spread of harmful free-radical chain reactions. Supplementation at 100% of the recommended dietary allowance appears to be safe.[15]

Boron

Boron is a trace element that influences calcium and magnesium metabolism.

CLAIM

Increases serum testosterone levels, enhances muscle growth and strength.

FACT

These claims were based on a US Department of Agriculture (USDA) study that showed that boron supplementation increased estrogen and testosterone levels in postmenopausal women.[23] However, another study found that boron supplementation altered serum mineral levels but did not affect circulating hormone levels or strength in female athletes.[43] At present, there is insufficient information to conclude that boron supplementation will increase muscle mass in female athletes.

Branched Chain Amino Acids: Leucine, Isoleucine, and Valine

Branched chain amino acids (BCAAs) are primary amino acids used for energy during prolonged endurance exercise.

CLAIM

Supplementation with BCAAs during endurance exercise delays central fatigue and improves performance by preventing increases in brain serotonin levels.

FACT

The available data supporting BCAA supplementation are limited and equivocal. Since

BCAA supplements may not be safe or effective, and since it is easy to obtain adequate quantities from food, supplements currently are not recommended. Unlike BCAA supplementation, carbohydrate feedings during exercise are recommended because their safety and performance benefits are well established.[8]

Caffeine

Caffeine is an alkaloid found in coffee, tea, the herb guarana, and some medications that increases serum levels of epinephrine.

CLAIM

Improves endurance.

FACT

Caffeine is a central nervous system stimulant that increases alertness and decreases the perception of fatigue. Consuming 3 to 6 mg/kg 1 hour before exercise improves endurance performance without raising urinary caffeine levels above the International Olympic Committee doping threshold.[12] Although caffeine is a diuretic, none of the studies that have evaluated caffeine's metabolic and performance effects have suggested that caffeine increased the risk of heat-related illness.[12] Side effects of high caffeine consumption include nausea, muscle tremors, palpitations, and headache. Combining caffeine with ephedra greatly increases the adverse effects.[11]

Carnitine

Carnitine is a compound synthesized in the body from lysine and methionine.

CLAIM

Increases fat metabolism and decreases body fat.

FACT

Carnitine facilitates the transfer of fatty acids into the mitochondria for oxidation. There is no evidence that carnitine supplementation increases the use of fatty acids during exercise or decreases body fat. There is no dietary requirement for carnitine.[47]

Choline

Choline is an amine precursor for the neurotransmitter acetylcholine and lecithin.

CLAIM

Increases strength and decreases body fat by increasing acetylcholine and lecithin levels, respectively.

FACT

There is no dietary requirement for this substance. Choline can be synthesized from methionine, an essential amino acid. There is no evidence that increasing choline intake will increase strength or reduce body fat.[47]

Chromium Picolinate

Chromium picolinate is an active component of the glucose tolerance factor, which facilitates the action of insulin.

CLAIM

Increases muscle mass, decreases body fat, promotes weight loss.

FACT

The success of chromium picolinate is due to a well-orchestrated marketing campaign. Independent research by the USDA Human Nutrition Research Centers in Beltsville, Maryland, and Grand Forks, North Dakota, found that 200 µg chromium picolinate daily and weight training for 8 to 12 weeks did not increase strength or muscle mass or decrease body fat.[14,21] In November 1996, the FTC ordered a cessation of unsubstantiated weight-loss and health claims for chromium picolinate.

Coenzyme Q10

Coenzyme Q10 is a coenzyme in the aerobic energy system.

CLAIM

Optimizes adenosine triphosphate (ATP) production to increase energy and stamina.

FACT

There is no dietary requirement for this substance. Supplementation with coenzyme Q10 does not improve endurance performance or VO_2max.[4]

Creatine

Creatine combines with phosphate to form creatine phosphate (CP), a high-energy compound stored in muscle.

CLAIM

Increases CP content in muscles, improves high-power performance, increases fat-free mass.

FACT

Research suggests that consuming 20 to 25 g/day (5 g consumed 4 to 5 times daily) for 5 to 7 days increases CP stores in trained subjects by 20% to 40%, delays fatigue during explosive sprint performance, and facilitates ATP resynthesis following sprint-type exercise.[13]

Long-term creatine supplementation (the loading dose followed by 2 to 5 g/day for several months) enhances repetitive sprint performance and promotes greater gains in muscular strength and fat-free mass during training. The gains in strength and sprint performance are typically 5% to 8% following creatine supplementation and the gains in fat-free mass are about 3 to 7 pounds.[16]
Not all studies have found that creatine improves strength, sprint performance, or fat-free mass.[16] Creatine may not improve all high-power activities, since the majority of the studies have evaluated activities such as running, swimming, cycling sprints, and weight lifting.[13,16,42] Female athletes are less likely to take creatine than male athletes because of the increase in body weight associated with creatine supplementation.

DHEA

DHEA, or dehydroepiandrosterone, is an adrenal hormone that functions as a metabolic precursor for the production of testosterone, estrogen, and other hormones.

CLAIM

Increases testosterone levels, legal alternative to anabolic steroids, anti-aging hormone.

FACT

DHEA is called the "steroid of youth" since levels decrease with age. There is no evidence that DHEA produces anabolic effects (eg, increased muscle mass or strength), or decreased body fat in healthy, young adults.[30] Side effects include oily skin, acne, extra growth of body hair, liver enlargement, and aggressiveness.[30] The hormone's long-term safety has not been established and, as with other hormones, adverse effects may not appear for years. Individuals who have a family history of breast or prostate cancer should not take DHEA.[30]

Mexican yam contains a plant sterol ring called diosgenin that is a processor for the semisynthetic production of DHEA and other steroid hormones, but this conversion only takes place in the laboratory.

Ephedra (Ma Huang)

Ephedra, or ma huang, contains ephedrine, a central nervous system stimulant and decongestant.

CLAIM

Improves athletic performance, enhances weight loss.

FACT

Ephedrine is effective for relieving bronchial asthma, but has been banned by the International Olympic Committee and National Collegiate Athletic Association. Ephedrine is structurally similar to the amphetamines and increases heart rate and blood pressure. The adverse effects of ephedrine range from clinically significant effects such as heart attack, stroke, seizures, psychosis, and death, to clinically less significant effects (dizziness, headache, gastrointestinal distress, irregular heartbeat, and heart palpitations) that may indicate the potential for more serious problems. Side effects from ephedrine intake can vary and do not always depend on the dose consumed. Serious adverse effects can occur within susceptible persons with low doses.[11]
An athlete may not realize that an herbal product contains ephedrine or another stimulant because the stimulant is not included in the ingredient listing or an unfamiliar name for the stimulant is used. At the very least, the unwitting use of such herbal products may result in a doping suspension.

Gamma-Oryzanol

Gamma-oryzanol is a plant sterol, a ferulic acid ester derived from rice bran oil.

CLAIM

Increases serum testosterone and growth hormone levels, enhances muscle growth.

FACT

Oryzanol is composed of ferulates of the phytosterols stigmasterol, beta-sitosterol, campesterol, and cycloartenol. The structural similarity of oryzanol and its plant sterols to cholesterol has led to numerous claims that these plant sterols, like cholesterol, can be converted to testosterone. Oryzanol and its components are purported to provide the same benefits as anabolic steroids, but without the side effects. Oryzanol is not anabolic because it cannot be converted to testosterone by the human body.[44] Because of the poor absorption characteristics of oryzanol and plants sterols (less than 5%), the risks appear to be minimal.[44]

Ginseng

Ginseng is an extract of the root of the *Panax* genus.

CLAIM

Adaptogen (enhances the immune system to increase resistance to stress and disease), improves performance, and is a "cure-all."

FACT

A recent study found that ginseng supplementation at the clinically recommended dosage (200 mg/day), as well as twice that dosage, did not improve aerobic work capacity or oxygen uptake.[9]

No drug has all the healthful properties that are attributed to ginseng. The existence of a genuine "cure-all" is unlikely. Until proper research has been conducted, claims that ginseng has medicinal value should be considered unproven.[38] Triterpenoid saponins are thought to be responsible for whatever pharmacologic activity ginseng might possess.[38] Since ginseng root is expensive, the commercial preparations (extracts, powders, teas, or paste) may contain little or no ginseng. The best-documented side effects of ginseng are insomnia and, to a lesser degree, diarrhea and skin eruption.[38] The prolonged use of ginseng by adults seems to be relatively safe.

Glucosamine

Glucosamine is a naturally occurring aminosugar found in glycoproteins and glycosaminoglycans (GAG).

CLAIM

Rebuilds cartilage, cures arthritis.

FACT

The theory is that supplementing with glucosamine salts (1.5 g/day in divided doses) ensures rapid synthesis of GAG, helping to overcome the degradation that occurs during joint diseases and cartilage diseases such as arthritis. There is some support for the efficacy and safety of glucosamine supplementation from both animal and human studies in the treatment of arthritis.[37] Glucosamine salts are standard therapy for osteoarthritis in Europe. In the United States, the jury is still out on the effectiveness of glucosamine sulfate.[37]

Glutamine

Glutamine is a nonessential amino acid.

CLAIM

Speeds up recovery, enhances immune system.

FACT

Glutamine is a major energy source for gut enterocytes, lymphocytes, and brain cells and has been called "the essential nonessential amino acid" because of its numerous other functions. Skeletal muscle synthesizes, stores, and releases glutamine at a high rate. Glutamine helps to reduce immunosuppression and catabolism after major stress or surgery. Plasma glutamine concentration may be decreased in overtrained athletes and after a marathon run.[27] In theory, decreased glutamine concentrations may impair immune function and increase the risk of infection. Further research is required to determine whether supplemental glutamine enhances immune function during prolonged, intense exercise.

Glycerol

Glycerol is an alcohol that combines with fatty acids to form triglyceride.

CLAIM

Improves thermoregulation and endurance performance.

FACT

The US Olympic Committee added glycerol to the banned substances list in 1997. The ban is based on glycerol being classified as a diuretic, since in high doses (1 to 2 g/kg) it can be used to "make weight." Glycerol hyperhydration may also confer an unfair athletic advantage by reducing heat stress.

Glycerol hyperhydration may increase plasma volume and sweat rate, thereby reducing body temperature and improving performance during prolonged exercise in warm weather. Montner and colleagues found that glycerol hyperhydration (1.2 g/kg glycerol with 26 mL/kg water) was associated with a significantly longer endurance time (93.8 minutes) and lower heart rate (2.8 beats/min) compared to water hyperhydration (77.4 minutes).[25]

Latza and colleagues evaluated the effect of euhydration, water hyperhydration, and glycerol hyperhydration on sweat rate and core temperature during exercise. Glycerol hyperhydration did not alter core temperature, skin temperature, sweat rate, or heart rate compared with euhydration or water hyperhydration, suggesting that glycerol hyperhydration was ineffective.[18]

HMB

HMB, or beta-hydroxy beta-methylbutyrate, is a downstream metabolite of the essential amino acid leucine.

CLAIM

Increases muscle mass and strength, decreases muscle breakdown after exercise.

FACT

Supplementation with 1.5 and 3.0 g HMB daily during resistance training for 3 weeks increased muscle mass (not statistically significant) and strength (statistically significant) in a dose-dependent manner.[24] HMB also decreased the exercise-induced rise in muscle proteolysis. HMB may protect against muscle damage and improve muscle repair. These results have not been reproduced by other researchers in other laboratories and the subjects were untrained, so the results cannot be applied to athletes.[24]

Inosine

Inosine is a nucleoside involved in the formation of purines.

CLAIM

Increases ATP production, increases strength, and enhances recovery.

FACT

There are no research studies to support these claims for strength trained athletes.[47] Inosine may actually impair endurance performance.[45]

Medium-Chain Triglycerides

Medium-chain triglycerides, or MCTs, are fats that are water soluble and readily absorbed.

CLAIM

Promote muscularity and body fat loss, increase thermic effect, improve endurance.

FACT

MCTs are an inefficient energy source during aerobic exercise. There is no proof that MCTs increase muscularity or enhance body fat loss in strength-trained athletes. Consuming large amounts can cause gastrointestinal distress and diarrhea.[47]

Omega-3 Fatty Acids

Omega-3 fatty acids are highly polyunsaturated fatty acids found mostly in fish oils.

CLAIM

Stimulate release of growth hormone.

FACT

Omega-3 fatty acids (eicosapentaenoic acid, docosahexaenoic acid, and linolenic acid) may be converted to prostaglandins (hormone-like substances) in the body. A specific prostaglandin called PGE_1 may stimulate growth hormone release. However, there is no proof that omega-3 fatty acids improve aerobic endurance or have an ergogenic effect in strength-trained athletes.[47]

Phosphates

Phosphates are components of ATP and CP.

CLAIM

Improve endurance.

FACT

Phosphate loading may increase intracellular phosphate levels and thereby increase oxidative metabolism. Kreider and colleagues found that phosphate loading (1 g sodium phosphate, taken 4 times a day for 3 days) increased VO_2Max, blood lactate threshold, and maximum oxidative capacity, and enhanced endurance.[17] More research on phosphate loading is needed.

Protein Supplements

CLAIM

Support muscle growth, increase muscle mass and strength.

FACT

Exercise increases protein requirements, but the protein intake of most athletes meets or exceeds needs. Novice athletes require more protein than experienced athletes, and protein needs are elevated when energy or carbohydrate intake is inadequate.[7]

Currently, the research does not support a protein intake above 2 g/kg/day to increase muscle mass.[19] An intake of protein above 2 g/kg/day (from food or supplements) is not incorporated into new muscle protein; rather, amino acid oxidation is increased.[19] "High-tech" protein supplements contain a variety of additives purported to boost weight gain, however, no research is available to support the claims made by these products. Protein supplements are not superior to dietary protein; powdered milk is as effective and costs less.[7]

Pyruvate

Pyruvate is a 3-carbon sugar produced at the end stages of glycolysis from the breakdown of glucose.

CLAIM

Increases endurance, enhances fat loss.

FACT

Two studies of untrained men suggest that consuming 25 g pyruvate and 75 g dihydroxyacetone (DHA), another 3-carbon sugar produced in the breakdown of glucose, for 7 days improves both arm endurance and leg endurance by 20%.[32,33]

The claims of greater weight and fat loss are supported by two studies done by Stanko on very obese, sedentary women who took 22 to 28 g pyruvate daily and ate only 500 to 1000 calories for 21 days.[34,35] In one study, the supplemented subjects lost 37% (3.5 pounds) more body weight and 48% (2.9 pounds) more fat than the placebo group.[35] The deceptively large percentage differences in weight loss amounted to only a couple of pounds in this short-term study.

William Sukala notes that the female athlete should consider several points before taking pyruvate supplements to improve performance or promote fat loss[36]: Stanko's results have not been reproduced by other researchers in other laboratories. His subjects were untrained men or obese women, so the results cannot be applied to lean, active women. His subjects also experienced side effects in the form of intestinal gas, flatus, and diarrhea. The performance benefits were observed with 25 g pyruvate and 75 g DHA and weight loss was obtained with 22 to 28 g pyruvate; however, commercial pyruvate preparations only contain 500 mg to 1 g pyruvate and may not contain DHA.[36]

Smilax

Smilax is a genus of desert plants comprising several species of sarsaparilla.

CLAIM

Increases serum testosterone levels, increases muscle growth and strength, legal alternative to anabolic steroids.

FACT

Smilax does contain saponins (sarsasapogenin and smilagenin) that serve as precursors for the semisynthetic production of certain steroids, but this conversion takes place only in the laboratory. There is no evidence that *Smilax* is anabolic, or functions as a "legal replacement" for anabolic steroids.[39] The saponins in sarsaparilla have a strong diuretic action as well as some diaphoretic, expectorant, and laxative properties.[39]

Sodium Bicarbonate

Sodium bicarbonate buffers lactic acid in the blood.

CLAIM

Augments the body's buffer reserve, counteracts the buildup of lactic acid in the blood, improves anaerobic performance.

FACT

Several studies have supported improved anaerobic performance (400- and 800-meter runs) with bicarbonate administration. Taking 0.3 g/kg sodium bicarbonate with water over a 2- to 3-hour period may improve 800-meter run time by several seconds.[46] However, as many as half of those individuals using sodium bicarbonate experienced urgent diarrhea 1 hour after the soda loading was completed.[36] The effects of repeated ingestion are unknown and caution is advised.

Succinate

Succinate is a metabolite of the Krebs cycle of the aerobic energy system.

CLAIM

Metabolic enhancer; reduces lactic acid buildup and maintains ATP production.

FACT

Succinate is an intermediary in aerobic metabolism. Supplemental succinate will not reduce lactic acid buildup or accelerate the process of ATP production, as this is controlled by rate-limiting enzymes within the pathway.

Vanadyl Sulfate

Vanadyl sulfate is a trace mineral for which there is no dietary requirement.

CLAIM

Promotes anabolic effects similar to those of insulin.

FACT

Vanadyl sulfate has well-documented insulin-mimetic activity in non-insulin-dependent diabetes. Administration of 0.5 mg/kg daily for 12 weeks did not increase strength or muscle mass during a weight-training program. Mild gastrointestinal symptoms and other side effects have been reported with vanadyl sulfate supplementation.[10]

Vitamin B_{12}

Vitamin B_{12} is essential for DNA synthesis.

CLAIM

Enhances DNA synthesis, increases muscle growth.

FACT

Vitamin B_{12} is essential in the synthesis of DNA. Dibencobal (a coenzyme form of vitamin B_{12}) supposedly stimulates muscle growth by increasing DNA synthesis, however, there is no evidence that dibencobal or vitamin B_{12} promotes muscle growth or enhances strength.[47]

Vitamin/Mineral Supplements

CLAIM

Provide "nutritional insurance," increase energy, and improve performance.

FACT

Vitamins are metabolic regulators that help govern the processes of energy production and tissue growth, maintenance, and repair. Contrary to what many athletes believe, vitamins do not provide energy, although some vitamins are important for the release of energy from food. Only protein, carbohydrate, and fat provide energy (calories). This means that, in general, the vitamin requirements of an active woman are no greater than those of a sedentary woman.[41]

Supplementation at levels exceeding the recommended dietary allowance does not improve the performance of well-nourished individuals.[6,41] Although vitamin and mineral deficiencies can impair athletic performance, it is unusual for active women to have such deficiencies.[6,41] Although iron-deficiency anemia impairs athletic performance, it is no more prevalent in female athletes than in sedentary women.[6] There is a close relationship between caloric intake and vitamin intake: the more food eaten, the greater the vitamin intake.[41] Active people generally eat more than sedentary people and so tend to get more vitamins and minerals relative to their needs.[6,41]

Female athletes who limit their caloric intake are at risk for nutritional deficiencies.[6,41] These athletes usually compete in sports that emphasize leanness for enhanced performance (running, lightweight crew) or for appearance (gymnastics, figure skating, diving, ballet dancing). Weight-conscious active women may also be at risk. A vitamin/mineral supplement supplying no more than 100% of the recommended dietary allowances may be appropriate for some of these individuals.

Most health authorities agree that there is no harm in a simple vitamin/mineral supplement, provided that it does not exceed 100% of the recommended dietary allowances for nutrients. Keep in mind there is also no evidence that this supplementation is beneficial.

Yohimbine

Yohimbine, an alkaloid extracted from the bark of a West African tree, functions as a monoamine oxidase inhibitor, thereby increasing serum levels of norepinephrine. It is available by prescription only.

CLAIM

Increases serum testosterone levels, enhances muscle growth and strength, lowers body fat; also promoted as an aphrodisiac.

FACT

There is no proof that yohimbine is anabolic and its value as an aphrodisiac is inconclusive.[40] To prevent a hypertensive crisis, tyramine-containing foods (red wine, liver, cheese) and nasal decongestants or diet aids containing phenylpropanolamine should be rigorously avoided when this monoamine oxidase inhibitor is used. People who have diabetes or disease of the cardiovascular, hepatic, or renal system should not take yohimbine.[40] Yohimbine's effects make it unsuitable for over-the-counter sale.

WORKING WITH ATHLETES

New ergogenic aids for athletes are constantly emerging. Often these products are marketed without any scientific research to support potential benefits or indicate possible harmful side effects. Some products come on and go off the market before studies are done to establish or refute their claims. Prosecutions or other legal actions take years, allowing the promoter to reap huge profits during the delay.[1]

Under our consumer protection laws, a substance is considered a drug if a medical claim is made for it, even though it is a dietary supplement. The reality, however, is that just about anything can be sold as long as it is called a dietary supplement. The DSHEA allows dietary supplements and ergogenic aids to be marketed without proof of efficacy, safety, or potency.[1,2]

Unfortunately, most athletes (as well as the general public) think that advertisements and anecdotes are proof of efficacy.[31] They also think that the products on the market are safe.[31] Short notes that most athletes do not understand the inherent risks in using untested products, nor are they concerned about future health problems that may be caused by these products.[31]

Discussing supplements with athletes is not easy. In many cases, the health professional is concerned about safety and cost, while the athlete is concerned with immediate athletic success.[29] If the product is ineffective but safe, the health professional should consider working with the athlete to find a way to use the product on a trial basis.[31] This helps to improve the health professional's credibility with the athlete.[31]

Butterfield recommends four tactics when discussing supplement use with an athlete[5]:

- Gain an understanding of the athlete's motives and beliefs. Determine who or what influences the athlete (eg, coaches, popular sports magazines, celebrity endorsements) and realize that athletes usually care about short-term benefits more than long-term risks.
- Assess the athlete's knowledge. Discussing sound nutrition practices and supplements demonstrates concern in helping the athlete to reach her goals—with or without supplements.
- Evaluate the overall diet. By definition, a supplement is a substance to augment the diet. Supplements alone will not enable an athlete to reach her goals. Rather, supple-

ments must be used as part of a sound nutritional and training program.

- Promote healthful dietary practices as the cornerstone to improved athletic performance. Give the athlete positive feedback for the sound nutrition practices already followed. Educate the athlete about healthy dietary practices, from choosing healthier fast foods to optimizing fluid intake.

References

1. Barrett S: Don't buy phony "ergogenic aids." Nutr Forum 14(3):17, 1997.
2. Barrett S: The "dietary supplement" mess. Nutr Forum 14(4):2, 1997.
3. Barrett S, Herbert V: How athletes are exploited. In The Vitamin Pushers. Amherst, Mass, Prometheus Books, 1994, p 236.
4. Braun B, Clarkson PM, Freedson, PS, et al: Effect of coenzyme Q-10 supplementation on exercise performance, VO$_2$Max, and lipid peroxidation of trained cyclists. Int J Sport Nutr 1(4):353–65, 1991.
5. Butterfield G: Ergogenic aids: evaluating sports nutrition products. Int J Sport Nutr 6(2):191–7, 1996.
6. Clarkson PM: Minerals, exercise performance, and supplementation in athletes. J Sports Sci 9:91–116, 1991.
7. Clarkson PM: Nutritional supplements for weight gain. Sport Sci Exch 11(1):1, 1998.
8. Davis JM: Carbohydrates, branched chain amino acids, and endurance: the central fatigue hypothesis. Int J Sport Nutr 5(suppl):S29–S38, 1995.
9. Engels, HJ, Wirth, JC: No ergogenic effects of ginseng (Panax ginseng C.A. Meyer) during graded maximal aerobic exercise. J Am Diet Assoc 97(10):1110–5, 1997.
10. Fawcett JP, Farquhar SJ, Walker RJ, et al. The effect of oral vanadyl sulfate on body composition and performance in weight-training athletes. Int J Sport Nutr 6(4):382–9, 1996.
11. Food and Drug Administration Center for Food Safety and Applied Nutrition: Adverse events associated with ephedrine-containing Products. August 16, 1996. FDA webpage: http://vm.cfsan.fda.gov/~dms/ephedrin.html
12. Graham TE, Spriet LL: Caffeine and exercise performance. Sport Sci Exch 9(1):1, 1996.
13. Greenhaff, PL: Creatine and its application as an ergogenic aid. Int J Sport Nutr 5(suppl):S100–10, 1995.
14. Hallmark MA, Reynolds TH, DeSouza CA, et al: Effects of chromium and resistive training on muscle strength and body composition. Med Sci Sports Exerc 28(1):139–44, 1996.
15. Kanter MM: Free radicals, exercise, and antioxidant supplementation. Int J Sports Nutr 4(3):205–220, 1994.
16. Kreider RB: Creatine: the next ergogenic supplement? Sportscience webpage: http://www.sportsci.org/traintech/creatine/rbk.html.
17. Kreider RB, Miller GM, Schenck D, et al: Effects of phosphate loading on metabolic and myocardial responses to maximal and endurance exercise. Int J Sport Nutr 2(1)20–47, 1992.
18. Latzka WA, Sawka MN, Montain SJ, et al: Hyperhydration: thermoregulatory effects during compensable exercise-heat stress. J Appl Physiol 83(3):860–6, 1997.

19. Lemon PWR: Do athletes need more dietary protein and amino acids? Int J Sport Nutr (suppl) S39–S61, 1995.

20. Lightsey DM, Attaway JR: Deceptive tactics used in marketing purported ergogenic aids. Nat Strength Conditioning Assoc J 14(2):26–31, 1991.

21. Lukaski HC, Bolonchuk WW, Siders WA, et al: Chromium supplementation and resistance training: effects on body composition, strength, and trace element status of men. Am J Clin Nutr 63(6):954–65, 1996.

22. New York City Department of Consumer Affairs: Magic Muscle Pills! Health and Fitness Quackery in Nutrition Supplements. New York, May 1992.

23. Nielson FH, Hunt CD, Mullen LM, et al: Effects of dietary boron on mineral, estrogen, and testosterone metabolism in post-menopausal women. FASEB J 1(5): 394–7, 1987.

24. Nissen, S, Sharp R, Ray M, et al: Effect of leucine metabolite beta-hydroxy beta-methylbutyrate on muscle metabolism during resistance exercise-training. J Appl Physiol 81(5):2095–104, 1996.

25. Montner P, Stark DM, Riedesel ML, et al: Pre-exercise glycerol hydration improves cycling endurance time. Int J Sports Med 17(1):27–33, 1996.

26. Noble HB: Questions surround performance enhancer. NY Times Sept. 8, 1998.

27. Parry-Billings M, Budgett R, Koutedakis Y, et al: Plasma amino acid concentrations in the over-training syndrome: possible effects on the immune system. Med Sci Sports Exerc 24(12):1353–8, 1992.

28. Philem RM, Ortiz DI, Auerback SB, et al: Survey of advertising for nutritional supplements in health and body building magazines. JAMA 268(8):1008–11, 1991.

29. Rosembloom C, Storlie J: A nutritionist's guide to evaluating ergogenic aids. SCAN's Pulse 17(4):1, 1998.

30. Skerrett, PJ: Helpful hormone or hype? Healthnews 2(16):1, 1996.

31. Short SH, Marquart LF: Sports nutrition fraud. NY State J Med 93(2):112–6, 1993.

32. Stanko RT, Robertson RJ, Spina RJ, et al: Enhancement of arm exercise endurance capacity with dihydroxyacetone and pyruvate. J Appl Physiol 68(1): 119–24, 1990.

33. Stanko RT, Robertson RJ, Galbreath RW, et al: Enhancement of leg exercise endurance with a high-carbohydrate diet and dihydroxyacetone and pyruvate. J Appl Physiol 69(5):1651–6, 1990.

34. Stanko RT, Tietze DL, Arch JE, et al: Body composition, energy utilization, and nitrogen metabolism with a severely restricted diet supplemented with dihydroxyacetone and pyruvate. Am J Clin Nutr 55(4):771–6, 1992.

35. Stanko RT, Tietze DL, Arch JE, et al: Body composition, energy utilization, and nitrogen metabolism with a 4.25-MJ/d diet supplemented with pyruvate. Am J Clin Nutr 56(4):630–5, 1992.

36. Sukala W: Pyruvate: beyond the marketing hype. Int J Sport Nutr 8(3):241–9, 1998.

37. Reginster JY, Deroisy R, Rovati LC, Lee RL, et al: Long term effects of glucosamine sulfate on osteoarthritis progression: a randomized, placebo-controlled clinical trial. Lancet 357, 2001.

38. Tyler VE: Ginseng and related herbs. The Honest Herbal, 3rd edition. Binghamton, NY, Pharmaceutical Products Press, 1993, p 153.

39. Tyler VE: Sarsaparilla. The Honest Herbal, 3rd edition. Binghamton, NY, Pharmaceutical Products Press, 1993, p 277.

40. Tyler VE: Yohimbe. The Honest Herbal, 3rd edition. Binghamton, NY, Pharmaceutical Products Press, 1993, p 327.

41. Van Der Beek EJ: Vitamin supplementation and physical exercise performance. J Sports Sci 9:77–90, 1991.

42. Volek JS, Kraemer WJ, Bush JA, et al: Creatine supplementation enhances muscular performance during high-intensity resistance exercise. J Am Diet Assoc 97(7):765–70, 1991.

43. Volpe SL, Taper LJ, Meachum S: The effect of boron supplementation on bone mineral density and hormonal status in college female athletes. Med Exerc Nutr Health 2:323–30, 1993.

44. Wheeler KB, Garleb KA: Gamma oryzanol-plant sterol supplementation: metabolic, endocrine, and physiologic effects. Int J Sports Nutr 1(2):178–87, 1991.

45. Williams MH, Kreider RB, Hunter DW, et al: Effect of oral inosine supplementation on 3-mile treadmill run performance and VO_2 peak. Med Sci Sports Exerc 22(4): 517–22, 1990.

46. Williams MH: Bicarbonate loading. Sports Sci Exch 5(1):1, 1992.

47. Williams MH: Nutritional supplements for strength trained athletes. Sports Sci Exch 6(6):1, 1993.

48. Williams MH: Introduction to nutrition for fitness and sport. Nutrition for Fitness and Sport, 4th edition. Dubuque, Iowa, Brown & Benchmark, 1995, p 13.

Chapter 11

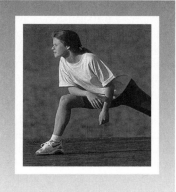

Substance Abuse

Wade F. Exum, M.D., M.B.A.
Joan M. Price, B.S.N.

In line with today's increasingly popular desire for quick fixes, it is not surprising that a growing number of female athletes look to the world of science for performance enhancement. Many of the substances that are prohibited by the International Olympic Committee (IOC), the United States Olympic Committee (USOC), and/or the National Collegiate Athletic Association (NCAA) are classified under the legal system as controlled substances and/or have debilitating side effects.

Along with health considerations, the risks of using prohibited substances include disqualification, suspension from competition, loss of awards, dishonor or disgrace, and the threat of sanctions or penalties upon the detection of such prohibited substances.[16]

HISTORY

Use of prohibited performance-enhancing substances by athletes is condemned because it violates the principle of fair play and because of concerns for the athlete's health and safety. Headline stories relating the abuse and misuse of drugs among athletes are almost commonplace today.

Gladiators benefited from stimulants, mushrooms were investigated by Greeks, Romans mixed strychnine with wine, and 19th-century athletes experimented with alcohol, caffeine, nitroglycerin, and opium.[41] It is speculated that athletes observed the treatment of World War II casualties with anabolic steroids and exploited their actions to heighten aggression and develop muscle mass.

Exposure of amphetamine use by American football players and the death of Knud Jensen, Denmark's elite cyclist, illuminated abuse of central nervous system stimulants in the mid-1900s.[1] Such drug abuse among athletes cast a dark shadow over the ideals of fair play, prompting the introduction of drug testing at the Summer and Winter Olympic Games of 1968. By 1988, the IOC, in considering the scope of doping, noted the potential for doping in every sport. Issues relating to athlete health and safety, the integrity of sport, rights and roles of the athlete, and the desire for fair play were all addressed in the International Olympic Charter Against Doping in Sport and later in the IOC Medical Code.[8,9] The IOC belief that doping contravenes the ethics of both sport and medical science is widely accepted.[17] Also of consideration is a potential relationship between performance-enhancing drugs and an *adverse* effect on performance and health.[10] Recent disclosure of anabolic steroid use by East German athletes such as triple Olympic gold medalist Rica Reinisch, and Christiane Knacke, the first woman to break a minute in swimming the 100-meter butterfly, prove that abuse of performance-enhancing substances is not limited to the male gender. In 1993, Chinese women swimmers stunned the world with their climb from obscurity to dominance in all but the distance events. A year following the detection of the anabolic steroid, methandrostenolone (Dianabol), in swimmer Zhou Xin, another female Chinese swimmer, Zhong Wieyue, tested positive for the same substance at the 1994 World Cup competition.[43] Zhang Yi and 3 other Chinese swimmers found positive for diuretic use were expelled from the 1998 World Championships and given 2-year suspensions.[5]

Years ago, societal expectations differed for what was then considered to be the gentler sex, and the belief that females did not use drugs was prevalent. With increases in competitive opportunities and sports participation incentives, outstanding female athletes emerged, and problems of drug abuse surfaced as well. Along with opportunity came greater pressures to win and increased vulnerability to drug abuse. The temptation to achieve immediate success caused the weak and susceptible to yield, regardless of the costs or risk of detection and exposure.[13,14]

In 1989, Gael Martin, an Australian Olympic team runner, reported that she and 30% of the track and field athletes used steroids to stay competitive, believing that not doing so would place them behind the rest of the world.[2] Women today should disregard such testimony and look to positive images. There are top athletes to serve as role models for upcoming generations of athletes as well as fans and the general population. Some of the many women that might come to mind as representing drug-free athletic achievement and success include Janet Evans, Picabo Street, Amy VanDyken, Shannon Miller, Dominique Dawes, Tara Lipinski, Michelle Kwan, Mia Hamm, Bonnie Blair, Nancy Lopez, Wilma Rudolf, Cheryl Miller, Dorothy Hammel, Peggy Flemming, Chris Evert, and Mary Lou Retton, among others.[14]

Drug use among females can essentially be divided into 3 categories: drugs used for performance enhancement, for recreational purposes, and for the treatment of medical ailments and injuries. In this chapter, various performance-enhancing substances and the reasons for their use will be addressed,[4] along with brief remarks about the unique effects they may have in females.[20]

DRUG ABUSE IN THE FEMALE ATHLETE: CAUSES AND GENDER DIFFERENCES

It is well documented that drug abuse is a problem for the population at large. It would be unrealistic to believe that females, including athletes, are immune to this type of problem. In a 1991 survey by Anshel, 42% of the women athletes reported teammates' use of prohibited or illegal substances. This report rate was substantially higher than that seen in the early studies of English and Pope in 1987 and 1988. Along with the stress associated with being in the public eye, reasons stated for use included management of the tension, anxiety, and depression that accompanied expectations for success in sport.[2] Competitive athletes do not just gain direct performance enhancements, they also see improvement in ability as a result of maintaining a lowered stress level.[41]

Drugs used for the purpose of enhancing performance can also increase strength and aggression, relieve or mask pain, control weight, and improve endurance. They may also be used for their emotional or psychological value to enhance self-esteem and overcome fear, among other things. Certain types of drugs are misused solely to attempt to improve physical appearance.

There have been a few studies that stratify risk of drug and alcohol use as well as other risk-taking behaviors in athletes by gender.[19,25,31] In the 2001 NCAA study of substance use and abuse by Green and colleagues, female student-athletes reported significantly lower usage rates for 6 of the 8 categories studied (alcohol, amphetamines, anabolic steroids, cocaine, ephedrine, marijuana, psychedelics, and smokeless tobacco) compared to male athletes. The exceptions were alcohol and amphetamines use, which were not significantly different in female and male athletes.[19] In the multicenter study by Nattiv et al[31] and the study by Kokotailo et al,[25] which both assessed lifestyle and health risk behaviors of collegiate athletes compared to nonathletes, female athletes demonstrated fewer risk-taking behaviors overall compared to male athletes and female nonathletes. However, the multicenter study found that female athletes consumed alcohol at greater frequency and quantity per sitting than their nonathletic peers, as well as more smokeless tobacco use.[31]

DRUGS OF ABUSE

Stimulants

In sports, sympathomimetics comprise the largest class of drugs used as central nervous system stimulants. Included in this classification are decongestants and diet aids (phenylpropanolamine, phenylpropanolol, pseudoephedrine), and certain supplements (natural ephedrine such as ma huang).

A 1985 survey of female collegiate athletes indicated that 32% practiced pathologic weight control, including use of diet pills, laxatives, and/or diuretics. There was a higher prevalence of these practices among Caucasians than African Americans. More than half of those surveyed reported using performance-enhancing substances for achieving weight control rather than for enhancing athletic performance. Weight control substance abuse was highest in young women participating in gymnastics and long-distance running. It was not surprising to find that males used stimulants for weight loss at a substantially lower rate.[37] It is common knowledge that females in the general population more frequently use weight-loss medications than males. In a recent study, pathogenic weight-control behavior differences were seen in female athletes versus female nonathletes when identified by sport. Female track, cross-country, gymnastics, and lacrosse athletes exhibited the highest rate of pathogenic weight-control behaviors. Male athletes exhibited these behaviors to the highest extent in wrestling, track, cross-country, and football.[31] Athletes have a higher incidence of use of amphetamines and anabolic agents to obtain the various ergogenic effects. Females, during puberty, may experience body-image conflict and indulge in stimulant and other drug use (laxatives, diuretics, and diet pills) in an effort to control weight gained as part of the normal physical maturation process.[14]

In addition to an appetite-suppression effect, moderate doses of amphetamine commonly produce mood elevation and increased energy and alertness. Improvement of performance that is impaired because of fatigue is attractive to athletes seeking to heighten concentration and energy. Amphetamines affect many aspects of athletic performance, but performance is especially improved in sports involving strength, speed, and endurance.[20,41]

Of the substances that are classified as stimulants, cocaine produces the most profound psychic dependence among drugs that are abused recreationally. Historically, males have tended to abuse cocaine far more than females. A 3% cocaine usage rate was observed in the 1980s,[13] increasing to 5% to 17% in the 1990s, according to various studies.[42] At the 1996 Olympic Games in Atlanta, use of a new stimulant, bromantan, was detected in the urine of a number of Eastern European athletes. This substance, while new to the Olympics, had reportedly been used by Russian troops to enhance alertness and adaptation to extreme temperatures.[3]

Diuretics

Another class of drugs that may be heavily abused by women is diuretics.[13] The rapid water weight loss that results from use of this type of drug enables an athlete to artificially drop to a lower weight class, thus gaining an unfair advantage over lower-weight-class competitors.[2] The IOC prohibited diuretics for the 1988 Games.[10] They continue to be prohibited for 2 purposes: (1) artificial weight reduction for sports involving weight categories, and (2) interference with the detection of prohibited substances as a result of a diluting effect on the urine.[40]

Anabolic Agents

Anabolic agents is the term used by the IOC to describe a category of substances that includes androgenic anabolic steroids (AAS), substances that are chemically or pharmacologically related to AAS, and other substances with anabolic effects. Women have traditionally been undereducated with respect to anabolic agents.[33] Even so, surveys show that female athletes do use anabolic steroids. Usage rates of 1% of high school females and 5% at elite and professional levels have been documented.[6,45] A 1990 study found more athletes than nonathletes reporting anabolic use, with the incidence of male use being 3.5 times higher than that of females.[7] At least one female death has been attributed to anabolic use, that of Birgit Dressel, a West German heptathlete, in 1987.[33]

These drugs are readily available on the black market in the United States. Frequent international travel offers opportunities for elite athletes to purchase or obtain anabolic agents in countries that have lax regulations prohibiting the sale or distribution of these substances. Physicians in the United States must exercise caution in prescribing these and other ergogenic drugs in order to avoid contributing to the problem and because many ergogenics also happen to be controlled substances.[13,35] The most commonly used injectable anabolic, androgenic steroid is testosterone cypionate. Methandrostenolone, oxymetholone, oxandrolone, ethylestrenol, and fluoxymesterone are popular oral agents that are used by athletes. Dosages vary, often dependent upon the advice of a favored guru, and are estimated to be as much as 40 times the dose given for therapeutic treatment.[35,45] A new substance, androstenedione, a precursor to testosterone, has entered the scene of performance enhancement. It became popular following disclosure that it was used by Mark McGwire, then baseball's single-season home run leader.[5]

As early as the 1970s, physicians warned that female steroid users could be risking the loss of normal sexual function and childbearing ability.[34] At the same time, women were being warned of the undesirable effects of exogenous anabolic-androgenic steroids, including masculinization, hirsutism, deepening of the voice, acne, baldness, and clitoral enlargement.[26] Warnings were given that many of the effects were not reversible.[29]

In 1973, suspicion of steroid use by East German female swimmers surfaced when the team dominated the world championships. A lighter team by 20 pounds per athlete had been overtaken a year before by the US Women's Olympic team. At the 1976 Olympic Games, the IOC prohibited anabolic steroids for the first time.[14] They were first tested for at the 1983 Pan American Games in Caracas, Venezuela. Within 19 years, a study of 10 weight-trained women proposed that women have a better chance than men to increase muscle mass from steroid use since natural levels of testosterone in females are lower.[14,39,41]

In a study of 9 steroid-using female weight-lifters, 7 experienced menstrual disturbances. Increases were also seen in acne, aggressiveness, appetite, clitoral size (clitoromegaly), body hair (hirsutism), irritability, sexual drive, and voice deepening.[25]

Other disturbing effects noted following use by females include liver damage, sterility and fetal defects, virilization such as beard development and baldness, blood dyscrasias, edema, nervousness, headache, depression, rashes, shrinking of breast tissue, and uterine atrophy.[14,35] Many of the effects are not reversible following cessation. Life-threatening consequences to be considered are hepatic dysfunction (liver function abnormalities), hepatocellular carcinoma (liver tumors), and peliosis hepatis (blood-filled cysts in the liver).[19,35,41]

Peptide and Glycoprotein Hormones and Analogues

Erythropoietin

Prohibited by the IOC in 1990,[11] erythropoietin (EPO) is a naturally occurring hormone that is primarily produced in the kidneys for the regulation of the production of red blood cells by bone marrow. EPO infusion or stimulation results in an increase in the red blood cell mass and in the hemoglobin and hematocrit levels. The increase in red blood cells expands the oxygen-carrying capacity of the blood, which is a desirable effect for endurance athletes. Red cell production may continue for up to 2 weeks, providing the benefits of blood doping, without the risks associated with blood transfusion.[24] Recombinant erythropoietin (rEPO) is the currently available synthetic form.[40] Presently approved uses are for treatment of anemia in dialysis patients and anemia associated with AZT treatment in AIDS patients.[18]

Sluggish blood flow from the rise in the hematocrit to dangerously high levels is believed to place the athlete at risk for cardiovascular events. Dangers include such thromboembolic events as stroke or heart attack, as well as venous stasis in small vessels and deep venous thrombosis and pulmonary embolism.[38] Fluid loss through dehydration due to extensive exercise is believed to contribute to the danger of the condition.[18] Connie Meyer, a Dutch woman cyclist, is counted among those who died from coronary maladies similar to those that are possible with abuse of EPO.[27]

Methods to distinguish the synthetically produced EPO from that produced by the body are progressing. Although means of detection are not perfected, several studies have been undertaken to identify a recombinant glycoprotein by immunologic means, based on the difference in carbohydrate structure. This technology may make it possible to detect exogenous EPO in the presence of endogenous EPO.[30]

It is hoped that support for this or some other type of research will result in an effective test for exogenous EPO use in the near future. Without such an effective test there is a risk that athletes' lives will continue to be jeopardized.

Exogenous Growth Hormone (Somatrem and Somatropin)

The actions of endogenous human growth hormone (hGH) are duplicated by the exogenous forms. Somatrem and somatropin are purified polypeptide hormones with a primary action of stimulating linear growth in all bodily tissues. Treatment with hGH produces an increase in muscle cell size and number. Adverse reactions reported include the development of leukemia and diabetes mellitus. High doses over a long period of time could lead to gigantism or acromegaly along with metabolic and endocrine disorders.[18,23,41]

Abuse of growth hormone in sport has been reported with application of megadoses at 20 times the therapeutic dose. The use of hGH from human cadavers carries with it the risk of viral contaminant-induced diseases such as Creutzfeldt-Jakob disease, a fatal neurologic condition.[18,40] Administered by physicians for the treatment of dwarfism and a condition called small for gestational age (SGA) in children, hGH is abused by athletes to increase bulk and to speed recovery of muscles following intensive workouts, thereby making it possible to increase the duration and frequency of training.[3] Although detection of hGH is not possible by current testing methods, a potential breakthrough has been reported. The process involves analyses of blood from the ear lobe or finger.[5]

Human Chorionic Gonadotropin

In December of 1987, the IOC approved the addition of human chorionic gonadotropin (hCG) to the list of prohibited substances, stating that "Due to the frequent misuse of this substance in order to increase the production of androgenic steroids, the use of hCG or compounds with related activity is now pro-hibited."[12] hCG is a hormone secreted by the placenta and found in the urine of pregnant women. In women, it is used medically to induce ovulation in the treatment of infertility.

Some of the minor side effects that have been encountered with hCG use include headache, fatigue, restlessness, changes in mood, irritability, depression, edema, precocious puberty, and pain on injection. The primary serious adverse reactions are ovarian hyperstimulation (sudden ovarian enlargement), ascites (accumulation of serous fluid in the peritoneal cavity or the membrane lining the abdominal cavity), rupture of ovarian cysts, multiple births, and arterial thromboembolism (blocking of the blood vessel by a blood clot). Males experiment with this substance in an attempt to avoid the testicular atrophy (shrinkage of the testicles) and gynecomastia (abnormally large mammary glands) that often accompany anabolic steroid use.[18,22,41] In December 1987, it was reported by the Rocky Mountain Drug Consultation Center in Denver that a counterfeit product was being sold as hCG. The product was determined to be both pyrogenic (fever producing) and nonsterile (potentially infectious).

Adrenocorticotropic Hormone

Adrenocorticotropic hormone (ACTH), secreted by the anterior pituitary, stimulates the adrenal cortex to produce and secrete adrenocortical hormones.[23] It has been used to increase blood levels of endogenous corticosteroids in order to obtain a euphoric effect. Its use is considered by the IOC to be equivalent to the prohibited systemic administration of corticosteroids by the oral, intramuscular, or intravenous routes.

Insulin

Abuse of natural hormones is predicted to be a major problem at future Olympic Games. Insulin, a protein hormone, has anabolic and anticatabolic actions. Its stimulatory effects on glucose and amino acid uptake follow ingestion of carbohydrates and protein.[22] Whether insulin use actually results in increased muscle mass is currently being studied. It is known that it increases protein synthesis in the muscles by increasing amino acid transport and by stimulating ribosomal protein synthesis. There is no known current test for insulin abuse. The detection of low levels of C-peptide in the urine is one technique that may have promise.

Insulin is widely available and therefore subject to abuse. The athlete involved with insulin abuse may suffer adverse reactions such as hypoglycemia, which can result in confusion, convulsions, and coma, as well as vasoconstriction, tachycardia, and profuse sweating from ephedrine release.[21] Other risks include lipodystrophy or lipoatrophy (distortion and shrinkage of fat cells) from prolonged injection without rotation of sites, insulin allergy, insulin resistance, and immunologic response.[44] Of course, insulin shock can be fatal.

Narcotics

Although not specifically ergogenic, narcotics are misused in sport mainly to enable continuation of effort required while training and competing in spite of injury. Side effects of these drugs include sedation, mood changes, nausea and vomiting, altered thought processes, visual impairment, and apathy.[41]

Pain relief is seen as the major motivation for narcotic abuse in sport. A perception of psychological stimulation along with a false feeling of invincibility and illusions of athletic prowess beyond inherent ability is also often seen. The raised pain threshold provided may result in an athlete sustaining further damage from failing to recognize signs and symptoms of initial injury.[40] These painkillers may place an athlete in a state of euphoria, with the psychological stimulation resulting in impaired judgment. The user's perception of danger may be clouded, placing both the athlete and his or her fellow competitors in unsafe situations.[18,40] Abusers also risk complications of physical dependence, including addiction and withdrawal, as well as side effects such as respiratory depression and sudden death.

Heroin, a semisynthetic opiate with higher potency than morphine, is the most widely known "street" drug and the most addicting of the class.[41] The IOC presently prohibits all drugs of this class for use in competition except codeine, dextromethorphan, ethylmorphine, dextropropoxyphene, diphenoxylate, and propoxyphene.[9] The NCAA bans only heroin under this classification at this time.[32]

Beta Blockers

Widespread abuse of beta blockers is not evident, especially with the range of alternative medications available to treat angina pectoris, cardiac arrhythmias, hypertension, and migraine. They are unlikely to be used in endurance sports necessitating high cardiac output such as basketball, cycling, and running, where they would impair performance.[40] Since beta blockers antagonize epinephrine-induced tremor, they may be beneficial to decrease heart rate, control tremor, and promote hand steadiness in sports such as shooting and archery.[18,20]

Recreation and Leisure Drugs

For more than 2 decades, marijuana has been publicized as being a commonly used illegal drug among young adults. Along with psychotropic effects, marijuana smoking precipitates sinus tachycardia, bronchodilation, and an increase in limb blood flow. A decrease in peak exercise performance, reported following marijuana smoking, is possibly due to a premature achievement of maximum heart rate.[36]

Substances that are still believed to be the most abused for recreation and leisure are alcohol and marijuana, with alcohol being the drug of choice for female and male athletes and students alike. Reasons that have been given for alcohol use include socialization, recreation, mood enhancement, and reduction of stress. Reasons for nonuse include detrimental health effects, fear of adverse social or legal consequences, and the belief that use would impair athletic performance. Signs of anger and fatigue have been linked to alcohol abuse and may be helpful to those working with student and athlete populations as part of the abuse identification process.[15]

Pharmacologically, alcohol at high doses has a sedative action, inducing central nervous system depression. It has been reported that small amounts of alcohol may increase performance to a slight degree as a result of lowered stress, enhanced self-concept, and mild stimulation.[18]

Although side effects of alcohol ingestion are dose and frequency related, studies have shown a decrease in coordination, reaction time, and hand–eye coordination, along with impaired balance. The same is true for marijuana. Both are seen to have a negative affect on performance. Abuse of either of these substances, both of which are classified as "restricted" by the IOC, may adversely affect strength and alter thermoregulatory mechanisms.[20] Social acceptance and availability make restrictions difficult to enforce.[41]

CONCLUDING REMARKS

In the past, female as well as male athletes have indicated similar attitudes toward taking various drugs. Consistent with behavior exhibited by the general population, all were inclined to agree with the use of alcohol and tobacco, especially outside of their training and competition season. Of particular concern is the fact that performance-enhancing substances are becoming more widely used by both male and female athletes, particularly those substances that are undetectable. However, the majority of athletes continue to express disagreement with the abuse of anabolic steroids and are in favor of treatment programs for abusers.[28]

It is apparent that drug use in the female population, particularly athletes, is related to several factors. The sociological and physiologic aspects of being female contribute to their special drug concerns.[14] Of consideration is whether abuse is related to personal problems, societal stress, pressure to succeed, fear of losing, other factors, or a combination of influences. In order to provide effective coping skills, health care professionals, educators, and other concerned parties need to identify drug abuse as an ineffective means of coping.[13] Preventive health measures must be identified, and strategies for risk reduction must be put in place.[31]

References

1. Adams M: Coming soon to a little plastic cup near you. Fitness 7:62, 1995.
2. Anshel MH: A survey of elite athletes on the perceived causes of using banned drugs in sport. J Sport Behav 14:283–307, 1991.
3. Bamberger M, Yaeger D: Over the edge. Sports Illustrated 86:62–70, 1997.
4. Barnett NP, Wright P: Psychosocial factors and the developing female athlete. In Agostini R (ed): Medical and Orthopedic Issues of Active and Athletic Women. Philadelphia, Hanley & Belfus, 1994, pp 92–100.
5. Begley S, Brant M: The real scandal. Newsweek 133:48–54, 1999.
6. Buckley WE, Yesalis CE, Friedl KE, et al: Estimated prevalence of anabolic steroid use among male high school seniors. JAMA 260:3441–5, 1988.
7. Chng CL, Moore A: A study of steroid use among athletes: Knowledge, attitude and use. Health Educ 21:11–7, 1990.
8. Comite International Olympique: International Olympic Charter Against Doping in Sport. Ottawa, Canada, Comite International Olympique, 1988.
9. de Merode A: International Olympic Committee Medical Code: Prohibited Classes of Substances and Prohibited Methods. Letter 31 January. Lausanne, Comite International Olympique, 1998.
10. de Merode A: IOC Medical Commission—Doping in Sport. Letter 31 July. Lausanne, Comite International Olympique, 1998.
11. de Merode A: IOC Medical Commission—Erythropoitin. Letter 17 May. Lausanne, Comite International Olympique, 1990.
12. de Merode A: IOC Medical Commission-List of Doping Classes and Methods. Letter 11 December. Lausanne, Comite International Olympique, 1987.
13. Duda M: Documenting drug use among female athletes. Physician Sportsmed 16:44, 1988.
14. Duda M: Female athletes: Targets for drug abuse. Physician Sportsmed 14:142–6, 1986.

15. Evans M, Weinberg R, Jackson A: Psychological factors related to drug use in college athletes. Sport Psychol 6:24–41, 1992.
16. Exum WF, Price JM: Doping rules and the treatment of respiratory and allergic disease. In Weiler JM (ed): Allergic and Respiratory Disease in Sports Medicine. New York, Marcel Dekker, 1997, pp 377–88.
17. Exum WF, Spletzer S, Bodin G, et al (eds): United States Olympic Committee Drug Education Handbook. Colorado Springs, Colo, USOC National Anti-Doping Program, 1996.
18. Fuentes RJ, Rosenberg JM, Davis A (eds): Athletic Drug Reference 1996. Durham, NC, Clean Data, Inc, 1996.
19. Green GA, Uryasz FD, Petr TA, Bray CD: NCAA Study of substance use and use habits of college student-athletes. Clin J Sports Med 11:51–6, 2001.
20. Haupt HA: Substance abuse by the athletic female. In Pearl AJ (ed): The Athletic Female. Champaign, Ill, Human Kinetics, 1993, pp 125–40.
21. Honour JW: Misuse of natural hormones in sport. Lancet 349:1786, 1997.
22. Horswill CA, Zipf WB, Kien CL, et al: Insulin's contribution to growth in children and the potential for exercise to mediate insulin's action. Pediatr Exerc Sci 9:18–32, 1997.
23. Kastrup EK, Hebel SK, Threlkeld DS, et al (eds): Drug Facts and Comparisons. St Louis, Mo, Facts and Comparisons, Inc, 1998.
24. Knopp WD, Wang TW, Bach BR Jr: Ergogenic drugs in sports. Clin Sports Med 16:375–92, 1997.
25. Kokotailo PK, Henry BC, Koscik RE, et al: Substance use and other health risk behaviors in collegiate athletes. Clin J Sports Med 6:183–9, 1996.
26. Malarkey WB, Strauss RH, Leizman DJ, et al: Endocrine effects in female weightlifters who self-administer testosterone and anabolic steroids. Am J Obstet Gynecol 165:1385–90, 1991.
27. Mantell ME: EPO: Cycling's atomic bomb. VeloNews, December 17, 1990, pp 17–8.
28. Martin MB, Anshel M: Attitudes of elite adolescent Australian athletes toward drug taking: Implications for effective drug prevention programs. Drug Educ J Austr 5:223–38, 1991.
29. Munch LR: Drugs and the athlete. Sport Psychol 6:24– 41, 1992.
30. Murray AK: Determination of recombinant glycosylated proteins and peptides in biological fluids. Chem Abstr 129:521, 1998.
31. Nattiv A, Puffer JC, Green GA: Lifestyles and health risks of collegiate athletes: A multi-center study. Clin J Sports Med 7:262–72, 1997.
32. NCAA Sports Sciences: Drug Testing Program 1998–99 [Brochure]. Overland Park, Kan, NCAA Sports Sciences, 1998.
33. Otis CL: Women and anabolic steroids. Sports Med Dig 12:4, 1990.
34. Payne FE: The physiology of physical fitness. In Birrer RB (ed): Sports Medicine for the Primary Care Physician. Norwalk, Conn, Appleton-Century-Crofts, 1984, pp 42–54.
35. Perlmutter G, Lowenthal DT: Use of anabolic steroids by athletes. Am Fam Physician 32:208–210, 1985.
36. Renaud AM, Cormier Y: Acute effects of marijuana smoking on maximal exercise performance. Med Sci Sports Exerc 18:685–689, 1986.
37. Rosen LW, McKeag DB, Hough DO, et al: Pathogenic weight-control behavior in female athletes. Physician Sportsmed 14:79–86, 1986.
38. Sawka MN, Joyner MJ, Miles DS, et al: American college of sports medicine position stand: The use of blood doping as an ergogenic aid. Med Sci Sports Exerc 28:i–viii, 1996.
39. Strauss RH, Liggett MT, Lanese RR: Anabolic steroid use and perceived effects in 10 weight-trained women athletes. JAMA 253:2871–3, 1985.
40. United States Olympic Committee (USOC) National Anti-Doping Program: USOC Guide to Prohibited Substances and Methods [Pamphlet]. Colorado Springs, Colo, USOC National Anti-Doping Program, 1998.
41. Wadler GI, Hainline B: Drugs and the Athlete. Philadelphia, FA Davis, 1989.
42. Wagner JC: Enhancement of athletic performance with drugs: An overview. Sports Med 12:250–65, 1991.
43. Whitten P: Red star over Atlanta. Swimming World and Junior Swimmer 35:50–2, 1994.
44. Wiley JW II: Insulin as an anabolic aid? A danger for strength athletes. Physician Sportsmed 25:103–4, 1997.
45. Windsor R, Dumitri D: Prevalence of anabolic steroid use by male and female adolescents. Med Sci Sports Exerc 21:494–7, 1989.

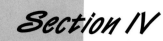

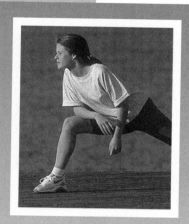

Obstetric/ Gynecologic Conditions

Chapter 12

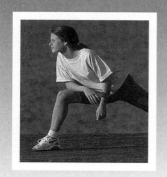

Common Gynecologic Problems

W. David Hager, M.D., F.A.C.O.G.

Male and female athletes alike experience the physiologic effects of vigorous training, have the potential for athletic-related injury, and deal with stress-related issues of competitive athletics. Female athletes, however, must also face the effects of training and competition on their menstrual cycles, ovulatory function, and pelvic floor musculature. In addition, inadequate nutrition and disordered eating can affect the menstrual cycle and subsequent bone health in women. This chapter will review some of these and other common gynecologic problems experienced by the pre- and postmenopausal female athlete.

MENSTRUAL DYSFUNCTION

One of the most common reasons female athletes seek gynecologic care is for diagnosis and treatment of a menstrual disorder. Young athletes who have trained vigorously, especially runners, gymnasts, and ballet dancers, may have delayed puberty, with a late onset of menarche and the development of secondary sexual characteristics. As long as vigorous training is pursued, they may maintain an amenorrheic state. In addition, these highly trained female athletes have higher rates of anovulation, luteal-phase defects, and oligomenorrhea or amenorrhea than controls.[15]

Ovarian function depends directly on secretion of hypothalamic gonadotropin-releasing hormone (GnRH). If there is a significant decline in pulsatile GnRH secretion, pituitary secretion of luteinizing hormone (LH) and follicle-stimulating hormone (FSH) is reduced. There is a resulting compromise in folliculogenesis or ovulation or both.[4] In addition to overexercise, inadequate energy availability and excessive stress may also be contributing factors in the occurrence of oligo- or amenorrhea.

Loucks and co-workers evaluated the disruption of LH pulsatility in exercising women.

Energy availability, as controlled by dietary intake, affected LH pulsatility more than stress did. This indicates that the GnRH "pulse generator" is disrupted by an as-yet unidentified signal that dietary energy intake is inadequate for the energy costs of both reproduction and locomotion.[14] This emphasizes the complex interactions affecting menstrual function in athletes. Giles and Berga have also demonstrated that stress and unrealistic expectations among female athletes affect the hypothalamic-pituitary-ovarian (HPO) axis.[7]

These effects of menstrual dysfunction, as well as the disordered eating habits seen in some female athletes, may lead to serious bone loss and its consequences. Jones has reported that women with weight loss-associated amenorrhea and women with premature menopause are at significant risk for cortical bone loss compared with normal controls, whereas women with exercise-associated amenorrhea without weight loss may not be at as much risk.[10]

Although there is some controversy in the literature, hormone replacement may be used in selected female athletes, over age 16, in the form of oral contraceptive pills to counteract the effects of low estrogen and attempt to reduce the incidence of stress fractures. Constantini and Warren discuss that this form of intervention may be indicated in cases in which reduction of exercise, dietary changes, and weight gain are not feasible or are unsuccessful.[3]

The energy efficiency of vigorously trained athletes has been studied extensively. Vigorous training does not lower energy requirements, but these women have low energy intake:energy expenditure ratios. This is often due to extensive efforts on the part of the athlete to control weight or to an under-reporting of actual intake.[6] Female athletes are not necessarily more energy efficient than nonathletes and their nutritional intake and weight gain/loss patterns must be monitored carefully.

DYSFUNCTIONAL UTERINE BLEEDING

Oligo- and anovulation may result in amenorrhea or may be factors in the development of dysfunctional uterine bleeding, abnormal bleeding that occurs in the absence of a pathologic cause. When the HPO axis is altered, women may bleed heavily with a period (menorrhagia), bleed between their periods (metrorrhagia), or have no menses. Since abnormal bleeding in young women is predominantly hormonal in etiology, sampling of the endometrium by biopsy is seldom necessary. Hormonal therapy is usually required to regulate the menstrual cycle when these conditions occur. Oral contraceptives or cyclic progestins will usually control dysfunctional uterine bleeding in the female athlete.

CONTRACEPTION

Sexual activity among young athletes has increased just as it has among young people in general in the United States. The Youth Risk Behavior Surveillance Survey from the Centers for Disease Control and Prevention evaluated the frequency of sexual intercourse of teens from all 50 states. Thirty-two and one tenth percent of ninth grade females and 66.0% of twelfth grade females admitted to having intercourse in the past year.[2] The rates among males are significantly higher.

If sexual activity is that prevalent, it is imperative that the topic be discussed with junior high school-, high school-, and college-aged women. If they are unmarried and currently sexually active, they should be encouraged to become abstinent. If they plan to continue sexual activity, the risks of nonmarital pregnancy and sexually transmitted diseases should be discussed and preventive measures offered.

Risks include not only pregnancy and sexually transmitted diseases (STDs) but also the emotional consequences of bonding and broken relationships. There are over a million teenage pregnancies in the country annually, 42% of which are electively aborted. There are over 30 specific STDs that may infect humans and have acute and chronic effects. Bacterial STDs can be cured with antibiotic therapy, but viral STDs have no known cure. The emotional consequences may interfere with performance by the female athlete.

Abstinence is the only sure way to avoid unwanted pregnancy and STDs. If the young athlete chooses to be sexually active, appropriate contraception should be used, including method(s) that minimize the risk of pregnancy—oral contraceptive steroids afford the best protection—and also may decrease the chance of acquiring STDs. Condoms offer some risk reduction from certain STDs but are not totally protective, especially against diseases transmitted by secretions, such as human papilloma virus and syphilis. Only 3% of young women who take birth control pills will also insist on the use of condoms by their partner.

Oral contraceptives may possess an added benefit for some athletes as opposed to nonathletes who use them. The vigorously trained female athlete may benefit from the estrogenic effect of oral contraceptives to help protect her bones from hypoestrogenic sequelae. However, in the female athlete with hypoestrogenic amenorrhea, attention to lifestyle factors, including optimal caloric intake, and a possible decrease in training are important factors to address. Additional beneficial effects of birth control pills include regulation of the menstrual cycle, relief of dysmenorrhea, a decrease in the chance of developing functional cysts of the ovary, and moderation of the emotional swings that may occur during a normal cycle in some individuals.

MENOPAUSE

Menopause may have been a time when many women became less active athletically in the past, but no longer. In caring for female athletes, it is important to understand the physiologic and psychological effects of menopausal change as well as treatment regimens to minimize the adverse effects of this time in a woman's life. There are currently over 32 million postmenopausal women in the United States, and an estimated 700 million women 45 years of age and older in the world.[24] The principal symptoms of menopause are hot flushes, sweats, irritability, vaginal dryness, skin changes, and difficulty sleeping. Most of the symptoms can be improved or alleviated with the use of estrogen/progestin therapy, which can be administered cyclically or continuously. If the uterus has been removed surgically, progestins are not needed since their primary function is to protect the endometrium from hyperplasia and carcinoma.

In addition to the symptoms of menopause, changes occur in a woman's body that can result in damage over time. At menopause, the rates of heart attack and stroke begin to increase because there is no longer adequate estrogen present to inhibit the deposition of atherosclerotic plaque on the intima of arteries. A sedentary lifestyle and poor physical fitness both lead to a higher risk of cardiovascular disease, especially coronary artery disease.[1] Estrogen also acts to increase high-density lipoprotein (HDL) and decrease low-density lipoprotein (LDL). Myocardial infarction is the leading cause of death among postmenopausal women. Until recently, hormonal replacement therapy was recommended for many postmenopausal patients for prevention of heart disease, as well as for its other benefits.[22] However, recent data exploring the protective effect of estrogen replacement on atherosclerosis have questioned this recommendation, specifically with regard to prevention of heart disease.[8]

Bone loss is a normal part of the aging process. From menopause on, untreated women lose 1% to 2% of their bone mass each year. Estrogen acts to help keep calcium in the bony matrix to maintain strength. Weight-bearing exercise, calcium, and vitamin D do not prevent osteopenia/osteoporosis in the majority of postmenopausal women, unless estrogen is also consumed. Seventy-five percent or more of the bone loss that occurs in women during the first 15 years after menopause is attributable to estrogen deficiency rather than aging itself. Combined estrogen replacement and calcium therapy can result in an 80% decrease in compression fractures of the spine during menopause.[20] Studies have shown that the minimum effective dose of estrogen necessary to prevent postmenopausal bone loss is 0.625 mg conjugated estrogens, or the equivalent thereof.[13,16] Hormonal replacement therapy can be administered orally or in the form of skin patches.

A newer product, raloxifene hydrochloride, which is a selective estrogen receptor modulator, can prevent and treat osteoporosis, lower LDLs, and raise HDL2 without exposing the patient to an increased risk of breast cancer.[15] Chapter 26 describes additional strategies for prevention and treatment of osteoporosis in women.

With appropriate counseling, adequate training, and timely medical therapy, women can continue to remain physically active and competitive. There is no evidence that athletic participation accelerates or delays the time of menopause. Preparticipation medical evaluation, as well as ongoing medical care for gynecologic problems when they occur, is essential for girls and women of all ages. Menopausal women should take 1000 to 1500 mg calcium daily, but as discussed, calcium and exercise alone will not prevent osteoporosis in the majority of postmenopausal women. Estrogen is necessary to keep calcium in the bony matrix and keep bones strong. Appropriate exercise and a well-balanced diet are necessary to maintain weight control.

STRESS

The response to stress can influence performance, alter the athlete's sense of self-esteem, affect hormonal production, and influence the susceptibility to injury. All athletes experience stress from a multitude of sources, some external, some internal. The circumstances or events that cause stress are known as *stressors*. Seyle has developed the concept of *positive and negative stressors*. Certain situations may be a positive stressor to one female athlete, whereas the same conditions would adversely affect a different athlete and result in negative stress.[21]

Kamal compared the self-esteem of 18- to 25-year-old male and female athletes after they were provided positive or negative verbal feedback on a nonathletic task. Female athletes responded more adversely to negative feedback than did males. Both groups were more influenced by negative than positive feedback.[11]

Vigorous training increases the production of cortisol from the adrenal glands, which is a vigilance or maintenance reaction to moderate stress effects. Recent research in female long-distance runners has shown that they produce less estradiol and androgen. Tsia studied these effects in vitro and concluded that direct effects of cortisol were not responsible for these lowered sex hormone levels but rather inadequate gonadotrophic stimulation, related to hypothalamic amenorrhea, and/or a selective decrease in the adrenal secretion of precursor steroids were causative.[23]

Studies have shown a correlation between anxiety and injury in athletes. Data indicate that more-injured gymnasts, for example, were more anxious and tired than those less-injured and they reported higher scores on the Competitive-State Anxiety Inventory-2 scale (CSI-2).[12]

EATING DISORDERS

The presence of an eating disorder (ED) in a female athlete is often of significance to the gynecologist because of its potential to disturb the menstrual cycle. The pressure to improve performance by having lower weight and the desire to maintain a socially acceptable physique may result in disordered eating behaviors, amenorrhea, and osteoporosis—the so-called female athletic triad.[9] Instead of weight reduction in this fashion improving performance, however, it may actually decrease performance and result in a greater chance for injury.

The presence of an ED in an athlete is not always obvious; this behavior can be hidden very easily. Frequently, the ED is first discovered by the gynecologist or primary care physician when the patient presents with complaints of a menstrual disorder or another gynecologic problem. A careful physical examination, laboratory workup, and appropriate referral for counseling are indicated.

STRESS URINARY INCONTINENCE

When genuine stress urinary incontinence (SUI)—leakage of urine with coughing, straining, sneezing, or exercise—is discussed, one usually thinks of it occurring in an older woman who has given birth to several children delivered vaginally, or to a woman with a strong family history of pelvic support problems. When questioned about leakage of urine, 28% of 144 female athletes indicated that they had experienced SUI. In decreasing order, the activities during which SUI occurred in these subjects were gymnastics (67%), basketball (66%), tennis (50%), and field hockey (42%). Two thirds of the women who noted urine loss during athletics were incontinent more often than rarely. Incontinence is not infrequent in female athletes[19] and is more prevalent in higher-impact sports.

Although it has been proposed that women with conditions involving chronic straining and persistently increased intra-abdominal pressure have an increased prevalence of genital prolapse as a result of connective tissue damage,[17] this has not been well documented. In a retrospective study of female olympic athletes, Nygaard found that participation in regular strenuous, high-impact activity when younger did not predispose women to a markedly higher rate of clinically significant urinary incontinence in later life.[18]

Since experiencing stress incontinence while participating in certain sports does not necessarily predict a need to deal with the problem in later life, the key is to control symptoms acutely. The physician should recommend that the athlete empty her bladder prior to athletic participation and thereafter as breaks in competition or training allow.

CONCLUDING REMARKS

Gynecologic care of female athletes is interesting and rewarding. In the chapters that follow, experts will expand on the various topics reviewed in this chapter. This information will assist the primary care physician and gynecologist, as well as other health care providers, in managing the unique problems of female athletes.

References

1. Blair SN, Kohl HW III, Paffenbarger RS Jr, et al: Physical fitness and all-cause mortality: A prospective study of healthy men and women. JAMA 262:2395–2401, 1989.
2. Centers for Disease Control and Prevention: Youth Risk Behavior Surveillance Survey—United States, 1997. CDC Surveillance Summaries. MMWR 47:No. SS–3, 1998.
3. Constantini NW, Warren MP: Special problems of the female athlete. Baillieres Clin Rheumatol 8:199–219, 1994.
4. Cumming DC: Physical activity and control of the hypothalamic-pituitary-gonadal axis. Semin Reprod Endocrinol 8(1):15, 1990.
5. Delmas PD, Bjarnason NH, Mitlak BH, et al: Effects of raloxifene on bone mineral density, serum cholesterol concentrations, and uterine endometrium in menopausal women. N Engl J Med 337:1641–7, 1997.
6. Edwards JE, Lindeman AK, Mikesky AE: Energy balance in highly trained female endurance runners. Med Sci Sports Exerc 25:1398–404, 1993.
7. Giles DE, Berga SL: Cognitive and psychiatric correlates of functional hypothalamic amenorrhea: a controlled comparison. Fertil Steril 60:486–92, 1993.
8. Herrington DM, Reboussin DM, Brosnihan KB, et al: Effects of estrogen replacement on the progression of coronary-artery atherosclerosis. N Engl J Med 343(8):522–9, 2000.
9. Johnson MD: Disordered eating in active and athletic women. Clin Sports Med 13:355–69, 1994.
10. Jones KP, Ravmikar VA, Tulchinsky D, et al: Comparison of bone density in amenorrheic women due to athletics, weight loss and premature menopause. Obstet Gynecol 66:5–8, 1985.
11. Kamal AF, Blais C, McCarrey M, et al: Informational feedback and self esteem among male and female athletes. Psychol Rep 70:955–60, 1992.
12. Kolt GS, Kirkby RJ: Injury, anxiety and mood in competitive gymnasts. Percept Motor Skills 78:955–62, 1994.
13. Lindsay R, Hart DM, Clark DM. The minimum effective dose of estrogen for the prevention of postmenopausal bone loss. Obstet Gynecol 63:759–63, 1984.
14. Loucks AB, Verdun M, Heath EM: Lower energy availablility, not stress of exercise, alters LH pulsatility in exercising women. Appl Psysiol 84:37–46, 1998.
15. Marshall LA: Clinical evaluation of amenorrhea in active and athletic women. Clin Sports Med 13:371–87, 1994.
16. Michaelsson K, Baron JA, Farahmand BY, et al: Hormone replacement therapy and risk of hip fracture: Population based case control study. Br Med J 316:1858–63, 1998.
17. Nichols HD, Randall CL: Vaginal Surgery, 3rd edition. Baltimore, Williams & Wilkins, 1989, p 69.

18. Nygaard IE: Does prolonged high-impact activity contribute to later urinary incontinence? A retrospective cohort study of female olympians. Obstet Gynecol 90:718–22,1997.
19. Nygaard IE, Thompson FL, Svengalis SL, et al: Urinary incontinence in elite nulliparous athletes. Obstet Gynecol 84:183–7, 1994.
20. Riggs BL, Seeman E, Hodgson SF, et al: Effect of the fluoride/calcium regimen on vertebral fracture occurrence in postmenopausal osteoporosis. N Engl J Med 306:446, 1982.
21. Seyle H: Stress in Health and Disease. Boston, Butterworth, 1976.
22. Speroff L, Glass RH, Kase HG: Menopause and postmenopausal hormonal therapy. Clinical Gynecologic Endocrinology and Infertility,5th edition. Baltimore, Williams & Wilkins, 1994, pp 583–4.
23. Tsia L, Pousette A, Johansson C, et al: Effect of cortisol on the secretion of testosterone and estradiol-17 beta by human granulosa-luteal cell cultures. A model system for analyzing hormonal alterations in female athletes. Acta Obstet Gynecol Scand 71:502–5, 1992.
24. US Bureau of the Census Projection of the Population of the United States, 1977–2050. Current Population Reports Series No. 704, p 25.

Chapter 13

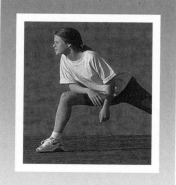

Menstrual Dysfunction

Joseph S. Sanfilippo, M.D., M.B.A.
Joseph S. Bird, Jr., M.D.

The menstrual cycle is a compilation of intricate interactions among the hypothalamus, the pituitary gland, and the ovaries. The physiologic development of this axis begins in the fetus at 10 to 12 weeks after conception. The hypothalamic stimulus, gonadotropin-releasing hormone (GnRH), is present in the fetal circulation as early as 10 weeks gestation.[42] The appropriate release of GnRH is mandatory for the initiation of regular ovulatory menstrual cycles. As a prerequisite, an understanding of the endocrinology of a normal menstrual cycle allows for appropriate evaluation of problematic states, including infertility, dysfunctional uterine bleeding, and disruption of menses caused by athletic activity, as well as effective contraception.

HORMONAL REVIEW OF THE FIRST MENSTRUAL CYCLE

The hypothalamus, an organ strategically located at the base of the brain just above the junction of the optic nerves, is responsible for both production and release of the neurohormone GnRH, which ultimately stimulates release of follicle-stimulating hormone (FSH) and luteinizing hormone (LH). The interaction between the hypothalamus and pituitary occurs through an intricate web of vascular channels commonly referred to as the *portal vessel system*. Alterations in the pulsatile frequency and amplitude of GnRH release determine whether gonadotropin secretion is suppressed or stimulated. Ultimately, FSH and LH via the hematogenous route reach the ovarian prenatal follicle. This developmental process includes an initial recruitment phase of a cohort of ovarian follicles and, ultimately, selection of one dominant follicle destined to ovulate. (Fig. 13-1) The process is repeated with each menstrual cycle.[36]

The corpus luteum, a product of ovulation, develops from the site of ovum release on the

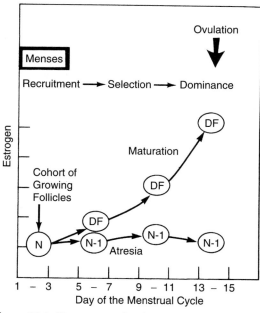

Figure 13-1. Time course for the recruitment, selection, and ovulation of the dominant ovarian follicle (DF) with onset of atresia among other follicles of the cohort (N1). (From Hodgen GD: The dominant ovarian follicle. Fertil Steril 1982, 38: 281–300, with permission.)

ovary. Progesterone production and release is the predominant product of the corpus luteum.

The circulating levels of gonadotropins, human chorionic gonadotropin (HCG), and sex steroids are presented in Figure 13-2. The gonadotropin levels increase dramatically after delivery, ultimately developing a nadir between 6 months and 2 years of age, and remain quiescent until age 8. Very little is known concerning the suppression of the pituitary during this period, but many theories have been proposed.[65] The two most widely accepted concepts deal with a sex steroid-dependent feedback system versus an intrinsic central nervous system inhibitory mechanism independent of the presence of sex steroid. Ultimately, hypothalamic inhibition occurs in the arcuate nucleus,

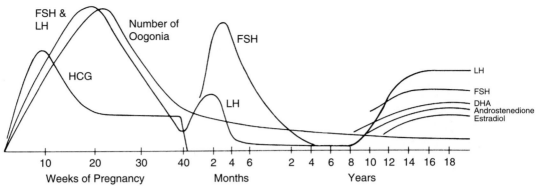

Figure 13-2. Serum levels of FSH, LH, human chorionic gonadotropin (HCG), dehydroepiandrosterone (DHEA), androstenedione, and estradiol in females from prenatal state to 18 years of age. (From Speroff L, Glass RH, Kase NG: Clinical Gynecologic Endocrinology and Infertility, 5th edition. Baltimore, Williams & Wilkins 1994, p 173, with permission.)

preventing release of GnRH from the pulse generator. The suppression of pulse frequency and amplitude of GnRH release prevents pituitary gonadotropes from releasing FSH and LH. Despite our current level of uncertainty about the impetus required for onset of puberty, it is well understood that around 8 or 9 years of age, the anterior pituitary begins secreting gonadotropins in response to the pulsatile secretion of GnRH from the medial basal hypothalamus. The fact that GnRH is required for initiation of puberty is well accepted.[23]

What is understood at present is that sleep and adequate body fat are considered essential elements for initiation of secondary sexual development. Boyar, Katz, and coworkers[7,43] described gonadotropin secretory patterns in prepubertal, pubertal, and mature stages of growth. Their findings are consistent with a sleep-entrained release of LH, which occurs during stage IV sleep. As secondary sexual maturation reaches completion, the relationship between sleep and gonadotropin release ceases to exist.

An association between critical body weight, lean:fat ratio, and secondary sexual development with subsequent menarche was proposed by Frisch.[29] The initiation of menarche is followed by a period of oligo-ovulation. The frequency of ovulation, though, appears to increase from its beginning in adolescence to what is considered complete hypothalamic—pituitary–ovarian axis maturation in the early to mid 20s.[1] A general understanding of the endocrine patterns that often persist during early puberty (ie, oligo-ovulation or anovulation) may increase our knowledge of pathologic entities that occur among certain populations.[26]

Recent research focusing on the issues of low energy availability and its relationship to LH pul-

satility in exercising women has been performed by Loucks and colleagues.[54] Their research demonstrates that there appears to be a reduction in LH pulse frequency and an increase in LH pulse amplitude in exercising women with low energy availability. When appropriate energy stores were available to the exercising women (through diet) and exercise stress was induced, the participants showed a reduction in neither LH pulse frequency nor amplitude.[54] These results suggest a potential etiology for athletic amenorrhea, based upon energy availability, which is currently an active area of research.

SPECIFIC HORMONAL CHANGES IN THE FEMALE ATHLETE

Follicle Stimulating Hormone–Luteinizing Hormone–Inhibin

Exercise is associated with release of pituitary and hypothalamic hormones and a decline in the concentration of circulating levels of LH; however, FSH generally is not affected by exercise.[26] Serum inhibin concentrations, which have a direct negative feedback, specifically on FSH, are increased in animal models; however, when studied in human males there appears to be no significant alteration in serum levels of inhibin. Furthermore, it is hypothesized that the decline in LH may be an integral part of the "fight and flight" reaction to conserve energy and enhance survival following exercise.[26] GnRH appears to be altered from the perspectives of both the pulse frequency and the pulse amplitude, especially in women who have developed amenorrhea; thus, there is an apparent effect on LH output.

In athletes who did not experience menstrual disturbances, a study was conducted by Pirke and coworkers in which 31 young female athletes 13 years of age or older were matched with sedentary controls; all subjects were evaluated during 1 menstrual cycle or over a 6-week period. The "episodic gonadotropin secretion" was measured during the early follicular phase as well as during the late luteal phase by taking samples over a 12-hour period at 15-minute intervals. The end result was that during this time 8 athletes developed anovulatory cycles, all of which were associated with impaired progesterone secretion during the luteal phase. Those athletes who maintained normal menstrual cycles had shorter cycles, lower circulating estradiol levels mid-cycle, and lower estrone (E_1), as well as serum progesterone, concentrations during the luteal phase than did the sedentary controls. Episodic pulsatile release of LH was impaired, especially during the early follicular phase, when the athlete was anovulatory. Overall, there was minimal change with respect to FSH.[61] The work of Loucks, Williams, and coworkers[54,78] has led to a better understanding of caloric restriction and energy availability and its role in LH secretion activity. Current thinking favors low energy availability as having the primary effect on LH output.

Gonadotropin- and Corticotropin-Releasing Hormones

Another hypothesis has been that the altered LH secretion may be associated with increased corticotropin-releasing hormone (CRH) secretion, which also inhibits GnRH release.[46] The increase in CRH tone "results" in increased ß-endorphin levels, which also contributes to the GnRH inhibition. A third contribution is that of the "continuous activation of the adrenals" with resultant higher production of catecholamine, which may be converted to catecholestrogens. The latter compounds are potent inhibitors of GnRH secretion.[46] Overall, it is believed that the high-intensity endurance exercise exerts a "central inhibitory" effect on hypothalamic GnRH secretion that precedes the alteration of the menstrual cycle. The defect in pulsatile LH release in "normal menstruating runners" is primarily a reflection of reduction in pulsatile LH frequency in accordance with increased amplitude of the pulsation in comparison with sedentary controls.[16,79]

Prolactin

Prolactin has been more thoroughly evaluated with respect to response to exercise in both eumenorrheic and amenorrheic runners. One group of researchers concluded that control for menstrual phase in eumenorrheic athletes is important in assessing prolactin responses following exercise, but not in studies of adrenal corticotropic hormone (ACTH) and cortisol responses following exercise.[21] Furthermore, cortisol responses following submaximal and maximal exercise in amenorrheic runners are blunted at the "adrenal level"; prolactin response following submaximal and maximal exercise is also blunted in amenorrheic runners. Prolactin responses following exercise may be mediated by adrenal activation.

Steroid Hormones

Serum free testosterone and estradiol have been evaluated in both trained (marathon runners) and untrained athletes, all of whom were eumenorrheic.[45] The estradiol levels of the groups were not significantly different; however, there was an increase in the percentage of free testosterone in the untrained group using a standardized bicycle ergometer or treadmill test in luteal and follicular phases of the menstrual cycle. The free testosterone increase was noted in the marathon runners as well as in the untrained group of runners.

Endogenous Opioid Peptide and Catecholestrogens in Association With Menstrual Irregularity

Endogenous opioid peptides (EOP), as well as catecholestrogens, have been implicated in association with menstrual irregularity. Specifically, ß-endorphins, which have an "opiate-like activity," contribute to the decrease in LH by suppressing hypothalamic GnRH. The phenomenon is only observed during the late follicular and mid-luteal phases of the menstrual cycle.[19] ß-Endorphins exert a "tonic inhibition" on the secretion of GnRH and, as a result, LH release. Prolactin regulation is also under the control of endorphins interfering through the dopaminergic pathway; that is, dopamine is the primary prolactin-inhibiting factor.[18] DeCree hypothesized that the increase in circulating concentrations of ß-endorphins that occurs following physical activity is involved in the frequent menstrual irregularities in female athletes.[18]

Naloxone infusion inhibits endogenous opiate output. Amenorrheic runners, when given naloxone (infusion), do not have consistent alteration of basal, postexercise, or stimulated hormonal levels compared with eumenorrheic runners.[68]

Catecholestrogens are the 2- and 4-hydroxy derivatives of estrone and estradiol. The catecholestrogens suppress LH and "potentiate as well as induce" the LH surge.[19] Catecholestrogens also play a role in suppression of prolactin release, in all probability by interfering with dopamine, and also may be involved in luteolysis via an effect on prostaglandin $F_{2\alpha}$ activity.[68] From a historical perspective, catecholestrogens were first identified by Niederal and Fogel in 1949.[59] In addition to the 2- and 4-hydroxyestrone, 2- and 4-hydroxyestradiol and 2- and 4-methoxy metabolites contribute to the family of catecholestrogens. This group of hormones exerts its estrogenic activity in a manner similar to that of estrone and estradiol in that they bind to estrogen receptors.[57] 2-Hydroxycatecholestrogens stimulate LH release and 4-hydroxyestradiol inhibits LH release. Another factor in the chain is ß-lipotropin, which appears to be increased following exercise in a manner similar to that of ß-endorphins.

As alluded to previously, catecholestrogens may play a role with respect to corpus luteum demise. Prostaglandin $F_{2\alpha}$ is involved with respect to luteolysis from the perspective of an "anti-LH action," resulting in destruction of the LH receptors in the corpus luteum.[3] Exercise is associated with an increase in plasma prostaglandin $F_{2\alpha}$ levels.[20] Both 2- and 4-hydroxyestrone are able to provoke prostaglandin $F_{2\alpha}$ release.[32]

Another significant effect with respect to catecholestrogens is that of the extent of estradiol 2-hydroxylation; that is, conversion to catecholestrogens is inversely related to the total fat content of the athlete. Changes in regional fat deposits of both subcutaneous and internal fat may be involved in menstrual dysfunction.[31]

Thyroid Hormones

Several studies have reported that low-T_3 syndrome, a sign of energy deficiency, occurs in amenorrheic and not eumenorrheic athletes. In one study, the resting metabolic rate was significantly lower in amenorrheic compared with eumenorrheic runners and sedentary women, even though the daily caloric intakes of the groups did not differ significantly.[58] Loucks and colleagues, in their randomized prospective cohort study, found that the low-T_3 syndrome was induced by the energy cost of exercise and prevented in exercising women by increasing their dietary energy intake.[22] These studies support the premise that reproductive disorders are caused by failure to compensate dietary energy intake for the energy cost of exercise (an "energy drain") rather than by exercise itself.

Glucose Metabolism

Glucose homeostasis appears to be impaired during the mid-luteal phase of the menstrual cycle; however, this finding remains somewhat controversial.[22] The inter-relationship between glucose metabolism and the menstrual cycle has several aspects: (1) the effect of menstrual phase (ovarian steroids) on glucose metabolism; (2) the effect of exercise on glucose metabolism; and (3) the effects on the menstrual cycle of glucose metabolism during exercise in female athletes.

Using a hyperglycemic hyperinsulinemic clamp model, researchers have concluded that endurance exercise training results in a slower decline in muscle glycogen depletion during exercise. In addition, the uptake of glucose by working muscles is decreased during exercise after a 12-week training program.[12] Thus, exercise training overall results in a carbohydrate-sparing effect.

Diet and insulin-like growth factor I (IGF-I) have been assessed with respect to body composition in women with exercise-induced hypothalamic amenorrhea. In this study, IGF-I and fat-free mass as well as fat mass were assessed in matched groups of exercising women with and without secondary "hypothalamic" amenorrhea. The investigators concluded that differences in body composition between exercising women with and without exercise-induced hypothalamic–pituitary dysfunction were related to an alteration in IGF-I secretion.[11]

Insulin-like growth factor binding protein (IGF-BP-I) appears to be a "metabolic signal" associated with exercise-induced amenorrhea. This hepatic protein is acutely and inversely regulated by insulin and is believed to modulate the peripheral actions of IGF-I. Thus, IGF-BP-I may also be involved in the metabolic regulation of reproductive activities.[38]

Melatonin

Exercise of sufficient intensity during daylight hours results in an acute elevation of circulating melatonin levels.[48] This increase is independent of menstrual status, whereas nocturnal melatonin secretion demonstrates a twofold amplification in amenorrheic but not eumenorrheic athletes.[48] Neither naloxone infusion nor metoclopramide had a significant effect on melatonin secretion.

Leptin

The discovery of the hormone leptin, of the obesity gene, has provided a better understanding of the inter-relationships among nutritional status, energy balance, and the reproductive axis. Laughlin and Yen demonstrated an absense of the normal diurnal pattern of 24-hour leptin levels in amenorrheic athletes.[49] Warren and colleagues found significantly lower levels of leptin and thyroid function in amenorrheic women and reported a link with disordered eating, low bone mass, and hypoleptinemia.[76] The specific mechanisms of leptin's action linking the metabolic and reproductive axes, however, have not been fully elucidated.

AMENORRHEA

Prior to any discussion of amenorrhea, it is important to define the criteria used to classify individuals who would benefit from an initial evaluation. Absence of growth and development of secondary sexual features in the absence of menarche by age 14 should prompt an initial investigation. The patient with normal growth and development of secondary sexual characteristics who has not menstruated by age 16 warrants a medical evaluation for *primary amenorrhea*. Any female patient with absence of menses for greater than 3 months who has already begun menstruating would benefit from an evaluation for *secondary amenorrhea*. The patient with intermittent or frequent oligomenorrhea (menstrual cycle longer than 36 days) also requires further workup. Realizing that there are exceptions to every rule, these criteria generally identify patients who would likely benefit from diagnostic evaluation. It is important to note that exercise-associated amenorrhea is a diagnosis of exclusion. Female athletes with amenorrhea should have a complete workup to exclude other potential causes for their menstrual dysfunction and should receive appropriate counseling about nutrition and bone health as well as contraception.[60]

As with any disorder, it is essential to perform a careful history and physical examination to establish a differential diagnosis. A compartmental classification, shown in Table 13-1, permits a structured understanding of the physiologic and anatomic disorder.[72] This in no way precludes simultaneous evaluation of different compartments during the initial visit.

The initial phase of the amenorrhea workup should include serum evaluation of thyroid-stimulating hormone, FSH, and prolactin levels, a pregnancy test, and a progestational challenge test. Withdrawal bleeding after progestin administration (medroxyprogesterone acetate 10 mg daily for 10 days) and normal prolactin and TSH levels indicate anovulation is the primary cause of amenorrhea. A lack of withdrawal bleeding after administration of a progestational agent indicates some form of end-organ dysfunction. Further treatment with conjugated estrogens (1.25 mg daily for 21 days), complemented by a progestin such as medroxyprogesterone acetate (10 mg daily for 10 days), may be necessary to achieve withdrawal bleeding. Performing multiple cyclic attempts to achieve withdrawal bleeding is a wise precaution prior to making the diagnosis of end-organ dysfunction. Conversely, withdrawal bleeding in response to estrogen and progestin therapy is indicative of an intact outflow tract and appropriate end-organ function. It is therefore imperative to focus on ovarian disorders, the second compartment, for identification of specific abnormalities.

Ovarian disorders are evaluated initially by FSH assay. Serum FSH levels above 30 mIU/mL indicate ovarian failure. A number of cases of ovarian failure have been associated with other causes, such as autoimmune disorders, which should prompt selected laboratory testing to rule out this entity.

The absolute age associated with a high yield from chromosomal evaluation in patients with ovarian failure is not certain. Many authors suggest that a FSH level above 30 mIU/mL at age 30 years identifies ovarian failure. The rare patient with a testicular component within the gonadal area is identified by the presence of a Y chromosome. Patients with a testicular component have a significant tendency to develop malignant tumors such as gonadoblastoma, yoke-sac tumor, dysgerminoma, and choriocarcinoma. Therefore, it is clinically prudent to intervene operatively prior to development of malignancy.

The relationship between exercise and amenorrhea has been elucidated to a great extent by our observations of competitive female athletes as well as women engaged in other demanding activities, such as modern dance and ballet. One study showed anovulatory cycles as well as short-luteal-phase dysfunction in two thirds of

Table 13-1. Compartmental Classification of Amenorrhea

Compartment 1: Disorders of outflow tract or uterine target organ
Compartment 2: Ovarian disorders
Compartment 3: Anterior pituitary disorders
Compartment 4: Hypothalamic / CNS disorders

From Speroff L, Glass RH, Kase NG: Clinical Gynecologic Endocrinology and Infertility, 5th edition. Baltimore, Williams & Wilkins, 1994, pp 402–6, with permission.

runners.[62] In the past, the major influences contributing to normal menstrual function were thought to be critical body fat levels and a stressful environment. These theories have given way to a new theory that indicates a more critical role of energy availability in LH output.[54] These issues are addressed below.

EXERCISE-ASSOCIATED AMENORRHEA

Incidence

The incidence of amenorrhea and oligomenorrhea in the athlete is higher than that in the general population, although the exact incidence in the athlete remains a point of discussion. An incidence of secondary amenorrhea in the general population has been noted to be 2% to 5%.[53] The incidence of amenorrhea in endurance athletes has been noted to be as high as 50%.[71] Furthermore, 10% of women who competed in the Tokyo Olympics of 1964 reported menstrual abnormalities, as opposed to 59% of those who competed in the 1976 Montreal Olympics.[66] Another study involving New York City Marathon runners demonstrated an overall 7% incidence of menstrual aberrations. It was noted that the incidence was more frequent in women who "weighed less" and were younger and/or nulliparous.[74]

Calabrese and coworkers noted that professional and student ballet dancers consumed fewer calories (1358 calories) than the recommended dietary allowance (2030 calories) established by the National Research Council.[9] Of interest, Frisch noted the collegiate women who began athletic training prior to menarche consumed less fat (65 g) and protein (71 g) than a group who began training after menarche (95 g fat and 92 g protein).[30] It is important to remember the interrelationships of disordered eating, amenorrhea, and osteoporosis, better known as the female athletic triad, when considering the potential long-term medical effects on the female athlete.

A number of female athletes participate in pathologic eating behaviors. There appears to be some overlap of features of anorexic patients with amenorrhea with those of highly active female athletes with exercise-associated amenorrhea (Fig. 13-3).[15] The pathophysiology

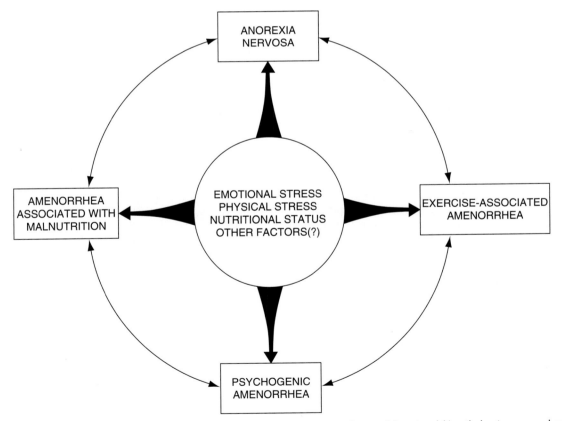

Figure 13-3. Theoretical representation of the associations among various forms of functional hypothalamic amenorrhea. These disorders appear to be closely related. (Adapted from Rebar RW: The reproductive age: Chronic anovulation. In Serra G (ed): Comprehensive Endocrinology. The Ovary. New York, Raven Press, 1983, pp 241–56, with permission.)

revolves around a hypoestrogenic state in association with suppression of the GnRH pulse generator. Another consideration is that the young athlete may fail to achieve peak bone mass, with reduction in bone mineral density, scoliosis, and stress fractures occurring as a result of the prolonged hypoestrogenic state. In some female athletes, an abnormal preoccupation with weight and pursuit of being thin may occur. The clinician must realize the symptoms and signs of disordered eating, which may be life threatening and can be clearly overlooked. (Chapter 25 presents a detailed discussion of disordered eating in athletes.)

In 1978, Feicht and coworkers conducted a survey in which a questionnaire was distributed to collegiate runners.[27] These researchers concluded that the incidence of amenorrhea was in direct proportion to the "training mileage." (Fig. 13-4) In women competing in activities such as ballet and gymnastics, a "particularly increased incidence of both primary and secondary amenorrhea" was noted. In addition, problems such as decreased bone mineral density, stress fractures, and symptoms of anorexia nervosa were also reported.[14]

As mentioned previously, weight loss and changes in body composition are factors that may contribute to amenorrhea in athletes. Amenorrheic athletes, in general, are considered to have a lower level of body fat and a lower weight, and oftentimes lose more weight following initiation of training than athletes with regular menstrual cycles.[53] It is thought that this alteration of body composition may be associated with changes in circulating estrogen and androgen levels.

Controversy abounds as to whether there is a single mechanism or multiple associated causes for amenorrhea related to exercise. Predisposition revolves around training, nutritional status, body composition changes, and stress hormone effects during exercise, as well as "reproductive axis immaturity." The type of exercise as well as psychologic background also appears to play a role.[53]

The incidence of amenorrhea has been reported in Olympic marathon runners.[66] This intensively exercising group of runners averaged 70 miles/week in association with the 1984 Olympics; 19% were amenorrheic. That specific cohort (amenorrheic) was younger (24.8±1.2 vs 30.8±0.8 years; p=0.05), lighter (108.4±2.5 vs 114.6±1.7 lbs), and leaner (11.2±0.5 vs 12.5±0.3% body fat) than those with normal menstrual cycles. There was no difference between the two groups with respect to weekly training mileage, proportion

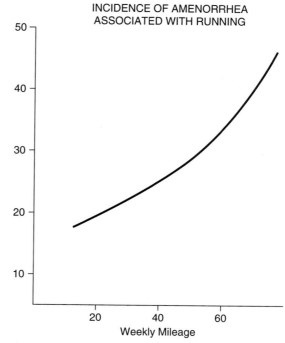

Figure 13-4. The relationship between the incidence of amenorrhea (defined as fewer than 3 cycles in the preceding 12 months) and weekly running mileage of from 20 to 80 miles. (Adapted from Feicht et al,[27] reprinted from Cumming DC, Rebar RW: Exercise and reproductive function in women: A review. Am J Ind Med 4: 113, 1983. Copyright 1993. Reprinted by permission of Wiley-Liss, a division of John Wiley and Sons, Inc.)

completing the marathon, and basal serum or postmarathon prolactin levels. Of interest, the basal serum cortisol level was slightly higher in the amenorrheic group (p=0.05). The authors concluded that training intensity above a certain threshold had little effect on the alterations in the menstrual cycle. Furthermore, vigorously trained "national-caliber" marathon runners had a lower incidence of amenorrhea than previously predicted.[33] Menstrual aberrations in endurance runners may thus be classified into three types of reproductive dysfunction: (1) delayed menarche or primary amenorrhea; (2) secondary amenorrhea; and (3) more subtle cycle-phase abnormalities, including prolonged follicular phase and abnormal luteal function in association with altered LH pulsatility.[53,74]

Athletic amenorrhea can occur with or without weight loss. Menses may return without significant alteration in body weight or lean:fat mass ratio,[67] as is often noted with interruption of training through injury. It may be difficult to explain this phenomenon given the work of Feicht and coworkers,[27] who emphasized the effect of percent body fat on menstrual function. Research emphasized earlier by Loucks and coworkers[54] would more aptly explain the menstrual aberration with no weight loss since their study identified the low energy availability as the primary reason for abnormal LH output.

The effect of running on menstrual function was investigated in a group of "habitual" runners (ie, those running more than 30 miles/week). The researchers found that "pre-running" menstrual irregularity was a more significant reflection of the potential to develop menstrual aberration than the exact number of miles run per week. The controversy still remains over the effect of training intensity and the incidence of amenorrhea. Confounding factors included stress, diet, and other lifestyle changes.[13]

Pathophysiology

Exactly why athletes have altered menstrual cycles is not completely understood. There are a number of major factors that should be considered, including (1) energy availability, (2) lean body mass (3) stress as related to the physical endeavor, (4) changes at the hypothalamic–pituitary axis, (5) type of athletic endeavor, and (6) previous history of interval between menses (Fig. 13-5). With respect to lean body mass, while not a completely accepted hypothesis, there does appear to be a "link" between body fat and circulating levels of estrogen.

A minimal body fat threshold has been professed to be necessary for onset of menarche (17%) and for maintenance of regular menstrual cycles (22%).[28] Over time, measurement of percent body fat has not always correlated with nutritional status and menstrual aberration, as reported by Loucks and coworkers in their evaluation of energy availability and LH output.[54] Wentz found that a 30% decrease in body fat resulted in significant menstrual dysfunction.[77] Among athletes who developed secondary amenorrhea, percent body fat (18.9%) was lower than the average percentage body fat in athletes without amenorrhea[67] (ie, 20.5% body fat was noted among those with normal menstrual cycles or oligomenorrhea). Other factors include overall nutritional status and stress; furthermore, a compilation of factors appears to be the most feasible explanation.

The effect of leptin on the reproductive status of the female athlete is an area of ongoing research.[49,55,76] Low leptin levels in female athletes who exercise strenuously as well as in women with anorexia have been found to be closely associated with neuroendocrine abnormalities. Leptin may monitor the body's fat content and inhibit ovulation when nutritional reserves drop below a certain level.

It has been understood that the reproductive system "adapts" to a number of effects, including environmental, nutritional, emotional, and physical stresses, with resultant "downregula-

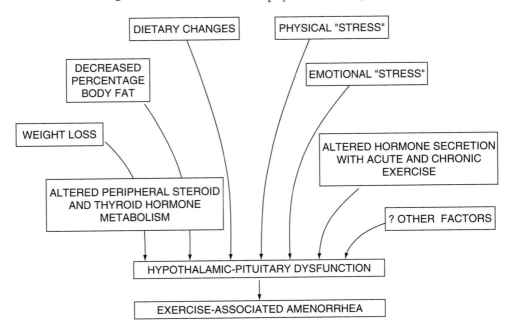

Figure 13-5. Diagrammatic representation of some of the factors involved in the pathophysiology of exercise-associated amenorrhea. (Adapted from Rebar RW: Effects of exercise on reproductive function in females. In Givens JR (ed). The Hypothalamus. Chicago, Year Book Medical, 1984, pp 245–62, with permission.)

tion" to a pattern similar to that of a premenarcheal female.[63] One must also consider the theory that athletic women may become amenorrheic if their hypothalamic–pituitary–ovarian axis has not "fully matured," thus reflecting aberrations such as emotional stress and nutritional status.

An interesting survey was conducted by Cavanaugh and coworkers in which age at menarche, incidence of menstrual irregularity, whether training occurred before or after menarche, specific personality traits (ie, anxiety, curiosity, anger), and type of athletic activity were assessed in 161 "highly competitive" female athletes.[10] This study included professional dancers, basketball players, fencers, gymnasts, field hockey players, and swimmers, all of whom were compared with age-matched nonathletic women. The resultant findings were that, indeed, the traits anxiety, curiosity, and anger, as well as age at menarche, had a significant effect on whether or not the athlete developed a menstrual aberration.

Exercise-associated amenorrhea has been considered to be a form of hypothalamic amenorrhea. An adverse effect on the hypothalamic hormonal output has been associated with physical and/or emotional (stress) factors, all of which can affect the GnRH pulse generator located in the hypothalamus. This sensitive "generator" can be affected by changes in body composition (ie, percent body fat), diet, and nutritional status. Vegetarian (vegan) diets as well as diets low in calories, fat, and protein have been correlated with a higher risk of amenorrhea.[70] In addition, specific changes with respect to circulating levels of LH, estradiol, prolactin, endorphins, prostaglandins, dopamine, epinephrine, norepinephrine, cortisol, and other hormones during and after exercise play a role in menstrual alteration. The circulating levels of these hormones can affect the frequency and amplitude of GnRH output, thus having a direct effect on LH pulses and ovarian hormone output. This all translates for the clinician into the importance of obtaining a dietary history and weight history, complementing the menstrual and athletic endeavor history. During the physical examination, an attempt should be made to assess the presence of any endocrinopathy.

Yen has summarized the pathophysiology of exercise-associated menstrual dysfunction, which appears to induce progressive dysfunction of ovarian cyclicity: (1) luteal-phase defects, (2) anovulatory cycles and amenorrhea, and (3) delayed onset of menarche in prepubertal girls.[79]

Effects of Menstrual Phase, Amenorrhea, and Oral Contraceptives on Performance

While overall there is a paucity of information addressing the relationships among menstrual phase, amenorrhea, oral contraceptives, and performance, one study conducted by DeSouza and coworkers evaluated selected physiologic and metabolic responses to maximal and submaximal exercise during the follicular and luteal phases of the menstrual cycle in eumenorrheic and in amenorrheic runners.[21] The amenorrheic runners performed maximal (40 minutes at VO_2max) and submaximal treadmill runs. The result revealed a decrease in urinary LH and progesterone levels as well as circulating estradiol and progesterone levels. Of interest, oxygen uptake, minute ventilation, heart rate, respiratory exchange ratio, and plasma lactate levels were not significantly altered between the 2 phases in both the eumenorrheic and the amenorrheic runners. The investigators concluded that neither menstrual phase (follicular vs luteal) nor menstrual status (eumenorrheic vs amenorrheic) alters or limits exercise performance in female athletes. A more comprehensive review of this topic was performed by LeBrun, who found that neither the phase of the menstrual cycle nor the use of birth control pills had a significant effect on athletic performance.[50]

DELAYED MENARCHE AND PUBERTY

Normal developmental milestones are somewhat difficult to define because of the wide variation of "normal" development. The average age of puberty in the United States is 12.8 years of age.[34] Many young female athletes, such as gymnasts, fail to show changes of puberty by this age. *Delayed puberty* is defined as absence of secondary sexual characteristics by age 14 or of menarche by age 16 with secondary sex characteristics being present. Clinicians must realize that 5 years may be required between initial onset of puberty (ie, thelarche) and menarche. A history and physical examination are appropriate as the initial workup phase of delayed puberty. Special attention should be paid to the pubertal history of older siblings and parents, general health, and pertinent behavior patterns such as abnormal eating habits or extreme exercise routines. The physical examination offers an opportunity to identify clinical stigmata associated with specific disorders responsible for delayed puberty. For example, failure of growth and age-inadequate stature have causes ranging from isolated growth hormone deficiency to gonadal dysgenesis (45X); and visual field defects and absence of olfactory function are often associated with intracranial lesions.

It is helpful to categorize the causes of delayed puberty in relation to the level of gonadotropins identified during the evaluation. The delayed pubertal abnormalities are classified into three types: (1) hypergonadotropic hypogonadism, (2) hypogonadotropic hypogonadism, and (3) eugonadism (Table 13-2).[64] Minimal laboratory assessment for delayed puberty centers around laboratory testing for gonadotropin and prolactin levels, skull imaging, roentgenography for bone age, thyroid function testing, and appropriate adrenal and gonadal steroid assessment for systemic disorders often evaluated with general laboratory screening methods. Certainly patients with elevated gonadotropin levels deserve karyotyping owing to the concern for underlying gonadal dysgenesis and gonadal carcinomas.

Hypergonadotropic hypogonadism is associated predominantly with ovarian failure, most commonly gonadal dysgenesis. Other possibilities include 17-α-hydroxylase deficiency, resistant ovary syndrome, pure gonadal dysgenesis,

and ovarian destruction whether by torsion or an inflammatory process.

Hypogonadotropic hypogonadism is associated with depressed levels of LH and FSH. Many conditions, ranging from physiologic delay (the most common single cause of this subgroup) to malignant pituitary tumor, have been identified.[72] Only in the face of normal olfactory function, normal prolactin levels, and appropriate neuroradiologic procedures to exclude pituitary/hypothalamic tumors can the diagnosis of physiologic delay of puberty be established.

Eugonadism, the last classification group, is associated primarily with anatomic defects such as müllerian agenesis, vaginal septum, and imperforate hymen. Normal gonadotropin levels should stimulate focused evaluation for anatomic defects as well as mechanisms contributing to inappropriate positive feedback of the hypothalamic–pituitary–gonadal axis. These conditions could include androgen-producing adrenal disease as well as chronic anovulation syndrome, more commonly termed *polycystic ovarian syndrome*, which can present with primary amenorrhea as a chief complaint.

The primary therapeutic interest revolves around correcting the underlying etiologic factor. This may be as easy as thyroid hormone replacement for hypothyroidism or as complex as appropriately timed gonadectomy in 46XY individuals. Physiologic hormone replacement to reduce psychosocial stress by maintaining normal pubertal development and a state of positive energy balance and perhaps recommending a reduction in training are the first steps to take in treating the female athlete with delayed menarche. Integrity of bone development (ie, preventing premature closure of the growth plates) may be achieved by hormone replacement therapy in girls who have reached 16 years of age.[41] One caveat: in patients with hypothalamic–pituitary–ovarian dysfunction leading to delayed puberty who are sexually active, it is prudent to administer oral contraceptives in lieu of physiologic estrogen replacement regimens in order to protect against an unwanted pregnancy.

Table 13-2. Relative Frequency of Delayed Pubertal Abnormalities

HYPERGONADOTROPIC HYPOGONADISM	**43.0%**
Ovarian failure, abnormal karyotype	26.0%
Ovarian failure, normal karyotype	17.0%
46, XX	15.0%
46, XY	2.0%
HYPOGONADOTROPIC HYPOGONADISM	**31.0%**
Reversible	18.0%
Physiologic delay	10.0%
Weight loss/anorexia	3.0%
Primary hypothyroidism	1.0%
Congenital adrenal hyperplasia	1.0%
Cushing's syndrome	0.5%
Prolactinomas	1.5%
Irreversible	13.0%
GnRH deficiency	7.0%
Hypopituitarism	2.0%
Congenital CNS defects	0.5%
Other pituitary adenomas	0.5%
Craniopharyngioma	1.0%
Malignant pituitary tumor	0.5%
EUGONADISM	**26.0%**
Müllerian agenesis	14.0%
Vaginal septum	3.0%
Imperforate hymen	0.5%
Androgen insensitivity syndrome	1.0%
Inappropriate positive feedback	7.0%

From Speroff L, Glass RH, Kase NG: Clinical Gynecologic Endocrinology and Infertility, 5th edition. Baltimore, Williams & Wilkins, 1994, p 384, with permission.

LUTEAL-PHASE DEFECT

Luteal-phase defect, caused by progesterone deficiency, is of special concern to individuals who have an active interest in fertility. The issue was first brought to light in the 1970s with the report of 4 teenage swimmers who were noted to have shorter luteal phases than a control group composed of nonexercising teens and adults.[6,69] If a pregnancy occurs, the corpus luteum remains active for a minimum of 7 to 10 weeks. Thus, the degree of athletic endeavor takes on increased significance in the athlete who is attempting to conceive.

As the physiologic aspects unfold, it is both frequency and amplitude of LH pulses that are critical in maintaining the "lifespan" (average of 14 days) of the corpus luteum. Current thinking is that corpus luteum physiology is directly related to the granulosa cell component of the developing follicle. The granulosa cell component has the following functions: (1) synergy with thecal androgen production resulting in increased estrogen production, (2) development of LH receptors enhancing progesterone production, and (3) "cytoplasmic" egg maturation.[39] The thecal component is associated with induction of an angiogenesis factor to increase follicular blood supply and facilitate response to the LH pulse. When pregnancy occurs, HCG assumes the role of LH receptor occupancy, since LH and HCG are virtually identical molecules, except that the latter has an additional 21 amino acids. Thus, either hormone is capable of LH receptor occupancy and stimulation.

As defined, luteal-phase defect is associated with a normal duration of the corpus luteum, but a low to inadequate amount of progesterone production—the result of either inadequate granulosa cell production and/or inadequate LH surge in light of a normal LH pulse and thecal cell response.

A "short" luteal phase is related to a poor LH surge and absent or inadequate LH pulse and lower progesterone production. Assessment can occur by determination of serum progesterone levels or, ideally, by bioassay (ie, endometrial biopsy). Progesterone is released in a pulsatile manner, and thus serum assessment has significant shortcomings; ideally, multiple serum samplings should be undertaken.

In a broad sense, luteal-phase defect has 2 components (1) a short luteal phase with associated overall decrease in progesterone production, and (2) a normal luteal phase with inadequate progesterone production. A hypothalamic–pituitary defect with resultant inadequate LH surge is currently thought to be the primary cause rather than a distinct ovarian factor per se.

The apparent question is whether exercise induces luteal-phase dysfunction. Bullen, Beitins, and coworkers observed untrained young women with previously documented ovulatory menstrual cycles who underwent 2

months of "strenuous" exercise and developed both a luteal-phase defect and secondary oligomenorrhea.[4,8] Within 6 months of termination of the study, all subjects had normal menstrual cycles. The investigators concluded that vigorous exercise, especially when associated with weight loss, can reversibly disturb reproductive function in women and may lead to corpus luteum dysfunction associated with insufficient progesterone secretion and, in the case of short luteal cycles, to decreased luteal-phase length. Other investigators associate calorie restriction and an energy deficit to menstrual dysfunction, rather than strenuous exercise itself and the stress associated with exercise.[54,78]

RISK FOR OSTEOPOROSIS

While it is not a main focus of this chapter, it must be pointed out that amenorrhea and oligomenorrhea in the athlete have been associated with low bone density[24,51,56] and an increased risk of stress fractures.[2,52] Warren has found that delayed menarche has been associated with scoliosis and an increase in stress fractures in young ballet dancers.[75] The amenorrheic and oligomenorrheic athlete should be counseled appropriately and precautions taken. This is particularly of concern in the adolescent who has not attained peak bone mass. The exact mechanism by which physical stress affects bone mass in the amenorrheic athlete is not completely understood, although it is hypothesized that the primary effect may be on the osteoblast, affecting bone formation. Further discussion on this topic can be found in Chapters 24 and 26.

TREATMENT OF MENSTRUAL DISORDERS IN THE ATHLETE

There appear to be multiple factors associated with menstrual aberration in the athlete, including emotional stress and nutritional factors with resultant endocrinologic abnormalities. The chronic hypoestrogenemic state associated with amenorrhea and even oligomenorrhea may be detrimental to the skeleton, with increased risk of osteoporosis and stress fractures. Furthermore, when there is evidence of significant weight loss, appropriate counseling should be provided. Addressing energy balance is essential to ensure that calories consumed by the athlete are adequate to meet the demands of exercise energy expenditure. If reduction of exercise activity is not feasible, additional calories may be needed. Deuck and coworkers addressed the important issues relating to treatment of the athletic amenorrheic patient, including dietary factors and decreasing training intensity.[25] Other lifestyle changes may be necessary to facilitate appropriate weight increase and resumption of menses.

Until the mechanisms of bone loss (or inadequate bone formation) are better understood in this population, consideration should be given to hormone supplementation. Specifically, use of oral contraceptive pills (preferable) or physiologic hormone replacement therapy (conjugated estrogen 0.625 mg daily for 25 days each month with the addition of a progestin such as medroxyprogesterone acetate 10 mg/day during the latter 10 to 13 days of each 25-day treatment cycle) should be considered.

Estrogen Replacement Therapy: Pros and Cons

Our basic understanding of the hypoestrogenemic state as it relates to amenorrhea and its impact on preventive health issues has been greatly enhanced over the past 10 years. Many excellent studies have identified a close interdependence between bone density and adequate levels of estrogen and progesterone during normal reproductive development. No level of exercise can counterbalance the bone loss encountered in a hypoestrogenemic state.[25,51,56] The rate of bone loss over time that occurs in the postmenopausal hypoestrogenemic women emphasizes the importance of early detection, since rapid loss occurs within the first few years of hypoestrogenism. Sadly, adolescent menstrual irregularities suggesting a hypoestrogenemic state have been associated with significant bone loss only partially correctable with hormone replacement therapy or spontaneous resumption of menstrual flow.[40] Generally, there has been some debate as to whether prolactin offers an independent effect on bone loss irrespective of estrogen status. This debate has finally been laid to rest with the recognition that hyperprolactinemic amenorrheic women experience bone density changes due to their hypoestrogenemic state.[5] The accepted beneficial effect of regular exercise on lipid profiles can reverse in an estrogen-deficient environment.[17]

Occasionally, an elite or recreational athlete may choose to avoid menstrual bleeding. Cessation of menses can be obtained quite easily

through administration of 0.625 mg conjugated estrogen and 2.5 mg medroxyprogesterone acetate daily (without a break). One crucial point to remember when utilizing estrogen replacement therapy is that it offers no contraceptive benefits. In a patient whose return of normal hypothalamic function is in question, a low-dose oral contraceptive should be used preferentially to replace the inadequate estrogen production. Athletes who wish to prevent menstrual flow could ignore the pill-free interval and take oral contraceptives on a daily basis. Ultimately, there will be some patients who will refuse hormone replacement therapy. There is some controversy as to the effect of hormone replacement therapy on bone in young amenorrheic women, as outlined in the articles by Hergenroeder and coworkers, Keen and Drinkwater, and Lamon-Fava and coworkers.[35,44,47] More prospective, randomized studies are needed to assess this further in this population. Nevertheless, supplemental calcium therapy (1000 to 1500 mg daily) should be strongly recommended since high levels of exercise complimented by high calcium intake have been shown to be better than exercise or calcium alone in maintaining vertebral bone density.

FERTILITY- AND PREGNANCY-ASSOCIATED CONCERNS

There is no evidence that athletic females with a history of menstrual dysfunction have a higher incidence of infertility. However, anovulation in association with menstrual aberration is a concern, especially in the young competitive female athlete. In the athlete with menstrual dysfunction desiring pregnancy, decreased training intensity and improved dietary intake are the first steps to take in the effort to induce normal menstrual function. Ovulation induction may be required if pregnancy is desired, usually with the use of clomiphene citrate, a medication whose exact mechanism of action is unknown but is believed to cause increased pituitary gland output of both FSH and LH. In addition, assessment for luteal-phase defect must be considered, especially when infertility is a concern. This is best evaluated either with serum progesterone levels or with a bioassay in the form of an endometrial biopsy. Other pharmacologic agents for ovulation induction include gonadotropins, gonadotropin-releasing hormone, and bromocriptine. Further discussion of fertility concerns and treatment of infertility can

DYSMENORRHEA–PREMENSTRUAL SYNDROME AND SPORTS ACTIVITIES

Primary dysmenorrhea, defined as painful menses in the absence of any anatomic abnormality, was evaluated in a study by Izzo and Labriola[37] in which 483 athletes were assessed. One group initiated its athletic endeavor prior to onset of menarche; a second group began after menarche. It was noted that primary dysmenorrhea was identified in a lower percentage of patients who had initiated their athletic activities prior to onset of menarche. The investigators concluded that athletic activity of almost any type or level had a positive influence on dysmenorrheic symptoms, while at the same time causing minimal disturbance in the interval between menses per se.

Premenstrual symptoms and the effect of aerobic activity has been assessed by Steege and Blumenthal.[73] In 23 healthy premenopausal females, premenstrual symptoms were assessed initially and after 3 months of participation in aerobic exercise. The investigators concluded that participation in exercise-related activities was associated with an overall improvement in premenstrual symptoms, especially premenstrual depression.

CONCLUDING REMARKS

Menstrual dysfunction indeed plagues a high percentage of young female athletes. Our understanding of the pathophysiology of these abnormalities is growing as new information becomes available that ultimately challenges our knowledge of the etiology of these conditions. A good example is the work by Loucks and associates, who challenged the belief that body weight, percent body fat, and stress-inducing exercise routines were primarily responsible for these aberrations. It appears now that energy availability to a greater extent controls LH production and its ultimate effect on the menstrual pattern as well as on fertility. More work will need to be done in this area to confirm those initial findings, but it appears that research is headed in a whole new direction that may elucidate this question further. Nevertheless, the long-term implications of amenorrhea on the female athlete and therapeutic interventions to prevent sequelae such as heart disease, osteoporosis, and skeletal fractures are worthy of our attention.

There appears to be no increased risk of future infertility in the female athlete with a history of menstrual dysfunction. In athletes with exercise-associated menstrual dysfunction desiring pregnancy, a decrease in exercise intensity combined with improved dietary intake, may restore regular menses and ovulation.

References

1. Apter D, Vihko R: Hormonal patterns of first menstrual cycles. In Flamignic Venturoli S, Givens JR (eds): Adolescence in Females. Chicago, Year Book Medical, 1985.
2. Barrow GW, Saha S: Menstrual irregularity and stress fractures in collegiate female distance runners. Am J Sports Med 16(3):209–16, 1988.
3. Behrman HR: Prostaglandins in hypothalamo-pituitary and ovarian function. Ann Rev Physiol 41:685–700, 1979.
4. Beitins IZ, McArthur JW, Turnbull BA, et al: Exercise induces two types of human luteal dysfunction: confirmation by urinary free progesterone. J Clin Endocrinol Metab 72(6):1350–8, 1991.
5. Biller BM, Baum HB, Rosenthal DI, et al: Progressive trabecular osteopenia in women with hyperprolactinemic amenorrhea. J Clin Endocrinol Metab 75(3):690–7, 1992.
6. Bonen A, Belcastro AN, Ling WY, Simpson AA: Profiles of selected hormones during menstrual cycles of teenage athletes. J Appl Physiol 50:545, 1981.
7. Boyar RM, Finkelstein JW, David R, et al: Twenty-four hour patterns of plasma luteinizing hormone and follicle-stimulating hormone in sexual precocity. N Engl J Med 289:282–6, 1973.
8. Bullen BA, Skrinar GS, Beitins IZ: Induction of menstrual disorders by strenuous exercise in untrained women. N Engl J Med 312:1349, 1985.
9. Calabrese LH, Kirkendall DT, Floyd M, et al: Menstrual abnormalities, nutritional patterns and body composition in female classical ballet dancers. Physician Sports Med 11(2):86–98, 1983.
10. Cavanaugh DJ, Kanonchoff AD, Bartels RL: Menstrual irregularities in athletic women may be predictable based on pre-training menses. J Sports Med Phys Fitness 29(2):163–9, 1989.
11. Christ DM, Hill JM: Diet and insulin like growth factor I in relation to body composition in women with exercise induced hypothalamic amenorrhea. J Am Col Nutr 9(3):200–4, 1990.
12. Coggan AR: Plasma glucose metabolism during exercise in humans. Sports Med 11(2):102–24, 1991.
13. Cokkinades VE, Macrea CA, Pate RP: Menstrual dysfunction among habitual runners. Women Health 16(2):59–69,1990.
14. Committee on Sports Medicine 1986–89: Amenorrhea in adolescent athletes. Pediatrics 4(2):394–5,1989.
15. Constantini N, Warren MP: Special problems with a female athlete. Baillieres Clin Rheumatol 8(1):199–219, 1994.
16. Cumming DC, Vickovic MM, Wall SR, et al: Defects in pulsatile LH release in normally menstruating runners. J Clin Endocrinol Metab 60:810–12, 1985.
17. Cumming DC: Exercise associated amenorrhea, low bone density, and estrogen replacement therapy. Arch Intern Med 156:2193–5, 1996.

18. De Cree C: Endogenous opioid peptides in the control of the normal menstrual cycle and their possible role in athletic menstrual irregularities. Obstet Gynecol Surv 44(10):720–32, 1989.

19. De Cree C: The possible involvement of endogenous opioid peptides and catechol estrogens in provoking menstrual irregularities in women athletes. Int J Sports Med 11:329–48, 1990.

20. Demers LM, Harrison TS, Halbert DR: Effective prolonged exercise on plasma prostaglandin levels. Prostaglandins 6:413–8, 1981.

21. DeSouza MJ, Maguire MS, Maresh CN, et al: Adrenal activation and the prolactin response to exercise in eumenorrheic and amenorrheic runners. J Appl Physiol 70(6):2378–87, 1991.

22. DeSouza MJ, Sequenzia LC: Menstrual phase and exercise: intermediary effects on glucose metabolism. Semin Reprod Endocrinol 12(2):97–109, 1994.

23. Disorders of ovary and female reproductive tract. In Wilson JD, Foster DW (eds): Williams Textbook of Endocrinology, 7th edition. Philadelphia, WB Saunders, 1985, p 206.

24. Drinkwater BL, Bruemner B, Chestnut CH III: Menstrual history as a determinant of current bone density in young athletes. JAMA 263(4):545–8, 1990.

25. Dueck C, Matt KS, Manore MM, et al. Treatment of athletic amenorrhea with a diet and training intervention program. Int J Sports Nutr 6:24–40, 1996.

26. Elias AN, Wilson AF: Exercise and genital function. Hum Reprod 8(10):1747–61, 1993.

27. Feicht CB, Johnson JS, Martin BJ, et al: Secondary amenorrhea in athletes. Lancet 2:1145–6, 1978.

28. Frisch RE: Body fat, puberty and fertility. Biol Rev 59:161–88, 1984.

29. Frisch RE: Body weight and reproduction. [Letter] Science 246(4929):432, 1989.

30. Frisch RE, Gotz-Welbergen AV, McArthur JW, et al: Delayed menarche and amenorrhea of college athletes in relation to age of onset of training. JAMA 246(14): 1559–63, 1981.

31. Frisch RE, Snow RC, Johnson LA, et al: Magnetic resonance imaging of overall and regional body fat, estrogen metabolism, and ovulation of athletes compared to controls. J Clin Endocrinol Metab 77(2):471–7, 1993.

32. Gambert SR, Hagen TC, Garthwaite TL: Letter to the Editor. N Engl J Med 305:1590–1, 1981.

33. Glass AR, Deuster PA, Kyle MA, et al: Amenorrhea in olympic marathon runners. Fertil Steril 48:740–5, 1987.

34. Harlan WR, Harlan EA, Grillo GP: Secondary sex characteristics of girls 12 to 17 years of age: the US health examination survey. J Pediatr 96:1074–8, 1980.

35. Hergenroeder AC, Smith EO, Shypailo R, et al: Bone mineral changes in young women with hypothalamic amenorrhea treated with oral contraceptives, medroxyprogesterone, or placebo over 12 months. Am J Obstet Gynecol 176:1017–25, 1997.

36. Hodgen GD: The dominant ovarian follicle. Fertil Steril 38(3):281–300, 1982.

37. Izzo A, Labriola D: Dysmenorrhea and sports activities in adolescence. Clin Exp Obstet Gynecol 18(2): 109–16, 1991.

38. Jenkins PG, Ibanez-Santos X, Holly J, et al: IGF BP-I: a metabolic signal associated with exercise-induced amenorrhea. Neuroendocrinol 57(4):600–4, 1993.

39. Jones GS: Luteal phase defect: a review of pathophysiology. Curr Opin Obstet Gynecol 3(5):641–8, 1991.

40. Jonnavithula S, Warren MP, Fox RP, et al: Bone density is compromised in amenorrheic women despite return of menses: a 2-year study. Obstet Gynecol 81(5):669–74, 1993.

41. Kanders BS, Lindsay R: The effect of physical activity and calcium intake on the bone density of young women aged 24 to 35. Med Sci Sports Exerc 17:284, 1985.

42. Kaplan S, Grumbaugh M: Physiology of puberty. In Flamigni C, Givens J (eds): The Gonadotropins: Basic Science and Clinical Aspects in Females. New York, Academic Press, 1982, p 167.

43. Katz J, Boyar RM, Roffwarg H, et al: Weight and circadian luteinizing hormones secretory pattern in anorexia nervosa. Psychosomat Med 40(7):549–67, 1978.

44. Keen AD, Drinkwater BL: Irreversible bone loss in former amenorrheic athletes. Osteoporosis Int 7:311–5, 1997.

45. Keizer HA, Beckers E, deHaan J, et al: Exercise-induced changes in the percentage of free testosterone and estradiol in trained and untrained women. Int J Sports Med 8(Suppl 3):151–3, 1987.

46. Keizer HA, Rogol AD: Physical exercise and menstrual cycle alterations. What are the mechanisms? Sports Med 10(4):218–35, 1990.

47. Lamon-Fava S, Fisher EC, Nelson ME, et al: Effect of exercise in menstrual cycle status on plasma lipids, low density lipoprotein particle size and apolipoproteins. J Clin Endocrinol Metab 68:17, 1989.

48. Laughlin GA, Loucks AB, Yen SSC: Marked augmentation of nocturnal melatonin secretion in amenorrheic athletes but not in cycling athletes: unaltered by opioidergic or dopaminergic blockade. J Clin Endocrinol Metab 73:1321–6, 1991.

49. Laughlin GA, Yen SSC: Hypoleptinemia in women athletes: absence of a diurnal rhythm with amenorrhea. J Clin Endocrinol Metab 82(1):318–21, 1997.

50. LeBrun CM: The effect of the phase of the menstrual cycle and the birth control pill on athletic performance. Clin Sports Med 13(2):419–41, 1994.

51. Lindberg JS, Fears WB, Hunt MM, et al. Exercise induced amenorrhea and bone density. Ann Intern Med 101:647–8, 1984.

52. Lloyd T, Triantafyllou SJ, Baker ER, et al: Women athletes with menstrual irregularity have increased musculoskeletal injuries. Med Sci Sports Exerc 18(4):374–9, 1986.

53. Loucks AB, Horvath SM: Athletic amenorrhea: a review. Med Sci Sports Exerc 17(1):56–72, 1985.

54. Loucks AJ, Verdun M, Heath EM. Low energy availability, not stress of exercise, alters LH pulsatility in exercising women. J Appl Physiol 84(1):37–46, 1998.

55. Mantzoros CS: The role of leptin in human obesity and disease: a review of current evidence. Ann Intern Med 130:671–80, 1999.

56. Marcus R, Cann C, Madvig P, et al: Menstrual function and bone mass in elite women distance runners. Endocrine and metabolic features. Ann Intern Med 102(2):158–63, 1985.

57. Merriam GR, Maclusky NJ, Picard MK: Comparative properties of the catechol estrogens. I: Methylation by catechol-O-methyltransferase and binding to cytosol estrogen receptors. Steroids 36:1–11, 1980.

58. Myerson M, Gutin B, Warren MP, et al: Resting metabolic rate and energy balance in amenorrheic and eumenorrheic runners. Med Sci Sports Exerc 21(1):15–22, 1991.

59. Neideral JB, Fogel HJ: Estracatechol. J Am Chem Soc 71:2566–8, 1949.

60. Otis CL: Exercise associated amenorrhea. Clin Sports Med 11(2):351–62, 1992.

61. Pirke KM, Schweiger U, Vroocks A, et al: LH and FSH secretion patterns in female athletes with and without menstrual disturbances. Clin Endocrinol 33(3):345–53, 1993.

62. Prior JC: Luteal phase defects and anovulation: adaptive alterations occurring with conditioning exercise. Semin Reprod Endocrinol 3:27–33, 1985.

63. Prior JC, Vigna YM, McKay DW: Reproduction for the athletic women: New understandings of physiology and management. Sports Med 14(3):190–9, 1992.

64. Reindollar RH, Tho SPT, McDonough PG: Delayed puberty: an updated study of 326 patients, Trans Am Gynecol Obestet Soc 8:146, 1989.

65. Reiter EO, Grumbach MM: Neuroendocrine control mechanisms and the onset of puberty. Annu Rev Physiol 44:595–613, 1982.

66. Rockainen H, Pakarinen A, Kirkinen P, et al: Physical exercise induced changes and season-associated differences in the pituitary–ovarian function of runners and joggers. J Clin Endocrinol Metab 60(3):416–22, 1985.

67. Saldi V, Nagwekar SL, Patel DN: Exercise induced delayed menarche and amenorrhea. J Postgrad Med 34(4):211–5, 1988.

68. Samuels MH, Sanborn CF, Hofeldt F, Robbins R: The role of endogenous opiates in athletic amenorrhea. Fertil Steril 55(3):507–12, 1991.

69. Shangold M, Freeman R, Thysen B, Gatz M: The relationship between long distance running, plasma progesterone and luteal phase length. Fertil Steril 31:130, 1979.

70. Shangold M, Rebar RW, Wentz AC, Schiff L: Evaluation and management of menstrual dysfunction in athletes. JAMA 263(12):1665–9, 1990.

71. Shangold MM: Causes, evaluation, and management of athletic oligomenorrhea/amenorrhea. Med Clin North Am 69(1):83–95, 1985.

72. Speroff L, Glass RH, Case NG: Clinical Gynecologic Endocrinology and Infertility. Baltimore, Williams & Wilkins, 1994, pp 402–6.

73. Steege JE, Blumenthal JA: The effects of aerobic exercise on premenstrual symptoms in middle age women: preliminary study. J Psychosomat Res 37(2):127–33, 1993.

74. Warren MP: Amenorrhea in endurance runners. J Clin Endocrinol Metab 75(6):1393–7, 1992.

75. Warren MP, Brooks-Gunn J, Hamilton LH, et al: Scoliosis and fractures in young ballet dancers. Relation to delayed menarche and secondary amenorrhea. N Engl J Med 314:1348–53, 1986.

76. Warren MP, Voussoughian F, Geer EB, et al: Functional hypothalamic amenorrhea: hypoleptinemia and disordered eating. J Clin Endocrinol Metab 84(3):873–7, 1999.

77. Wentz AC. Body weight and amenorrhea. Obstet Gynecol 56:482–7, 1980.

78. Williams NI, Young JC, McArthur JW, et al: Strenuous exercise with caloric restriction: Set on luteinizing hormone secretion. Med Sci Sports Exerc 27:1390–8, 1995.

79. Yen SSC. Hypogonadotropic/hypogonadism. Endocrinol Metab Clin North Am 22(1):29–8, 1993.

Chapter 14

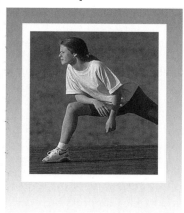

Updates in Exercise-Associated Amenorrhea and Leptin

Michelle P. Warren, M.D.
Russalind Ramos, M.D.
Lauren Bari Davis, B.A.

Women have become increasingly physically active over the past few decades. In 1970 the only woman who ran in the New York City Marathon did not finish. Twenty years later 5249 women entered and 4500 finished; in 2000 over 8300 women finished the marathon. However, as women became more involved in athletics, physicians noted that intense exercise could pose a unique set of risks to the health of the female athlete. In 1992, the American College of Sports Medicine stated that female athletes were in danger of developing one or more of 3 inter-related disorders within the so-called female athlete triad, which refers to amenorrhea, osteoporosis, and disordered eating. Reproductive dysfunction seen in female athletes and women with eating disorders results from a disturbance of the gonadotropin-releasing hormone (GnRH) pulse generator, which leads to a hypoestrogenic state. One of the major risks associated with hypoestrogenic amenorrhea is compromised bone density, putting women at great risk for osteopenia, osteoporosis, scoliosis, and bone fractures.

Original theories attempting to explain the well-documented association between hypoestrogenic amenorrhea and bone loss focused on the role of estrogen as a mediator of bone resorption. However, accumulating evidence suggests that metabolic factors associated with nutritional insult and energy drain may be more important in regulating bone activity. In particular, the hormone leptin, discovered in 1994, may play a significant role in the mediation of reproductive function as it responds to a negative energy balance found in women with exercise-induced hypothalamic amenorrhea. Leptin has been found to be a regulator of the basal metabolic rate and a critical indicator of nutritional status.[10,31,41] Leptin levels are also directly proportional to the body fat mass and there appears to be a critical leptin level necessary to maintain normal menstrual cycles.[19,44] In general, amenorrheic athletes are found to have abnormal leptin secretion and low metabolic rates.[31,21] This response may trigger the changes seen in GnRH pulsatility since leptin receptors have been found on the hypothalamic neurons believed to be involved in the control of the GnRH pulse generator.[6]

Interestingly, leptin receptors have also been found on bone[3,8] which suggests that the hormone may function as a physiologic regulator of bone mass as well as GnRH pulsatility. Therefore, the leptin–metabolic axis may represent a mechanism, other than hypoestrogenism, that could account for the low bone density and high stress fracture rates seen in women with amenorrhea associated with caloric deficiency, nutritional insults, and intense exercise. This chapter reviews the pathophysiology of exercise-associated amenorrhea and the evidence supporting its link to metabolic parameters, as well as some of the more recent evidence that suggests that leptin may be partially responsible for the homeostasis of both bone maintenance and normal menstrual cycles. Understanding the role of leptin as a metabolic signal that connects the neuroendocrine, reproductive, and metabolic systems may give doctors and scientists a better understanding of how the 3 components of the female athlete triad are inter-related and how best to treat them.

EXERCISE-ASSOCIATED AMENORRHEA

Although the specific hormonal profiles of athletes with reproductive irregularities may vary depending on the kind of athletic discipline a woman participates in (sports emphasizing low weight versus sports emphasizing strength), exercise-associated reproductive abnormalities usually stem from dysfunction at the hypothalamic level. Women with low body weight and low body fat due to excessive exercise or disordered eating frequently develop amenorrhea. *Amenorrhea* is defined as the lack of a regular menstrual period and may be classified as either primary or secondary in nature. Primary amenorrhea is diagnosed if menstrual bleeding has never occurred by age 14 with no appearance of secondary sex characteristics; or age 16 with the appearance of secondary sex characteristics. Secondary amenorrhea is the absence of menstruation for 3 months if previous menses were regular, or for 6 months if previous menses were irregular.[34]

The most common hormonal pattern seen in amenorrheic athletes includes low gonadotropins and hypoestrogenism, resulting from the disruption of the hypothalamic–pituitary–ovarian axis. Specifically, there is a suppression of the pulsatile release of GnRH, which normally occurs every 60 to 90 minutes. This GnRH suppression thus limits the pituitary secretion of luteinizing hormone (LH) and, to a lesser extent, follicle-stimulating hormone (FSH), which, in turn, limits ovarian stimulation and the production of estradiol. A wide spectrum of abnormalities, from decreased frequency and amplitude of pulses to a pattern of sporadic pulses or nocturnal entrainment of LH pulses, can occur. A prolonged follicular phase, or the absence of the critical LH or estradiol surge mid-cycle, is what leads to the mild or intermittent suppression of menstrual cycles in many athletic women. Very low LH levels also result in delayed menarche or primary or secondary amenorrhea.[27,42]

The amenorrhea associated with sports requiring low body weight (such as ballet dancing, long-distance running, and figure skating) is very similar to that seen in women with anorexia nervosa.[38,45] Previously, it was believed that the cause of this type of amenorrhea was the presence of body fat below a certain critical level.[16] However, this body composition hypothesis has been increasingly challenged over the years as researchers have confirmed that there is no specific body fat percentage below which regular menses cease[26,43] and that this specific hypothesis is based entirely on correlation rather than experimental evidence.[37] In fact, regular menstrual cycles have been seen in female athletes with less than 17% body fat and amenorrheic and eumenorrheic runners have

been found to have the same percentage of body fat.

Another theory as to the cause of exercise-associated amenorrhea is the exercise stress hypothesis, which states that intensive athletic training activates the hypothalamic–pituitary–adrenal axis, which is thus the cause of the suppression of GnRH pulsatility and subsequently the menstrual cycle. However, this theory has also been challenged recently as experiments attempting to induce menstrual dysfunction in women have shown that exercise alone has no effect on LH suppression, but when exercise is coupled with caloric restriction, LH suppression does occur.[24,25] Therefore, the stress of exercise is not a direct cause of reproductive dysfunction among female athletes but rather an additive factor. This evidence suggests that GnRH pulsatility may be affected by metabolic parameters, specifically energy drain and nutritional insults, and that the suppression of normal reproductive function in female athletes may be a neuroendocrine adaptation to caloric deficit.[42,46]

Many athletes become highly concerned with their body composition and weight and participate in strict dieting, while at the same time maintaining intense training schedules. They often eat a low-fat diet with little or no red meat and thus may also have iron deficiency. A negative caloric balance and energy deficit is often the result of this kind of lifestyle.[27,31] The depleted energy stores stimulate the body to increase food efficiency by decreasing metabolic rate. Studies of women with eating disorder-induced hypothalamic amenorrhea are generally in a severe hypometabolic state, which usually reverses with weight gain. However, hypothalamic and reproductive dysfunction may persist if disordered eating is still present, which also suggests the persistence of metabolic factors inhibiting reproduction that may be independent of weight. In fact, amenorrhea may persist in up to 10% to 30% of recovered anorectics despite a return to normal weight. These findings suggest that metabolic abnormalities may remain in these women and that a factor other than weight must be responsible for the hypothalamic dysfunction.[14,18,20]

However, it is important to note that the energy drain hypothesis may not be the sole explanation for reproductive dysfunction seen among women across all athletic disciplines. In athletes involved in sports in which low body weight is not required and the emphasis is on strength and endurance, the incidence of complete amenorrhea is low and menstrual cycles are more likely to be irregular.[35] These athletes may be participating in strenuous exercise, but are not as likely to be restricting their caloric intake. Their hormone profiles may show elevated LH levels, increased LH:FSH ratios, normal estrogen levels, and higher androgen levels. This type of hyperandrogenism with anovulation may be seen in swimmers and this hormonal profile resembles polycystic ovarian syndrome.[36] Activation of the hypothalamic–pituitary–adrenal axis may be what is occurring in this situation, which results in increased levels of androgens (in particular dehydroepiandrosterone sulfate (DHEA-S)). Chronically high levels of DHEA-S may impair follicular development and result in the anovulation or amenorrhea seen in these particular female athletes. Alternatively, because high levels of androgens positively affect muscle mass and may be therefore advantageous in sports where power is a major determinant of performance, naturally elevated levels of androgens may be self selected in these sports.[9] The syndrome observed in these athletes is less common and has been much less extensively studied than that observed in athletes participating in sports emphasizing thinness. Therefore more research is necessary to determine whether the hormonal profile of these women is genetically determined or secondary to activation of the adrenal axis.

In summary, although women may participate in different athletic disciplines with emphasis on different ideal body types, it is generally accepted that exercise-associated amenorrhea stems from a dysfunction at the hypothalamic level, specifically the suppression of the GnRH pulse generator. The question that remains a source of interest in the field of medicine is what specifically causes the GnRH pulse generator to switch off. More and more evidence indicates that metabolic parameters are associated with hypothalamic amenorrhea, suggesting that a pathway or signal somehow connects the metabolic and reproductive systems. One possible signal that has been implicated in this role is the hormone leptin, a small polypeptide secreted mainly by the adipocyte and which has receptors located on the hypothalamus. The next section looks at leptin as a possible mechanism that signals metabolic changes and deficiencies to the neuroendocrine and reproductive systems, influencing not only menstrual cycles, but also bone formation.

THE ROLE OF LEPTIN

The exact mechanism resulting in GnRH/LH pulsatility suppression, which characterizes the menstrual disturbances among female athletes,

remains unclear. Peripheral signal(s) capable of relating nutritional status to the hypothalamic regulators of reproduction has been implicated to provide a potential link,[24] and the hormone leptin has been suggested to play a role in the interactions between nutrition and reproduction. Leptin, a protein product from the *obesity (ob)* gene is synthesized by adipocytes[13] and placenta.[47] Leptin is secreted into the blood, crosses the blood–brain barrier, and acts in the hypothalamic nuclei to regulate food intake, energy expenditure, growth, and sexual maturation.[5] In addition, recent studies have shown that leptin is also involved with the regulation of bone metabolism.[4,12] Leptin receptors are located primarily in the hypothalamus, and have been found on hypothalamic neurons involved in control of the GnRH pulse generator,[6] thus leptin may be a potential factor involved in signaling low energy availability to the reproductive axis. The potential mechanism by which leptin links the metabolic– reproductive axis is presently unknown. Leptin appears to be regulated by total energy intake and fat stores, and significantly correlates with the body mass index (BMI) in humans.[28] Leptin also regulates the basal metabolic rate and is disproportionately lowered in the presence of fasting.[29]

In addition to its metabolic function, leptin has been shown to affect reproductive and neuroendocrine systems. Low leptin levels have been reported in amenorrheic women who exercise regularly at a high level. The typical diurnal pattern of leptin concentrations found in the normal menstrual cycle is shown to be absent in amenorrheic athletes.[21] The relationship between leptin and the integrity of the reproductive axis does not seem to be related to leptin levels per se, rather it is the absence of a diurnal rhythm that identifies the arrested cyclic reproductive axis (ie, amenorrhea).[21] Recent reports suggest, however, that this diurnal rhythm is mediated by food and is eliminated when feeding does not occur.[17] In this sense, nutritional deficiencies may directly lead to changes in leptin regulation. This also provides further support for the idea that one of leptin's major roles is to aid the body via neuroendocrine changes in adjusting to energy deprivation, which leads to the cessation of menses. There appears to be a threshold leptin level of 1.85 mg, below which menstruation will not occur, although there is considerable variation.[2,19]

Leptin has been implicated in the neuroendocrine response to fasting and has been found to blunt the starvation-induced responses of the gonadal–thyroid–adrenal axis when administered to male mice.[1] Other studies in rats show that the hypothalamic–pituitary–thyroid axis may serve as a critical locus to mediate the central actions of leptin by regulating pro-thyroid stimulating hormone (TSH) gene expression,[22],[23] and reports of leptin mutations in humans indicate lack of pubertal development and suppression of TSH.[7] Thus, leptin's essential roles may be not only to serve the control of body mass but also to be involved in the initiation of puberty. Furthermore, leptin may play a role in enabling the body to respond to starvation by shutting down reproduction.[28] Mammals partition energy among 5 major metabolic activities—cellular maintenance, thermoregulation, locomotion, growth, and reproduction—therefore suppression of reproductive function may be a mechanism that allows the body to adapt to a chronic energy deficit.

One of the most disastrous consequences of exercise-associated amenorrhea is the compromise of bone mineral density, leading to the development of osteopenia or more severely, osteoporosis with increased risk for fractures. Physical activity is important in maintaining bone mass, however, a great number of women tend to exercise excessively, leading to hormonal changes that predispose them to loss of bone mass. At present, not much is known about the effects of leptin on bone, but the interest is certainly increasing, and there is growing evidence for 2 possible mechanisms: one is central regulation, likely by the hypothalamus, and the second is direct effects on bone.

Recent studies[11],[12] have shown that mice deficient in leptin (ob/ob) or its receptor (db/db) have increased bone mass despite hypogonadism and hypercortisolism. Moreover, intracerebroventricular infusion of leptin causes bone loss in leptin-deficient mice. Considering that these animals do not have any circulating leptin in their serum, this result demonstrated that bone formation and therefore bone remodeling, may be centrally regulated, likely by the hypothalamus. This regulatory loop is especially significant because if bone remodeling has a central regulation, then diseases of bone remodeling such as osteopenia and osteoporosis may also be centrally regulated. The researchers of these studies postulated that leptin is a potential inhibitor of bone formation acting through the central nervous system.

Some studies suggest a direct mechanism for leptin's effect on bone. In a study investigating the role of leptin as a hormonal regulator of bone growth,[40] leptin administration led to a significant increase in femoral length, total-body bone area, bone mineral content, and bone density in ob/ob mice. The demonstration of the presence of the signaling or long form (Ob-Rb) of the leptin receptor in both primary adult osteoblasts and chondrocytes suggests that the promoting effects of leptin could be direct. These findings indicate a significant role for leptin in skeletal bone growth and development. In yet another study involving rats, leptin administration was found to be effective at reducing trabecular bone loss and trabecular architectural changes,[4] which further signifies leptin's protective role in bone metabolism.

The findings of these studies on possible central mechanism and direct bone effects have been controversial, with contrasting results. The route of leptin administration is a crucial factor, and it is postulated that leptin's effects on bone may result from a balance between negative central effects and positive peripheral effects depending on serum levels or blood–brain barrier permeability.[4]

Human studies involving leptin have been promising. In a study investigating the relationship between leptin concentration and bone metabolism in the human fetus, it has been found that leptin may decrease bone resorption with the overall effect of increasing bone mass[32]; hence, leptin may play a role in fetal bone metabolism as part of its effect on fetal growth and development. A study on premenarcheal girls revealed leptin's association with periosteal envelope expansion, which led to the hypothesis that leptin might mediate the effects of obesity on bone mass.[30] Furthermore, recombinant leptin therapy given for a year in a child with congenital leptin deficiency induced a decrease in body fat by 15.6 kg and a decrease in lean mass by 0.82 kg, but increased bone mineral mass by 0.15 kg.[15] Moreover, leptin's effect on bone in adult women aged 40 to 60 years has been studied[33] and results indicated that leptin's influence is less significant for the mature than for the growing skeleton, which suggests that leptin influences modeling of growing bones rather than remodeling of the mature skeleton.

Researchers traditionally attributed the bone loss in women with exercise-associated amenorrhea to estrogen deficiency leading to increased bone turnover and excessive bone resorption, as is observed in postmenopausal women. However, more recent research has challenged the notion that hypoestrogenism is the primary cause of bone loss in active amenorrheic women, and we now understand that undernutrition and its metabolic consequences appear to result directly in a reduction in bone turnover[48] and, more importantly, reduced bone formation,[39] thereby causing osteopenia. These data suggest that undernutrition may underlay the bone remodeling imbalance and bone loss in active amenorrheic women, and furthermore, that nutritional factors may counteract or override the stimulatory effects of an estrogen deficiency on bone turnover. In addition, a potential metabolic factor such as leptin may also play a role. In fact, a recent study on rats with ovariectomy-induced bone loss has shown that a combination of estrogen and leptin further decreased bone turnover compared with estrogen treatment alone.[4]

In conclusion, there is growing evidence to suggest that there is a metabolic relay of homeostasis of bone metabolism and maintenance of normal menstrual cycle. The limited number of data on leptin's role in metabolic and reproductive physiology has provided us some important, yet still preliminary information. Further studies are warranted and it is hoped that future protocols will be designed to evaluate the direct effects of leptin administration in humans.

References

1. Ahima RS, Prabakaran D, Mantzoros C: Role of leptin in the neuroendocrine response to fasting. Nature 382:250–2, 1996.
2. Ballauff A, Ziegler A, Emons G, et al: Serum leptin and gonadotropin levels in patients with anorexia nervosa during weight gain. Mol Psychiatry 4(1):71–5, 1999.
3. Bradley, SJ, Taylor MJ, Rovet JF, et al: Assessment of brain function in adolescent anorexia nervosa before and after weight gain. J Clin Exper Neuropsych 19(1):20–33, 1997.
4. Burguera B, Hofbauer LC, Thomas T, et al: Leptin reduces ovariectomy-induced bone loss in rats. Endocrinology 142(8):3546–53, 2001.
5. Casanueva FF, Dieguez C: Neuroendocrine regulation and actions of leptin. Front Neuroendocrinol 20(4):317–63, 1999.
6. Cheung CC, Thornton JE, Kuijper JL, et al: Leptin is a metabolic gate for the onset of puberty in the female rat. Endocrinology 138(2):855–8, 1997.
7. Clement K, Vaisse C, Lahlou N, et al: A mutation in the human leptin receptor gene causes obesity and pituitary dysfunction. Nature 392:398–401,1998.
8. Constantini NW, Warren MP: Physical activity, fitness, and reproductive health in women: Clinical observations. In Bouchard C, Shephard RJ, Stephens T (eds): Physical Activity, Fitness, and Health: International Proceedings and Consensus Statement. Champaign, Ill, Human Kinetics, 1994, pp 955–66.
9. Constantini NW, Warren MP: Menstrual dysfunction in swimmers: a distinct entity. J Clin Endocrinol Metab 80:2740–4, 1995.
10. Cunningham MJ, Clifton DK, Steiner RA: Leptin's actions on the reproductive axis: perspectives and mechanisms. Biol Reprod 60(2):216–22, 1999.
11. Ducy P, Schinke T, Karsenty G: The osteoblast: a sophisticated fibroblast under central surveillance. Science 289(5484):1501–4, 2000.
12. Ducy P, Amling M, Takeda S, et al: Leptin inhibits bone formation through a hypothalamic relay: a central control of bone mass. Cell 100(2):197–207, 2000.
13. Elmquist JK, Maratos-Flier E, Saper CB, Flier JS: Unraveling the central nervous system pathways underlying responses to leptin. Nature Neurosci 1(6):445–50, 1998.
14. Falk JR, Halmi KA: Amenorrhea in anorexia nervosa: examination of the critical body weight hypothesis. Biol Psych 17:799–806, 1982.
15. Farooqi IS, Jebb SA, Langmack G, et al: Effects of recombinant leptin therapy in a child with congenital leptin deficiency. N Engl J Med 341(12):879–84, 1999.
16. Frisch RE, McArthur JW: Menstrual cycles: fatness as a determinant of minimum weight for height necessary for their maintenance or onset. Science 185:949–51, 1974.
17. Frusztajer NT, Dhuper S, Warren MP, et al: Nutrition and the incidence of stress fractures in ballet dancers. Am J Clin Nutr 51:779–83, 1990.
18. Kohmura H, Miyake A, Aono T, Tanizawa O: Recovery of reproductive function in patients with anorexia nervosa: a 10-year follow up study. Eur J Obstet Gynecol Reprod Biol 22:293–6, 1986.
19. Kopp W, Blum WF, von Prittwitz S, et al: Low leptin levels predict amenorrhea in underweight and eating disordered females. Mol Psychiatry 2(4):335–40, 1997.
20. Kreipe RE, Churchill BH, Strauss J: Long-term outcome of adolescents with anorexia nervosa. Am J Dis Child 143:1322–7, 1989.
21. Laughlin GA, Yen SSC: Hypoleptinemia in women athletes: absence of a diurnal rhythm with amenorrhea. J Clin Endocrinol Metab 82(1):318–21, 1997.
22. Legradi G, Emerson CH, Ahima RS, Flier JS, Lechan RM: Leptin prevents fasting-induced suppression of prothyrotropin-releasing hormone messenger ribonucleic acid in neurons of the hypothalamic paraventricular nucleus. Endocrinology 138:2569–76, 1997.
23. Legradi G, Emerson CH, Ahima RS, et al: Arcuate nucleus ablation prevents fasting-induced suppression of ProTRH MRNA in the hypothalamic paraventricular nucleus. Neuroendocrinology 68:89–97, 1998.
24. Loucks AB, Verdun M, Heath EM: Low energy availability, not stress of exercise, alters LH pulsatility in exercising women. J Appl Physiol 84(1):37–46, 1998.
25. Loucks AB: Exercise training in the normal female. In Warren MP, Constantini NW: Sports Endocrinology. Totowa, NJ, Humana Press, 2000, pp 165–80.
26. Loucks AB, Horvath SM: Athletic amenorrhea: a review. Med Sci Sports Exerc 17(1):56–72, 1985.
27. Loucks AB, Mortola JF, Girton L, Yen, SSC: Alterations in the hypothalamic-pituitary-ovarian and the hypothalamic-pituitary-adrenal axes in athletic women. J Clin Endocrinol Metab 68:402–11, 1989.
28. Macut D, Micic D, Pralong FP, et al: Is there a role for leptin in human reproduction? Gynecol Endocrinol 12(5):321–6, 1998.
29. Maffei M, Halaas J, Ravussin E, et al: Leptin levels in human and rodent: measurement of plasma leptin and Ob RNA in obese and weight-reduced subjects. Nature Med 1(11):1155–61, 1995.
30. Matkovic V, Ilich JZ, Skugor M, et al: Leptin is inversely related to age at menarche in human females. J Clin Endocrinol Metab 82(10):3239–45, 1997.
31. Myerson M, Gutin B, Warren MP, et al: Resting metabolic rate and energy balance in amenorrheic and eumenorrheic runners. Med Sci Sports Exerc 23(1):15–22, 1991.
32. Ogueh O, Sooranna S, Nicolaides KH, Johnson MR: The relationship between leptin concentration and bone metabolism in the human fetus. J Clin Endocrinol Metab 85(5):1997–9, 2000.

33. Rauch F, Blum WF, Klein K, et al: Does leptin have an effect on bone in adult women? Calcif Tissue Int 63(6):453–5, 1998.
34. Sakala E: Obstetrics & Gynecology: Board Review Series. Baltimore, MD, Williams & Wilkins, 1997, pp 266–272.
35. Sanborn CF, Martin BJ, Wagner WW Jr: Is athletic amenorrhea specific to runners? Am J Obstet Gynecol 143:859–61, 1982.
36. Sanborn CF, Albrecht BH, Wagner WW Jr: Athletic amenorrhea: lack of association with body fat. Med Sci Sports Exerc 19(3):207–12, 1987.
37. Schneider JE, Wade GN: Letter to the editor. Am J Physiol (Endocrinol Metab) 273(36):E2331–2, 1997.
38. Schweiger U: Menstrual function and luteal-phase deficiency in relation to weight changes and dieting. Clin Obstet Gynecol 34(1):191–7, 1991.
39. Soyka LA, Grinspoon S, Levitsky LL, et al: The effects of anorexia nervosa on bone metabolism in female adolescents. J Clin Endocrinol Metab 84(12):4489–96, 1999.
40. Steppan CM, Crawford DT, Chidsey-Frink KL, et al: Leptin is a potent stimulator of bone growth in Ob/Ob mice. Regul Pept 92(1–3):73–8, 2000.
41. Thong FS, McLean C, Graham TE: Plasma leptin in female athletes: relationship with body fat, reproductive, nutritional, and endocrine factors. J Appl Physiol 88(6):2037–44, 2000.
42. Warren MP: The effects of exercise on pubertal progression and reproductive function in girls. J Clin Endocrinol Metab 51(5):1150–7, 1980.
43. Warren MP: Eating, body weight and menstrual function. In Brownell KD, Rodin J, Wilmore JH: Eating, Body Weight and Performance in Athletes: Disorders of Modern Society. Philadelphia, Lea & Febiger, 1992, pp 222–34.
44. Warren MP, Voussoughian F, Geer EB, et al: Functional hypothalamic amenorrhea: hypoleptinemia and disordered eating. J Clin Endocrinol Metab 84(3):873–7, 1999.
45. Wilmore JH, Wambsgans KC, Brenner M, et al: Is there energy conservation in amenorrheic compared with eumenorrheic distance runners? J Appl Physiol 72(1):15–22, 1992.
46. Winterer J, Cutler GB Jr, Loriaux DL: Caloric balance, brain to body ratio, and the timing of menarche. Med Hypotheses 15:87–91, 1985.
47. Yura S, Sagawa N, Mise H, et al: A positive umbilical venous-arterial difference of leptin level and its rapid decline after birth. Am J Obstet Gynecol 178(5):926–30, 1998.
48. Zanker CL, Swaine IL: Bone turnover in amenorrhoeic and eumenorrhoeic distance runners. Scand J Med Sci Sports 8:20–6, 1998.

Chapter 15

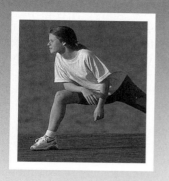

Hormonal Disorders

James W. Akin, M.D.

Hormonal disorders commonly affect women of all ages. Because the female athlete is at increased risk for menstrual dysfunction and its associated sequelae, physicians and other health professionals working with female athletes should be familiar with the various types of hormonal disorders that may arise and their treatment options. This chapter reviews treatment strategies for common menstrual disorders seen in the female athlete, as well as other hormonal disorders in women.

AMENORRHEA AND OLIGOMENORRHEA

Hypothalamic amenorrhea, as is commonly seen in the female athlete, results in decreased ovarian hormone production and hypoestrogenemia, which can contribute to a decrease in bone mineral density. As discussed in other chapters, female athletes commonly have irregular or absent menstrual cycles due to alterations within the normal hypothalamic–pituitary–ovarian axis. One hypothesis for these alterations is that they are a response to excessive stress from strenuous exercise and training. The theory suggests that stress leads to an elevation in the serum cortisol level as a result of increased cortisol-releasing hormone from the hypothalamus and adrenal corticotropin hormone (ACTH) from the pituitary gland. Cortisol-releasing hormone has been demonstrated to have a depressive effect on the arcuate nucleus within the hypothalamus, which controls the reproductive hormones via the simultaneous release of endogenous central nervous system opioids. The arcuate nucleus within the hypothalamus is responsible for pulsatile gonadotropin-releasing hormone (GnRH). GnRH modulates the release of follicle-stimulating hormone (FSH) and luteinizing hormone (LH) from the anterior pituitary. FSH and LH control ovarian hormonal activity to achieve normal ovulatory cycles, which are regular and estrogen producing in the follicular phase and progesterone producing after ovulation.[3,7,14]

A more widely accepted hypothesis for amenorrhea in exercising women is known as the *energy-availability hypothesis*.[18] The energy-availability hypothesis suggests that the initial trigger in the above hypothalamic–pituitary pathway is not stress but rather a direct result of a low amount of available energy. The low amount of available energy results in the shutting down of the GnRH pulse generator directly by some yet to be determined signal. Whether or not dietary intervention to increase available energy would completely reverse this hypothalamic–pituitary disruption and subsequent menstrual disturbance remains to be fully determined.[18]

As the level of hypothalamic suppression increases in athletes, normal menstrual cycles initially become irregular, then frequently stop altogether. Amenorrhea, oligomenorrhea, anovulation, and luteal-phase defect all may lie on the same spectrum, representing varying degrees of hypothalamic dysfunction, although luteal-phase dysfunction has been hypothesized to represent adaptation to physical stress in some individuals.[23]

Estrogen-breakthrough bleeding is the most common cause of abnormal uterine bleeding in women less than 35 years of age.[24] In nonathletic women, generally if the patient is having estrogen-breakthrough bleeding she most likely has enough estrogen to prevent osteoporosis or adverse cardiovascular changes, although progestin treatment to control the bleeding may be considered. However, in the athletic patient, the decreased amount of estrogen seen with amenorrhea and, in some cases, oligomenorrhea, may not be enough to prevent adverse bone effects.[8] In the female athlete with amenorrhea or prolonged oligomenorrhea, bone density should be measured, especially in those with disordered eating, low weight, and/or a history of stress fracture.

If a female athlete has had a complete diagnostic workup for her amenorrhea or oligomenorrhea and other causes of menstrual dysfunction have been ruled out, she may initially benefit from a trial of nutritional intervention (calcium supplementation in the range of 1200 to 1500 mg/day and increased caloric intake) and/or a reduction in exercise intensity to restore a positive energy balance, with the goal of achieving normal menstrual function.[9] The appropriate duration of this nonpharmacologic intervention varies and needs to be individualized. Female athletes 16 years of age and older who do not respond to this nonpharmacologic treatment, especially if low bone density has been noted, may benefit from estrogen-replacement therapy (ERT) or low-dose oral contraceptive pills (OCPs) in the effort to maintain or improve bone mineral density.[11] Use of ERT and OCPs in this population, however, is still controversial and may not result in increased bone density.[13,19,27] In fact, Weaver and colleagues have found that exercising women using OCPs actually had a lower spine bone mineral density and bone mineral content after 24 months compared to nonexercising women using OCPs.[28] Additional treatments for osteoporosis prevention in young female athletes and postmenopausal women may also be considered and are discussed further in Chapters 24 and 26. In those women identified as having nutritional concerns and disordered eating patterns, referral to a nutritionist and psychologist should be considered. If significantly underweight, weight gain may be recommended.

Athletes with anovulation or luteal-phase defects and some athletes with oligomenorrhea may not be hypoestrogenic and may respond to a progesterone challenge. Medroxyprogesterone acetate 10 mg/day for 5 to 10 days per month may prevent irregular menses as well as the possible risk of endometrial hyperplasia. If there is no withdrawal bleeding with estrogen, then OCPs or ERT can be prescribed.

The management of young female athletes with delayed menarche is more controversial. The aim is to resume normal menses in order to avoid the potential risk of osteopenia and future fractures. Nutrition should be optimized, including adequate calcium and caloric intake, and exercise training decreased if indicated, with the goal of restoration of adequate weight.[1] In order to prevent premature closure of the epiphyses, linear growth should be completed (usually after 16 years of age) before consideration of hormonal therapy.

LUTEAL-PHASE DEFECT

Luteal-phase defect usually manifests as short cycle lengths caused by inadequate luteal phase of the menstrual cycle due to insufficient progesterone support of the endometrium. It may be difficult to diagnose, however, as menstrual periods may occur regularly. A number of factors may contribute to luteal-phase defect, including decreased production of progesterone by the ovary, decreased levels of FSH in the follicular phase, abnormal LH surging, or decreased response of the endometrium to progesterone.

Exercising women may develop luteal-phase defect from impaired folliculogenesis, with decreased progesterone during periods of training and reduced LH pulse frequency.[17] Although euestrogenic, exercising women with luteal-phase defect may be at risk for osteopenia,[21] however, more research is needed in this area.

Methods to test for luteal-phase defect include basal body temperature monitoring, use of ovulation predictor kits to test for LH surge, and checking serum progesterone levels, as well as obtaining an endometrial biopsy. By strict definition, luteal-phase defect is diagnosed when 2 endometrial biopsies are abnormal.[24]

Luteal-phase defect in the exercising women need only be treated if pregnancy is desired and needs to be considered as a possible diagnosis in women with recurrent spontaneous abortion. The first step toward treatment is to decrease exercise and improve caloric and nutritional intake. If luteal-phase defect persists and pregnancy is desired, pharmacologic treatment options include progesterone supplementation, clomiphene citrate therapy, and gonadotropin therapy. The latter 2 treatments will stimulate ovulation and increase progesterone after ovulation. There is an increased risk for multiple births with these treatments.

Progesterone supplementation is usually started 3 days after ovulation and can be given as a vaginal suppository, a twice-daily oral dosage, or intramuscularly. Progesterone supplementation is continued until menses starts or pregnancy is diagnosed. If pregnancy is achieved, the progesterone is often continued for 8 to 10 weeks, by which time the placenta has achieved adequate production of progesterone independent of the ovaries.

DISORDERS OF EXCESSIVE ANDROGEN PRODUCTION

Hirsutism and Irregular Menses

The presence of excessive hair in women usually results from excess production of androgens. Androgens are normally produced in 2 endocrine glands, the adrenal cortex and the ovarian stroma. Androgens are precursors of certain estrogen compounds and also play a role in female libido. Normal male levels of the androgen testosterone are 300 to 800 ng/dL, whereas normal female levels are 20 to 80 ng/dL. Typically, levels in women with hirsutism fall in between these values.[24]

The adrenal gland mainly produces the weaker androgens androstenedione and dehydroepiandrosterone sulfate (DHEAS), making a smaller amount of the more potent testosterone. The ovary does not produce DHEAS but does produce both androstenedione and testosterone.[24]

Although androgens have an effect on hair growth in both men and women, the total number of hair follicles is determined prior to birth and does not differ according to sex. The number of hair follicles does differ depending on ethnic background, with persons of Mediterranean decent having more follicles than those of Nordic descent, and Caucasians having more hair follicles than Asians.[16] Testosterone, from either the ovary or the adrenal gland, is converted at the level of the hair follicle to the more potent androgen, dihydrotestosterone, which is directly responsible for converting hair from a lanugo pattern to a coarse terminal pattern.

Females ordinarily have a predominance of lanugo hair, with the exception of the axillae and pubic area. Conversion of the fine lanugo hair to the coarse terminal hair in other places such as the face, chest, and abdomen results in clinical hirsutism. As the testosterone level rises, there is more conversion of hair to the terminal type. This conversion is not reversible and the only option for removal of existing terminal hair is electrolysis. Still, treatment of androgen overproduction is important in order to prevent further conversion of remaining lanugo hair. The most common preventive treatment is through the use of OCPs, as will be discussed later in this chapter.

Medical treatment for hirsutism can also be directed at the hair follicle. Spironolactone, a mild diuretic, is known to interfere with 5-α-reductase, which converts testosterone to dihydrotestosterone at the hair follicle. The conversion of testosterone to dihydrotestosterone is necessary for stimulation of hair growth. Therefore, spironolactone has some ability to slow conversion of lanugo hair to terminal hair.[31] Antiandrogens such as flutamide and cimetidine are antagonist at the androgen receptor on the hair follicle and are also used in the treatment of hirsutism.

Chronic Anovulation

Patients with chronic anovulation or irregular menses frequently have elevated androgen levels from an ovarian source. In patients who are not ovulating, continued LH stimulation results in increased ovarian stromal androgen production in the form of androstenedione and testosterone.[5]

Appropriate ways to manage the overproduction of ovarian androgen are by suppressing ovarian hormonal production entirely by giving OCPs and by breaking the cycle of excess LH stimulation by inducing ovulation.[4] Ovulation can be induced by the introduction of fertility medications such as clomiphene citrate or by human menopausal gonadotropin therapy. However, such fertility medications are a poor choice for the chronic management of anovulation in an athlete because of their high cost and side effects, including the predisposition to ovarian cyst development and the possible long-term increased risk of ovarian cancer.[22,30] OCPs are a very good choice for female athletes who do not have any of the contraindications to them (see Chapter 17). Almost all OCPs contain the synthetic estrogen ethinyl estradiol in various amounts, while most of the pills differ in their synthetic progestin component. Many of the newer pills contain the progestins desogestrel and norgestimate. Desogestrel and norgestimate have the least androgenic side effects of all the synthetic progestins. OCPs containing these synthetic progestins should be considered as first-line therapy in patients with hirsutism.

Polycystic Ovarian Disease

Polycystic ovarian disease (PCOD) is a very common disorder. Classic patients with PCOD were described as obese and hirsute with irregular or absent menses. However, many women of normal weight suffer from PCOD.

Controversy exists over the starting point of PCOD. The argument mirrors the old riddle: which came first, the chicken or the egg? Some investigators believe the cause of PCOD exists within the arcuate nucleus within the hypothalamus.[26] The arcuate nucleus in PCOD patients releases too much GnRH too frequently, which leads to a predominance of LH over FSH release, favoring excess androgen production from the follicle. Excess androgen production poisons follicular development and causes arrest at an early stage. These small follicles are numerous, hence the term *polycystic ovarian disease*. A lack of ovulation results in a lack of proper feedback to the hypothalamus, and thus repetition of the cycle.

Some investigators believe the problem starts in the ovary with the overproduction of androgens, which then results in the same vicious cycle.[6] This theory is plausible since giving a normal patient exogenous androgen will precipitate the same clinical picture as seen with PCOD. Another argument in favor of an ovarian origin is the fact that excising portions of the ovary that produce androgens improves the syndrome and may result in ovulation. An old surgical technique called *ovarian wedge resection* did just that. The removal of ovarian stroma resulted in lowered production of ovarian androgen, causing the patient to ovulate. The problem with this treatment is that the surgery frequently caused adhesions to the ovarian surface, which can itself be a source of infertility. This procedure is only rarely performed today since drugs are available to induce ovulation in most patients.

A more recent theory about the etiology of PCOD suggests that these patients have an abnormal insulin receptor. The pancreas compensates for an abnormal insulin receptor by increasing the amount of circulating insulin in the bloodstream, thus lowering glucose levels down to normal. These higher than normal blood levels of insulin cross react with insulin-like growth factor type 1 (IGF-1) receptors on the ovary, which causes the release of excessive ovarian androgens. The excess circulating ovarian androgens such as androstenedione and testosterone result in the pattern of PCOD described above.[10]

Testosterone levels in patients with PCOD are frequently elevated but these levels are not usually within the normal range for males. Testosterone levels over 200 ng/mL require a search for neoplasia, but only about 20% of the time is an ovarian neoplasm, such as an arrhenoblastoma, diagnosed.[24]

DHEAS is a specific androgen secreted by the adrenal gland. When it is elevated it usually implies an adrenal problem. Patients with PCOD, however, may have an elevated DHEAS level, thought secondary to an estrogen-induced 3-β-hydroxysteroid dehydrogenase insufficiency.[15]

Female athletes are not at increased risk for PCOD but certainly may suffer from this disorder. Long-term sequelae of PCOD include irregular bleeding, which at times may require dilatation and curettage to control and may even require transfusion. Other health risks if the condition is untreated are an increased risk of developing endometrial cancer from the prolonged unopposed estrogen effect and potential coronary heart disease from the elevated insulin levels.[20] Infertility is also seen from the lack of ovulation, although some patients with PCOD occasionally do ovulate.

The main treatment is OCPs to suppress ovarian androgen production and provide progesterone-induced menses on a regular basis. This treatment reduces the risk of endometrial cancer to baseline. Patients with PCOD wanting to achieve a pregnancy usually have to take fertility drugs such as clomiphene citrate or human menopausal gonadotropins. The infertility treatments are very effective if no other cause of infertility is present once ovulation is achieved.

A much newer treatment for PCOD is the use of the insulin-lowering drug metformin. Metformin is a biguanide antihyperglycemic drug that enhances insulin sensitivity and insulin-mediated glucose disposal. Upon taking metformin, insulin levels are reduced, which in turn lessens the cross reactivity with IGF-1 receptors on the ovary, thus lowering ovarian androgen production. The long-term treatment of PCOD patients with metformin could also reduce the serious health risks seen with PCOD such as adult-onset diabetes and coronary heart disease.[29]

Excessive Adrenal Androgen Production

Excess adrenal androgen production represents a rare problem usually resulting from an adrenal-producing adenoma or hyperplasia. The hyperplasia may result from a congenital enzyme disorder of 21-hydroxylase deficiency, also referred to as *congenital adrenal hyperplasia* (CAH).

Congenital adrenal hyperplasia is a common genetic abnormality. It usually presents at birth or in childhood but rarely can go undetected and results in adult-onset CAH.[29] CAH in the adult results in elevated 17-hydroxyprogesterone and adrenal androgen levels since there is a decreased ability to produce glucocorticoids such as cortisol. In order to produce adequate amounts of cortisol, increased amounts of other adrenal steroids are made.

Adult-onset CAH usually presents with hirsutism and irregular periods. Treatment is directed at replacing cortisol, which lowers the ACTH, which in turn lowers other adrenal steroids.

A screening test for adult-onset CAH is measurement of the 17-hydroxyprogesterone level. If the level is less than 300 mg/mL, adult-onset CAH is ruled out. If the level is greater than 800 mg/mL, CAH is diagnosed. For patients falling in between, an ACTH-stimulation test measuring 17-hydroxyprogesterone levels must be performed.

HYPERPROLACTINEMIA/ GALACTORRHEA

Patients experiencing irregular menses sometimes have an elevated serum prolactin level. Prolactin is released from the anterior pituitary gland. Its most understood action is stimulating milk production. Prolactin levels are high in pregnancy and these high levels are maintained after pregnancy by nipple stimulation from suckling. In the absence of suckling or breastfeeding the prolactin levels return to normal rapidly.

Some patients with abnormally high levels of prolactin will have galactorrhea, while others do not. Prolactin is considered a stress hormone and can be released at times of abnormal stress. Other causes of hyperprolactinemia include benign pituitary adenomas.

Pituitary adenomas are suspected with elevated levels of prolactin. Magnetic resonance imaging of the pituitary gland is the best diagnostic study available and is very accurate. Some patients with larger tumors will complain of headaches and blurry vision, but most complain only of galactorrhea or irregular menses.

In a patient with irregular menses, measurement of prolactin levels along with thyroid evaluation should be performed. In the past, treatment of an abnormal prolactin level or even a pituitary adenoma required transsphenoidal sinus surgery, which had a high morbidity. Fortunately, almost all such patients may now be treated medically with bromocriptine or cabergoline.

Bromocriptine and cabergoline are dopamine-receptor agonists, which lower prolactin levels.[2] Shrinkage of prolactin-secreting pituitary adenomas is seen with bromocriptine or cabergoline use, but on stopping the drug the adenoma returns.

Hyperprolactinemia may lead to estrogen deficiency via disturbance of the nucleus, much like the disturbance produced by cortisol-releasing hormone. Patients with symptoms of estrogen deficiency need to be treated. Patients not having symptoms may need no treatment for this common problem. Based on autopsy data, pituitary adenomas are found in approximately 5% of the population.

Side effects of bromocriptine treatment include nausea and vomiting, which may not be compatible with the daily schedule of a committed athlete in training. Cabergoline is the newer and more expensive alternative, but it is less likely to cause nausea and vomiting. Bromocriptine is for daily use, while cabergoline is only taken twice per week.

THYROID DISEASE

Thyroid hormone has an effect on just about every organ system within the body. While the incidence of thyroid disease is not increased in athletes, females are more likely to have thyroid disorders than men.

Symptoms of hypothyroidism include lethargy, weight gain, and cold intolerance. Symptoms unique to women include irregular or absent menses, lack of ovulation, and infertility. Women with irregular menses usually should be tested for thyroid disease. Treatment is with thyroid hormone replacement therapy.

Symptoms of hyperthyroidism include heat intolerance, irritability, impatience, weight loss, tachycardia, and hypertension. One of the most common causes of hyperthyroidism is Graves disease, an autoimmune disorder in which long-acting antibodies stimulate release of thyroxine, the active thyroid hormone. The antibodies may also produce exophthalmos with time. Treatment is usually administration of radioactive iodine.

Hashimoto's thyroiditis has components of both hyperthyroidism and hypothyroidism. Hashimoto's disease is also an autoimmune problem. Most of the disease is spent in the hypothyroid component. Women are commonly affected. Treatment is directed at replacing thyroid hormone.

PREMENSTRUAL SYNDROME

Premenstrual syndrome (PMS) can be defined as the cyclic appearance of numerous symptoms, including bloating, anxiety, depression, fatigue, and irritability just prior to menses that affects the person's ability to perform her usual routines. The classic patient with PMS feels fine the first 2 weeks of her menstrual calendar but develops symptoms 2 weeks prior to her period. The PMS symptoms then usually rapidly improve within the first day or so of starting menses.[24]

Many symptoms of depression are similar to those of PMS and many clinicians can confuse the disorders. The treatment of these disorders usually differs although selective serotonin reuptake inhibitors (SSRIs) such as fluoxetine

(Prozac) have been used with success in each disease state.

PMS seems to be worse in women in their thirties and improves in their forties. PMS has been cited as reason for some acts of violence. However, most patients with PMS usually only talk about becoming violent and never actually do so.

Many treatment options have been proposed for PMS, with varying degrees of success for limited amounts of time since there appears to be a large placebo effect associated with PMS treatment. Treatments that have been tried with questionable results include administration of progesterone, vitamin B_6, OCPs, and bromocriptine, as well as numerous others.

Other treatment options include the use of GnRH agonists.[12] GnRH agonists shut down the menstrual cycle completely, and if a patient does not cycle she cannot suffer from PMS. GnRH agonists have even been touted for use as a diagnostic tool to distinguish patients with depression from patients with PMS.

The problem with GnRH agonist therapy is that the drug cannot be used long term because of the induced estrogen-deficiency state. With some exceptions, treatment is usually limited to 6 months unless small amounts of estrogen are added back to prevent osteoporosis and adverse lipid effects.

While many drug therapies have been tried as treatment options for PMS, many work only temporarily or in selected patients. Nondrug therapies such as aerobic exercise may improve the symptoms of PMS, thereby lessening its theoretical incidence among athletes.[25]

CONCLUDING REMARKS

Certainly, the treatment of hormonal disorders is important to all women, and the female athlete is no exception. Highly competitive and driven female athletes are at unique risk for menstrual dysfunction, especially involving a hypoestrogenic state, compared to nonathletic women of the same age. Preservation of bone density and prevention of stress fractures remain important goals in the treatment of menstrual dysfunction. Attention to energy balance and nutritional concerns, as well as optimal weight are important factors in treatment. Use of estrogen-replacement therapy and OCP use are still controversial with regard to bone health issues and fracture reduction in the female athlete with menstrual dysfunction. Understanding the significance of the various hormonal disorders reviewed and the treatment thereof can positive-

ly impact the future health of athletic individuals long after their competitive athletic days have ended.

References

1. American Academy of Pediatrics Committee on Sports Medicine and Fitness: Medical concerns in the female athlete. Pediatrics 106:610–3, 2000.
2. Bevan JS, Webster J, Burke CW, Scanlon MF: Dopamine agonists and pituitary tumor shrinkage. Endocrinol Rev 13:220, 1992.
3. Biller BMK, Federoff HJ, Koenig JI, Klibanski A: Abnormal cortisol secretion and responses to corticotropin-releasing hormone in women with hypothalamic amenorrhea. J Clin Endocrinol Metab 70:311, 1990.
4. Cassidenti DL, Paulson RJ, Serafini P, et al: Effects of sex steroids on skin 5 alpha reductase activity in vitro. Obstet Gynecol 78:103, 1991.
5. Chang RJ: Ovarian steroid secretion in polycystic ovarian disease. Semin Reprod Endocrinol 2:244, 1984.
6. Chang RJ, Mandel FP, Lu JK, Judd HL: Enhanced disparity of gonadotropin secretion by estrone in women with polycystic ovarian disease. J Clin Endocrinol Metab 54:490, 1982.
7. Chrousos GP, Gold PW: The concepts of stress and stress system disorders. JAMA 267:1244, 1992.
8. Drinkwater BL, Bruemmer B, Chester CH III: Menstrual history as a determinant of current bone density in young athletes. JAMA 263:545, 1990.
9. Dueck CA, Matt KS, Manore MM, et al: Treatment of athletic amenorrhea with a diet and training intervention program. Int J Sport Nutr 6:24, 1996.
10. Dunaif A: Molecular mechanisms of insulin resistance in the polycystic ovary syndrome. Semin Reprod Endocrinol 12:15, 1994.
11. Hergenroeder AC, Smith EO, Shypailo R, et al: Bone mineral changes in young women with hypothalamic amenorrhea treated with oral contraceptives, medroxyprogesterone, or placebo over 12 months. Am J Obstet Gynecol 176:1017–25, 1997.
12. Hussain SY, Massil JH, Matta WH, et al: Buserelin in premenstrual syndrome. Gynecol Endocrinol 6:57, 1992.
13. Keen AD, Drinkwater BL: Irreversible bone loss in former amenorrheic athletes. Osteoporosis Int 7:311–5, 1997.
14. Knobil E: Neuroendocrine control of the menstrual cycle. Rec Prog Horm Res 3:363, 1980.
15. Lobo RA, Goebelsmann U, Brenner PF, Mishell DR Jr: The effects of estrogen on adrenal androgens in oophorectomized women. Am J Obstet Gynecol 142:471, 1982.
16. Lookingbill DP, Demers LM, Wang C, et al: Clinical and biochemical parameters of androgen action in normal and healthy caucasian versus Chinese subjects. J Clin Endocrinol Metab 72:1242, 1991.
17. Loucks AB, Mortola JF, Girton L, et al: Alterations in the hypothalamic—pituitary—ovarian and the hypothalamic—pituitary—adrenal axis in athletic women. J Clin Endocrinol Metab 68:402, 1989.
18. Loucks AB, Verdun M, Heath EM: Low energy availability, not stress of exercise, alters LH pulsatility in exercising women. J App Physiol 84:37, 1998.
19. Miller KK, Klibanski A: Amenorrheic bone loss: J Clin Endocrinol Metab 176:1017–25, 1999.
20. Morin-Papunen LC, Koivunen RM, Ruokonen A, et al: Metformin therapy improves the menstrual pattern with

minimal endocrine and metabolic effects in women with polycystic ovary syndrome. Fertil Steril 69:691, 1998.

21. Prior JC, Vigna YM, Scheehter MT, et al: Spinal bone loss and ovulatory disturbances. N Engl J Med 323, 1221, 1990.

22. Rossing MA, Daling JR, Weiss NS, et al: Ovarian tumors in a cohort of infertile women. N Engl J Med 331:771, 1994.

23. Shangold M: Menstruation. In: Shangold M, Mirkin G (eds): Women and Exercise. Philadelphia, FA Davis, 1988, pp 129–45.

24. Speroff L, Glass RH, Kase NG (eds): Clinical Gynecologic Endocrinology and Infertility, 5ᵗʰ edition, Baltimore, Williams & Wilkins, 1994, p 535.

25. Steege JF, Blumenthal JA: The effects of aerobic exercise on premenstrual symptoms in middle-aged women: a preliminary study. J Psychosom Res 37:127, 1993.

26. Waldstreicher J, Santoro NF, Hall JE, et al: Hyperfunction of the hypothalamic–pituitary axis in women with polycystic ovarian disease: indirect evidence for partial gonadotroph desensitization. J Clin Endocrinol Metab 66:165, 1988.

27. Warren MP, Shantha, S: The female athlete. Bailliere's Clin Endocrinol Metab 14(1):37–53, 2000.

28. Weaver CM, Teagarden D, Lyle RM, et al. Impact of exercise on bone health and contraindication of oral contraceptive use in young women. Med Sci Sports Exerc 33:873–80, 2001.

29. White PC, New MI, Dupont B: Congenital adrenal hyperplasia. N Engl J Med 316:1519, 1987.

30. Whittemore AS, Harris R, Itnyre J, et al: Characteristics relating to ovarian cancer risk: collaborative analysis of 12 U.S. case controlled studies. Am J Epidemiol 136:1184, 1992.

31. Young RL, Goldzieher JW, Elkind-Hirsch K: The endocrine effects of spironolactone used as an antiandrogen. Fertil Steril 48:223, 1987.

Chapter 16

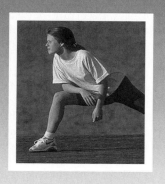

Fertility

Robert J. Homm, M.D.

The benefits of exercise are undisputed. General fitness achieved through reasonable diet and exercise helps maintain ideal body weight and performance. Additionally, regular exercise benefits cardiovascular health, weight control, muscle strength and control, flexibility and strength of the skeleton, and coordination. Although the specifics of an exercise program may change depending on the patient's health status and age, exercise is to be encouraged as a healthy part of a lifestyle at all ages.

REVIEW OF THE EFFECTS OF EXERCISE ON REPRODUCTIVE FUNCTION

Strenuous exercise, endurance training in particular, has been associated with an increased frequency of reproductive dysfunction in women.[14] Even moderate or recreational exercise has been shown to impact menstrual function in some women.[2] The various disorders of reproductive function that have been associated with exercise include delayed menarche, inadequate luteal phase, anovulatory cycles, oligomenorrhea, and amenorrhea. The focus of this chapter will be on the effects that exercise may have on ovulation and regular menstrual function in reproductive-age women, and associated concerns of fertility and ultimate pregnancy. Additional concerns, including menstrual dysfunction and effect on bone health, are reviewed in other chapters.

Effect of Exercise on Menstrual Function in Reproductive-Age Women

Exercise may alter both the flow and frequency of menses. The exact mechanisms are not known, but a number of theories have been proposed. The "exercise stress hypothesis" holds that athletic training is a stressor that activates the hypothalamic—pituitary—adrenal axis. One or more of the central and peripheral mediators of the axis disrupts the gonadotropin-releasing hormone (GnRH) pulse generator, causing aberrations in the pulsatility and amplitude of the gonadotropins luteinizing hormone (LH) and follicle-stimulating hormone (FSH) signaling. If this hypothesis is true, the appropriate intervention to prevent or reverse menstrual dysfunction would be to modulate exercise.

A more recent theory gaining acceptance is the "energy availability hypothesis," which holds that the GnRH pulse generator is disrupted by a putative signal or signals as yet not totally known. Dietary energy intake is inadequate for the energy costs of ovulation, menstruation, reproduction, and the exercise pursuits. This theory is supported by findings that athletic women consume less energy than would be expected for their activity levels, by endocrine signs of chronic energy deficiency in amenorrheic athletes, and by reversal of this abnormality when a state of positive energy balance results, specifically when dietary energy intake is sufficient to meet the energy costs of exercise.[8,9,18,19] If this hypothesis is true, athletes may be able to prevent or reverse menstrual dysfunction by increasing dietary and energy intake without necessarily altering their exercise protocol.

The exact cause of menstrual dysfunction in an individual patient may differ from another exercising female. Indeed, multiple causes may be operative that, in synergy, culminate in an exercising female becoming less regular with regard to ovulation and thereby menstrual function. The various contributing factors include disordered eating or other changes in diet and energy requirements in the exercising female,[3] changes in body composition and weight (especially abrupt loss), stress, an increase in training intensity (especially without compensatory increases in dietary energy intake), and altered levels of endorphins and other neuroregulatory substances with effects centrally and possibly directly on the ovary.

In women who excessively diet to control their weight, there is noted hypothalamic–pituitary dysfunction in the form of loss of normal pulsatility of LH and FSH. Low to normal levels of LH and FSH are seen in amenorrheic women who have had extreme weight loss and in amenorrheic women exercising to the extreme. The 24-hour secretory pattern of these hormones lacks the requisite episodic variation and in the extreme even may revert to a prepubertal state much below normal adult or mature levels. Weight gain, nutritional intervention, or modulation in exercise may lead to correction of these patterns.[7] As mentioned, there are still as yet unknown mediators that may help to signal the energy deficit and low nutritional reserve and effect a subsequent response of a cascade of feedback mechanisms to the brain, resulting in inhibition of ovulation. It is possible that leptin, the hormone product of the obesity gene, may play a role as this mediator.[17] This is discussed further in Chapters 13 and 14.

Disruption of hypothalamic–pituitary function is essential to understand. Normal menstrual homeostasis requires the appropriate signal generation (GnRH) from the hypothalamus to the pituitary, which in turn causes appropriate LH and FSH to be secreted, thereby resulting in the orderly events of folliculogenesis and ovulation. Only with the appropriate function of this complicated feedback cascade will the reproductively competent female maintain ovulation, regular menstrual function, and pregnancy potential.

As a matter of a more practical nature to the female athlete, she may indeed be placing herself at undue risk of additional medical complications in that the disruption of the normal feedback mechanisms associated with ovulation and regular menses may signal low and, in some cases, profoundly low estrogen levels. Long-term deficiency in estrogen in women will often place them at risk for osteopenia and osteoporosis, even while actively engaged in athletic endeavors. More importantly, peak bone mass is attained during the adolescent and early adult years. Even catch-up bone building in later years many not adequately compensate for this inadequate bone formation in early years. Therefore some of these young women may be at a substantial risk for osteoporosis in their later years.

Abnormalities of GnRH secretion from the hypothalamic areas of the brain seem to be the primary defects in patients with exercise-induced menstrual dysfunction. The common thread in almost every study that has explored this phenomenon hormonally has found this "athletic amenorrhea" to be hypothalamic in nature, with low or low-normal levels of the gonadotropins and estradiol. This in turn is thought to be due to disruption of the normally occurring release of GnRH from the hypothalamus at regular intervals. Normally menstruating women show a pulsatility of GnRH and resultant pulsatility of LH and FSH every 60 to 120 minutes. This pulsatility of GnRH, LH, and FSH is controlled by elaborate feedback mechanisms, primarily estrogens secreted from the ovary, and varies with the phase of the menstrual cycle. A detailed discussion is beyond the scope of this review, but the reader is referred to the excellent review by Speroff.[16]

When subjected to elaborate hormonal survey studies during the periods of training, these patients have been shown to have aberrant pulsatile LH frequency and amplitude. The LH and FSH pulsatility also has been shown to vary from month to month as well when assayed repeatedly in the same individual.[8]

The fact that the hypothalamic–pituitary axis is not centrally deficient in patients with exercise-induced oligoamenorrhea is shown by the fact that infusion of exogenous GnRH at appropriate intervals from 60 to 120 minutes apart will restore normal adult levels of LH and FSH and raise estrogen levels appropriately. In fact, this type of therapy is occasionally required in patients who do not respond to simpler forms of ovulation induction or enhancement if pregnancy is desired. Thankfully, with appropriate nutritional intervention, weight gain, and/or reduction in exercise intensity many female athletes will not need this extreme of therapy unless they have had true underlying hypothalamic–pituitary dysfunction prior to their exercise endeavors.

Fertility Concerns of the Exercising Female

It is not surprising that a regularly exercising female may from time to time experience menstrual dysfunction as a consequence of ovulatory dysfunction. She may also experience subclinical luteal-phase abnormalities. Luteal-phase insufficiency and defect have been inferred by increased cycle length and reduction in luteal-phase length and documented by inadequate mid-luteal-phase progesterone levels, abnormalities in basal body temperature charting, and endometrial biopsy. Ovulatory and menstrual dysfunction has been associated with athletes in a variety of sports, especially runners, gymnasts, and dancers. Lesser degrees of dysfunction have been documented with female athletes in other sports, including swimmers, cyclists, weight lifters, and "recreational athletes."[2]

As discussed, ovulatory dysfunction has been linked to changes in weight, body composition, nutritional factors, stress—physical and emotional—and alterations in hormonal concentration and feedback mechanisms. An energy-deficit state, with dietary factors seeming to play a more significant role than exercise per se,[4] has been demonstrated to be a likely mechanism contributing to menstrual dysfunction. A vegetarian diet in conjunction with regular exercise seems to place some women at risk for reproductive dysfunction. Schweiger and others have shown calorie-restricted, vegetarian diets to be associated with luteal-phase cycles consistent with luteal-phase insufficiency. These defects were manifested by shortened cycles, inadequate thermogenic shift in basal body temperature, and low progesterone levels. Not surprisingly, menstrual irregularities were also more frequent with this vegetarian diet than with a nonvegetarian diet of equal calories.[13]

Prior to treatment of the exercising woman desiring to become pregnant with fertility medications, a thorough workup of likely causes for menstrual dysfunction and infertility should be undertaken. Optimizing nutrition and energy balance and/or modifying exercise should be the first steps to take in the effort to induce normal menstrual function.

Ovulation induction may be required if infertility persists and pregnancy is desired.

EVALUATION OF EXERCISE-INDUCED MENSTRUAL DYSFUNCTION AND INFERTILITY

The health-care provider challenged by the exercising patient with menstrual irregularities should not assume the changes in menses to be due to exercise without a thorough consideration of other factors. The diagnosis of exercise-associated menstrual dysfunction is made by the exclusion of other more serious causes. A detailed history and physical examination, including a pelvic examination, is indicated, as is laboratory testing. Additionally, current or past sexually transmitted diseases, a history of pelvic inflammatory disease, and prior surgical procedures should be detailed. Additional causes of menstrual irregularity in young women include thyroid disease, prolactin excess, polycystic ovary disease, adrenal hormone excess, and hypothalamic or pituitary tumors. These conditions can only be detected by appropriate laboratory and/or radiologic studies.

An initial workup for screening of any patient with menstrual dysfunction, whether exercising or not, includes obtaining a thyroid-stimulating hormone (TSH) level and thyroid function studies, prolactin level, LH, and FSH levels, and a pregnancy test. Thyroid disorders—both hypothyroidism and hyperthyroidism—can cause ovulatory irregularity and subsequent problems with fertility. Prolactin excess is associated with interference in the generation of appropriate GnRH signals from the hypothalamus to the pituitary gland and subsequently, abnormal secretory patterns of LH and FSH. Some regularly exercising females have transient increases in prolactin immediately after exercising. Chronic elevations of prolactin are rarely seen in athletes. Elevations in prolactin can be associated with hyperplasia of the prolactin-secreting cells of the pituitary gland and may be visualized on a computed tomography (CT) or magnetic resonance imaging (MRI) scan as microadenomas. These benign tumors can be controlled with dopamine receptor agonist medication such as bromocriptine and cabergoline and rarely require surgery.

The evaluation of LH and FSH is important to document the presence of these hormones and infer secretion. While a single assay obviously does not ensure appropriate dynamics of secretion or appropriate feedback mechanisms, it may rule out a brain tumor of the hypothalamus or pituitary if the levels are normal and the prolactin level is normal. Very low or nonmeasurable levels should heighten the suspicion of a tumor. Very high levels of LH and FSH are seen in premature ovarian failure. Although not seen with any increased frequency in exercising females, ovarian failure can occur at any age, from before pubertal development up to the expected age of menopause of 45 to 50 years. This diagnosis is important to begin appropriate estrogen replacement therapy or other therapy to prevent osteoporosis.

Patients presenting with hirsutism, a condition presenting with abnormal masculinizing hair growth or acne, should also be screened for adrenal abnormalities with total testosterone and dehydroepiandrosterone sulfate (DHEA-S) determinations. Random screening for serum cortisol is rarely helpful. A better test for cortisol excess is the rapid screening overnight dexamethasone suppression test. Dexamethasone 1 mg is given at 11 PM and a serum cortisol is drawn the next morning at 8 AM. A normal response is for the cortisol level to be less than 5 µg/dL. Patients with Cushing syndrome will have levels greater than 10 µg/dL. These studies should exclude most serious endocrinologic causes of ovulatory and menstrual dysfunction.

There is no evidence that the female athlete with a history of menstrual dysfunction has a higher incidence of future infertility compared to the nonathlete. However, problems related to ovulation are a concern and represent the most frequent cause of infertility in women. In men, problems with sperm account for the majority of problems. Therefore, in the exercising female desiring pregnancy, the physician should obtain a detailed past and current menstrual cycle history, including ovulatory pattern, and a sperm sample from the male partner to assess for count, motility, and other factors if pregnancy is desired.

If no detectable ovulatory or sperm problem is identified, assessment of cervical mucus or interaction of mucus and sperm should be undertaken. If problems still are not identified, assessment of structural problems of the fallopian tubes and/or uterus should be undertaken. This usually involves hysterosalpingography. If the cause of infertility is still not discovered after the above workup, testing the pelvic environment for evidence of adhesions or pelvic endometriosis would be considered, although this involves a more invasive laparoscopic procedure.

Common causes of menstrual dysfunction in the female athlete and related concerns with fertility, as well as their treatment, will be reviewed below.

LUTEAL-PHASE DEFECTS

A normal menstrual cycle is expected every 25 to 35 days and should lead to an orderly flow lasting 1 to 5 days. A woman experiencing menses more frequently than every 23 days or at intervals longer than 35 days should be evaluated. Short cycle lengths are likely with anovulatory cycles or may be due to luteal-phase defects, which are caused by an inadequate luteal phase of the menstrual cycle that is due to insufficient progesterone support of the endometrium. Although luteal-phase defect is often a result of decreased hormone production of progesterone by the ovary, the underlying causes may be multiple. Decreased levels of FSH in the follicular phase, abnormal LH surging, and decreased response of the endometrium to progesterone may all be causative of luteal-phase defect. Many of the patients with luteal-phase defects are thought to have inadequate follicular development begetting the poorer luteal function.

A luteal-phase defect, presumably due to inadequate progesterone secretion or action on the endometrium, can be found in up to 30% of isolated menstrual cycles of normal women. Only if the defect is found in more than 2 cycles is it considered to be a possible factor in infertility. Patients with recurrent pregnancy loss are found to suffer from luteal-phase defects more frequently.[12]

Tests of the luteal phase include basal body temperature charting, ovulation predictor kits for confirmation of the LH surge, serum progesterone levels, and endometrial biopsy. The basal body temperature charting relies on the thermogenic shift in body temperature induced after ovulation by the secretion of progesterone. In a normally ovulating patient, the body temperature will elevate by 0.5° to 1° after ovulation has occurred and remain elevated while progesterone is secreted sufficiently. If a patient becomes pregnant in the testing cycle, her temperature will remain elevated beyond the expected 11 to 14 days. An elevation of less than 10 days before the onset of the next menses implies the possibility of luteal inadequacy. Most patients find the basal body temperature charting technique unreliable and tedious to perform and therefore abandon it.

Testing for the signal for ovulation, the LH surge, can be used similarly to infer luteal-phase deficiency. If the patient starts menses 11 days or sooner after a positive surge of LH in the urine, the luteal phase may be too short. Also, with analysis of the LH surge, the patient trying to conceive may have prospective information of impending ovulation. This method is superior to the basal body temperature charting technique, in which the thermogenic shift may not be discriminated until after ovulation has already occurred.

A serum progesterone determination or series of determinations has been utilized to confirm the occurrence of ovulation and the adequacy of mid-luteal secretion of this important hormone. While a normal level (more than 15 ng/dL) 7 days after the LH surge or a rise in basal temperature is reassuring, one must remember that the secretory pattern of progesterone varies throughout the day and is pulsatile in nature. A low value may not be truly reflective of inadequacy. Obtaining serial low levels over several days adds diagnostic certainty of luteal-phase defect but also adds cost and discomfort. One should also be aware that an adequate serum level does not necessarily guarantee correlation with adequate endometrial development.[15]

Although all of the above screening tests for luteal-phase defects infer inadequate progesterone production, the best test for confirmation is the endometrial biopsy. Generally, the biopsy is performed 1 to 3 days before the expected onset of menses and is evaluated histologically. With strict adherence to the criteria for "dating" the endometrium the biopsy should agree with the date of the biopsy within 2 days. If the biopsy is out of phase by 2 or more days, a luteal-phase defect is confirmed.[11] Essential to this confirmation is to know the presumed day of ovulation, the day of the biopsy from the first day of the previous menses, and the first day of the subsequent menses.

Treatment of Luteal-Phase Defect

Luteal-phase defect in the exercising female need only be treated if pregnancy is desired. If the defect is due to extremes of exercise or an energy-deficit state, alteration of diet and caloric consumption and/or modulation of the exercise program may be all that is necessary. In some cases, however, treatment may be necessary and must be individualized. Many athletes are reticent to take hormonal medications. A thorough and honest discussion of the risks and benefits of hormonal therapy is usually appreciated and ensures more likely compliance.

Treatment options for luteal-phase defect in women desiring pregnancy include clomiphene citrate, progesterone supplementation, and gonadotropin therapy. Based on the assumption that poor follicular development begets poor luteal phase, clomiphene citrate and gonadotropin therapies are both appropriate to consider. Both will increase the stimulus to ovulate and increase progesterone levels after ovulation. Each has its respective risks and benefits.

Clomiphene citrate is an orally administered synthetic antiestrogen with a known central effect of blocking the estrogen-receptor feedback mechanisms within the hypothalamus and pituitary gland. In doing so, the brain "perceives" a low-estrogen state and is stimulated to generate more intense signals of GnRH to the pituitary to secrete higher levels of LH and FSH. This in turn produces more and presumably better follicular-phase development. Indeed, estrogen levels tend to be higher in clomiphene cycles than in normal ovulatory cycles. Likewise, most patients will have improvement in the progesterone secretion dynamics when clomiphene is utilized.

Clomiphene therapy is a logical first step in the treatment of luteal-phase defect. Its only significant risk is an increase in the rate of multiple pregnancies to 4% to 5% compared to the normal rate of twin pregnancies of 1 in 90 conceptions. Multiple gestations greater than twins are rare but can occur. Persistent ovarian cysts can develop in patients taking clomiphene. This usually represents only a nuisance side effect since such cysts usually resolve within 1 to 3 months with no therapy except reassurance. Recurrent cyst formation on clomiphene may represent the so-called Luteinized Unruptured Follicles Syndrome. In this situation, follicles develop but do not release, presumably because of intraovarian receptor defects not allowing recognition of the LH surge or inadequate LH surge dynamics. Progesterone and even endometrial biopsy may suggest correction of the luteal-phase defect but pregnancy does not occur. This is a rare occurrence but may indicate an underlying problem of inappropriate LH surge generation, the signal for ovulation to occur. In these cases, the addition of a 10,000-IU injection of human chorionic gonadotropin (HCG) when the follicles are appropriately developed, as determined by ultrasonography, may ensure actual ovulation of the oocyte or egg. HCG is very similar in biochemical structure to LH and can trigger ovulation. This protocol has an additional benefit. HCG is an additional stimulus to the corpus luteum to secrete greater levels of progesterone after ovulation has occurred. Downs and Gibson have shown conception rates of 79% when clomiphene was utilized to correct severe luteal-phase defect. More subtle degrees of luteal-phase defect, however, did not show such profound improvement.[5]

While administration of human menopausal gonadotropins (LH and FSH) will produce the same results as clomiphene with greater certainty, it is reserved for nonresponders. Gonadotropin therapy has the potential for hyperstimulation of the ovaries, which in the severest presentation may be life threatening. It also puts the patient at more extreme risk for multiple births (in the range of 15% to 20%). Add to these considerations the expense of the medication ($50 to $150/day minimum), the fact that it must be given by injection, and the stringent monitoring costs (estradiol levels and ultrasonography) to utilize it safely, it is clear why gonadotropins are seldom used for luteal-phase defect.

Since the primary defect in luteal-phase defect is the inadequate effect of progesterone on the endometrium, addition of progesterone after ovulation may be presumed to be effective, and, indeed, in many cases will be. A vaginal suppository of 50 to 100 mg of progesterone once or twice daily started 3 days after ovulation will result in adequate increases in progesterone in many patients. This is continued until menses start or pregnancy is diagnosed. Progesterone in these dosage ranges will not prevent menses from starting if pregnancy does not occur but may delay it to a more "normal" luteal length of 12 to 15 days after ovulation. In cases where luteal-phase defect had been diagnosed, if pregnancy is achieved, supplementation is usually continued for 9 to 10 weeks, at which time the placenta has achieved adequate production of progesterone independent of the ovary's production and the supplementation can be discontinued. Studies comparing the efficacy of clomiphene to progesterone in the treatment of luteal-phase defect are difficult to compare because of differences in methodology. However, it can be said that both work if well chosen and the patient employs the therapy appropriately. A review of the comparative benefits is presented by Murray and associates.[10] Oral therapy with progesterone has proponents but suffers from erratic absorption in many patients owing to gastrointestinal degradation of the progesterone. Daily intramuscular injection of 25 to 50 mg progesterone in oil is an alternative for patients experiencing irritation utilizing the progesterone vaginally. Once pregnancy is achieved, progesterone supplementation can also be provided by a weekly depot preparation of 17-hydroxyprogesterone caproate (250 mg), again continued through 10 weeks of pregnancy.

OLIGO-OVULATION AND ANOVULATION

Patients with very short cycles or very long cycles with monophasic basal body temperature charts and low serum levels of progesterone are usually anovulatory. These patients produce estrogen but inadequate levels of progesterone. They are probably not at the greatest risk for osteoporosis in that they will generally respond to a progestin challenge by evidencing a withdrawal flow. Those at great risk are women with long-standing amenorrhea and very low estrogen levels as determined either by direct serum measurement or by inference by lack of menstrual withdrawal flow with a progestin challenge of medroxyprogesterone acetate 10 mg/day for 5 to 10 days. Although comparative studies have not been done, Shangold has proposed a serum estradiol of more than 50 pg/mL to be needed to prevent the exercising female with menstrual dysfunction from being at significant risk for osteoporosis.[14]

Osteopenia or osteoporosis should be of concern to the exercising female with menstrual dysfunction, as well as to her physician. Regular spontaneous menstrual cycles are the ideal for osteoporosis prevention. Drinkwater and associates have shown correlation of current bone density with the menstrual cycle. Their data support the importance of the cumulative effectiveness of estrogen status on bone density. Women with an extended history of oligomenorrhea or amenorrhea had significant bone loss despite weight-bearing exercise and weight maintenance.[6]

Treatment of Oligo-Ovulation and Anovulation

The patient wishing to conceive and evidencing anovulation or oligo-ovulation presents a real challenge. Discussion of the pathophysiology of ovulatory mechanisms, and the effect of weight and exercise on them, should be part of the early evaluation and preconceptual treatment planning. Profoundly hypoestrogenic females generally will not respond to clomiphene. Low body weight, low body fat, and exercise-induced impact on the hypothalamic-pituitary–ovarian axis all make the use of clomiphene less likely to be successful. However, given its safety profile, ease of use, and relative low cost, clomiphene citrate should be tried initially. Occasionally, estrogen "priming" for several months prior to the trial of clomiphene citrate will be successful in allowing a response by "up-regulating" estrogen receptors necessary for the clomiphene actions as described previously. This is done in the usual fashion for estrogen replacement utilizing conjugated estrogens 0.625 mg/day or esterified estrogen 1 mg/day for several months with monthly withdrawal induced by medroxyprogesterone acetate 10 mg for 5 days. The patient is counseled to not conceive during the exposure to progestin. Clomiphene is initiated with the onset of menses at a starting dose of 50 mg/day on the third day of menses and continued for 5 days. Dosage is increased in subsequent attempts if ovulation is not confirmed. Most conceptions occur at dosages less than 150 mg/day and within 6 ovulatory cycles. If conception does not occur, a thorough re-evaluation of causes of infertility in the female and male partner should be pursued in a timely fashion as previously reviewed.

LH and FSH are purified preparations of gonadotropins from the urine of menopausal women, hence the generic name *menotropins*. The recombinant preparations now available represent an advance over the urine-derived products because of their higher potency and batch-to-batch consistency. These features have allowed their consistent use by subcutaneous administration with reliable absorption, contrasted with the older medications that needed to be given as an intramuscular injection. The recombinant gonadotropins also greatly reduce the problem of availability seen in the past with urine-derived products. Their cost, however, is still very high, with average treatment cycles costing between $1000 and $2000.

Gonadotropins stimulate the ovary exogenously and do not rely on feedback mechanisms to be intact to be effective. Therefore, a patient with profound anovulation will respond to this medication. The medications are usually begun after withdrawal flow has been induced and continued until one or more appropriate-sized follicles have been developed. Ovulation is triggered exogenously with an injection of HCG. Monitoring of the effects of the drugs on the follicular development is assayed by serum estradiol and ultrasonography. Most practitioners also supplement the luteal phase after ovulation has occurred with progesterone, similar to the protocols outlined for luteal-phase defects. Because of the complexity of their use, need for stringent monitoring, and risk for complications, the gonadotropins generally should be reserved for use under the direction of a medical or reproductive endocrinologist.

An alternative method of ovulation induction in patients with hypothalamic anovulation is the GnRH infusion pump. The defect, in some of these patients, is absent or inappropriate GnRH secretion from the hypothalamus. With the development of microdelivery systems, it has been possible to induce ovulation by the infusion of GnRH either subcutaneously or intravenously in a pattern that mimics the normal secretory patterns within the hypothalamic–pituitary axis. Theoretically, the pituitary and ovary in these patients are competent to respond if the signal generation from the pump "artificial hypothalamus" is appropriate. Ovarian hyperstimulation and multiple gestations are rare because the response should be no more follicle growth than a normally ovulating female. Although expensive, this form of therapy is less expensive than gonadotropins because the elaborate monitoring with estradiol levels and ultrasonography is not imperative. Luteal support is important to manage as outlined previously. Pregnancy rates for pure hypothalamic anovulation treated with this modality have been similar to those with gonadotropin cycles and average 20% to 30% per cycle.[4]

PREGNANCY IN THE EXERCISING FEMALE

Although this topic is covered in detail elsewhere in this book, a few comments are relevant to the present discussion. Preconceptual good health is paramount to the health of the pregnant patient and her child. Concern for appropriate diet, calcium supplementation, vitamin supplementation, and weight should be discussed with the female athlete trying to conceive. While not all athletes have a problem with very low weight, enough do to warrant counseling of all patients regarding expectations of weight gain during pregnancy to assess their likely compliance and discern any problems with body image. Any patient steadfastly resistant to exercise modification or weight gain requirements of pregnancy may need psychological counseling preconceptually. It is well recognized that there is a correlation between maternal weight prepregnancy and intrapregnancy weight gain and the infant's size. Any patient with an undiagnosed disorder who is pregnant is in a high-risk pregnancy for mother and infant. A review of 14 women recovering from an eating disorder or compulsive exercise, failing to respond to clomiphene citrate and needing advanced help to conceive, showed a high incidence of low-birth-weight infants (less than 2500 g).[1]

CONCLUDING REMARKS

There are many reasons to recommend regular exercise in the reproductive-age woman. In this chapter we have covered salient factors with regard to the effects of exercise on reproductive physiology, menstrual dysfunction, and fertility. Exercise incorporated into a healthy lifestyle generally promotes gynecologic well being as well as a general sense of wellness.

However, exercise may have impact on the "normalcy" of menstrual function and reproduction. The exercising female who seeks help with reproductive or gynecologic complaints generally can be managed initially with non-pharmacologic measures, including nutritional intervention and/or exercise modification to maintain a positive energy balance. If the patient is willing and able to modulate her nutrition and exercise endeavors, the cure may be "tincture of time."

Fertility concerns in the exercising female must be evaluated initially as it would in any patient presenting with these challenges. For some female athletes, a combination of nutritional intervention, modulation of exercise, and fertility-enhancing strategies may be indicated. Strategies that have been employed and reviewed include estrogen supplementation, progesterone supplementation, ovulation induction with clomiphene, gonadotropins, and GnRH agonists.

Correction of infertility and poor pregnancy outcome should be directed at the specific problems identified. Not infrequently in the exercising female, this should initially be directed at excellent preconceptual counseling with special regard to nutrition and energy balance. With conception, aggressive luteal support has much to be recommended. Survey for appropriate growth of the fetus and maternal weight gain should be paramount throughout pregnancy.

References

1. Abraham S, Mira M, Llewellyn-Jones D: Should ovulation be induced in women recovering from an eating disorder or who are compulsive exercisers? Fertil Steril 53:566, 1990.
2. Broocks A, Pirke KM, Schweiger U, et al: Cyclic ovarian function in recreational athletes. J Appl Physiol 68(5): 2083, 1990.
3. Brooks-Gunn J, Warren MP, Hamilton L: The relationship of eating disorders to amenorrhea in ballet dancers. Med Sci Sports Exerc 19(1):41, 1987.
4. Carr JS, Reid RL: Ovulation induction with gonadotropin releasing hormone (GnRH). Semin Reprod Endocrinol 8:174, 1990.
5. Downs KA, Gibson M: Clomiphene citrate for luteal phase defect. Fertil Steril 39:34, 1983.
6. Drinkwater BL, Bruemner B, Chestnut CH: Menstrual history as a determinant of current bone density in young athletes. JAMA 263(4):545–8, 1990.
7. Laughlin GA, Yen SSC: Nutritional and endocrine-metabolic aberrations in amenorrheic athletes. J Clin Endocrinol Metab 81:4301–9, 1996.
8. Loucks AB, Mortola JF, Girton L, Yen SSC: Alterations in the hypothalamic-pituitary–ovarian and hypothalamic–pituitary–adrenal axes in athletic women. J Clin Endocrinol Metab 68:402–11, 1989.
9. Loucks AB, Verdun M, Heath EM: Low energy availability, not stress of exercise, alters LH pulsatility in exercising women. J Appl Physiol 84(1):37–46, 1998.
10. Murray DL, Reigh L, Adashi EY: Oral clomiphene citrate and vaginal progesterone suppositories in the treatment of luteal phase dysfunction: a comparative study. Fertil Steril 51:35, 1989.
11. Noyes RW, Hertig AT, Rock J: Dating the endometrial biopsy. Fertil Steril 1:23, 1950.
12. Peters AJ, Lloyd RP, Coulam CP: Prevalence of out of phase endometrial biopsy specimens. Am J Obstet Gynecol 166:1738, 1992.
13. Schweiger U, Laessle R, Pfister H, et al: Diet induced menstrual irregularities: effects of age and weight loss. Fertil Steril 48:746, 1987.
14. Shangold M, Rebar RW, Wentz AC, Schiff I: Evaluation and management of menstrual dysfunction in athletes. JAMA 263:1665, 1990.
15. Soules MR, McLachlan RI, Ed M, et al: Luteal phase deficiency: characterization of reproductive hormones over the menstrual cycle. J Clin Endocrinol Metab 69:804, 1989.
16. Speroff L, Glass RH, Kase NG (eds): Regulation of the Menstrual Cycle. In Clinical Gynecologic Endocrinology and Infertility, 6th edition. Baltimore, Lippincott-Williams & Wilkins, 1999, pp 201–46.
17. Warren MP, Voussoughian F, Geer EB, et al. Functional hypothalamic amenorrhea: hypoleptinemia and disordered eating. J Clin Endocrinol Metab 84(3):873–7, 1999.
18. Williams NI, Young CJ, McArthur JW, et al: Strenuous exercise with caloric restriction: effect on luteinizing hormone secretion Med Sci Sports Exerc 27:1930–8, 1995.
19. Zanker CL, Swaine IL: The relationship between serum oestradiol concentration and energy balance in young women distance runners. Int J Sports Med 19:104–8, 1998.

Chapter 17

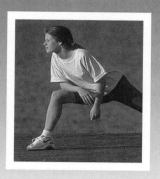

Contraception

James W. Akin, M.D.

Various methods of contraception are available today. These methods differ in their effectiveness, convenience, costs, reduction in exposure to sexually transmitted diseases, and alteration in menstrual symptoms such as amount of bleeding, timing of flow, bloating, and cramping. Other factors of importance to the female athlete also include positive or negative impact on performance, endurance, and overall well being.

The focus of this chapter is to discuss the various options for contraception available as related to the female athlete bringing out the benefits and drawbacks of each method. As with most areas of medicine, ultimately the female athlete along with her physician must choose the most appropriate method for her. Contraception is not a "one size fits all" matter.

HORMONAL CONTRACEPTION

Combination Oral Contraceptive Pills

One of the most popular and reliable forms of birth control is the combination pill. The oral contraceptive pill was introduced in the 1960s and has revolutionized contraceptive therapy. Since that time, several generations of the pill have been developed and improved. Much of the previous concerns about using the pill no longer apply.

Today's combination pill contains both estrogen and progestin given together in daily doses. The estrogen present in almost all combination pills sold is the synthetic ethinyl estradiol and it is the progestin component that varies. Most of the progestin compounds used are chemical derivatives of testosterone. These compounds have been modified so that the testosterone effect is almost nonexistent especially with the newer progestins available such as desogestrel and norgestimate.[19]

There are several potential mechanisms of action for the combination pill such as preventing ovulation, increasing cervical mucus so as to retard sperm penetration, altering uterotubal transport timing of the ova and sperm, and disrupting endometrial gland development to decrease the likelihood of successful embryo implantation. Preventing ovulation is primarily an estrogen effect through interference with the release of gonadotropin-releasing hormone (GnRH). This effect becomes less as the amount of estrogen is reduced. The other mechanisms of contraception listed above are mainly due to the progestin component of the pill.[19]

The combination pill is a very effective contraceptive if taken properly. However, its effectiveness is totally dependent on patient compliance. A very compliant patient can expect a failure rate of 0.1% per year (Table 17-1).[13] However, failure rates rise as compliance decreases. The average cost of the pill is less than $30 per month.

Rates of pelvic inflammatory disease (PID) are decreased with pill use probably due to thickened cervical mucus impairing bacterial ascent into the reproductive tract.[36] Still, oral contraceptive pills should be considered little protection against sexually transmitted diseases such as human immunodeficiency virus (HIV).

Metabolic Effects

The more common adverse effects of today's combination pill are relatively mild. Symptoms attributed to the estrogen within the pill include nausea, breast tenderness, and fluid retention. The fluid retention is a result of decreased sodium excretion and rarely exceeds 3–4 extra pounds of body weight. Clinically significant changes in circulating vitamin levels are no longer a concern. Chloasma, or pigmentation of the face with sun exposure, is rarely seen. The overall incidence of cholelithiasis is no longer increased. Some women still develop headaches although this side effect is less common with lower dose pills.[20]

Progestin side effects include possible increase in depression, irritability, and fatigue. The progestin component may also cause an anabolic

Table 17-1. Percentage of Women Experiencing a Contraceptive Failure During the First Year of Typical Use and the First Year of Perfect Use and the Percentage Continuing Use at the End of the First Year, United States

Method (1)	% OF WOMEN EXPERIENCING AN ACCIDENTAL PREGNANCY WITHIN THE FIRST YEAR OF USE		% OF WOMEN CONTINUING USE AT 1 YEAR[c]
	Typical Use[a] (2)	Perfect Use[b] (3)	(4)
Chance[d]	85	85	
Spermicides[e]	21	6	43
Periodic abstinence	20		67
Calendar		9	
Ovulation method		3	
Symptothermal[f]		2	
Postovulation		1	
Withdrawal	19	4	
Cap[g] Parous women	36	26	45
Nulliparous	18	9	58
Sponge			
Parous women	36	20	45
Nulliparous	18	9	58
Diaphragm[h]	18	6	58
Condom[i]			
Female (Reality)	21	5	56
Male	12	3	63
Pill	3		72
Progestin only		0.5	
Combined		0.1	
IUD			
Progesterone T	2.0	1.5	81
Copper T 380A	0.8	0.6	78
LNg 20	0.1	0.1	81
Depo-Provera	0.3	0.3	70
Norplant (6 capsules)	0.09	0.09	85
Female sterilization	0.4	0.4	100
Male sterilization	0.15	0.10	100
Emergency contraceptive pills			
Treatment initiated within 72 hours after unprotected intercourse reduces the risk of pregnancy by at least 75%[j]			
Lactational amenorrhea method			
A highly effective, temporary method of contraception[k]			

[a]Among typical couples who initiate use of a method (not necessarily for the first time), the percentage who experience an accidental pregnancy during the first year if they do not stop use for any other reason.
[b]Among typical couples who initiate use of a method (not necessarily for the first time), and who use it perfectly (both consistently and correctly), the percentage who experience an accidental pregnancy during the first year if they do not stop use for any other reason.
[c]Among couples attempting to avoid pregnancy, the percentage who continue to use a method for 1 year.
[d]The percents failing in columns (2) and (3) are based on data from populations where contraception is not used and from women who cease using contraception in order to become pregnant. Among such populations, about 89% become pregnant within 1 year. This estimate was lowered slightly (to 85%) to represent the percent who would become pregnant within 1 year among women now relying on reversible methods of contraception if they abandoned contraception altogether.
[e]Foams, creams, gels, vaginal suppositories, and vaginal film.
[f]Cervical mucus (ovulation) method supplemented by calendar in the preovulatory and basal body temperature in the postovulatory phases
[g]With spermicidal cream or jelly.
[h]Without spermicides.
[i]The treatment schedule is 1 dose as soon as possible (but no more than 72 hours) after unprotected intercourse, and a second dose 12 hours after the first dose. The hormones that have been studied in the clinical trials of postcoital hormonal contraception are found in Nordette, Levlen, Lo/Ovral (1 dose is 4 pills), Triphasil, Tri-Levlen (1 dose is 4 yellow pills), and Ovral (1 dose is 2 pills).
[j]However, to maintain effective protection against pregnancy, another method of contraception must be used as soon as menstruation resumes, the frequency or duration of breastfeeds is reduced, bottle feeds are introduced, or the baby reaches 6 months of age.
From Hatcher RA, Trussell J, Stewart F, et al: Contraceptive Technology. New York, Irvington Publishers, 1994, with permission.

effect with a resultant increase in weight. Synthetic progestins suppress endometrial growth, which causes a decrease in menstrual flow but can also lead to breakthrough bleeding. If present, breakthrough bleeding usually only lasts a few months but can persist longer in a small percentage of women.[20]

Protein Effects. Synthetic estrogens increase hepatic production of several globulins, some of which are involved in the coagulation cascade. The increases in clotting factors are insignificant in nonsmokers less than 40 years of age and smokers less than 35 without active venous thrombotic disease or previous thrombosis with oral contraceptives.[10]

Another protein that is elevated with combination pill usage is angiotensinogen. Angiotensinogen is converted to angiotensin, which is involved in blood pressure control. Historically, increases in blood pressure were observed in some users, however, decreases in estrogen within the pill has made this less of a problem.[18]

Carbohydrate Effect. Progestins may alter carbohydrate metabolism but there is disagreement whether this is of significance in the general population. This effect may be of importance to the female athlete as discussed later. If there is a history of glucose intolerance, combination pills may worsen the situation. However, there is no increased risk of developing diabetes among users or former users.[39]

Lipid Effect. Estrogens are known to elevate high-density lipoprotein (HDL) cholesterol and decrease low-density lipoprotein (LDL) cholesterol. This is considered a beneficial effect on cardiovascular status. Many progestins have just the opposite effect, raising LDL cholesterol and lowering HDL cholesterol. Overall, the net effect on lipid metabolism with the majority of oral contraceptive pills is about zero. Some of the newer pills that contain the less-androgenic progestins norgestimate and desogestrel may have an overall positive benefit on the lipid profile.[1,15]

Cardiovascular Effects

Adverse cardiovascular effects are primarily thrombotic rather than lipid for reasons as was just discussed. The increase in clotting factors becomes an issue with smokers over age 35 and in nonsmokers over 40. If there is a history of cardiovascular disease in the person, consideration should be given to using another method of contraception. In an appropriate patient for oral contraceptive use, the risk of thrombosis or myocardial infarction is very small.[32] Chances for death are greater with childbirth than from complications of oral contraceptive use in nonsmokers less than 40.[27]

Reproductive Effects

There are no adverse consequences on future fertility from using oral contraceptives.[4,34] Women can begin trying to get pregnant immediately after stopping the pill. Some physicians ask their patients to wait for the first menstrual cycle off oral contraceptives prior to starting to get pregnant. This is to be more accurate in dating the pregnancy which has become less important with the proliferation of fetal sonography for dating purposes.

Neoplastic Effects

Oral contraceptive pills (OCPs) have been shown to decrease the incidence of ovarian cancer later in life.[7,12] If a women takes OCPs for as many as 3 months, her risks of developing ovarian cancer are reduced in half. This effect is thought secondary to one theory of ovarian cancer development called the theory of incessant ovulation. Incessant ovulation and subsequent repair of the epithelial surface of the ovary after disruption from ovulation is thought to increase the risk for ovarian cancer. Events preventing ovulation such as OCP use or pregnancy are thereby thought to be protective.

There have been numerous reports concerning oral contraceptive use and breast cancer. Many of these individual reports have conflicting conclusions. Two respected meta-analyses of such studies have reached different conclusion. A meta-analysis by Rushton et al.[28] of 27 epidemiological studies from 1980–1989 of breast cancer and oral contraceptive use found that breast cancer risk may be increased by 20% in younger, nulliparous patients and with long-term use. A similar meta-analysis by Schlesselman[29] using studies from 1980–1994 found no significant difference in breast cancer risk. The controversey surrounding breast cancer risk and oral contraceptive use will continue for now.

Less controversial is the fact that oral contraceptive use does decrease benign breast lesions such as fibroadenomas and fibrocystic disease.[5]

Endometrial cancer risks are reduced in anovulatory women taking oral contraceptives. The periodic withdrawal of progestin-induced menses reduces an anovulatory patient's chances for developing endometrial cancer by at least 40%.[6,30]

Contraindications to Oral Contraceptive Use

Oral contraceptives should not be used by women with active thrombophlebitis or a history of deep venous thrombophlebitis or thromboembolic disorders, cerebral vascular or coronary artery disease, breast cancer, endometrial cancer, undiagnosed abnormal vaginal bleeding, cholestatic jaundice of pregnancy or previous pill use, hepatic adenoma or carcinoma, or pregnancy.

Relative contraindications include smokers over age 35, uncontrolled hypertension or migraine headaches with previous pill use.

Effect on Athletic Performance

In some athletes, menstrual disturbances can develop as a consequence of the intensity of their training. The hypothalamic-pituitary axis which controls ovarian function, can become suppressed either due to low energy availability or due to stress (see Chapter 15). This depression of ovarian function leads to a hypoestrogenic state subjecting the athlete to potential harm due to calcium loss. Appropriate management in such athletes includes a reduction of the intensity of the training, an increase in caloric intake or initiation of estrogen therapy.

Combination oral contraceptive pills are generally considered a good source of estrogen for the estrogen-deficient individual. However, the effect of oral contraceptives on bone density in the amenorrheic athlete remains controversial due to a lack of prospective studies of their use.

One report by Myburgh et al.[26] concluded that stress fractures are more common in athletes with lower bone density, lower calcium intake, menstrual dysfunction, and lower use of oral contraceptives. Yet, a conflicting report by Bennell et al.[3] found no benefit of oral contraceptives on reducing stress fractures. A study of soccer players by Moller-Nielsen et al.[24] indicated that musculoskeletal injuries are reduced in women on oral contraceptive pills for reasons that are unclear.

Oral contraceptives can be adjusted and given so that the timing of the menses is possible. Menstrual flow is a result of progestin withdrawal bleeding from an estrogen primed uterus. Stopping the oral contraceptive pills will lead to a period in 2–3 days in most women. Much data has been accumulated looking at menstrual phases and athletic performances. An excellent review of dozens of studies over the last few decades was done by Lebrun.[16] In her conclusions of the extensive review it appears that there generally is no significant effect of the timing of the menstrual phases on athletic performances. These conclusions are further supported by a prospective controlled trial of exercise performance in runners as related to menstrual phase and amenorrhea.[8]

Still, high progesterone levels during the luteal phase of the menstrual cycle as in pregnancy stimulate ventilation and ventilatory responses to hypoxia and hypercapnia. Since success in endurance sports is correlated with blunted respiratory drives, the progesterone effect may be detrimental in some athletes. The combination oral contraceptive pill provides a progestin 3 out of 4 weeks. There is also an increase in oxygen consumption with oral contraceptive use perhaps through a cellular mechanism at the level of the mitochondria.[9,17,25]

Athletes on oral contraceptives have also been noted to have lower blood glucose levels during prolonged exercise with an associated decrease in carbohydrate utilization. Fat burning was not affected. Thus, sparing of carbohydrates is a theoretical competitive advantage.[2]

Women taking oral contraceptives typically have a decreased amount of menstrual flow which translates into less blood and iron loss making anemia less common.[14] Pill users also report less severe menstrual cramps which may be a competitive advantage for some athletes. Combination oral contraceptives will continue to be a popular choice of contraception for the female athlete.

Progestin-Only Contraceptives

As stated in the discussion of the combination oral contraceptive pill, much of its contraceptive effect is due to the progestin component. Progestins alone are an effective means of contraception. If progestins are given alone, the incidence of irregular breakthrough bleeding is higher than with the combination pill. However, after the first few months on progestins alone, the patient frequently becomes amenorrheic. There is also a reduced likelihood of suppressing the hypothalamic-pituitary axis without the exogenous estrogen component making ovulation more likely. Progestins as contraceptives are presently available in three forms—a daily pill, every-3-month injection and every-5-year subdermal implant. None of this class effectively prevents sexually transmitted diseases. Much of the discussion for combination oral contraception also applies here.[21]

Progestin-only pills have been available for some time. As with the combination pill, the effectiveness depends on patient compliance. Missing even a single pill markedly reduces the effectiveness. Progestin-only pills sold in the United States contain either norethindrone or norgestrel. The price of progestin-only pills is similar to the combination pill.

Depo-Provera is a long-acting medroxyprogesterone acetate given as an every-3-month intramuscular injection. It is a true progesterone compound and not a testosterone derivative like all the other progestin agents discussed.[21] Depo-Provera has been available for several years for treatment of hormonal disorders but only recently received U.S. Food and Drug Administration (FDA) approval for contraception use. Since the contraceptive effect of each injection lasts 3 months, day-to-day compliance is not an issue as is reflected in the similarity in the typical use and perfect use failure rate as noted in Table 17-1. Still, many patients will not tolerate the breakthrough bleeding and discontinue Depo-Provera after the first injection.

Norplant was FDA approved for contraception as a long-acting subdermal implant in the United States in 1991. It has been used successfully for over 20 years in other countries. Norplant contains levonorgestrel as its progestin agent and it is released slowly into the bloodstream in very small amounts. The implants are placed subdermally under local anesthesia in an office setting. The implants are effective for contraception for 5 years. As with the other progestin-only contraceptives, there is a higher incidence of breakthrough bleeding within the first few cycles.

Some patients using Norplant become amenorrheic while others continue to have menses.[31] Day-to-day compliance is not a problem with Norplant and patients choosing to stop Norplant for bleeding irregularities or restoration of fertility can have the implants removed earlier than the 5 years. Recently, there have been some questionable litigation suits filed in the United States over difficulty in removing the Norplant implants, which have not been seen abroad. The total cost of having the Norplant inserted can be several hundred dollars but this cost is minimized when spread out over a 5-year period of contraceptive effect.

Metabolic Effects

Progestin-only contraceptives have little effect on liver proteins. As with the combination pill, glucose metabolism may be slightly altered, but these pills do not cause diabetes. The major effects of progestins are on lipids. Generally, the more androgenic the progestin compound then the more unfavorable the effect of lipid metabolism with a rise in LDL-cholesterol and a decrease in HDL-cholesterol.

Unlike estrogen containing compounds, progestin-only contraceptives do not elevate clotting factors therefore risk of vascular thrombosis is reduced.[33]

Effects on Athletic Performance

Most of the discussion on the combination pill and effect on athletic performance also applies with the progestin-only pill. With progestin-only contraceptives, the timing of the menstrual cycle cannot be controlled as well. As previously discussed, timing of the menstrual phases has little effect on athletic performance.[16] Patients on long-acting progestin compounds frequently become amenorrheic due to the progestin thinning the endometrial lining after a few months. Still, the amenorrhea is not universally seen and some patients will continue to have break-through vaginal bleeding at unpredictable times which can be annoying even if not detrimental to athletic performance. Patients on progestin-only daily pills usually have regular menses. Supplemental estrogen can be used to temporarily treat the breakthrough bleeding when needed. Progestin-only pills will not treat estrogen deficiency and its potential consequences.

Postcoital Contraception

This has historically been reserved for the patient who has been sexually assaulted or when a barrier method of contraception fails such as a condom breaking. High doses of estrogen given with 24–72 hours of coital exposure will inhibit pregnancy via inhibiting implantation. It should not be considered a routine form of birth control.[11]

Various doses and compounds of estrogen are effective.[37] One commonly used method is Ovral, 4 tablets (2 given 12 hours apart). Each Ovral tablet contains 50 micrograms of ethinyl estradiol and 0.5 mg of norgestrel. Recently, Preven received FDA approval as an emergency contraceptive kit containing 4 birth control tablets each with 50 micrograms of ethinyl estradiol and 0.25 mg of levonorgestrel.

This high dose of estrogen can be associated with gastrointestinal side effects. It should be reserved for one-time protection and not considered a long-term strategy for contraception.

INTRAUTERINE DEVICES

Intrauterine devices (IUDs) were a widely used form of contraception until the 1980s when litigation forced many of the manufacturers to stop. Today, there is one IUD on the United States market, the Para Guard T 380A which is a copper device. IUDs are an effective form of contraception but they are not for everyone.

IUDs work by inhibiting implantation of the early embryo within the uterine cavity. Because of the foreign object within the uterine cavity, the patient is at increased risk of developing infection and pelvic inflammatory disease. IUDs should therefore only be used in stable monogamous couples.[22]

IUDs may occasionally cause increased uterine cramping and bleeding. They have been known to migrate through the uterine wall and sometimes have to be surgically removed. Approximately, 10% of IUDs are expelled and another 15% are removed within the first year for pain or bleeding problems.[38]

Contrary to popular opinion, IUDs do not increase the rate of ectopic pregnancies compared to women on no form of contraception. Pregnancies with an IUD in place are ectopic 3–4% of the time, which is increased from the normal 1% rate in women using no form of contraception. The total number of ectopics is still reduced since women using IUDs do not become pregnant as often.[35]

BARRIER CONTRACEPTION

Male Condoms

Male condoms are a very old and reliable form of birth control. While no method provides 100% effectiveness against sexually transmitted diseases including HIV, condoms are the best defense secondary to abstinence. Like all forms of contraception, condoms are only effective if they are used correctly. Some condoms contain spermacidal jelly which further increase their effectiveness, particularly if the condom breaks or comes off inside the vagina. The major drawback of the condom is lack of convenience and compliance problems.

Female Condoms

The concept is the same as with the male condom. These are polyurethane reservoirs placed within the vagina to create a barrier to sperm and sexually transmitted diseases. They are more awkward than male condoms and widespread use of female condoms is yet to be seen. The failure rate is 20% per year (Table 17-1).

Diaphragm

The diaphragm acts as a barrier against the cervix, but needs spermacidal jelly to be an effective contraceptive. The diaphragm must be fitted properly by a physician trained in its use. An improper fit may decrease the effectiveness. The diaphragm is inferior to the condom in protection against sexually transmitted diseases. Fewer patients are choosing this method today compared to the past perhaps because of safer oral contraception.

The diaphragm should be inserted into the vagina no longer than 6 hours prior to intercourse with about a teaspoonful of spermicidal jelly. The diaphragm needs to be left in place approximately 6 hours after coitus but no more than 24 hours. Additional spermicide should be used with each additional episode of intercourse while the diaphragm is in place.

Cervical Cap

A small cap is placed on the cervix to block sperm. Contraceptive jelly need not be used with the cervical cap. It should be applied to the cervix at least 20 minutes before intercourse but no more than 4 hours. It should be left in place for a minimum of 6 hours after intercourse but can be left in for up to 36 hours.

Proper fitting of the cap can be difficult and accomplished successfully in only 50% of women. Women must become proficient in placing the cap properly on the cervix which can be difficult. Dislodgement of the cap can occur during intercourse and is a cause of the failures with this method.[23]

SPERMICIDES

Spermicides used include nonoxynol-9, octoxynol-9, and menfegol. These agents are available as jellies, creams, foams, melting suppositories, and vaginal film. Spermicides require application 10–30 minutes prior to sexual intercourse. They are inexpensive and provide some protection against sexually transmitted diseases, but should not be considered protective against HIV.

Contraceptive effect is listed in Table 17-1. The principal side effect with this method is an allergy to the spermacidal agent in about 5% of the population.

STERILIZATION

Female tubal sterilization is a highly effective form of contraception. However, it is only to be used when child bearing is complete. Effectiveness is very high and compliance is not a problem. The sterilization procedure may be reversed at a later date depending on how much tube has been destroyed. A patient asking about reversal prior to the tubal sterilization procedure may not be the best candidate as sterilization should be considered permanent going into the procedure.

CONCLUDING REMARKS

Contraception is an issue important to all sexually active women not seeking pregnancy and female athletes are no exception. When determining mode of contraception, the female athlete should consider what is more important for their contraceptive choice, prevention of sexually transmitted diseases, ease of use or as a method of hormone replacement. Lastly, all contraceptives are only as good as the compliance factor.

References

1. Anderson FD: Selectivity and minimal androgenicity of norgestimate in monophasic and triphasic oral contraceptives. Acta Obstet Gynecol Scand 156 (Suppl):15, 1992.
2. Bemden DA, Boileau RA, Bahr JM, et al: Effects of oral contraceptives on hormonal and metabolic responses during exercise. Med Sci Sports Exerc 24:434–441, 1992.
3. Bennell KL, Malcolm SA, Thomas SA et al. Risk factors for stress fractures in track and field athletes, a twelve-month prospective study. Am J Sports Med 24:810, 1996.
4. Bracken MB, Hellenbrand KG, Holford TR. Conception delay after oral contraceptive use: the effect of estrogen dose. Fertil Steril 53:21, 1990.
5. Brinton LA, Vessey MP, Flavel R, Yeates D. Risk factors for benign breast disease. Am J Epidemiol 1981; 113:203.
6. The Cancer and Steroid Hormone Study of the CDC and NICHD. Combination oral contraceptive use and the risk of endometrial cancer. JAMA 1987; 257:796.
7. The Cancer and Steroid Hormone Study of the CDC and NICHD. The reduction in risk of ovarian cancer associated with oral-contraceptive use. New Engl J Med 1987; 316:650.
8. De Souza MJ, Maguire MS, Rubin KR et al. Effects of menstrual phase and amenorrhea on exercise performance in runners. Med Sci Sports Exerc 1990; 22:575.
9. Dombovy ML, Bonekat HW, Williams TJ, Staats BJ. Exercise performance and ventilatory response in the menstrual cycle. Med Sci Sports Exerc 1987; 19:111.
10. Goldbaum GM, Kendrick JS, Hogelin GC, Gentry EM. The relative impact of smoking and oral contraceptive use on women in the United States. JAMA 1987; 258:1339.
11. Gray MJ, Norton P, Yuhasz B. Emergency Contraception. The Female Patient 1991; 16:33.
12. Hankinson SE, Colditz GA, Hunter DJ, Spencer TL, Rosner B, Stampfer MJ. A quantitative assessment of oral contraceptive use and risk of ovarian cancer. Obstet Gynecol 1992; 80:708.
13. Hatcher RA, Trussell J, Stewart F, et al: Contraceptive Technology. New York: Irvington Publishers, 1994,113–114.
14. Kay CR. The Royal College of General Practitioners' Oral Contraception Study: some recent observations. Clin Obstet Gynaecol 1984; 11:759.
15. Kloosterboer HJ. Selectivity in progesterone and androgen receptor binding of progestogens used in oral contraception. Contraception 1988; 38:325.
16. Lebrun CM. The effect of the phase of the menstrual cycle and the birth control pill on athletic performance. Clin Sports Med 1994; 13:419.
17. Martin BJ, Sparks KE, Zwillich CW, Weil JV. Low exercise ventilation in endurance athletes. Medicine and Science in Sports and Exercise 1979; 11:181.
18. Meade TW, Greenberg G, Thompson SG. Progestogens and cardiovascular reactions associated with oral contraceptives and a comparison of the safety of 50- and 30

microgram oestrogen preparations. Br Med J 1980; 280:1157.
19. Mishell DR: Family Planning. In Mishell DR, Stenchever MA, Droegmueller W, et al (eds): Comprehensive Gynecology, 3rd edition, pp 291–296. St. Louis, Mosby, 1997.
20. Mishell DR: Family Planning. In Mishell DR, Stenchever MA, Droegmueller W, et al (eds): Comprehensive Gynecology, 3rd edition, pp 297–299. St. Louis, Mosby, 1997.
21. Mishell DR: Family Planning. In Mishell DR, Stenchever MA, Droegmueller W, et al (eds): Comprehensive Gynecology, 3rd edition, pp 317–325. St. Louis, Mosby, 1997.
22. Mishell DR: Family Planning. In Mishell DR, Stenchever MA, Droegmueller W, et al (eds): Comprehensive Gynecology, 3rd edition, pp 331–333. St.Louis, Mosby, 1997.
23. Mishell DR: Family Planning. In Mishell DR, Stenchever MA, Droegmueller W, et al (eds): Comprehensive Gynecology, 3rd edition, pp 289. St.Louis, Mosby, 1997.
24. Moller-Nielsen J, Hammar M. Women's soccer injuries in relation to the menstrual cycle and oral contraceptive use. Med Sci Sports Exerc 1989; 21:126.
25. Moore LF, McCullough RE, Weil JV. Increased HVR in pregnancy: relationship to hormonal and metabolic changes. J Appl Physiol 1987; 62:158.
26. Myburgh KH, Hutchins J, Fataar AB et al. Low bone density is an etiologic factor for stress fractures in athletes. Ann Intern Med 1990; 113:754.
27. Ory HW. Mortality associated with fertility and fertility control: 1983. Family Planning Perspectives 1983; 15:50.
28. Rushton L, Jones DR. Oral contraceptive use and breast cancer risk: a meta-analysis of variations with age at diagnosis, parity and total duration of oral contraceptive use. Br J Obstet Gynecol 1992; 99:239.
29. Schlesselman JJ. Net effect of oral contraceptive use on the risk of cancer in women in the United States. Obstet Gynecol 1995; 85:793.
30. Schlesselmann JJ. Oral contraceptives and neoplasia of the uterine corpus. Contraception 1991; 43:557.
31. Shoupe D, Mishell DR, Bopp BL et al. The significance of bleeding patterns in Norplant implant users. Obstet Gynecol 1991; 77:256.
32. Thorogood M, Mann J, Murphy M et al. Is oral contraceptive use still associated with an increased risk of fatal myocardial infarction? Report of a case-control study. Br J Obstet Gynaecol 1991; 98:1245.
33. Van der Vange N, Blankenstein MA, Kloosterboer HJ et al. Effects of seven low-dose combined oral contraceptives on sex hormone binding globulin, corticosteroid binding globulin, total and free testosterone. Contraception 1990; 42:345.
34. Vessey MP, Smith MA, Yates D. Return of fertility after discontinuation of oral contraceptives: influence of age and parity. Br J Fam Plann 1986; 11:120.
35. WHO Special Programme of Research, Development and Research Training in Human Reproduction. Task Force on Intrauterine Devices for Fertility Regulation. A multinational case-control study of ectopic pregnancy. Clin Reprod Fertil 1985; 3:131–143.
36. Wolner-Hanssen P, Svensson L, Mardh PA, et al. Laparoscopic findings and contraceptive use in women with signs and symptoms suggestive of acute salpingitis. Obstet Gynecol 1985; 66:233.
37. Woodward J, Schnare S, Stewart F. Time to spread the word about postcoital contraception. Contemp Ob Gynecol-NP 1993; 1:12.

38. World Health Organization (WHO). The Tcu220C, multiload 250 and Nova T IUDs at 3.5 and 7 years of use: results from three randomized multicentre trials. Contraception 1990; 42:141.

39. Wynn V, Godsland I. Effects of oral contraceptives and carbohydrate metabolism. J Reprod Med 1986; 31(9)(Supplement):906.

Chapter 18

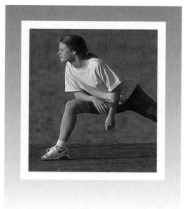

Sexually Transmitted Diseases

W. David Hager, M.D., F.A.C.O.G.

Sexually transmitted diseases (STDs) are those infections that are spread by direct intimate human sexual contact. Rather than the original five "venereal diseases" (syphilis, gonorrhea, chancroid, granuloma inguinale, lymphogranuloma venereum) we now have a lengthy list of diseases that are spread in this manner. Many of these infections have been present for years but only recently has their prevalence increased. There are many reasons for this, including improved laboratory diagnostic testing, increased transmission due to a larger number of young people in the sexually active age range, greater freedom of sexual expression, including multiple sexual partners, and expanded use of drugs and alcohol. The Centers for Disease Control and Prevention (CDC) estimates that there are over 15 million new diagnoses of STDs in the United States. One of every 5 teens has been exposed to a viral STD.[5]

Obviously, we face a tremendous problem in diagnosing and treating all of these individuals. It is not the purpose of this chapter to describe each STD in detail, but to focus on the basic information about each of the major STDs.

Female athletes are at risk for any and all of the STDs if they engage in intimate sexual contact. There is a tendency to focus attention on other causes of rashes, sores, and abdominal and pelvic pain and neglect the possibility of a sexually transmitted etiology. Each gynecologic evaluation should include questions about sexual activity and possible symptoms of STDs. Unfortunately, most of the major STDs may not cause symptoms until sequelae of disease begin to emerge.

VAGINITIS

Although 2 of the 3 infectious causes of vaginitis are not considered to be sexually transmitted, it is appropriate to consider them in this section.

Candidal Vulvovaginal Infections

Candidal vaginitis is now less frequent than bacterial vaginosis as a cause of vaginal infection in women. Candidiasis accounts for 20% to 30% of diagnosed vaginitis.[15] Since candidal species may normally be present in the rectum and vagina of women, it is not considered an STD. It has been estimated that 75% of women will experience at least one episode of vulvovaginal candidiasis during their reproductive years.[18] The fungal organisms causing infection may be isolated from 20% of asymptomatic women.[26]

Candida albicans causes approximately 85% of candidal vaginitis, while 15% of cases are caused by other species such as *Candida glabrata* and *Candida tropicalis*. Although these organisms may exist in the vagina as normal commensals, it usually requires an increased inoculum or altered immunity to induce infection. These species gain access to the vagina from the anal and perianal regions.[2]

There are several predisposing factors associated with candidal vaginitis (Table 18-1). Among these, the female athlete may be predisposed because of exposure to excessive moisture and use of tight-fitting underclothing. Avoidance of extended wear of wet uniforms or swimwear and adequate drying of the genital area should be emphasized to all athletes.

Table 18-1. Predisposing Factors for Candidal Vaginitis

Diabetes mellitus	Antibiotic treatment
Excessive intake of "sweets"	Poor hygiene
Anal contact sexually	Diarrhea
Tight-fitting synthetic garments	Corticosteroid treatment

Candidal vaginitis is diagnosed by performing a microscopic examination of vaginal secretions. Although a saline wet mount is adequate for identifying pseudohyphae, they may be seen more readily on a 10% potassium hydroxide (KOH) wet preparation. Culture is not cost effective unless one is dealing with resistant infections. The vaginal pH is acidic in these women (Table 18-2).

Yeast infections cause increased, turbid vaginal discharge, as well as vulvar pruritus and burning. On examination, a thick, white vaginal discharge is commonly seen and the vulva may be erythematous or, in some cases, pallid.

The treatment of candidiasis is usually initiated with a vaginal cream or suppositories. Butoconazole, clotrimazole, and miconazole are now over-the-counter preparations. Unfortunately, resistance to these medications is increasing. Terconazole 2% cream or suppositories daily in 3- or 7-day regimens and fluconazole (150 mg) orally are the first lines of prescribed therapy. If patients have severe pruritus, a nonfluorinated steroid cream, such as desonide, may be used on the vulva. In resistant cases or individuals with multiple recurrences, oral antifungals such as fluconazole or ketoconazole may be prescribed. We have used boric acid suppositories (600 mg), in a suppressive dose of one, 3 times a week to control the vaginal pH and suppress growth of candida.

Trichomonas vaginalis Vaginitis

Trichomoniasis is a sexually transmitted vaginal infection caused by Trichomonas vaginalis. It is estimated that 3 to 8 million cases occur in the United States annually.[10] T. vaginalis causes approximately 20% of all cases of vaginitis.

As an STD, having multiple sexual partners is the principal risk factor for this infection. Ninety percent of the male sexual partners of infected women and 90% to 100% of the female sexual partners of infected men are found to harbor the organism.[22] Trichomonas vaginitis causes abnormal vaginal discharge, vaginal discomfort,

pruritus, dyspareunia, and dysuria. Sampling the vaginal discharge with a saline wet mount reveals motile trichomonads (flagellated protozoans) and increased white blood cells. Vaginal pH is in the alkaline range (Table 18-2).

The treatment is with the 5-nitrimidazole, metronidazole. Various doses have been used successfully, with a single 2-g oral dose equivalent to 500 mg twice daily for 5 or 7 days.[11] Relatively resistant organisms have been recovered and require extended therapy with oral metronidazole, or combined oral therapy 500 mg twice daily for 10 to 14 days, and vaginal suppositories 500 mg daily for 14 days.

Bacterial Vaginosis

The form of vaginal infection formerly known as *Haemophilus* vaginitis, or nonspecific vaginitis or anaerobic vaginitis, is now known as bacterial vaginosis (BV). The condition is called vaginosis because there is a decrease in leukocytes in the vaginal discharge, indicating that this is not an infection but an inflammatory condition of the vagina.[9] Forty to fifty percent of all vaginal infections are associated with BV.

Bacterial vaginosis is not caused by a single organism, but by several different bacteria, particularly anaerobes. *Gardnerella vaginalis*, *Mobiluncus* species, and anaerobic rods are the principal isolates when cultures are done.[31]

The diagnosis is made when the vaginal secretions of a patient complaining of vaginal discharge, pruritus, and burning are evaluated with a wet mount that reveals clue cells, curved motile rods known as *Mobiluncus* species, a vaginal pH of >4.5, an amine (fishy) odor when KOH is added to the slide, and a paucity of lactobacilli. There should be at least 1 clue cell per high-power field on 10 consecutive fields to diagnose BV. Cultures are not beneficial in making the diagnosis (see Table 18-2).

The treatment of BV has evolved from use of broad-spectrum antibiotics to specific therapy for anaerobes. Metronidazole 500 mg twice daily for 7 days is the gold standard for treatment.[28]

Table 18-2. Diagnosis of Vaginitis/Vaginosis

DIAGNOSTIC CRITERIA	NORMAL	BACTERIAL VAGINOSIS	CANDIDA	TRICHOMONIASIS
Vaginal pH	3.8–4.2	>4.5	>4.5	>4.5
Discharge	White, clear, floculant	Thin, white to gray, homogeneous, adherent, often increased	White, curdy, "cottage cheese"-like, sometimes increased	Yellow, green, frothy, adherent increased
Amine odor	Absent	Present	Absent	Present sometimes
Microscopic	Lactobacilli	Clue cells, coccoid bacteria, no WBCs	Mycelia, budding yeasts, pseudohyphae	Motile trichomonads, WBCs >10/hpf

More recently, clindamycin cream 2% administered as a 5-g dose daily for 7 days and metronidazole gel 0.75% administered daily for 5 days have been introduced and are well accepted for treatment. Oral clindamycin also may be used.

Although BV is not considered a STD, if symptoms recur within 30 days of treatment, the possibility that it is sexually transmitted should be considered and the sexual partner(s) treated with doxycycline.

Syphilis

Syphilis is a sexually transmitted infection that has been described for centuries. The development of antibiotics was heralded as an opportunity to eradicate the infection, however, that did not occur, and with the epidemic of human immunodeficiency virus (HIV) infection, a concomitant increase in syphilis cases occurred. The incidence has decreased in the past 3 years. Over 75,000 cases occur each year, with approximately 35,000 being primary or secondary disease.[35]

Syphilis is caused by the bacterial spirochete *Treponema pallidum*. The organism is thin and cannot be seen by routine Gram stain or light microscopy and requires darkfield microscopy to visualize it.

When *T. pallidum* is transmitted from an infected person by direct intimate contact, it can penetrate tiny breaks in the host's skin or mucous membranes, infect the host, and cause a chancre. The chancre is a painless ulcer with raised, rounded borders and an indurated base. Chancres may become secondarily infected with bacteria and become suppurative and painful. The chancre appears 10 to 90 days after exposure and heals within 2 to 6 weeks even when not treated with antibiotics.

Six weeks to 6 months after the appearance of a chancre, secondary syphilis may occur if treatment was not administered earlier. Secondary syphilis is characterized by a maculopapular rash over the entire body, with emphasis on the palms of the hands and soles of the feet. Lymphadenopathy, malaise, and weight loss may occur.

Tertiary syphilis involving the cardiovascular, musculoskeletal, and central nervous systems may occur 1 to 20 years after the disease becomes latent. Chronic degenerative disease results.

Syphilis is categorized as a latent disease if it is not diagnosed in its acute phase. If the latency is less than 1 year's duration, it is staged as early latent disease; if more than 1 year, late latent.

The diagnosis is made by examination of the primary chancre contents under darkfield microscopy, or by serologic evaluation of the host's blood. The rapid plasma reagin (RPR) and Venereal Disease Research Laboratory (VDRL) tests are screening serologic tests. The fluorescent treponemal antibody (FTA) test becomes positive with any true diagnosis of syphilis and remains positive for a lifetime. The screening tests may become negative or low-titer positive after treatment.

The treatment of syphilis is penicillin. Benzathine penicillin 2.4 million units intramuscularly in one dose is the treatment for early syphilis (primary, secondary, and early latent disease). For penicillin-allergic persons, doxycycline or tetracycline may be used. The treatment for late latent syphilis is 7.2 million units of benzathine penicillin given as three, 2.4-million unit doses each week for 3 weeks.

With the surge of syphilis occurring with the acquired immunodeficiency syndrome epidemic, it is important to screen any HIV-positive patient for syphilis.

Chlamydia

Chlamydia trachomatis is 1 of 3 species of the genus *Chlamydia*, the others being *Chlamydia psittaci* and *Chlamydia pneumoniae*. Chlamydiae also possess some viral characteristics, including an obligate need to remain intracellular to survive. They do contain both DNA and RNA and are sensitive to antibiotic therapy. The life cycle of the organisms includes a genetic or reproductive phase and an infectious phase.

Chlamydia trachomatis infection is the most common bacterial STD in the United States and is one of the leading infectious causes of pelvic inflammatory disease (PID). More than 4 million cases of chlamydia are diagnosed each year,[29] 70 to 80% of women and 20 to 30% of men are asymptomatic. The highest prevalence rates are found among unmarried, sexually active, adolescent women, of whom 10% to 40% are positive.[3] In a recent prospective, longitudinal study of 3202 sexually active females ages 12 to 19 attending family planning, STD, or school-based clinics, 24.1% were infected at their first visit and 13.9% on repeat visits.[4] Because chlamydial infections have numerous sequelae that can result in chronic pain and infertility, infected teens are at great risk for chronic problems.

Like most STDs, chlamydia is transmitted by direct, intimate contact with an infected partner. Male-to-female transmission is more efficient than female-to-male transmission. The bacterium has a propensity to infect columnar epithelial cells, like those in the conjunctivae, urethra, endocervix, endometrium, and fallopian tubes.

Risk factors for infection include black race, unmarried state, and multiple sexual partners.[13] Infections are also more frequent among patients who have coexisting *Neisseria gonorrhoeae* or *Trichomonas vaginalis* infection.[20]

Common clinical syndromes in women include urethritis, endocervicitis (mucopurulent cervicitis), endometritis, PID, and perihepatitis (Fitz-Hugh–Curtis syndrome).

Fifteen to twenty-five percent of female sexual partners of chlamydia-infected men have positive chlamydial urethral cultures.[38] Classically, females will have dysuria and/or urgency but will have negative urine cultures in 65% of cases.[32]

Endocervicitis is the most frequent female genital infection caused by chlamydia. Over half of these women are asymptomatic.[14] Classically, there is mucopurulent discharge from the cervix, tenderness with motion of the cervix, and friability of the cervix resulting in spotting with examination or with coitus. The infection of the cervix can result in marked inflammation and atypical cells on Pap smear.

Because of the propensity of *C. trachomatis* to infect columnar epithelial cells, infection may spread to the endometrium and, subsequently, the fallopian tubes. Chlamydiae and *N. gonorrhoeae* are the most common initiating pathogens in infection of the fallopian tubes.[34] Disease initiated by chlamydiae may result in fewer acute symptoms than that caused by the gonococcus. These women may present later in their course of disease and have more significant damage to the fallopian tubes.[33]

Women who have spread of disease beyond the pelvis due to spillage of bacteria into the peritoneal cavity and up the right paracolic gutter from the fallopian tubes may develop perihepatitis. *Chlamydia trachomatis* is a frequent cause. In addition to the symptoms and signs of PID, these women have right-upper-quadrant pain and hepatic tenderness.

Cell culture on mammalian cell lines such as McCoy cells is the definitive diagnostic test against which all others are compared. Other diagnostic techniques include the direct fluorescent antibody (DFA) test, the enzyme immunoassay (EIA), the polymerase chain reaction (PCR), and the ligase chain reaction (LCR). Because young sexually active women are at significant risk for chlamydial infection, screening should be done at least annually at the time of the Pap smear, or whenever symptoms of increased vaginal discharge or abdominal/pelvic pain occur. The treatment of *C. trachomatis* infections is listed in Table 18-3). Azithromycin 1 g orally as a single dose and

Table 18-3. Treatment of Chlamydial Infections

RECOMMENDED REGIMENS
Azithromycin 1 g PO in a single dose, *or* Doxycycline 100 mg PO twice a day for 7 days

ALTERNATIVE REGIMENS
Erythromycin base 500 mg PO 4 times a day for 7 days, *or* Erythromycin ethylsuccinate 800 mg PO 4 times a day for 7 days, *or* Ofloxacin 300 mg PO twice a day for 7 days *or* Levofluxacin 500 mg PO once daily for 7 days

From Centers for Disease Control and Prevention: 1998 Guidelines for Treatment of Sexually Transmitted Diseases. MMWR 47(No. RR-1): 1–111, 1998, with permission.

doxycycline 100 mg orally twice daily for 7 days are equally effective in eradicating the organism in nonpregnant women. Of the alternative drugs listed, only ofloxacin 300 mg orally twice daily for 7 days or levofloxacin 500 mg daily for 7 days are reliably effective. Erythromycin base and amoxicillin are the treatments of choice in pregnant women.[6]

There is no significant resistance of the organism to tetracyclines. Azithromycin is equally effective and with its single-dose regimen allows for near-guaranteed compliance, but it is much more expensive than generic doxycycline.

Gonorrhea

Infection with the bacterium *Neisseria gonorrhoeae* is among the most ancient of the STDs. There are just under 1 million reported cases and an estimated 2 million total cases of gonorrhea in the United States annually.[6]

Neisseria gonorrhoeae is a gram-negative coccus that is spread by direct, intimate contact with an infected partner. The risk of transmission from male to female is 80% to 90%, whereas the risk from female to male is only 20% to 25%.[17] The organism infects columnar and transitional epithelial cells, therefore the genital tract is primarily affected.

When the gonococcus infects the female lower genital tract it may remain undetected in an asymptomatic state. These women may spread the disease without knowing they are infected. If an infected woman fails to seek diagnosis and treatment or receives inadequate treatment, 10% to 20% will develop acute PID.[16]

The gonococcus can cause similar infections to those caused by chlamydiae, including acute urethritis, cervicitis, endometritis, salpingitis, and perihepatitis. Gonorrhea is a more common infection in the rectum and pharynx than chlamydia. In addition, 0.5% to 1.0% of women who have anogenital infection will develop disseminated gonococcal infection (DGI). This infection may involve the skin and joints (dermatitis–tenosynovitis syndrome, septic arthritis syndrome) and rarely the heart (endocarditis) and meninges (meningitis).

The diagnosis is made by plating discharge containing the organism onto selective media containing antibiotics (such as modified Thayer–Martin medium). Duplicate endocervical specimens or consecutive endocervical and anal swabs improve recovery rates. Gram staining is helpful in making the diagnosis among males with urethritis but is less sensitive in females. Combination DNA-probe devices are available for detecting chlamydia and gonorrhea.

The treatment regimens for uncomplicated urethral, endocervical, or rectal gonococcal infections are given in Table 18-4. The rising incidence of infection due to penicillinase-producing or tetracycline-resistant *N. gonorrhoeae* and strains with chromosomally mediated resistance to multiple antibiotics have led the Centers for Disease Control and Prevention to alter treatment recommendations.

Pelvic Inflammatory Disease

Infection of the fallopian tubes from ascending infection of the lower genital tract is a major consequence of chlamydial and gonococcal infection. There are an estimated 1.5 million cases in the United States annually, with the majority being managed as outpatients.

Although *C. trachomatis* and *N. gonorrhoeae* may initiate the process of PID, other bacteria, including Enterobacteriaceae and anaerobes, as well as mycoplasmas may infect the tubes secondarily.

The principal diagnostic findings among women with PID are abdominal tenderness, tenderness with motion of the cervix, and adnexal tenderness. A history of fever (41%) and a history of abnormal vaginal discharge (55%) are not frequently reported.[19] The most frequent symptom is that of abdominal pain.

The diagnosis is made on clinical grounds. Obtaining endocervical and rectal cultures, doing a saline wet prep to look for leukocytes, and obtaining an endometrial culture via biopsy or using a sterile double-lumen brush may help to isolate the causative organisms. Whenever there is any question about the diagnosis, laparoscopy should be performed to visualize the tubes. The differential diagnosis of PID includes appendicitis, ovarian cysts, inflammatory bowel disease, urinary tract infection, and ectopic pregnancy.

Treatment guidelines for PID are listed in Table 18-5. Coverage is intended for *N. gonorrhoeae*, *C. trachomatis*, and anaerobes.

Indications for hospitalization include inability to comply with oral medication, failure to respond to oral antibiotics within 48 to 72 hours, uncertain diagnosis, young age (teenage), the presence of a pelvic abscess, and pregnancy. The author believes that all young women with PID who desire future pregnancy should be hospitalized and treated with parenteral antibiotics.

The consequences of infertility, tubal pregnancy, and chronic pelvic pain make it essential that PID be diagnosed appropriately and treated aggressively with antibiotics.

VIRAL SEXUALLY TRANSMITTED DISEASES

Herpes Simplex Virus

Genital herpes infections are caused by the DNA virus herpes simplex. Infection with this virus is acquired by direct, intimate contact with an individual who is shedding virus.

Estimates of the prevalence of herpes simplex virus (HSV) infections are based on surveys of physicians' practices in the United States through the National Disease and Therapeutic Index. According to the Index, there are over 175,000 initial visits to physicians' offices annually for diagnosis and treatment of genital HSV infections.[5] There has been a steady increase in the number of cases since the mid-1960s and current estimates are 1 million new cases annually.

Table 18-4. Treatment Guidelines for Uncomplicated Urethral, Endocervical, or Rectal Infection with Gonorrhea

RECOMMENDED REGIMENS
Cefixime 400 mg PO in a single dose,
or
Ceftriaxone 125 mg IM in a single dose,
or
Ciprofloxacin 500 mg PO in a single dose,
or
Ofloxacin 400 mg PO in a single dose,
plus
Azithromycin 1 g PO in a single dose,
or
Doxycycline 100 mg PO twice a day for 7 days

From Centers for Disease Control and Prevention: 1998 Guidelines for Treatment of Sexually Transmitted Diseases. MMWR 47(No. RR-1): 1–111, 1998, with permission.

Table 18-5. Treatment Guidelines for Pelvic Inflammatory Disease

INPATIENT TREATMENT

Regimen A
Cefotetan 2 g IV every 12 hours, *or* cefoxitin 2 g IV every 6 hours,
plus
Doxycycline 100 mg IV or PO every 12 hours

Regimen B
Clindamycin 900 mg IV every 8 hours,
plus
Gentamicin loading dose IV or IM (2 mg/kg of body weight), followed by a maintenance dose (1.5 mg/kg) every 8 hours (single daily dosing may be substituted)

OUTPATIENT TREATMENT

Regimen A
Ofloxacin 400 mg PO twice a day for 14 days,
plus
Metronidazole 500 mg PO twice a day for 14 days

Regimen B
Ceftriaxone 250 mg IM once,
or
Cefoxitin 2 g IM plus probenecid 1 g PO in a single dose concurrently once,
or
Other parenteral third-generation cephalosporin (eg, ceftizoxime or cefotaxime),
plus
Doxycycline 100 mg PO twice a day for 14 days (include this regimen with one of the above regimens)

From Centers for Disease Control and Prevention: 1998 Guidelines for Treatment of Sexually Transmitted Diseases. MMWR 47(No. RR-1): 1–111, 1998, with permission.

Genital herpes may be caused by either of two viral subtypes, HSV-1 or HSV-2, however, HSV-2 is certainly the most frequent cause in the United States. There are many strains of each major type of HSV and this has made the development of a vaccine or prevention very difficult. Although HSV-1 causes most oral-labial herpes, the type-1 strain may be transmitted to the genitalia by oral–genital contact or by genital–genital contact if the infected partner already has HSV-1 on the genitals.

The incubation period for HSV is 3 to 5 days. Many infections are asymptomatic. Patients experiencing their first-ever HSV infection or their first symptomatic infection will often develop symptoms of a flu-like illness initially, with low-grade fever, malaise, myalgia, and fatigue. The occurrence of vulvar burning, tingling, or pruritus usually precedes the occurrence of papular lesions, which become fluid-filled blisters called vesicles and then break down into shallow ulcerative areas that are painful and tender.[7] With primary HSV infection, the duration of lesions and

pain is approximately 9 to 13 days and the mean time to crusting is 9 to 15 days. Complete healing requires 10 to 22 days. Patients may shed virus for a mean of 8 to 14 days.[12] Unfortunately for diagnostic purposes, many patients are asymptomatic and yet transmit the virus.

Herpes infections are categorized as primary, nonprimary first episode, and recurrent disease (Table 18-6). After the initial infection, the frequency of recurrences varies. Some patients may never have another episode; others may suffer recurrences as often as every month. Recurrences are usually not nearly as symptomatic as primary outbreaks.

Herpes infections may be diagnosed by clinical appearance only but at least one definitive diagnosis by culture, the gold standard, is recommended.[8] Viral transport media may be used to swab an unroofed vesicle or an ulcer. The specimen is then transported to the laboratory, where it is inoculated onto tissue culture for isolation. Results are usually returned within 48 to

Table 18–6. Categorization of Genital Herpes Infections

CATEGORY	IgG STATUS	KNOWN PREVIOUS STATUS	VIRAL SHEDDING
True primary	Negative	Negative	8–14 days
Nonprimary, first episode	Positive	Negative	3–7 days
Recurrent	Positive	Positive	3–7 days

72 hours. FAB tests and PCR techniques are also available. Three antiviral medications provide clinical benefit for genital herpes: acyclovir, valacyclovir, and famciclovir.[6] Although acyclovir can be administered topically, orally, or intravenously, oral therapy is the preferred mode of therapy in a dosage of 200 mg, 5 times a day for 7 to 10 days, or 400 mg, 3 times daily for 7 to 10 days. Several studies have evaluated the efficacy of acyclovir, including that of Mertz and coworkers, which reported a 78% decrease in duration of viral shedding and a 25% enhancement of lesion healing compared to placebo.[23]

Valacyclovir is a valine ester of acyclovir with enhanced absorption after oral administration.

In the first clinical episode, the dosage for valacyclovir is 1 g orally twice daily for 7 to 10 days, while episodic recurrent infection is treated with 1 gram orally twice daily for 5 to 10 days. Famciclovir, a prodrug of penciclovir, is also highly bioavailable in an oral dose. In the first clinical episode, the dosage for famciclovir is 250 mg orally 3 times daily for 7 to 10 days, while episodic recurrent infections are treated with 500 mg orally twice daily for 5 to 10 days.[6]

In order to diminish the frequency of recurrences, these agents may be administered prophylactically. Several doses have been used, however, with acyclovir at a dosage of 400 mg twice a day approximately 45% of patients will not have recurrences.[24] In addition, famciclovir 500 mg twice daily or valacyclovir in dosages of 500 mg twice daily, or 1000 mg once daily are accepted regimens for suppressive therapy.[6]

Hepatitis B Virus

Hepatitis B virus (HBV) is one of the major causes of acute and chronic liver disease in the world today. There are an estimated 1 million chronic carriers of HBV in the United States.[1] It is now recognized that sexual transmission is a major mechanism of spread of this virus.

Hepatitis B virus infection is caused by a DNA virus that preferentially infects humans. The virus can be transmitted directly through contaminated blood or blood products, contaminated needles or syringes, tattoos, ear piercing, intimate sexual contact, and exchange of bodily secretions, and perinatally from an infected mother to her newborn infant.

Hepatitis B virus infection is diagnosed by serology. The presence of surface (s) antigen indicates previous infection, envelope (e) antigen indicates high infectivity, core (c) antibody indicates healing, and surface (s) antibody indicates immunity.

There is no definitive treatment for either acute or chronic HBV infection. Supportive therapy in the form of fluids, rest, adequate nutrition, and treatment of nausea and vomiting or bowel-related symptoms is essential. Immunization with a 3-dose series of HBV vaccine is recommended for persons in at-risk groups, including sexually active homosexual and bisexual males, men and women diagnosed as having recently acquired another STD, persons who have had more than one sex partner in the preceding 6 months, and persons working with or around blood or blood products. Universal immunization is encouraged for all newborn infants.

Human Papillomavirus

Although lesions called genital warts have been recognized for centuries, it was not until 1949 that the causative agent, human papillomavirus (HPV), was identified. Since that time there has been a dramatic increase in the number of reported cases. HPV is the most common viral STD in the United States, with estimates of over 4 million cases annually.[21] Infection is especially frequent among college coeds.

Since 1977, over 60 different HPVs have been typed. Certain types such as 6 and 11 are generally associated with benign cervical changes, whereas types 16, 18, 31, 33, 35, and 45 are more frequently associated with malignant potential.[30] Over 95% of all cases of cervical cancer and dysplasia in women are associated with HPV.

It is not uncommon for HPV to cause subclinical lesions that are detected at the time of colposcopy after the patient has had an abnormal Pap smear. Clinically evident lesions are classically raised excrescences with lobulated, finger-like projections. They are usually found on the vulva, perineum, or perianal region, or within the vagina or anus. The application of a 5% acetic acid solution will cause these lesions to appear as pearly white on colposcopic examination.

The diagnosis may be made clinically with identification of classic wart-like lesions or cytologically with the detection of HPV changes on Pap smear. Colposcopy with visual or biopsy identification of the viral changes confirms the diagnosis. Use of DNA hybridization or antigen-detection studies to identify the exact HPV type is not essential since cervical dysplasia is managed by its occurrence rather than by the specific type and its prognosis for causing malignant change. Any patient with HPV change on Pap smear should be colposcoped and biopsies done as indicated. If only HPV change is diagnosed, Pap smears should be repeated every 6 months. The treatment of cervical dysplasia is beyond the scope of this chapter.

Genital warts may be treated with the direct application of the caustic agents bi- or trichloracetic acid (80% to 90% solution). It may be necessary to reapply the solution every 2 weeks for several sessions until the warts have resolved. It is important to continue to look for new crops of lesions. Lesions can be excised if they are unresponsive to topical treatment by using a wire loop cautery or laser vaporization. Interferon injections may be used for persistent lesions.

Patients may apply podofilox solution with a cotton swab, or podofilox gel with a finger, to visible genital warts twice a day for 3 days, followed by 4 days of no therapy. This cycle may be repeated as necessary for a total of 4 cycles. The total wart area treated should not exceed 10 cm^2, and the total volume of podofilox should not exceed 0.5 mL/day. If possible, the health-care provider should apply the initial treatment to demonstrate the proper application technique and identify which warts should be treated. The safety of podofilox during pregnancy has not been established. In addition, imiquimod 5% cream may be applied by the patient at bedtime, 3 times a week for as long as 16 weeks. The treatment should be washed with mild soap and water 6 to 10 hours after the application. Many patients may be clear of warts by 8 to 10 weeks or sooner. As with podofilox, the safety of this agent during pregnancy has not been established.[6]

Recurrences of HPV infection may be related to incomplete treatment of initial lesions or by delayed activation of viral particles in the submucosa. The sexual partners of women with HPV infection should be examined and treated if they have visible lesions. Condoms are not totally protective since lesions or subclinical areas may be present outside the covered area on the penis.

Human Immunodeficiency Virus Infection

It is beyond the scope of this chapter to describe in detail the history and pathophysiology of human immunodeficiency virus type 1 (HIV-1) infection or its ultimate consequence, acquired immunodeficiency syndrome (AIDS). Athletes may acquire HIV if they engage in behaviors that place them at risk. These include having sex with multiple partners, sexual exposure to bisexual males, and intimate exposure to IV drug users, as well as exposure to a known HIV-infected individual.

The first case of AIDS in the United States was reported in June of 1981. Since that time, there have been over 900,000 individuals found to be HIV positive and over 300,000 cases of AIDS diagnosed.[37] Of 79,674 adults diagnosed with HIV infection in 1994, 14,081 (18%) were women. This is a drastic increase from the rate of 7% in 1985.[37]

Infection requires exposure to HIV by direct intimate contact, or direct exposure to contaminated body fluids or blood. HIV infects most readily when there are breaks or abrasions on the skin or mucosal surfaces. HIV antibody is detectable in over 95% of patients within 6 months of infection. The time until development of frank AIDS may be as long as 10 to 14 years.[6]

The diagnosis of HIV is made by using HIV-1 antibody tests. Screening is initiated after informed consent is obtained, and risks and benefits explained. The enzyme-linked immunosorbent assay (ELISA) is a sensitive screening test. If exposure is suspected and the initial screen is negative, the test should be repeated in 4 weeks. If the test is positive, it may be repeated or one may proceed to a confirmatory test such as the Western-blot assay. If the confirmatory test is positive, the patient is infected with HIV and has the potential to transmit the virus to other persons.

At the time of the initial infection with HIV, the individual will usually have a flu-like illness with low-grade fever, myalgias, and malaise. After this initial episode, the patient will remain asymptomatic until becoming ill with the manifestations of AIDS. Progressive decompensation of the immune system then results in overwhelming secondary infection(s) and death within 18 to 24 months.

The rates of heterosexual transmission of HIV have increased drastically in the past few years. As women are infected more frequently, they have the potential of transmitting HIV to their unborn children. Studies indicate that 25% to 30% of mothers transmit the infection to their offspring.

Should female athletes who are HIV positive participate in contact sports? While the chance of transmission during typical athletic contact is low, gloves should be worn and adequate protection used when treating open wounds. An occlusive dressing may be applied and the athlete returned to action if there is no further bleeding. One must assume that all athletes are potentially infected and use universal precautions in managing any injury, especially open wounds. Any spillage of blood should be handled with precautions noted elsewhere.

Since 1994, advances have been made in the understanding of the pathogenesis of HIV-1 infection and in the treatment and monitoring of HIV-1 disease. The rapidity and magnitude of viral turnover during all stages of HIV-1 infection are greater than previously recognized; plasma virions are estimated to have a mean half-life of only 6 hours,[27] thus, current therapeutic interventions focus on early initiation of aggressive combination antiretroviral regimens to maximally suppress viral replication, preserve immune function, and reduce the development of resistance. New potent antiretroviral drugs that inhibit the protease enzyme of HIV-1 are now available. When a protease inhibitor is used in combination with nucleoside analogue reverse-transcriptase inhibitors, plasma HIV-1 RNA levels may be reduced for prolonged periods to levels that are undetectable using current assays. Improved clinical outcome and survival have been observed in adults receiving such regimens.[9]

Most people infected with HIV will eventually develop symptoms related to the infection, particularly secondary infections such as pneumonia, tuberculosis, and fungal infections. Prophylactic therapy for these infections may be indicated. Appropriate regimens are listed in the 1998 Guidelines for the Treatment of Sexually Transmitted Diseases published by the CDC.[6]

Athletes who engage in behavior that places them at risk for STDs should be encouraged to undergo appropriate screening. All STD reports, including HIV infection, are to be held in the strictest confidence. The identification and timely reporting of STDs form an integral part of successful disease control. Syphilis, gonorrhea, and HIV infection are reportable diseases in every state.

CONCLUDING REMARKS

Female athletes who choose to engage in sexual intercourse face the same consequences as female nonathletes. Abstinence is the only sure way to prevent STDs. If an athlete chooses to be sexually active, she should be advised to have sex with only one partner who is also monogamous, and to use a reliable means of contraception. Although oral contraceptives are effective in preventing pregnancy, they do not prevent STDs. Women must insist that their partners use a condom. Even with the use of condoms, there is ineffective protection against HPV, syphilis, and certain other STDs.

It is important for those providing health care to female athletes to remember that young people are "risk takers." The Youth Risk Behavior Surveillance Survey conveys the alarming fact that although men take more risks than women, females place themselves at risk frequently.[39]

Nattiv, looking at risk-taking behavior in collegiate athletes, found that athletes demonstrated significantly more risk-taking behaviors than their nonathletic peers in the following areas: seatbelt use; consistent use of helmets when riding motorcycles and bicycles; being a passenger riding with a driver under the influence of alcohol or drugs; consumption of alcoholic beverages; use of smokeless tobacco and anabolic steroids; adherence to safe-sex guidelines; number of sexual partners; contraceptive use; and physical fighting. Males reported more risk-taking behaviors than did female athletes, and athletes in contact sports demonstrated more risk-taking behaviors than athletes in noncontact sports.[25]

When an athlete is a risk-taker, she is likely to engage in multiple risk-taking behaviors.[25]

It is important then to counsel female athletes about avoiding risk-taking behavior to protect themselves from the potential adverse consequences of such behavior, particularly pregnancy and STDs; the emotional consequences of bonding to an individual must be considered as well.

When the female athlete has a gynecologic examination, she should be questioned about sexual activity and risk factors for STDs, including multiple sexual partners and frequent sexual intercourse, as well as contact with an infected partner. Screening for STDs should include a Pap smear, vaginal wet preps, endocervical cultures for gonorrhea and chlamydia, and serologic tests for syphilis and HIV infection. Patients who are diagnosed with an STD should be treated with appropriate antibacterials, antifungals, or antivirals as indicated. A careful follow-up examination is essential.

References

1. Alter MJ, Hadler SC, Margolis HS, et al: The changing epidemiology of hepatitis B in the United States. JAMA 263:1218–22, 1990.
2. Bertholf ME, Stafford MJ: Colonization of *Candida albicans* in vagina, rectum, and mouth. J Fam Pract 16:919–24, 1983.
3. Blythe M: Historical and clinical factors associated with *Chlamydia trachomatis* genitourinary infection in female adolescents. J Pediatr 112:1000, 1988.
4. Burstein GR, Gaydos CA, Diener-West M, et al: Incident *Chlamydia trachomatis* infections among inner-city adolescent females. JAMA 280:521–26, 1998.

5. Centers for Disease Control and Prevention, Division of STD: STD Surveillance 1994, United States Department for Health and Human Services. Atlanta, Centers for Disease Control and Prevention, September 1995.

6. Centers for Disease Control and Prevention: 1998 Guidelines for Treatment of Sexually Transmitted Diseases. MMWR 47(No. RR–1):1–111, 1998.

7. Corey LC, Adams HG, Brown ZA, et al: Genital herpes simplex virus infection: clinical manifestations, course and complications. Ann Intern Med 98:958, 1983.

8. Corey L, Holmes KK: Genital herpes simplex virus infections: current concepts in diagnosis, therapy and prevention. Ann Intern Med 98:973, 1983.

9. Gulick RM, Mellors JW, Havlir D, et al: Treatment with indinavir, zidovudine, and lamivudine in adults with HIV infection and prior anti-retroviral therapy. N Engl J Med 337:734–9, 1997.

10. Hager WD: Trichomonas vaginalis infection. In Pastorek JG (ed): Obstetrics and Gynecologic Infectious Disease. New York, Raven Press, 1994, pp 537–43.

11. Hager WD, Brown ST, Kraus SJ, et al: Metronidazole for vaginal trichomoniasis: Seven-day versus single dose regimens. JAMA 244:1219–20, 1980.

12. Harger JH, Pazin GJ, Breinig MC: Current understanding of the natural history of genital herpes simplex infections. J Reprod Med 31:365, 1986.

13. Harrison HR, Alexander ER, Weinstein L, et al: Cervical *Chlamydia trachomatis* and mycoplasmal infections in pregnancy. Epidemiology and outcomes. JAMA 250:1721–27, 1983.

14. Harrison HR, Costin M, Meder JB, et al: Cervical *Chlamydia trachomatis* infection in university women: relationship to history, contraception, ectopy, and cervicitis. Am J Obstet Gynecol 153:244–51,1985.

15. Hirsch HA: Candidal vaginal infections. In Mead PB, Hager WD (eds): Infection Protocols for Obstetrics and Gynecology. Montvale, NJ, Medical Economics, 1992, pp 143–6.

16. Holmes KK, Eschenbach DA, Knapp JS: Salpingitis: overview of etiology and epidemiology. Am J Obstet Gynecol 138:893–900, 1980.

17. Hook EW III, Handsfield HH: Gonococcal infections in the adult. In Holmes KK, Mardh PA, Sparling PA, et al (eds): Sexually Transmitted Diseases. New York, McGraw-Hill, 1990, pp 149–65.

18. Hurley R, DeLouvois J: Candida vaginitis. Postgrad Med J 55:645–7, 1979.

19. Jacobson L, Westrom L: Objectivized diagnosis of acute pelvic inflammatory disease: diagnostic and prognostic value of routine laparoscopy. Am J Obstet Gynecol 105:1088,1969.

20. Judson FN: The importance of coexisting syphilitic, chlamydial, mycoplasmal, and trichomonal infections in the treatment of gonorrhea. Sex Transm Dis 6(Suppl 2):112–9, 1979.

21. Koutsky LA, Galloway DA, Holmes KK: Epidemiology of genital human papilloma virus infection. Epidemiol Rev 10:122–63, 1988.

22. Latif AS, Mason PR, Marowa E: Urethral trichomoniasis in men. Sex Transm Dis 14:9–11, 1987.

23. Mertz GJ, Critchlow CW, Benedetti J, et al: Double-blind placebo controlled trial of oral acyclovir in first episode genital herpes simplex virus infection. JAMA 252:1147, 1984.

24. Mertz GJ, Jones CC, Mills J, et al: Long-term acyclovir suppression of frequently recurring genital herpes simplex virus infections: a multicenter double-blind trial. JAMA 260:201, 1988.

25. Nattiv A, Puffer JC, Green GA: Lifestyles and health risks of collegiate athletes: A multi-center study. Clin J Sport Med 7:262–72, 1997.

26. Odds FC: Candidiasis of the genitalia. In Candida and Candidiasis. A Review and Bibliography, 2nd edition. London, Ballière-Tindall, 1988, p 124.

27. Perelson AS, Neumann AU, Markowitz M, et al: HIV-1 dynamics in vivo: virion clearance rate, infected cell life-span, and viral generation time. Science 271:1582–6, 1996.

28. Pheifer TA, Forsyth PS, Durfee MA, et al. Nonspecific vaginitis: Role of *Haemophilus vaginalis* and treatment with metronidazole. N Engl J Med 298:1429–34, 1978.

29. Recommendations for the prevention and management of *Chlamydia trachomatis* infections. MMWR 42 (No. RR–12): August 6, 1993.

30. Reid R, Greenburg M, Jenson AB, et al: Sexually transmitted papillomaviral-infections. I. The anatomic distribution and the pathologic grade of neoplastic lesions associated with different viral types. Am J Obstet Gynecol 156:212–22, 1987.

31. Roberts MC, Hillier SL, Schoenknecht FD, et al: Comparison of gram stain, DNA probe and culture for the identification of species of *Mobiluncus* in female genital specimens. J Infect Dis 152:74–7, 1985.

32. Stamm WE, Wagner KF, Amsel R, et al: Causes of the acute urethral syndrome in women. N Engl J Med 303:409–15, 1980.

33. Svenson L, Westrom L, Ripa KT, et al: Differences in some clinical and laboratory parameters in acute salpingitis related to culture and serologic findings. Am J Obstet Gynecol 138:1017–21, 1980.

34. Sweet RL, Draper DL, Schacter J, et al: Microbiology and pathogenesis of acute salpingitis as determined by laparoscopy: what is the appropriate site to sample? Am J Obstet Gynecol 138:985–9, 1980.

35. Sweet RL, Gibbs RS:Infectious Diseases of the Female Genital Tract, 2nd edition. Baltimore, Williams & Wilkins, 1990, pp 119–26.

36. Thomason JL, Gelbart SM, Broekhvizen FF: Advances in the understanding of bacterial vaginosis. J Reprod Med 34(8S):581–7, 1989.

37. Update: AIDS among women—United States, 1994. MMWR 44:February 1081–4, 1995.

38. Wallin JE, Thompson SE, Saidi A, et al: Urethritis in women attending an STD clinic. Br J Vener Dis 57:50, 1987.

39. Youth Risk Behavior Surveillance Survey—United States, 1997. Centers for Disease Control and Prevention. CDC Surveillance Summaries. MMWR 47 (No. SS–3): August 14, 1998.

Chapter 19

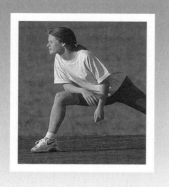

Disorders and Injuries of the Breast

William H. Hindle, M.D.

Into the early 1900s, law courts in England continued to judge trauma to the breast as a cause (if not *the* cause) of breast cancer. Industrial companies and others were found liable when acute trauma to a woman's breast preceded her cancer diagnosis. In some cases, the interval between the trauma and the diagnosis was less than a few weeks. Subsequent scientific inquiry has found no correlation between breast trauma and breast cancer, much less any evidence of causality. However, breast trauma can be the precipitating event for a woman to examine her breast and incidentally find a palpable mass that in all probability had been present for years. Many breast cancers are first noticed by the woman herself.

Until recently, little has been published on injuries to the female breast and the interrelation of the female breast and athletic activities.[27] With the rapid and continuing expansion of women's athletic activities, particularly contact sports, female athletes are experiencing "breast problems" and are now coming forward with their breast-related concerns and experiences. Like all women, female athletes are interested in breast health and comfort and are apprehensive about the possibility of developing breast cancer, with its grave prognosis and potentially defeminizing treatments. Thus, breast disorders and injuries are of keen interest to female athletes, their coaches, their trainers, and their physicians.

Review of pertinent medical textbooks, Medline searches, and conversations with coaches, trainers, and competitive athletes (eg, aerobics instructors and competitive runners) reveal a paucity of information about breast problems of female athletes or about female breast injuries. Female sports injury surveys published in 1975 and 1976 reported breast injuries to be one of the least common types of sports injuries.[20,25] However, with changes in the attitude of physicians, athletes, and women, and within our culture, there is emerging willingness to discuss female breast problems openly. This chapter sets forth a summary of the currently available data about the female breast and useful background information for the orientation of physicians, coaches, trainers, and athletes involved with women's athletics.

Fear of breast cancer is a pervasive and powerful emotion. Physicians and other health care providers for women can be authoritative resources of current and accurate information about breast cancer and breast care.[26]

DEVELOPMENT

The male and female breasts are essentially similar until puberty, when the female breasts develop from modified sweat glands into endocrine end organs capable of lactation and breast-feeding. Complex interactions of adrenal glucocorticoids, estrogen, growth hormone, insulin, progesterone, and prolactin produce the differentiation and maturation of the alveoli, ducts, lobules, stroma, and surrounding adipose tissue that make up the developing female breast. The mean age range for the full maturation of the female breast is between 11 to 15 years, with a normal range of 9 to 19 years. Accessory nipples, often rudimentary, and ectopic breast tissue can occur along the embryologic "milk ridge." These abnormally located tissues can become symptomatic during pregnancy and subsequent lactation.

ANATOMY

The breast extends from the second or third rib to the sixth or seventh rib. The primary blood supply is from internal thoracic, lateral thoracic, thoracodorsal, and intercostal perforating arteries. Lymphatic drainage is through the axillary lymph nodes with some drainage to the substernal lymph nodes. For surgical descriptive purposes, the axillary lymph nodes are designated as level I, from the lateral aspects to the insertion of the pectoralis minor muscle; level II, underneath the insertion of the pectoralis minor muscle; and level III, medial to the insertion of the pectoralis minor muscle. Sensory innervation to the breast is provided by the lateral and anterior cutaneous branches of the second through sixth intercostal nerves. The superficial and deep layers of the superficial pectoralis fascia encapsulate the breast glandular and stromal tissues.

Most of the breast is adipose tissue (fat) within which glandular tissue is organized into separate lobes with no anatomic connection between them. There are usually 10 to 15 lobes, each with a single opening (galactophore) on the nipple. The structure of the ductal system of each lobe resembles the intertwined branches of a tree, with the terminal duct lobular units (TDLUs) as the peripheral leaves of the tree branch. The diagrammatic anatomy of the mature human female breast is depicted in Figure 19-1.

Cooper's ligaments are thin irregular fascial bands that form a random pattern of fine sheets throughout the breast (Fig. 19-2). Historically described as "suspensory," they do not actually support the breast but do limit the motion of the breast by their attachments between the pectoralis fascia and the skin. However, Cooper's ligaments are clinically important as they can contract when invaded by carcinoma, thus producing secondary signs of breast cancer (eg, skin dimpling, nipple retraction, and peau d'orange of the skin).

The size of a woman's breast is genetically predetermined. The fat that composes most of the breast volume is "sex specific" and not directly affected by changes in the body's "essential" fat,[6] which varies markedly with changes in body weight. Even with rigorous exercise, body-weight fat loss has little effect on breast volume.[39] Focused exercise can increase the mass of the pectoralis muscle, but the increase has minimal effect on breast size per se.

When a woman reaches about age 25, progressive fatty replacement of the glandular tissue of the breast begins. This results in progressively clearer mammographic contrast between the fat and any lesions that may be present. Thus, accuracy of mammographic detection of breast cancer increases with aging. These changes

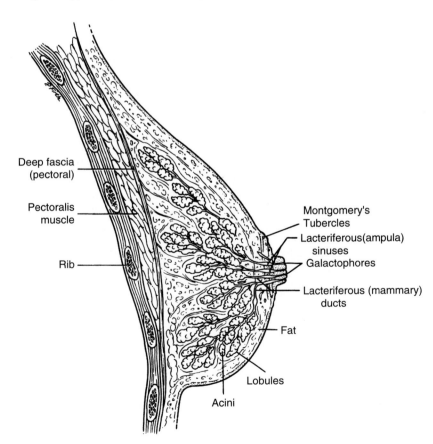

Figure 19-1. Diagrammatic anatomy of the female breast. (From Breast disease. In Morrow CP, Curtin JP (eds): Synopsis of Gynecologic Oncology. New York, Churchill Livingstone, 1998, p 371, with permission.)

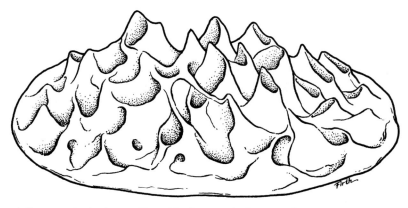

Figure 19-2. Cooper's ligaments in the breast. (From Hindle WH: The breast and exercise. In Hale RW (ed): Caring for the Exercising Woman. New York, Elsevier Science, 1991, p 86, with permission. Redrawn from the original in Cooper AP: The Anatomy and Disease of the Breast. Philadelphia, Lea & Blanchard, 1845.)

accelerate after the menopause along with decreasing numbers of TDLUs and atrophy of the ductules, which further result in increased radiolucency.[13]

The inframammary fold is an anatomic curved ridge at the lower dependent aspect of the breast. A pendulous breast hangs over this area. Erythema, maceration, excoriation, and infection can occur in this fold if the area is not kept clean and dry. Sweating predisposes to these symptoms. For large-breasted women, effective uplifting bra support is essential for proper skin care in this area.

PHYSIOLOGY

During the reproductive years, the breasts respond to the cyclic hormonal changes of the menstrual cycle. Swelling and tenderness are common prior to menstruation and sometimes at ovulation. The increase in breast volume prior to menstruation may be as much as 40%.[23] Palpation often reveals tender diffuse nodularity during the late-luteal phase of the menstrual cycle. The optimum time in the menstrual cycle for breast examinations (breast self-examination and clinical breast examinations), including mammography, is during the mid-follicular phase. The equivalent to what would be mid-cycle is also the optimum time for breast examinations for women on oral contraceptive therapy or hormone replacement therapy. Exogenous estrogen, such as oral contraceptives or estrogen replacement therapy, can induce breast tenderness, swelling, and palpable nodularity. These symptoms usually subside with continuing hormonal therapy.

The cells of the ductal epithelium (the source of 80% of carcinomas of the breast) undergo replication (mitosis) and deletion (apoptosis) in response to the hormonal (ie, estrogen and progesterone) changes during the menstrual cycle. However, the breast glandular epithelium is in an "endocrinologic resting state" until lactation occurs.[5]

COMFORT

Although the wearing of a bra has no proven intrinsic medical or health value, most women, particularly if they have large breasts, are more comfortable wearing a supportive bra, especially during vigorous athletic activity. The "athletic" bra should be designed to restrict up and down motion of the breasts and have wide shoulder straps and no wires or metallic hooks and fasteners.[35] A wide crisscross design in the back gives support and is usually the most comfortable. Fabric with limited stretch (particularly laterally), which produces diffuse compression is the most effective, especially for women with small breasts. Large breasts require support and limitation of upward motion. There should be no seams or ridges in the area over the nipple–areolar complex. For women engaging in contact sports, bras with nonelastic straps and padded cups are advised.[35]

With vigorous exercise the primary motion of the breast is up and down. Thus, compression of the upper portion of the breast is essential for comfort during intense athletic activity. With an ideal athletic bra, upward motion should be limited to about 1 inch. Again, this support of the upper portion of the breast is especially important for large-breasted women.

Discomfort from the up-and-down motion of large breasts is such that many women avoid athletic activities that create vigorous motions, such as jogging and running.[19] Effective athletic bras often have to be custom fitted for large-breasted women. Padding built into the athletic bra and seamless cups over the nipple area are recommended for contact sports such as football, hockey, and martial arts.[42,51] Large breasts, no matter how well supported, can slow the competitive times of female swimmers.[34]

Which athletic bra is best? Each active woman should choose her own type and brand of bra, preferably after trying it during her athletic activities.

INJURIES

Soft-tissue injury, often with ecchymosis (bruising with discoloration), is the most common breast injury both in female athletes and in women in general. Significant trauma to the breast is a rare occurrence.

The breasts are superficially located soft-tissue organs that are susceptible to blunt trauma, which usually results in tenderness, swelling, ecchymosis, and sometimes deep hematoma formation. With severe blunt trauma, torn arteries within the breast may require surgical ligation.[31] Fat necrosis with fibrosis and calcification may follow breast trauma, as may oil cysts.[49] Fat necrosis, as revealed by both palpation and mammography,[24] can mimic invasive carcinoma. However, when associated with a history of trauma, findings of fat necrosis can be followed for a reasonable period as they tend to subside over time. However, if ever doubt on the part of the patient, clinician, or mammographer persists, tissue-core needle or open surgical biopsy is indicated for confirmation by histologic diagnosis.

When there is evidence of ecchymosis and a clinical question of a hematoma deeper in the breast tissue, particularly if the hematoma is painful, ultrasonography can be useful in identifying and draining the liquid center of a symptomatic hematoma. A 7.5-mHz handheld linear-array near-field transducer is utilized for visualization of the hematoma. Drainage of the liquid center can be performed with local anesthesia and aspiration using a #18 needle and syringe. Pain relief and more rapid healing is achieved by drainage of a breast hematoma that contains liquefied blood.

Lacerations to the breasts can be treated, as are skin lacerations elsewhere on the body, by cleansing and suture closure of the skin defect. A cosmetically acceptable closure of a wound is desirable. Some severe lacerations require a second operation with revision of the scar by a qualified plastic surgeon. Similar extensive scar revision and skin grafting may be necessary for plastic reconstruction after severe burns to the breasts.[22]

Seat belts have caused the most severe recorded traumas to the female breast,[12,31,40,41,43] of which some have even resulted in "traumatic mastectomy."[32] Typical band-shaped mammographic findings after seat-belt injuries have been described.[14]

Recent awareness of spousal and similar abuse has led to the correlation of some breast lacerations and ecchymoses/hematomas with that etiology. Injuries related to nipple piercing and tassel dancing have been reported.[11]

NIPPLES

The prominence of the nipples cause them to be susceptible to abrasion such as when repeatedly rubbed by a shirt during jogging. "Runner's nipples" is a well-known phenomenon of this type of irritation. A firm compressive athletic bra can usually prevent this; in some cases, it may be necessary to place adhesive strips over the nipples. A well-fitted athletic bra can also prevent "bicyclist's nipples," a condition related to prolonged exposure to cold, by providing needed warmth.

IMPLANTS

Rupture or displacement of breast prosthetic implants (ie, silicone or saline-filled silicone bags) has been reported with severe trauma directly to the breast, such as in auto accidents. Rare cases of similar displacement or rupture have occurred with intense blunt trauma in contact sports. Firm compressive supporting athlete bras are essential for women with implants who engage in strenuous athletics. Since added body weight and breast movement can affect efficiency, implants are not advised for female elite athletes who are swimmers or runners.

MASTITIS

Most breast infections occur in pregnant or lactating women (puerperal mastitis). Infections are usually acute in onset and respond rapidly to appropriate antibiotic therapy. *Staphylococcus aureus* is the most common etiologic agent.[17] Treatment with dicloxacillin (500 mg by mouth every 6 hours for 7 days), or a similar antibiotic effective against the same bacterial spectra, is effective. The breast should be re-evaluated every 3 days to be certain that the signs and symptoms are responding to therapy and that there is no evidence of abscess formation.

Needle aspiration or ultrasonography can verify the formation of a breast abscess. Small abscesses can be drained with syringe suction using a #18 gauge needle. Local anesthesia (eg, 1% lidocaine) should be used. The aspiration may have to be repeated every 3 days for several times until the abscess clears completely.[15] Large abscesses require surgical incision and drainage under general anesthesia with placement of a dependent drain in the incision.

Nonpuerperal mastitis is usually caused by *S aureus*, *Peptostrepococcus magnus*, or *Bacteriodes fragilis*.[17] Amoxicillin/clavulanate 400 mg by mouth every 8 hours for 7 days (or equivalent) is appropriate therapy. Mixed aerobic and anaerobic bacteria (eg, coagulase-negative staphylococci and *Peptostreptococcus proprioni*) usually cause chronic nonpuerperal mastitis. Dicloxacillin 500 mg by mouth every 6 hours with metronidazole 500 mg by mouth every 8 hours for 10 days is appropriate therapy for chronic breast infections. Recurrent subareolar fistulae require surgical excision for definitive treatment.

If a clinically diffuse breast infection or area of erythema and induration does not respond to antibiotic therapy, an adequate sample of skin, obtained by punch biopsy, should be obtained to rule out the rare inflammatory carcinoma characterized histologically by extensive invasion of the dermal lymphatics by infiltrating ductal carcinoma.

MASTALGIA

Most menstruating women are aware of occasional breast pain (mastalgia/mastodynia) prior to the onset of menstruation. For many women the pain can be severe and can interfere with athletic and other activities.[1] At some point during their lifetimes, many women consult a physician about breast pain. Typically, the pain is cyclic, premenstrual, and diffuse. Such discomfort is usually an exaggeration of the physiologic changes in the breasts of menstruating women. On the other hand, pathologic breast pain is usually localized and often constant or occasionally intermittent. As many as 75% of women presenting with the chief complaint of breast pain are found to have no pathologic abnormality and may be reassured that the pain is not a sign of breast cancer. Evaluation of mastalgia consists of a careful history, complete bilateral breast examination, mammography (if the woman is over 30), and fine-needle aspiration (if there is a palpable dominant mass). If cysts are suspected (eg, multiple bilateral tender mobile cystic masses with definite borders identified by either palpation or mammography), the diagnosis can be confirmed by ultrasonography of a nonpalpable mass or fine-needle aspiration of a palpable mass.

The therapy for mastalgia begins with the simplest measures and then proceeds, if the initial treatment is not effective, in stepwise fashion: (1) reassurance that there is no evidence of significant pathology; (2) use of mechanical aids, such as a fitted bra; (3) premenstrual salt restriction (which is just as effective as diuretics); (4) nonsteroidal analgesia; (5) low-dose oral contraceptives; and (6) danocrine (Danazol),which is rarely prescribed because of its potential masculinizing side effects.[7,29,48] Clinical trials in Europe have demonstrated the efficacy of linoleic acid therapy (500 mg by mouth 3 times per day) for the treatment of cyclic and noncyclic mastalgia.[29,30] Minimal side effects have been reported. The optimum response to therapy may take several months. In addition, linoleic acid therapy for mastalgia is not approved by the US Food and Drug Administration. However, most health food stores carry 500-mg linoleic acid capsules.

Although occasionally a woman with breast pain may respond to restriction of methylxanthine-containing foods (caffeine, coffee, chocolate, cola, peanuts, and tea) because of her particular end organ-sensitivity, multiple double-blinded crossover studies have failed to demonstrate a measurable therapeutic effect of methylxanthine restriction upon cyclic mastalgia, diffuse breast pain, or associated diffuse nodularity of the breasts.[18,37,38,44,46] Furthermore, there is no correlation between caffeine intake and the incidence of breast cancer.[2]

FIBROCYSTIC CHANGES

Autopsy studies reveal that more than 90% of women have fibrocystic changes in their breast tissue.[36] These histologic changes are physiologic and normal. Historically the misused term "fibrocystic disease" covered a multitude of specific histologic findings and diagnoses. Many patients, some physicians, and most insurance companies mistakenly came to believe that "fibrocystic disease" was a premalignant condition and a clinically significant risk factor for breast cancer. Of the many histologic diagnoses that used to be lumped together under the title of "fibrocystic disease," only atypical epithelial hyperplasia of the breast is a clinically meaningful risk factor for invasive carcinoma.[16] (Unfortunately, there are no characteristic symptoms, physical findings, or mammographic signs for atypical epithelial hyperplasia, either lobular or ductal.) Wisely, in 1985, the College of American Pathologists officially discarded the term "fibrocystic disease."[10] The Dupont and Page data, supported by other published works, categorizes the relative risk of breast cancer for the individual histologic diagnoses that used to be covered by the inappropriate historical term "fibrocystic disease."[16]

There is a general nonspecific correlation between diffuse palpable nodularity, which is often tender cyclically, and both mammographic density and histologic fibrocystic changes. If confirmation by histologic diagnosis is necessary, tissue biopsy is required.

NIPPLE DISCHARGE

Most women, certainly during their reproductive years, can express discharge from their nipples with repeated squeezing. This is physiologic fluid. Pathologic nipple discharge is spontaneous and occurs without stimulation. Except with periductal mastitis (mammary duct ectasia), pathologic discharge is unilateral and from a single duct opening on the nipple. The discharge may be clear, serosanguineous, or bloody. Intraductal papillomas are the cause of most cases of pathologic spontaneous nipple discharge. The diagnosis is confirmed by surgical excision after the lesion is localized by galactography (ductography).[47] Histologic diagnosis is mandatory to identify the rare papillary carcinoma. Most cytologic smears of nipple discharge fail to provide diagnostic cytology and are not cost effective.

Milky discharge from multiple duct openings on the nipple is not caused by intrinsic breast pathology. If the milky discharge is not pregnancy related, galactorrhea should be considered with serum prolactin and thyroid-stimulating hormone levels ordered as clinically indicated.

Excoriation of the nipple can cause staining inside the bra. If a weepy, moist, erythematous or dry, scaly lesion of the nipple persists in spite of corrective measures and treatment, a biopsy should be performed to check for possible Paget's disease of the nipple, a variant of ductal carcinoma in situ with or without associated invasive carcinoma.

CYSTS

Breast cysts can be appropriately diagnosed, treated, and followed in the office setting. Microcysts (nonpalpable) are normal in female breast tissue. Typically, numerous microcysts are present within areas of fibrocystic changes of the breast. Macrocysts (palpable) are often multiple and frequently bilateral. However, a symptomatic cyst, that is, one that is painful and tender to touch, is usually single. Palpable breast cysts occur most commonly during the late reproductive years.

Microcysts can be perceived upon mammography and the diagnosis confirmed by ultrasonography. A macrocyst can be definitively diagnosed and treated by fine-needle aspiration. Aspirated cyst fluid should be discarded, as cytology of breast cyst fluid is unrewarding and not cost effective. The rare intracystic carcinoma will become clinically apparent by one or more of the following: (1) grossly bloody aspirated fluid; (2) a residual palpable mass after complete aspiration of the cyst fluid; or (3) refilling of the cyst within 3 months. If necessary, a nonpalpable cyst can be aspirated with ultrasound guidance.

DOMINANT BREAST MASSES

Women and their health care providers are most concerned with the identification and evaluation of a palpable breast mass. Although not always specifically verbalized, fear of breast cancer underlies the intense anxiety women have about all breast symptoms and findings.

A persistent dominant breast mass must be definitively diagnosed.[28] By definition, a dominant breast mass is a 3-dimensional distinct mass that is different from the remainder of the breast tissue. A definitive diagnosis can be made by fine-needle aspiration cytology or by tissue-core needle or open surgical biopsy and histology. In a menstruating woman, an indistinct "mass" with benign characteristics can be re-evaluated during a following menstrual cycle. However if a palpable mass persists, even though it seems smaller, a definitive diagnosis is required.

A diagnosis can be obtained in the office or clinic setting when there is concordance of the diagnostic triad of (1) clinical breast examination; (2) mammography; and (3) fine-needle aspiration cytology. If the clinician is not personally prepared to bring about the definitive diagnosis, the patient must be referred to a physician trained and experienced in breast diagnostic techniques. Furthermore, any woman presenting with a breast problem should be instructed in breast self-examination and told to return for re-evaluation if her symptoms or findings persist or progress.

Many palpable dominant breast masses removed by surgical excision are configurations of fibrocystic changes. A fibroadenoma typically presents as a firm, mobile, nontender mass with distinct borders. Mammography of a fibroadenoma typically reveals a mammographically benign mass with distinct borders. Focused ultrasound examination can confirm that the mass is solid with benign characteristics. Fibroadenomas occur most commonly during the early reproductive years. Given an adequate cell sample, fine-needle aspiration can establish a definitive cytologic diagnosis of a fibroadenoma.

SURVEILLANCE FOR BREAST CANCER

The guidelines of the American College of Obstetricians and Gynecologists for breast cancer surveillance are: (1) breast self-examination monthly beginning at age 18; (2) annual clinical breast examination by a health care professional beginning at age 18[4]; and (3) screening mammography every 1 to 2 years during the ages of 40 to 49 and annually after age 50.[3] The goal is to detect nonpalpable breast cancers, for which current methods of treatment offer an excellent prognosis. Mammography remains the only proven effective breast cancer screening tool for finding nonpalpable breast cancers.

Although the cost effectiveness of screening mammography prior to age 50 continues to be debated,[45] the benefit to the individual woman whose breast cancer is detected before it is palpable is substantial at any age since many such small breast cancers may indeed be "cured" with current methods of therapy. The age-related cost of detecting nonpalpable breast cancers is an economic issue appropriately addressed by health care policy decision-makers. The American Cancer Society recommends annual screening mammography beginning at age 40.[33] Swedish studies specifically designed to evaluate the effectiveness of screening mammography in the 40- to 49-year-old age group have provided statistically significant results that approximate the benefit in decreasing the mortality from breast cancer for women 50 years of age and older.[8,50]

ESTROGEN REPLACEMENT THERAPY AND BREAST CANCER

Since the incidence rate of invasive breast cancer is more than 170 times more for women than for men, it may seem logical that the major female hormones, estrogen and progesterone, play an important role. However, the incidence rate for women continues to rise after the menopause, when estrogen falls to low levels. After 50 years of medical research and clinical investigation, the role of estrogen and progesterone in the etiology and growth of breast cancer in women is not defined. There is no consensus as to the effects of these female hormones upon the origin and biologic behavior of breast cancer. However, it is clear from review of the published data that alterations of the relative risk of breast cancer associated with estrogen or progesterone therapy can result in statistically significant epidemiologic low levels of increased risk in selected groups of patients. None of the data approach the acknowledged relationship of estrogen and the incidence and progression of endometrial cancer (eg, a 1.4 relative risk for breast cancer[9] compared to a 5.9 increased relative risk for endometrial cancer with 5 to 10 years of estrogen therapy).[21] Furthermore, the relative risk of a woman dying from breast cancer is decreased among even users of estrogen replacement therapy.[52] Since prospective randomized clinical trials of long duration have not been carried out and published, the relationship of estrogen and progesterone to breast cancer remains controversial.

CONCLUDING REMARKS

The breast concerns of all women (including female athletes) should be properly acknowledged and thoroughly evaluated. A breast "lump" requires urgent attention and a definitive diagnosis if found to be a dominant breast mass. Although the incidence of breast cancer increases with advancing age, women of all ages are intensely concerned that any perceived breast abnormality may be a sign of breast cancer. Screening mammography is the most effective available technique for the detection of nonpalpable breast cancer, which has an excellent prognosis with current methods of therapy. Other breast problems should be evaluated systematically, treated as indicated, and followed. A woman with an unresolved breast problem should be referred to an appropriate medical breast specialist.

It cannot be overemphasized that a persistent dominant breast mass must be diagnosed definitively; otherwise breast cancers will be missed. When there is doubt as to the precise diagnosis of a dominant breast mass, an open surgical biopsy should be performed and a definitive histologic diagnosis obtained.

References

1. Ader DN, Browne MW: Prevalence and impact of cyclic mastalgia in a United States clinic-based sample. Am J Obstet Gynecol 177:126–32, 1997.
2. Allen SS, Froberg DC: The effect of decreased caffeine consumption on benign proliferative breast disease: a randomized clinical trial. Surgery 101:720–30, 1986.
3. American College of Obstetricians and Gynecologists: Report of the task force on routine cancer screening. ACOG Committee Opinion 68. Washington, DC, American College of Obstetricians and Gynecologists, 1989.
4. American College of Obstetricians and Gynecologists: Standards for Obstetric-Gynecologic Services, 7th edition. Washington, DC, American College of Obstetricians and Gynecologists, 1989.
5. Anderson TJ, Ferguson DJP: Cell turnover in the "resting" human breast: influence of parity, contraceptive pill, age and laterality. Br J Cancer 46:376–82, 1982.
6. Behnke A, Wilmore J: Evaluation and Regulation of Body Build and Composition. Englewood Cliffs, NJ, Prentice-Hall, 1974.
7. BeLieu RM: Mastodynia. Obstet Gynecol Clin North Am 21:461–77, 1994.
8. Bjurstam N, Bjorneld L, Duffy SW, et al: The Gothenburg breast screening trial: first results on mortality, incidence, and mode of detect for women ages 39–49 years at randomization. Cancer 80–2091–9, 1997.
9. Collaborative Group on Hormonal Factors in Breast Cancer: Breast cancer and hormone replacement therapy: collaborative reanalysis of data from 51 epidemiologic studies of 52,705 women with breast cancer and 108,411 women without breast cancer. Lancet 350:1047–59, 1997.
10. College of American Pathologists: Is "fibrocystic disease" of the breast precancerous? Arch Pathol Lab Med 110:171–2, 1986.
11. Collins RE: Breast disease associated with tassel dancing. Br Med J 283:1660, 1981.
12. Dawes RF, Smallwood JA, Taylor I: Seat belt injury to the female breast. Br J Surg 73:106–7, 1986.
13. de Paredes ES: Atlas of Film-Screen Mammography. 2nd edition. Baltimore, Williams & Wilkins, 1992, pp 1–26.
14. DiPiro PJ, Meyer JE, Frenna TH, et al: Seat belt injuries of the breast: findings on mammography. AJR 164:317–20, 1995.
15. Dixon JM: Repeated aspiration of breast abscesses in lactating women. Br Med J 297:1517–8, 1988.
16. Dupont WD, Page DL: Risk factors for breast cancer in women with proliferative breast disease. N Engl J Med 312:146–51, 1985.
17. Edmiston CE Jr, Walker AP, Krepel CJ, Gohr C: The nonpuerperal breast infection: aerobic and anaerobic microbial recovery from acute and chronic disease. J Infect Dis 162:695–9, 1990.
18. Ernester VL, Mason L, Goodson WH III, et al: Effects of caffeine free diet on benign breast disease: a randomized trial. Surgery 91:263–7, 1982.
19. Fardy HJ: Women in sport. Aust Fam Physician 17:185–6, 1988.
20. Gillette JV: When and where women are injured in sports. Phys Sports Med 3:61–3, 1975.
21. Grady D, Gebretsadik T, Kerlikowske K, et al: Hormone replacement therapy and endometrial cancer risk: a meta-analysis. Obstet Gynecol 85:304–13, 1995.
22. Guan WX, Jin YT, Cao HP: Reconstruction of postburn female breast deformity. Ann Plast Surg 21:65–9, 1988.
23. Hamilton T, Rankin ME: Changes in volume of the breast during the menstrual cycle. Br J Surg 62:600, 1975.
24. Harnist KS, Ikeda DM, Helvie MA: Abnormal mammogram after steering wheel injury. Western J Med 159:504–6, 1993.
25. Haycock CE, Gillette JV: Susceptibility of women athletes to injury: myths vs reality. JAMA 236:163–5, 1976.
26. Hindle WH: The breast and exercise. In Hale RW (ed): Caring for the Exercising Woman. New York, Elsevier Science, 1991, pp 83–92.
27. Hindle WH (ed): Breast Care. New York, Springer-Verlag 1999.
28. Hindle WH: The diagnostic evaluation. In Marchant DJ (ed): Breast Disease. Philadelphia, WB Saunders, 1997, pp 69–82.
29. Holland PA, Gateley CA: Drug therapy of mastalgia: What are the options? Drugs 48:709–16, 1994.
30. Hughes LE, Mansel RE, Webster DJT: Breast pain and nodularity. In Hughes LE, Mansel RE, Webster DJT (eds): Benign Disorders and Diseases of the Breast. London, Baillière-Tindall, 1989, pp 75–92.
31. Johnstone BR, Wasman BP: Transverse disruption of the abdominal wall—a tell-tale sign of seat belt related hollow viscous injury. Aust NZ J Surg 57:455–60, 1987.
32. Larson S, Svane S: Subcutaneous avulsion of the breast caused by a seat belt injury. Report of a case requiring emergency mastectomy. Eur J Surg 159:131–2, 1992.
33. Leitch M, Dodd GD, Costanza M, et al: American Cancer Society guidelines for the early detection of breast cancer: Update 1997. CA Cancer J Clin 47:150–3, 1997.
34. Levine NS, Buchanan RT: Decreased swimming speed following augmentation mammaplasty. Plast Reconstr Surg 71:255–9, 1983.
35. Lorentzen D, Lawson L: Selected sports bra: a biomechanical analysis of breast motion while jogging. Phys Sports Med 15:128–39, 1987.
36. Love SM, Gelman SR, Silem W: Sounding board. Fibrocystic "disease" of the breast—a nondisease? N Engl J Med 307:1010–4, 1982.
37. Lubin F, Ron E, Wax Y, Black M, et al: A case-control study of caffeine and methylxanthines in benign breast disease. JAMA 253:2388–92, 1985.
38. Marshall J, Graham S, Swanson M: Caffeine consumption and benign breast disease: a case-control comparison. Am J Public Health 72:610–2, 1982.
39. Mayhew JL, Gross PM: Body composition changes in young women with high resistance weight training. Res Q 45:433–40, 1974.
40. McInerney PD: Breast lumps and seat belt injury. Br J Surg 74:231, 1987.
41. Murday AJ: Seat belt injury of the breast—a case report. Injury 14:276–7, 1982.
42. Otis CL: Women and sports: breast and nipple injuries. Sports Med Dig 10:7, 1988.
43. Pennes DR, Phillips WA: Auto seat restraint soft-tissue injury. AJR 148:458, 1987.
44. Rohan TE, Cook MG, McMichael AJ: Methylxanthines and benign proliferative epithelial disorders of the breast in women. Int J Epidemiol 18:626–33, 1989.
45. Salzmann P, Kerlikowske K, Phillips K: Cost-effectiveness of extending screening mammography guidelines to include women 40 to 49 years of age. Ann Intern Med 127:955–65, 1997.
46. Schairer C, Brinton LA, Hoover RN: Methylxanthines and benign breast disease. Am J Epidemiol 124:603–11, 1986.

47. Tabar L, Dean PB, Pentek Z: Galactography: the diagnostic procedure of choice for nipple discharge. Radiology 149:31–8, 1983.
48. Tavaf-Motamen H, Ader DN, Browne MW, Shriver CD: Clinical evaluation of mastalgia. Arch Surg 133:211–3, 1998.
49. Templeton PA: Breast mass in a farm woman. Invest Radiol 23:144–6, 1988.
50. The organizing committee and collaborators, Falun meeting: Breast-cancer screening with mammography in women aged 40–49 years. Int J Cancer 68:693–9, 1996.
51. Wilkerson LA: The female athlete. Am Fam Practitioner 29:233–7, 1984.
52. Willis DB, Calle EE, Miracle-McMahill HL, Health CW Jr: Estrogen replacement therapy and the risk of fatal breast cancer in a prospective cohort of postmenopausal women in the United States. Cancer Causes Control 7:449–57, 1996.

Chapter 20

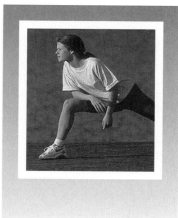

Pregnancy
PHYSIOLOGY AND EXERCISE

Jeffrey S. Christian, M.D.
Stefanie Schupp Christian, M.D.
Carol A. Stamm, M.D.
James A. McGregor, M.D.

Planning for and managing pregnancy are special challenges for the athlete and her caregiver. The normal physiologic changes of pregnancy are dramatic and complex, and involve every organ system. Some athletic women may be unnecessarily cautious during pregnancy because of concerns that these physiologic changes would make exercise difficult, or even dangerous. Advice from the medical profession has tended to reinforce these concerns, and may unnecessarily limit types and quantity of exercise in pregnancy. If recommendations from practitioners are unjustified or unnecessarily restrictive, they might result in an unnecessary reduction in conditioning; or worse, if the athlete continues vigorous training against medical advice, communication and trust may be disrupted between the caregiver and patient, resulting in feelings of guilt and reduced compliance with other aspects of care.

The goal of this chapter is to review the physiologic changes of pregnancy, focusing on adaptations to exercise and training of the well-conditioned athlete. Knowledge concerning the consequences of exercise and training on the course of pregnancy and labor and delivery is also presented, along with the effect of pregnancy on athletic conditioning. A practical approach to continuing exercise and physical conditioning during gestation is presented to provide guidelines for the practitioner to ensure the safety of both mother and fetus.

PHYSIOLOGIC CHANGES OF PREGNANCY

Cardiovascular System

Many physical changes occur throughout pregnancy that affect athletic conditioning and exercise. The heart and circulatory system are affected by the substantial increases in blood volume that occur early in pregnancy. The expansion of blood volume and cardiac output precedes the growth of the uterus and the fetus and has an impact on the maternal response to exercise even in the first trimester. By the end of pregnancy, blood volume has increased by almost 50% compared to prepregnancy levels. Both red cell mass and plasma volume increase, but the increase in plasma volume occurs first and exceeds the increase in cellular mass, resulting in a dilutional anemia in early and mid-pregnancy. The plasma volume peaks at about 32 weeks of gestation, but red cell mass continues to increase during the third trimester, so this dilutional anemia is partially corrected at term.[3]

Blood volume expansion in pregnancy results in a greater oxygen-carrying capacity and increased cardiac work. Stroke volume and cardiac output both increase. The resting pulse rate also increases by 10 to 15 beats per minute. The chambers of the heart dilate and the position of the heart changes, rotating outward to the left.[8] In well-conditioned athletes, blood volume increases are greater than in sedentary women.[13] This additional increase may help ensure adequate blood flow to the uterus during exercise and improves heat dissipation.

Blood pressure usually falls slightly during pregnancy, reaching its lowest levels in mid-pregnancy and climbing slowly thereafter to prepregnancy levels. There is a redistribution of resting blood flow, with increased circulation to the uterus, intestines, kidneys, skin, and breasts. As the uterus and placenta grow, an increasing percentage of the cardiac output perfuses these organs, and the blood flow through the uterine arteries at term is approximately 500 mL/min.[9] The increased blood volume and cardiac output of pregnancy is accompanied by a reduction in venous tone. Further, the increasing size of the uterus decreases venous return to the heart, especially in the supine position. Supine hypotension can occur any time in late pregnancy if the uterus impairs venous return by partially occluding the inferior vena cava. Therefore, exercise requiring long periods of time spent in the supine position should be avoided after 20 weeks' gestation.

Pulse, cardiac output, and blood pressure all increase with exercise, although during pregnancy, these increases are slightly blunted. Most of this increased blood flow goes to the working muscles, resulting in some shunting of blood flow away from the uterus and developing fetus during vigorous exercise.[1] These observations raise concern about the potential risks of intense and/or prolonged exercise in pregnancy. Evidence for such concern, however, is lacking.

Respiratory System

The anatomy of the chest wall changes in pregnancy, allowing for increased oxygen transport and utilization. There is increased elasticity, expansion, and flaring of the ribcage and elevation of the diaphragm. The tidal volume and minute ventilation increase, as does oxygen consumption. Reserve volumes, such as residual volume and functional residual capacity, are decreased, so the overall vital capacity is unchanged. Progesterone increases the sensitivity of carbon dioxide feedback centers in the medulla, which leads to increased ventilation, resulting in lower blood levels of carbon dioxide and slightly more alkaline pH.[8] The mild maternal alkalosis that results helps facilitate placental gas exchange and prevent fetal acidosis. The net effect of these physical and biochemical changes allows the pregnant woman to be more aware of her breathing and, occasionally, to feel short of breath. Despite this sensation, pregnant women are able to achieve increased levels of oxygen consumption during exercise just as efficiently as nonpregnant women.[1]

The respiratory changes of pregnancy facilitate gas exchange between the mother and fetus through the placenta. Changes in maternal oxygenation are amplified in the fetus. Sustained maternal acidosis or hypoxia will eventually induce fetal acidosis and hypoxia; therefore, it is reasonable to avoid prolonged anaerobic exercise. On the other hand, aerobic exercise in pregnant subjects results in greater increases in minute ventilation than in nonpregnant women. This hyperventilation helps protect against the harmful shifts in blood oxygenation or pH that

might be encountered in intense aerobic exercise otherwise.[12]

Musculoskeletal System

The physical changes of pregnancy result in changes in posture, gait, and balance. The uterus and breasts enlarge significantly, causing the center of gravity to move forward and upward. This results in a tendency toward spinal lordosis (extension of the lower back and curvature). Pregnant women abduct the shoulders and flex the cervical spine to compensate for this.[1] The pregnancy hormone progesterone induces ligamentous laxity, which increases the mobility of all joints. The protein hormone relaxin, produced by the placenta during pregnancy, also increases pelvic laxity and joint laxity all over the body. The combined effects of progesterone and relaxin on the pelvic girdle can cause the characteristic maternal "waddling" of late pregnancy. As weight increases during pregnancy, impact forces on the vertebral column and joints increase and chronic lower back pain is common. Consequently, musculoskeletal concerns in pregnancy include the possibility of excess torque forces on lax joints causing sprains as well as a greater propensity to falling. Severe falls can cause placental abruption or rupture of the membranes.[3] To minimize the risk of orthopaedic injury, a pregnant woman may prefer swimming, stationary bicycling, treadmills, and stair-climbing machines over prolonged running or physical sports.[1]

Weight Gain and Nutrition

Changes in weight and body mass are potentially important during pregnancy. The average weight gain in pregnancy is about 25 to 30 pounds. Forty percent of the weight gain comes from growth of the fetus, amniotic fluid, and placenta. Increased blood volume, growth of the breasts and uterus, and a slight increase in body fat account for the remainder. Most of this weight gain occurs in the second half of pregnancy; normally, only 5 to 10 pounds accumulate in the first 20 weeks. A modest decline in weight is easily tolerated in the first trimester, especially in patients who start pregnancy at or above their ideal body weight. Adequate weight gain is essential in patients who start pregnancy underweight: low-birthweight infants are significantly more likely to be born to women who start pregnancy at least 15% underweight.[1] Female athletes tend to be underweight and have a lower percentage of body fat than nonathletes. Weight loss in early pregnancy and poor weight gain in later pregnancy are cause for concern about fetal well being. Prospective studies of pregnant women who continue vigorous training and maintain adequate nutrition confirm that a normal rate of pregnancy weight gain occurs in healthy pregnant athletes. Although pregnant athletes tend to gain slightly less weight in the third trimester, this deficiency is accounted for by less subcutaneous fat deposition, and overall weight gain is well within normal limits.[5]

Pregnancy results in increased nutrient requirements in all women. The pregnant athlete needs to respond by increasing water and electrolyte intake appropriately, and should increase caloric intake by approximately 300 calories a day.[8] As the level of physical activity increases, so will the caloric needs, so the pregnant athlete will have to increase her food intake further. Dehydration should be avoided, as it can exacerbate nausea, vomiting, and possible ketosis as well as exercise-induced hyperthermia. Dehydration is also associated with preterm contractions. Frequent, liberal adequate water intake is always advisable.[1,3] A diet rich in complex carbohydrates, for example, potatoes, rice, corn, and other whole grains, is best suited to the pregnant athlete because carbohydrates will most readily replenish the glycogen stores lost during strenuous exercise over a period of hours. Starvation should be avoided because prolonged catabolism is associated with significant ketone production, which can be harmful to the fetal nervous system.

Sustained vigorous exercise such as long-distance running can cause a significant increase in maternal core temperature. High maternal core temperature at elevation very early in fetal development has been associated with the development of neural tube defects,[7] such as spina bifida and meningoencephalocele. Because fetal temperatures are always higher than maternal temperatures, multiple metabolic difficulties also may be encountered in the fetus with high maternal temperatures.

Many of the physiologic changes of pregnancy work to help keep maternal temperature lower. Temperature at rest and sweating threshold are lower in pregnancy, and decreased venous tone in the skin facilitates greater heat exchange across the skin. These changes result in smaller elevations in temperature during moderate exercise in pregnancy. Indeed, the greater the gestational age, the less the effect of exercise on temperature.[2] Training programs for athletes who are pregnant therefore should be designed to help keep maternal temperature near normal, especially during the first trimester,

when the risk of fetal anomalies is highest. Sauna or hot tub use after exercise should be avoided. Strenuous exercise in a woman with a low fitness level, exercise-induced dehydration, and exercise-induced hyperthermia, all of which are associated with significant increases in core temperature, should be avoided.[3]

EXERCISE AND PREGNANCY OUTCOME

Effect on Fetal Growth

The pregnant athlete may have well-founded concerns about whether past intense exercise and training will affect fetal growth and birth weight. For as-yet unexplained reasons, women who begin pregnancy underweight, as many athletes do, are at risk for delivering an underweight or preterm newborn. With attention to nutrition and appropriate weight gain, this concern is minimal. Data from pregnant athletes about the effects of training on birth weight, though, are inconclusive. Evidence shows that moderately intense training throughout pregnancy, especially if pregnancy training intensities do not exceed prepregnancy levels, does not compromise fetal growth.[3] If exercise levels in the third trimester increase, birth weight may be decreased in proportion to the intensity of work.[3]

When aerobic conditioning in late pregnancy exceeds prepregnancy levels, reduced infant birth weight may result, from a combination of two factors. First, mothers who exercise intensely deliver approximately 1 week earlier than do those who are sedentary or exercise moderately. This relative shorter gestation may account for the approximately 100-g difference in birth weight compared to full-term infants. The remainder of the weight difference (about 220 g) is mostly accounted for by the decreased deposition of brown fat in the neonate.[2] This type of adipose tissue is found only in newborn infants and is important for energy and heat regulation, especially if the infant is premature; thus decreased fat deposition may have adverse consequences in the preterm infant.

Pregnant women with gestational diabetes may find that exercise improves glucose control.[1]

Acute Effects

Recent reports confirm that exercise has relatively little effect on the acute status of the fetus and uterus when the mother and the unborn baby are healthy. The finding that intense exercise shunts blood flow away from the pregnant uterus in late pregnancy has led to concern that exercise could cause transient fetal hypoxia. Prospective data from athletes, however, have shown that during intense exercise fetal heart rates remain normal.[14] Fetal oxygenation, as measured by cord blood and amniotic fluid erythropoietin, is not affected by maintaining intense exercise during the third trimester up to the onset of labor.[6] The placenta plays an important role in women who exercise and in women who reside at higher altitudes. Women who exercise regularly have placentas that consistently measure larger than those of nonexercising control women. Additionally, athletes demonstrate improved placental blood flow and placental gas exchange efficiency.[10]

Labor

Occasionally, intense physical activity induces contractions, however, moderate- to high-intensity regular exercise does not increase the pregnant athlete's risk of premature labor and delivery.[3] Strong regular contractions prior to term must be evaluated, even if the patient has recently exercised, because preterm labor can occur in the pregnant athlete as in any other patient. A pregnant athlete with findings of preterm labor may require additional care provider and family support in adjusting to reduced activity.

Although the risk of preterm delivery is not increased in athletes, patients who exercise regularly tend to deliver about 1 week earlier than patients who do not exercise who have otherwise uncomplicated pregnancies. Analysis of the impact of athletic conditioning on labor shows consistent benefits. Prospective data indicate that training decreases the rate of medical intervention, such as pitocin use, forceps delivery, and cesarean section. Additionally, maternal pain perception is decreased in women who exercise regularly. Patients who exercise up to the end of pregnancy may have a shorter labor and push for a shorter time for delivery.[3] Women who exercise regularly are more than twice as likely to progress from 4 cm dilation to full cervical dilation in less than 4 hours, and their second stage averages 36 minutes versus 60 minutes in controls.

PREGNANCY AS AN OPPORTUNITY FOR IMPROVED CONDITIONING

Much of the current research on exercise and training in pregnancy has focused on the effect that pregnancy has on conditioning and per-

formance. The growing uterus and progressive weight gain of pregnancy provide a natural increase in exercise resistance.[4,15] Pregnant women who exercise regularly therefore experience an increased tolerance for physical work and enjoy the same conditioning benefits that anyone who works out regularly will achieve.

PSYCHOLOGICAL BENEFITS OF EXERCISE DURING PREGNANCY AND THE PUERPERIUM

Exercise during and after pregnancy has been shown to have a positive effect on psychological state. Twenty women volunteered to complete the State-Trait Anxiety Inventory and the Profile of Mood States before and following either an exercise session ($N = 10$) or a quiet rest session ($N = 10$). Exercise consisted of 60 minutes of low-impact aerobic activity at an intensity between 60% and 70% of maximal heart rate reserve. Quiet rest consisted of sitting quietly in a room free from distractions for 60 minutes. Results indicated that state anxiety and depression decreased significantly ($p < 0.05$) following exercise and quiet rest. Furthermore, exercise was associated with significant decreases ($p < 0.05$) in total mood disturbance, as well as significant increases ($p < 0.05$) in vigor in physically active postpartum women.[11]

DEVELOPMENT OF A RATIONAL STRATEGY FOR EXERCISE IN PREGNANCY

Preconception Planning

As data about the beneficial effects of athletic training during pregnancy accumulates, physicians are now encouraging their pregnant patients to exercise. Athletic women should plan for exercise in pregnancy before conception. Adopting a new exercise routine or exercise of significantly increased intensity is not recommended in pregnancy. Therefore, the athlete who is planning a pregnancy should modify her training schedule and activities to suit the pregnant state prior to conception. Intense dieting prior to or during pregnancy also should be avoided because being underweight will result in poor fetal weight gain or severe malnutrition.

American College of Obstetricians and Gynecologists Guidelines

The most recent guidelines published by the American Academy of Obstetricians and

Recommendations for Exercise in Pregnancy and Postpartum

There are no data in humans to indicate that pregnant women should limit exercise intensity and lower target heart rates because of potential adverse effects. For women who do not have any additional risk factors for adverse maternal or perinatal outcome, the following recommendations may be made:

1. In the absence of either medical or obstetric complications, 30 minutes or more of moderate exercise a day on most, if not all, days of the week is recommended for pregnant women.
2. Women should avoid exercise in the supine position after the first trimester. Such a position is associated with decreased cardiac output in most pregnant women; because the remaining cardiac output will be preferentially distributed away from splanchnic beds (including the uterus) during vigorous exercise, such regimens are best avoided during pregnancy. Prolonged periods of motionless standing should also be avoided.
3. Women should be aware of the decreased oxygen available for aerobic exercise during pregnancy. They should be encouraged to modify the intensity of their exercise according to maternal symptoms. Pregnant women should stop exercising when fatigued and not exercise to exhaustion. Weight-bearing exercises may under some circumstances be continued at intensities similar to those prior to pregnancy throughout pregnancy. Non-weight-bearing exercise such as cycling or swimming will minimize the risk of injury and facilitate the continuation of exercise during pregnancy
4. Morphologic changes in pregnancy should serve as a relative contraindication to types of exercise in which loss of balance could be detrimental to maternal or fetal well-being, especially in the third trimester. Further any

type of exercise involving the potential for even mild abdominal trauma should be avoided.
5. Pregnancy requires an additional 300 kcal/d in order to maintain metabolic homeostasis. Thus, women who exercise during pregnancy should be particularly careful to ensure an adequate diet.
6. Pregnant women who exercise in the first trimester should augment heat dissipation by ensuring adequate hydration, appropriate clothing, and optimal environmental surroundings during exercise.
7. Many of the physiologic and morphologic changes of pregnancy persist 4–6 weeks postpartum. Thus, prepregnancy exercise routines should be resumed gradually based on a woman's physical capability.

Contraindications to Exercise

The aforementioned recommendations are intended for women who do not have any additional risk factors for adverse maternal or perinatal outcome. A number of medical or obstetric conditions may lead the obstetrician to recommend modifications of these principles. The following conditions should be considered contraindications to exercise during pregnancy.

- Pregnancy-induced hypertension
- Preterm rupture of membranes
- Preterm labor during the prior or current pregnancy or both
- Incompetent cervix/cerclage
- Persistent second- or third-trimester bleeding
- Intrauterine growth retardation

In addition, women with certain other medical or obstetric conditions, including chronic hypertension or active thyroid, cardiac, vascular, or pulmonary disease, should be evaluated carefully in order to determine whether an exercise program is appropriate.

Figure 20-1. Guidelines for exercise in pregnancy. (From American College of Obstetricians and Gynecologists: Exercise during pregnancy and the postpartum period. ACOG Technical Bulletin 189. Washington, DC, ACOG, 1994, with permission.)

Gynecologists (Fig. 20-1) reflect a more positive attitude about vigorous exercise in pregnancy. These guidelines recognize the safety and benefits of exercise during pregnancy. Pregnancy causes significant physiologic changes, to which the pregnant athlete should adapt. Intense exercise in pregnancy should be undertaken with the supervision of care providers, keeping in mind fetal well being. With attention to adequate weight gain, prevention of hyperthermia, and

avoidance of injury, the pregnant athlete can remain conditioned and expect to have a more healthy pregnancy than the unconditioned woman.

CONCLUDING REMARKS

In summary, the female athlete can continue athletic pursuits during pregnancy. The form and intensity of exercise may change as the pregnancy progresses and the patient responds physiologically to these changes. Because many health benefits accrue from regular exercise, the pregnant woman should participate in a wide variety of activities.

References

1. Artal R: Exercise and pregnancy. Clin Sports Med 11:363–77, 1992.
2. Clapp JF 3rd: The changing thermal response to endurance exercise during pregnancy. Am J Obstet Gynecol 165:1684–9, 1991.
3. Clapp JF 3rd: A clinical approach to exercise during pregnancy. Clin Sports Med 13:443–58, 1994.
4. Clapp JF 3rd, Capeless E: The VO2 of recreational athletes before and after pregnancy. Med Sci Sports Exerc 23:1128–33, 1991.
5. Clapp JF 3rd, Little KD: Effect of recreational exercise in pregnancy weight gain and subcutaneous fat deposition. Med Sci Sports Exerc 27:170–7, 1995.
6. Clapp JF 3rd, Little KD, Appleby-Wineberg SK, Widness JA: The effect of regular maternal exercise on erythropoetin in cord blood and amniotic fluid. Am J Obstet Gynecol 172:1445–51, 1995.
7. Clarren SK, Smith DW, Harvey MA, et al: Hyperthermia: A prospective evaluation of a possible teratogenic agent in man. J Pediatr 95:81–4, 1979.
8. Cunningham, FG, MacDonald PC, Gant, NF, et al: Maternal adaptations to pregnancy. In Williams Obstetrics, 19th edition. Norwalk, Conn, Appleton & Lange, 1993.
9. Edman CD, Toofanian A, McDougal PC, Gant NF: Placental clearance rate of maternal plasma androstenedione through placental estradiol formation: An indirect method of assessing uteroplacental blood flow. Am J Obstet Gynecol 131:1029–37, 1981.
10. Jackson MR, Gott P, Lye SJ, et al: The effects of maternal aerobic exercise on human placental development: placental volumetric composition and surface areas. Placenta 16:179–91, 1995.
11. Koltyn KF, Schultes SS: Psychological effects of an aerobic exercise session and a rest session following pregnancy. J Sports Med Phys Fitness 37:287–91, 1997.
12. Pivarnik JM, Lee W, Spillman T, et al: Maternal respiration and blood gases during aerobic exercise performed at moderate altitude. Med Sci Sports Exerc 24:868–72, 1992.
13. Pivarnik JM, Mauer MB, Ayres NA, et al: Effects of chronic exercise on blood volume expansion and hematologic indices during pregnancy. Obstet Gynecol 83:265–9, 1994.
14. van Doom NIB, Lotgering FK, Struijk PC, et al: Maternal and fetal cardiovascular responses to strenuous bicycle exercise. Am J Obstet Gynecol 166:854–9, 1992.
15. Wolfe LA, Walker RMC, Bonen A, McGrath MJ: Effects of pregnancy and chronic exercise on respiratory responses to graded exercise. J Appl Physiol 76:1928–36, 1994.

Chapter 21

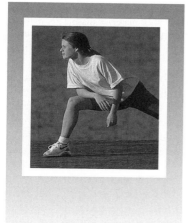

Return to Activity Postpartum

Stefanie Schupp Christian, M.D.
Jeffrey S. Christian, M.D.
Carol A. Stamm, M.D.
James A. McGregor, M.D.

Women who have just given birth may be driven, or feel obligated, to lose the weight gained during pregnancy. Exercise is often recommended as an alternative or adjunct to dieting because of its known benefits of maintaining lean body mass, enhancing fat loss, and improving cardiovascular fitness, as well as the proposed benefits of reducing stress, promoting good posture, and improving mood and body image.[7] Each of these goals is particularly important to the female athlete. However, many women question when to resume exercise and what duration and level of exertion is desirable. In addition, women who are lactating have concerns about the possible impact of vigorous exercise on breast milk production and palatability. Other women may worry about pelvic relaxation or be bothered by transient urinary stress incontinence with vigorous exercise in the postpartum period.

Care providers frequently recommend unnecessarily conservative exercise regimens to postpartum patients; however, research on exercise in the puerperium is providing a sound scientific basis for encouraging less cautious programs.

GUIDELINES FOR EXERCISE POSTPARTUM

Following an uncomplicated vaginal delivery, exercise may be restarted as soon after delivery as the woman feels able to exercise, often within a few days. Athletes desiring to continue training or reinitiate training should engage in exercise programs that include aerobic conditioning and strength training as well as exercises designed to correct pregnancy-induced changes such as pelvic floor laxity and relaxed or stretched abdominal wall tissues, including separation of the rectus muscles, diastasis recti.[26]

Pelvic-floor strengthening exercises, Kegel exercises, should be resumed as soon after the birth as possible because this may increase circulation and aid healing. Kegel exercises have been advocated routinely since 1948[18] when they were first described in the medical literature. A sustained program of voluntary isometric contractions of the pubococcygeus muscle and pelvic sphincter system can strengthen the pelvic diaphragm and help prevent or mitigate symptoms of mild stress urinary incontinence as well as enhance sexual functioning. The patient should carry out at least a series of 15 rapid pelvic floor contractions, followed by 15 sustained contractions, each of which is held for 3 seconds and released for 3 seconds, 5 or 6 times per day. The patient should be instructed to perform Kegel exercises with an empty bladder and not while on the commode in order to prevent the development of abnormal voiding patterns. A perineometer or vaginal weighted cones can assist the patient in identifying the correct muscles for the exercise.[2] A recent study shows that women who attended an 8-week pelvic muscle exercise group achieved greater strengthening and practiced more often than women who received written instructions only.[27]

We recommend that corrective exercises for diastasis recti begin as soon as one is comfortable after delivery, often within 3 days. Patients can begin with simple head lifts. The mother lies in a supine position with knees bent, feet flat on the floor, and hands crossed over the midline at the diastasis to support the area. As she exhales, she lifts only her head off the floor until just before a bulge appears. Her hands should gently pull the rectus muscles toward midline. She then lowers her head slowly and relaxes. A simultaneous posterior pelvic tilt can be added to the head lift. The head lift with or without pelvic tilt is the only abdominal strengthening exercise that should be performed until the diastasis is corrected to 2 cm. At that time, more vigorous abdominal exercise can be initiated.[20] These may include sit-ups or abdominal crunches.

Aerobic and strengthening exercises can be resumed as soon as the postpartum woman feels able. Hormone-induced joint laxity may be present for 4 to 6 weeks after delivery, especially if the mother is breast-feeding. Precautions should be taken to protect the joints during exercise. No joint should be taken beyond its normal physiologic range. Hamstring and adductor stretches should be done cautiously. Overstretching of these muscle groups may increase pelvic girdle instability or hypermobility. Activities that require balancing or single-leg weight bearing can promote sacroiliac or pubic symphysis discomfort.[38] Muscle or joint pain indicates that the particular exercises should be discontinued.

Following a cesarean section, a patient should wait 6 to 8 weeks before beginning any type of abdominal exercises owing to the need for healing of fascial structures as the body dissolves surgical sutures. However, during these first 2 months, she should advance aerobic conditioning by walking or cycling, as long as she positions herself for cycling in such a way that avoids undo tension on her abdominal wall incision.

Psychological benefits of exercise in the puerperium are considerable and well-established. Anxiety and depression were significantly reduced in 10 women who volunteered to participate in 60 minutes of low-impact aerobics at an exercise intensity of 60% to 70% of maximal heart rate and completed the State-Trait Anxiety Inventory and the Profile of Mood States before and after exercise compared with 10 women who participated in a quiet rest session and completed the same inventories.[22] Depression and anxiety were significantly reduced in pregnant women who completed an exercise session in comparison to pregnant women who simply attended a prenatal education session.[21] This suggests that exercise can be an effective and safe nonpharmacologic method of mood regulation in the puerperium.

EXERCISE AND LACTATION

The effect of vigorous exercise on the quantity and quality of breast milk produced by lactating women is a common concern in the postpartum period. Experiments in various animal models have yielded conflicting results. Exercise has shown no adverse effects on milk production in rats.[17,38] On the other hand, forced exercise in dairy cows reduces the amount of milk produced.[23]

Several investigators have studied the effects of exercise on milk production in lactating women. Dewey and coworkers conducted a randomized trial to assess the effects of an exercise program on the lactation performance in previously unconditioned women.[6] Thirty three women who were feeding their babies exclusively with breast milk at 6 weeks postpartum were randomly assigned to 1 of 2 groups. The exercise group undertook a program of aerobic exercise for 45 minutes per day, 5 days per week for 12 weeks. The control group undertook no vigorous exercise more than once a week during the same 12-week period. The intervention had no adverse effects on lactation performance or infant weight gain. There were no differences between the 2 groups in basal serum prolactin levels, infant intake of breast milk, or breast milk concentrations of lipid, protein, or lactose. This study shows that breast-feeding women can safely undertake a moderate exercise program postpartum without jeopardizing breast-milk volume or composition.

Health-care providers can suggest the following guidelines to healthy lactating women who are initiating an exercise program or resuming training. We recommend that healthy postpartum mothers exercise at least 3 times per week, do warm-up activities before exercising, increase exercise frequency and intensity gradually, and maintain an adequately high fluid intake.

Wallace and colleagues studied the effects of exercise on lactation in women who were already exercising regularly.[40,41] Wallace and coworkers studied 26 lactating women between 2 and 6 months postpartum who exercised during pregnancy and the puerperium. The subjects expressed milk before and after a maximal treadmill test. The investigators evaluated both the lactic acid concentration and the infants' acceptance of the milk. They found significantly higher concentrations of lactic acid and significantly lower mean acceptance scores for the postexercise milk than for the pre-exercise milk. Presumably, milk with a higher lactic acid concentration tastes different from normal breast milk. However, no infant ever refused to nurse following maximal maternal exercise. Concentration of lactic acid in breast milk is likely to be much higher following maximal treadmill exertion than after the moderate exercise levels needed to maintain fitness or even the strenuous levels that are required for aerobic training.

Wallace and colleagues also performed a subsequent study evaluating the influence of the fullness of milk in the breasts on the concentration of lactic acid in postexercise milk. They found that milk lactic acid concentrations reached their peak more rapidly when the breasts were filled with milk prior to exercise (peak within 10 minutes) than if the breast had been emptied pre-exercise (peak within 30 minutes). They also showed that for both groups lactic acid concentrations remained elevated at more than twice their normal level 90 minutes postexercise.[39]

Based on these results, we can make the following suggestions to breast-feeding mothers who engage in maximally vigorous exercise programs. Even a strenuous exercise program will not alter the infant's acceptance of her milk to a clinically significant degree. However, if she finds that her infant refuses to nurse after exercise, she should nurse or collect milk for later feedings before exercising. In addition, the mother may find it necessary to express milk after exercising and discard it, but only if her child refuses to nurse. Nursing or expressing milk before vigorous exercise has the additional benefit of improving breast comfort during exercise.

WEIGHT LOSS POSTPARTUM

Three recent studies report that postpartum women retain an average of 1.5 kg (3.3 pounds) at 6 to 12 months after delivery.[15,19,33] However, in 1 study, fully 25% of the Caucasian women and more than 40% of the African-American women retained 9 or more pounds postpartum.[31] Commonly, weight loss is rapid within the initial 2 weeks after delivery but slows thereafter. Fewer than 25% of mothers have lost all of their pregnancy weight by 6 weeks postpartum.[33] Figure 21-1 depicts the cumulative weight loss in the first 6 months postpartum. The graph demonstrates that following the rapid initial fluid readjustment, weight loss is usually gradual. Clearly, neither patient nor the practitioner should expect a return to prepregnancy weight by the time of the 6-week postpartum visit.

Weight gain during pregnancy is the variable most highly correlated with weight loss after delivery.[33] A multivariate study of normal-weight women from the 1988 National Maternal and Infant Health Survey found that women who gained more than 35 pounds during pregnancy were more than twice as likely to retain 20 or more pounds postpartum than were those women whose weight gains did not exceed the 25- to 35-pound guidelines established in 1990 by the Institute of Medicine.[15,19] Careful dietary and exercise counseling before and during prenatal care are important interventions in attaining successful postpartum weight loss (see Chapter 20). Certain patterns of eating behavior (binge eating, frequent snacks, and missing meals) have been associated with the inability to lose weight postpartum. Not surprisingly, women who do not modify

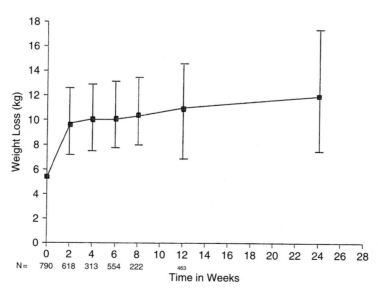

Figure 21-1. This graph shows that weight loss after delivery is very gradual after the initial 2 weeks and can take as long as 6 months. (From Schauberger C, Rooney B, Brimer L: Factors that influence weight loss in the puerperium. Obstet Gynecol 79: 424–9, 1992, with permission.)

their pregnancy eating habits postpartum fail to lose weight. Eating patterns that rely on frequent snacks and skipping lunch are also specifically associated with poor weight loss.[29] Women who stopped smoking during pregnancy have more retained weight postpartum.[28] Their decision to stop smoking should be intensively encouraged and supported both during and after pregnancy.

Physical activity during the first 12 months postpartum, especially between months 6 and 12, is also important for facilitating postpartum weight loss.[29] The guidelines set forth above for the resumption or institution of an exercise program following delivery should assist both patient and care provider in establishing a plan for healthy weight loss in the postpartum period.

Lactation may also have an impact on postpartum weight loss by increasing energy intake and reducing physical activity.[1,37] Results show that breast-feeding between 6 and 12 months postpartum contributes to weight loss.[5] These investigators hypothesize that previous studies were hampered by methodologic problems as well as by selection bias. By providing individualized exercise and dietary counseling to lactating athletes, health-care providers theoretically should be able to assist these women in achieving their desired weight loss. The daily energy required for lactation is estimated to be 640 kcal each day during the first 6 months. The recommended daily allowance for extra maternal intake during lactation is 500 kcal. This potential energy deficit should safely facilitate moderate weight loss during the breast-feeding period.[33]

Patients who have had gestational diabetes in pregnancy need to be encouraged to exercise and maintain normal body weight to delay or prevent development of adult-onset (type II) diabetes. Persistent obesity and continued weight gain have been shown to be modifiable risk factors for the potential development of type II diabetes.[30] Weight loss appears to reduce this risk.[32] Insulin sensitivity increases with weight loss.[13] Exercise also increases insulin sensitivity and decreases abdominal fat.[10] Data from longitudinal studies suggest that women can lower their risk of acquiring type II diabetes with regular exercise.[8,12,25] Women with gestational diabetes should be encouraged to normalize their weight postpartum.

The following guidelines for weight loss during lactation are provided by the Institute of Medicine.[14] Lactating women should consume at least 1800 kcal/day in order to avoid possible problems with breast-milk production and maternal nutritional deficiencies. Women who begin pregnancy with a normal body mass index should not lose more than 1 to 2 pounds per month after the first month postpartum; however, most overweight mothers can lose up to 4.5 pounds per month without jeopardizing lactation. Dieting during the first 2 to 3 weeks, when the milk supply is being established, is not recommended because of a possible decrease in milk volume. And finally, liquid diets and weight-loss medications should be avoided during lactation.

LACTATION-ASSOCIATED BONE LOSS

Lactation is associated with suppression of estrogen production by the ovaries, which may result in reduced bone mass and calcium loss. Calcium loss of approximately 200 to 400 mg occurs through milk production each day.[24] Approximately 3% to 6% of axial bone may be lost during lactation.[3,4,9,11,16,34–36] Such physiologic lactation-associated osteopenia is reversed with weaning.[3,4,9,11,16,34–36] Exercise is associated with improved bone mineralization but it is not yet determined if exercise can reduce the magnitude of lactation-associated osteopenia.

CONCLUDING REMARKS

The guidelines outlined in this chapter are meant to assist health-care providers who take care of female athletes in the postpartum period. The female athlete can encounter many obstacles to resuming exercise in the puerperium, such as the cost of childcare, fatigue, and lack of time. Care providers can counteract these barriers by encouraging and supporting the female athlete to return to a safe and healthy exercise regimen following delivery. The normal and healthy process of lactation should be encouraged and supported in all postpartum women, including athletes.

References

1. Abrams B, Berman C: Women, nutrition, and health. Curr Probl Obstet Gynecol Fertil 16:30–5, 1993.
2. American College of Obstetricians and Gynecologists: Precis V. Washington DC, ACOG, 1994, p 240.
3. Cross NA, Hillman LS, Allan SH, Krause GF: Changes in bone mineral density and bone remodeling during lactation and postweaning in women consuming high amounts of calcium. J Bone Miner Res 10:1312–1320, 1995.
4. Cross NA, Hillman LS, Allan SH, et al: Calcium homeostasis and bone metabolism during pregnancy, lactation, and postweaning; a longitudinal study. Am J Clin Nutr 61:514–23, 1995.

5. Dewey K, Heinig M, Nommsen L: Maternal weight loss patterns during prolonged lactation. Am J Clin Nutr 58:162–6, 1993.

6. Dewey KG, Lovelady CA, Nommsen-Rivers LA, et al: A randomized study of the effects of aerobic exercise by lactating women on breast-milk volume and composition. N Engl J Med 330:449–53, 1994.

7. Dewey KG, McCrory MA: Effects of dieting and physical activity on pregnancy and lactation. Am J Clin Nutr 59(suppl):446S–53S, 1994.

8. Dornhorst, A Rossi M: Risk and prevention of type 2 diabetes in women with gestational diabetes. Diabetes Care 21 (Suppl 2):B43–9, 1998.

9. Drinkwater BL, Chestnut CH: Bone density changes during pregnancy and lactation in active women. Bone Miner 14:153–60, 1991.

10. Eriksson J, Taimda S, Koivisto VA: Exercise and the metabolic syndrome. Diabetologia 40:125–35, 1997.

11. Hayslip CC, Kline TA, Wray HL, Duncan WE: The effects of lactation on bone mineral content in healthy postpartum women. Obstet Gynecol 73:588–92, 1989.

12. Helmrich SP, Ragland DR, Lueng RW, Dalfenbarger RSJ: Physical activity and reduced occurrence of non-insulin dependent diabetes mellitus. N Engl J Med 325:147–52, 1991.

13. Holte J, Bergh T, Berne C, et al: Restored insulin sensitivity but persistently increased early insulin secretion after weight loss in obese women with polycystic ovary syndrome. J Clin Endocrinol Metab 80:2586–93, 1995.

14. Institute of Medicine, Committee on Nutritional Status during Pregnancy and Lactation, Subcommittee on Nutrition during Lactation: Nutrition during lactation. Washington, DC, National Academy Press, 1991.

15. Institute of Medicine, Subcommittee on Dietary Intake and Nutrient Supplements During Pregnancy, Committee on Nutritional Status During Pregnancy and Lactation: Nutrition during pregnancy, weight gain and nutrient supplements. Washington, DC, National Academy Press, 1990.

16. Kalkwarf HJ, Specker BL: Bone mineral loss during lactation and recovery after weaning. Obstet Gynecol 86:26–32, 1995.

17. Karasawa K, Suwa J, Kimura S: Voluntary exercise during pregnancy and lactation and its effect on lactational performance in mice. J Nutr Sci Vitaminol (Tokyo) 27:333–9, 1981.

18. Kegel AH: Progressive resistance exercise in the functional restoration of the perineal muscles. Am J Obstet Gynecol 56:238–48, 1948.

19. Keppel K, Taffel S: Pregnancy-related weight gain and retention: Implications of the 1990 Institute of Medicine guidelines. Am J Public Health 83:1l00–3, 1993.

20. Kisner C, Colby LA: Therapeutic Exercise, 2nd edition. Philadelphia, FA Davis, 1990, pp 562–3.

21. Koltyn KF: Mood Changes in pregnant Women following an exercise session and a prenatal information session. Women's Health Issues 4:191–5, 1994.

22. Koltyn KF, Schultes SS: Psychological Effects of an aerobic exercise session and a rest session following pregnancy. J Sports Med Phys Fitness 37:287–91, 1997.

23. Lamb RC, Sbarder BO, Anderson MJ, Walters JL: Effects of forced exercise on two-year-old Holstein Heifers. J Dairy Sci 62:1791–7, 1979.

24. Little KD, Clapp JF: Self-selected recreational exercise has no impact on early postpartum lactation-induced bone loss. Med Sci Sports Exerc 30:831–6, 1998.

25. Manson JE, Rimm EB, Stampfer MJ, et al: Physical activity and incidence of NIDDM women. Lancet 338:774–8, 1991.

26. Markowiz E, Brainen H: Baby Dance: A Comprehensive Guide to Prenatal and Postpartum Exercise. Englewood Cliffs, NJ, Prentice-Hall, 1980.

27. Morkved S, Bo K: The effect of post-natal exercises to strengthen the pelvic floor muscles. Acta Obstet Gynecol Scand 75:382–5, 1996.

28. Ohlin A, Rosner S: Maternal body weight development after pregnancy. Int Obesity 14:159–73, 1990.

29. Ohlin A, Roessner S: Trends in eating patterns, physical activity and socio-demographic factors in relation to postpartum body weight development. Br J Nutr 71:457–70, 1994.

30. O'Sullivan JB: The Boston gestational diabetes studies: review and perspectives. In Sutherland HW, Stowers JM, Pearson DWM (eds): Carbohydrate Metabolism in Pregnancy and the Newborn. London, Springer-Verlag, 1989, pp 287–94.

31. Parker J, Abrams B: Differences in postpartum weight retention between black and white mothers. Obstet Gynecol 81:768–74, 1993.

32. Peters RK, Kjos SL, Xiang A, Buchanan TA: Long-term diabetogenic effect of single pregnancy in women with previous gestational diabetes mellitus. Lancet 347:227–30, 1996.

33. Schauberger C, Rooney B, Brimer L: Factors that influence weight loss in the puerperium. Obstet Gynecol 79:424–9, 1992.

34. Sowers M, Corton G, Shapiro B, et al: Changes in bone density with lactation. JAMA 269:3130–5, 1993.

35. Sowers M, Eyre D, Hollis BW, et al: Biochemical markers of bone turnover in lactating postpartum women. J Clin Endocrinol Metab 80:2210–6, 1995.

36. Sowers M, Randolph J, Shapiro B, Jannausch M: A prospective study of bone density and pregnancy after an extended period of lactation with bone loss. Obstet Gynecol 85:285–9, 1995.

37. Spaaij C, Raaij J, Groot L, et al: Effect of lactation on resting metabolic rate and on diet- and work-induced thermogensesis. Am J Clin Nutr 59:42–7, 1994.

38. Treadway JL, Lederman SA: The effects of exercise on milk yield, milk composition, and offspring growth in rats. Am J Clin Nutr 44:481–8, 1986.

39. Wallace JP, Ernsthausen K. Inbar G: The influence of the fullness of milk in the breasts on the concentration of lactic acid in postexercise breast milk. Int J Sports Med 13:395–8, 1992.

40. Wallace JP, Inbar G, Ernsthausen K: Infant acceptance of postexercise breast milk. Pediatrics 89:1245–7, 1992.

41. Wallace JP, Rabin J: The concentration of lactic acid in mothers milk following maximal exercise. Int J Sports Med 12:328–31, 1991.

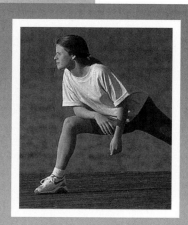

Section V

General Medical Conditions

Chapter 22

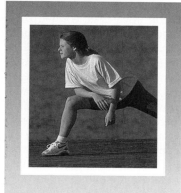

Growth and Development

Sabrina M. Strickland, M.D.
Jordan D. Metzl, M.D.

INTRODUCTION

In the past 15 years, we have witnessed a youth sports explosion in the United States. Currently there are approximately 30 million American children and adolescents, under the age of 18, playing on some form of sports team. The greatest changes in demographics have occurred among females. In 1972, there were 20,000 girls playing on high school sports teams. In contrast, in 1999 there were almost 3.5 million.

On every level, from neighborhood soccer leagues to Olympic-level teams, the increased participation of female athletes has changed the very nature of sports. Whereas four years ago Olympic women's soccer or softball received passing mention in Olympic broadcasting, the Sydney Olympiad of 2000 featured women's sports with equal billing compared to men. For the young female athlete, emulating famous women athletes has changed the tenor of female sports. Today, girls in local soccer programs dream of being the next star for the Women's World Cup team.

Sports participation in girls is certainly favorable. There are many considerations, however, that make caring for the young female athlete different than caring for the male athlete. This chapter will review the growth and development of the female athlete and explain how this affects both sports performance and injury risk. Specific injury pattern prevention in female athletes will also be discussed.

GROWTH AND DEVELOPMENT OF THE FEMALE ATHLETE

Female athletes face different hurdles as they mature compared to their male counterparts. Sports performance improves with increasing chronological age both as a result of skeletal growth and maturation of the endocrine, nervous, muscular, and cardiovascular systems. Awareness of issues pertinent to the growth and development of athletes is important as girls engage in an ever-widening selection of sports.

Childhood

In general, there are relatively few differences between boys and girls during childhood. Dehydroepiandrosterone-sulfate (DHEA-S) is a weak adrenal androgen with high serum concentrations. DHEA-S concentrations begin to increase around the age of 6 to 8 (adrenarche) and may play a minor role in bone growth and maturation. During childhood there are no gender differences in testosterone and estradiol concentrations. Some girls experience a short mid-childhood growth spurt with adrenarche with a corresponding increase in bone age.[27]

An increase in growth hormone binding protein (GHBP) activity occurs throughout childhood. In children GHBP influences growth hormone (GH) action by enhancing growth promoting effects. GH concentrations are modulated to accommodate the prevailing GHBP environment to assure that genetically programmed growth continues. Most important to the regulation of GH release are genetics, nutrition, and absence of debilitating disease. Increasing levels of body fat increases GHBP levels and vice versa; this may partially account for the frequently seen greater growth velocities of obese children. In contrast, children lacking sufficient GH go on to have growth failure at puberty.[27]

Experimental data suggests that anaerobic performance is lower in children than in adolescents or adults. Increasing gender differences occur in absolute anaerobic power during pubertal progression owing to the acceleration in boys and the plateau in girls.[8,15,27] Anaerobic power increases with increasing testosterone concentrations, perhaps due to changes in myofibrillar density or neuromuscular development.[15] Study of children less than 8 years of age is limited because maximal oxygen uptake cannot be accurately measured in this age group. Anaerobic power may be particularly important to sport performance in children as many children compete in sports where maximal aerobic capacity is not of primary importance like football and volleyball. Children tend to play with short bursts of exertion followed by rest, which relies on stored glycogen and therefore anaerobic glycolysis rather than aerobic energy.

Aside from performance, clinicians have worried that young athletes may be particularly at risk for injury. For example, concern for growth plate injury has kept some physicians from recommending strength-training programs. It is now clear that prepubescent children can make significant gains in muscle strength in response to progressive resistive training. Nevertheless, close supervision with emphasis on specific stretching exercises, slow controlled motions and avoidance of excessive weights is mandatory in all strength training programs, especially those involving prepubescent athletes.[29]

Children can benefit from physical activity in terms of level of fitness and social development. Recently, research has demonstrated that a structured aerobic exercise-training program influences the lipoprotein profile of apparently healthy, prepubertal children. Tolfrey et al were able to effect a 9.3% increase in HDL and a 17.2% decline in LDL/HDL ratio. They concluded that it is possible to influence the prepubertal lipoprotein profile independent of the alterations in confounding variables such as body composition, cardiorespiratory fitness, and habitual physical activity.[33] Whether or not these changes are lasting has yet to be determined, however, structured exercise may become a lifetime habit in these individuals.

Adolescence

The most dramatic changes in physical growth and development occur during the adolescent years. During a six to seven year period from nine to sixteen years of age, girls quickly become young women. Adolescent growth and development is best viewed by examining the different categories of development, including sexual, skeletal, and physiologic development.

Sexual Development

Sexual development has historically been the basis for the determination of maturation level,

and also for predicting remaining growth and development. Most girls start puberty approximately two years before their male counterparts. The appearance of the breast bud is the first manifestation of puberty in approximately 85% of girls with a range from 8 to 13 years.[34] A combination of sex steroids and growth hormone appears to be responsible for the pubertal growth spurt. DHEA-S concentration and the age of onset of pubertal maturation are inversely correlated. A complex interaction occurs between the age of onset of puberty and final height. Sexual precocity increases the immediate growth rate and the total pubertal height gain as compared with average maturers. In fact, there is an increased duration of puberty in these children compensated for by an increased rate of bone maturation. Bone maturation, however, ends the period of skeletal growth. Unfortunately, the increase in total pubertal height gain is not sufficient to counter balance the markedly reduced

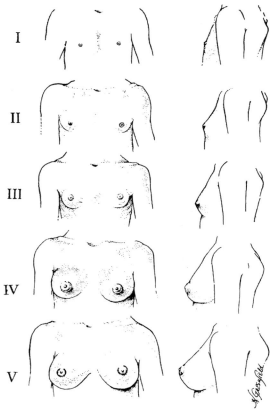

Figure 22-1. Tanner staging of adolescent female development. (From Marshall WA, Tanner JM: Variations in patterns of pubertal changes in girls. Arch Dis Child 1969; 44:291. Reprinted from Ross GT, Vande Wiele RL, Frantz AG: The normal ovary. In: Williams RH (ed): Textbook of Endocrinology, 6th ed. Philadelphia, WB Saunders, 1981, p 362.)

period of prepubertal growth and thus these children usually are shorter.

The Tanner staging system (Fig. 22-1) is widely utilized to assess developmental stage based on secondary sexual characteristics. The Tanner stage can estimate skeletal maturity and reflect the hormonal status of the young athlete. In girls, breast and pubic hair development are rated separately on a scale from 1 to 5. Pubic hair stages are categorized as follows:

- Stage 1 is preadolescent without pubic hair;
- Stage 2 consists of sparse growth of long, slightly pigmented downy hair which is straight or only slightly curled appearing chiefly along the labia;
- Stage 3 is marked by considerably darker, coarser and more curled hair spread sparsely over the junction of the pubes;
- Stage 4 is when hair resembles adult in type but the area covered is smaller than that of the adult without spread to the medial surface of the thighs;
- Stage 5 is typified by adult quantity and type of hair.

The transition from stage 2 to stage 5 takes about 4 years on average. Axillary hair usually appears two years after the beginning of pubic hair growth.

Breast development stages are classified as follows:

- Stage 1 (preadolescent) is characterized as no breast development;
- Stage 2 is the breast bud stage with elevation of the breast and papilla as a small mound with enlargement of areolar diameter;
- Stage 3 involves further enlargement and elevation of the breast and areola without separation of their contours;
- Stage 4 is differentiated by projection of areola and papilla to form a secondary mound above the level of the breast; and finally;
- Stage 5 is the mature stage with projection of papilla only due to recession of the areola.

After breast stage 3, estradiol concentrations increase most dramatically. Deming in 1957 determined that there was a .93 correlation between menarche and peak height velocity.[31]

Musculoskeletal Development

In general, the velocity of growth decreases from the fourth month of fetal life onward. However this trend is interrupted between 6 and 8 years of age and once again between ages 13 and 15. The adolescent growth spurt occurs in all children, though it varies in intensity and duration. In girls, this spurt begins coincident with breast budding about 2 years earlier than in boys and on average lasts from age 10.5 to 13. The standard deviations around the mean ages are about 1 year in most studies. There is a tendency for children who experience an early growth spurt to have a somewhat higher peak height velocity (PHV), and vice versa. There is no relationship between age at PHV and adult stature. Maximum growth in body weight during adolescence occurs after PHV.[6] The female PHV is somewhat smaller in magnitude than boys with an average of about 8cm per year. An average girl of 14 years has already reached 98% of her adult height. The adolescent growth spurt is all encompassing with growth of every muscular and skeletal component, including head diameter.

Strength differences between boys and girls become more pronounced during adolescence, making inter-gender sports participation less safe during the teen years than during childhood. Girls increase muscular endurance in a linear fashion throughout childhood and adolescence without a definite pubertal acceleration.[27] Muscle mass peaks at menarche and then diminishes. A pre-adolescent fat wave exists in both sexes in which skin folds show an increase in fat prior to the PHV. By the time maturation is complete the total amount of body fat in girls is almost twice that in boys. The peak in strength gain as measured by dynamometers is about 14 months after the height peak and 9 months after the weight peak. This demonstrates a delay in strength gains compared to muscle mass.[31] There exists an interval where strength has not caught up to height and weight; this is a fact that can complicate categorization of young athletes.

Paralleling the changes in sexual development, skeletal development also follows a regular order in which the various skeletal dimensions accelerate. Leg length generally reaches its peak first, followed four months later by hip width and chest breadth. Several months later, shoulder breadth peaks. Finally, trunk length and chest depth reach their peak. Within the leg, the foot accelerates in growth 6 months before the calf and thigh. In fact, foot length is often the first of all skeletal dimensions below the head to cease growing. Foot breadth at heel and sole continues growing for a year or more after foot length has stopped. The calf length accelerates a little before the thigh.

Similarly, in the arm the forearm peaks in growth velocity 6 months ahead of the upper arm. Surprisingly, the height spurt is due more to an increase in length of trunk than length of leg. Characteristically, broadening of the hips relative to the shoulders and waist occurs during female adolescence. For equal stature, girls on the average have shorter legs than boys. Age at PHV is a maturity indicator that can be used in both sexes.

Meanwhile, the commonly used Risser sign is not an accurate predictor of vertebral growth nor accurate for estimation of skeletal age; in fact it is less accurate than chronological age.[21]

Physiologic Development

Girls, relatively, decline in aerobic function as they mature. Maximal aerobic power relative to body weight decreases with age in girls from 6 to 16 years, whereas an increase occurs in boys. The most commonly offered explanation for the discrepancy between boys and girls is the greater accumulation of fat in girls. Maximal aerobic power in girls has been shown in longitudinal studies to increase linearly until age 12 to 13 or until peak height velocity is reached at which time it plateaus or may slightly increase. Strength improves linearly through about 15 years of age with no clear evidence of an adolescent spurt in girls. The increase in strength during childhood and adolescence is more than that predicted from growth in stature. Performances in a variety of motor tasks also improve in girls to about 13 or 14 years of age. In addition, girls show greater flexibility at virtually all ages than boys.[6]

Girls lack the increase in number of red blood cells and amount of hemoglobin in the blood that occurs in boys. This difference is due to lack of secretion of testosterone. Intracellular water component of total body water decreases in girls during adolescence from 36% to 29%.[34] Other physiological changes important in sustained physical exercise also occur at adolescence. The heart grows faster during the growth spurt and increases in strength.[31] There is a marked increase in heart and lung size, a higher systolic pressure and a lower resting heart rate, and an increased ability to contract an oxygen debt. Creatinine excretion per 24 hours rises, although considerably less in girls than in boys. There is an increased excretion of hydroxyproline, the values paralleling the velocity curve for height.[32] As children grow, oxygen availability increases, raising the capacity for adenosine triphosphate production (ATP) from aerobic respiration. The increase in ATP allows muscles to contract for longer periods; this capacity enables adolescents to exercise for longer peri-

ods of time than children. Increased endurance can lead to overly long periods of exercise and overuse injuries.

Peak oxygen uptake, otherwise known as VO_2max, is defined as heart rate times stroke volume times arterial-venous oxygen difference, and is the most frequently used predictor of physiologic fitness. There is no relationship between peak oxygen uptake and habitual physical activity of 11- to 16-year-olds when estimated from continuous heart rate monitoring and computerized on-line gas analysis. Physical activity of children and adolescents does not appear to overload the cardiopulmonary system enough to initiate significant increases in peak oxygen uptake. Very few children or adolescents appear to satisfy the recommended criteria for the improvement of peak oxygen uptake through exercise, and this may be the simple explanation for the lack of relationship between peak oxygen uptake and habitual physical activity.[4]

During puberty there is no relationship between the concentrations of GHBP and degree of sexual maturation or bone age. In fact, GH itself does not influence GHBP levels. During the pubertal growth spurt GH concentrations peak but GHBP concentrations do not increase to as great an extent. This leads to an increased relative amount of free, biologically active GH. The amplitude of spontaneously circulating GH pulses, as modified by increasing levels of the sex-steroid hormones, is an important biological signal for growth of the organism, especially at puberty. Some actions of GH are direct, and others are indirect, through increasing levels of insulin like growth factor I (IGF-I). GH and IGF-I act via (1) stimulation of lipolysis; (2) increased circulating levels of free fatty acids; (3) antagonism of insulin action; (4) increased circulating phosphorus levels; and (5) increased urinary excretion of calcium. The net effect is anabolism and growth.[27]

Growth and Development in the Post-Adolescent Years

Minimal increases in growth have been reported at maturity. Buchi in 1950 demonstrated that stature increased from age 20 to 29 half a centimeter entirely due to growth of the trunk and then remained stationary until age 45, decreasing thereafter.[31]

Physical performance upon reaching maturity is thought to plateau until the fourth decade and subsequently diminish with time. Basic science studies have looked at the influence of age on skeletal muscle glucose transport and glycogen metabolism. There is considerable evidence linking the availability of muscle glycogen with endurance performance. In one study, young and old rats were compared, exaggeration of creatine phosphate depletion and muscle lactate accumulation occurred during exercise in the aged rats. Greater muscle glycogen depletion during contractile activity occurs in old compared to young rats. Additionally, there is evidence for reduced blood flow during contractile activity by older male rats and humans. Muscle mass declines with advancing age in both species. Sedentary rats and humans have an age-related decline in muscle oxidative capacity. All of these changes combined with increased blood catecholamine levels during exercise and lower resting muscle glycogen concentration would be expected to contribute to a reduced endurance capacity in old, untrained people. The metabolic responses and adaptations of skeletal muscle to exercise are, in most respects, qualitatively similar across a large portion of the life span, yet there may be an age-related decline in the adaptive capacity of muscle.[12]

The Effect of Sports Participation on Developing Bone

Cross-sectional studies of athletes and non-athletes show that training results in increased bone mineral density (BMD) and prospective exercise programs conducted with girls and premenopausal women have shown that strength training and high impact activities lead to increased bone densities. Lloyd et al have demonstrated in a prospective study of 112 premenarchal females that cumulative sports-exercise scores between ages 12 and 18 years were associated with increased hip BMD at age 18.[22] Witzke and Snow observed trends in bone mass suggesting that *plyometric* jump training continued over a long period of time during adolescent growth may increase peak bone mass.[35] Enhancement of bone mineral acquisition during growth may be a useful preventative strategy against osteoporosis. Morris et al. demonstrated an osteogenic effect was associated with exercise. Their results suggest that high-impact, strength building exercise is beneficial for premenarchal strength, lean mass gains, and bone mineral acquisition. The premenarchal years appear to be an opportune time to gain osteogenic benefits from exercise, corresponding to a time of greatest bone modeling, increasing concentrations of estrogen, and high growth hormone concentrations, and possibly an ideal time to establish positive attitudes toward exercise participation. If the 10% net increase in femoral neck BMD in the exercise group is sus-

tained into adulthood, the higher peak bone mass translates into a substantial reduction in relative hip fracture risk.[24]

In a study of 200 girls age 3 to 16 years dual-energy x-ray absorptiometry (DEXA) was utilized to determine at what age adult hip geometry is achieved and to examine possible influences of anthropometry and body composition on the development of femur axis length and femur width during growth. Adult values were achieved by age 14 years. Twin studies indicate that 20% of adult hip axis length is associated with environmental factors. They concluded that any environmental effects of physical activity or nutrition on hip geometry must occur before early adolescent years.[18]

MUSCULOSKELETAL INJURIES IN THE DEVELOPING FEMALE ATHLETE

Overuse Injury

Some types of overuse injuries can occur in both growing and adult athletes. Chronic overloading of bone can result in stress fracture, of tendons may lead to tendonitis, and at bone-tendon junctions a bursitis can occur. Growing cartilage in children and adolescents is susceptible to injury at the epiphyseal plate, the articular surface, and the apophyses. Training errors are the most common cause of overuse injury in athletes. Injuries may occur in the early phase of training program when tissues or groups of tissues are unused to such stresses. Children today may be accustomed to sitting in front of the television or computer, and therefore, may be rather de-conditioned compared to their forebears who played outdoors and performed chores. Injury can occur any time that new skills are introduced or the intensity increases, not just at the beginning of the season. A second major scenario in which overuse injury occurs is when the stress placed upon musculoskeletal tissue reaches the ultimate breakdown stress. This may occur when the athlete is considered to be in peak condition, but injury is caused either from muscular imbalance or poor technique.[26]

Stress fractures most frequently involve the tibia, fibula, and pars interarticularis. Normal x-rays do not rule out these injuries and bone and SPECT scanning is required for confirmation of the diagnosis. Spondylolysis or pars interarticularis stress fracture is frequently seen in athletes that perform excessive spinal extension such as gymnasts and *ballerinas*. Postural hyperlordosis

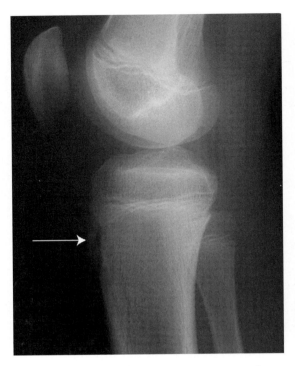

Figure 22-2. Osgood-Schlatter's disease (jumper's knee): Radiograph of skeletally immature knee.

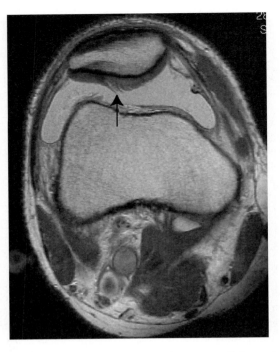

Figure 22-3. Coronal MRI of knee showing patellofemoral joint.

also contributes to this injury. As long as there is no evidence of spondylolisthesis the treatment is conservative, bracing and hamstring stretching usually suffice. The presence of a stress fracture in a young female athlete should warrant concern regarding underlying bone health. This point is especially important in young athletes since bone mass peaks at 32 years of age, and the bone development during adolescence is a strong predictor of eventual bone density.

Apophysitis often occurs in skeletally immature athletes. The most common site is the tibial tubercle, which is referred to as Osgood-Schlatter's disease or jumper's knee (Fig. 22-2). Patients with markedly symptomatic Osgood-Schlatter's disease who engage in activities involving rapid deceleration or vigorous vertical acceleration are in a relatively high-risk category for disruption of the extensor mechanism. Ogden and Southwick described Osgood-Schlatter's disease as an avulsion of a portion of the developing ossification center.[25] This insult stimulates callus formation increasing the size of the tuberosity without changing the growth plate. A case report by Bowers described a male athlete with symptoms and x-rays consistent with Osgood-Schlatter's disease that suffered a patellar tendon avulsion.[9] The region of failure corresponds to the zone of callus formation as described by Ogden and Southwick.[9,25]

Iliac crest apophysitis is typically seen in runners during the adolescent growth spurt with concomitant intensive training. Symptoms described include pain over the anterior iliac crest with running and with palpation, pain also occurs with resisted abduction of the hip. Contractures around the hip may coexist; tightness is elicited in Ober's (iliotibial band), Thomas's (hip flexor), and Ely's (rectus femoris) tests. Occasionally, x-rays will demonstrate widening of the iliac crest apophysis. Treatment consists of 3 to 4 weeks of rest, ice and gentle range of motion exercises.[26]

Patellofemoral stress syndrome is the most common complaint in the adolescent female athlete (Fig. 22-3). Patients complain of aching anterior knee pain that is exacerbated with activities or after sitting with the knee flexed. The adolescent growth spurt can result in superior and lateral migration of the patella with patella alta. Anatomic malalignments can contribute to patellofemoral stress syndrome, especially genu valgum, excessive pronation of the feet, and femoral anteversion. Diagnosis is based on classic findings including pain with patellofemoral compression, tightness of the lateral patellar retinacular structures, and patellar facet tenderness. Chondromalacia of the patellar articular cartilage is rare. Treatment is based on physical therapy to stretch the quadriceps, hamstrings, and iliotibial band while strengthening the vas-

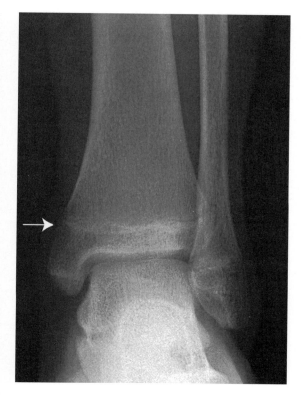

Figure 22-4. Radiograph of skeletally immature ankle.

from 0.7/100 in club athletes to 5/100 at the Olympic level. Chronic wrist pain in gymnasts is a common complaint especially related to hand-springs, round offs, and uneven parallel bar maneuvers. Several authors have reported radial growth plate injury in female gymnasts. Unlike most other sports, gymnastics requires use of the upper extremities as weight-bearing limbs, causing high-impact loads to be distributed through the elbow and wrist. The use of dowel grips, which are leather straps which act like mini-splints to maintain the fingers in flexion at the metacarpophalangeal, proximal inter-phalangeal and distal interphalangeal joint, may increase the compression applied to the distal radius during parallel bar routines.[28] In one study, 13 of 14 gymnastic wrist injuries were chronic and four of the nine physician-seen wrist injuries involved the distal radial physis.[10,11] Compressive loading of the wrist with the fore-arm out of full pronation or with some supina-tion may thus lead to disproportionate loading of the physis of the distal radius and selected premature closure at this site. Stress-related dis-tal radius physeal arrest with secondary ulna-radial-length difference may exist although the evidence is as of yet inconclusive.[1, 11]

tus medialis obliquus and quadriceps in terminal extension.[26]

An uncommon type of overuse injury of the ankle is medial malleolar ossification center pain. Medial ankle pain is brought on by repetitive athletic activities such as soccer or cross-country running. Swelling and point tenderness occur over the medial malleolus and radiographs show areas of ossification without acute changes (Fig. 22-4). The symptoms subside with growth and fusion of the ossification center.[26]

The types of injuries that occur in sports dif-fer based on age. DeHaven and Lintner looked at the age distribution of patients presenting to a sports medicine center over a 7-year period. The peak age group for injuries was 16 to 19. In general, the most common diagnoses were patellofemoral pain syndrome and internal derangement of the knee, increasing in frequen-cy as the stage of adolescence progressed.[13]

SPORT-SPECIFIC CONSIDERATIONS IN THE YOUNG FEMALE ATHLETE

Gymnastics

Female athletic participation in gymnastics has grown in the past 20 years. Injury rates range

Swimming

There is evidence to support an increased inci-dence of scoliosis among female swimmers. Repetitive swimming activity can cause adapta-tion of the primary structures and musculature, with the possibility that a secondary adaptation can occur in the vertebral column. Biomechanical assessment of stroke technique among swimmers will likely elucidate whether kinesthetics or hand dominance plays a role in the etiology of scoliosis in swimmers.[5]

Figure Skating

Skaters must maintain "the axis of rotation," an individualized sense of equilibrium, that each figure skater develops. This becomes difficult when young women develop secondary sexual characteristics that deposit fat tissue in the breast and around the hips. Maintaining spins and achieving adequate rotation and height dur-ing jumps becomes harder, predisposing the skater to injury. Gymnasts also can face similar risks when their sense of balance is affected, particularly on the balance beam. With the development of increased strength throughout growth, gymnasts are at increased risk for injury while vaulting and somersaulting.

Unfortunately, in an attempt to avoid these growth related problems, skaters and gymnasts might limit their caloric intake.[23]

Clinicians treating young performance sport athletes, such as ballerinas, gymnasts, and figure skaters, need to be mindful of the increased incidence of eating disorders as female athletes enter adolescence. Often, the first sign of disordered eating is menstrual dysfunction, either in the form of primary amenorrhea, absence of menses until age 16, or secondary amenorrhea defined as the absence of menses for greater than 3 months after the onset of menstruation. If these symptoms become evident, referral to a nutritionist who is familiar with female athletes is warranted. If symptoms persist, an adolescent medicine specialist or primary care sports medicine physician and/or a psychologist are often helpful resources. These issues are of paramount importance to the young female athlete since the bone mineral density loss in adolescence can have significant deleterious effects on adult peak bone density values.

Soccer

Soccer is the fastest growing team sport among female athletes. Although this is generally favorable, increased concern has been raised regarding the increased propensity towards rupture of the anterior cruciate ligament (ACL) among female athletes.

Anterior cruciate ligament injuries in female athletes have been reported to exceed that of male athletes at similar levels of athletic competition.[3,7, 14,16,17] The disparity in injury rates have been attributed to intrinsic causes, specifically generalized laxity, hormonal differences, and notch dimensions. Extrinsic factors blamed for the gender inequality are body mechanics, muscular strength and timing, and inferior conditioning. Recent research has led to the institution of plyometric training for female athletes in order to decrease ACL injury rates. These types of programs are gaining increasing amounts of popularity among junior high and high school level sports programs.

PSYCHOLOGICAL INFLUENCES ON THE YOUNG FEMALE ATHLETE

There are many developmental benefits of participation in youth sports for young girls including increased self-esteem, body image, tangible experiences of competency and success, as well as increased self confidence.[14] Participation in sports also provides opportunities for leadership and socialization, as well as coping skills in dealing with success and failure.[2] Studies on the young female athlete have found that the primary reason female children and adolescents engaged in physical activity were to have fun, followed by positive health benefits.[19,20] Higher grades and lower high school dropout rates have also been reported for high school girls participating in sports, as well as a higher enrollment in college.[14]

Increased pressures, however, are being placed on the young female athlete to "win at all costs" from coaches, parents, and others during vulnerable developmental stages. This competitive stress has been shown to contribute significantly to drop out rates in the young athlete and may cause impaired performance, increased risk of injury and sleep disturbances. Fear of failure has been found to be the main source of anxiety in the young athlete. An inverse relationship between fun and anxiety has been noted in the young athlete which is independent of victory or defeat.[30]

Parents and coaches can help facilitate enjoyment from sport participation for the young female athlete by emphasizing process and effort instead of outcome, providing realistic expectations, positive reinforcement and predictability. In addition, the young athlete needs to know that love and identity are not linked to their performance or whether or not they win.[30] Parents, coaches and teachers must be aware of girls' motives for participating in sport and physical activity—not only for competitive reasons, but to get in shape, improve skills, socialize and have fun.[14]

SUMMARY

Young female athletes are participating in organized sports in record numbers around the world. Historically cast as the "weaker" sex, girls and women have shown that they can excel in athletics. Significant differences, however, exist in growth and development between male and female athletes. These differences are important for the clinician treating the young athlete to recognize.

Research focusing on injury prevention and gender specific body mechanics promises to improve training methods in the future. Female athletes engaged in classic female sports such as skating, gymnastics and ballet face pressures to maintain a preadolescent physique and are at risk for eating disorders, amenorrhea and osteoporosis. Although there are many developmental benefits of participation in youth sports, there are increasing pressures for the young female athlete to "win at all costs." Coaches and parents need to help the young female athlete find enjoyment from sport participation and refrain from focusing only on winning. Education of coaches, parents, and athletes is vitally important in order to prevent medical and orthopaedic problems related to sports participation in the developing female athlete.

References

1. Albanese SA, Palmer AK, Kerr DR, Carpenter CW, Lisi D, Levinsohn EM: Wrist pain and distal growth plate closure of the radius in gymnasts. J Pediatr Orthop 1989;9:23–28.
2. American Academy of Pediatrics, Committee on Sports Medicine and Fitness: Fitness, activity and sports participation in the preschool child. Pediatrics 1992;90: 1002–1004.
3. Arendt E, Dick R: Knee injury patterns among men and women in collegiate basketball and soccer. NCAA data and review of literature. Am J Sports Med 1995;23:694–701.
4. Armstrong N, Balding J, Gentle P: Peak oxygen uptake and physical activity in 11- to 16-year-olds. Pediatr Exerc Sci 1990;2:349.
5. Becker T: Scoliosis in swimmers. Clin Sports Med 1986;5:149–158.
6. Beunen G, Malina R: Growth and physical performance relative to the timing of the adolescent growth spurt. Exerc Sport Sci Rev 1988;16:503–540.
7. Bjordal JM, Arnly F, Hannestad B, Strand T: Epidemiology of anterior cruciate ligament injuries in soccer. Am J Sports Med 1997;25:341–345.
8. Blimkie C, Roche P, Hay J: Anaerobic power of arms in teenage boys and girls: Relationship to lean tissue. Eur J Appl Physiol 1988;57:677–683.
9. Bowers K Jr: Patellar tendon avulsion as a complication of Osgood-Schlatter's disease. Am J Sports Med 1981;9:356–359.
10. Caine D, Cochrane B, Caine C, Zemper E: An epidemiologic investigation of injuries affecting young competitive female gymnasts. Am J Sports Med 1989;17:811–820.
11. Caine D, Roy S, Singer KM, Broekhoff J: Stress changes of the distal radial growth plate. A radiographic survey and review of the literature. Am J Sports Med 1992;20:290–298.
12. Cartee GD: Influence of age on skeletal muscle glucose transport and glycogen metabolism. Med Sci Sports Exerc 1994;26:577–585.
13. DeHaven KE, Lintner DM: Athletic injuries: comparison by age, sport, and gender. Am J Sports Med 1986;14: 218–224.
14. Executive Summary—The President's Council on Physical Fitness and Sports Report: Physical Activity and Sport in the Lives of Girls. Supported by The Center for Mental Health Services/Substance Abuse and Mental Health Services Administration, U.S. Department of Health and Human Services, May 1997.
15. Falk B, Bar O: Longitudinal changes in peak aerobic and anaerobic mechanical power of circumpubertal boys. Pediatr Exerc Sci 1993;5:318.
16. Ferretti A, Papandrea P, Conteduca F, Mariani PP: Knee ligament injuries in volleyball players. Am J Sports Med 1992;20:203–207.
17. Gomez E, DeLee JC, Farney WC: Incidence of injury in Texas girls' high school basketball. Am J Sports Med 1996;24:684–687.
18. Goulding A, Gold E, Cannan R, Williams S, Lewis-Barned NJ: Changing femoral geometry in growing girls: A cross-sectional DEXA study. Bone 1996;19:645–649.
19. Jaffe L, Manzer R: Girls' perspectives: Physical activity and self-esteem. Melpomene: A Journal for Women's Health Research 1992;11:19–26.
20. Jaffe L, Wu P: After school activities and self-esteem in adolescent girls: The teen years. Melpomene: A Journal for Women's Health Research 1996;15:18–25.
21. Little DG, Sussman MD: The Risser sign: A critical analysis. J Pediatr Orthop 1994;14:569–575.
22. Lloyd T, Chinchilli VM, Johnson-Rollings N, Kieselhorst K, Eggli DF, Marcus R: Adult female hip bone density reflects teenage sports-exercise patterns but not teenage calcium intake. Pediatrics 2000;106:40–44.
23. Metzl J: Caring for the young dancer (gymnast, figure skater). Contemp Pediatr 1999;16:135–147.
24. Morris FL, Naughton GA, Gibbs JL, Carlson JS, Wark JD: Prospective ten-month exercise intervention in premenarcheal girls: positive effects on bone and lean mass. J Bone Miner Res 1997;12:1453–1462.
25. Ogden JA, Southwick WO: Osgood-Schlatter's disease and tibial tuberosity development. Clin Orthop 1976; 116:180–189.
26. Outerbridge AR, Micheli LJ: Overuse injuries in the young athlete. Clin Sports Med 1995;14:503–516.
27. Roemmich JN, Rogol AD: Physiology of growth and development: Its relationship to performance in the young athlete. Clin Sports Med 1995;14:483–502.
28. Ruggles DL, Peterson HA, Scott SG: Radial growth plate injury in a female gymnast. Med Sci Sports Exerc 1991;23:393–396.
29. Sewall L, Micheli LJ: Strength training for children. J Pediatr Orthop 1986;6:143–146.
30. Smoll FL, Smith RE: Psychology of the young athlete: Stress-related maladies and remedial approaches. Pediatr Clin North Am 1990;37:1021–1046.
31. Tanner JM: Growth at Adolescence, 2nd ed. Oxford, UK, Blackwell Science, 1962.
32. Tanner JM: Normal growth and techniques of growth assessment. Clin Endocrinol Metab 1986;15411–451.
33. Tolfrey K, Campbell IG, Batterham AM: Exercise training induced alterations in prepubertal children's lipid-lipoprotein profile. Med Sci Sports Exerc 1998;30:1684–1692.
34. Wheeler MD: Physical changes of puberty. Endocrinol Metab Clin North Am 1991;20:1–14.
35. Witzke KA, Snow CM: Effects of *plyometric* jump training on bone mass in adolescent girls. Med Sci Sports Exerc 2000;32:1051–1057.

Chapter 23

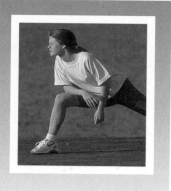

The Preparticipation Physical Examination

John D. Perrine, M.D.

With an estimated 25 to 50 million women participating in organized athletics in this country, it is important that some form of evaluation of their physical condition be done prior to their participation. The preparticipation physical examination (PPE) has been criticized by some for being too expensive for the amount of information obtained, as only about 1% of those examined are found to have a medical condition considered to be severe enough to exclude athletic participation.[43] Also, those conditions that are likely to lead to sudden death are usually missed on the physical examination.[21] However, the purpose of the examination is not only to exclude persons from athletic competition, but to make training and competition as safe as possible for the athlete.

The PPE should help identify those athletes who are most at risk and find pre-existing physical conditions that would limit athletic participation or predispose an athlete to injury or sudden death. Also, it should establish a baseline for comparison if the athlete develops a problem during participation and help determine if treatment is needed for an existing condition.

The report of the Board of Trustees of the American Medical Association stated that while the PPE is helpful in identifying adolescents at risk for orthopaedic injury, there was no evidence from the literature that it is of value in identifying those at risk for sudden cardiac death or for diagnosing previously undiagnosed medical disorders.[35] For the school, it fulfills legal and insurance needs. For the medical team, it provides a valuable foundation for providing care during the period of the athlete's participation, and may become the foundation on which future participation in a sports career is built.

The PPE is not intended to replace a comprehensive general history and physical examination by the athlete's personal physician.

However, since the PPE is the only periodic health examination for a majority of athletes, careful attention to general health maintenance and counseling would be helpful if time allows. For the female athlete, special concerns include screening for disordered eating, menstrual irregularities, premature osteoporosis, and stress fractures. In addition, iron and calcium requirements may need to be addressed.

Although there is some controversy about the frequency of the PPE, most agree that the PPE should be performed annually. The National Collegiate Athletic Association recommends that a complete exam be done on those entering a program, such as entering freshmen or transfer students, with annual updates thereafter. If the athlete remains with the same school or team, any subsequent medical information should be included in the medical chart and forms the basis for future annual evaluations. This allows for concentration on the pertinent areas and avoids collection of redundant, superfluous information.

Ideally, the initial PPE is performed at least 6 weeks prior to the beginning of the athletic season. This allows for the completion of any subsequent examination or referral prior to the beginning of practice and allows adequate time for athletic trainers to complete strengthening programs that may be deemed necessary.

The PPE may be performed by the athlete's private physician, by the team physician, or by a group of physicians using the station method of examination. Each option has advantages and disadvantages. The private physician has the advantages of knowing the athlete and having access to the past history, but has the disadvantage of being generally more expensive. Frequently the private physician has little interest or knowledge of sports medicine. Having the team physician perform the PPE is more cost effective, establishes a relationship between the team physician and the athlete, and allows for continuity in the coordination of care if rehabilitation is needed. However, past medical records are generally not available to the team physician. The station approach is the most commonly used and least expensive method of mass PPE. The exam is usually performed by primary care physicians, but specialists can be used for portions of the exam if they are available. More abnormalities are identified by using the station method of examination, but usually the conditions found are no more severe or disqualifying than those found by the other methods. This form of PPE has the advantages of expediency and getting most of the athletes examined at one time, but the disadvantages of requiring many support personnel and a larger area for the examination.

HISTORY

The most productive portion of the PPE is the medical history. The history concentrates on prior diseases and injuries, with particular emphasis on the cardiovascular and musculoskeletal systems as well as pertinent family history. Of all the problems disclosed from the PPE, 75% are detected by the history.[17] Although the PPE rarely reveals conditions that could lead to sudden death, if these are detected, they are more likely found in the history rather than in the physical examination.

A sports-related health questionnaire for athletes provides an opportunity to obtain concise information, which includes pertinent medical problems, past history, prior injuries, and relevant family medical history. It should be informative, yet brief and easy to review. It gives the examining physician the opportunity to quickly scan the medical history prior to the physical examination and target specific areas of concern. Ideally, the history form should be completed jointly by the parents and the athlete, as the childhood history and the immunization history may be more accurate with the aid of the parents. When parents and athletes give separate histories, they agree only 40% of the time.[37]

Figure 23-1 is a copy of a concise, complete history form. This form was most recently revised in 1997 through the efforts of the American Academy of Family Physicians, the American Academy of Pediatrics, the American Medical Society for Sports Medicine, the American Orthopaedic Society for Sports Medicine, and the American Osteopathic Society for Sports Medicine. Each question is designed to obtain specific information concerning the athlete's health and is reviewed in more detail below:

1. *Have you had a medical illness or injury since your last check up or sports physical?* This information will tune the examiner into more recent illnesses or injury.

2. *Have you ever been hospitalized or had surgery?* This question also helps identify those past illnesses or injuries that may be significant.

3. *Are you currently taking any prescription or nonprescription medications or pills or using an inhaler? Have you ever taken any supplements or vitamins to help you gain or lose weight or improve your performance?* Many athletes take over-the-counter medicines that may be contraindicated or cause complications if other medicines are ordered by the team physician. Some medications that female athletes may take in an effort to lose weight, such as diuretics, laxatives, and stimulants, may make prolonged exercise hazardous. The team physician may want to communicate with the private physician about whether to continue a prescription medication that may place the athlete at risk.

4. *Do you have any allergies (for example, to pollen, medicine, food, or stinging insects)? Have you ever had a rash or hives develop during or after exercise?* Medication allergies can be serious and even potentially life threatening. With bee sting and other allergies, it is helpful to keep epinephrine available (usually in the form of an autoinjector, such as EpiPen), particularly when participating in outdoor sports. If past reactions have been severe, desensitization may be considered. Allergies to foods also can be life threatening and should be made known to the team physician.

5. *Have you ever passed out during or after exercise? Have you ever been dizzy before or after exercise? Have you ever had chest pain during or after exercise?* Syncope or near syncope may be a presentation of hypertrophic cardiomyopathy (HCM) and should be further evaluated, as the majority of sudden deaths in athletes less than age 30 are due to structural cardiac problems. Chest pain may be due to angina from arteriosclerotic cardiovascular disease in the older athlete or to aberrant coronary arteries or HCM in younger athletes. If chest pain is recurrent or persistent, further workup, including an electrocardiogram, echocardiogram, and/or a graded exercise test, may be indicated.

Athletes with exercise-induced asthma (EIA) may have shortness of breath with exercise or may have only a cough that may occur only after completion of exercise. EIA occurs in 40% of persons with an allergic history,[19] and in 60% if those with a history of asthma. In a 1984 screening of Olympic athletes, 11% were found to have EIA, over half of whom were not diagnosed prior to the screening.[36] Since EIA may impair athletic performance and generally responds well to treatment, it is important to make this diagnosis in the PPE.

Do you get tired more quickly than your friends do during exercise? This is not often a complaint of the seasoned athlete, but is more common with the younger or casual athlete. If the elite athlete complains of unusual fatigue or decreased exercise tolerance, acute illnesses such as mononucleosis and myocarditis should be considered.

Have you ever had racing of your heart or skipped heartbeats? A positive answer would suggest the possibility of an arrhythmia. An electrocardiogram may be indicated to determine if an arrhythmia is present and, if so, the nature of the arrhythmia. Further workup, including a Holter monitor or event recorder, may be indicated based upon further history and examination.

Have you had high blood pressure or high cholesterol? Have you ever been told you have a heart murmur? A history of high blood pressure may be a tip-off to underlying cardiovascular disease, and should alert the examiner to focus on the cardiac exam. A history of a heart murmur occurs frequently, as up to 85% of children will have a flow murmur sometime during their lives. Although a careful cardiac exam should be a part of every entry examination, a history of a murmur in the past will alert the examining physician to listen carefully for this specific problem. Murmurs that have been heard previously may have been thoroughly evaluated or referred to a cardiologist, and having this information could avoid studies that may not be necessary. Previous evaluations should be verified, however, by obtaining copies of the original reports of echocardiograms, stress tests, and other diagnostic tests or reports from cardiologists, rather than accepting the athlete's history.

Has any family member or relative died of heart problems or of sudden death before age 50? This question probes for a family history that might suggest a congenital cardiac problem, such as hypertrophic cardiomyopathy, aberrant coronary arteries, Marfan syndrome, and familial hyperlipidemia.

Have you had a severe viral infection (for example, myocarditis or mononucleosis) within the last month? Recent viral infections may lead to myocarditis, which can cause chest pain or fatigue.

Has a physician ever denied or restricted your participation in sports for any heart problem? A thorough review of prior disqualifications is necessary, especially those from cardiac conditions.

6. *Do you have any current skin problems (for example, itching, rashes acne, warts, fungus, or blisters)?* Acne is the most common skin condition of athletes and is not a cause for concern. However, recurrent herpes simplex type I (herpes gladiatorum), or furunculosis in contact sports such as wrestling may pose an exposure risk for other athletes.

7. *Have you ever had a head injury or concussion? Have you ever been knocked out, become unconscious, or lost your memory?* A history of previous concussion is important information for the athletic trainer and team physicians to know, as athletes with this history have a greater potential risk of intracerebral hemorrhage compared to the athlete without this history.[16] The prior number of concussions, grading, and neuropsychological testing, if known, are important for consideration, especially in athletes involved in contact sport participation.

Have you ever had a seizure? Do you have frequent or severe headaches? If the athlete has had seizures, it is important to know how well the seizures are controlled and what medications she may be taking for control. If seizures are not well controlled, athletes should be withheld from contact sports, as well as potentially hazardous sports such as swimming, diving, gymnastics, archery, and weight or power lifting, until their seizure disorder is under control. Frequent or severe headaches need further evaluation.

Have you ever had a stinger, burner, or pinched nerve? Have you ever had numbness or tingling in your arms, hands, legs, or feet? A history of stingers or burners helps pinpoint brachial plexus injuries or cervical spine injuries and is more often helpful in evaluating the male athlete, as it is much more common in contact sports such as football. If the athlete has this history, a thorough neurologic exam is necessary. Additional studies may be needed, such as cervical spine radiography, and additional imaging, depending on the patient's history, frequency of symptoms, and physical examination, should be considered.

8. *Have you ever become ill from exercising in the heat?* The athletic trainers and team physicians need to be alerted to a history of potential heat problems, as these disorders are often recurrent. Athletes with a prior history of heat illness should have their weight loss monitored closely during hot weather, with a prepractice weigh-in and a postpractice weigh-out, and should be encouraged to replace fluids during practice and games. Exercise in hot and humid environments should be discouraged, especially for individuals with a prior history of heat illness.

9. *Do you cough or wheeze, or have trouble breathing during or after activity? Do you have asthma? Do you have seasonal allergies that require medical treatment?* Athletes with EIA should be identified and optimal prevention and treatment reviewed.

10. *Do you use any special protective or corrective equipment or devices that aren't usually used for your sport or position (for example, knee brace, special neck roll, foot orthotics, retainer on your teeth, hearing aid)?* Health-care personnel should take advantage of the athlete's past experience in injury prevention as well as any measures that have worked well in the past. Special equipment required may alert the physician to a problem not as yet identified.

11. *Have you had any problems with your eyes or vision? Do you wear glasses, contacts, or protective eyewear?* Athletic trainers will often keep on hand a second pair of contact lenses or a prescription in case they are needed. A positive response alerts the trainer in the event of injury that the athlete is wearing contact lenses. In addition, the physician needs to be aware of athletes with significant loss of vision in one eye.

12. *Have you ever had a sprain, strain, or swelling after injury? Have you broken or fractured any bones or dislocated any joints? Have you had any other problems with pain or swelling in muscles, tendons, bones, or joints?* This history alerts the team physician and the orthopaedic consultant to potential problems, as athletes who give a positive response to this question are more apt to suffer recurrent injuries. Most athletic injuries are actually a reinjury of a previously damaged joint,[22] especially the knee and ankle. This question also helps to identify those athletes who may need special evaluation by the orthopaedic consultant.

13. *Do you want to weigh more or less than you do now? Do you lose weight regularly to meet weight requirements for your sport?* These questions are designed to help detect disordered eating patterns, which are more common in the female athlete compared to the male athlete. Although all female athletes are at risk for disordered eating, female athletes in certain sports that emphasize thinness for appearance or performance, such as gymnastics,[40] swimming, and diving, as well as cross-country and track, may be at higher risk.[24] The athlete will often not admit to an eating disorder but her response may reveal an abnormal self image and drive for abnormal thinness.

If the answer to these questions arouses suspicion, the physician may want to ask further questions regarding the use of diuretics, laxatives, diet pills, a history of self-induced vomiting, prolonged fasting, or excessive exercise. Further follow-up is indicated if disordered eating behaviors are noted.

14. *Do you feel stressed out?* If the athlete answers "yes" to this question, the physician has the opportunity to ask more direct questions as the history suggests regarding stress, psychosocial issues, depression, and thoughts of suicide.

15. *Record the dates of your most recent immunizations (shots) for tetanus, hepatitis B, measles, chickenpox.* Tetanus immunization should be up to date on all athletes, and should be obtained every 10 years. Adult athletes should have received their second measles shot (MMR). The Centers for Disease Control and Prevention recommends that all adolescents receive the hepatitis B series, especially high-risk patients. If the patient has not had a history of chickenpox or does not have a documented varicella vaccination, the varicella vaccine is recommended. After age 12, a second dose is recommended. These simple precautions could prevent an outbreak in the middle of the athletic season. Parents' input can be quite helpful in this part of the history.

16. *When was your first menstrual period? When was your most recent menstrual period? How much time do you usually have from the start of one period to the start of another? How many periods have you had in the last year? What was the longest time between periods in the last year?* Menstrual irregularities, including amenorrhea, oligomenorrhea, and delayed menarche, are quite common in the athlete, especially in sports emphasizing leanness and thin

physique, such as gymnastics and running.[7,39] This part of the history is extremely important in evaluating the female athlete.

In the past, loss of body fat was thought to be the primary culprit contributing to amenorrhea, but studies have shown a poor correlation of body fat with athletic amenorrhea. The etiology of athletic amenorrhea is more likely multifactorial, including dietary deficiency, a negative energy balance, stress, and training intensity, as well as other factors.[41] Athletic amenorrhea is hypothalamic in origin and results in low levels of estrogen, which is necessary for proper bone mineralization. Since the majority of bone mineralization in girls occurs by the middle of the second decade and usually does not recover in spite of therapy, osteopenia or osteoporosis may result. Stress fractures have been reported to be more common in athletes with amenorrhea compared to those with normal periods.[27] Early identification and correction of this condition may prove to be extremely important to the athlete, as future problems with osteoporosis may be avoided. Eating disorders may also contribute to an abnormal menstrual history, as discussed. The physician should be screening for all components of the female athlete triad (disordered eating, amenorrhea, and osteoporosis).[2]

All questions answered "yes" must be explained by the athlete at the bottom of the page.

PHYSICAL EXAMINATION

The physical examination is usually performed at predetermined stations. The athlete should be appropriately attired in shorts and halter to allow easy access but preserve modesty.

A preprinted physical examination form is convenient and promotes consistency. The attached form categorizes the examination by body systems and is useful in either the station-type examination or with 1 physician doing the complete exam. The orthopaedic examination is performed separately for clarity and convenience.

The height, weight, and vital signs are recorded by a nurse or other support personnel. If the blood pressure is found to be elevated, it should be repeated on several other occasions. If desired, the percentage of body fat can be determined by any of several methods and is a better indication of body composition than weight. Many institutions are de-emphasizing the

importance of weight and percentage of body fat in the female athlete in an effort to decrease the prevalence of disordered eating. However, a baseline measurement may be helpful, should problems arise in the future.

The skin, scalp, and hair can be scanned rapidly during the physical examination and any abnormalities noted.

The neurologic examination should test for weakness, loss of sensation, and any other neurologic condition that might be indicated by the history. It is important to record anisocoria for future reference in the event of head injury.

The ears, nose, and throat exam is usually superficial if the exam is sport focused rather than comprehensive. Teeth should be examined for dental erosion, an irreversible consequence found in two thirds of persons who induce vomiting with bulimia.[25,42] Airway obstruction from enlarged tonsils or a deviated nasal septum should be noted if present.

The cardiovascular examination is one of the most important portions of the PPE. Although previously undetected cardiac problems are rarely found, a careful exam may identify the high-risk athlete with a potentially life-threatening condition. Bradycardia and lower blood pressure are to be expected in the well-conditioned athlete owing to increased ventricular stroke volume and increased vagal tone.[8] Innocent murmurs are also quite common. A soft systolic ejection murmur frequently is heard, due to increased pulmonary flow.[14] Mild regurgitation murmurs of the tricuspid and mitral valves are also commonly heard in athletes.[46] With pulsed Doppler, at least 1 regurgitant jet may be found in over 90% of athletes, and triple-valve regurgitation in 20%.[23] These innocent murmurs are typically best heard in the supine position and soften or disappear in the upright position. It is important to separate significant murmurs from these "innocent" murmurs. Suspicious systolic murmurs should be further evaluated. Since the most common cause of atraumatic sudden death in young athletes is hypertrophic cardiomyopathy (HCM), the examiner should listen specifically for this murmur. Characteristically, this is a systolic ejection murmur best heard at the left sternal border shortly after the first heart sound. Maneuvers that reduce blood return to the left side of the heart, such as standing or performing a Valsalva maneuver, will accentuate the murmur.[15] An echocardiogram may be necessary to exclude this diagnosis, if suspected.

Rhythm abnormalities found on examination, such as irregular pulse or tachycardia, as well as a history of an arrhythmia, should be evaluated with an electrocardiogram. Athletes with a history of chest pain on exertion suggestive of angina should also have an electrocardiogram and/or stress test, as even young athletes can have myocardial ischemia as a result of coronary artery disease, HCM, or aberrant coronary arteries. An electrocardiogram may also be helpful to evaluate syncope with exercise.

The pulmonary examination is rarely abnormal unless the history is suggestive. An athlete with EIA will usually have no abnormal findings at rest and may require special testing for confirmation, such as a methacholine challenge test or spirometry before and after 6 to 8 minutes of exercise or with symptoms. A 12% to 15% decrease in the expiratory flow volume in 1 minute (FEV_1) or a 25% decrease in the mid forced expiratory flow (FEF_{25-75}) is considered positive for EIA. A therapeutic trial of albuterol or cromolyn via inhaler may help confirm the diagnosis and establish an effective treatment.

The abdomen should be checked for any organomegaly, especially spleen enlargement in a patient with recent mononucleosis. Auscultation of the abdomen is seldom beneficial and bruits heard in young athletes are common and are rarely pathologic.

Pelvic and rectal examinations are not done routinely unless the history suggests some abnormality. In a female athlete with amenorrhea or prolonged oligomenorrhea, further workup and examination are indicated at a follow-up appointment.

ORTHOPAEDIC EXAMINATION

A careful orthopaedic examination should be done during the initial examination. The orthopaedic exam often is directed by the history of previous injuries, with those muscles or joints involved being closely scrutinized. If there is no history of previous injury, a quick screening examination may be sufficient, including a check for symmetry of extremities and muscle groups, laxity and range of motion of joints, muscle strength, and "duck walking" (walking in a squatted position) as advocated by Dyment.[10] However, some abnormalities are subtle and there may be no history of previous injury. Anatomic defects such as an abnormally long arm span, arachnodactyly, and pectus carinatum or excavatum may suggest Marfan syndrome, and the patient should be worked up further if this diagnosis is suspected. If abnormalities are not detected during the initial examination and become apparent subsequently

during an athletic event, the institution may find itself responsible for an injury that, in fact, may have been pre-existing.

Female athletes have been found to have a higher incidence of anterior cruciate ligament injuries compared to their male athletic counterparts, especially in the sports of soccer and basketball. Other musculoskeletal concerns commonly seen in the female athlete include patellofemoral pain syndrome and bone stress injuries.

LABORATORY STUDIES

Laboratory studies are rarely of benefit in the asymptomatic athlete. Studies routinely done in the past and found not to be cost effective include the urinalysis,[11] complete blood count, chem-20, chest roentgenography, and electrocardiogram.[20] Abnormalities found on routine testing in the asymptomatic athlete are usually found to be normal when repeated. The cost of proving some studies to be inconsequential may be prohibitive. Some examiners have performed routine echocardiography in the hope of identifying that individual who may be at risk for sudden death due to cardiomyopathy. Routine echocardiography may detect cardiac hypertrophy in athletes who do not have HCM. Also, distinguishing between the hypertrophied heart of the athlete and HCM may be difficult. Many elite athletes will be found to have physiologic hypertrophy, more so in males than in females with the same level of training.[34] Athletes with echocardiograms that fall outside the parameters of accepted normal limits might be excluded from sports participation without just cause. There may also be legal ramifications if borderline or abnormal parameters are detected and the athlete is not restricted from participation. Since individuals with some mutations of the β-myosin heavy chain (the defect in HCM) are found to be more susceptible to sudden death than others, molecular genetic screening may prove in the future to be a more effective way of identifying those athletes with HCM who are at risk of sudden death.

Routine electrocardiography has not proven to be beneficial or cost effective.[29] Stress-testing the asymptomatic athlete often results in a false-positive test, especially in females.

Testing for sickle cell trait (SCT) has been a routine part of the PPE at some centers. Although the incidence of sudden death is significantly higher in athletes with SCT,[12] most cases have occurred in conditions of high temperature and high altitude and are extremely rare. Since approximately 8% of the black population are positive for SCT, many athletes would have to be excluded from competition to prevent an extremely rare complication. Since athletes are not excluded because of this finding, there seems to be little advantage in knowing if the athlete is SCT positive; therefore, the test is not recommended. However, educating those with known SCT regarding appropriate hydration and acclimatization is important.

Presently, there are no routine laboratory tests that have proved to be a helpful and cost-effective component of the PPE.

DISQUALIFYING CONDITIONS

There are no accepted standards for what conditions should be disqualifying. The 16th Bethesda Conference in 1985 and the update presented at the 26th Bethesda Conference in 1994 have helped establish standards that are acceptable for cardiovascular diseases.[32] Some conditions are obvious, but others are within the purview of the team physician, taking into consideration the nature of the sport to be played.

Very few athletes are disqualified by the PPE. About 89% pass without qualification, and another 10% pass after further tests or evaluation by specialists. The disqualification rate ranges from 0.2% to 1.3%, and most of these are conditions known to be present from the medical history.[28]

Cardiac Conditions

Hypertension, unless grade III (180/110 mm Hg) or greater, is not a disqualifying finding. There is no evidence that levels even higher than this are made worse or increase risk with exercise, although those persons with hypertension at rest usually experience a greater increase of both systolic and diastolic pressures with exercise than those who are normotensive.[3] Levels higher than grade II (160/100 mm Hg), although not a cause for exclusion, warrant referral to a primary care physician for evaluation and treatment. Athletes with target organ involvement should be evaluated before being allowed to participate. Vigorous weight lifting is not recommended in an athlete with uncontrolled hypertension. If on oral contraceptive medication, this should be discontinued and the blood pressure rechecked after several weeks. Also, the possibility of the hypertension being caused by the use of anabolic steroids should be considered.

Most athletes with congenital heart lesions are aware of their problem and can report it in the medical history. Those with mild defects are allowed to participate in competitive sports.[18] Those with symptomatic defects should be referred for further studies before being allowed to participate. The athlete who is suspected of having cardiomyopathy or Marfan syndrome should not be allowed to participate until cleared by further studies or cardiac consultation. Although the athlete with mitral valve prolapse has an increased propensity for sudden death, such incidences are rare and, if asymptomatic, the athlete should not be excluded from athletics.[23]

Cardiac arrhythmias are common in athletes and are not in themselves reason for exclusion. Sinus bradycardia is seen in most athletes,[5,33] although it is less marked in the female athlete than in the male.[45] Premature atrial contractions and premature ventricular contractions, as well as second-degree heart block, are common.[4] Any questionable arrhythmia should be evaluated with an electrocardiogram or additional testing if indicated by history and examination. Here, too, there may be findings in the athlete that are insignificant but considered problematic in the general population. Care must be taken to avoid excluding athletes on the basis of electrocardiographic findings alone. Increased QTc (which is more common in the female than in the male athlete), negative T waves, and "abnormal" mean QRS vectors in athletes may not have the same implications as in sedentary individuals.[6] ST-segment elevation due to early repolarization is present in up to 50% of athletes,[47] but is not as common or as marked in the female athlete as in the male athlete.[45]

Athletes with a history of chest pain, dizziness, or syncope with exertion should be further evaluated with appropriate studies (electrocardiography, echocardiography, exercise testing, Holter monitoring, etc) before being cleared for participation. Echocardiographic findings of HCM would exclude the athlete, as this is the most common cause of sudden cardiac death in young athletes.[31] Since some athletes with HCM may not be prone to cardiac arrhythmias and sudden death with extreme exercise,[30] genetic screening and the identification of those mutations known to make the athlete prone to sudden death may be the method of the future for elimination of susceptible athletes.[38]

Neurologic Conditions

Uncontrolled seizures, paralysis, or weakness may cause exclusion from participation, and need thorough evaluation. A history of recurrent concussions, especially if grade III, may preclude participation in contact sports.[26] Any history of transient paraplegia or quadriplegia would require neurologic consultation before approval.

Genitourinary Conditions

Athletes are rarely excluded for genitourinary problems unless they are known to have only one functioning kidney and desire to play a contact sport. Even in this situation, the chance for injury to the remaining kidney is slight.

Ocular Conditions

Few eye problems justify exclusion from sports. A history of prior retinal detachment or recent eye surgery would require approval of the attending ophthalmologist. If the athlete has only 1 functioning eye, eye protection may be required.

Pulmonary Conditions

Asthma, especially EIA, usually can be controlled sufficiently to allow sports participation.

Orthopaedic Conditions

Exclusion for orthopaedic reasons should be the decision of an orthopaedic consultant unless the defect is obvious. Loss of muscle strength, decreased flexibility, swollen or lax joints, or joint pain may respond to physical therapy and muscle-strengthening exercises, allowing the athlete to participate. Often, orthopaedic exclusions are conditional and the athlete may improve to the point of acceptance with an intense strengthening or mobility program.

Other Conditions

Other conditions that may lead to exclusion from athletic endeavors include recent infections, unexplained tachycardia, fever, undue or unexplained fatigue, recent surgery, and hepatomegaly. These exclusions are temporary until the etiology is determined and corrective measures taken, if possible. Diabetes is not in itself an exclusion if blood sugar levels can be maintained at an acceptable level.

CLEARANCE FOR PARTICIPATION

The last step in the examination is clearance for participation. The reviewing team physician should have a working knowledge of sports medicine and the physical requirements of the sport involved. After reviewing all information gleaned from the history and physical examinations, a decision is made to approve the athlete, to refer for other studies and/or treatment, or to deny participation. Approval may be deferred until the athlete is re-examined after therapy. Such conditions as orthopaedic problems, murmur evaluation, asthma evaluation, and neurologic testing may require a review of results before final approval is given. These results, as well as the final approval, should be transmitted to the athletic trainer for documented clarification of the athlete's status and inclusion in the medical record.

LEGAL CONSIDERATIONS

Who has the authority to make the final decision as to whether an athlete may participate? The team physician should form his/her opinion independently, with the athlete's best interest in mind, without pressure from the team, school, or other organization. There may be conflicting opinions from the athlete, her family, or the school. The more elite the athlete, the more conflict there may be. Some athletes will seek other opinions, in the hope of finding a clinician who will find a way for them to participate. On several occasions, this has occurred with devastating results.[1,13] The ideal situation is an agreement among the physician, the athlete, her family, and the school or organization. The physician must remember that he/she is the advocate of the athlete and make a decision on the basis of his/her best judgment after all information is reviewed.

Does the athlete have the right to require her physician to not reveal her physical status to the school or organization? If the physician is a representative of the school or organization, it is generally assumed that whatever information is obtained will be relayed to that organization. If no school is involved, but the physician and the athlete, there is no unspoken contractual agreement with the school and the situation is not as clear. In either situation, there could be legal ramifications if medical information were released that the athlete feels is damaging and should remain confidential.

Does the athlete have the right to ignore the advice of the team physician, accept whatever risk there is, and participate anyway? Can the athlete or her family sign a waiver exonerating the organization of any responsibility, accepting all responsibility herself? The Americans with

Text continued on page 12

Preparticipation Physical Evaluation

HISTORY

DATE OF EXAM _____

Name _____ Sex _____ Age _____ Date of birth _____

Grade _____ School _____ Sport(s) _____

Address _____ Phone _____

Personal physician _____

In case of emergency, contact

Name _____ Relationship _____ Phone (H) _____ (W) _____

Explain "yes" answers below.
Circle questions you don't know the answers to.

	Yes	No
1. Have you had a medical illness or injury since your last check up or sports physical?	☐	☐
Do you have an ongoing or chronic illness?	☐	☐
2. Have you ever been hospitalized overnight?	☐	☐
Have you ever had surgery?	☐	☐
3. Are you currently taking any prescription or nonprescription (over-the-counter) medications or pills or using an inhaler?	☐	☐
Have you ever taken any supplements or vitamins to help you gain or lose weight or improve your performance?	☐	☐
4. Do you have any allergies (for example, to pollen, medicine, food, or stinging insects)?	☐	☐
Have you ever had a rash or hives develop during or after exercise?	☐	☐
5. Have you ever passed out during or after exercise?	☐	☐
Have you ever been dizzy during or after exercise?	☐	☐
Have you ever had chest pain during or after exercise?	☐	☐
Do you get tired more quickly than your friends do during exercise?	☐	☐
Have you ever had racing of your heart or skipped heartbeats?	☐	☐
Have you had high blood pressure or high cholesterol?	☐	☐
Have you ever been told you have a heart murmur?	☐	☐
Has any family member or relative died of heart problems or of sudden death before age 50?	☐	☐
Have you had a severe viral infection (for example, myocarditis or mononucleosis) within the last month?	☐	☐
Has a physician ever denied or restricted your participation in sports for any heart problems?	☐	☐
6. Do you have any current skin problems (for example, itching, rashes, acne, warts, fungus, or blisters)?	☐	☐
7. Have you ever had a head injury or concussion?	☐	☐
Have you ever been knocked out, become unconscious, or lost your memory?	☐	☐
Have you ever had a seizure?	☐	☐
Do you have frequent or severe headaches?	☐	☐
Have you ever had numbness or tingling in your arms, hands, legs, or feet?	☐	☐
Have you ever had a stinger, burner, or pinched nerve?	☐	☐
8. Have you ever become ill from exercising in the heat?	☐	☐

	Yes	No
9. Do you cough, wheeze, or have trouble breathing during or after activity?	☐	☐
Do you have asthma?	☐	☐
Do you have seasonal allergies that require medical treatment?	☐	☐
10. Do you use any special protective or corrective equipment or devices that aren't usually used for your sport or position (for example, knee brace, special neck roll, foot orthotics, retainer on your teeth, hearing aid)?	☐	☐
11. Have you had any problems with your eyes or vision?	☐	☐
Do you wear glasses, contacts, or protective eyewear?	☐	☐
12. Have you ever had a sprain, strain, or swelling after injury?	☐	☐
Have you broken or fractured any bones or dislocated any joints?	☐	☐
Have you had any other problems with pain or swelling in muscles, tendons, bones, or joints?	☐	☐

If yes, check appropriate box and explain below.

☐ Head	☐ Elbow	☐ Hip
☐ Neck	☐ Forearm	☐ Thigh
☐ Back	☐ Wrist	☐ Knee
☐ Chest	☐ Hand	☐ Shin/calf
☐ Shoulder	☐ Finger	☐ Ankle
☐ Upper arm		☐ Foot

	Yes	No
13. Do you want to weigh more or less than you do now?	☐	☐
Do you lose weight regularly to meet weight requirements for your sport?	☐	☐
14. Do you feel stressed out?	☐	☐
15. Record the dates of your most recent immunizations (shots) for:	☐	☐

Tetanus _____ Measles _____

Hepatitis B _____ Chickenpox _____

FEMALES ONLY

16. When was your first menstrual period? _____
When was your most recent menstrual period? _____
How much time do you usually have from the start of one period to the start of another? _____
How many periods have you had in the last year? _____
What was the longest time between periods in the last year? _____

Explain "Yes" answers here: _____

_____

_____

_____

_____

_____

I hereby state that, to the best of my knowledge, my answers to the above questions are complete and correct.

Signature of athlete _____ Signature of parent/guardian _____ Date _____

© 1997 American Academy of Family Physicians, American Academy of Pediatrics, American Medical Society for Sports Medicine, American Orthopaedic Society for Sports Medicine, and American Osteopathic Academy of Sports Medicine.

Figure 23-1. This preparticipation physical evaluation form. (© 1997 American academy of Family physicians, American Academy of pediatrics, American Medical Society for sports Medicine, Society for Sport Medicine, and American Osteopathic Academy of Sports Medicine.

Preparticipation Physical Evaluation

PHYSICAL EXAMINATION

Name _____ Date of birth _____

Height _____ Weight _____ % Body fat (optional) _____ Pulse _____ BP ___/___ (___/___, ___/___)

Vision   R 20/_____ L 20/_____   Corrected: Y N   Pupils: Equal _____ Unequal _____

	NORMAL	ABNORMAL FINDINGS	INITIALS*
MEDICAL			
Appearance			
Eyes/Ears/Nose/Throat			
Lymph Nodes			
Heart			
Pulses			
Lungs			
Abdomen			
Genitalia (males only)			
Skin			
MUSCULOSKELETAL			
Neck			
Back			
Shoulder/arm			
Elbow/forearm			
Wrist/hand			
Hip/thigh			
Knee			
Leg/ankle			
Foot			

* Station-based examination only

CLEARANCE

❏ Cleared

❏ Cleared after completing evaluation/rehabilitation for: _____

_____

_____

❏ Not cleared for: _____ Reason: _____

Recommendations: _____

_____

_____

Name of physician (print/type) _____ Date _____

Address _____ Phone _____

Signature of physician _____, MD or DO

© 1997 American Academy of Family Physicians, American Academy of Pediatrics, American Medical Society for Sports Medicine, American Orthopaedic Society for Sports Medicine, and American Osteopathic Academy of Sports Medicine.

Figure 23-1 *(Continued)*

Preparticipation Physical Evaluation
CLEARANCE FORM

❏ **Cleared**

❏ **Cleared after completing evaluation/rehabilitation for:** _____

_____

_____

_____

❏ **Not cleared for:** _____ **Reason:** _____

Recommendations: _____

_____

_____

_____

Name of physician (print/type) _____ **Date** _____

Address _____ **Phone** _____

Signature of physician _____ **, MD or DO**

© 1997 American Academy of Family Physicians, American Academy of Pediatrics, American Medical Society for Sports Medicine, American Orthopaedic Society for Sports Medicine, and American Osteopathic Academy of Sports Medicine.

Preparticipation Physical Evaluation
CLEARANCE FORM

❏ **Cleared**

❏ **Cleared after completing evaluation/rehabilitation for:** _____

_____

_____

_____

❏ **Not cleared for:** _____ **Reason:** _____

Recommendations: _____

_____

_____

_____

Name of physician (print/type) _____ **Date** _____

Address _____ **Phone** _____

Signature of physician _____ **, MD or DO**

© 1997 American Academy of Family Physicians, American Academy of Pediatrics, American Medical Society for Sports Medicine, American Orthopaedic Society for Sports Medicine, and American Osteopathic Academy of Sports Medicine.

Figure 23-1 (*Continued*)

Disabilities Act and the Rehabilitation Act of 1973 both prohibit discrimination on the basis of physical disability. Several cases have been taken to court, with variable results. In general, the court will allow the athlete to assume some risks if reasonable, but will not go against expert testimony if the evidence is conclusive for excessive risk of sudden death. The physician must make his/her opinion clear to the court and be certain of its substantiation. The physician should be liable only if he/she deviates from professional standards, does not perform indicated testing, misinterprets tests, or withholds pertinent information.

RETESTING

After a complete PPE on entry into a program, a complete annual exam is not usually necessary. An interval history giving medical and surgical events that have occurred since the last exam and an examination based on that history will usually be sufficient. However, the team physician should, before each season, review the medical record before approval for athletic participation.

References

1. Altman LK: The doctor's world: an athlete's health and a doctor's warning. New York Times March 13:C3, 1990.
2. American College of Sports Medicine: Position stand on the female athlete triad. Med Sci Sports Exerc 9(5): i-ix, 1997.
3. Anders DL: Sound treatment strategies for active hypertensives. Physician Sportsmed 20(11):108, 1992.
4. Bjornstad H, Storstein L, et al: Ambulatory electrographic findings in top athletes, athletic students, and control subjects. Cardiology 84:43–50, 1994.
5. Bjornstad H, Storstein, et al: Electrocardiographic findings according to level of fitness and sport activity. Cardiology 83(4):268–79, 1993.
6. Bjornstad H, Storstein L, Meen HD, Hals O: Electrographic findings of repolarization in athletic students and control subjects. Cardiology 84(1):51–60, 1994.
7. Claessens A L, Marlina RM, Lefevre J, et al: Growth and menarcheal status of elite female gymnasts. Med Sci Sports Exerc 24(7):755–63, 1992.
8. Crawford MH: Physiologic consequences of systematic training. Cardiol Clin 10:209–18, 1992.
9. Douglas PS, Berman GO, et al: Prevalence of multivalvular regurgitation in athletes. Am J Cardiol 64:209–12, 1989.
10. Dyment PG: The orthopedic component of the preparticipation examination. Pediatr Ann 21(3):157–62, 1992.
11. Dyment PG: The preparticipation examination. In American Academy of Pediatrics: Sports Medicine: Health Care of the Young Athlete, 2nd edition. Elk Grove Village, Ill, American Academy of Pediatrics, 1991, p 49.
12. Eichner ER: Sickle cell trait, heroic exercise, and fatal collapse. Physician Sportsmed 21(7):51, 1993.
13. Fainaru S, Foreman J, Golden D, et al: The death of Reggie Lewis. A search for answers. Boston Globe September 12:70–6, 1993.
14. Farenbach MC, Thompson PD: The preparticipation sports examination. Cardiol Clin 10:319–28, 1992.
15. Fields KB, Delaney M: Focusing the preparticipation sports examination. J Fam Pract 30(3):304–12, 1990.
16. Geber SG: Concussion incidence and severity in secondary school varsity football players. Am J Public Health 73:1370–5, 1983.
17. Golberg B, et al: Preparticipation sports assessment—an objective evaluation. Pediatrics 66:736–45, 1980.
18. Graham TP, Bricker JT, James FW, Strong WB: Congenital heart disease. Med Sci Sports Exerc 26 suppl(10):S246–53, 1994.
19. Guidelines for the Diagnosis and Management of Asthma. Bethesda, Md, National Asthma Education Program, 1991.
20. Henderson JM: The preparticipation screening evaluation. J Med Assoc Ga 81:277–82, 1992.
21. Hoekelman RA: A pediatrician's view. Pediatr Ann 21:3, 1992.
22. Hulse E, Strong WB: Preparticipation evaluation for athletics. Pediatr Rev 9(6):1–10, 1987.
23. Jerseaty R: Mitral valve prolapse: definition and implication in athletes. J Am Coll Cardiol 7:231–5, 1986.
24. Johnson MD: Disordered eating in active and athletic women. Clin Sports Med 13(2):355–69, 1994.
25. Jones RR, Cleaton-Jones P: Depth and area of dental erosions, and dental caries in bulimic women. J Dent Res 68:1275–8, 1989.
26. Kelly JP, Nichols JS, Filley CM, et al: Concussion in sports: guidelines for prevention of catastrophic outcome. JAMA 166:2867–9, 1991.
27. Lloyd T, Triantafyllou SJ, Baker ER, et al: Women athletes with menstrual irregularity have increased musculoskeletal injuries. Med Sci Sports Exerc 18(4):374–9, 1986.
28. Magnes SA, Henderson JM, Hunter SC: What conditions limit sports participation? Physician Sportsmed 20(5):143, 1992.
29. Maron BJ, Bodison SA, Wesley YE, et al:Results of screening a large group of intercollegiate competitive athletes for cardiovascular disease. J Am Coll Cardiol 10:1214–21, 1987.
30. Maron BJ, Klues HG: Surviving competitive athletics with hypertrophic cardiomyopathy. Am J Cardiol 73(15):1098–104, 1994.
31. Maron BJ, Roberts WC, et al: Sudden death in young athletes. Circulation 62:218–29, 1980.
32. Mitten MJ, Maron BJ: Legal considerations that affect medical eligibility for competitive athletes with cardiovascular abnormalities and acceptance of Bethesda Conference recommendations. Med Sci Sports Exerc 26(suppl 10):S238–41, 1994.
33. Oalkey CM: The electrocardiogram in the highly trained athlete. Cardiol Clin 10:295–302, 1992.
34. Pelliccia A: Outer limits of physiologic hypertrophy and relevance to the diagnosis of primary cardiac disease. Cardiol Clin 10:267–97, 1992.
35. Report of the Board of Trustees: Athletic preparticipation examinations for adolescents. Arch Pediatr Adolesc Med 148:93, 1994.
36. Risser WL: Exercise for children. Pediatr Rev 10(5):131–9, 1988.

37. Risser WL, Hoffman HM, Bellah GG: Frequency of preparticipation sports examinations in secondary school athletes: are university interscholastic league guidelines appropriate? Texas Med 81:35–9, 1985.

38. Roberts R: What clinicians need to know about molecular genetics of the cardiomyopathies. Williamsburg Conference on Heart Disease, December 1994

39. Robinson TL, Snow-Harter C, Taaffee DR, et al: Gymnasts exhibit higher bone mass than runners despite similar prevalence of amenorrhea and oligomenorrhea. J Bone Miner Res 10(1):26–35, 1995.

40. Rosen LW, Hough DO: Pathogenic weigh-control behaviors of female college gymnasts. Physician Sportsmed 16(9):141–4, 1988.

41. Sanborn CF, Albrecht BH, Wagner WW Jr: Athletic amenorrhea: lack of association with body fat. Sci Sports Exerc 19(3):207–12, 1987.

42. Schroeder PL, Filler SJ, Ramirez B, et al: Dental erosion and acid reflux disease. Ann Intern Med 122(11): 809–15, 1995.

43. Smith J, Laskowski ER: The preparticipation physical examination: Mayo Clinic experience with 2,739 examinations Mayo Clin Proc 73:419–29, 1998.

44. Storstein L, Bjornstad H, et al: Cardiology 79:227–36, 1991.

45. Storstein L, Bjornstad H, Hals O, Meen HD: Electrocardiographic findings according to sex in athletes and controls. Cardiology 79:227, 1991.

46. Wright JN, Salem D: Sudden cardiac death and the "athlete's heart." Arch Intern Med 155:1473, 1995.

47. Zehander M, Meinertz T, Keul J, Hansjorg J: EKG variants and cardiac arrhythmias in athletes: clinical relevance and prognostic importance. Am Heart J 119:1378–91, 1990.

Chapter 24

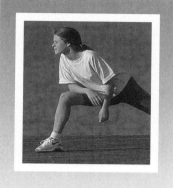

The Female Athlete Triad

Aurelia Nattiv, M.D.
Lisa R. Callahan, M.D.
Ariella Kelman-Sherstinsky, M.D.

In the last decade there has been an explosion of sport and exercise participation by girls and women of all ages, and as such, the sports medicine physician and health scientist has had the opportunity to learn much about the many health benefits of involvement in these sporting activities, as well as the medical and orthopaedic concerns more specific to the female athlete. One of the primary medical concerns for women in sport is that of the *female athlete triad*, which was initially defined at the Triad Consensus Conference in 1992,[103] as including the interrelationship of disordered eating, amenorrhea, and osteoporosis among physically active girls and women. The problems of the female athlete triad collectively, as well as its individual components, have since been recognized as potentially serious problems for girls and women in sport worldwide.[62,68,92,103]

Interest in and concern about the female athlete triad over the last decade has led to numerous national and international task forces, health initiatives, and committees with focused efforts on the prevention and recognition of the triad disorders. Despite these efforts, there continues to be a lack of prospective epidemiologic data assessing prevalence and causes, as well as a lack of outcome studies assessing the efficacy of preventive and treatment programs of the triad disorders in young athletic women. There have, however, been a number of studies on one or more components of the triad that have helped us to better understand and manage the spectrum of female athlete triad disorders. This chapter presents an overview of current research, controversies, and recommendations in prevention and management of the components of the female athlete triad. Areas of study in need of research will also be discussed.

ADVANCES IN TRIAD RESEARCH AND UNDERSTANDING

Recent research on the pathogenesis of amenorrhea in female athletes[105,106] and exercising women[52] with amenorrhea has lent support to metabolic and hormonal pathways involving a state of energy deficit. Although the specific mechanisms linking an energy deficit to reproductive dysfunction are still being elucidated, research has focused on the role of leptin as being a possible metabolic mediator. Decreased levels of leptin have been demonstrated in female athletes with disordered eating,[96] as well as in female athletes with amenorrhea.[47]

Research in the area of bone health in the female athlete has helped uncover important mechanisms resulting in lower bone mineral density (BMD) in some female athletes with amenorrhea and/or disordered eating. A decrease in markers of bone formation have been demonstrated in female athletes with amenorrhea and an energy deficit[104] as opposed to mechanisms involved in postmenopausal estrogen-deficient women, involving primarily bone loss. These mechanisms are important in that they represent a shift in our understanding and therefore management of athletes with the triad disorders. As stated in the American College of Sports Medicine Position Stand on the Female Athlete Triad, the components of the triad are likely interrelated in their etiology, pathogenesis, and health consequences.[68] These recent findings support the interrelated mechanisms and metabolic pathways which will need to be further elucidated with ongoing research.

The true prevalence of the triad is not entirely known, and most likely varies by age, sport, ethnicity, and other factors. Striving to be thin and maintain a low body weight underlies the development of the triad. Although one or more of the components of the triad can occur in girls and women in any sport, adolescents, elite athletes, and young women training in sports that emphasize a thin physique for appearance reasons or improved performance are at greatest risk.[83,104] Because the triad can result in significant medical and psychological morbidity as well as mortality in the female athlete, further research is imperative.

It is important to realize that each of the triad disorders occurs on a spectrum. Early detection is critical in the prevention and treatment of these disorders as each of the components of the triad are more easily managed when diagnosed earlier in the spectrum. From the available research, it appears that disordered eating and osteoporosis in the female athlete setting are more typically identified at an intermediate or earlier point on the spectrum. For example, disordered eating patterns appear to be more common in female athletes, as opposed to the extremes of anorexia nervosa or bulimia nervosa criteria, as identified by the Diagnostic and Statistical Manual of Mental Disorders, 4th Edition (DSM-IV).[1] Similarly, most of the studies to date that have detected low BMD in the female athlete with amenorrhea and disordered eating, although limited, have demonstrated bone density levels in the osteopenic versus osteoporotic range as defined by the World Health Organization (Table 24-1).[102] Female athletes with menstrual dysfunction often present at various points along the spectrum of menstrual dysfunction, including hypothalamic amenorrhea. The problems of the triad emphasize the potential manifestation for more serious disorders along the spectrum, and the importance of early detection and intervention.

Disordered Eating

Eating disorders are characterized by a serious disturbance in eating, such as restriction of intake or bingeing, as well as excessive concern about body shape or body weight. As reviewed, *disordered eating* refers to the spectrum of abnormal eating behaviors that may not necessarily fit the DSM-IV criteria for eating disorders (Table 24-2).[1] Most female athletes will not have frank anorexia or bulimia nervosa, but many may have a clinically significant variant associated with dissatisfaction with their body size or shape or may fit the DSM-IV criteria for eating disorders not otherwise specified (Table 24-2).[1] Methods for weight loss commonly utilize practices that include restricting food intake, fasting, self-induced vomiting, diet pills, laxatives, diuretics and excessive exercise. In addition to the potentially devastating effects of disordered eating on psychological well-being, there is also significant concern of the effects on skeletal health[74] and other physiologic sequelae of restrictive eating or purging.[4,69,70,72] An athlete experiencing excessive weight loss can demonstrate dehydration, a loss of fat-free mass, and subsequent decrease in performance.[100]

Eating disorders affect an estimated 3% of young women in the general United States population,[1,4] although probably twice this number have clinically important variants.[40,81,84] Although the actual prevalence of disordered eating in the female athlete is not known, it is clear that it is a significant problem that affects many young female athletes and places them at significant risk to their psychological and medical well-being.

The adolescent girl or young woman is most commonly affected, although eating disorders are increasingly seen in young children,[11] and 5% to 15% of cases of anorexia and bulimia[2] and 40% of binge-eating disorders occur in boys and men.[1] Eating disorders are most prevalent in industrialized societies and occur in all socioeconomic classes and major ethnic groups in the United States.[18,29]

A combination of interactive factors most likely contribute to the development of eating disorders and disordered eating behaviors, including genetic,[44,85] neurochemical,[13] sociocultural,[30] and psychodevelopmental factors.[14]

Although there have been a number of studies assessing disordered eating behaviors in the

Table 24-1. World Health Organization Diagnostic Guidelines for Osteoporosis[a]

Normal bone	BMD < 1 SD below the mean peak bone mass[b]
Osteopenia	BMD > 1 and <2.5 SD below the mean peak bone mass
Osteoporosis	BMD > 2.5 SD below the mean peak bone mass
Severe osteoporosis	Osteoporosis criteria plus one or more fragility fractures

[a]WHO guidelines were established for postmenopausal women.
[b]These measurements are for mean peak bone mass in normal young women. BMD, bone mineral density; SD, standard deviation.
From WHO Study Group. Assessment of fracture risk and its application to screening for postmenopausal osteoporosis: Report of WHO study group. Geneva, Switzerland, WHO Technical Report Series 843:6, 1994, with permission.

Table 24-2. Diagnostic Criteria for Anorexia Nervosa, Bulimia Nervosa, and Eating Disorder Not Otherwise Specified

DIAGNOSTIC CRITERIA FOR 307.1 ANOREXIA NERVOSA

A. Refusal to maintain body weight at or above a minimally normal weight for age and height (eg, weight loss leading to maintenance of body weight less than 85% of that expected; or failure to make expected weight gain during period of growth, leading to body weight less than 85% of that expected).
B. Intense fear of gaining weight or becoming fat, even though underweight.
C. Disturbance in the way in which one's body weight or shape is experienced, undue influence of body weight or shape on self-evaluation, or denial of the seriousness of the current low body weight.
D. In postmenarcheal females, amenorrhea, ie, the absence of at least three consecutive menstrual cycles. (A woman is considered to have amenorrhea if her periods occur only following hormone, eg, estrogen, administration.)

Specify type:
   Restricting Type: during the current episode of Anorexia Nervosa, the person has not regularly engaged in binge-eating or purging behavior (ie, self-induced vomiting or the misuse of laxatives, diuretics, or enemas)
   Binge-Eating/Purging Type: during the current episode of Anorexia Nervosa, the person has regularly engaged in binge-eating or purging behavior (ie, self-induced vomiting or the misuse of laxatives, diuretics, or enemas)

DIAGNOSTIC CRITERIA FOR 307.51 BULIMIA NERVOSA

A. Recurrent episodes of binge eating. An episode of binge eating characterized by both of the following:
   (1) eating, in a discrete period of time (eg, within any 2-hour period an amount of food that is definitely larger than most people would eat during a similar period of time and under similar circumstances.)
   (2) a sense of lack of control over eating during the episode (eg, feeling that one cannot stop eating or control what or how much one is eating)
B. Recurrent inappropriate compensatory behavior in order to prevent weight gain, such as self-induced vomiting; misuse of laxatives, diuretics, enemas, or other medications; fasting; or excessive exercise.
C. The binge eating and inappropriate compensatory behaviors both occur on average, at least twice a week for 3 months.
D. Self-evaluation is unduly influenced by body shape and weight.
E. The disturbance does not occur exclusively during episodes of Anorexia Nervosa.

Specify type:
   Purging Type: during the current episode of Bulimia Nervosa, the person has regularly engaged in self-induced vomiting or the misuse of laxatives, diuretics, or enemas
   Nonpurging Type: during the current episode of Bulimia Nervosa, the person has used other inappropriate compensatory behaviors, such as fasting or excessive exercise, but has not regularly engaged in self-induced vomiting or the misuse of laxatives, diuretics, or enemas

307.50 EATING DISORDER NOT OTHERWISE SPECIFIED

The Eating Disorder Not Otherwise Specified category is for disorders of eating that do not meet the criteria for any specific Eating Disorder. Examples include
1. For females, all of the criteria for Anorexia Nervosa are met except that the individual has regular menses.
2. All of the criteria for Anorexia Nervosa are met except that, despite significant weight loss, the individual's current weight is in the normal range.
3. All of the criteria for Bulimia Nervosa are met except that the binge eating and inappropriate compensatory mechanisms occur at a frequency of less than twice a week or for a duration of less than 3 months.
4. The regular use of inappropriate compensatory behavior by an individual of normal body weight after eating small amounts of food (eg, self-induced vomiting after the consumption of two cookies).
5. Repeatedly chewing and spitting out, but not swallowing, large amounts of food.
6. Binge-eating disorder: recurrent episodes of binge eating in the absence of the regular use of inappropriate compensatory behaviors characteristic of Bulimia Nervosa.

From American Psychiatric Association. Diagnostic and Statistical Manual for Eating Disorders, 4th Edition. Washington, DC, American Psychiatric Association, 1994, with permission.

young female athlete,[25,37,42,65,67,76,77,86,89] many of these studies have limitations that may preclude generalizations of prevalence of these behaviors in specific sports or in the general female athlete population. Many of the existing studies do not use validated diagnostic instruments for assessment of eating disorders or lack appropriate nonathlete controls. In addition, most of these studies have been in the collegiate female athlete, with few studies assessing the adolescent athlete or other age groups.

Smolak and colleagues, in their meta-analysis of 34 studies assessing disordered eating in female athletes (including 2459 athletes and 8858 controls), concluded that female athletes are at higher risk for disordered eating compared to nonathletes, and that elite athletes are at increased risk, especially in sports emphasizing thinness. Gymnasts, swimmers, and runners did not have a significant increased risk in this meta-analysis, although dancers were at higher risk. Nonelite athletes, especially those in high school, had reduced risk. This was especially noted in athletes in sports not emphasizing leanness.[83]

Of importance is that the majority of studies on eating disorders in the female athlete have assessed *symptoms* of eating disorders by questionnaire, such as the Eating Disorders Inventory (EDI), or the Eating Attitude Test (EAT), in the absence of an interview by a trained clinician using the DSM-IV[1] for a variety of eating disorders or other clinical screening tools to suggest disordered eating behaviors. These studies assessing eating disorder symptoms are still important because body image dissatisfaction, a drive for thinness, and preoccupation with weight are important risk factors for the development of eating disorders in the female athlete.[67,87] A more accurate diagnosis of eating disorders, however, would include an assessment by a clinician, in addition to completing a questionnaire, to help interpret the symptoms and signs.

A number of the studies assessing disordered eating in female athletes using validated psychometric instruments have found the female athlete to score higher on the Drive for Thinness (DFT) subscale of the EDI or EDI-2 compared to nonathlete controls (ie, to be more dissatisfied with their body image and more preoccupied with their weight).[37,67,86] In these same studies, the athletes, however, have not exhibited extreme scores on the EDI or EDI-2 compared to nonathlete controls.[8,35,37,67,93] It is important to note that estimates of symptoms of disordered eating prevalence from self-reports may also be underestimated. O'Connor and colleagues found that the EDI-2 can be easily faked in female college gymnasts,[67] and Wilmore and colleagues found that scores on the EDI were not related to the existence of frank eating disorders in elite female athletes.[99]

The young female athlete may be at additional risk for developing or perpetuating her disordered eating behaviors for a number of reasons. There is an underlying belief that being thin is equated with improved performance, whether it be because of faster speeds or improved marks from judges. Pressures to lose weight from coaches, parents, judges, and others may present additional risk factors for disordered eating behaviors.[41,62,87,103] Although there are no specific guidelines in judging regulations that relate specifically to body size or shape, gymnasts and athletes in other aesthetic sports often believe being thin is important to their overall success.[36]

Adolescence is a time of vulnerability to physical as well as psychological injury. Body height, weight, percent body fat, and shape often change significantly during this time as the result of puberty, and may present a challenge to the young female athlete who is striving to stay thin. Low self-esteem and depression may also be associated factors that perpetuate disordered eating behaviors.

The personality type of the successful competitive female athlete—perfectionist, high achiever, sometimes with obsessive/compulsive traits—is often similar to the personality type described in eating disorder patients. It is unclear if female athletes with these personality traits are most attracted to the sport and most successful or if involvement in the sport contributes to these behaviors.

As mentioned, studies have demonstrated that anorexia nervosa has profound negative effects on bone.[74] Athletes with disordered eating behaviors, especially with food restriction and low weight, can also experience negative consequences to bone health. However, Sundgot-Borgen demonstrated that normal-weight women with bulimia nervosa have normal bone mass.[88] These effects may, in part, be due to the effects of body weight on bone. Low body weight and lean body mass are independent predictors of low BMD. Lower dietary fat, common in the athlete who is striving for thinness, has been associated with risk for stress fractures in female track and field athletes.[7] As discussed, the mechanisms involving low BMD in this population appear to be related more to problems with decreased bone formation and energy deficit[104–106] than to an increased bone resorption, as seen in the hypoestrogenic postmenopausal woman. More research is needed in this area.

Secondary Amenorrhea

Secondary amenorrhea is defined as the lack of menses for 3 or more consecutive months after menarche has begun.[51,80] A spectrum of menstrual irregularities is often seen in the athletic setting, with hypoestrogenic amenorrhea at one end of the spectrum and periods of oligomenorrhea (menstrual cycles greater than 36 days in length) at an intermediate point along the spectrum.[80] Oligomenorrhea may be the result of anovulation or low estrogen and progesterone. Luteal-phase dysfunction is also commonly found in athletes, and is manifested by shortened luteal phase and inadequate progesterone production.[80] Female athletes with luteal-phase dysfunction may have regular menses.

In the general female population, the prevalence of secondary amenorrhea ranges from 2% to 5%. Amenorrhea is more frequent in athletes than in sedentary women[27,51,80] with a reported prevalence ranging from 15% to 66%, depending on sport and other factors.

The etiology of exercise-associated amenorrhea has been found to be hypothalamic in origin. Low levels of gonadotropins and ovarian steroids have been observed consistently.[48,79] One of the most well-accepted mechanisms of secondary amenorrhea in the female athlete is the energy-availability hypothesis proposed by Loucks and colleagues,[49,52] whereby *energy availability* is defined as dietary energy intake minus exercise energy expenditure. Loucks and colleagues propose that a reduction in luteinizing hormone and resultant menstrual dysfunction is caused by a lack of dietary energy intake meeting the demands of the energy cost of exercise, rather than by exercise itself.[52] Williams and colleagues also found that strenuous training, in and of itself, may not be a sufficient stimulus to disrupt the reproductive hormone secretion unless accompanied by dietary restriction.[98] This finding is important in that treatment may be directed at correction of the energy deficit, which may involve adjustment of dietary intake without necessarily altering exercise activity.

Much attention has been placed on leptin and its effect on the reproductive status of the female athlete.[58,96] Low leptin levels in patients with anorexia and in women athletes who exercise strenuously have been found to be associated closely with neuroendocrine abnormalities. Loucks and colleagues have demonstrated that low energy availability suppressed the normal diurnal rhythm of leptin in young women.[39] It is possible that an individual may sense her fat content through leptin, which in turn may inhibit ovulation when a certain amount of nutritional reserve is not present. The role of leptin and its relationship to menstrual disturbances is discussed further in Chapter 14.

A significant potential consequence of amenorrhea relates to negative effects on skeletal health. A decrease in BMD of the lumbar vertebrae,[23,56,60] as well as low bone density at multiple skeletal sites have been noted in young female athletes with extended periods of amenorrhea.[59,73] Of great concern is that there is evidence that decreased BMD in former oligoamenorrheic athletes may be irreversible,[43] emphasizing the important role of prevention. Grinspoon and colleagues found that the severity of osteopenia in estrogen-deficient women with hypothalamic amenorrhea (and nutritionally replete) was not as great as in nutritionally depleted, estrogen-deficient women with anorexia nervosa.[34] In their study, they demonstrated that lumbar bone density in women with hypothalamic amenorrhea was correlated to weight and duration of amenorrhea.[34]

In the anorexic women, lean body mass was an important predictor of amenorrhea, independent of the duration or degree of estrogen deficiency, emphasizing the role of nutritional factors on bone health in these women.[34]

Delayed Menarche

Delayed menarche is defined as the lack of menstruation by age 16 in a girl with secondary sexual characteristics.[80] Later mean ages of menarche are commonly reported in the female athlete. Most of the data on menarcheal age in the female athlete come from retrospective data on athletes in a variety of sports and events within a sport.[53] The actual prevalence of delayed menarche in the female athlete is not known.

The mechanisms underlying delayed menarche in the female athlete have not been fully elucidated. Premenarcheal training for sport has been indicated as a causative factor based on correlational data in a number of sports[28]; however, the association of delayed menarche and premenarcheal training does not imply causation. Data also suggest that this association is to a large part familial.[55] Most likely there is an interaction of both environmental and genetic factors.[54]

Warren and colleagues have associated delayed menarche with stress fractures and scoliosis in ballet dancers,[95] and runners with delayed menarche have also been found to have an increased risk for stress fractures.[3] In Bennell's prospective study assessing risk factors for stress fractures in track and field athletes, a later age of menarche was found to be one of the best predictors of stress fractures in women.[7]

In the young female athlete, does a delay in menarche affect the attainment of peak bone mass? This too is an important question that has not been answered. Nichols-Richardson and colleagues have found that child artistic gymnasts (ages 8 to 13) have significantly higher BMD compared to nongymnast controls,[66] suggesting that gymnastics training in childhood may help maximize peak BMD. Whether or not a delay in menarche affects this increase in BMD has not been determined.

Osteoporosis

The Consensus Development Conference on Osteoporosis defines *osteoporosis* as a disease characterized by low bone mass, microarchitectural deterioration of bone tissue leading to enhanced skeletal fragility, and an increased risk for fracture.[12]

The World Health Organization has established diagnostic criteria for postmenopausal osteoporosis using bone density measurements (Table 24-1)[102]; however, there are no similar diagnostic criteria that have been established for girls or young women using bone density criteria. Although osteoporosis may develop in young female athletes, bone density values in the osteopenic range are more typical, as previously mentioned. The concern in the young female is the possible progression to osteoporosis later in life and potential irreversible harm to current and future bone health.

Osteoporosis is a worldwide problem affecting an estimated 75 million people in the United States, Europe, and Japan combined, including 1 in 3 postmenopausal women.[17] The prevalence of osteopenia and osteoporosis in female athletes is not known. What is known is that the presence of the other triad disorders (disordered eating and amenorrhea) is often a precursor to the development of osteoporosis. The etiology of premenopausal osteopenia and osteoporosis in young athletic women is primarily a hypoestrogenic state resulting from hypothalamic amenorrhea,[23,56,74] involving an energy deficit[52,106] and potential for decreased bone formation.[104] In the young (pediatic or adolescent) female athlete, the primary problem relates to not adequately achieving peak BMD (as opposed to bone loss).

The consequences of osteopenia and osteoporosis in the female athlete are great. These include a possible increase in risk for stress fractures,[3,7,60,61,63,64] as well as the potential for hip, vertebral, and wrist fractures later in life. Studies have demonstrated lower BMD at multiple skeletal sites in the athlete with amenorrhea,[73] although vertebral bone density is usually more profoundly affected.

Greater than 90% of peak skeletal mass is likely present by 18 years of age, with skeletal ages from 10 to 14 being the most important years for bone acquisition.[10] A decrease in bone formation or bone loss during this time may decrease the attainment of peak bone mass in the young athlete, thus making her more prone to fractures later in life.

Site-specific increases in bone density have been demonstrated in athletes involved in higher-impact sports at specific skeletal sites.[75,82,101] The most striking studies illustrating this phenomenon have been in the female gymnast. These studies have shown that the female gymnast has significantly higher BMD at various weight-bearing skeletal sites compared to female athletes in other sports, as well as to nonathlete controls.[45,66,75] This appears to be true in the face of delayed menarche and secondary amenorrhea. The exact mechanisms resulting in a higher BMD in these athletes has not been fully elucidated. The higher-impact forces on specific skeletal sites seem to play a role in this increased BMD. An increase in bone formation has been postulated in higher- versus lower-impact sports.[19] The increased fat-free soft-tissue mass in the gymnast may also be a significant factor resulting in higher BMD.[66]

MEDICAL AND PSYCHOLOGICAL ASSESSMENT

History and Physical Examination

The assessment and management of an athlete with the triad disorders should address the nutritional, medical and psychological components of the problem, ideally with a multidisciplinary team that works closely together.[62,68,103]

All female athletes should be screened for symptoms, signs, and risk factors for the triad disorders at the preparticipation physical examination or at their annual physical examination by their primary care physician. Other opportunities for screening for disordered eating by physicians may also present themselves when the athlete is being evaluated for other medical problems, such as stress fractures or recurrent illness or injury, that may be suggestive of an underlying eating disorder, menstrual dysfunction, or low bone density. If one component of the triad is present in an athletic girl or woman, she should be screened for the other components.

A careful history of dietary patterns, weight changes, preoccupation with weight, and frequency and severity of purging behavior should be evaluated. An assessment of the presence of specific purging behaviors should be reviewed with the athlete, including excessive exercise, abuse of laxatives, enemas, diuretics, caffeine, or other stimulants. A detailed menstrual history should include age of menarche and specific menstrual pattern since menarche to the present. This is very important, as menstrual history is one of the most important predictors of current BMD.[21,31] Any history of stress fractures, low-impact fractures or frequent injury should be assessed.

The athlete's appropriateness of weight for height, age, and sex should be determined according to the percentage of expected body weight or body mass index (BMI).[4] Typically a weight or BMI *range* is used in the athletic setting to take into account individual variability in body frame and other factors, as well as methodologic error.[99]

The physical examination should include an assessment of vital signs and general nutritional status. In athletes with very low weight, bradycardia, hypotension, and hypothermia are often seen. With bulimia, weight is often normal but lightheadedness and hypotension can be associated with electrolyte disturbances and dehydration. Table 24-3 includes common physical signs and symptoms and medical complications of eating disorders that the clinician should be aware of. A complete physical examination should be performed, including an assessment of the Tanner stage.

A pelvic examination is helpful in the evaluation of amenorrhea to assess pelvic anatomy and possible aberrations, and to help assess the cause of the disorder. The American College of Obstetricians and Gynecologists and the American Academy of Pediatrics recommend screening all sexually active women and all women over 18 years with an annual pap smear and pelvic examination.[15,16,33] There is some controversy regarding when the otherwise asymptomatic adolescent or young adult needs a pelvic examination if she is not sexually active. Some clinicians recommend screening asymptomatic women only over 20 years of age.[78]

The psychological assessment of patients with disordered eating should focus on an initial assessment from a physician, psychologist, or psychiatrist. The clinician should assess the psychosocial context of the symptoms, establish a diagnosis, and identify any concurrent psychiatric illness, as well as assess the risk of suicide.[4] Suicidal behavior is important to assess in the athlete with anorexia or bulimia, as it is one of the main contributors to the increase in mortality among patients with anorexia nervosa.

Laboratory Studies and Electrocardiography

Routine laboratory studies for the athlete being evaluated for disordered eating include measurements of serum electrolytes, a complete

Table 24-3. Signs, Symptoms, and Medical Complications of Eating Disorders

OROFACIAL	
Perimolysis	Hypoglycemia
Dental caries	Hypothermia
Cheilosis	Euthyroid sick syndrome
Enlargement of the parotid gland	Hypercortisolism, elevated free cortisol level in urine
Submandibular adenopathy	Low serum estradiol level
	Decreased serum testosterone level
CARDIOVASCULAR	Amenorrhea, oligomenorrhea
Postural and nonpostural hypotension	Delay in puberty
Acrocyanosis	Arrested growth
Electrocardiographic abnormalities: low voltage, prolonged QT interval, prominent U waves	Osteoporosis
Sinus bradycardia	Lipid abnormalities
Atrial and ventricular arrhythmias	Obesity
Left ventricular changes: decreased mass, decreased cavity size	**RENAL**
Mitral-valve prolapse	Renal calculi
Cardiomyopathy (due to ipecac poisoning)	**REPRODUCTIVE**
GASTROINTESTINAL	Infertility
Esophagitis, hematemesis (including the Mallory–Weiss syndrome)	Insufficient weight gain during pregnancy
Delayed gastric emptying	Low-birth-weight infant
Decreased intestinal motility	**INTEGUMENTARY**
Constipation	Dry skin and hair
Rectal prolapse	Hair loss
Gastric dilatation and rupture	Lanugo
Abnormal results on liver-function tests	Yellow skin due to hypercarotenemia
Elevated serum amylase level	Hand abrasions
ENDOCRINE AND METABOLIC	**NEUROLOGIC**
Hypokalemia (including hypokalemic nephropathy)	Peripheral neuropathy
Hyponatremia, (rarely) hypernatremia	Reversible cortical atrophy
Hypomagnesemia	Ventricular enlargement
Hyperphosphatemia	**HEMATOLOGIC**
	Anemia, leukopenia, neutropenia, thrombocytopenia

From Becker A, Grinspoon SK, Klibanski A, Herzog DB: Eating disorders. N Engl J Med 340:1092–8, 1999, with permission.

blood count, and serum glucose levels. Thyroid function tests may be obtained if symptoms suggest possible thyroid disease. Laboratory tests and findings on physical examination may be normal, especially in patients of normal weight who have bulimia nervosa.[4]

Prolongation of the QT interval is a concern with anorexia nervosa, even in the absence of abnormal serum electrolytes. An electrocardiogram should therefore be obtained in the athlete with clinically significant food restriction and/or purging.

In the workup of amenorrhea, a urine pregnancy test should be obtained, as pregnancy is the most likely cause for missed menses in the adolescent and young adult. Thyroid-stimulating hormone, follicle-stimulating hormone, and prolactin levels are necessary to exclude other common causes of amenorrhea. A serum estradiol level can also be helpful, especially if the phase of the menstrual cycle is known. A progesterone challenge test with medroxyprogesterone acetate 10 mg/day for 7 to 10 days can serve as an indirect assessment of estrogen status. A positive response includes menstrual bleeding, which usually indicates adequate estrogen levels. If androgen features are present or polycystic ovarian syndrome is a possibility, luteinizing hormone, free testosterone, and dehydroepiandrosterone sulfate may be obtained. Further details are discussed in Chapter 13.

If the athlete is osteopenic or osteoporotic, bone markers, including a urine N-telopeptide level for assessing bone resorption and a serum osteocalcin level for bone formation, may be helpful. More studies are needed to evaluate the clinical utility of bone markers in the female athlete with the triad disorders. Other metabolic causes for the bone loss, such as underlying thyroid disease, should also be assessed to rule out secondary causes for bone loss. Assessment of metabolic markers for an energy-deficit state may also be beneficial depending upon the clinical presentation, such as assessment of thyroid function. Loucks and colleagues have demonstrated a low-T_3 syndrome in exercising women that may occur at a certain threshold of low energy availability, independent of the level of exercise.[50]

Bone Density Studies

Inadequate bone formation and bone loss are serious problems that may be a result of disordered eating, oligomenorrhea, or amenorrhea. With frank anorexia nervosa, bone density should be assessed as 50% of the girls and women actually have bone density measurements greater than 2 standard deviations (SD) below normal,[9,74] affecting both cortical and trabecular bone.

Drinkwater has demonstrated that there is a linear relationship with the degree of bone loss and the degree of menstrual dysfunction.[21] A recent study found that athletic females with stress fractures sustained in cancellous bone (such as in the femoral neck) had a higher likelihood of having osteopenia than athletes who sustained stress fractures in cortical bone (such as in the tibia or metatarsal bone).[57] Although there are currently no established guidelines for assessment of bone density in the athlete with triad disorders, the authors recommend determining bone density in athletes with a history of clinically significant disordered eating, amenorrhea, or oligomenorrhea for more than 6 months or a history of stress fractures. Although more studies are needed, the authors recommend bone density testing in any female athlete with a history of a stress fracture of the femoral neck, sacrum or pelvis.

TREATMENT

Disordered Eating

The focus of treatment for disordered eating includes recognition of the problem, identification and resolution of psychosocial precipitants, stabilization of medical and nutritional conditions, and re-establishment of healthy patterns of eating.[4] Eating disorders respond to a variety of psychotherapeutic approaches, including individual, group, and family therapy. Often a combination of these therapies is beneficial. The use of behavioral strategies early in treatment to control symptoms is often helpful.[4] Coaches and parents need to be educated about prevention of disordered eating and be aware of signs and symptoms. Sundgot-Borgen has found that education of coaches and athletes has a positive effect on the prevention of disordered eating behaviors.[90] In another study, Sundgot-Borgen found that cognitive behavioral therapy was more effective than nutritional therapy alone in female athletes with disordered eating.[91] More outcome studies assessing treatment strategies in athletes with disordered eating are needed.

In the athletic setting, a multidisciplinary team including a physician, psychologist, nutritionist, and often an athletic trainer working closely with the athlete is recommended. An important goal of the nutritionist and physician is to keep the athlete in a state of a positive energy balance to avoid the potential negative effects of an energy-deficit state on menstrual dysfunction and bone health. In the more serious cases of disordered eating, a psychiatrist is consulted.

Medication is generally not helpful in treating the primary symptoms of anorexia, but fluoxetine may stabilize recovery in individuals with anorexia who have attained 85% of their expected body weight.[4] In patients with bulimia, psychopharmacologic therapy is moderately effective in treatment. Fluoxetine is the only drug, however, currently approved by the US Food and Drug Administration (FDA) for the treatment of bulimia. Other selective serotonin reuptake inhibitors are used routinely as well, but have not been studied to date in controlled trials. Desipramine and imipramine have also been found to be helpful in the treatment of bulimia.

The large majority of athletes may be treated as outpatients. Candidates for inpatient care include those with very low weight (75% or less of expected body weight), rapid weight loss, cardiac arrhythmias, severe electrolyte imbalances, severe or intractable purging, or suicidal ideation, and those who are not responding to adequate outpatient therapy.[4]

Amenorrhea

The focus of the treatment of amenorrhea or oligomenorrhea is to treat the problem that most likely contributed to the menstrual disorder and institute normal menstrual function. Optimizing nutritional and calcium status and adjusting exercise to maintain a state of positive energy balance is the goal. Often a 3- to 6-month or longer period of observation with nonpharmacologic agents is initiated,[24] especially if the athlete is not osteopenic or osteoporotic. The optimal energy balance for an athlete needs to be individualized and may vary depending upon the sport, body composition, genetics, and other factors. If this nonpharmacologic treatment does not result in normal menses, hormonal intervention in the hypoestrogenic female may be considered. However, research supporting estrogen replacement therapy (ERT) or oral contraceptive pills (OCPs) for improving or maintaining bone density is still controversial.[20,32,38,43,94,97] This is likely due to the different mechanisms involving inadequate bone formation in the premenopausal hypoestrogenic amenorrheic athlete, as compared to the postmenopausal hypoestrogenic woman with increased bone resorption. Some studies report a dose related effect, with OCPs being more effective than ERT in maintaining BMD in this population. Treatment should be individualized and the athlete should be followed closely.

Of note is that ERT has not shown to have significant effect on bone density in women with anorexia nervosa and can not be recommended for anorexic patients.[46]

Osteoporosis

In the female athlete with osteopenia or osteoporosis, treating the underlying problem is the initial step of the treatment plan. There may be a need to focus on weight gain (if significantly underweight), as well as optimizing nutritional and calcium status, including attention to energy balance. Resumption of normal menses to optimize bone health is an important goal. Avoidance of excessive exercise is important. Weight-bearing exercise and resistive exercises, however, may be helpful in some athletes with low bone density who are in non-weight-bearing sports, such as swimming. Adding plyometrics to the exercise regimen may also be beneficial.

If the athlete is osteopenic, serial bone density examinations 1 year (initial follow-up) or 2 years apart can be helpful to monitor treatment. In the young athlete with osteopenia and amenorrhea, OCPs or ERT may be used (if greater than 16 years of age), although, as discussed, there is controversy regarding the resultant effect on bone density.[20,32,38,43,94] Prospective longitudinal data that demonstrate an increase in BMD in the athletic woman with amenorrhea is clearly lacking. In fact, Weaver and colleagues demonstrated a decrease in BMD in female athletes on OCPs.[97] The emphasis, therefore, is focused primarily on maximizing peak bone mass with adequate nutrition, calcium supplementation, prevention of disordered eating and amenorrhea, achieving and maintaining a state of positive energy balance, and consideration of plyometric or higher-impact exercise if appropriate.

No specific criteria have as yet been developed regarding when to treat athletic women with osteopenia or osteoporosis. The authors recommend starting with nonpharmacologic intervention in all female athletes with disordered eating, menstrual dysfunction, and/or osteopenia or osteoporosis. The National Osteoporosis Foundation has established guidelines for pharmacologic treatment of osteopenia or osteoporosis in postmenopausal women based on bone density criteria. Pharmacologic treatment of osteopenia or osteoporosis in the female athlete, however, is not well studied and can not be uniformly recommended based on the available data. Treatment needs to be individualized based on the athlete's risk profile. Further research and outcome studies are needed in this area.

There are currently no guidelines available regarding withholding an athlete from competition because of very low bone density levels. These decisions need to be individualized depending upon the athlete's risk profile, sport, and compliance with recommended treatment.

Pharmacologic treatment with miacalcin nasal spray (200 IU/day) has been found to be beneficial in one study, with resultant bone density increase in the spine and proximal femur.[22] Other pharmacologic agents, such as the bisphosphonates used in postmenopausal women, are not approved for premenopausal women of childbearing age and are not recommended in this age group because of their potential teratogenic effects. This is especially true with alendronate (Fosamax), which has a long half life. The selective estrogen receptor modulator (SERM) raloxifene is currently approved for the prevention and treatment of osteoporosis in the postmenopausal woman,[26] but not in the premenopausal woman. In fact, tamoxifen, which is also a SERM, has been associated with a decrease in bone density in premenopausal women, even though it has been shown to increase bone density in postmenopausal women.[71]

All pharmacologic treatments available for the prevention and treatment of osteoporosis in postmenopausal women work primarily by decreasing bone resorption. Since evidence suggests that the primary problem in the female athlete with amenorrhea and osteopenia appears to be a decrease in bone formation, these agents may not be targeting the appropriate mechanism involved. This may explain why ERT has not consistently shown improvements in bone density in the female athlete with amenorrhea and osteopenia. There are currently no pharmacologic treatments approved by the FDA for premenopausal women that improve bone formation.

CONCLUDING REMARKS

The majority of girls and women benefit greatly from involvement in sports and exercise. For some female athletes, the triad of disordered eating, amenorrhea, and osteoporosis may be a significant problem that can lead to increased morbidity and mortality, as well as decreased performance. Current research supports the important role of maintaining a positive energy balance in the efforts to avoid amenorrhea and the negative effects on bone health and decreased bone formation. All female athletes should be assessed to determine their risk for the

triad disorders, and be aware of the spectrum of problems that exist. The presence of one component of the triad should alert the clinician to evaluate for the other disorders. Prevention and recognition of the triad disorders should be a priority in those who work closely with female athletes. There is a lack of well-controlled research at this time in a number of areas, including prevalence of the triad disorders, prevention, and treatment in the athletic setting. Treatment currently focuses on maximizing peak bone mass and optimizing energy intake and nutrition, with the goal of achieving a positive energy balance. Working with a multidisciplinary team is important, especially in the athlete with disordered eating. There is no uniform support at this time for pharmacologic management in the female athlete with amenorrhea and osteopenia or osteoporosis. There is an urgent need for more research on the prevalence of the triad disorders and the mechanisms involved in its pathogenesis, as well as for outcome studies that identify optimal strategies for prevention and treatment.

References

1. American Psychiatric Association: Diagnostic and Statistical Manual of Mental Disorders, 4th Edition. Washington, DC, American Psychiatric Association, 1994.
2. Anderson AE: Eating disorders in males. In Brownell KD, Fairburn CG (eds): Eating Disorders and Obesity: A Comprehensive Handbook. New York, Guilford Press, 1995, pp 177–87.
3. Barrow GW, Saha S: Menstrual irregularity and stress fractures in collegiate female distance runners. Am J Sports Med 16:209–16, 1988.
4. Becker A, Grinspoon SK, Klibanski A, Herzog DB: Eating disorders. N Engl J Med 340:1092–8, 1999.
5. Becker AE, Hamburg P: Culture, the media, and eating disorders. Harv Rev Psychiatry 4:163–7, 1996.
6. Becker AE, Hamburg P, Herzog DB: The role of psychopharmacologic management in the treatment of eating disorders. In Dunner DL, Rosenbaum JF (eds): Annual of Drug Therapy. Philadelphia, WB Saunders, 1998, pp 17–51.
7. Bennell KL, Malcolm SA, Thomas SA, et al: Risk factors for stress fractures in track and field athletes: A twelve-month prospective study. Am J Sports Med 24:810–8, 1996.
8. Benson JE, Allemann Y, Thienz GE, Howard H: Eating problems and caloric intake levels in Swiss adolescent athletes. Int J Sports Med 11:249–52, 1990.
9. Biller BMK, Saxe V, Herzog DB, et al: Mechanisms of osteoporosis in adult and adolescent women with anorexia nervosa. J Clin Endocrinol Metab 68:548–54, 1989.
10. Bonjour JP, Theinz G, Buchs B, et al: Critical years and stages of puberty for spinal and femoral bone mass accumulation during adolescence. J Bone Miner Res 73:555–63, 1991.
11. Bostic JQ, Muriel AC, Hack S, et al: Anorexia nervosa in a 7-year-old girl. J Dev Behav Pediatr 18:331–3, 1997.

12. Bouillon P, Burckhardt P, Christiansen C, et al: Consensus development conference: Prophylaxis and treatment of osteoporosis. Am J Med 90:107–10, 1991.
13. Brewerton TD: Toward a unified theory of serotonin dysregulation in eating and related disorders. Psychoneuroendocrinology 20:561–90, 1995.
14. Brush H: Eating Disorders: Obesity, Anorexia Nervosa, and the Person Within. New York, Basic Books, 1973.
15. Committee on Professional Standards, American College of Obstetricians and Gynecologists: Guidelines for Women's Health Care. Washington, DC, American College of Obstetricians and Gynecologists, 1995.
16. Committee on Sports Medicine, American Academy of Pediatrics: Amenorrhea in adolescent athletes. Pediatrics 84:394, 1989.
17. Consensus Development Conference: Who are candidates for prevention and treatment for osteoporosis? Osteoporos Int 7:1–6, 1997.
18. Crago M, Shisslak CM, Estes LS: Eating disturbances among American minority groups: a review. Int J Eat Disord 19:239–48, 1996.
19. Creighton DL, Morgan AL, Boardley D, Brolinson G: Weight-bearing exercise and markers of bone turnover in female athletes. J Appl Physiol 90:565–70, 2001.
20. Cummings DC: Exercise-associated amenorrhea, low bone density, and estrogen replacement therapy. Arch Intern Med 156:2193–5, 1996.
21. Drinkwater BL, Bruemmer B, Chestnut CH III: Menstrual history as a determinant of current bone density in young athletes. JAMA 263:545, 1990.
22. Drinkwater BL, Healy NL, Rencken ML, et al: Effectiveness of nasal calcitonin in preventing bone loss in young amenorrheic women. [Abstr]. J Bone Miner Res 8:S264, 1993.
23. Drinkwater BL, Nilson K, Ott S, et al: Bone mineral content of amenorrheic and eumenorrheic athletes. N Engl J Med 311:277–81, 1984.
24. Dueck CA, Matt KS, Manore MM, Skinner JS: Treatment of athletic amenorrhea with a diet and training intervention program. Int J Sport Nutr 6:24–40, 1996.
25. Dummer GM, Rosen LW, Heusner WW, et al: Pathogenic weight-control behaviors of young competitive swimmers. Physician Sportsmed 15:75–86, 1987.
26. Ettinger B, Black DM, Mitlak BH, et al: Reduction of vertebral fracture risk in postmenopausal women with osteoporosis treated with raloxifene: results from a 3-year randomized clinical trial. JAMA 282:637–45, 1999.
27. Feight CB, Johnson TS, et al: Secondary amenorrhea in athletes. Lancet 2:1145, 1978.
28. Frisch RE, Gotz-Welbergen AV, McArthur JW, et al: Delayed menarche and amenorrhea of college athletes in relation to age of onset of training. JAMA 246:1559–63, 1981.
29. Gard CME, Freeman CP: The dismantling of a myth: A review of eating disorders and socioeconomic status. Int J Eat Disord 20:1–12, 1996.
30. Garner DM, Garfinkel PE, Schwartz D, Thompson M: Cultural expectations of thinness in women. Psychol Rep 47:483–91, 1980.
31. Georgious EK, Ntalles K, Papageorgiou A, et al: Bone mineral loss related to menstrual history. Acta Orthop Scand 60:192–4, 1989.
32. Gibson JH, et al: Treatment of reduced bone mineral density in athletic amenorrhea: a pilot study. Osteoporos Int 10:284–9, 1999.
33. Green M (ed): Bright Futures: Guidelines for Health Supervision of Infants, Children, and Adolescents. Arlington, VA, National Center for Education in Maternal and Child Health, 1994.
34. Grinspoon S, Miller K, Coyle C, et al: Severity of osteopenia in estrogen-deficient women with anorexia nervosa and hypothalamic amenorrhea. J Clin Endocrinol Metab 84:2049–55, 1999.
35. Harris MB, Greco D: Weight control and weight concerns in competitive female gymnasts. J Sport Exerc Psychol 12:427–33, 1990.
36. Hecht S, Nattiv A, Balague G, Marshall N: Gymnastics and the female athlete triad. In Marshall N (ed): The Athlete Wellness Book. Indianapolis, Ind, USA Gymnastics, 1999.
37. Hecht S, Nattiv A, Puffer JC: Disordered eating in female collegiate gymnasts. [Abstr]. Presented at the American Medical Society of Sports Medicine Annual Meeting, San Diego, April 2000.
38. Hergenroeder AC, Smith EO, Shypailo R, et al: Bone mineral changes in young women with hypothalamic amenorrhea treated with oral contraceptives, medroxyprogesterone, or placebo over 12 months. Am J Obstet Gynecol 176:1017–25, 1997.
39. Hilton LK, Loucks AB: Low energy availability, not exercise stress, suppresses the diurnal rhythm of leptin in healthy young women. Am J Physiol Endocrinol Metab 278:E43–9, 2000.
40. Hoek HW: The distribution of eating disorders. In Brownwell KD, Fairburn CG (eds): Eating Disorders and Obesity: A Comprehensive Handbook. New York, Guilford Press, 1995, pp 207–11.
41. Johnson M: Disordered eating in active and athletic women. Clin Sports Med 13:355–69, 1994.
42. Karlson KA, Black Becker C, Merker A: Prevalence of eating disordered behavior in collegiate lightweight women rowers and distance runners. Clin J Sport Med 11:32–7, 2001.
43. Keen AD, Drinkwater BL: Irreversible bone loss in former amenorrheic athletes. Osteoporos Int 7:311–5, 1997.
44. Kendler KS, MacLean C, Neale M, et al: The genetic epidemiology of bulimia nervosa. Am J Psychiatry 148:1627–37, 1991.
45. Kirchner EM, Lewis RD, O'Connor PJ: Bone mineral density and dietary intake of female college gymnasts. Med Sci Sports Exerc 27:543–7, 1995.
46. Klibanski A, Biller BMK, Schoenfeld DA, et al: The effects of estrogen administration on trabecular bone loss in young women with anorexia nervosa. J Clin Endocrinol Metab 80:898–904, 1995.
47. Laughlin GA, Yen SSC: Hypoleptinemia in women athletes: absence of a diurnal rhythm with amenorrhea. J Clin Endocrinol Metab 82:318–21, 1997.
48. Loucks AB: Alterations in the hypothalamic—pituitary–ovarian and the hypothalamic—pituitary–adrenal axes in athletic women. J Clin Endocrinol Metab 68:402–11, 1989.
49. Loucks, AB: Effects of exercise training on the menstrual cycle: existence and mechanisms. Med Sci Sports Exerc 22:275, 1990.
50. Loucks, AB, Heath EM: Induction of low T3 syndrome in exercising women occurs at a threshold of energy availability. Am J Physiol 266:R817, 1994.
51. Loucks AB, Horvath SM: Athletic amenorrhea: a review. Med Sci Sports Exerc 17:56–72, 1985.
52. Loucks AB, Verdun M, Heath EM, et al: Low energy availability, not the stress of exercise, alters LH pulsatility in exercising women. J Appl Phys 84:37, 1998.
53. Malina RM: Menarche in athletes: a synthesis and hypothesis. Ann Hum Biol 10:1–24, 1983.
54. Malina RM: Physical growth and biological maturation of young athletes. Exerc Sports Sci Rev 22:389–433, 1994.

55. Malina RM, Ryan RC, Bonci CM: Age at menarche in athletes and their mothers and sisters. Ann Hum Biol 21:417–22, 1994.

56. Marcus R, Cann C, Madvig P, et al: Menstrual function and bone mass in elite women distance runners. Ann Intern Med 102:158–163, 1985.

57. Marx RG, Saint-Phard D, Callahan LR, et al: Stress fracture sites related to underlying bone health in athletic females. Clin J Sport Med 11:73–6, 2001.

58. Montzoros CS: The role of leptin in human obesity and disease: a review of current evidence. Ann Intern Med 130:651–7, 1999.

59. Myburgh KH, Bachrach LK, Lewis B, et al: Low bone mineral density at axial and appendicular sites in amenorrheic athletes. Med Sci Sports Exerc 25:1197–202, 1993.

60. Myburgh KH, Hutchins J, Fataar AB, et al: Low bone density is an etiologic factor for stress fractures in athletes. Ann Intern Med 113:754–9, 1990.

61. Nattiv A: Stress fractures and bone health in track and field athletes. J Sci Med Sport 3(3):267–78, 2000.

62. Nattiv A, Agostini R, Drinkwater BL, Yeager KK: The female athlete triad: the inter-relatedness of disordered eating, amenorrhea and osteoporosis. Clin Sports Med 13:405–18, 1994.

63. Nattiv A, Armsey TD Jr: Stress injury to bone in the female athlete. Clin Sports Med 16:197–224, 1997.

64. Nattiv A, Puffer JC, Casper J, et al: Stress factor risk factors, incidence and distribution: A 3-year prospective study in collegiate runners. Med Sci Sports Exerc 32(Suppl 5):S347, 2000.

65. Nattiv A, Puffer JC, Green G: Lifestyles and health risks of collegiate athletes: A multi-center study. Clin J Sports Med 7:262–72, 1997.

66. Nichols-Richardson SM, O'Connor PJ, Shapses SA, Lewis RD: Longitudinal bone mineral density in female child artistic gymnasts. J Bone Miner Res 14:994–1002, 1999.

67. O'Connor PJ, Lewis RD, Kirchner EM: Eating disorder symptoms in female college gymnasts. Med Sci Sports Exerc 27:550–5, 1995.

68. Otis CL, Drinkwater B, Johnson MD, et al: American College of Sports Medicine Position Stand on the Female Athlete Triad. Med Sci Sports Exerc 29:i–ix, 1997.

69. Palla B, Litt IF: Medical complications of eating disorders in adolescents. Pediatrics 81:613–23, 1988.

70. Pomeroy C, Mitchell JE: Medical issues in the eating disorders. In Brownell KD, Rodin J, Wilmore JH (eds): Eating, Body Weight and Performance in Athletes: Disorders of Modern Society. Philadelphia, Lea & Febiger, 1992, pp 202–21.

71. Powles TJ, Hickish T, Kanis JA, et al: Effect of tamoxifen on bone mineral density measured by dual-energy x-ray absorptiometry in healthy premenopausal women. J Clin Oncol 14:78–84, 1996.

72. Ratnasuriya RH, Eisler I, Szmuckler GI: Anorexia nervosa: Outcome and prognostic factors after 20 years. Br J Psychiatry 158:495, 1991.

73. Rencken M, Chesnut CH, Drinkwater BL: Decreased bone density at multiple skeletal sites in amenorrheic athletes. JAMA 276:238–40, 1996.

74. Rigotti NA, Nussbaum SR, Herzog DB, Neer RM: Osteoporosis in women with anorexia nervosa. N Engl J Med 311:1601–6, 1984.

75. Robinson TL, Snow-Harter C, Taafe DR, et al: Gymnasts exhibit higher bone mass than runners despite similar prevalence of amenorrhea and oligomenorrhea. J Bone Miner Res 10:26–35, 1995.

76. Rosen LW, Hough DO: Pathogenic weight-control behaviors of female college gymnasts. Phys Sports Med 16:141–5, 1988.

77. Rosen LW, McKeag DB, Hough DO, Curley V: Pathogenic weight-control behavior in female athletes. Physician Sportsmed 14:79–86, 1986.

78. Schachter J, Shafer M, Young M, et al: Routine pelvic examinations in asymptomatic young women. New Engl J Med 335:1847, 1996.

79. Schwartz B, Cumming DC, Riordan E, et al: Exercise-associated amenorrhea: a distinct entity? Am J Obstet Gynecol 141:662–70, 1981.

80. Shangold MM, Rebar RAW, Wentz AC, Schiff I: Evaluation and management of menstrual dysfunction in athletes. JAMA 263:1665–9, 1990.

81. Shisslak CM, Crago M, Ests LS: The spectrum of eating disturbances. Int J Eat Disord 18:209–19, 1995.

82. Slemenda CW, Johnson CC: High intensity activities in young women: Site-specific bone mass effects among female figure skaters. Bone Miner 20:125–32, 1993.

83. Smolak L, Murnen SK, Ruble AE: Female athletes with eating problems: A meta-analysis. Int J Eat Disord 27:371–80, 2000.

84. Spitzer RL, Yanovski S, Wadden T, et al: Binge eating disorder:its further validation in a multisite study. Int J Eat Disord 13:137–53, 1993.

85. Strober M: Family-genetic studies of eating disorders. J Clin Psychiatry 52:S9–S12, 1991.

86. Sundgot-Borgen J: Prevalence of eating disorders in elite female athletes. Int J Sport Nutr 3:29–40, 1993.

87. Sundgot-Borgen J: Risk and trigger factors for the development of eating disorders in female elite athletes. Med Sci Sports Exerc 26:414–19, 1994.

88. Sundgot-Borgen J, Bahr R, Falch JA, Sundgot Schneider L: Normal bone mass in bulimic women. J Clin Endocrinol Metab 83:3144–9, 1998.

89. Sundgot-Borgen J, Larsen S: Pathogenic weight-control methods and self-reported eating disorders in female elite athletes and controls. Scand J Med Sci Sports 3:150–5, 1993.

90. Sundgot-Borgen J: The female athlete triad and the effect of preventive work. Med Sci Sports Exerc 30 (Suppl 5):S181, 1998.

91. Sundgot-Borgen J: The long-term effect of CBT and nutritional counseling in treating bulimic elite athletes: A randomized controlled study. Med Sci Sports Exerc 33 (Suppl 5):S97, 2001.

92. Warren MP, Shantha S: The female athlete. Baillieres Clin Endocrinol Metab 14:37–53, 2000.

93. Warren BJ, Stanton AL, Blessing DL: Disordered eating patterns in competitive female athletes. Int J Eat Disord 9:565–9, 1990.

94. Warren MP, Brooks-Gunn J, Fox RP, et al: Osteopenia in hypothalamic amenorrhea: a 3 year longitudinal study [Abstr]. Proceedings from the Endocrine Society, 1994.

95. Warren MP, Brooks-Gunn J, Hamilton LF, et al: Scoliosis and fractures in young ballet dancers. N Engl J Med 314:1348–53, 1986.

96. Warren MP, Voussoughian F, Geer EB, et al: Functional hypothalamic amenorrhea: hypoleptinemia and disordered eating. J Clin Endocrinol Metab 84:873–7, 1999.

97. Weaver CM, Teegarden D, Lyle RM, et al: Impact of exercise on bone health and contraindication of oral contraceptive use in young women. Med Sci Sports Exerc 33:873–80, 2001.

98. Williams NI, Young JC, McArthur JW, et al: Strenuous exercise with caloric restriction: effect on luteinizing hormone secretion. Med Sci Sports Exerc 27:1390–8, 1995.

99. Wilmore JH: Body weight standards and athletic performance. In Brownell KD, Rodin J, Wilmore JH (eds): Eating, Body Weight and Performance in Athletes: Disorders of Modern Society. Philadelphia, Lea & Febiger, 1992, pp 315–329.

100. Wilmore JH: Eating and weight disorders in the female athlete. Int J Sports Nutr 1:104–17, 1991.

101. Wolman RL, Clark P, McNally E, et al: Menstrual state and exercise as determinants of spinal trabecular bone density in amenorrheic and oestrogen-replete athletes. Br Med J 301:518–21, 1990.

102. World Health Organization (WHO) Study Group: Assessment of fracture risk and its application to screening for postmenopausal osteoporosis: Report of WHO study group technical report series 843. Geneva, Switzerland, WHO Technical Report Series, 843:6, 1994.

103. Yeager KK, Agostini R, Nattiv A, Drinkwater BL: The female athlete triad: disordered eating, amenorrhea, osteoporosis. [Commentary]. Med Sci Sports Exerc 25:775–7, 1993.

104. Zanker CL, Swaine IL: Bone turnover in amenorrheic and eumenorrheic women distance runners. Scand J Med Sci Sports 8:20–6, 1998.

105. Zanker CL, Swaine IL: Relation between bone turnover, oestradiol, and energy balance in women distance runners. Br J Sports Med 32:167–71, 1998.

106. Zanker CL, Swaine IL: The relationship between serum oestradiol concentration and energy balance in young women distance runners. Int J Sports Med 19:104–8, 1998.

Chapter 25

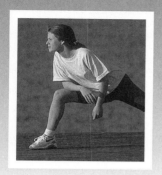

Disordered Eating

Jorunn Sundgot-Borgen, Ph.D.

Some female athletes and nonathletes do not consider training or exercise as sufficient to accomplish their idealized body shape or level of thinness. Therefore, to meet their goals, a significant number of them diet and use harmful—and ineffective—weight-loss practices such as extremely restrictive eating, vomiting, and use of laxatives and diuretics to meet their goals.[38] These patterns may lead to menstrual dysfunction, subsequent bone loss, and osteoporosis.

Disordered eating, amenorrhea, and osteoporosis are interrelated conditions referred to as the *female athlete triad*. Each component of the triad increases the chance of morbidity and mortality, but the dangers of the conditions together are synergistic.[31]

DISORDERED EATING

Eating disorders are characterized by disturbances in eating behavior, body image, emotions, and relationships. Athletes constitute a unique population, and special diagnostic considerations should be made when working with this group.[38,42,43]

Anorexia nervosa is the extreme of restrictive eating behavior in which an individual continues to starve and feel fat in spite of being 15% or more below an ideal body weight. Bulimic behavior refers to a cycle of food restriction or fasting followed by bingeing and purging.

Not all persons with disordered eating meet the American Psychiatric Association's definitions of anorexia nervosa or bulimia nervosa. *Eating disorders not otherwise specified* (EDNOS) is also included in the DSM-IV criteria. Athletes who meet the criteria for EDNOS also suffer serious short- and long-term medical and psychosocial problems if their pathologic eating habits continue.

The DSM-IV[1] diagnostic criteria for anorexia nervosa, bulimia nervosa, and EDNOS are listed in Tables 25-1, 25-2, and 25-3, respectively. These DSM-IV[1] criteria formalize overlapping conventions for subtyping anorexia nervosa into restricting and binge eating/purging types based on the presence or absence of bingeing and/or purging (ie, self-induced vomiting or the misuse of laxatives or diuretics). Most athletes alternate between these 2 subtypes of eating disorders.[41]

The EDNOS category[1] refers to disorders of eating that do not meet the criteria for any specific eating disorder. This category acknowl-

Table 25-1. Diagnostic Criteria for Anorexia Nervosa

A. Refusal to maintain body weight at or above a minimally normal weight for age and height (eg, weight loss leading to maintenance of body weight less than 85% of that expected; or failure to make expected weight gain during period of growth, leading to body weight less than 85% of that expected).
B. Intense fear of gaining weight or becoming fat, even though underweight.
C. Disturbance in the way in which one's body weight or shape is experienced, undue influence of body weight or shape on self-evaluation, or denial of the seriousness of the current low body weight.
D. In postmenarcheal females, amenorrhea, ie, the absence of at least 3 consecutive menstrual cycles. (A woman is considered to have amenorrhea if her periods occur only following hormone, eg, estrogen, administration.)

Specify type:

Restricting type: During the episode of anorexia nervosa, the person has not regularly engaged in binge eating or purging behavior (ie, self-induced vomiting or the misuse of laxatives, diuretics, or enemas).

Binge eating/purging type: During the current episode of anorexia nervosa, the person has regularly engaged in binge eating or purging behavior (ie, self-induced vomiting or the misuse of laxatives, diuretics, or enemas).

From American Psychiatric Association: *Diagnostic and Statistical Manual of Mental Disorders,* 4th edition. Washington, DC, American Psychiatric Association, 1994, with permission.

Table 25-2. Diagnostic Criteria for Bulimia Nervosa

A. Recurrent episodes of binge eating. An episode of binge eating is characterized by both of the following: (1) eating, in a discrete period of time (eg, within any 2-hour period), an amount of food that is definitely larger than most people would eat during a similar period of time in similar circumstances; and, (2) a sense of lack of control over eating during the episode (eg, a feeling that one cannot stop eating or control what or how much one is eating).
B. Recurrent inappropriate compensatory behavior in order to prevent weight gain, such as self-induced vomiting; misuse of laxatives, diuretics, or other medications; fasting; or excessive exercise.
C. The binge eating and inappropriate compensatory behaviors both occur, on average, at least twice a week for 3 months.
D. Self-evaluation is unduly influenced by body shape and weight.
E. The disturbance does not occur exclusively during episodes of anorexia nervosa.

Specify type:

Purging type: The person regularly engages in self-induced vomiting or the misuse of laxatives, diuretics, or enemas.

Nonpurging type: The person uses other inappropriate compensatory behaviors, such as fasting or excessive exercise, but does not regularly engage in self-induced vomiting or the misuse of laxatives, diuretics, or enemas.

From American Psychiatric Association: *Diagnostic and Statistical Manual of Mental Disorders*, 4th edition. Washington, DC, American Psychiatric Association, 1994, with permission.

edges the existence and importance of a variety of eating disturbances (Table 25-3).

PREVALENCE OF EATING DISORDERS IN FEMALE ATHLETES

It has been claimed that female athletes are at increased risk for developing eating disorders.[39,48] In some studies, anorexia nervosa, bulimia nervosa, and EDNOS have been found to be more prevalent in both female and male elite athletes when compared to female and male nonathletes.[39,41,45] Furthermore, eating disorders are significantly more frequent among young female elite athletes competing in aesthetic and weight-class sports than among other sport groups in which leanness is considered less important (Fig. 25-1).

FACTORS ASSOCIATED WITH THE DEVELOPMENT OF EATING DISORDERS

The etiology of eating disorders is multifactorial.[16,22] Because of additional stress associated with the athletic environment, female elite athletes appear to be more vulnerable to eating disorders than the general female population.[41,43]

Caloric Deprivation

One retrospective study indicated that a sudden increase in training load may induce a caloric deprivation in endurance athletes, which in turn may elicit biologic and social reinforcements leading to the development of eating disorders.[39] However, longitudinal studies with close monitoring of a number of sport-specific factors (ie, type, duration, and intensity of the training) in athletes representing different sport-specific factors (ie, clothing, weight classes, physical and psychological demands, roles, subjective judging and coaching behavior) are needed to answer questions regarding the role played by different sports in the development of eating disorders.

Starting Sport-Specific Training at Prepubertal Age

Athletes with eating disorders have been shown to start sport-specific training at an earlier age

Table 25-3. Diagnostic Criteria for Eating Disorders Not Otherwise Specified

1. For females, all of the criteria for anorexia nervosa are met except that the individual has regular menses.
2. All of the criteria for anorexia nervosa are met except that, despite significant weight loss, the individual's current weight is in the normal range.
3. All of the criteria for bulimia nervosa are met except that the binge eating and inappropriate compensatory mechanisms occur at a frequency of less than twice a week or for a duration of less than 3 months.
4. The regular use of inappropriate compensatory behavior by an individual of normal body weight after eating small amounts of food (eg, self-induced vomiting after the consumption of 2 cookies).
5. Repeatedly chewing and spitting out, but not swallowing, large amounts of food.
6. Binge-eating disorder: recurrent episodes of binge eating in the absence of the regular use of inappropriate compensatory behaviors characteristic of bulimia nervosa.

From American Psychiatric Association: *Diagnostic and Statistical Manual of Mental Disorders*, 4th edition. Washington, DC, American Psychiatric Association, 1994, with permission.

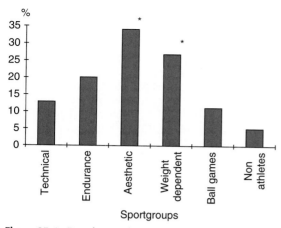

Figure 25-1. Prevalence of eating disorders in female elite athletes representing technical sports (N = 98), endurance sports (N = 119), aesthetic sports (N = 64), weight-dependent sports (N = 41), ball games (N = 183), power sports (N = 17), and nonathletes (N = 522). The data are shown as mean. *, p < 0.05 compared to endurance sports, technical sports, and ball games sports.

than athletes without eating disorders.[39] Another factor to consider is that starting sport-specific training at a prepubertal age may result in athletes not choosing the sport most suitable for their adult body type.

Traumatic Events

From subjective experience, female athletes have reported that they developed eating disorders as a result of what they call a traumatic event such as the loss or change of a coach, or an injury or illness that left them temporarily unable to continue their normal level of exercise.[22,39] An injury can curtail the athlete's exercise and training habits. As a result, the athlete may gain weight in response to less energy expenditure, which in some cases may develop into an irrational fear of further weight gain. Then, the ath-

lete may begin to diet to compensate for the lack of exercise.[41,43]

Pressure to Reduce Weight and Weight Cycling

Pressure to reduce weight has been the common explanation for the increased prevalence of eating-related problems among athletes. The important factor may, however, not be dieting per se, but rather the situation in which the athlete is told to lose weight, the words used, and whether the athlete received guidance or not. The various reasons for the development of eating disorders reported by eating-disordered high-level athletes are presented in Table 25-4. In addition to the pressure to reduce weight, athletes are often pressed for time, and they have to lose weight rapidly to make or stay on the team. As a result they often experience frequent periods of restrictive dieting or weight cycling.[39] Weight cycling has been suggested as an important risk or trigger factor for the development of eating disorders in athletes.[5,39]

Most researchers agree that coaches do not cause eating disorders in athletes, although through inappropriate coaching, the problem may be triggered or exacerbated in vulnerable individuals.[39,48] In most cases, then, the role of coaches in the development of eating disorders in athletes should be seen as a part of a complex interplay of factors.

To sum up, then, there is no hard evidence for sport-specific risk factors for eating disorders. The use of longitudinal quantitative and qualitative studies is clearly needed.

The Attraction to Sport Hypotheses

On the other hand, some investigators have argued that specific sports attract individuals who are anorectic before commencing their

Table 25-4. Reasons for the Development of Eating Disorders Reported by Athletes

	N	EATING-DISORDERED ATHLETES (%)
Prolonged periods of dieting	29	37
New coach	23	30
Injury/illness	18	23
Casual comments	15	19
Leaving home/failure at school/work	8	10
Problem in relationship	8	10
Family problems	5	7
Illness/injury to family members	5	7
Death of significant others	3	4
Sexual abuse (by coach)	3	4

Multiple answers were allowed. 15% did not give any specific reason.
From Sundgot-Borgen J: *Risk and trigger factors for the development of eating disorders in female elite athletes.* Med. Sci. Sports Exerc 4:414–9, 1994, with permission.

participation in sports, at least in attitude, if not in behavior or weight.[36,43] It is the author's opinion that the attraction to sport hypotheses might be true for the general population, while athletes do not achieve the elite level if the only motivation is weight loss. Therefore, this hypothesis most likely applies to lower-level athletes.

MEDICAL ISSUES

For both athletes and nonathletes, eating disorders may cause serious medical problems and can even be fatal. Most complications of anorexia nervosa occur as a direct or indirect result of starvation, whereas complications of bulimia nervosa occur as a result of binge eating and purging. The loss of fluids and electrolytes during purging may lead to serious medical problems like dehydration, acid-base abnormalities, and cardiac rhythm disturbances. Dehydration and electrolyte abnormalities may decrease coordination, balance, and muscle function. Therefore, the behavior is dangerous to their health and counterproductive to improving their athletic performance.

The long-term effects of weight cycling and eating disorders in athletes are unclear. Biologic maturation and growth have been studied in girl gymnasts before and during puberty, suggesting that young female gymnasts are smaller and mature later than females from sports that do not require extreme leanness, such as swimming.[26,44] It is, however, difficult to separate the effects of physical strain, energy restriction, and genetic predisposition to delayed puberty. Some studies have found a strong relationship between abnormal dietary behaviors and menstrual dysfunction.[3,28,33]

Anorexia nervosa patients display a standard mortality rate 6 times that of the general population.[29] Death is usually attributable to fluid and electrolyte abnormalities, or suicide.[5] Mortality in bulimia nervosa is less well studied, but deaths do occur, usually secondary to the complications of the binge–purging cycle or suicide. Mortality rates of eating disorders among athletes are not known. However, a number of death cases of top-level athletes representing gymnastics, running, alpine skiing, and cycling have been reported in the media. Five (5.4%) of those diagnosed in the Norwegian study[39] reported suicide attempts.

Stress Fractures in Amenorrheic Athletes

Studies report a higher incidence of injuries and stress fractures among amenorrheic and oligomenorrheic athletes as compared to eumenorrheic athletes.[3,11,25] However, it should be noted that a number of the female athletes who suffer from menstrual dysfunction and disordered eating are exercising compulsively and do not stop training in spite of an injury or injury symptoms. Therefore, it may be the stresses of overtraining that lead to an increased prevalence of injury in this population[6,32] and/or a decrease in bone density.[11]

Besides increasing the likelihood of stress fractures, disordered eating and amenorrhea may result in an inability to achieve maximal peak bone mass. Athletes with frequent or longer periods of amenorrhea and/or a long history of disordered eating may be at high risk of sustaining fractures.

Long-Term Effect of Menstrual Irregularities on Vertebral Bone Mineral Density

To date, no long-term study has shown that amenorrheic individuals can fully regain lost bone mineral density, despite returning to a normal reproductive status.[6,21] This risk is especially critical for the adolescent or young adult athlete as peak bone mass is reached by the third decade of life.[21] Therefore, further studies are needed to determine the long-term effects of resumption of menses on bone mineral density.

THE EFFECT OF EATING DISORDERS ON ATHLETIC PERFORMANCE

The nature and the magnitude of the effect of eating disorders on athletic performance are influenced by the severity and chronicity of the eating disorder and the physical demands of the sport. For example, anorexia nervosa will probably have different effects on an endurance athlete, such as a distance runner, as compared to an athlete in a less aerobic sport such as gymnastics.

A number of studies have shown that "healthy" athletes and athletes suffering from eating disorders who need to keep lean to improve performance consume surprisingly low amounts of calories.[13,27,40] Athletes with eating disorders, except for some of the athletes with bulimia nervosa, consume diets low in energy and key nutrients.[40] However, the effects of the low energy intake on protein balance have not been studied in detail. Athletes know that the quickest way to lose weight is by losing body water. Water is essential for the regulation of body temperature, and a dehydrated athlete becomes overheated and fatigued more easily. It has been shown that loss of endurance and coordination as a result of dehydration impairs exercise performance.[46]

Reduced plasma volume, impaired thermoregulation and nutrient exchange, decreased glycogen availability, and decreased buffer capacity in the blood are plausible explanations for reduced performance in aerobic, anaerobic, and muscle endurance work, especially after rapid weight reduction. It is more difficult to explain decreased muscle strength found in some studies.[14,17] Absolute maximal oxygen uptake (measured in liters per minute) is unchanged or decreased after rapid weight loss, but maximal oxygen uptake expressed in relation to body weight (milliliters per kilogram body weight per minute) may increase after gradual weight reduction.[4,19] Anaerobic performance and muscle strength are typically decreased after rapid weight reduction with or without 1 to 3 hours of rehydration. When tested after 5 to 24 hours of rehydration, performance is maintained at euhydrated levels.[15,24]

Psychological factors may also affect performance. Many young wrestlers feel mood alterations (increased fatigue, anger, or anxiety) when attempting to lose weight rapidly.[2]

The psychological and medical features and consequences of eating disorders among athletes and nonathletes have been described and discussed in detail elsewhere.[5,23,43] Laboratory abnormalities and characteristic endocrine abnormalities of eating disorders are discussed by Katz.[23] A drawback of studies on weight reduction in athletes is that the relationship between performance test results and actual competitive performance is not clear.[14] Most investigators have used athletes in weight class events as study participants. More longitudinal data on gradual weight reduction in endurance athletes and aesthetic sports is clearly needed.

HOW TO IDENTIFY ATHLETES AT RISK FOR EATING DISORDERS?

Since athletes often are evaluated by their coach every day, changes in behavior and physical symptoms should be easily observed. However, symptoms of eating disorders in competitive and elite athletes are too often ignored or not "detected" by coaches. One reason for this is a lack of knowledge about symptoms of eating disorders.

Most individuals with eating disorders do not realize that they have a problem, and therefore do not seek treatment on their own. Athletes, however, might consider seeking help only if they experience a decrease in their performance level.

Figure 25-2 illustrates an etiologic model for the development of eating disorders in female athletes.

In contrast to the athletes with anorectic symptoms most athletes suffering from bulimia nervosa are at or near normal weight and therefore their eating disorder is difficult to detect. Hence, the team staff and parents learn to recognize the physical signs and psychological characteristics listed in Tables 25-5 and 25-6. It should be noted that the presence of some of these characteristics does not necessarily indicate the presence of disordered eating or the female athlete triad. However, the likelihood of 1 or more of the components of the triad being present increases as the number of presenting characteristics increases.

TREATMENT OF EATING DISORDERS

Female athletes with a single component of the female athlete triad should be screened for the other components. Screening for the triad can be done at the time of the preparticipation examination and during clinical evaluation of menstrual change, disordered eating patterns, weight change, cardiac arrhythmias (including bradycardia), depression, or stress fracture.[20,31,35]

Eating-disordered athletes seem more likely to accept the idea of going for a single consultation than committing themselves to prolonged treatment.[43] Athletes with eating disorders usually resist treatment until they reach a point of despair, at which time they are more willing to accept help.[7] The treatment of athletes with eating disorders ideally should be undertaken by health care professionals with expertise in working with athletes with disordered eating. It is the author's experience that it is easier to establish a trusting relationship when the eating-disordered athlete works with a therapist who knows their sport, in addition to being trained in treating eating-disordered patients. Therapists who are thoroughly knowledgeable about eating disorders and know the various sports will better understand the athlete's training setting, daily demands, and relationships that are specific to the sport/sport event and competitive level. The treatment team needs to accept the athlete's fears and irrational thoughts about food and weight, and then present a rational approach to achieving self-management of a healthy diet, weight, and training program.[7]

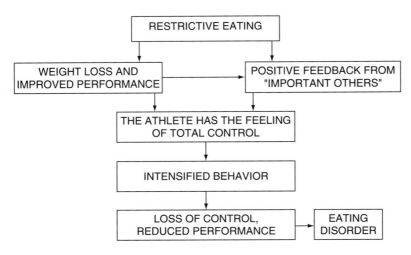

Figure 25-2. Etiologic model for the development of eating disorders in female athletes.

It is the author's experience that a total suspension of training during treatment is not a good solution. Therefore, unless severe medical complications are present, training at a lower volume and at a decreased intensity should be allowed. In general, athletes are not encouraged to compete during treatment to avoid communicating a message of sport performance being more important than the athlete's health. Nevertheless, competitions during treatment might be considered for individuals with less severe eating disorders engaged in low-risk sports. The athlete who continues to participate in her sport while in treatment must have close medical follow-up and not be placed at further medical or psychological risk.[43]

Exercise-associated amenorrhea is a diagnosis of exclusion, and all other causes of amenorrhea must be excluded by a thorough medical evaluation.[30,37] Eating-disordered athletes with amenorrhea should be encouraged to ingest at least 1500 mg of elemental calcium daily to ensure calcium balance.[30] In some studies, amenorrheic athletes using hormone replacement therapy in doses used for menopausal women have shown maintenance of bone mineral density but no gains.[31] Use of hormone replacement therapy by amenorrheic athletes remains controversial. Women with amenorrhea and less severe bone loss may prefer to adjust training and nutritional patterns to resume their normal reproductive cycle.[8–10,30,37] Eating-disordered athletes with amenorrhea and osteopenia or osteoporosis may be better off choosing hormone replacement therapy or other pharmacologic treatment for their

Table 25-5. Physical Symptoms of Eating-Disordered Athletes

• *Dermatologic/Dental*	• *Thermoregulation*
Hair loss[a]	Hypothermia[a]
Dry skin, brittle hair and nails[a]	• *Hematologic*
Lanugo[a]	Anemia
Callus or abrasion on back of	• *Fluids and electrolytes*
hand (from inducing vomiting)[a]	Dehydration
Dental and gum problems[a]	Edema
• *Cardiovascular*	Electrolyte abnormalities
Bradycardia	Hypokalemia
Hypotension	Muscle cramps
• *Metabolic/Gastrointestinal*	Metabolic alkalosis
Gastrointestinal problems (ie, constipation,	• *Others*
diarrhea, bloating, postprandial	Significant weight loss (beyond that necessary for
distress) Swollen parotid glands[b]	adequate sport performance)[a]
• *Endocrine*	Frequent and often extreme weight fluctuations[b]
Hypoglycemia	Low weight despite eating large volumes[b]
Low female sex hormone levels	Fatigue (beyond that normally expected in training or
Delayed onset of puberty[a]	competition)
Amenorrhea or menstrual dysfunction	Muscle weakness
Reduced bone mineral density	Hyperactivity
Stress fractures	

[a]Especially for anorexia nervosa.
[b]Especially for bulimia nervosa.

Table 25-6. Psychological and Behavioral Characteristics of Eating-Disordered Athletes

Anxiety	Exercising while injured (despite prohibitions by medical and training staff)
Dieting (unnecessary for, health, sport performance, or appearance)	Restlessness: relaxing is difficult or impossible
Avoidance of eating and eating situations	Change in behavior from open, positive, and social to suspicious, untruthful, and sad
Claims of "feeling fat" despite being thin[a]	Social withdrawal
Self-critical, especially concerning body, weight, and sport performance	Depression and insomnia
Resistance to weight gain or maintenance recommended by sport support staff	Secretive eating
Unusual weighing behavior (ie, excessive weighing, refusal to weigh, negative reaction to being weighed)	Binge eating[b]
Compulsiveness and rigidity, especially regarding eating and exercise	Agitation when bingeing is interrupted[b]
	Evidence of vomiting unrelated to illness[b]
Excessive or obligatory exercise beyond that recommended for performance enhancement	Excessive use of the restroom or "disappearing" after eating[b]
	Use of laxatives or diuretics (or both) that is unsanctioned by medical or training staffs[b]
	Substance abuse, whether legal, illegal, prescribed, or over-the-counter drugs, medications, or other substances[b]

[a]Especially for anorexia nervosa.
[b]Especially for bulimia nervosa.

osteopenia, in addition to the treatment received for the eating disorder, since treatment for eating disorders usually requires a period of time. As the rate of bone loss in hypoestrogenic women is greatest in the 5 to 6 years following the decrease in levels of endogenous estrogen, there may be only a brief window of opportunity to initiate intervention therapy to prevent irreversible bone loss.[31]

Once coaches, teammates, or health care staff suspect that an athlete has an eating disorder, questions about referral and arrangements for treatment, implementation of the therapeutic regimen, monitoring of specific therapeutic strategies, and arrangements for follow-up should arise.[43] The formal treatment of athletes with eating disorders should be undertaken by health care professionals. Ideally, these individuals should also be familiar with, and have an appreciation for, the sport environment.[7,43]

It has been our experience that in some ways, admitting to having an eating disorder is more threatening for athletes with bulimia nervosa or bulimic symptoms than for those suffering from anorexia nervosa. Many athletes with bulimic symptoms have binged and purged for years, and regard their disorder as a disgusting habit.

Refusal of Medical Examination

If the athlete refuses a medical evaluation and examination, training should be prohibited until she undergoes such an examination. The athlete should be given information concerning a healthier weight if weight is significantly low for

height and body frame. She should be asked if she is having difficulty sleeping, or is feeling depressed, weak, tired, or irritable, and if she has lost her menstrual cycle. If she admits to these problems, it should be suggested that they may all be related to her eating or weight control behavior.

Suspension from training is not a good solution for several reasons. First, if the athlete is suspended she may train on her own, which in some cases may be more dangerous because no one will be monitoring her training. Second, not allowing the athlete to participate in her sport may further reduce her self-esteem. Third, control is a key issue for the individual with an eating disorder. She may view the suspension as an attempt by others to control.[43]

The athlete's family may be involved in the process of getting the athlete into treatment. One factor affecting this involvement is the athlete's age. One would anticipate more family involvement with younger athletes.[43]

Inpatient Versus Outpatient Therapy

Many individuals with true anorexia nervosa require inpatient treatment at some point during their illness, although the health care provider may try outpatient treatment if the individual's weight is stable and not extremely low and she is not purging.[18] Most individuals with bulimia nervosa and EDNOS can be treated on an outpatient basis. The most common reasons for hospitalization in patients with bulimia nervosa is significant electrolyte disturbances, dehydration, and/or related cardiac arrhythmias.

Types of Treatment

Whether the athlete is in inpatient or outpatient treatment, he or she is likely to be involved in several modes of treatment. Typically these include individual, group, and family therapy. Nutritional counseling and pharmacotherapy may also be included as adjuncts to the treatment regimen (Table 25-7).

Treatment Goals and Expectations

The primary focus of treatment includes normalizing weight and eating behaviors, modifying unhealthy thought processes that maintain the disorder, and dealing with the emotional issues in the individual's life that in some cases create a need for the disorder. Athletes have the same general concerns as nonathletes about increasing their weight, but they also have concerns from a sport standpoint. What they think is an ideal competitive weight, one that they believe helps them be successful in their sport, may be significantly lower than their treatment goal weight. As a result, athletes may have concerns about their ability to perform in their sport following treatment.

Regardless of the type of disordered eating, the severity and chronicity of the disorder affect the length of treatment, as do complicating personality factors. It may take months or years to recover from an eating disorder. Generally anorexia nervosa requires a longer treatment time than bulimia nervosa. For athletes to complete treatment successfully, they must be able to trust the individuals involved in managing and treating their difficulties. A violation of confidentiality can destroy that trust. Some athletes may not want anyone associated with their sport to be involved in or receive any information about their treatment. These athletes may need to have a special relationship with their therapist in which only the therapist is privy to certain information.[43]

The author has found that most athletes are willing to allow a coach or other support staff at least minimal contact with the therapist. Some others very much want the coach involved and view this as evidence of caring and concern on the part of the coach. Teammates of an athlete with an eating disorder are often aware of the problem and may also know that the athlete is in treatment. Information about the eating disordered athlete should be handled as the affected athlete desires. Some athletes may not want their parents to know about their disorder. Therapists cannot release information even to parents without the individual's consent, except under special circumstances and in the case of minors.

Athletes in Treatment

Athletes with an eating disorder should not compete until the health care professionals working with him/her decide it is safe to do so. This decision can come at any point during the treatment process. Thompson and Trattner-Sherman[43] state a number of reasons why the athlete should not compete until cleared to do so. First, depending on the nature and severity of the disorder, competing while eating disor-

Table 25-7. Treatment of Athletes with Eating Disorders

TYPES OF TREATMENT	CONTENTS
Individual pschotherapy	• The therapist works with the eating-disordered athlete and intends to: Determine the nature of the individual's eating difficulties and how they might be most effectively changed. Implement a change process. Teach the athlete to deal with how her sport or sport participation may be contributing to the maintenance of the eating disorder.
Group therapy	• The athlete is part of a group made up of other eating-disordered athletes. Athletes discover that others have a similar problem. Gives the individual a support group that understands her feelings and eating problem. Provides a safe environment for the athlete to practice the new skills and attitudes she has learned.
Family therapy	• Includes the patient and her immediate family. The family is the focus of treatment. A goal is to modify maladaptive family interactions, attitudes, and dynamics to decrease the need for, or the function of, the eating disorder in the family.
Nutritional counseling	• Often part of a multimodal treatment approach. Eating-disordered athletes do not remember what constitutes a balanced meal or "normal" eating. The dietician's primary roles involve providing nutritional information and assisting in meal planning.
Pharmacotherapy	• Can be useful in some cases, especially with patients with bulimic behaviors.

dered may place the athlete at greater risk medically or psychologically. Second, sport may play a significant role in the disorder such that the athlete's participation in sport may help to maintain or perpetuate the disorder. In addition, allowing an athlete to compete while affected by an eating disorder may give him/her the message that sport performance is more important than his/her health.

Health Maintenance Standards

If it is determined by the medical staff that the athlete is safe to compete, a management plan regarding health maintenance must be implemented to protect the athlete. The treatment staff determines these and individually tailors them according to the athlete's particular condition. These standards may vary between individual athletes and by sport. Often times a written contract is used.

According to the author, athletes should maintain a weight of no less than 90% of "ideal" weight, not sport related, but health related. The athlete should eat at least 3 balanced meals a day, consisting of enough calories to sustain the pre-established weight standard the dietician has proposed. Athletes who have been amenorrheic for 6 months or more should undergo a medical examination to evaluate the need for hormone replacement therapy or other management.[37] In addition, bone mineral density should be assessed.

The following list represents what Thompson and Trattner-Sherman[43] believe are the minimal criteria to continue competition and training: (1) The athlete must agree to comply with all treatment strategies as best he/she can; (2) the athlete must genuinely want to compete; (3) the athlete must be closely monitored on an ongoing basis by the medical and psychological health care professionals handling treatment and by the sport-related personnel who are working with him/her in his/her sport; (4) treatment must always take precedence over sport; and (5) if any question arises at any time regarding whether the athlete is meeting or is able to meet the preceding criteria, competition should be denied while the athlete is in treatment.[43]

Limited Training While in Treatment

If the criteria mentioned above for competing cannot be met, or if competition rather than physical exertion is a problem, some athletes who are not competing may still be allowed to engage in limited training. The same criteria used to assess the safety of competition (ie,

diagnosis, problem severity, type of sport, competitive level, and health maintenance) apply. We believe that continuing in training and competition can have advantages for some athletes. Some athletes will be motivated in treatment by the opportunity to continue training. If the athlete is ready for treatment, allowing her to continue with her sport with minimal risk when she really wants to continue can enhance the motivation for and the effect of treatment. For some athletes, allowing them to train or compete may help their state of well-being and self-esteem.[43]

Decision to Compete

Some athletes may be allowed to compete while in aftercare if not medically or psychologically contraindicated. It is extremely important to examine whether the athlete really desires to go back to competitive sport. If so, participation should be allowed as soon as the athlete feels ready to compete and is healthy, and the medical team has cleared her.[43]

PREVENTION OF EATING DISORDERS IN ATHLETES

In contrast to the findings from previously reported studies in the general adolescent population,[34] education of competitive athletes and coaches regarding eating disorders and related problems such as menstrual dysfunction and bone loss may help prevent these problems in this population.[41] Therefore, within the sport arena, coaches, trainers, administrators, and parents should receive information about eating disorders and related issues, such as growth and development, the relationship between body composition, health, and performance, and nutrition. In addition, coaches should realize that they can strongly influence their athletes. Coaches or others involved with young athletes should not comment on an individual's body size, or require weight loss in young and still-growing athletes. Without offering further guidance, dieting may result in unhealthy eating behavior or eating disorders in highly motivated and uninformed athletes.[12] Early intervention is also important, since eating disorders are more difficult to treat the longer they progress. Therefore, professionals working with athletes should be informed about the possible risk factors for the development, early signs and symptoms of the medical, psychological, and social consequences of disordered eating, how to approach the problem if it occurs, and what treatment options are available.

Teammates, coaches, and parents who are aware of these signs of disordered eating are likely to notice them. Those who provide medical care for athletes should be alerted to athletes presenting with irregular periods, disordered eating patterns, and stress fractures as possible signs of the triad, particularly noting unusual fractures that occur from minimal trauma.[31]

References

1. American Psychiatric Association: Diagnostic and Statistical Manual of Mental Disorders, 4th edition. Washington, DC, American Psychiatric Association, 1994.
2. Armstrong LE, Costill DL, Fink WJ: Influence of diuretics induced dehydration on competitive running performance. Med Sci Sports Exerc 17:456–61, 1985.
3. Barrow GW, Saha S: Menstrual irregularity and stress fractures in collegiate female distance runners. Am J Sports Med 16:209–16, 1988.
4. Brownell KD, Rodin J: Prevalence of eating disorders in athletes. In Brownell, KD, Rodin J, Wilmore JH (eds): Eating, Body Weight and Performance in Athletes. Disorders of Modern Society Philadelphia, Lea & Febiger, 1992, pp. 128–43.
5. Brownell KD, Steen SN, Wilmore JH: Weight regulation practices in athletes: analysis of metabolic and health effects. Med Sci Sports Exerc 6:546–60, 1987.
6. Carbon RJ: Exercise, amenorrhea and the skeleton. Br Med Bull 48:546–59, 1992.
7. Clark N: How to help the athlete with bulimia: Practical tips and case study. Int J Sport Nutr 3:450–60, 1993.
8. Drinkwater BL, Bruemer B, Chesnut CH: Menstrual history as a determinant of current bone density in young athletes. JAMA 263:545–8, 1990.
9. Dueck CA, Matt KS, Manore MM: Treatment of athletic amenorrhea with a diet and training-intervention program. Int J Sport Nutr 6:24–40, 1996.
10. Dueck CA, Manore MM, Matt KS: The role of energy balance in athletic menstrual dysfunction. Int J Sport Nutr 6:165–90, 1996.
11. Dugowson CE, Drinkwater BL, Clark JM: Nontraumatic femur fracture in oligomenorrheic athlete. Med Sci Sports Exerc 23:1323–5, 1991.
12. Eisenman PA, Johnson SC, Benson JE: Coaches Guide to Nutrition and Weight Control. 2nd edition. Champaign, Ill, Leisure Press, 1990.
13. Erp-Bart AMJ, et al: Energy inntake and energy expenditure in top female gymnasts. In Brinkhosts et al (eds): Children and Exercise XI. Champaign, Ill, University Park Press, 1985, pp 218–23.
14. Fogelholm M: Effects of bodyweight reduction on sports performance. Sports Med 4:249–67, 1994.
15. Fogelholm GM, Koskinen R, Laakso J: Gradual and rapid weight loss: effects on nutrition and performance in male athletes. Med Sci Sport Exerc 25:371–7, 1993.
16. Garfinkel PE, Garner DM, Goldbloom DS: Eating disorders implications for the 1990s. Can J Psych 32: 624–31, 1987.
17. Housten ME, Marrin DA, Green HJ: The effect of the rapid weight loss on physiological functions in wrestlers. Physician Sportsmed 9:73–8, 1981.
18. Hsu LKG: Eating Disorders. New York, Guilford Press, 1990.
19. Ingjer F, Sundgot-Borgen J: Influence of body weight reduction on maximal oxygen uptake in female elite athletes. Scand J Med Sci Sports 1:141–6, 1991.
20. Johnson MD: Tailoring, the preparticipation exam to female athletes. Physician Sportsmed 20:61–72, 1992.
21. Jonnavithula S, Warren MP, Fox RP, et al: Bone density is compromised in amenorrheic women despite return of menses: A 2-year study. Obstet Gynecol 81:669–74, 1993.
22. Katz JL: Some reflections on the nature of the eating disorders. Int J Eat Disord, 4:617–26, 1985.
23. Katz JL: Eating disorders in women and exercise. In Shangold MM, Mirken G (eds): Physiology and Sports Medicine. Philadelphia, FA Davis, 1988, pp 248–63.
24. Klinzing JE, Karpowicz W: The effect of rapid weight loss and rehydration on a wrestling performance test. J Sports Med Phy Exerc 26:149–56, 1986.
25. Lloyd T, Triantafyllou SJ, Baker A, et al: Women athletes with menstrual irregularity have increased musculoskeletal injuries. Med Sci Sports Exerc 18:374–9, 1986.
26. Mansfield MJ, Emans SJ: Growth in female gymnasts: should training decrease during puberty? Pediatrics, 122:237–240, 1993.
27. Mitchell JE: Bulimia Nervosa. Minneapolis, University of Minnesota Press, 1990.
28. Nelson ME, Fisher EC, Catsos PD, et al: Diet and bone status in amenorrheic runners. Am J Clin Nutr 43: 910–6, 1986.
29. Nielsen S, Møller-Madsen S, Isager T, et al: Standardized mortality in eating disorders—a qualitative summary of previously published and new evidence. J Psychosom Res 44:413–34, 1998.
30. Otis CL: Exercise associated amenorrhea. Clin Sports Med 11(2):351–62, 1992.
31. Otis CL ACSM position stand on the female athlete triad. Med Sci Sports Exerc 295: ppi–ix, 1997.
32. Prior JC, Vigna YM, McKay DW: Reproduction for the athletic woman: New understandings of physiology and management. Sports Med 14:190–9, 1992.
33. Rigotti NA, Neer RM, Skates SJ, et al: The clinical course of osteoporosis in anorexia nervosa: longitudinal study of cortical bonemass. JAMA 263:1133–8, 1991.
34. Rosenvinge JH, Gresko RB: Do we need a prevention model for eating disorders? Eat Disord J Treatm Prevent 5:110–8, 1997.
35. Ryan R: Management of eating problems in athletic settings. In Bronwell KD, Rodin J, Wilmore JH (eds): Eating, Body Weight and Performance in Athletes: Disorders of Modern Society. Philadelphia, Lea & Febiger, 1992, pp 344–60.
36. Sacks MH: Psychiatry and sports. Ann Sports Med 5: 47–52, 1990.
37. Shangold MM, Rebar RW, Wentz AC, et al: Evaluation and management of menstrual dysfunction in athletes. JAMA 263:1665–9, 1990.
38. Sundgot-Borgen J: Prevalence of eating disorders in female elite athletes. Int J Sport Nutr 3:29–40, 1993.
39. Sundgot-Borgen J: Risk and trigger factors for the development of eating disorders in female elite athletes. Med Sci Sports Exerc 4:414–9, 1994.
40. Sundgot-Borgen J, Larsen S: Nutrient intake and eating behavior of female elite athletes suffering from anorexia nervosa, anorexia athœtica and bulimia nervosa. Int J Sport Nutr 3:431–42, 1993.

41. Sundgot-Borgen J, Klungland M: The female athlete triad and the effect of preventive work. Med Sci Sports Exerc Suppl 5:181, 1998.

42. Szmuckler GI, Eisler, I, Gillies C, Hayward ME: The implications of anorexia nervosa in a ballet school. J Psychiatr Res 19:177–81, 1985.

43. Thompson, RA, Trattner-Sherman R: Helping Athletes with Eating Disorders. Champaign, Ill, Human Kinetic, 1993.

44. Theintz MJ, Howald H, Weiss U. Evidence of a reduction of growth potential in adolescent female gymnasts. J Pediatr 122:306–13, 1993.

45. Torstveit G, Rolland, CG, Sundgot-Borgen J: Pathogenic weight control methods and self-reported eating disorders among male elite athletes. Med Sci Sports Exerc Suppl 5:181, 1998.

46. Webster S, Rutt R, Weltman A: Physiological effects of weight loss regimen practiced by college wrestlers. Med Sci Sports Exerc 22:229–33, 1990.

47. Welch PK, Zager KA, Endres J: Nutrition education, body composition and dietary intake of female college athletes. Physician Sportsmed 15:63–74, 1987.

48. Wilmore JH: Eating and weight disorders in female athletes. Int J Sports Nutr 1:104–17, 1991.

Chapter 26

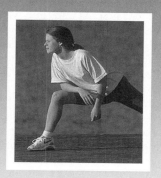

Osteoporosis

Joseph M. Lane, M.D.

Osteoporosis is a common human bone disease characterized by decreased bone mass, microarchitectural deterioration, and fragility fractures.[32] Based on World Health Organization (WHO) criteria, it is estimated that 15% of postmenopausal Caucasian women in the United States and 35% of women over 65 years have frank osteoporosis.[48] Up to 50% have some degree of low bone density in the hip. One out of every 2 Caucasian women will experience an osteoporotic fracture at some point in her lifetime. There is also a significant, although lower risk for men and non-Caucasian women to sustain osteoporotic fractures. The fragility fractures create a significant economic burden, requiring over 400,000 hospital admissions and 2.5 million physician visits per year.

BASIC PATHOPHYSIOLOGY

The hallmark of osteoporosis is deficient bone density and connectivity.[16,33] The trabecular bone in an osteoporotic individual will be thinner and have evidence of osteoclastic resorption, leading to disconnectivity of the trabecular elements. Thus, there is both a deficiency of bone and a deterioration of the structural integrity of the underlying trabecular bone. Since trabecular bone has a much greater surface area, it is more readily affected by osteoporosis than the cortical bone.[24,25] The major elements of cortical osteoporosis are tunneling resorption, which can lead to stress fractures, and the gradual thinning of the cortical thickness. The body expands the cortical dimensions away from the epicenter of the bone with aging. A 10% outward shift of bone can compensate for a 30% decrease bone mass in terms of torque and bending, but it will not compensate for axial loading.

Both males and females increase their bone mass with growth, achieving a peak bone mass by approximately the age of 25. Thereafter, bone will be lost at a slow rate for men. Women will have a precipitous drop around menopause, but after 60 their rate of loss will mirror that of men. In both sexes, there will be a significant decrease in total mass as the age of 80 is approached, leading to a marked deficiency in mechanical properties. The total strength of a given bone is related to the mass plus distribution, the relative ratio of trabecular to cortical bone, and the structural integrity and connectivity of the trabecular and cortical elements.

Bone is a living tissue.[24] It is constantly undergoing remodeling and repair. The process involves the identification of a molecular structural defect, followed by osteoclastic resorption and the development of a pit. The pit is then repaired with an ingrowth of osteoblasts replacing the bone. After the age of 40 osteoblastic repair rarely restores the original bone surface, and, thus every remodeling cycle leaves a small deficit of bone. The discrepancies in the rates of bone resorption and formation lead to the gradual onset of osteoporosis.

A bone has a number of functions.[16,24] Besides providing structural support for the human, it is the main mineral bank in which 98% of the calcium is maintained, and is also the site at which blood elements are produced. The body has developed a complex system for maintaining calcium levels within the body, of which bone is the major mineral repository. Vitamin D, a fat-soluble vitamin that is used in the absorption of calcium, is produced in the skin following exposure to sunlight. One hour of sunlight on a Caucasian face is sufficient to produce 400 units of vitamin D. This store of vitamin D lasts for approximately 2 months. Inadequate exposure to sunlight such as occurs in housebound individuals will compromise this process; the presence of a high amount of melanin in the skin also decreases production of vitamin D. Vitamin D is converted in the liver to 25-hydroxy (25-OH) vitamin D, an inactive metabolite having a 3-day half-life. When the calcium level is low, parathyroid hormone

(PTH) is released, stimulating the kidney to convert the inactive metabolite to the active component, $1\alpha,25$-dihydroxy (1α, 25-OH) vitamin D. The kidney retains calcium from the glomerular filtrate. The $1\alpha,25$-OH vitamin D sets off a process in the intestine that leads to calcium absorption from the gut. This active metabolite, in conjunction with PTH, ultimately leads to the resorption of bone. The cessation of this process results in an elevation of serum calcium. Children are extremely capable of squeezing calcium out of their diet. However, as one gets older, the efficiency of the intestinal system decreases. In the elderly, calcium deficiency often will preferentially lead to resorption of bone rather than increased absorption of calcium from the intestine.

Peak bone mass is achieved at the approximate age of 25.[35] Individuals who become deficient in calcium during their adolescence will not achieve this peak bone mass. Bone mass accretion depends not only on the presence of adequate calcium in the diet but also on an adequate array of all essential nutritional components. Calcium requirements depend on the age. A dairy portion (milk, cheese, ice cream, or yogurt) contains about 250 to 300 mg calcium. Children require at least 800 mg/day, or 3 dairy portions. Adolescents between the ages of 10 and 25, during which peak bone mass is achieved, require 1300 mg/day. Premenopausal women require at least 1000 mg/day if normally menstruating, and 1200 to 1500 mg/day if oligomenorrheic or amenorrheic. Pregnant and lactating women should obtain 1500 mg/day; postmenopausal women, 1500 mg/day. Patients recovering from a major fracture require 1500 mg/day. Studies have demonstrated that 95% of young women at the age of 13 have a calcium intake inadequate to achieve peak bone mass.

A number of drugs can decrease calcium retention; a short illustrative list would include isoniazid, corticosteroids, heparin, tetracycline, furosemide, and caffeine. Drugs that are detoxified in the liver by the P450 hydrolase system are similarly suspect, particularly barbiturates.

Hormonal status is critical in achieving and maintaining peak bone mass.[24] Women who are premenopausal lose about 0.3% of their skeleton per year, unless they are taking in normal physiologic amounts of calcium, in which case their bone density may be maintained. At the point of menopause, or for every year that they are amenorrheic or oligomenorrheic, they will lose approximately 2% of their skeleton. Women who are postmenopausal by surgical hysterectomy and oophorectomy or who are postmenopausal

naturally will demonstrate equal amounts of bone loss when matched by years. Thus, the clock for rapid bone loss is set at the time when women loose normal menstrual cycles.

Bone is extremely sensitive to exercise and mechanical load.[33] In a no-load situation, bone will be lost; low loads will maintain bone; and high loads will remodel bone to withstand the new loads. Very high loads will lead to bone failure. Impact exercise programs and activities such as walking and dancing, when coupled with calcium supplementation, have been demonstrated in the elderly to maintain or increase the appendicular skeleton. Exercise alone is inadequate to protect the spinal trabecular bone in perimenopausal women, though it can clearly decrease the rate of loss as compared to nonexercising individuals. Overexercise leading to amenorrhea is another issue: in one study by Drinkwater,[9,10] amenorrheic women runners had a bone mass of 1.12 g/cm^2, while eumenorrheic women who ran half the distance of the amenorrheic subjects, but maintained normal menstrual cycles, had a bone mass of 1.30 g/cm^2 and statistically had more bone. In fact, women who did not exercise but maintained normal nutrition and menstrual cycles had a higher bone mass (1.2 g/cm^2) than amenorrheic exercising women. This demonstrated that exercise to the point of developing amenorrhea is deleterious. Male long-distance runners may also have low bone mass, however, it is not clear whether their hormonal state is the cause or just a co-marker. Most investigators believe that, in women, just re-establishing menstrual cycles without adequate calories and nutrition is an ineffective approach to treatment.

DEFINITION AND DIAGNOSIS

Low bone mass is the single most accurate predictor for increased fracture risk.[32,44] An individual whose bone mass is 1 standard deviation below that of his or her peers will have a 1.9 increased risk of spine fracture and a 2.4 increased risk of hip fracture. These data are based on a slowly changing skeletal state. Acute changes in bone status, such as produced by steroids, can profoundly weaken bone before the bone mass reflects that finding. Bone mass is determined by a number of methods. The technique utilized by most bone centers is dualbeam x-ray absorptiometry, or DEXA. In this technique, the amount of mineralized tissue within an aerial section of the spine or hip bone is analyzed and expressed as grams per square centimeter.

Comparisons can be made both to the individual's peer group and to a young, normalized adult population with peak bone mass. If the individual is more than 1.5 standard deviations below her age-corrected peer group (derived from cross-sectional studies in the United States), that individual may have a secondary cause of osteoporosis that needs further evaluation. By comparing the individual's bone mass to the young-adult peak bone mass, an assessment of fracture risk may be made.[48.] The WHO have established guidelines for the diagnosis of osteoporosis using bone density criteria for postmenopausal women. If the individual is within 1 standard deviation, she is considered normal. If she is between 1 and 2.5 standard deviations below peak bone mass, she is considered to have significant bone loss and is osteopenic. If she is more than 2.5 standard deviations below peak bone mass, she is considered frankly osteoporotic, and if she has a fragility fracture, plus the above criteria for osteoporosis, she is defined as severely osteoporotic.

There are other methods to determine bone mass besides DEXA. These include single-energy x-ray absorptiometry and peripheral dual-energy absorptiometry. These measure bone density in the forearm and finger, and sometimes the heel. A second method is radiographic absorptiometry (RA). This technique is based on a standard roentgenogram or a computer-generated roentgenogram of the hand with a metal wedge in the field as a reference standard. Quantitative computed tomography, or QCT, measures the trabecular bone at several sites, but is most commonly used to evaluate the area of the spine. It uses 20 times the radiation used by DEXA and is less precise. Ultrasound densitometry assesses the heel, patella, tibia, and peripheral sites. It measures several properties of bone. The peripheral sites are at a distance from the hip and the spine and results have only a 0.75 correlation, at best, with central readings. In addition, their ability to recognize change with pharmacologic treatment is much more limited. These methods are excellent for identifying people who are osteopenic and at risk. However, for treatment and follow-up of individuals, at this time the consensus is to utilize DEXA.

Bone density determination[15,36] is indicated for both perimenopausal and postmenopausal women to determine their need for hormonal replacement therapy as well as other antiosteoporotic therapies, for individuals with known metabolic bone disorders and on agents that affect bone mass, for individuals with low-energy fractures, and for individuals with a high number of osteoporotic risk factors. It is also indicated to monitor efficacy of treatment. Table 26–1 lists the National Osteoporosis Foundation (NOF) guidelines for bone density assessment. (A discussion of bone density assessment recommendations for the young, premenopausal female athlete is addressed further in Chapter 24.)

Although bone density indicates the current skeletal mass, it does not provide information about metabolic activity.[13] Several markers have been developed for both bone formation and bone resorption. Bone formation markers are bone-specific alkaline phosphatase and osteocalcin. Markers for bone resorption are based on collagen breakdown products released into the urine. The most common products measured are the N- and C-telopeptides of the collagen cross-link area, and the pyridinium cross-links, pyridinoline and deoxypyridinoline. They provide an extremely sensitive determination of the rate of bone turnover.

RISK FACTORS

Osteoporosis is associated with a number of risk factors, some modifiable and some nonmodifiable.[1,32] Major nonmodifiable factors are a personal history of a fracture as an adult or a history of a fracture in a first-degree relative. Minor factors include Caucasian race, advanced age, female sex, dementia, and poor health or frailty. The potentially major modifiable risk factors are current cigarette smoking and low body weight. The minor modifiable factors are estrogen defi-

Table 26-1. National Osteoporosis Foundation Guidelines for BMD Assessment

All women ≥ 65 years of age (regardless of risk factors) willing to accept treatment if BMD is low
All postmenopausal women < 65 years of age who have at least one additional risk factor for osteoporosis
All postmenopausal women who present with fractures
All women who are considering therapy for osteoporosis and for whom BMD test results would influence this decision
All women who have been receiving hormone replacement therapy for a prolonged period

BMD, bone mineral density
(Adapted from the National Osteoporosis Foundation Physician's Guide to Prevention and Treatment of Osteoporosis. Belle Mead, NJ: Excerpta Medica, Inc., 1998.)

252 V General Medical Conditions

ciency, low calcium intake, alcoholism, impaired eyesight, recurrent falls, inadequate physical activity, and poor health and frailty. Health and frailty can be related to either modifiable or nonmodifiable factors.

There is clear evidence of genetic predisposition. The most commonly identified at-risk individuals are those with blond or red hair, fair skin, and freckles, those with easy bruisability, hypermobility, and small build, and those with adolescent scoliosis.[24] The major risk factors—low body weight and recent loss of bone, a personal history of fracture (or a history of fracture in a first-degree relative), and smoking—are independent of bone mass and their presence should raise the level of concern regardless of bone mass.

MEDICAL EVALUATION

Over 65% of individuals presenting with a compression fracture will be asymptomatic.[16,24] Most individuals will lose up to 2 inches in height due to narrowing of the discs. Any height loss greater than 2 inches should raise suspicion of a compression fracture. The etiology of fractures includes trauma, a localized lesion, and underlying metabolic bone disease. The predominant forms of underlying metabolic bone disease other than osteoporosis are bone marrow abnormality, endocrinopathy, and osteomalacia.

It is important for the clinician to assess for secondary causes of osteoporosis. A low hemoglobin level, an elevated erythrocyte sedimentation rate, and an abnormal serum protein electrophoresis indicate multiple myeloma. About 1% of osteoporotic patients will present with this disorder. Other than an early menopause, the major endocrinopathies are Cushing's disease, type I diabetes, hyperparathyroidism, and hyperthyroidism. Primary Cushing's disease is rare. Iatrogenic Cushing's disease, widespread because of steroid use in the treatment of a number of medical disorders, can easily be determined by history. Osteoporosis associated with type I diabetes is worse in individuals whose diabetes is poorly controlled. Hyperparathyroidism is best identified by an intact PTH assay and an elevation in urinary N-telopeptide. Most patients are diagnosed prior to the development of kidney stones and brown tumors. Hyperthyroidism is often associated with overmedication and is a common presenting state for women of large girth with osteoporosis. Studies indicate that these individuals frequently are hypothyroid and take enhanced

doses of thyroid medication in part to control their weight. They can best be identified with a suppressed thyroid stimulating hormone assay. Osteomalacia is commonly seen in the urban northern United States. At New York Presbyterian Hospital, 8% of individuals with hip fractures have frank osteomalacia, and well over 40% have some degree of malnutrition. The common laboratory abnormalities associated with osteomalacia are low calcium, low phosphate, low 1,25-OH vitamin D, high alkaline phosphatase, and high PTH levels. Alkaline phosphatase will rise with a fracture, but it takes 5 days to do so. Therefore, a patient presenting with a fragility fracture and an initial high alkaline phosphatase level should be suspected of having an underlying high-turnover-state disease until proven otherwise. Once the secondary causes of osteoporosis have been eliminated, the clinician is then left with a decision as to whether this osteoporosis is high- or low-turnover type. Use of bone marker assessment, especially the N-telopeptide level, is a helpful tool for assessment of bone turnover.

CONSEQUENCES OF HIP FRACTURES

Hip fractures are the single most debilitating problem in osteoporotic individuals, with two thirds of the osteoporotic money spent on the treatment of this disorder.[32] Sixteen percent of women will experience a hip fracture in their lifetime. It leads to a 15% increase in mortality within the first year, with over 70% of survivors having a profound diminution of function. Men have less than 50% the risk of women for hip fracture but twice the mortality rate.

The load:fracture ratio correlates well with the femoral bone density.[17,21] Therefore, decreased bone density profoundly increases the risk of weakening the bone. An older individual's femur has half the strength and one third the energy of absorption of a younger individual's femur. Given a direct blow to the trochanter, a young individual still has 20% more bone strength than the injury will impart. However, an elderly individual has passed her mechanical capability by 50%. Studies have demonstrated that over 90% of fractures occur from falls and that the majority of falls occur in the home between the hours of noon and 6:00 o'clock. Falls, in fact, are the primary risk factor for hip fracture. The reason that there are fewer fractures than falls is that most individuals do not directly injure their trochanter. A fall to the side would increase the risk of a hip fracture by

5.7-fold in an ambulatory patient and 21.7-fold in a nursing-home patient. A decrease of 1 standard deviation of bone density will increase the femoral neck fracture risk about 2.4-fold. The lower the body mass index, the higher the risk of a hip fracture, particularly in the nursing-home population. Thus, a fracture is related to the initial bone mass, the type of trauma to the bone, the ability to repair a microfracture before it becomes a macrofracture, the quality of the bone, the general health of that individual, and the age of the individual.

CLASSIFICATION OF OSTEOPOROSIS

Riggs and Melton have defined two forms of osteoporosis.[42] Type 1 osteoporosis occurs more frequently in women than men (6:1 female:male ratio). It is related to estrogen deficiency associated with vertebral fractures and is usually unrelated to calcium intake. Type 2 osteoporosis occurs in an elder age group, around 75 years, and affects women more frequently than men (2:1 female:male ratio). Trabecular and cortical bone hip fractures are the main fracture types and are related to a lifetime of inadequate calcium intake. It was presumed by Riggs and Melton that type 1 osteoporosis involved a high rate of turnover and type 2 a low rate, although we now recognize that both types can occur in either age group. In high-turnover osteoporosis, there is an increased number and depth of osteoclastic resorption sites and the normal osteoblast effort during repair is insufficient to totally fill the defect. In low-turnover osteoporosis, there are normal or decreased osteoclastic resorption sites, however, the osteoblasts are markedly inactive. This could be brought on by genetic predisposition, senility, or drugs such as methotrexate. An excellent way to differentiate these types of osteoporosis is to measure the collagen breakdown products.[13,25,40,43] In the N-telopeptide assay, the normal range is from 5 to 65 nmol bone collagen equivalents/mmol creatinine, depending on the assay. However, in the normal, younger individual, most N-telopeptide values are below 35. Values over 35 indicate a higher resorption rate. Those values on the order of 50 or higher reflect a relative increase in this resorption rate.

THERAPY

A number of agents have been developed to treat postmenopausal osteoporosis. The antiresorptive agents include estrogens, selective estrogen receptor modulators, calcitonin, and bisphosphonates. The bone stimulators, which include the fluorides, PTH, and PTH-related peptide analogs, are experimental and have not been approved by the US Food and Drug Administration (FDA), but demonstrate excellent promise. Table 26-2 lists the guidelines established by the NOF for initiation of pharmacologic treatment in postmenopausal women.

The general recommendation for all patients with osteoporosis as well as for osteoporosis prevention, is to ensure intake of physiologic levels of calcium and vitamin D, follow an appropriate exercise program, and adopt measures to prevent falls. Cessation of smoking and excessive alcohol consumption is also recommended.

Calcium and Vitamin D

Calcium and vitamin D will decrease bone resorption and will mineralize the osteoid. Studies have demonstrated that patients on calcium and vitamin D have a lower fracture rate.[3] Particularly in the nursing home aged populations, calcium and vitamin D have been associated with a 18% decrease in the hip fracture rate and lower mortality. Calcium and vitamin D alone, however, usually will not prevent spinal bone loss in the postmenopausal woman not on estrogen therapy (or other antiresorptive agent). Conversely, the appendicular skeleton will be

Table 26-2. National Osteoporosis Foundation Guidelines for Initiation of Pharmacologic Treatment in Postmenopausal Women for Fracture Reduction

Initiate therapy to reduce fracture risk
   In women with BMD T-scores below -2.0 SD in the absence of risk factors
   In women with BMD T-scores below -1.5 SD if other risk factors are present
   In women with vertebral or hip fractures
   In high risk women (age > 70 years with multiple risk factors) without BMD testing

BMD, bone mineral density; SD, standard deviations; T-score, comparison to young-adult peak bone mass
(Adapted from The National Osteoporosis Foundation Physician's Guide to Prevention and Treatment of Osteoporosis. Belle Mead, NJ: Excerpta Medica, Inc., 1998.)

maintained in all age groups, in premenopausal women and in the elderly who obtain physiologic levels of calcium and vitamin D and get adequate exercise. There are various forms of calcium preparations; the most commonly utilized are calcium carbonate and calcium citrate.[21] Calcium carbonate requires gastric acidity to be dissolved. A number of medications, including H_2-blockers, may interfere with this function. Calcium citrate, on the other hand, is easily digested in all age groups and gastric conditions. Calcium carbonate may increase the risk of kidney stones; calcium citrate actually is protective.[28] It is therefore recommended that calcium citrate be used in the elderly, in individuals with dyspepsia, in men with a history of kidney stones, and in states of constipation. Magnesium is usually readily available in the normal diet, however, in compromised individuals, alcoholics, or the malnourished, magnesium may be beneficial. Moreover, magnesium does lead to amelioration of constipation, and, therefore, 400 to 500 mg magnesium over the course of the day may prevent constipation in calcium takers.

Estrogen

Estrogen has been the most studied and utilized agent for prevention of osteoporosis.[11,12,18,24,25,28,29,34,49] Estrogen will decrease bone resorption in most women. Estrogen in the dose equivalent of 0.625 mg conjugated equine estrogen will increase bone mass approximately 2% per year. Once estrogen is stopped the individual will lose 2% per year, and 7 years after terminating estrogen all benefit will have been lost. Estrogen has been shown at this dose to decrease fractures at all sites by approximately 50% in prevention studies. Recent studies indicate that a lower dosage of 0.3 mg/day was unable to demonstrate within 3 years any efficacy in terms of hip fracture prevention. There are a lack of estrogen treatment studies demonstrating fracture reduction in postmenopausal women with established osteoporosis.

Estrogen has a number of nonosseous effects, in particular, a favorable modification of the cardiolipid profile, which has been thought to represent a decreased risk for heart disease, although a recent study has shown no evidence of a decreased risk of atherosclerosis.[22] In another study of postmenopausal women with established coronary artery disease, starting estrogen was associated with an increase in myocardial infarction and stroke the first year, whereas those already on estrogen had a favorable pattern of coronary events after several years.[23]

Estrogen has been shown to have several benefits. It protects teeth from migration. It improves the genitourinary physiology, leading to fewer urinary tract infections and better vaginal function. There is some suggestion that it may ameliorate, to some degree, the effects of Alzheimer's disease and improve cognitive functioning.

Estrogen is associated with an increased risk of thrombophlebitis. It increases the risk for uterine cancer if taken without progesterone.[24] The concomitant use of progesterone can eliminate this increased risk.

Although there is still controversy regarding the risk of breast cancer with estrogen therapy, some studies have shown a 2.5% annual increased rate of breast cancer over the baseline, which translates after 10 years to a 30% increased risk. Thus, rather than having a 10% to 11% risk of getting breast cancer, the rate will rise to 14% to 15%.[11,18] The Women's Health Initiative study was terminated early (in 2002) for those women with a uterus receiving conjugated equine estrogen plus medroxyprogesterone acetate daily, due to a 26% increased risk of invasive breast cancer. Risks and benefits of estrogen therapy need to be discussed thoroughly with patients.

There are various forms of estrogen. Most are beneficial forbone, and equivalent doses of 0.625 mg conjugated equine estrogen are effective in about 80% of patients. After a woman has been on estrogen for 3 to 6 months, the N-telopeptide assay should have declined by 30% (if initially elevated.) If it has not, the dosage of estrogen should be reconsidered. Very thin individuals may require a higher dose. To avoid breast engorgement, a slow buildup of estrogen may be required. A combination of estrogen with 2.5 mg progestin continuously can provide effective bone protection and avoid provoking menstrual cycles in the postmenopausal woman. There may be breakthrough bleeding within 5 years of menopause, however, when one starts beyond that point, breakthrough bleeding is less common. Postmenopausal women on estrogen require yearly follow-up by their gynecologist or primary care physician, as well as yearly mammograms. The combination of estrogen with other antiresorptive agents may be synergistic.

Selective Estrogen Receptor Modulators

A series of estrogen-like agents have been developed. Tamoxifen, originally utilized as an antiestrogen, particularly in the management of breast cancer, has been shown to have a positive effect on bone mineral density.[39] The benefit of tamoxifen in maintaining bone mass in post-menopausal women is 70% of that of estrogen. Tamoxifen has not been used therapeutically in osteoporosis because 70% of women taking tamoxifen developed significant post-menopausal symptoms and their risk of uterine cancer increased. This observation gave rise to the development of selective estrogen receptor modulators, or SERMs.[8,14,19] These agents compete for the estrogen-binding site and seem to function more like estrogens at bone. The bone cells consider these agents to be estrogens. They work quite effectively as antiresorptive agents. They can alter the lipid profile, particularly the total and low-density lipoprotein cholesterol, but effect very little change in the high-density lipoprotein fraction. They cause no uterine hypertrophy and the risk of uterine cancer appears to be no more than normal. Data suggest that there is a significantly decreased risk of invasive breast cancer in postmenopausal women during 3 years of treatment with raloxifene.[7] A trial is now underway comparing the preventive action against breast cancer of SERMS and tamoxifen. Raloxifene, which was the first SERM released, has been shown to decrease the risk of vertebral fracture by approximately 40% to 50%, however, no protective effect has been reported in the hip. An increase in bone mass, similar to the improvement related to estrogen, has been found.

Raloxifene is associated with hot flashes and leg cramps, and with an increased risk of thrombophlebitis comparable to that with estrogen. A number of oncologic groups are now considering the use of raloxifene for protection against breast cancer and it is currently being studied for this indication.

Calcitonin

Calcitonin is a nonsex, nonsteroid hormone that may play a role in development. It has been used effectively in the treatment of hypercalcemia and Paget's disease.[25,26,37,38,41,45] Studies have demonstrated that subcutaneous calcitonin, about 100 units/day, has been effective in treating osteoporosis. A more recently introduced nasal form (Miacalcin), at a dosage of 200 units/day, increases bone mass in the spine, comparable to estrogen, and decreases spinal fractures by 37% independent of known major pretreatment risk factors.[4–6] No benefit with regard to hip fractures has been seen after 5 years. Lower and higher doses of calcitonin may not be as effective in protecting against fractures. Whether this is a peculiarity of the study is not clear. Calcitonin does have the added benefit of providing some analgesia. It has been utilized in painful osteoporotic fractures and does not interfere with fracture healing. Two percent of patients complain of dry nares. Nasal ulcerations are less common, but have been reported.

Bisphosphonates

Bisphosphonates are pyrophosphate analogs in which the linking central oxygen molecule is replaced by a long carbon chain with either hydroxyl groups or a nitrogen group.[2,24–27,46,47] The bisphosphonates are nondegradable analogs. They function by binding to the resorbing surface of the osteoclast and act as a nondegradable shield. If absorbed by the osteoclast they inhibit the osteoclast function secondarily. Short-chain bisphosphonates, such as in chlondronate, lead to interference with the ATP pathway. The long-chain nitrogen-containing bisphosphonates, such as alendronate, interfere with the prenylation of the lipid membrane. Bisphosphonates have a very low bioavailability and less than 1% is absorbed by the oral route. The first FDA-approved bisphosphonate, alendronate (Fosamax), has been demonstrated to increase bone mass in both the hip and the spine. It decreases the risk of all fractures by approximately 50% after 1 year of treatment.[2,6,27] Regardless of the degree to which the bone mass is enhanced, there is an equal protection for all patients against fractures. Those individuals with the lowest bone mass gain and those with the highest bone mass gain had equal protection against fractures by alendronate, suggesting an improvement in bone quality. Alendronate has been associated with esophageal irritation, with up to 30% of individuals developing esophagitis. However, in carefully controlled studies, the rate seems to be comparable to that in the placebo group. The slow buildup of alendronate (1 10-mg pill the first week, 2 pills the second, etc., until once-daily dosing is reached) has led to significantly increased compliance at the Hospital for Special Surgery. A lower dosage of alendronate, of 5 mg/day, is used as a preventive dose. The higher dosage (10 mg/day) is utilized successfully for the treatment of osteoporosis. A weekly regimen of alendronate (70 mg once/week) has also proven effective and may improve compliance. Alendronate, in animal studies, appears to inhibit osteolysis around prostheses and at higher doses has been used quite effectively in the treatment of Paget's disease.

A series of new bisphosphonates that have been approved for the treatment of Paget's disease are awaiting approval as osteoporotic agents; these include intravenous agents that have very short administration times as well as a number of new oral agents. Risedronate (Actinol), an oral agent recently approved by the FDA for the treatment of postmenopausal osteoporosis,[20] has been demonstrated to reduce fractures in the spine[20] and hip.[31] Risedronate is approved for both prevention and treatment of postmenopausal osteoporosis in the dosage of 5 mg/day. A weekly dosage of 35 mg/week is also available to enhance compliance. Risedronate has less gastrointestinal side effects compared to alendronate. Other new bisphosphonates will most likely be utilized in this arena within the next few years.

Pamidronate has not been approved for treatment of osteoporosis, but has been used to treat metastatic disease or hypercalcemic malignancy and Paget's disease. Intravenous doses of pamidronate have been quite effective in treating osteoporosis in this population group, but fracture reduction has not been demonstrated.

The first-generation bisphosphonate, etidronate, when used at 400 mg daily for 2 weeks followed by 11 weeks of just calcium and multivitamin and an intermittent cyclical etidronate regimen, has been reported to decrease fractures and increase bone mass.[46,47] The etidronate regimen does not have the gastric side effects associated with alendronate. However, the regimen is best followed for only 2 years, as long-term use may produce a mineralization defect. A question remains about its utility, and the FDA has never approved it for use in osteoporosis in the United States, although it is used in Canada and some other countries.

Combination Therapy

Combination agents have been tried. Ninety percent of individuals who have failed on estrogen therapy have improved when switched to alendronate. Twenty percent of individuals who failed on alendronate therapy, when switched to estrogen have shown improvement. Recent studies indicate that, in terms of bone density augmentation, a combination of alendronate and estrogen is superior to estrogen alone.[30] There were no data on fracture healing protection.

Therapeutic Considerations

Estrogen, raloxifene, alendronate, risedronate, and calcitonin (injectable and nasal spray) have been approved for the treatment of osteoporosis. The FDA has also approved low-dose alendronate and raloxifene for the prevention of osteoporosis. None of these have been labeled specifically for men, however, the bisphosphonates and calcitonin have been quite effective in men. Drug choices, including calcium and vitamin D, have to be made very carefully in premenopausal women. If menstrual cycles become slightly irregular, birth control pills or an estrogen/progesterone combination may be prescribed, although the benefits on bone in amenorrheic and osteopenic premenopausal women are controversial. Alendronate or risedronate have not been approved for premenopausal women, particularly pregnant women or those considering pregnancy due to potential teratogenicity, and long half life of these medications. However, when pregnancy is not an issue, alendronate has been used by a number of centers, either in a low dose for prevention or in a higher dose for treatment, as well as risedronate for prevention or treatment. As mentioned, both are available as a weekly dosage regimen.

At this time, there is no approved method for bone stimulation, but trials of fluoride, PTH, and PTH-related peptides are under way. PTH, however, will most likely be approved soon, for osteoporosis treatment.

A treatment algorithm has been proposed by the National Osteoporosis Foundation based on fracture risk.[36] In an individual with a known vertebral fracture, they recommend the use of estrogen, raloxifene, a bisphosphonate, or calcitonin, depending on the patient's bone density and risk profile. If there is no fracture and the patient is not willing to consider pharmacologic treatment, the recommendations are calcium, vitamin D, exercise, and smoking cessation. In the patient older than 65 years who is willing to consider treatment, bone density should be measured and treatment given depending on the level of bone loss. In the osteoporotic patient, osteoporosis is treated, and in the osteopenic patient, preventive measures are indicated. If the patient is less than 65 and has positive risk factors, particularly low body weight, personal history of fracture or a fracture in a first-degree relative, or a history of smoking, a bone density determination is indicated. If the patient has no risk factors, then calcium, exercise, and smoking cessation are recommended. Bone mineral density determination can be taken after menopause as an optional measure.

PREVENTION

In summary, recommendations to prevent osteoporosis include physiologic calcium according to the patient's age and vitamin D, on the order of 400 to 800 IU/day. Appropriate exercise should be carried out, including impact and strengthening exercises and balance training. Effective balance training programs include impact and weight-bearing sports, dancing, and tai chi. A study done at Emory University demonstrated a 47% decrease in falls in subjects practicing tai chi. In addition to risk factors, the major determinants of the status of osteoporosis, are apparent bone mass as determined by bone density examination, and bone marker levels, notably the collagen breakdown products, which demonstrate bone turnover. Treatments should be based appropriately. Finally, because hip fractures are the major consequence of osteoporosis, efforts should be directed at preventing osteoporosis and, equally important, preventing falls. The triad of disordered eating, amenorrhea, and osteoporosis in the female athlete is discussed elsewhere in this book. Clearly, preventing osteoporosis is much preferred to treating it. The young woman with the potential for developing osteoporosis should be counseled aggressively so this can be prevented from becoming a reality. With the tools to diagnose, prevent, and treat osteoporosis now readily available, morbidity from this potentially debilitating disorder should significantly decrease.

References

1. Bernstein DS, Sadowsky N, Hegsted DM, et al: Prevalence of osteoporosis in high- and low-fluoride areas in North Dakota. JAMA 198:499–504, 1966.
2. Black DM, Cummings SR, Karpf DB, et al: Randomized trial of effect of alendronate on risk of fracture in women with existing vertebral fractures. Lancet 348:1535–41,1996.
3. Chapuy MC, Arlot ME, Duboeuf F, et al: Vitamin D3 and calcium to prevent hip fractures in the elderly woman. N Engl J Med 327:1637–42, 1992.
4. Cardona JM, Pastor E: Calcitonin versus etidronate for the treatment of postmenopausal osteoporosis: a meta-analysis of published clinical trials. Osteoporos Int 7:165–174, 1997.
5. Chestnut CH, Silverman SL, Andriano K, et al: Salmon calcitonin nasal spray reduces the rate of new vertebra fractures independently of known major pre-treatment risk factors: accrued 5 year analysis of the PROOF study. Bone 23(5) Abstract T373:S290, 1998.
6. Cummings SR, Black DM, Thompson DE, et al: Effect of alendronate on risk of fracture in women with low bone density but without vertebral fractures. JAMA 280:24:2077–82, 1998.
7. Cummings SR, Eckert S, Krueger KA, et al: The effect of raloxifene on risk of breast cancer in postmenopausal women: results from the MORE randomized trial. JAMA 281:2189–97, 1999.
8. Delmas PD, Bjarnason NH, Mitlak BH, et al: Effects of raloxifene on bone mineral density, serum cholesterol concentrations, and uterine endometrium in postmenopausal women. N Engl J Med 337:1641–47, 1997.
9. Drinkwater BL, Nilson K, Chestnut CH III, et al: Bone mineral content of amenorrheic and eumenorrheic athletes. N Engl J Med 311:277–81, 1994.
10. Drinkwater BL, Nilson K, Ott, S, Chestnut CH III: Bone mineral density after resumption of menses in amenorrheic athletes. JAMA 256:380–2, 1986.
11. Eriksen EF, Kassem M. Lang Dahl B: European and North American experience with HRT for the prevention of osteoporosis. Bone 19:197S–83S, 1996.
12. Ettinger B: Overview of estrogen replacement therapy: a historical perspective. Proc Soc Exp Biol Med 217: 2–5, 1998.
13. Eyre DR: Bone biomarkers as tools in osteoporosis management. Spine 22:24S:17S–24S, 1997.
14. Fuleihan GE: Tissue-specific estrogens—the promise for the future. N Engl J Med 337:1686–7, 1997.
15. Genant HK, Engelke K, Fuerst T, et al: Noninvasive assessment of bone mineral and structure: State of the art. J Bone Miner Res 11:707–30, 1996.
16. Glaser DL, Kaplan FS: Osteoporosis: Definition and clinical Presentation. Spine 22:24S:12S–6S, 1997.
17. Greenspan S, Myers E, Maitland L, et al: Fall severity and bone mineral density as risk factors for hip fracture in ambulatory elderly. JAMA 271:128–33, 1994.
18. Grodstein F, Stampfer MJ, Colditz GA, et al: Postmenopausal hormone therapy and mentality. N Engl J Med 336:1769–75, 1997.
19. Gustafsson JA: Raloxifene: magic bullet for heart and bone? Nat Med 4:152–3, 1998.
20. Harris ST, Watts NB, Genant HK, et al: Effects of risedronate treatment on vertebral and nonvertebral fractures in women with postmenopausal osteoporosis: a randomized clinical trial. JAMA 282:1344–52, 1999.
21. Hayes WC, Myers ER, Morris JN, et al: Impact near the hip dominates fracture risk elderly nursing home residents who Fall. Calcif Tissue Int. 52:192–8, 1993.
22. Herrington DM, Reboussin DM, Brosnihan KB, et al: Effects of estrogen replacement on the progression of coronary-artery atherosclerosis.N Engl J Med 343(8): 522–9, 2000.
23. Hulley S, Grady D, Bush T, et al: Randomized trial of estrogen plus progestin for secondary prevention of coronary heart disease in postmenopausal women. JAMA 280:605–13, 1998.
24. Lane JM: Osteoporosis: Medical prevention and treatment. Spine 22(24S):32S–7S, 1997.
25. Lane JM, Riley EH, Wirganowizc PZ: Osteoporososis: Diagnosis and treatment. J Bone Joint Surg (Am) 78: 618–32, 1996.
26. Lane JM, Riley EG, Wirganowizc PZ: Letter on osteoporosis. J Bone Joint Surg Am 79:634–35, 1997.
27. Leiberman UA, Weiss SR, Broll J, et al: Effect of oral alendronate on bone mineral density and the incidence of fracture in postmenopausal osteoporotic women. N Engl J Med 333:1437–43, 1995.
28. Levine B, Rodman JS, Weinerman ST, et al: Effect of calcium citrate supplementation on urinary calcium oxalate saturation in female stone formers: Implications

for prevention of osteoporosis. Am J Clin Nutr 60: 592–6, 1994.

29. Lindsay R, Bush TL, Graly D, et al: Therapeutic controversy. Estrogen replacement in menopause. J. Clin Endocrinol Metab 81:3829–38, 1996.

30. Lindsay R, Cosman F, Lobo R, et al: Addition of alendronate to ongoing hormone replacement therapy in the treatment of osteoporosis: a randomized, controlled clinical trial. J Clin Endocrinol Metab 84: 3076–81, 1999.

31. McClung MR, Geusens P, Miller PD, et al: Effect of risedronate on the risk of hip fracture in elderly women. N Engl J Med 344:333–40, 2001.

32. Melton LJ III: Epidemiology of spinal osteoporosis. Spine 22:24S:2S–11S, 1997.

33. Myers ER, Wilson SE: Biomechanics of osteoporosis and vertebral fracture. Spine 22(24S):25S–31S, 1997.

34. Nadelovitz M: Estrogen therapy and osteoporosis: Principles and practice. Am J Med Sci 313:2–12, 1997.

35. National Institutes of Health (NIH): Consensus development panel on optimal calcium intake. Optimal calcium intake. JAMA 272:1945–8, 1994.

36. National Osteoporosis Foundation: Osteoporosis: Physician's Guide to Prevention and Treatment of Osteoporosis. NOF, Washington, DC. Belle Mead, NJ, Excerpta Medica, 1998.

37. Overgaard K, Riis BJ, Christiansen C: Effect of calcitonin given intra-nasally on early postmenopausal bone loss. Bone Miner J 299:477–9, 1989.

38. Overgaard K, Hansen NA, Jensen SB, et al: Effect of calcitonin given intranasally on bone mass and fracture rates in established osteoporosis. A dose response study. Bone Miner J 305:556–61, 1992.

39. Powels TJ, Hicklish T, Kanis JA, et al: Effect of tamoxifen on bone mineral density measured by dual energy x-ray absorptiometry in healthy premenopausal and postmenopausal women. J Clin Oncol 18:78–84, 1995.

40. Price CP, Thompson PW: The role of biochemical tests in the screening and monitoring of osteoporosis. Ann Clin Biochem 32:244–60, 1995.

41. Reginster JY: Calcitonin. Curr Opin Orthop 7:31–4, 1996.

42. Riggs BL, Melton LJ III: Involutional osteoporosis. N Engl J Med 326:357–62, 1992.

43. Sanchez CP, Salusky IB: Biochemical markers in metabolic bone disease. Curr Opin Orthop 5:43–9, 1994.

44. Seeger LL: Bone density determination. Spine 22: 24S:49S–57S, 1997.

45. Silverman SL: Calcitonin. Am J Med Sci 313:13–16, 1997.

46. Storm T, Thamsborg G, Steinich T, et al: Effect of intermittent cyclical etidronate therapy on bone mass and fracture rate in women with postmenopausal osteoporosis. N Engl J Med 32:1265–71, 1990.

47. Watts NB, Harris ST, Genant HK, et al: Intermittent cyclical Etidronate treatment of postmenopausal osteoporosis. N Engl J Med 323:73–9, 1990.

48. World Health Organization: Assessment of fracture risk and its application to screening for postmenopausal osteoporosis: Report of a WHO study group. World Health Organization Tech Rep Ser. 843:1–129, 1994.

49. Yaffe K, Sawaya G. Lieburburg I, Grady D: Estrogen therapy in postmenopausal women. Effects on cognitive function and dementia. JAMA 279:688–95, 1998.

Chapter 27

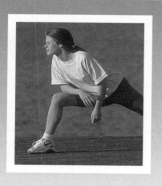

Anemia

Suzanne S. Hecht, M.D.

Is anemia a special concern for the female athlete? It appears that prevalence of anemia in female athletes is similar to the prevalence in the general female population.[3,72,88,90] Despite a similar prevalence, identifying anemia in the female athlete is crucial, since even mild anemia can adversely affect performance and well-being.

This chapter will not attempt to cover all of the causes of anemia, but rather will focus on hematologic issues that have special importance to the health and performance of the female athlete.

DIAGNOSING ANEMIA

The approach to evaluating the female athlete for anemia is similar to that used for the general patient population. The diagnosis of anemia is based on a lower than normal hemoglobin concentration. To narrow the extensive differential diagnosis, anemia is classified on either red blood cell (RBC) morphology or RBC kinetics. The classification of anemia based on RBC morphology involves the measurement of the mean corpuscular volume (MCV). The MCV represents the mean volume of the RBCs. This classification includes three groups: microcytic (MCV < 80 fL), normocytic (MCV 80 to 100 fL), and macrocytic (MCV > 100 fL). Table 27-1 lists a complete differential diagnosis of anemia based on RBC morphology. The RBC kinetic classifi-

cation system includes 3 divisions: (1) increased RBC destruction, (2) decreased RBC production, and (3) blood loss.

HEMOGLOBIN CONCENTRATIONS FOR FEMALE ATHLETES

As will be discussed further, mildly low hemoglobin concentrations in athletes do not necessarily represent true anemia. Determining when an athlete with borderline low hemoglobin concentrations is truly anemic is sometimes difficult for the clinician. Guidelines have been published for hemoglobin concentrations in athletes. In the elite female aerobic athlete, a hemoglobin concentration less than 11.0 g/dL has a 95% chance of being a true anemia. For moderate female exercisers, a hemoglobin concentration of less than 11.5 g/dL is probably abnormal.[34]

PSEUDOANEMIA

Even in the face of normal iron studies, athletes, particularly endurance-trained athletes, often have relatively lower hemoglobin concentrations than nonathletes. This phenomenon goes by many terms, including sports anemia, athlete's anemia, runner's anemia, postexercise anemia, and pseudoanemia.[4] Eichner suggests that the most appropriate term for this phenomenon is

Table 27-1. Classification of Anemia According to RBC Morphology

MICROCYTIC (< 80 fL)	NORMOCYTIC (80–100 fL)	MACROCYTIC (> 100 fL)
Iron deficiency	Iron deficiency	Megaloblastic anemia
Anemia of chronic disease	Anemia of chronic disease	Reticulocytosis
Lead poisoning	Acute blood loss	Sideroblastic anemia
Hemoglobinopathy	Hemolysis	Acute blood loss
Thalassemia	Chemotherapy/drugs	Hypothyroidism
Sideroblastic anemia	Aplastic anemia	Chronic liver disease
		Hemolytic anemia
		Chemotherapy
		Aplastic anemia
		Down syndrome

pseudoanemia, since this term accurately reflects that this is a false anemia caused by an expanded plasma volume and not a true anemia.[37] True anemia is defined as an absolute decrease in RBC mass, while pseudoanemia is defined as a relative (dilutional) decrease in the hemoglobin concentration.[104]

Physiology

It is known that routine exercise will expand plasma volume by as much as 6% to 25%, depending on the frequency and intensity of the exercise.[4] The more frequent and intense the exercise, the greater the degree of plasma volume expansion. Weight and coworkers showed that the mean plasma volume of female distance runners is 18.1% greater than that of controls.[117] Increased plasma volume is thought to be an early adaptation in response to the decrease in plasma volume seen during and immediately following exercise. Initially, plasma volume decreases 8% to 20%[37,122] with exercise, due to 3 factors: (1) increased capillary hydrostatic pressure, (2) formation of osmotically active tissue metabolites, and (3) sweating. Capillary hydrostatic pressure increases as a result of increased mean arterial pressure and venule muscle contractions. Osmotically active tissue metabolites, such as lactic acid, are formed during exercise and draw fluid out of the vascular system and into the tissues. Plasma volume is also lost in the form of sweat.[37]

In order to restore blood volume, the body conserves water and salt by releasing renin, aldosterone, and vasopressin, and increases plasma oncotic pressure by increasing levels of plasma proteins. Convertino and coworkers found a 9-fold increase in plasma renin activity and vasopressin, and a steady increase in plasma albumin levels in response to exercise.[22] A study that included 20 female runners found significant increases in total protein levels and albumin immediately following the completion of a marathon. At 24 and 48 hours after exercise, total protein levels remained significantly increased.[116] Relative anemia from plasma volume expansion appears to resolve 3 to 5 days following exercise.[3]

The physiologic benefit of an expanded plasma volume with resultant lower hemoglobin concentration remains unclear. The fact that increasing hemoglobin concentrations with RBC transfusions results in improved performances speaks against a physiologic advantage of an expanded plasma volume.[13,18] Proposed benefits from an expanded plasma volume include decreased viscosity and increased cardiac output from increased stroke volume.[87,105]

IRON-DEFICIENCY ANEMIA

Normal Iron Values

Iron is an essential trace element. Most, 33% or more, of the body's iron is found in hemoglobin, which is critical for transporting oxygen to tissues. One gram of hemoglobin contains 3.4 mg of iron. Smaller amounts of iron are found in myoglobin, cytochromes, and other iron-containing enzymes. In adult females, the average total amount of iron in the body is approximately 2 to 3 g. The typical distribution of iron in a 60-kg female is 1.9 g in hemoglobin, 0.125 g in myoglobin, 0.008 g in heme enzymes, and 0.3 g of iron stores.[100] Less than 0.1% of total body iron is found in the plasma.

Excess iron is stored in the bone marrow, liver, and spleen as either ferritin or hemosiderin. Men store approximately 1 g of iron, while women store an average of 0.3 g.

The recommended daily allowance (RDA) for iron in menstruating females is 15 mg/day, while premenarchal and postmenopausal females need only 10 mg/day. Adolescent and adult females in the United States average a daily iron intake of only 11.8 to 12.7 mg/day, which falls short of the RDA.[1]

Remember that the RDA for vitamins and minerals is based on the general population and is not specific for athletes. Whether female athletes have a daily iron requirement higher than the RDA is unknown.

Iron Metabolism

The typical American diet contains 6 mg of iron per 1000 calories. Under normal conditions, 0.6 to 2 mg of the total dietary iron is absorbed per day.[89] Iron is absorbed from the gut in the duodenum and proximal jejunum. Absorption is regulated at the level of the intestinal mucosal cell and is dependent on the following factors: the amount of dietary iron consumed, iron bioavailability, iron stores, the need for RBC production, and dietary components that either inhibit or improve iron absorption.

The absorbed iron is handled in 1 of 3 ways: it is sent to the bloodstream for transport, it is retained inside the mucosal cell bound to ferritin, or it is excreted back into the gut lumen. Iron retained inside the mucosal cell is eventually lost when the mucosal cell is sloughed. Generally, less than 4% of the absorbed iron is transferred to the bloodstream.[100] This iron binds to apotransferrin, a plasma protein, for bloodstream transport to the tissues. Apotransferrin can bind 2 ferric molecules.

Once apotransferrin is fully saturated with iron, it is called transferrin. Upon reaching the cell, transferrin binds to a receptor and is internalized within the cell. Inside the cell, iron is released from transferrin and apotransferrin is recycled and released back into the plasma. The released iron then combines with protoporphyrin to form the heme portion of hemoglobin, which is essential for normal erythropoiesis. Iron not needed for erythropoiesis is stored as ferritin or hemosiderin. Reticuloendothelial cells and hepatocytes store iron as ferritin.[12]

Ferritin

Prior to the development of serum ferritin testing, it was difficult to diagnose depleted iron stores. The most sensitive and specific test for depleted iron stores was and still is a bone marrow biopsy stained for hemosiderin granules. The clinical utility of a bone marrow biopsy is limited by the fact that it is an invasive and uncomfortable procedure. Serum ferritin testing provides an attractive alternative, since it generally reflects the amount of stored iron that is available for hemoglobin synthesis.[24] A serum ferritin of 1 μg/L is equal to approximately 10 mg of iron stores.[12] The clinical test for serum ferritin is a radioimmunoassay, which measures the transport of iron, bound to apoferritin, between reticuloendothelial cells and hepatocytes.

Normal serum ferritin values range from 12 to 135 μg/L, although there is variability as to what is considered the low end of normal. Classically, a value less than 12 μg/L is considered to reflect depleted iron stores. Some authors consider values less than 20 μg/L as diagnostic of low iron stores, while others use 30 to 35 μg/L as their cutoff.[83]

When interpreting serum ferritin values, it is important to remember that ferritin is an acute-phase reactant. Ferritin increases in response to infection, inflammation, cancer, liver disease, and exercise. Lampe and coworkers found that serum ferritin in female runners remains significantly elevated up to 3 days after a marathon,[61] although another study of female runners found no change.[116] If iron deficiency in an athlete is suspected, it is probably best to test the serum ferritin level 2 to 3 days after the last workout to avoid a falsely elevated value.[104]

Iron Losses

In women, less than 1 mg of iron is lost daily from the urine (0.45 mg/day), skin (0.24 mg/day), and gastrointestinal tract (0.1 mg/day).[48] Average iron loss from menses accounts for an additional 0.5 to 1 mg/day, although this amount may be highly variable, with some women losing as much as 2.8 mg/day. Women on oral contraceptive pills tend to have less menstrual bleeding (approximately 50% less), thus decreasing the monthly loss of iron. Intrauterine devices (IUDs) almost double the menstrual blood loss.[47] The estimated loss of iron during pregnancy and lactation is 500 to 700 mg.[12]

It takes about 20 mg of iron per day to synthesize new hemoglobin to replace the hemoglobin lost in the normal breakdown of RBCs. As RBCs are degraded, transferrin binds and transports some of the released iron back to the bone marrow for erythropoiesis. A small percentage (about 10%) of normal RBC breakdown occurs in the plasma, with either haptoglobin or hemopexin binding the hemoglobin to prevent it from being lost in the urine.[89]

Incidence

Iron-deficiency anemia (IDA) is the most common type of anemia in the United States and also worldwide. Women are at greater risk of suffering from IDA, since they generally consume fewer calories than do men and also lose additional iron during menstruation. The incidence of IDA in the general female population is 5% to 6%. Cook and coworkers reported the prevalence of IDA to be 2.6% in premenopausal women and 1.9% in postmenopausal women, based on body iron estimates from data collected in the second National Health and Nutrition Examination Survey.[23] Up to 25% of healthy college females have depleted iron stores as determined by bone marrow staining.[101]

Although it is common for female athletes to have low iron stores,[61,69,86] as a group, female athletes do not appear to be at greater risk than the general female population.[3,20,37,90,96,118] In the United States, 21% of women have low ferritin levels.[23] The prevalence of low ferritin levels in female athletes ranges from 3% to 50%,[28,95,107,119] with higher values found in distance runners.[28,49,94]

Studies in male athletes suggest that intense exercise leads to low serum ferritin levels, increased iron absorption and excretion, and depleted liver and bone marrow iron stores.[83] Whether exercise, by itself, is a risk factor for the development of IDA in female athletes remains to be seen. A longitudinal study of female college field-hockey players found that serum ferritin levels steadily decreased over 3 years.[29] A decrease in serum ferritin and hemoglobin was seen in synchronized swimmers over 2 seasons of training.[91] In contrast, 12 weeks of endurance training in previously inactive women caused no change in serum ferritin levels.[11] Sixteen female swimmers demonstrated no significant differences between preseason and postseason hemoglobin, ferritin, total iron-binding capacity (TIBC), and transferrin saturation values.[65]

Low dietary iron intake due to inadequate caloric consumption is associated with IDA in female athletes, just as it is in the general female population. Since a typical American diet contains 6 mg of iron per 1000 kcal, a female athlete who consumes 2000 kcal/day would only get 12 mg of iron from her diet, leaving her short of the minimal RDA of 15 mg/day. A review of 22 dietary intake studies revealed that 88% of aerobic and 100% of anaerobic elite female athletes were not meeting the minimal recommended caloric intake. Iron intake, in addition to zinc, magnesium, calcium, and vitamin B_{12}, was below the RDA, particularly in female athletes consuming less than 2000 kcal/day.[31] A study that included 10 elite female ballet dancers demonstrated that they were deficient in caloric consumption and iron intake.[21] Only female basketball players met the RDA for iron intake in a study that included female athletes in karate, handball, and middle- and long-distance running.[85]

Female distance runners have been reported to have poor iron status.[28,52,61,82] A nutritional survey of 51 female marathoners, who had qualified to compete in the United States Olympic Trials, found that 43% of these athletes were not meeting the RDA for iron intake. The mean serum ferritin level was 22.8 ± 2.7 ng/mL and more than 35% of the runners had a serum ferritin below 12 ng/mL, suggesting low iron stores. Forty-seven percent were taking iron supplements.[28]

In addition to the quantity of iron ingested, the source of iron intake is also an important variable in preventing IDA.[65,106,107] Female runners who minimize meat in their diet are more likely to be iron deficient than female athletes who include meat in their diet.[106]

Thus, female athletes who restrict caloric intake and limit meat from their diet appear to be at greater risk of developing IDA than female athletes who consume adequate calories and include meat in their diets.

Diagnosis

Iron deficiency anemia (IDA) is commonly divided into 3 stages based on laboratory evaluation (Table 27-2). Stage I represents a depletion of iron stores without anemia. Laboratory evaluation reveals only a low serum ferritin level. The hemoglobin concentration, TIBC, percent transferrin saturation, and serum iron concentration will be normal. The TIBC measures the total amount of transferrin, whether or not iron is bound to it (apotransferrin + transferrin = TIBC). The proportion of transferrin that has iron bound to it is measured by the percent transferrin saturation. Stage II represents impaired erythropoiesis secondary to impaired hemoglobin synthesis. The liver increases transferrin synthesis in order to transport more iron to the bone marrow. This results in an increased TIBC. In addition to a low serum ferritin level, the percent transferrin saturation and the serum iron concentration may be decreased. The hemoglobin concentration will still be normal. Stage III IDA is diagnosed when the hemoglobin concentration drops below normal. All iron studies will be abnormal, including an elevated TIBC and low ferritin, percent transferrin saturation, and serum iron concentration.[25] At this stage, a peripheral blood smear reveals RBCs that are smaller (microcytic) and paler (hypochromic) than normal.

IDA and Performance

Stage III IDA decreases maximal oxygen uptake.[99] The degree of maximal oxygen uptake decrease depends on the degree of anemia. Since the maximum amount of oxygen that can combine with hemoglobin is 1.34 mL, a female athlete with a hemoglobin concentration of 13 g would have an oxygen-carrying capacity of 17.4 mL versus 14.7 mL in a female athlete with a hemoglobin concentration of 11 g.

Table 27-2. IDA Stages and Laboratory Values

IDA STAGE	HB	MCV	FERRITIN	TIBC	% TRANSFERRIN SATURATION	SERUM IRON CONCENTRATION	IRON MARROW STORES	FREE ERYTHROCYTE PROTOPORPHYRIN LEVEL
I	nl	nl	↓	nl	nl	nl	↓ or absent	nl or ↑
II	nl	nl or ↓	↓	↑	nl or ↓	nl or ↓	↓ or absent	↑
III	↓	↓	↓	↑	↓	↓	absent	↑

nl, normal.

Animal[26,27,73] and human[18,39,44,114] studies have demonstrated that stage III IDA results in decreased performances. Davies and coworkers showed a 50% reduction in whole-animal maximal oxygen consumption (VO_2max) and a 90% lower maximal endurance capacity in anemic, iron-deficient rats as compared to controls.[27] In humans, female laborers with hemoglobin concentrations between 11.0 and 11.9 g/dL have approximately 20% less exercise tolerance compared to those with a hemoglobin concentration above 13 g/dL.[44]

As discussed above, research has clearly demonstrated that anemia diminishes performance. Are athletes with stage I or II IDA at risk of compromised athletic performance? Animal studies showing impaired performance in iron-deficient, nonanemic rats provided the first evidence that iron depletion in the face of a normal hemoglobin concentration may be detrimental to athletic performance.[26,27,40] Finch and coworkers studied nonanemic, iron-deficient rats (stage I or II IDA) and found diminished treadmill performance, decreased mitochrondrial cytochromes, and reduced rates of oxidative phosphorylation. Treadmill performance normalized within 4 days of iron therapy.[40]

Although animal studies suggested a relationship between stage I or II IDA and endurance performance, human studies have demonstrated mixed results.[17,42,57,59,60,67,69,81,94,123] In a classic study by Celsing and coworkers, an iron-deficient, nonanemic state was induced in 9 males by repeated phlebotomy and correction of the anemia with RBC transfusion. Exercise in this state did not decrease endurance, maximal aerobic power, or muscle enzyme activity.[17] Additionally, a recent review of 10 studies, which evaluated the relationships between serum ferritin levels, iron supplementation, and endurance performance, concluded that low serum ferritin without anemia is not associated with diminished aerobic performance.[45] Overall, it appears that stage I or II IDA in humans does not decrease endurance performance, but further research in this area is warranted.

Etiology

In general, IDA may develop from inadequate iron intake, decreased iron absorption, increased iron requirements, or blood loss. Additional and more specific exercise-related causes have been proposed for athletes. These include footstrike hemolysis, gastrointestinal and urinary tract blood loss, and iron losses in sweat.

Footstrike Hemolysis

It has been known for over a century that repeated footstrikes on hard surfaces can cause blood loss via intravascular hemolysis. This condition was first termed *march hemoglobinuria* because of reports of soldiers urinating red to brown-black urine following long marches. March hemoglobinuria, also known as footstrike hemolysis or runner's macrocytosis, has been proposed as a theoretical cause of chronically depleted iron stores in distance runners.[33]

The pathophysiology of footstrike hemolysis is thought to involve the premature destruction of older RBCs from the repeated trauma of the feet striking the ground.[4,33,34,75] The hemoglobin released from the RBCs is bound to the plasma protein, haptoglobin. Haptoglobin transports the hemoglobin to the liver, where the iron is recycled. If the amount of RBC hemolysis exceeds the capacity of haptoglobin to bind the released hemoglobin, then the hemoglobin and its iron is excreted by the kidney. It is difficult to totally deplete haptoglobin, since it regenerates quickly,[111] but haptoglobin levels may be chronically depressed in elite endurance athletes.

Footstrike hemolysis may have a genetic component. There is evidence to suggest that athletes prone to footstrike hemolysis may have a defect in the proteins of the RBC membrane.[5] Swimmers have been shown to exhibit hematologic findings consistent with mild intravascular hemolysis. This finding calls into question the extent of the relationship of external impact forces to intravascular hemolysis.[102]

Other factors, such as increased RBC fragility with exercise, increased body temperature shortening the RBC life span, and increased susceptibility of older RBC to hemolysis, have been suggested as potential causes of footstrike hemolysis.[4]

A peripheral blood smear of an athlete with footstrike hemolysis will reveal a mild macrocytosis and reticulocytosis. She may have a low serum haptoglobin level, in addition to the changes seen on the peripheral blood smear.[33] Marathon running has been shown to increase hemolysis, but this is generally mild and the amount of iron lost is probably clinically insignificant.[37] Eichner suggests that runners should try to minimize footstrike hemolysis, since it may adversely affect performance by suppressing the degree of RBC mass increase seen in elite runners.[37]

Treatment of footstrike hemolysis includes wearing quality running shoes with good padding, running on softer terrain, decreasing mileage, correcting gait abnormalities, and reducing weight.[34] Iron replacement therapy for footstrike hemolysis is not recommended,[37] unless there is evidence of IDA.

Gastrointestinal Tract Blood Loss

Chronic gastrointestinal tract blood loss is thought to contribute to the low ferritin levels seen in some distance runners. Exercise-related gastrointestinal tract bleeding may arise from the upper or lower gastrointestinal tract and may be acute or chronic. The degree of blood loss may range from clinically insignificant amounts to life-threatening acute blood loss. During exercise, blood is shunted away from the gastrointestinal tract, in order to provide more blood flow to the exercising muscles. Splanchnic blood flow has been shown to decrease by 70% to 80% when exercising at maximal oxygen capacity.[14] Mean gut transit time was significantly increased in 15 female runners during and following a marathon as compared to prerace times.[62] The pathophysiology of exercise-related gastrointestinal tract bleeding appears to be the result of ischemia. Ischemia results from decreased blood flow to the gastrointestinal tract, secretion of vasoactive substances, and mechanical stress.[14]

Fisher and coworkers reported a case series of 4 distance runners with IDA and exercise-related gastrointestinal tract bleeding. No identifiable gastrointestinal pathology was found, despite extensive evaluation.[41] Two of the more commonly seen pathologies are hemorrhagic gastritis and colitis, which tend to be mild and self-limited.[77] Nevertheless, severe ischemic colitis requiring surgical intervention has been reported in a female distance runner[8] and 2 Ironman triathletes.[38] Also bear in mind that exercise-related gastrointestinal tract bleeding may be a signal of an underlying gastrointestinal disease, such as inflammatory bowel disease, infection, or malignancy.

It appears that gastrointestinal tract bleeding in runners is fairly common, with a reported incidence of 8% to 83% of runners having guaiac-positive stools after completing a marathon.[41,70,97,109] Stewart and coworkers found a significant increase in fecal hemoglobin concentrations in 20 of 24 (83%) runners postrace (10 to 42.2 km) as compared to prerace values.[109] The study by McCabe and coworkers, which included female runners, found that 17.5% of female runners had guaiac-positive stools premarathon and 31.6% had guaiac-positive stools postmarathon.[70] In contrast, 15 female runners showed no significant difference in fecal hemoglobin concentrations before and after a marathon.[62]

Most exercise-related gastrointestinal tract bleeding is probably self-limited, as suggested by the results of a study by McMahon and coworkers. In 6 marathon runners who developed guaiac-positive stools after a marathon, 5 of the stool samples reverted to normal within 72 hours.[74]

The intensity of exercise may play a role in the degree of exercise-related gastrointestinal tract blood loss.[79,92,97] Thirty-five ultramarathoners had an 85% incidence of guaiac-positive stools following a 100-mile race. The ultramarathoners with guaiac-positive stools experienced more nausea, diarrhea, bloating, and abdominal cramping during the race.[7] A study of 20 male triathletes, followed during intense training, prerace taper, and postcompetition, found that gastrointestinal tract blood loss appeared to be related to exercise intensity.[97] Fecal iron excretion in 45 distance runners was found to increase 3- to 4-fold during a period of intense training versus no training. Iron excretion in urine and sweat was also measured and was negligible, suggesting that iron losses via the gastrointestinal tract play a greater role in the depletion of iron stores in runners.[80] Finally, Robertson and coworkers showed that walking for 37 km on 4 consecutive days had no effect on gastrointestinal tract blood loss.[92]

Urinary Tract Blood Loss

Exercise-related hematuria, also known as *athlete's pseudonephritis*, appears to be a common and benign condition. It may also be a source of chronic blood loss in some athletes. Siegel and coworkers analyzed urine samples from 50 healthy, male marathoners 48 hours before and immediately following the completion of a marathon. Additional urine samples were collected 24, 48, and 72 hours after completion of the marathon. All prerace samples were normal. The incidence of hematuria was 18%, with 9 of the immediate postrace samples showing at least microscopic hematuria. Eight of the 9 samples reverted to normal within 48 hours of race completion.[103] A study of 45 ultra-long-distance runners, males and females, found 24.4% had hematuria following race completion.[54]

The mechanism of exercise-related hematuria has not been fully elucidated, but footstrike hemolysis[36,75] and bladder trauma[10] are 2 of the most frequently cited causes. A cystoscopic evaluation of 18 runners with microscopic hematuria, following the completion of at least a 10,000-meter run, revealed bladder contusion as the cause of hematuria in 8 cases.[10] Other proposed causes of exercise-related hematuria include dehydration, mechanical kidney trauma, renal vascular ischemia, hypoxic injury to the kidney, release of potentially renal toxic myoglobin from muscles, and nonsteroidal anti-inflammatory drugs (NSAIDs).[53]

Although hematuria in the athletic population is generally a common and self-limited phenomenon, there are case reports of bladder cancer presenting as exercise-related hematuria.[78] Persistent microscopic hematuria or gross hematuria requires a complete urologic evaluation.

Iron Loss in Sweat

The amount of iron lost in sweat is minimal and is probably clinically insignificant. Brune and coworkers studied 11 males, using meticulous methodology to avoid skin cell contamination, to determine the amount of iron lost in sweat. They found that the amount of iron lost was 22.5 μg of iron per liter of sweat. Based on these findings, in order to lose 1 mg of iron, one would have to sweat 50 L.[16] Waller and Haymes reported that estimating iron losses during exercise based on resting sweat iron concentration may actually overestimate the amount of iron lost during prolonged exercise or exercise performed in a hot environment, but is accurate for 1 hour of exercise in a thermoneutral environment. They also found that females lose less sweat iron at rest and during exercise than males.[115]

Symptoms

The symptoms of IDA relate to the acuteness and severity of the anemia. Although the general population is likely to be asymptomatic with a chronic, mild anemia, an athlete may notice diminished performances and fatigue.[90] Decreased exercise tolerance may be the first and only symptom of mild IDA in an athlete.

The differential diagnosis of decreased exercise tolerance in an athlete is extensive. IDA should be considered in any athlete who complains of decreased exercise tolerance. Historical information and/or symptoms consistent with IDA and its underlying cause should be sought by the clinician. A recent history of NSAID use, bloody stools, abdominal discomfort, heavy menses, restricted caloric intake, and a vegetarian diet are examples of causes of IDA. Therefore, a thorough history, review of systems, and physical examination is essential.

Treatment

The treatment of IDA depends on the cause of the anemia. Once the cause has been determined, cause-specific medical interventions, dietary changes, and iron replacement therapy can begin. For example, oral contraceptive pills, iron supplementation, and dietary modifications may be the best treatment combination for a female athlete with IDA caused by poor dietary intake and heavy menstrual bleeding.

Dietary Modifications

Dietary modifications can improve the amount and type of iron ingested and absorbed from the diet. Iron from meat sources (heme iron) is more readily absorbed than iron from grains and vegetable sources (nonheme iron). The intestine is able to absorb 34% of heme iron as compared to only 5% of nonheme iron. A study of the dietary intake of 37 elite and 17 amateur athletes, representing 5 different sports, revealed that more than 90% of iron intake was from nonheme sources.[19] Spodaryk and coworkers found a positive correlation between serum ferritin level and the amount of heme iron intake in female athletes and controls.[107] Iron supplements and meat ingestion were both found to protect hemoglobin and iron stores in previously sedentary women during a 12-week exercise program, but meat ingestion was more effective.[66]

Certain dietary components, such as tannins (found in tea and coffee), carbonates, oxalates and phosphates, decrease nonheme iron absorption by complexing with iron. Various acids and sugars can improve nonheme iron absorption by forming complexes that are more soluble. Additionally, ascorbic acid (vitamin C) improves iron absorption by changing it from the ferric form to the ferrous form, which has better intestinal solubility.

In a state of iron deficiency, iron absorption from the diet is increased to 3 to 4 g/day with approximately 30% being transported to the bloodstream.[100] Unfortunately, the increased absorption and transport of dietary iron is insufficient to replace the body iron stores in a patient with a mild IDA. Supplemental iron should be recommended for these patients, in combination with enhanced dietary iron intake.

Iron Supplements

Typically, 150 to 200 mg of elemental iron per day is recommended for iron replacement therapy. Iron preparations are available in oral and injectable forms. Oral iron supplements vary in the amount of elemental iron that they contain. Ferrous gluconate contains 12% elemental iron, while ferrous sulfate and ferrous fumarate have 20% and 33% elemental iron, respectively.[12] Thus, a dose of 325 mg ferrous sulfate taken 3 times per day provides 195 mg of elemental iron, while the same dose of ferrous gluconate provides 108 mg of elemental iron.

Failure to see improved ferritin and hemoglobin concentrations after 1 to 2 months of iron replacement therapy should prompt the health care provider to review the diagnosis and consider reasons why the patient may be resistant to oral iron replacement therapy. Common reasons include poor compliance owing to side effects, continuing blood loss, and poor absorption. Iron-deficient athletes have been shown to absorb less iron than iron-deficient controls.[32] Certain medications, including antihistamines, antacids, proton pump inhibitors and tetracyclines, are known to reduce iron absorption.[64] A study of female distance runners suggested that zinc deficiency contributes to IDA.[84]

Compliance with oral iron replacement therapy may be limited by gastrointestinal side effects. Nausea, constipation, diarrhea, and abdominal distress are common complaints. Gradually increasing the dose, decreasing the dosing frequency to 2 times per day, trying a different iron salt preparation and/or taking the supplement with food may help minimize these side effects. Note that taking iron supplements with food may decrease the amount of iron absorbed. Sustained-release or enteric-coated iron preparations do not dissolve well in the stomach, thereby limiting their absorption.

Oversupplementing with iron can be dangerous once the iron binding capacity is full, since free iron is toxic. Excessive iron stores have been associated with an increased risk of myocardial infarction in Finnish men.[98] Iron supplements should be avoided in people with hereditary iron metabolism disorders, such as hemochromatosis.

If oral iron replacement therapy fails, then parenteral iron therapy may be warranted. The severity of iron deficiency is generally not an indication for parenteral iron treatment, since the route of delivery does not affect the time needed for the RBCs to incorporate the iron. It is indicated for malabsorption and noncompliance due to gastrointestinal side effects. Intravenous injection of iron dextran is preferred, owing to the variable absorption seen with intramuscular injection. The total iron deficit should be calculated and may be replaced at a rate of 100 mg/day.[64]

Total milligrams of iron to be replaced[6] is equal to (normal hemoglobin concentration − patient's hemoglobin concentration) × wt (kg) × 2.21 + 1000.

Adverse reactions to injectable iron dextran, such as anaphylaxis and seizures, can occur. Therefore, it is recommended that a small test dose (0.5 mL) be given. If the test dose is well tolerated, then the full dose may be administered.

Treatment of the Nonanemic Athlete With a Low Ferritin Level

Iron supplementation in nonanemic athletes with low serum ferritin levels is controversial. Research generally supports that a low ferritin level in a nonanemic athlete does not adversely affect performance.[45,72] This suggests that iron supplementation has limited value in the nonanemic athlete (stage I or II IDA). Conversely, others recommend supplementation to avoid development of anemia, which is known to diminish performance. Supplementation also corrects the upregulated gut absorption of iron that occurs when iron stores are low. Gut absorption of metal ions is not specific just for iron, but also increases the absorption of other ions such as lead.

It is also pertinent to recognize that a hemoglobin concentration in the low normal range may represent a lower than normal hemoglobin concentration for that individual. It is helpful to compare to a previous hemoglobin concentration, if one is available. Another strategy is to recommend oral iron therapy for 1 or 2 months. At the end of the treatment period, the ferritin and hemoglobin concentrations are rechecked. If the hemoglobin concentration has risen, then a relative anemia from iron deficiency was present.[45]

Ashenden and coworkers studied the hematologic responses of 6 female basketball players over 3 weeks to a 100-mg intramuscular injection of iron. The basketball players had normal hemoglobin concentrations and a mean serum ferritin level of 35.6 ± 15.6 µg/L. The results showed no change in blood counts, iron profiles, or reticulocyte parameters as compared to control athletes. Both groups showed a decrease in ferritin levels over 3 weeks of training. This study suggests that iron injections offer no hematologic benefits in nonanemic athletes with low ferritin levels.[2]

Nielsen and coworkers recommend using iron supplementation, at a dose of 100 mg/day for 3 months, in all athletes with a serum ferritin below 35 µg/L. They suggest rechecking ferritin levels after 6 months of treatment. They also recommend maintenance iron treatment for

1 week out of every month in endurance athletes in order to maintain their iron stores, once their serum ferritin has reached 60 μg/L.[82] Mirkin recommends that female athletes take 30 to 60 mg elemental iron daily, if their serum ferritin is below 25 μg/L.[76]

SICKLE CELL TRAIT

A person with sickle cell trait (SCT) is heterozygous for the sickle cell gene. SCT confers protection against malaria. The concentration of abnormal hemoglobin (HbS) in SCT is less than 50% and generally ranges from 25% to 45%. Sickle cell anemia and SCT result from a nucleotide mutation on the hemoglobin β chain that codes for valine instead of glutamate. This single amino acid substitution results in decreased solubility of hemoglobin in the deoxygenated state. Thus, under low oxygen conditions, HbS will precipitate and cause the cell to sickle.[110]

In the United States, the prevalence of SCT is approximately 8% in the black population and 0.8% in nonblacks. The prevalence increases to as much as 30% to 40% in some areas of Africa. In the athletic population, the prevalence of SCT is similar to the portion seen in the general population.[30,63,79,112] One study even found a higher prevalence of SCT in Ivory Coast track and field throw and jump champions (males and females) as compared to the general population.[9]

Several large studies have demonstrated the SCT carriers have a normal life span and no excess causes of morbidity or mortality,[50,108] although there appears to be an increased risk of splenic infarction at high altitudes in SCT carriers.[35,71] SCT carriers are generally not anemic.

Are SCT carriers at increased risk of morbidity and mortality during exercise? There have been numerous reports of exercise and SCT-associated collapse and death.[15,51,56,58] Kark and coworkers reported a 40-fold increased risk of sudden death during exertion in military recruits with SCT.[55] It is important to recognize that many of these case reports occurred in patients who were poorly conditioned and/or performed exercise under extreme environmental conditions.

Epidemiologic data suggest a similar prevalence of SCT among athletes and the general population,[30,63,79,112] which supports the position that SCT does not confer a selective disadvantage to athletic participation. The percentage of National Football League (NFL) players with SCT is similar to the percentage of SCT carriers in the United States African-American population.[79] Le Gallais and coworkers found that the percentage of runners with SCT competing in a semimarathon was similar to the general population, although none of the SCT runners had an international ranking.[63] Altitude may diminish athletic performance in athletes with SCT. Thiriet and coworkers found that runners with SCT had significantly slower times at very high altitudes (3800 to 4095 m) compared to runners without SCT, but similar times at lower altitudes.[113]

Evidence from physiologic studies generally suggests no difference in exercise capacity in SCT carriers as compared to controls.[46,68,93,120,121] Oxygen consumption during exercise at varying altitudes is similar in SCT carriers and controls,[46,93,120,121] although one study found a lower maximal oxygen consumption and higher lactate production in subjects with SCT.[43] The amount of RBC sickling has been demonstrated to markedly increase in SCT carriers at 4000 m compared to the slight sickling seen at 1250 m, but did not diminish performance.[68]

Although it appears that exercise does not impose health risks to SCT carriers under most conditions, the female athlete with SCT has not been well studied. Athletes with SCT should be warned of possible complications, particularly with regard to exercising at high altitudes and under extreme environmental conditions. They should be counseled to maintain adequate hydration and participate in preseason conditioning programs, which is good advice for all athletes to follow.[15,35]

References

1. Alaimo K, McDowell MA, Briefel RR, et al: Dietary intake of vitamins, minerals, and fiber of persons aged 2 months and over in the United States. Third National Health and Nutrition Examination Survey, Phase I, 1988–91. Adv Data 258:1, 1994.
2. Ashenden MJ, Fricker PA, Ryan RK, et al: The haematological response to iron injection amongst female athletes. Int J Sports Med 19(7):474, 1998.
3. Balaban EP, Cox JV, Snell P, et al: The frequency of anemia and iron deficiency in the runner. Med Sci Sports Exerc 21(6):643, 1989.
4. Balaban EP: Sports anemia. Clin Sports Med 11(2);313, 1992.
5. Banga JP, Gratzer WB, Pinder JC, et al: An erythrocyte membrane-protein anomaly in march hemoglobinuria. Lancet 2(8151):1048, 1979.
6. Barrios CH: Anemia and transfusion therapy. In Dunagan WC, Ridner ML (eds): Manual of Medical Therapeutics, 26th edition. Boston, Little, Brown, 1989, p 343.
7. Baska RS, Moses FM, Graeber G, et al: Gastrointestinal bleeding during an ultramarathon. Dig Dis Sci 35(2):276, 1990.

8. Beaumont AC, Teare JP: Subtotal colectomy following marathon running in a female patient. J R Soc Med 84(7):439, 1991.

9. Bile A, LeGallais D, Mercier J, et al: Sickle cell trait in Ivory Coast athletic throw and jump champions, 1956–1995. Int J Sports Med 19(3):315, 1998.

10. Blacklock NS: Bladder trauma in the long distance runner: "10,000 metres haematuria." Br J Urol 49(2):129, 1977.

11. Bourque SP, Pate RR, Branch JD: Twelve weeks of endurance exercise training does not affect iron status measures in women. J Am Diet Assoc 97(10):1116, 1997.

12. Bridges KR, Bunn HF: Anemia with disturbed iron metabolism. In Isselbacher KJ, Braunwald E, Wilson JD, et al (eds): Harrison's Principles of Internal Medicine (Harrison's CD-ROM), 13th edition, part 12, section 303. New York, McGraw-Hill, 1994.

13. Brien AJ, Simon TL: The effects of red blood cell infusion on 10-km race time. JAMA 257(20):2761, 1987.

14. Brouns F, Becker E: Is the gut an athletic organ? Digestion, absorption and exercise. Sports Med 15(4):242, 1993.

15. Browne RJ, Gillespie CA: Sickle cell trait: A risk factor for life-threatening rhabdomyolysis? Physician Sports Med 21(6):80, 1993.

16. Brune M, Magnusson B, Persson H, et al: Iron losses in sweat. Am J Clin Nutr 43(3):438, 1986.

17. Celsing F, Blomstrand E, Werner B, et al: Effects of iron deficiency on endurance and muscle enzyme activity in man. Med Sci Sports Exerc 18(2):156, 1986.

18. Celsing F, Svedenhag J, Pihlstedt P et al: Effects of anaemia and stepwise-induced polycythaemia on maximal aerobic power in individuals with high and low haemoglobin concentrations. Acta Physiol Scand 129(1):47, 1987.

19. Chen JD, Wang KJ, Li KJ, et al: Nutritional problems and measures in elite and amateur athletes. Am J Clin Nutr 49(5 suppl):1084, 1989.

20. Clarkson PM, Haymes EM: Exercise and mineral status of athletes: calcium, magnesium, phosphorus, and iron. Med Sci Sports Exerc 27(6):831, 1995.

21. Cohen JL, Potosnak L, Frank O, et al: A nutritional and hematologic assessment of elite ballet dancers. Phys Sports Med 13(5):43, 1985.

22. Convertino VA, Brock PJ, Keil LC, et al: Exercise training-induced hypervolemia: role of plasma, albumin, renin, and vasopressin. J Appl Physiol 48(4):665, 1980.

23. Cook JD, Finch CA, Smith NJ: Evaluation of the iron status of a population. Blood 48(3):449, 1976.

24. Cook JD, Finch CA: Assessing iron status of a population. Am J Clin Nutr 32(10):2115, 1979.

25. Cook JD: Clinical evaluation of iron deficiency. Semin Hematol 19(1):6, 1982.

26. Davies KJ, Maguire JJ, Brooks GA, et al: Muscle mitochondrial bioenergetics, oxygen supply, and work capacity during dietary iron deficiency and repletion. Am J Physiol 242(6):E418, 1982.

27. Davies KJ, Donovan CM, Refino CJ, et al: Distinguishing effects of anemia and muscle iron deficiency on exercise bioenergetics in the rat. Am J Physiol 246(6 Pt 1):E535, 1984.

28. Deuster PA, Kyle SB, Moser PB, et al: Nutritional survey of highly trained women runners. Am J Clin Nutr 44(6):954, 1986.

29. Diehl DM, Lohman TG, Smith SC, et al: Effects of physical training and competition on the iron status of female field hockey players. Int J Sports Med 7(5):264, 1986.

30. Diggs LW, Flowers E: High school athletes with the sickle cell trait (HB A/S). J Natl Med Assoc 68(6):492, 1976.

31. Economos CD, Bortz SS, Nelson ME: Nutritional practices of elite athletes: Practical recommendations. Sports Med 16(6):381, 1993.

32. Ehn L, Carmark B, Hoglund S: Iron status in athletes involved in intense physical activity. Med Sci Sports Exerc 12(1):61, 1980.

33. Eichner ER: Runner's macrocytosis: a clue to footstrike hemolysis. Am J Med 78(2):321, 1985.

34. Eichner ER: The anemias of athletes. Physician Sports Med 14(9):122, 1986.

35. Eichner ER: Sickle cell trait, exercise and altitude. Physician Sports Med 14(11):144, 1986.

36. Eichner ER: Hematuria as a diagnostic challenge. Physician Sports Med 18(11):53, 1990.

37. Eichner ER: Sports anemia, iron supplements, and blood doping. Med Sci Sports Exerc 24(9):S315, 1992.

38. Eichner ER, Scott WA: Exercise as disease detector. Physician Sports Med 26(3):41, 1998.

39. Ekblom B, Goldbarg AN, Gullbring B: Response to exercise after blood loss and reinfusion J Appl Physiol 33(2):175, 1972.

40. Finch CA, Miller LR, Inamdar AR, et al: Iron deficiency in the rat. Physiological and biochemical studies of muscle dysfunction. J Clin Invest 58(2):447, 1976.

41. Fisher RL, McMahon LF Jr, Ryan MJ, et al: Gastrointestinal bleeding in competitive runners. Dig Dis Sci 31(11):1226, 1986.

42. Fogelholm M, Jaakkola L, Lampisjarvi T: Effects of iron supplementation in female athletes with low serum ferritin concentration. Int J Sports Med 13(2):158, 1992.

43. Freund H, Lonsdorfer J, Oyono-Enguelle S, et al: Lactate exchange and removal abilities in sickle cell trait carriers during and after incremental exercise. Int J Sports Med 16(7):428, 1995.

44. Gardner GW, Edgerton VR, Senewiratne B, et al: Physical work capacity and metabolic stress in subjects with iron deficiency anemia. Am J Clin Nutr 30(6):910, 1977.

45. Garza D, Shrier I, Kohl H, et al: The clinical value of serum ferritin tests in endurance athletes. Clin J Sports Med 7(1):46, 1997.

46. Gozal D, Thiriet P, Mbala E, et al: Effect of different modalities of exercise and recovery on exercise performance in subjects with sickle cell trait. Med Sci Sports Exerc 24(12):1325, 1992.

47. Hallberg L, Rossander-Hulten L: Iron requirements in menstruating women. Am J Clin Nutr 54(6):1047, 1991.

48. Haymes EM, Clarkson PM: Mineral and trace elements. In Berning JR, Nelson Steen S (eds): Nutrition for Sport & Exercise, 2nd edition. Gaithersburg, Md, Aspen, 1998, pp 88-91.

49. Haymes EM, Spillman DM: Iron status of women distance runners, sprinters and control women. Int J Sports Med 10(6):430, 1989.

50. Heller P, Best WR, Nelson RB, et al: Clinical implications of sickle-cell trait and glucose-6-phosphate dehydrogenase deficiency in hospitalized black male patients. N Engl J Med 300(18):1001, 1979.

51. Helzlsouer KJ, Hayden FG, Rogol AD: Severe metabolic complications in a cross-country runner with sickle cell trait. JAMA 249(6):777, 1983.

52. Hunding A, Jordal R, Paulev PE: Runner's anemia and iron deficiency. Acta Med Scand 209(4):315, 1981.

53. Jones GR, Newhouse I: Sport-related hematuria: A review. Clin J Sports Med 7(2):119, 1997.

54. Kallmeyer JC, Miller NM: Urinary changes in ultra long-distance marathon runners. Nephron 64(1):119, 1993.

55. Kark JA, Posey DM, Schumacher HR, et al: Sickle-cell trait as a risk factor for sudden death in physical training. N Engl J Med 317(13):781, 1987.

56. Kerle KK, Nishimura KD: Exertional collapse and sudden death associated with sickle cell trait. Mil Med 161(12):766, 1996.

57. Klingshirn LA, Pate RR, Bourque SP, et al: Effect of iron supplementation on endurance capacity in iron-depleted female runners. Med Sci Sports Exerc 24(7):819, 1992.

58. Koppes GM, Daly JJ, Coltman CA, et al: Exertion-induced rhabdomyolysis with acute renal failure and disseminated intravascular coagulation in sickle cell trait. Am J Med 63:313, 1977.

59. LaManca JJ, Haymes EM: Effects of low ferritin concentration on endurance performance. Int J Sport Nutr 2(4):376, 1992.

60. LaManca JJ, Haymes EM: Effects of iron repletion on VO2max, endurance and blood lactate in women. Med Sci Sports Exerc 25(12):1386, 1993.

61. Lampe JW, Slavin JL, Apple FS: Poor iron status of women training for a marathon. Int J Sports Med 7(2):111, 1986.

62. Lampe JW, Slavin JL, Apple FS: Iron status of active women and the effect of running a marathon on bowel function and gastrointestinal blood loss. Int J Sports Med 12(2):173, 1991.

63. Le Gallais D, Prefaut C, Mercier J, et al: Sickle cell trait as a limiting factor for high-level performance in a semi-marathon. Int J Sports Med 15(7):399, 1994.

64. Little DR: Ambulatory management of common forms of anemia. Am Fam Physician 59(6):1598, 1999.

65. Lukaski HC, Hoverson BS, Gallagher SK, et al: Physical training and copper, iron and zinc status of swimmers. Am J Clin Nutr 51(6):1093, 1990.

66. Lyle RM, Weaver CM, Sedlock DA, et al: Iron status in exercising women: the effect of oral iron therapy vs increased consumption of muscle foods. Am J Clin Nutr 56(6):1049, 1992.

67. Magazanik A, Weinstein Y, Abarbanel J, et al: Effect of an iron supplementation on body iron status and aerobic capacity of young training women. Eur J Appl Physiol 62(5):317, 1991.

68. Martin TW, Weisman IM, Zeballos RJ, et al: Exercise and hypoxia increase sickling in venous blood from an exercising limb in individuals with sickle cell trait. Am J Med 87(1):48, 1989.

69. Matter M, Stitfall T, Graves J, et al: The effect of iron and folate therapy on maximal exercise performance in female marathon runners with iron and folate deficiency. Clin Sci (Colch) 72(4):415, 1987.

70. McCabe ME, Peura DA, Kadakia SC, et al: Gastrointestinal blood loss associated with running a marathon. Dig Dis Sci 31(11):1229, 1986.

71. McCurdy PR: Sickle cell trait. Am Fam Physician 10(5):141, 1974.

72. McDonald R, Keen CL: Iron, zinc and magnesium nutrition and athletic performance. Sports Med 5:171, 1984.

73. McLane JA, Fell RD, McKay RH, et al: Physiological and biochemical effects of iron deficiency on rat skeletal muscle. Am J Physiol 241(1):C47, 1981.

74. McManon LF, Ryan MJ, Larson D, et al: Occult gastrointestinal blood loss in marathon runners. Ann Int Med 100(6):846, 1984.

75. Miller BJ, Pate RR, Burgess W: Foot impact forces and intravascular hemolysis during distance running. Int J Sports Med 9(1):56, 1988.

76. Mirkin G: Nutrition for sports. In Shangold MM, Mirkin G (eds): Women and Exercise: Physiology and Sports Medicine, 2nd edition. Philadelphia, FA Davis, 1994, p 116.

77. Moses FM: Gastrointestinal bleeding and the athlete. Am J Gastroenterol 88(8):1157, 1993.

78. Mueller EJ, Thompson IM: Bladder carcinoma presenting as exercise-induced hematuria. Postgrad Med 84(8):173, 1988.

79. Murphy JR: Sickle cell hemoglobin (Hb AS) in black football players. JAMA 225(8):981, 1973.

80. Nachtigall D, Nielsen P, Fischer R, et al: Iron deficiency in distance runners. A reinvestigation using Fe-labeling and non-invasive liver iron quantification. Int J Sports Med 17(7):473, 1996.

81. Newhouse IJ, Clement DB, Taunton JE, et al: The effects of prelatent/latent iron deficiency on physical work. Med Sci Sports Exerc 21(3):263, 1989.

82. Nickerson HJ, Holubets M, Tripp AD, et al: Decreased iron stores in high school female runners. Am J Dis Child 139(11):1115, 1985.

83. Nielsen P, Nachtigall D: Iron supplementation in athletes. Sports Med 26(4):207, 1998.

84. Nishiyama S, Inomoto T, Nakamura T, et al: Zinc status relates to hematological deficits in women endurance runners. J Am Coll Nutr 15(4):359, 1996.

85. Nuviala RJ, Castilli MC, Lapieza MG, et al: Iron nutritional status in female karatekas, handball and basketball players, and runners. Physiol Behav 59(3):449, 1996.

86. Parr RB, Bachman LA, Moss RA: Iron deficiency in female athletes. Physician Sports Med 12(4):81, 1984.

87. Pate R: Sports anemia: A review of the current research literature. Physician Sports Med 11:115, 1983.

88. Pate RR, Miller BJ, Davis CA, et al: Iron status of female runners. Int J Sports Med 3(2):222, 1993.

89. Ranny HM, Rapaport SI: The red blood cell. In West JB (ed): Best and Taylor's Physiological Basis of Medical Practice, 11th edition. Baltimore, Williams & Wilkins, 1985, pp 392–4.

90. Risser WL, Lee EJ, Poindexter HB, et al: Iron deficiency in female athletes: its prevalence and impact on performance. Med Sci Sports Exerc 20(2):116, 1988.

91. Roberts D, Smith D: Serum ferritin values in elite speed and synchronized swimmers and speed skaters. J Lab Clin Med 116(5):661, 1990.

92. Robertson JD, Mughan RJ, Davidson RJ: Faecal blood loss in response to exercise. Br Med J (Clin Res Ed) 295(6593):303, 1987.

93. Robinson JR, Stone WJ, Asendorf AC: Exercise capacity of black sickle cell trait males. Med Sci Sports 8(4):244, 1976.

94. Rowland TW, Deisroth MB, Green GM, et al: The effect of iron therapy on the exercise capacity of nonanemic iron-deficient adolescent runners. Am J Dis Child 142(2):165, 1988.

95. Rowland TW: Iron deficiency in the young athlete. Pediatr North Am 37(5):1153, 1990.

96. Rowland TW, Stagg L, Kelleher JF: Iron deficiency in adolescent girls. J Adolesc Health 12(1):22, 1991.

97. Rudzki SJ, Hazard H, Collison D: Gastrointestinal blood loss in triathletes: its etiology and relationship to sports anemia. Aust J Sci Med Sport 27(1):3, 1995.

98. Salonen JT, Nyyssonen K, Korpela H, et al: High stored iron levels are associated with excess risk of myocardial infarction in eastern Finnish men. Circulation 86(3):803, 1992.

99. Sanborn CF, Jankowski CM: Physiologic considerations for women in sports. Clin Sports Med 13(2):315, 1994.

100. Schrier SL: Hematology. In Rubenstein E, Federman DD (eds): Scientific American Medicine, vol 2, section II. New York, Scientific American, 1992, pp 1–10.

101. Scott DE, Pritchard JA: Iron deficiency in healthy young college women. JAMA 199(12):897, 1967.

102. Selby GB, Eichner ER: Endurance swimming, intravascular hemolysis, and iron depletion. New perspective on athlete's anemia. Am J Med 81 (5):791, 1986.

103. Siegel AJ, Hennekens CH, Solomon HS, et al.: Exercise-related hematuria. Findings in a group of runners. JAMA 241(4):391, 1979.

104. Siegel AJ: Medical conditions arising during sports. In Shangold MM, Mirkin G (eds): Women and Exercise: Physiology and Sports Medicine, 2nd edition. Philadelphia, FA Davis, 1994, pp 267–9.

105. Smith JA: Exercise, training and red blood cell turnover. Sports Med 19(1):9, 1995.

106. Snyder AC, Dvorak LL, Roepke JB: Influence of dietary iron source on measures of iron status among female runners. Med Sci Sports Exerc 21(1):7, 1989.

107. Spodaryk K, Czekaj J, Sowa W: Relationship among reduced level of stored iron and dietary iron in trained women. Physiol Res 45(5):393, 1996.

108. Stark AD, Janerich DT, Jereb SK: The incidence and causes of death in a follow-up study of individuals with haemoglobin AS and AA. Int J Epidemiol 9(4):325, 1980.

109. Stewart JG, Ahlquist DA, McGill DB, et al: Gastrointestinal blood loss and anemia in runners. Ann Intern Med 100(6):843, 1984.

110. Stryer L: Portrait of an allosteric protein. In Stryer L (ed): Biochemistry, 4th edition. New York, WH Freeman, 1995, p169.

111. Taylor C, Rogers G, Goodman C, et al: Hematologic, iron-related, and acute-phase protein responses to sustained strenuous exercise. J Appl Phyisol 62(2):464, 1987.

112. Thiriet P, Lobe MM, Gweha I, et al: Prevalence of the sickle cell trait in an athletic West African population. Med Sci Sports Exerc 23(3):389, 1991.

113. Thiriet P, LeHesran JY, Wouassi D, et al.: Sickle cell trait performance in a prolonged race at high altitude. Med Sci Sports Exerc 26(7):914, 1994.

114. Viteri FE, Torun B: Anaemia and physical work capacity. Clin Haematol 3:609, 1974.

115. Waller MF, Haymes EM: The effects of heat and exercise on sweat iron loss. Med Sci Sports Exerc 28(2):197, 1996.

116. Weight LM, Alexander D, Jacobs P: Strenuous exercise: analogous to the acute-phase response? Clin Sci (Colch) 81(5):677, 1991.

117. Weight LM, Darge BL, Jacobs P: Athlete's pseudoanaemia. Eur J Appl Physiol 62(5):358, 1991.

118. Weight LM, Jacobs P, Noakes TD: Dietary iron deficiency and sports anemia. Br J Nutr 68(1):253, 1992.

119. Weight LM, Klein M, Noakes TD, et al: "Sports anemia"—a real or apparent phenomenon in endurance-trained athletes. Int J Sports Med 13(4):344, 1992.

120. Weisman IM, Zeballos RJ, Johnson BD: Cardiopulmonary and gas exchange responses to acute strenuous exercise at 1270 meters in sickle cell trait. Am J Med 84(3 Pt 1):377, 1988.

121. Weisman IM, Zeballos RJ, Johnson BD: Effect of moderate inspiratory hypoxia on exercise performance in sickle cell trait. Am J Med 84(6):1033, 1988.

122. Wells CL, Stern JR, Hecht LH: Hematological changes following a marathon race in male and female runners. Eur J Appl Physiol 48(1):41, 1982.

123. Zhu YI, Haas JD: Iron depletion without anemia and physical performance in young women. Am J Clin Nutr 66(2):334, 1997.

Chapter 28

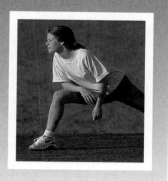

Cardiac Concerns

Elizabeth Joy, B.S., M.D.

Many of the cardiac concerns of female athletes are no different from those of their male counterparts; however, there are some important gender differences that physicians caring for athletes should be aware of. The objectives of this chapter are (1) to understand the cardiophysiologic differences between men and women; (2) to understand electrocardiographic testing in women; (3) to discuss cardiac conditions not uncommon in the female athlete; and (4) to discuss appropriate screening, diagnosis, and management guidelines for cardiac conditions in the female athlete.

CARDIAC PHYSIOLOGY

There are several gender differences in cardiovascular and respiratory physiology that account for some of the differences seen between men and women with respect to aerobic capacity. Women have a smaller thoracic cage than men, and thus have a smaller lung volume[28] (Table 28-1).

Women also have a smaller heart, resulting in lower stroke volume and thus a higher heart rate for the same oxygen consumption. Women have a smaller left ventricular mass both in absolute terms and relative to lean body mass.[29]

There are some age and gender differences relating to blood pressure as well. Both systolic and diastolic blood pressure increase as children age. Blood pressure in girls tends to plateau between 15 and 17 years of age, whereas blood pressure in boys plateaus at approximately 20 years of age. From 12 to 54 years, mean levels of blood pressure among females are lower than those among men, but from 55 to 74 years mean blood pressure levels of women are higher.[29]

Prepubescent girls and boys have similar aerobic power, or maximal oxygen consumption (VO_2max). The VO_2max peaks for both sexes between ages 16 and 20. Differences in body composition and oxygen transport system (lower blood volume, fewer red blood cells, lower hemoglobin content) account for many if not all of the sex differences in VO_2max. The large (52%) difference in VO_2max (expressed in liters per minute) between men and women decreases to 20% to 30% when VO_2 is expressed in milliliters per kilogram per minute, and then to 15% when VO_2 is expressed in milliliters per kilogram of fat-free mass per minute.[29]

Aging affects aerobic capacity of both sexes similarly. There is a decline in VO_2max, a decrease in maximal achievable heart rate, a decrease in mechanical performance of the myocardium, and limitations in the functioning of other organ systems that affect aerobic capacity.[10]

CARDIAC ADAPTATIONS TO TRAINING

The *athletic heart syndrome* is a benign condition that includes a number of physiologic adaptations to the increased demands of physical exercise on the heart. An understanding of these changes is imperative to enable the physician to differentiate the athletic heart syndrome from pathologic conditions.

Exercise leads to similar adaptations in the hearts of both men and women. The heart's response to training is directly related to the type of exercise being performed.[7] Aerobic-type exercise (running, cross-country skiing, cycling) requires greater cardiac output, and the heart

Table 28-1. Average Adult Lung Volumes

	WOMEN	MEN
Total lung capacity	4200 mL	6000 mL
Vital capacity	3200 mL	4800 mL
Residual volume	1200 mL	1000 mL

From Sanborn CF, Jankowski CM: Gender-specific physiology. In Agostini R (ed): Medical and Orthopedic Issues of Active and Athletic Women. Philadelphia, Hanley and Belfus, 1994, p 26, with permission.

responds by increasing stroke volume by increasing left ventricular end diastolic diameter. Athletes performing anaerobic activities, such as weight lifting, place large pressure loads on the heart. This results in heart muscle hypertrophy without an increase in volume or capacity. This type of cardiac conditioning allows athletes to sustain blood pressures above 320/250 mm Hg.[7]

Most athletes train both aerobically and anaerobically, and therefore may have cardiac features reflective of both pressure and volume overload.

CARDIAC ARRHYTHMIAS AND ELECTROCARDIOGRAPHIC CHANGES

Cardiac arrhythmias and electrocardiographic changes are not uncommon among certain athlete groups, although they are typically seen in aerobically trained athletes. Electrocardiographic changes can be classified into 4 groups: (1) changes in rate and/or rhythm; (2) changes in electrical conduction; (3) changes in the P wave and QRS complex; and (4) alteration in repolarization leading to changes in the ST segment or T wave.[27] The most common arrhythmia is sinus bradycardia. The degree of bradycardia correlates with the intensity of training, and is secondary to both increased vagal tone and decreased sympathetic tone. Resting heart rates less than 25 beats per minute and sinus pauses lasting more than 2 seconds are not uncommon in athletes, and are often of no significant concern.[38] Similarly, sinus arrhythmia, wandering atrial pacemaker, and junctional rhythms are not uncommon and may be seen in 14% to 69% of dynamically trained athletes.[38]

Atrioventricular (AV) blocks are the third most common form of rhythm change seen in athletes. AV block is secondary to increased vagal influence on the AV node. Cessation of training results in disappearance of the AV block. First-degree AV block is most common, detected in up to 33% of resting and ambulatory electrocardiograms (ECGs) in competitive athletes.[38] Second-degree AV block (Mobitz type I) is clearly related to training and has been observed in up to 8% of endurance athletes.[38] Long-term follow-up of these patients shows no association with evolving cardiac disease. Mobitz type II and third-degree blocks are rare and when discovered, should be evaluated thoroughly.

Premature ventricular contractions are no more common in athletes than nonathletes.[38] Incomplete right bundle branch block can be seen in up to 14% of athletes. It is thought to be related to an increase in right ventricular mass and often resolves when exercise activity is discontinued.[38]

Repolarization changes are common in athletes. ST-segment and T-wave changes are most common and correlate directly with the intensity of training. ST-segment elevation with peaked T waves, ST-segment depression with depressed J points, juvenile T-wave pattern (right precordial J-point elevation with inverted T waves), T-wave inversion in the lateral precordium, and biphasic T waves may all be seen in the ECGs of normal athletes.

Large voltages are often seen in athletes. This is a manifestation of the physiologic enlargement that occurs with conditioning. One can see increased P-wave amplitude as evidence of right ventricular hypertrophy (RVH), and increased R-wave amplitude as evidence of left ventricular hypertrophy (LVH). LVH in athletes has a prevalence of up to 80% in some surveys. In one study, R-wave amplitude increased by 25% after an 11-week training program. This effect however, disappeared with the cessation of training.[38]

ELECTROCARDIOGRAPHIC EXERCISE TESTING

Exercise testing is a useful tool to detect and evaluate patients with coronary artery disease (CAD). Indications for performing exercise testing include evaluation of chest pain, screening for ischemic heart disease in at-risk patients, evaluating dysrhythmias, determining functional capacity, and generating an exercise prescription.[11]

Recommendations for graded exercise testing for patients wanting to start a moderate exercise program (40% to 60% of VO_2max) include patients with known CAD and patients with 2 or more risk factors or signs of CAD. Recommendations for graded exercise testing for patients wanting to start a vigorous exercise program (above 60% VO_2max) are listed in Table 28-2.

Exercise testing in men is an excellent screening test that yields few false-positive results. Exercise testing in women is associated with a higher false-positive rate than in men. This difference lessens as women get older (over 50 years old).[11] Even with typical angina, the false-positive rate is 25% to 50%.[11] Pratt and coworkers[28] identified 4 independent variables that were helpful in predicting *true positive results* in women with chest pain: absence of mitral valve prolapse; exercise time less than 5 minutes on

Table 28-2. Current Recommendations for Graded Exercise Testing for Patients Wanting to Start a Vigorous Exercise Program ($> 60\%$ VO$_2$max)

Men over 40, women over 50
Patients with 2 or more risk factors or signs of CAD
Patients with known CAD
Establishing the severity/prognosis of ischemic heart disease to stratify those who may need additional intervention
Evaluating antianginal or antihypertensive therapy
Evaluating patients after myocardial infarction for risk stratification

Modified from American College of Sports Medicine: Guidelines for Exercise Testing and Prescription, 4th edition. Philadelphia, Lea & Febiger, 1991, p 8, with permission.

Bruce protocol; inability to reach target heart rate, and; ST-segment depression that persists longer than 6 minutes into recovery.

The specificity of exercise testing is equal in both genders after adjusting for the difference in the prevalence of CAD. Sensitivity (positive predictive value of a negative test) is equal among men and women. Clinical implications of women's higher false-positive rates are as follows: lower predictive value of a positive test, making it a poor screening test; greater expense, as further testing (stress echocardiography, stress nuclear testing) is often required; and potentially unnecessary use of medication due to misdiagnosis.

CORONARY ARTERY DISEASE

Epidemiology

The prevalence of CAD is greater in men than in women at all ages. However, the incidence of CAD after age 65 is actually higher in women. CAD accounts for 23% of all deaths and 52% of cardiovascular deaths in women. It is the leading cause of death in women over 50 years of age. Ninety percent of all CAD-related deaths occur in women aged 55 years and older.[1]

Among women aged 30 to 39 years, CAD is second only to breast cancer as the major cause of death. CAD-related mortality continues to rise in women until the age of 70, while it remains constant in men after the age of 60.[1] Women manifest symptoms of CAD at an older age than do men, typically 10 years later. Two reasons for this variance include gender differences in serum lipid concentrations, and a higher rate of silent ischemia in women. Sixty-seven percent of all sudden deaths in women occur in persons without previous clinical evidence of CAD, and a higher percentage of myocardial infarctions are fatal in women.[1] Women who suffer a myocardial infarction (MI) have a worse prognosis than men do. Women surviving their first MI have an increased risk of recurrent MI or cardiac death.[1] In the past, CAD was treated less aggressively in women, however, this trend is changing. Women are still less likely to utilize cardiac rehabilitation programs, and they have a higher rate of dropout.[1]

Risk Factors

There are some gender-related differences in CAD risk factors. Major CAD risk factors are listed in Table 28-3.

Men have a higher rate of CAD-related mortality when compared to women at all age groups; however, these gender-related differences diminish with advancing age. As discussed, 90% of all CAD-related deaths among women occur after the age of 55.[1]

Tobacco Use

Cigarette smoking is the most preventable risk factor for CAD. There is a direct correlation between the number of cigarettes smoked per day and the relative risk of developing CAD. Those who smoke 1 pack per day (PPD) have a 4-fold increase in their risk of developing CAD. For 2-PPD smokers, this risk increases 10-fold. These observations can be in part explained by the fact that smoking exerts an antiestrogenic effect in women. In women who smoke, menopause occurs at an earlier age. Once cigarette smoking is discontinued, one's risk of developing CAD declines progressively.[1]

Systemic Hypertension

Systemic hypertension is the most common cardiovascular disease in both men and women and is well recognized as a major risk factor for the development of CAD. However, hypertensive women appear to have a lower total and CAD-related mortality as compared to hypertensive men. Women with hypertension are at lower risk for stroke, CAD, congestive heart failure, and sudden death.[1] Reasons for this difference in

Table 28-3. Coronary Artery Disease Risk Factors

Age
Tobacco use
Systemic hypertension
Hyperlipidemia
Diabetes mellitus
Obesity

mortality and morbidity are unknown, but it is thought that the vascular response to elevated blood pressure may be tempered by hormonal factors in women.[1]

Serum Lipid Concentrations

The lower incidence of CAD in women, particularly at younger ages, is largely due to differences in serum lipid concentrations. Estrogen increases high-density lipid cholesterol (HDL-C) and lowers low-density lipid cholesterol (LDL-C). Within 30 months after natural menopause, a woman's HDL-C falls and her LDL-C rises so that her profile resembles that of a man. Within 10 years after menopause, the rate of CAD among women approaches that of men.

Diabetes Mellitus

In women, diabetes mellitus increases the risk of developing CAD by a factor of 3, thus placing them at the same risk as same-age men without diabetes mellitus.[1] The risk of experiencing a fatal cardiac event is higher among diabetic women compared to diabetic men.[1] Diabetic women are more likely to have other risk factors: obesity, hypertension, and lower HDL-C.[1]

Obesity

Obesity is an independent predictor of CAD in both men and women.[1] Thirty percent of white women and almost 50% of black women are obese (ie, more than 20% above ideal body weight). Altogether, about 32 million American women are overweight or obese. These women have a 3 times greater risk of CAD compared to nonobese women.[25]

Fat distribution patterns may be more important than overall obesity. Truncal obesity (apple shape) is associated with a higher risk of MI, angina, stroke, and overall cardiovascular mortality in women. In addition to a higher risk of CAD, obese women with truncal obesity are more likely to have hypertension and diabetes mellitus.[1]

Gender Differences in Diagnostic Testing and Interventional Strategies

Women with presumed CAD are less likely to undergo angiography and are less likely to undergo either revascularization or coronary artery bypass grafting.[1] When women are referred for either coronary artery bypass grafting or angioplasty, it is typically at a more advanced stage of

disease when compared to men. This practice has resulted in higher procedure-related morbidity and mortality rates for women.[1] Therefore, differences in referral patterns and outcome are related more to the stage of the disease than to gender.[1]

The Impact of Exercise on Coronary Artery Disease in Women

Exercise benefits both men and women with known CAD. There is a strong inverse relationship between cardiorespiratory fitness and total cholesterol, triglyceride, and HDL-C levels in women. Pre- and postmenopausal athletes have more favorable lipid profiles compared to age-matched sedentary or less active women.[37] Simply put, women who are cardiovascularly fit live longer than those who are not.[2]

MITRAL VALVE PROLAPSE

Pathophysiology and Epidemiology

Mitral valve prolapse (MVP) affects 5% of the general population and 17% of young women and girls.[30] More than 60% of adults with MVP are women. The prevalence of MVP in athletes is unknown.

MVP is, by definition, abnormal systolic displacement of the mitral valve leaflets superiorly and posteriorly from the left ventricle into the left atrium.[10] MVP is a heterogeneous disease, with affected patients demonstrating a continuum of both valvular disease severity and symptomatology.

MVP is most often an autosomal dominant condition.[10] Inherited abnormalities of valvular connective tissue result in redundancy and/or thickening of valve leaflets. This leads to various degrees of distensibility, poor leaflet opposition, and subsequent prolapse. These aberrations of leaflet microarchitecture may also be accompanied by widespread abnormalities of connective tissue elsewhere in the body.[3] MVP also may be present in people with other connective tissue diseases, such as Marfan syndrome and Ehlers-Danlos syndrome.[3,9]

In addition to the valvular changes, patients with *mitral valve prolapse syndrome* (MVPS) have associated neuroendocrine abnormalities and autonomic dysfunction. This results in a wide variety of symptoms, including fatigue, dyspnea, chest pain, palpitations, panic attacks, and other symptoms that cannot be explained on the basis of their valvular disease alone.[3]

People with MVPS have high adrenergic activity thought to be a result of increased serum levels of catecholamines coupled with adrenergic hyperresponsiveness.[3]

With respect to MVP symptomatology, 2 groups of patients emerge from the literature: those whose symptoms are directly related to their valvular disease and those whose symptoms cannot be explained on the basis of valvular disease alone.

The first group has been referred to as MVP-anatomic and the second, MVPS.[3,10]

Some symptom crossover occurs between groups. Palpitations are one of the few symptoms secondary to valve dysfunction alone.[10] Other symptoms reported by those patients with MVPS include exercise intolerance, headache, sleep disturbance, irritable bowel symptoms, and vascular symptoms such as flushing and tingling of extremities.

Complications

Most patients with MVP have a benign form and will have no significant complications.[30] Serious sequelae include mitral regurgitation, infective endocarditis, cerebrovascular accidents, and sudden death.[3,10,20]

Mitral Regurgitation

MVP is the most common cause of mitral regurgitation.[30] Those with leaflet thickening and redundancy seem to be at highest risk for developing regurgitation.[20]

The risk of progressing to regurgitation increases with age. Mitral regurgitation affects men more than women despite the preponderance of women with MVP.[30]

Elevated blood pressure and high body weight also increase the risk (this may explain greater risk for men).

Physical examination often reveals a holosystolic murmur. Doppler echocardiography can determine the severity of regurgitation. The larger the jet area, the more severe the regurgitation. A jet area of 4 to 8 cm^2 indicates moderate regurgitation, and a jet area of greater than 8 cm^2 indicates severe regurgitation.[32]

Infective Endocarditis

Leaflet thickening and redundancy increase the risk for infectious bacterial endocarditis. The risk of infective endocarditis in patients with MVP is low, 1% to 3.5%.[3,20] Antibiotic prophylaxis should be prescribed before invasive procedures.

Cerebrovascular Accident

The incidence of cerebrovascular accident, or stroke, in patients with MVP is higher than for the general population.[9] The reason for this is unknown. There are no known clinical clues to predict the risk of stroke in this population. However, those with severe regurgitation seem to be at greatest risk.[19,25] Several studies have concluded that leaflet thickening does not increase one's risk for stroke.[19]

Sudden Death

Sudden death is a rare, but devastating complication of MVP. Between 3% and 5% of cardiac-related sudden deaths during exercise are attributed to MVP.[21] Some factors have been identified that may increase the risk of sudden death[3,30]:

1. Severe mitral regurgitation
2. Severe valve abnormalities without regurgitation
3. Increased heart weight
4. Serious ventricular arrhythmia
5. Repolarization abnormalities
6. Convincing clinical symptoms of palpitations and/or syncope

Clinical Evaluation

Characteristic auscultatory findings are a midsystolic click followed by a late systolic murmur. The click results from tightening of the chord-leaflet structures at the time of maximum prolapse, and the murmur results from mitral regurgitation. Neither the presence nor the absence of these findings confirms or excludes the diagnosis of MVP.

Maneuvers that reduce left ventricular volume such as having the patient sit or stand cause the click and murmur to move closer to the first heart sound. Having the patient squat increases the left ventricular volume, causing the murmur to disappear or decrease in intensity.

When the click-murmur is present and responds to the aforementioned maneuvers, an auscultatory diagnosis of MVP can be made. A definitive diagnosis of MVP can be made only upon echocardiographic confirmation of auscultatory findings.

Echocardiography has markedly improved our ability to diagnose MVP. Patients with auscultatory findings should undergo echocardiography to further evaluate leaflet structure and identify regurgitation. Echocardiographic diagnosis is made when one or both valve leaflets protrudes or billows into the left atrium in the apical long-axis view.[10] Mild bowing of normal-appearing leaflets seen in the 4-chamber view probably represents a normal variant.

Echocardiography can help classify the patient as having low, mild, moderate, or high risk for complications of endocarditis and mitral regurgitation. At lowest risk are those patients with MVP without mitral valve thickening or regurgitation. Patients at mild risk for complications have MVP with valvular deformity and no regurgitation. At moderate risk are those with valvular deformity and mild regurgitation, and at highest risk are those with moderate to severe regurgitation, thickening of valve leaflets, enlargement of leaflets and annulus, and significant protrusion of one or more of the leaflets.[20,25] Other tests to consider in patients with MVP include:

1. Electrocardiography to screen for conduction disturbance
2. 24-hour Holter monitoring to evaluate those patients with palpitations
3. Graded exercise stress testing to monitor exercise tolerance
4. Stress echocardiography

Management and Risk Stratification

Management should be centered on patient education, symptom and risk management, and ongoing risk stratification. Table 28-4 lists the appropriate testing and management interventions for the various degrees of mitral valve dis-ease. In patients with MVPS, lifestyle modification is the key to reducing symptoms.

Dietary changes have been found to be helpful in alleviating symptoms and include avoidance of caffeine, which may reduce palpitations; restricting sugar, which may lessen fatigue; liberal fluid intake and minimal alcohol intake, which may improve the effect dehydration has on the hypovolemia experienced by some patients; and in those patients with symptomatic hypotension, adequate sodium chloride intake.

Medical Therapy

Medication use is fairly limited. In those with documented hemodynamically stable, nonsustained arrhythmias (usually premature ventricular contractions and premature atrial contractions), or in those who have distressing palpitations, a cardioselective β-blocker may be helpful. Patients with atrial fibrillation need anticoagulant therapy and may need rate control with digoxin or other medications.

Primary care physicians should seek cardiology consultation for anyone who has mitral valve disease with mitral regurgitation, significant arrhythmias, or a family history of sudden death due to MVP.[18]

Exercise Guidelines

Aerobic exercise should be encouraged for most patients with MVP.[16] Aerobic exercise has been shown to decrease anxiety and symptoms such

Table 28-4. Evaluation and Management of Mitral Valve Prolapse

RISK CATEGORY	EVALUATION	MONITORING	MANAGEMENT
Low MVP without valvular deformity or regurgitation	Echocardiography every 5 years	24-hour Holter Graded exercise stress testing	β-blocker Dietary changes Regular exercise
Moderate MVP with valvular deformity, no regurgitation	Echocardiography every 2–3 years	Same as above If stress echocardiography	Antibiotic dental prophylaxis Treat even mild hypertension Encourage weight loss if needed Treat palpitations as noted above
Moderate MVP with valvular deformity, mild regurgitation	Echocardiography every 2–3 years	Same as above	Antibiotic dental prophylaxis Treat even mild hypertension Encourage weight loss if needed Treat palpitations as noted above
High MVP with moderate to severe regurgitation	Doppler echocardiography every year	Same as above + others based on signs/symptoms	As above and closely monitor cardiac function and replace mitral valve when necessary
Further Evaluation	Initial electrocardiography	(+) Palpitations	

as chest pain, fatigue, dizziness, and mood swings, as well as improve overall well-being and functional capacity.[31]

The 26th Bethesda Conference[5,20] addressed the topic of exercise for athletes who have either MVP or mitral regurgitation and made the recommendations listed in Table 28-5.

SUDDEN DEATH IN CHILDREN AND YOUNG ADULTS

Epidemiology

Athletic-related sudden death is uncommon. One study estimated that an average of 11 sports-related cases of cardiac sudden death occur in the United States per year.[21] Males outnumber females (9:1) with respect to sudden death during sporting activities.[21]

Between 1 and 40 years of age, the most common cardiac causes of sudden death include hypertrophic cardiomyopathy, congenital coronary artery anomalies, conduction-system abnormalities, myocarditis, CAD, MVP, and aortic dissection.

Maron and coworkers[21] developed clinical, demographic, and pathologic profiles of young competitive athletes who died suddenly by examining the deaths of 134 athletes that occurred over 10 years (Table 28-6).

Pathophysiology

Incidence of prodromal symptoms among all people who die suddenly from cardiac causes is approximately 50%. The most common symptoms are chest pain and actual or near-syncope. Prompt cardiac evaluation is indicated for children and young adults with exertional chest pain not affected by movement, inspiration, or palpation, or without an apparent noncardiac cause, particularly if the patient has a high-risk cardiac disorder; a family history of sudden death; or exertion-related, unexplained syncope.[18]

Several cardiac conditions may be associated with a family history of sudden death, including hypertrophic or dilated cardiomyopathy, right ventricular cardiomyopathy, CAD, MVP, Marfan syndrome, or long-QT syndrome.[18] Therefore, a family history of sudden death should be obtained on any routine or sports-related physical examinations, and whenever evaluating symptoms of chest pain or syncope.[14]

Electrocardiographic abnormalities occur in association with a number of conditions that put young athletes at risk for sudden death. An ECG should be obtained when evaluating an athlete with chest pain, syncope, a known or suspected lesion associated with a high risk of sudden death, or a family history of sudden death.[18]

Table 28-7 lists electrocardiographic abnormalities often associated with an increased risk for sudden death.

Table 28-5. 26th Bethesda Conference Recommendations for Patients with Mitral Valve Prolapse or Mitral Regurgitation

MITRAL VALVE PROLAPSE

Athletes with MVP (having structurally abnormal valves manifested by leaflet thickening and elongation) and without any of the following criteria can engage in all competitive sports:
  History of syncope, documented to be arrythmogenic in origin.
  Family history of sudden death associated with MVP.
  Repetitive forms of sustained and nonsustained supraventricular arrythmias, particularly if exaggerated by exercise.
  Moderate to marked mitral regurgitation.
  Prior embolic event.
Athletes with MVP and one or more of the aforementioned criteria can participate in only low-intensity competitive sports.

MITRAL REGURGITATION

Athletes in sinus rhythm with normal left ventricular size and function can participate in all competitive sports.
Athletes in sinus rhythm or atrial fibrillation with mild left ventricular enlargement and normal left ventricular function at rest can participate in low and moderate static and moderate dynamic competitive sports.
Selected athletes can engage in some low and moderate static and low, moderate, and high dynamic competitive sports.
Athletes with atrial fibrillation should undergo exercise testing to evaluate ventricular rate response to exercise.
Athletes with definite left ventricular enlargement or any degree of left ventricular dysfunction at rest should not participate in any competitive sports.
Patients on chronic anticoagulation therapy should avoid sports involving body contact.

From Cheitlin M, Douglas PS, Parmley WW: 26th Bethesda Conference: Recommendations for determining eligibility for competition in athletes with cardiovascular abnormalities: Acquired valvular heart disease. Med Sci Sports Exerc 26(10 suppl):S254–60, 1994, and Maron BJ, Isner JM, Mckenna WJ: 26th Bethesda Conference: Recommendations for determining eligibility for competition in athletes with cardiovascular abnormalities. Task Force 3: Hypertrophic cardiomyopathy, myocarditis, and other myopericardial diseases and mitral valve prolapse. Med Sci Sports Exerc 26(10 suppl): S261–67, 1994, with permission.

Table 28-6. Characteristics and Probable Causes of Sudden Death Associated with Physical Exertion or Sports in Young Persons ($N = 134$)

Median age	17 years
Age range	12–40 years
Gender	
Male	120 (90%)
Female	14 (10%)
Race	
Caucasian	70 (52%)
Black	59 (44%)
Sport	
Basketball	47
Football	45
Prior history of symptoms thought to be cardiovascular in origin (chest pain, exertional dyspnea, syncope, or dizziness)	24 (18%)
Time of collapse	
Immediately after training	78
Immediately after formal athletic contest	43
Cause of sudden death	
Hypertrophic cardiomyopathy (HCM)	48 (36%)
Unexplained increase in cardiac mass (possible HCM)	14 (10%)
Aberrant coronary arteries	17 (13%)
Other coronary anomalies	8 (6%)
Ruptured aortic aneurysm Marfan syndrome: $N = 3$	6 (5%)
Tunneled left anterior-descending coronary artery	6 (5%)
Aortic valve stenosis	5 (4%)
Myocarditis	4 (3%)
Idiopathic dilated cardiomyopathy	4 (3%)
Arrhythmogenic right ventricular dysplasia	4 (3%)
Idiopathic myocardial scarring	4 (3%)
Mitral valve prolapse Marfan syndrome: $N = 1$	3 (2%)
Atherosclerotic coronary artery disease	3 (2%)
Other congenital heart disease	2 (1.5%)
Long-QT syndrome	1 (0.5%)
Sarcoidosis	1 (0.5%)
Sickle cell trait	1 (0.5%)
"Normal" heart	3 (2%)

From Maron BJ, Shirani J, Poliac LC, et al: Sudden death in young competitive athletes. JAMA 276(3): 199–204, 1996, with permission.

MYOCARDIAL DISORDERS

Obstructive Hypertrophic Cardiomyopathy

Hypertrophic cardiomyopathy (HCM) is uncommon in the general population (0.01% to 0.02%), but is associated with a high rate of sudden death—4.0% per year.[20] HCM is inherited in an autosomal dominant pattern. Sixty percent of patients have an affected first-degree relative.[20] The pathophysiology of HCM is ventricular hypertrophy leading to obstruction of left ventricular outflow. This often results in a systolic murmur heard at the left sternal border.

Symptoms of HCM include chest pain, dyspnea, and syncope on exertion.

Individuals at highest risk of sudden death are those with syncope, very young age at presentation, extreme degrees of ventricular hypertrophy, a strong family history of sudden death due to cardiac causes, and unsustained ventricular tachycardia.

The ECG may reveal lateral ST-T flattening or inversion, ventricular hypertrophy, and pathologic Q waves. Echocardiography is diagnostic in the vast majority of cases.[20] A septal diameter of 15 mm or more in an adult in conjunction with the appropriate findings obtained on history, physical examination, and electrocardiography is considered diagnostic.[20]

Treatment of HCM may include β-blockers or calcium channel blockers, but medications may not prevent sudden death. Amiodarone and an implantable defibrillator are appropriate in some patients. Strenuous physical exertion should be restricted.[14,20]

Myocarditis

Myocarditis accounted for only 3% of sudden death in the 134 athletes evaluated by Maron and coworkers.[21] However, in the general population of children and young adults, myocarditis accounts for up to 40% of sudden death from cardiac causes.[20] History may reveal a recent influenza-like illness prior to the onset of cardiac symptoms. It is most often due to infection with group B coxsackievirus.[15] Cardiac involvement is unpredictable and may involve the conduction system causing heart block, or the myocardium causing ventricular tachyarrhythmia. Thankfully, most patients with myocarditis have subclinical disease and a benign course, and go on to full recovery.[15] Electrocardiography may demonstrate low-voltage, diffuse, nonspecific ST-T changes, sinus tachycardia, premature ventricular contractions, heart block, or ventricular arrhythmia. Echocardiography may show dilat-

Table 28-7 Electrocardiographic Abnormalities That Can Be Associated with a Higher Risk of Sudden Death

Flat or inverted T waves in leads V5, V6, I, and a VL can accompany cardiomyopathy and coronary artery abnormalities
Prolonged QT interval
Ventricular pre-excitation
Ventricular tachycardia
Heart block: second degree type II, third degree

From Liberthson RR: Sudden death from cardiac causes in children and young adults. N Engl J Med 334(16): 1039–44, 1996, with permission.

ed chambers and decreased systolic function consistent with congestive heart failure.

Management is supportive. Rest and avoidance of exertion during the acute and healing stages are advised until the symptoms start to resolve. Patients with evidence of heart failure and/or rhythm disturbances are treated with conventional medical interventions.[15]

CORONARY ARTERY ANOMALIES

Atherosclerotic Coronary Artery Disease

Premature atherosclerotic coronary vascular disease (ASCVD) accounted for 3 of the 134 cases (2%) of sudden death in the cohort of Maron and coworkers[21]. All 3 were male and died at ages 14, 19, and 28 years, respectively.[21] Among nonathletes in the same age group (18 to 35 years), ASCVD may account for up to 23% of deaths.[18] Even in the second and third decades of life, aggressive management of coronary risk factors is warranted.

Ectopic Origin of the Left Coronary Artery on the Right Aortic Sinus of Valsalva

This is the most common congenital coronary artery anomaly causing sudden death in young people.[18,21] In this condition, the left main coronary artery arises at an acute angle, often from a slit-like, hypoplastic ostium, traverses the aortic wall obliquely, and emerges between the aorta and the right ventricular outflow before proceeding to its usual area of distribution. With exertion, proximal angulation or compression obstructs blood flow in the aberrant artery, leading to distal ischemia, ventricular tachycardia, and fibrillation.[18]

At highest risk for sudden death are those with a dominant aberrant artery that perfuses a large region of myocardium. The risk of sudden death is greatest during the first 3 decades of life. One third of patients have prior exertional syncope or angina.[18] Between 50% and 64% of deaths due to coronary artery anomalies are related to exertion.[33]

CONGENITAL HEART LESIONS

Marfan Syndrome and Aortic Dissection

Marfan syndrome is one of the most common inherited connective tissue disorders.[17] It is estimated to occur in 1 of every 10,000 Americans.[4]

It is inherited as an autosomal dominant trait with variable expression. No racial or gender differences are seen. Cardiovascular manifestations of Marfan syndrome include MVP and aortic dissection. Aortic root disease, dissection, rupture, and valvular disease are the most common causes of sudden death.[18]

The diagnosis of Marfan syndrome requires the presence of 3 of the following 4 features (Table 28-8): a family history of Marfan syndrome (this should prompt investigation in and of itself); cardiac signs (murmur or midsystolic click); skeletal anomaly (kyphoscoliosis, anterior thoracic abnormality, arm span greater than height, upper-to-lower-body ratio more than 1 standard of deviation below the mean); and ocular anomaly (myopia and a history of retinal detachment or lens dislocation).

Suggested Screening

All men over 6 feet and all women over 5 feet, 10 inches should be screened with electrocardiography, slit-lamp examination, and echocardiography when any 2 of the features of Marfan syndrome described above are found.[7]

Recommendations for Athletic Participation

Individuals with Marfan syndrome should avoid contact and collision sports, and those with

Table 28-8. Skeletal, Cardiac, and Ocular Findings in Marfan Syndrome

SKELETAL CHARACTERISTICS
Arachnodactyly
Chest wall deformity
High arched palate
Increased arm span relative to height
Joint hypermobility
Kyphosis
Lordosis
Scoliosis
Tall stature

OCULAR FINDINGS
Superior dislocation of the lens
Myopia
Retinal detachment

CARDIAC FINDINGS
Abnormal aortic root diameter
Aortic dissection
Aortic regurgitation
Mitral valve prolapse
Mitral regurgitation

From Lazar JM: Marfan syndrome: cardiovascular effects and exercise implications. Your Patient and Fitness 10(6): 6–15, 1996, with permission.

evidence of aortic root disease should participate in only low-intensity competitive sports (eg, golf).[14] Aortic root measurements should be undertaken every 6 months to allow continued sport participation.[14]

ARRHYTHMIA AND CONDUCTION ABNORMALITIES

Congenital Long-QT Syndrome

Congenital long-QT syndrome (LQTS) causes an estimated 3000 to 4000 deaths per year in the general population.[35] About two thirds of patients will have had at least 1 or 2 prior syncopal episodes.[35] It is generally inherited as an autosomal dominant condition. Patients with a corrected QT interval of longer than 0.50 second are at greatest risk for sudden death.[18]

Treatment for LQTS may include β-blockers, other anti-arrhythmic medications, implantable defibrillators, or pacemakers.[18,35] Competitive sports are prohibited for individuals with LQTS.[15]

Wolff-Parkinson-White Syndrome

In patients with Wolff-Parkinson-White (WPW) syndrome, there is a small risk of sudden death associated with short antegrade refractory periods and atrial fibrillation.[18] In addition to an ECG, patients should be evaluated with a 24-hour Holter monitor to record data during normal exercise activity, an exercise stress test, and an echocardiogram. Electrophysiologic testing may be necessary, especially in patients with a history of palpitations, syncope, or near-syncope.[15] Electrophysiologic ablation of the bypass tract is curative and the therapy of choice in patients with WPW syndrome. Athletes without either structural heart disease or arrhythmia can participate in all competitive sports without restriction. Athletes who undergo successful ablation of their accessory pathways, and are asymptomatic for 3 to 6 months, can also participate in all sports without restriction.[39]

HIGH-RISK BEHAVIORS

Cocaine

Len Bias's death from cocaine ingestion in 1986 highlighted the use of cocaine among athletes, and the potentially devastating consequences of such use. Cocaine increases heart rate and blood pressure, resulting in greater myocardial oxygen demand.[13] It causes coronary vasospasm, and acute MI has been seen in cocaine users without pre-existing atherosclerotic CAD. Cocaine may also provoke fatal arrhythmias. Sudden death can occur irrespective of the amount ingested, prior use, or route of administration.

Anorexia Nervosa

Cardiac sudden death related to anorexia nervosa may occur as a result of arrhythmia, electrolyte abnormalities, ipecac-induced cardiomyopathy, or CAD.[12]

Anorexia nervosa, which is more common in girls and young women, can result in certain cardiac changes caused by the restricted eating and severe caloric deprivation. These changes may include a decrease in left ventricular chamber dimension, a decrease in left ventricular mass, lower cardiac index secondary to low stroke index and heart rate, lower blood pressure (secondary to lower body mass and relative hypovolemia), bradycardia secondary to increased vagal tone, and a longer QT interval.[6] These changes revert to normal when normal weight is established.[8]

References

1. Becker RC, Corrao JM: Coronary heart disease in women: Medical science coming of age.
2. Blair SN, Kampert JB, Kohl 3rd HW, et al: Influences of cardiorespiratory fitness and other precursors on cardiovascular disease and all-cause mortality in men and women. JAMA 276(3):205–10, 1996.
3. Boudoulas H, et al: Mitral valve prolapse and the mitral valve prolapse syndrome: A diagnostic classification and pathogenesis of symptoms. Am Heart J 118(4):796–815, 1989.
4. Bracker MD, Jones KL, Moore BS: Suspected Marfan's syndrome in a female basketball player. Physician Sportsmed 16(2):69–77, 1988.
5. Cheitlin M, Douglas PS, Parmley WW: 26th Bethesda Conference: Recommendations for determining eligibility for competition in athletes with cardiovascular abnormalities: Acquired valvular heart disease. Med Sci Sports Exerc 26(10 suppl):S254–60, 1994.
6. Cooke RA, Chambers JB, Singh R, et al: QT interval in anorexia nervosa. Br Heart J 72(1):69–73, 1994.
7. Crown LA, Hizon JW, Rodney WM: The athlete's heart. In Mellion MB, Walsh WM, Shelton GL (eds): The Team Physician's Handbook, 2nd edition. Philadelphia, Hanley and Belfus, 1997, pp 294–302.
8. DeSimone G, Scalfi L, Galderisi M, et al: Cardiac abnormalities in young women with anorexia nervosa. Br Heart J 71(3):287–92, 1994.
9. Devereux RB: Mitral valve prolapse. J Am Med Womens Assoc 49(6):192–6, 1994.
10. Douglas PS: Cardiovascular disorders in women. In Agostini R (ed): Medical and Orthopedic Issues of Active and Athletic Women. Philadelphia, Hanley and Belfus, 1994, pp 265–9.

11. Evans CH, Karunaratne HB: Exercise stress testing for the family physician: Part I. Performing the test. Am Fam Physician 45(1):121–32, 1992.

12. Garcia-Rubira JC, Hidalgo R, Gomez-Barrado JJ, et al: Anorexia nervosa and myocardial infarction. Int J Cardiol 14(2):138–40, 1994.

13. Gradman AH: Cardiac effects of cocaine: A review. Yale J Biol Med 61:137–47, 1988.

14. Graham TP, Bricker JT, James, FW, Strong WB: 26th Bethesda Conference: Recommendations for determining eligibility for competition in athletes with cardiovascular abnormalities. Task Force 1: Congenital heart lesions. Med Sci Sports Exerc 26(10 suppl):S246–53, 1994.

15. Houghton JL: Pericarditis and myocarditis. Which is evil and which isn't? Postgrad Med 91(2):273–82, 1992.

16. Joy EA: Mitral valve prolapse in active patients: recognition, treatment, and exercise recommendations. Physician Sportsmed 24(7):78–86, 1996.

17. Lazar JM: Marfan syndrome: cardiovascular effects and exercise implications. Your Patient and Fitness 10(6):6–15, 1996.

18. Liberthson RR: Sudden death from cardiac causes in children and young adults. N Engl J Med 334(16):1039–44, 1996.

19. Marks AR, et al: Identification of high risk and low risk subgroups of patients with mitral valve prolapse. N Engl J Med 320(16):1031–6, 1989.

20. Maron BJ, Isner JM, Mckenna WJ: 26th Bethesda Conference: Recommendations for determining eligibility for competition in athletes with cardiovascular abnormalities. Task Force 3: Hypertrophic cardiomyopathy, myocarditis, and other myopericardial diseases and mitral valve prolapse. Med Sci Sports Exerc 26(10 suppl):S261–7, 1994.

21. Maron BJ, Shirani J, Poliac LC, et al: Sudden death in young competitive athletes. JAMA 276(3):199–204, 1996.

22. Mitchell JH, Haskell WL, Raven PB: 26th Bethesda Conference: Recommendations for determining eligibility for competition in athletes with cardiovascular abnormalities. Classification of sports. Med Sci Sports Exerc. 26(10 suppl):S242–5, 1994.

23. Mosca L: Cardiovascular disease in women. Clin Courier 16(31):1–8, 1998.

24. Mukerji B, Alpert MA, Mukerji V: Cardiovascular changes in athletes. Am Fam Physician 40(3):169–75, 1989.

25. Nishimura RA, McGoon MD, Shub C, et al: Echocardiographically documented mitral valve prolapse long-term followup of 237 patients. N Engl J Med 313(21):1305–09, 1985.

26. Pelliccia A, Maron BJ, Culasso F, et al: Athlete's heart in women: Echocardiographic characterization of highly trained elite female athletes. JAMA 276(3):211–5, 1996.

27. Pocock WA, et al: Sudden death in primary mitral valve prolapse. Am Heart J 107(2):378–82, 1964.

28. Pratt CM, Francis MJ, Divine GW, Young JB: Exercise testing in women with chest pain. Are there additional exercise characteristics that predict true positive results? Chest 95:139–44, 1989.

29. Sanborn CF, Jankowski CM: Gender-specific physiology. In Agostini R (ed): Medical and Orthopedic Issues of Active and Athletic Women. Philadelphia, Hanley and Belfus, 1994, p 26.

30. Savage DD, Garrison RJ, Devereux RB, et al:Mitral valve prolapse in the general population. I. Epidemiologic features: the Framingham Study. Am Heart J 106:571–6, 1983.

31. Scordo KA: Effects of aerobic exercise training on symptomatic women with mitral valve prolapse. Am J Cardiol 67:863–8, 1991.

32. Stoddard MF, et al: Exercise-induced mitral regurgitation is a predictor of morbid events in subjects with mitral valve prolapse. J Am Coll Cardiol 25(3):693–9, 1995.

33. Taylor AJ: Sudden cardiac death associated with coronary artery anomalies. J Am Cardiol 20:640–7, 1992.

34. Thomas RJ, Cantwell JD: Sudden death during basketball games. Physician Sportsmed 18(5):75–8, 1990.

35. Vincent GM: Sudden death in an athlete. Physician Sportsmed 26(7):59–62, 1998.

36. Weiner DA, Ryan TJ, Parsons L, et al: Long-term prognostic value of exercise testing in men and women from the Coronary Artery Surgery Study (CASS) registry. Am J Cardiol 75(14):865–70, 1995.

37. Wells CL: Physical activity and women's health. Phys Activity Fitness Res 2(5):1–6, 1996.

38. Zehender M, Meinertz T, Keul J, et al: ECG variants and cardiac arrhythmias in athletes: Clinical relevance and prognostic importance. Am Heart J 119(6):1378–91, 1990.

39. Zipes DP, Garson A: 26th Bethesda Conference: Recommendations for determining eligibility for competition in athletes with cardiovascular abnormalities. Task Force 6: Arrythmias. Med Sci Sports Exerc 26(10 suppl):S276–83, 1994.

Chapter 29

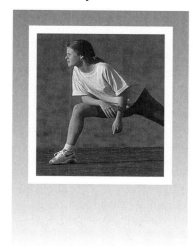

The Physically Challenged Athlete

Cindy J. Chang, M.D.
Katherine L. Dec, M.D.

"You gain strength, courage, and confidence by every experience in which you stop to look fear in the face. You must do the thing which you think you cannot do."

Eleanor Roosevelt

The myriad benefits of exercise for women are well documented and extensively discussed in other chapters. However, there remains a paucity of literature on exercise for people with disabilities, and for disabled women in particular. Although *disability* can be widely defined, in this chapter we will be focusing on physical challenges, or "visible" disabilities, rather than on disabilities associated with aging, medical diseases (eg, hypertrophic cardiomyopathy) or cognition (eg, mental impairment).

Many physicians are not knowledgeable about treating the various medical conditions of people with physical disabilities; there are also significant attitudinal barriers.[49] Many frequently underestimate the quality of life of people with disabilities, which can result in biased advice or limited options. For females with disabilities, this bias is seen most clearly in the areas of physical activity and reproductive health care services. A study by Warms in 1987 found that the services most commonly desired by individuals with physical disabilities but not obtained are planning for an exercise program (43%) and referral to a fitness center (26%).[74]

Even among the nondisabled population, women exercise less than men.[19] Of the approximately 10,000 to 11,000 spinal cord injuries that occur each year, 50% occur in individuals between the ages of 15 and 25. Of the total number of injuries, about 20% to 25% involve females.[4] With the encouragement of health care professionals, disabled females can experience the same great physical and emotional benefits of exercise and sports participation, especially when exercise is begun at a younger age, as women who are not disabled. In turn, increased participation by disabled athletes can heighten the awareness of health care professionals about the medical issues of the disabled female athlete.

A BRIEF HISTORY OF WOMEN IN SPORTS AND PHYSICALLY CHALLENGED FEMALE ATHLETES

The involvement of women in the Olympic games has been well documented since the time of the first women-only Herean games in Greece in 1000 BC. In 1896, at the first modern Olympic games, a Greek woman named Melpomene became the first female to run an unofficial marathon, completing the race in 4.5 hours. Other notable female participants in the Olympics include the American sprinter Wilma Rudolf, who won 3 gold medals in 1960 despite having worn leg braces for 6 years because of childhood polio.

It is more difficult to find information regarding the involvement of physically challenged women in sporting events. Organized competitive sports for athletes in wheelchairs began in England at the Stoke Mandeville Spinal Injuries Centre, where Sir Ludwig Guttman incorporated physical activities and sports into the rehabilitation program. This led to the founding in 1948 of the Stoke Mandeville Games for the Paralysed, in which 2 teams of 14 ex-servicemen and 2 ex-servicewomen competed in archery.[62] In 1960, the first Paralympic games were held in Rome following the Olympics, involving only spinal cord-injured athletes. Film from those 1960 games shows women competing in wheelchairs.[70]

The movement has grown dramatically since those first games in Rome, in which 400 athletes with spinal cord injuries from 21 countries competed. The 1976 Olympiad for the Physically Disabled in Toronto was the first with full competition for blind, paralyzed, and amputee athletes, with 1600 participants from 42 countries. The Paralympic games is now second in size only to the Olympic games. In parallel with the Olympics, these games now involve wheelchair athletes, amputees, *les autres* ("the others"— which includes athletes with various disabilities such as multiple sclerosis, Ehlers-Danlos syndrome, Friedreich's ataxia, dwarfism, arthrogryposis, osteogenesis imperfecta, and muscular dystrophy), visually impaired athletes, and athletes with cerebral palsy. Like the Olympics, the Paralympic games take place every 2 years, alternating summer and winter sports, immediately following the Olympics in the same host country. Events are Olympic events or equivalents, with appropriate changes in rules to allow for the functional ability of the athletes.

At the most recent Paralympic games in Nagano, Japan, in 1998, there were 571 total participants, with 123 (21.5%) being female.

The Olympic games that same year in Nagano had 2177 competitors, with 788 (36.2%) female. Twelve percent of the nations in the Atlanta Olympic games brought no women, compared to 48% of the nations in the Atlanta Paralympics.[30] One can see from Table 29-1 the upward trend in women's participation in the Olympic games. Unfortunately, the breakdown data for gender at the Paralympic games has been tabulated for only the most recent 1996 and 1998 Games.[30,71]

The United States Olympic Committee (USOC) is a member of the International Paralympic Committee (IPC). U.S. Paralympics, a division of the USOC, collaborates with the national governing bodies (NGBs) of the 21 Paralympic sports, as well as the disabled sports organizations (DSOs), member organizations of the USOC (Table 29-2). Together they work to develop high-performance plans and generate enhanced revenue to support the paralympic athletes. Support and resources to disabled athletes are also offered by many other specialized and local sports organizations, such as the Bay Area (San Francisco) Association of Disabled Sailors, the National Softball

Table 29-1. Breakdown of Participants in the Modern Olympic Games According to Gender

		WOMEN	MEN	TOTAL (NATIONS)
1976	Olympic Games	1247 (20.7%)	4781	6028 (92)
	Paralympic Games	?	?	1600 (42)
1980	Olympic Games	1124 (21.6%)	4093	5217 (80)
	Paralympic Games	?	?	2500 (42)
1984	Olympic Games	1567 (23.1%)	5230	6797 (140)
	Paralympic Games	?	?	4080 (42)
1988	Olympic Games	2186 (25.8%)	6279	8465 (159)
	Paralympic Games	?	?	3053 (61)
1992	Olympic Games	2708 (28.9%)	6659	9367 (169)
	Paralympic Games	?	?	3020 (82)
1996	Olympic Games	3523 (34.1%)	6797	10,320 (197)
	Paralympic Games	767 (24.0%)	2428	3195 (103)
2000	Olympic Games	4069 (38.2%)	6582	10,651 (199)
	Paralympic Games	978 (25.4%)	2867	3845 (127)
1976	Winter Olympic Games	231 (20.6%)	892	1123 (37)
	Winter Paralympic Games	?	?	250+ (14)
1980	Winter Olympic Games	233 (21.7%)	839	1072 (37)
	Winter Paralympic Games	?	?	350+ (18)
1984	Winter Olympic Games	274 (21.5%)	1000	1274 (49)
	Winter Paralympic Games	?	?	350+ (22)
1988	Winter Olympic Games	313 (22.0%)	1110	1423 (57)
	Winter Paralympic Games	?	?	397 (22)
1992	Winter Olympic Games	488 (27.1%)	1313	1801 (64)
	Winter Paralympic Games	?	?	475 (24)
1994	Winter Olympic Games	522 (30.0%)	1217	1739 (67)
	Winter Paralympic Games	?	?	1054 (31)
1998	Winter Olympic Games	814 (35.4%)	1488	2302 (72)
	Winter Paralympic Games	123 (21.5%)	448	571 (32)
2002	Winter Olympic Games	886 (36.9%)	1513	2399 (77)
	Winter Paralympic Games	N/A	N/A	421 (36)

Data from United States Olympic Committee Disabled Sports Services for Nagano; Olympic Museum Foundation of the International Olympic Committee; Kamper E, Mallon B: Who's Who at the Olympic Games 1896–1992 with updated data for 1996 and 1998. AGON: Sportverlas. http://www.paralympic.org

Table 29-2. Disabled Sports Organizations

Disabled Sports USA	Persons with physical disabilities, primarily amputation; also paraplegia and lower leg dysfunction
Dwarf Athletic Association of America	Persons 4'10" and under because of chondrodystrophy or related causes
Special Olympics International	Children and adults with mental impairment
United States Association for Blind Athletes	Blind/visually impaired
USA Deaf Sports Federation	Deaf and hearing impaired (> 55-dB loss in the better ear)
United States Cerebral Palsy Athletic Association	Persons with cerebral palsy, stroke, and closed head injuries with acquired vs. congenital motor dysfunction
Wheelchair Sports USA	Persons with permanent disability affecting mobility (eg, spinal cord injury, spina bifida, polio)

Association for the Deaf, and the American Wheelchair Bowling Association. On a community level, local rehabilitation hospitals may have community recreation departments that offer events and skill training in different sports of a less competitive nature such as golf, skiing, and kayaking.

INJURY PATTERNS AMONG PHYSICALLY CHALLENGED ATHLETES

Few epidemiologic studies have addressed the injury experience of athletes with disabilities. Most of the existing research has been limited to wheelchair athletes and athletes competing at large international events. Overall, these studies have shown that the most commonly reported injuries by athletes with disabilities are essentially the same as those in able-bodied athletes.[58] Furthermore, the injury rate for disabled athletes has been found generally to be within the same range as for athletes without disabilities.[7,10,21,22,31] However, most studies utilize survey data, which may introduce reporting bias.

A notable cross-disability retrospective survey was undertaken in 1989 by Ferrara and colleagues[21] of 426 athletes participating in the national competition of the National Wheelchair Athletic Association (NWAA) (now called Wheelchair Sports USA), United States Association for Blind Athletes (USABA), and the United States Cerebral Palsy Athletic Association (USCPAA). They found that 32% of all athletes suffered at least 1 injury during the 6 months prior to their respective national competitions that caused limitation in sport participation lasting for 1 day or more. The differences in injury type were also related to the type of disability. Fifty-seven percent of injuries in NWAA athletes involved the shoulder, arm, or elbow; 53% of injuries reported in blind athletes were of the lower extremities, with over half of these involving the ankle. Athletes with cerebral palsy were more likely than the other 2 groups

to suffer an injury, with the most commonly injured area the knee (21%). Overall, chronic injuries were only slightly more common than acute injuries. When comparing the reported injury rates experienced by nondisabled athletes in similar sports activities, this study found no significant difference in the percentage of disabled athletes reporting injuries.

At the 1976 Toronto Paralympics the same common medical problems were encountered, except that disabled athletes were found to be slightly more vulnerable to stress and fatigue than able-bodied athletes.[31] One half of the Canadian team at the 1988 Seoul Paralympics reported chronic musculoskeletal injuries, and the most common medical illnesses in descending order were upper respiratory tract infections, gastrointestinal disorders, and urinary tract infections in the catheter-dependent athletes.[10] A survey of disabled skiers at the Winter National Games in 1989 found the same distribution of injuries as in skiers without a disability.[22]

Only 1 study has examined the incidence of injury in pediatric disabled athletes. In a survey of competitors, mostly with spina bifida, at the 1990 Junior National Wheelchair Games, minor skin injuries were prevalent, most commonly blisters, wheel burns, abrasions, and bruises.[76] Ninety-seven percent of the athletes taking part in track events reported injuries in either training or competition. Nearly half of the track participants reported problems with hyperthermia and 9% of the swimmers reported hypothermia. Bladder infections were reported in 22% of respondents. More than a third of the track participants reported soft-tissue injuries such as sprains, strains, and tendinitis.

While these studies failed to distinguish between male and female injury types and injury rates, one can conclude that because of the similar rates and types of injuries as able-bodied athletes, the female athlete with a physical impairment should not be dissuaded from getting involved in an exercise program or sports for fear of further injury or illness.

Studies have noted that the participants needed to improve injury-prevention practices (eg, by becoming involved in a conditioning program or flexibility and strengthening program, and improving nutritional and fluid intake) and become more aware of the onset of fatigue and the need to discontinue activity.[21,22,76] Despite the above, the physically challenged female athlete is often faced with unique concerns specific to her impairment and/or use of adaptive equipment. With the increasing involvement of girls and women with disabilities in sports, in part due to the elimination of environmental barriers and increased availability of public recreation, it has become essential that sports medicine professionals be familiar with these concerns and their implications for injury prevention.

MEDICAL ASSESSMENT OF THE PHYSICALLY CHALLENGED FEMALE ATHLETE

In order to prescribe exercise regimens and prevent, diagnose, and treat sports-related injuries, the athlete's physician and other health care providers need some familiarity with the disability itself. For example, it is imperative that one knows the level and type of spinal cord injury (SCI) for an athlete in a wheelchair, as this can help predict her functional abilities, and in what type of activities and sports she can best participate. A chart developed by The American Academy of Orthopaedic Surgeons in 1983 lists major physical disabilities and major sporting activities that are possible for athletes with these disabilities.[16,17] Table 29-3 gives some examples from this chart. Although this template can be helpful as a guide, a large number of factors should be considered in addition to ability when recommending a particular sport, including age, skill level, level of interest, other motivational factors and goals, availability and costs, and the risk–benefit ratio.[16]

While there is limited information available regarding the medical assessment of the physically challenged female athlete, the concept of the "team" remains important in providing sports medicine care for this population. Most of these athletes will have been through some type of structured rehabilitation program following the initial diagnosis of their impairment and have had the benefit of working with a multidisciplinary team. This team will have managed the acute and continuing medical issues, in addition to assessing, modifying, and maintaining the adaptive equipment needs of the athlete. Information gathered from this team, which include various specialist physicians, therapists, and educators, can help the sports medicine physician determine the type of physical impairment, historical information (Table 29-4), and potential additional equipment needs related to the particular sport in question. Lastly, it is essential for the health care team to avoid focusing solely on the physical impairment. Although some of the health care needs of physically challenged women may be unique, to a large extent, their needs are also those common to all women. Engaging physically challenged women in a shared decision-making process about their reproductive needs, or their

Table 29-3. The American Academy of Orthopaedic Surgeons Participation Possibility Chart

	GOLF	DOWN-HILL SKIING	SWIMMING	WHEEL-CHAIR BASKETBALL	SOCCER	VOLLEYBALL
Amputations						
Upper extremity	RA	R	R		R	R
Lower extremity above knee	R	RA	R	R	I	R
Lower extremity below knee	R	R	R	I	R	R
Cerebral palsy						
Ambulatory	R	RA	R		R	R
Wheelchair	I		I	R		I
SCI						
Cervical		IA	R	I		IA
High thoracic: T1–5	RA	IA	R	R		RA
Thoracolumbar: T6–L3	RA	RA	R	R		RA
Lumbosacral: L4–below	R	R	R	I	R	R
Osteogenesis imperfecta	I	I	R	R	X	I

R, recommended; X, not recommended; A, adapted; I, individualized; blank, no information or not applicable.

Adapted from Clark MW: The physically challenged athlete. Adolesc Med 9(3): 491–9, 1998, with permission.

Table 29-4. Historical Information for the Physically Challenged Athlete

Prior secondary medical issues related to the impairment (eg, recurring pressure sores)
Concurrent systemic illnesses (eg, uncontrollable seizures, diabetes, arthritis, heart disease)
Presence of multiple impairments (eg, amputation and SCI)
Current medications (eg, seizure or spasticity medications)
History of previous surgeries (eg, past spinal fusion in an SCI may limit the truncal movement and strength necessary for certain sports chairs, or sports activities[25])
Success of current bowel/bladder management program
Level of functional independence (eg, independent in transfers from wheelchair, donning adaptive equipment)
Level of independence in mobility
Adaptive equipment needs
Prior training
Prior exercise program
Further questions specific to the individual's impairment should be asked as needed to clarify the athlete's ability to compete

possible use of hormone replacement therapy or other medications for prevention of fractures, is important, as is regular screening for breast and colorectal cancer. These simple interventions have the potential to delay the onset and improve the course of many chronic conditions that may beset them in later life.

Preparticipation Evaluation

The goals of the preparticipation evaluation are to *assess, educate,* and *prevent*—assess physical capability to participate; educate the athlete in the potential medical risks of the selected activity; and provide information on prevention of these medical risks. There may be disqualifying factors unique to the physically challenged, for example, poor pulmonary function in athletes with muscular dystrophy, infected pressure sores in wheelchair or amputee athletes, or congenital cardiac problems. Disqualification from sports participation should be considered on a case-by-case basis guided by recommendations in the sports literature of the able-bodied.

Certain physical impairments, such as hearing loss or amputation, may not preclude participation with able-bodied peers. Since 1978, athletes with below-knee amputations can compete in interscholastic sports with able-bodied peers, provided certain requirements are met.[1] Depending on the sport, athletes with upper-extremity amputations have also participated with able-bodied peers in athletic competition. Athletes with complete hearing loss have successfully competed in interscholastic sports. Since hearing loss and blindness are impairments of communication and not physical limitations in the sport's functional skill, they have sometimes not been considered under the classification of "physical challenge." Although the 1990 Americans with Disabilities Act

(ADA) does not specifically address the issue of sports participation,[40] it will likely affect the sports arena for the physically challenged by increasing their access to public recreation facilities and programs.

Classification systems are used in national and international competitions[45,65] to determine a competition class by utilizing functional criteria and, to a lesser extent, the medical impairment.[6] This chapter cannot do justice to the various classification systems used; more information can be obtained from the National Governing Body for that specific physical impairment.

As with the able-bodied preparticipation examination, the importance of the history is self-evident. Unique issues to review are included in Table 29-4. Additional areas of attention concerning medical impairments present in this population are noted in Table 29-5. The focus is to screen for medical impairments, with less emphasis on the functional classification specified in competition. The additional areas of evaluation should be tailored as appropriate to the athlete's physical impairment.

Several of these areas of attention require further discussion. The cardiac evaluation is similar to that of able-bodied athletes. The extensive medical literature reviewed has made no mention in case reports or scientific studies of an increased risk of sudden cardiac death in physically challenged or Special Olympics athletes, despite the high incidence of congenital heart problems in the latter.[32,53]

With regard to gastrointestinal and urologic issues of some physically challenged athletes, precompetition planning of management strategies [ie, intermittent urinary catheterization, continuous (indwelling) urinary catheter or bowel elimination] is helpful, especially in lengthy events such as marathons. The athlete should be informed that the various medications

Table 29-5. Additional Areas of Attention in the Physically Challenged Female Athlete

Vital signs	Orthostatic blood pressure, peripheral capillary refill, pulse; vital capacity in conditions with muscular or neurologic impairment affecting respiration
Skin	Insensate areas; skin breakdown and integrity; check for vasomotor changes in weak or painful limbs
Ears, nose, throat	Visual acuity, visual field deficits; hearing acuity; aspiration risk
Pulmonary	Diaphragmatic excursion (at nipple line, base of ribs, and at navel)
Gastrointestinal/urologic	Condition of necessary equipment for bowel/bladder control; urinary tract infection or bowel impaction; check skin condition at colostomy or feeding tube sites (gastrostomy or jejunostomy) when present
Neurologic	SCI level and classify degree of involvement: complete or incomplete; evaluate proprioception, deep and light touch, and pain sensation; evaluate balance (seated, standing)
Musculoskeletal	Manual muscle testing of joint stabilizing muscles (eg, shoulder in wheelchair athletes). Active and passive range of motion
Functional	Level of independence in transfers; mobility; and proficiency in use of adaptive equipment
Cognitive	As it pertains to skill acquisition and coaching; safety judgment

utilized for both are flexic (decreased tone and increased capacity, with urinary retention) and reflexic (increased tone and decreased capacity, with involuntary voiding). Neurogenic bladders can have side effects such as impaired sweating, drowsiness, hypotension, and gastrointestinal problems.

In assessing neurologic function, classifying hypertonicity using the Ashworth scale[3] (Table 29-6), in addition to eliciting provocative positions that cause increased or decreased tone or trigger primitive reflexes (eg, tonic labyrinthine reflex, startle reflex, extensor synergy, or flexor synergy) is important. Neutral head position and proper alignment during activities can help decrease hypertonicity in susceptible athletes.

As most injuries incurred are soft-tissue injuries, the musculoskeletal examination can also help the physician tailor the training and conditioning program to areas of potential injuries. For a wheelchair athlete with recurring shoulder impingement, with tight pectoralis muscle groups and weak scapular stabilizers, the physician can design a strength and flexibility program to enhance shoulder function. This area is of significant importance in wheelchair athletes, who tend to sustain overuse injuries to their shoulders in sports. Structural deformities (eg, genu valgum and associated foot pronation) are frequently seen in ambulatory athletes with cerebral palsy and can contribute to increased biomechanical stress during sports activities. Orthotics and other such devices should be considered during participation in order to minimize the risk of injury and to enhance performance.[21] Advanced surgical techniques for amputees, such as lengthening of stumps using the Ilizarov distraction technique, are being performed to help facilitate function.[51]

SPECIFIC MEDICAL ISSUES FACING THE PHYSICALLY CHALLENGED ATHLETE

Some of the specific medical areas of concern in the physically challenged population can be addressed during the preparticipation examination. Additional medical issues in this population can become more significant through sports participation than would occur in the physically challenged nonathlete. Being aware of the treatment options for the unique issues of physically challenged athletes is important. The most common concerns for physically challenged athletes are discussed below, as are aspects of these issues and other issues pertinent only to female athletes. As physically challenged females participate in sports in greater numbers, our understanding of the sports injury- and training-related issues of this population will grow as it has in able-bodied female athletes.

Table 29-6. Ashworth Scale for Measurement of Severity of Hypertonicity

0, normal

1, slight increase, "catch" with limb passive movement

2, mild increase, limb moves easily with passive range of motion

3, moderate increase, passive range of motion is difficult

4, severe tone—rigid muscle

From Ashworth B: Carisoprodol in multiple sclerosis. Practitioner 192:540–2, 1964, with permission.

Thermoregulation

Thermoregulation is an important issue because athletes compete away from their home in many climates and conditions. Hypothermia and hyperthermia are of special concern in athletes with SCI. These athletes are unable to generate sufficient body heat to maintain core temperature. Possible decreased input to the hypothalamic thermoregulatory centers,[60] the lack of muscle mass below the level of lesion, and the loss of vasomotor and sudomotor neural control likely impair this "shiver" response. Damp clothing also adds to the loss of body heat, however, the SCI athlete may not be able to perceive this dampness. It is crucial to monitor swimmers, endurance racers, and cold weather sports participants for hypothermia.

Bloomquist[7] points out that "hyperthermia presents an even greater danger to the [spinal cord injured] athlete than to the able-bodied one." Sweating is often impaired below the level of the spinal cord lesion, requiring the body to rely upon a smaller surface area (ie, arms and upper trunk) for evaporative cooling. Feeling the skin under the arms of a distressed athlete during competition can be a useful tactic. If it is hot, the athlete is likely to not be losing heat adequately, and lighter clothing, more fluids, or dousing the skin with water is necessary.[18] Mechanisms of local cooling are being studied but are currently found to be ineffective.[2]

Some female athletes may not want to share information about SCI-related hyperhidrosis, which can lead to uncomfortable and embarrassing social situations. The medications that are used for this condition, including propantheline, phenoxybenzamine, scopolamine, and atropine, block the muscarinic receptors responsible for sweat gland stimulation.[13] However, in exercise, their effects increase the risk of hyperthermia. They also need to be considered carefully in these athletes because of their potential effect on neurogenic bladder function.

Venous Blood Pooling and Exercise Capacity

In addition to the impairment of autonomic neural control and its effect on thermoregulation in preventing dehydration, impaired blood flow can restrict achievement of maximal exercise capacity in the SCI athlete, who may already be hypovolemic while training or competing. The partial or complete loss of innervation from the sympathetic nervous system results in the diminished reflexive control of blood flow.[55] Exercise capacity is further limited by the lack of venous pumping from active lower-extremity musculature in SCI. The risk of deep venous thrombosis should also be considered in the SCI athlete, especially in the premenopausal athlete. Strategies for minimizing venous blood pooling during exercise include the use of an abdominal binder[34] and wearing positive-pressure garments (stockings).[55] Lower-extremity functional electrical stimulation, while often impractical, can also be considered.

Autonomic Dysreflexia

Autonomic dysreflexia is most often a problem in SCI of the T6 vertebral level and above. Without supraspinal neurologic inhibition, the sympathetic nervous system is left unchecked. Symptoms of autonomic dysreflexia include headaches, piloerection, sweating, paroxysmal hypertension, and/or bradyarrhythmia. The cause is usually some form of noxious stimulus to the spinal cord below the level of the lesion, such as pressure sores, urinary tract infection, fracture, tight clothing, or a distended bowel or bladder. Thus, the first step in treatment is to eliminate the offending stimulus. In their review of treatment in autonomic dysreflexia, Braddom and Rocco[8] outlined a comprehensive treatment approach. Autonomic dysreflexia should be considered a medical emergency and treated quickly, as the rapidly developing hypertension can lead to cerebral hemorrhage, blindness, seizures, and even death.

The practice of self-inducing autonomic dysreflexia ("boosting") to improve race times is becoming more prevalent among SCI competitors.[11] It is proposed that increased cardiac output and vasoconstriction leads to increased venous return and increased muscle substrate, while the epinephrine acts to enhance glycogenolysis, lipolysis, pulmonary bronchodilation, and central nervous system (CNS) arousal. To some competitive athletes, this purported 10% improvement in athletic performance seems worth the risks of hypertension, hyperthermia, and urinary tract damage (eg, from a clamped Foley catheter).

Spasticity

Spasticity is a potential problem in any athlete with CNS injury, spina bifida, SCI, or cerebral palsy or other neuromuscular disorder, and it is often difficult to manage. Increase in tone is usually secondary to a nociceptive stimulus, such as urinary tract infection or distended viscera, as noted previously in the discussion of autonomic dysreflexia. Treatment involves elimination of the offending stimulus, changing posture position if this stimulated increased tone, and incorporating a stretching program if one has not already been commenced. The spasticity medications taken by the athlete should be reviewed and an appropriate, successful bowel and bladder program should be in effect.

Spasticity and intractable neuropathic pain are not infrequently related. A variety of pharmacologic and other approaches have been described for management of these problems in SCI, including oral medications such as dantrolene sodium (Dantrium) and baclofen (Lioresal), local anesthetic blocks, and even intrathecal administration of clonidine (Catapres) and baclofen.[39,45]

Heterotopic Ossification

Heterotopic ossification refers to ectopic bone formation, usually in the area of major joints. In SCI athletes it usually occurs below the level of the spinal lesion, but it is also a risk in athletes with traumatic brain injury. Localized pain, increased warmth, swelling, and contracture are some of the symptoms of ectopic bone growth. Heterotopic ossification should be considered in autonomic dysreflexia and when there is an unexplainable increase in spasticity. Sports participation does not increase the risk of ectopic bone formation.

Premature Osteoporosis

Women with physical disabilities appear to be at significantly higher risk for osteoporosis than nondisabled women.[33] The lack of weight bearing itself with immobilization is a known risk factor.[69] SCI athletes do not benefit from the forces applied to the bone from repetitive lower-extremity muscle-tendon pulling and thus are at risk for osteopenia. In contact sports, this decreased bone mass puts the paralyzed extremities at risk for fractures. Although electrically stimulated ambulation and other assisted ambulatory devices have proven benefits of increasing maximal oxygen consumption (VO_2max), decreasing heart rate, and increasing stroke volume at peak work efforts, the benefits for preventing osteoporosis are equivocal.[44,68]

In addition, those women with associated medical illnesses requiring chronic glucocorticoid use or certain anticonvulsants (severe asthma, rheumatoid arthritis, epilepsy) and those with digestive disorders or malabsorptive problems (Crohn's disease, colostomy, diabetes) have an increased risk of osteoporosis. The treatment and prevention of osteoporosis is similar to that in the able-bodied population. The challenges include emphasizing dietary calcium

and vitamin D while avoiding overuse of calcium supplements if one is already at risk for renal calculi, and finding alternatives such as calcitonin or bisphosphonates (if not of childbearing age) if risks outweigh the benefits of estrogen replacement therapy.[28,52]

Pressure Sores

Pressure sores can present in amputees with improperly fitting prosthetics or in wheelchair athletes from improper seating or from prolonged sitting. The correct seating system in wheelchair athletes, in addition to regular pressure relief, and proper fit of adaptive equipment and prosthetics will reduce the risk of pressure sores. Also, wearing absorbent fabric can reduce skin surface moisture and the potential for skin shear. In some sports, such as wheelchair racing, the positioning required by the chair (knees higher than the hips) can increase the risk of pressure sores over the sacrum and ischium.

Musculoskeletal Injuries

As mentioned throughout this chapter, soft-tissue injuries are the bane of physically challenged athletes. Wheelchair athletes are at particular risk for overuse injuries of the upper extremity, especially the shoulder complex, because of repetitive use of the upper extremities for propulsion. Wrist and forearm extensor tendonitis can result from the "backhand" wheelchair stroke, and carpal tunnel syndrome from repetitive compression and trauma to the heel of the hand. Also, compensatory muscle imbalances may develop at the shoulder from long-term wheelchair propulsion, or from a training program deficient in the strengthening of the rotator cuff and scapular stabilizer muscles.[9] This can lead to musculoskeletal injury in those athletes participating in sports requiring different movement patterns, such as swimming, throwing, or racquet sports. Quadriplegics suffer from a denervation of the shoulder adductors, as the latissimus dorsi, teres major, and lower fibers of the pectoralis major are all innervated by the C7 nerve root. This makes them less effective at counterbalancing the deltoid, which pulls the humerus cephalad.

Once again, there is a paucity of research examining the shoulder strength differences among men and women with physical disabilities, especially those that are wheelchair confined. In the able-bodied population, a study examining Masters' level swimmers found that men were significantly stronger than women in trunk extension and flexion, and in internal and external shoulder rotation.[37] The women performed significantly better in the supraspinatus muscle test. In another study testing shoulder isometric strength in men and women ages 17 to 70, the mean strength of females was 65% to 70% of men, but differences almost disappeared after accounting for weight.[5] While the wheelchair-dependent female athlete may also compare in a similar fashion to her male counterpart, research in this area would help in targeting shoulder rehabilitation issues specifically for this population.

Rehabilitation of these injuries follows a similar protocol to that in able-bodied athletes. Modifications may be needed in strengthening programs, such as provision of wheelchair-accessible weight machines or modifications of the free weights for limb deficiency or other functional impairment. Techniques addressing proprioceptive neuromuscular re-education and flexibility are also important. "Relative rest" in treatment recommendations will be difficult to follow, as there may be limited muscular function available to compensate for the injured area when performing daily tasks. Thus, prevention is the key.

BENEFITS OF EXERCISE

The risks of exercise have been discussed above. However, the risks of inactivity are potentially more far reaching. In the past, morbidity and mortality of the disabled population were due either to the acute phase of the acquired disability or to secondary urinary tract, respiratory tract, or skin infections, especially in those with SCI. With the advent of improved health care and prevention in these areas, the ultimate goal has shifted from an extension of life expectancy to the attainment of an optimal level of independent living and quality of life.[46] Lifestyle has now become the major factor in morbidity and mortality. The prevalence of diseases associated with obesity, such as cardiovascular disease and diabetes mellitus, is higher in the SCI population. For example, the mortality rate for cardiovascular disease is 228% higher in the SCI population.[35] Sedentary SCI individuals have "at-risk" levels of body fat (over 25% for men and over 32% for women). Physically active SCI men and women can decrease these percentages (16% to 24% and 24% to 32%), but still have an above-average fat mass, especially when compared with able-bodied men and women (15% and 23%).

The life expectancy of women currently exceeds that of men by almost 7 years, yet women spend about twice as many years disabled prior to death compared to men.[36]

Studies have shown that older women are weaker than men and become disabled and dependent in their later years at a much greater rate. Studies of both middle-aged and elderly women support a protective effect of physical fitness and physical activity on functional limitation.[12,29,56] Not surprisingly, disability and physical activity were inversely associated, with inactivity being most common among the most disabled women. Those with poorer strength reported more difficulties in motor activities; greater strength was found among the more physically active.

Another study testing functionally impaired community-dwelling elderly men and women found that strength loss was strongly associated with functional decline, but was reversible with exercise.[14] While lower-extremity strength gain was associated with gains in chair rise performance, gait speed, and mobility tasks such as gait and transfers, it did not result in improved endurance, balance, or disability. However, strength gain was associated with improvement in confidence in mobility. These results all support the idea of strength training as an intervention that could potentially improve physical health status in older women; perhaps these results could be extrapolated for the physically challenged female population.

For those with SCI, arm exercise is less efficient and less effective than lower-body exercise in developing and maintaining both central and peripheral aspects of cardiovascular fitness. The situation is further compounded in SCI because of poor venous return resulting from lower-limb blood pooling, a lack of sympathetic tone, and a diminished or absent venous "muscle pump" in the legs.[54] Despite this, obtaining a cardiopulmonary training effect in individuals with SCI is quite possible. However, the majority of these studies have been done in male subjects.

A 1998 study by Hjeltnes and Wallberg-Henriksson suggested that functional improvement in tetraplegic patients was not necessarily followed by aerobic metabolic improvement.[27] Male tetraplegic and paraplegic subjects participated in an arm cycling program. While the peak VO_2 improved in the paraplegic group, it did not change in the tetraplegic group. Mean heart rate and mean stroke volume also did not change in the tetraplegic patients, but both muscle strength and activities of daily living improved significantly.

Schmid and coworkers' study in 1998 of elite *female* wheelchair basketball players found that during graded wheelchair ergometry, wheelchair basketball players showed a higher maximal work rate, VO₂max, and maximal lactate level without a difference in maximal heart rate and workload than did SCI controls.[61] During the competitive basketball game, high cardiovascular stress was observed, indicating a high aerobic metabolism.

Various types of electrical stimulation-induced leg exercises have been introduced in attempts to further improve cardiovascular conditioning in SCI. In able-bodied humans, leg muscle afferents contributed to increased cardiac output during exercise, primarily via increased heart rate. In contrast, athletes with SCI were able to raise cardiac output only during electrically stimulated leg exercise, which increased venous return in the absence of any change in heart rate.[67] Combinations of functional electrically stimulated leg cycling with an upper-extremity training program have been shown to further improve aerobic capacity.[42,57]

Physical deconditioning can significantly decrease quality of life in individuals with SCI, ultimately placing them in a state of complete dependency. As shown in the studies above, and summarized in an extensive review by Noreau and Shephard,[46] exercise in this population can improve physical capacity, improve muscle strength and endurance, increase the high-density lipoprotein level, and normalize insulinemia. Exercise can also reduce or prevent secondary conditions of spasticity and contractures, chronic pain, and disuse osteoporosis. By reducing the physical strain of activities of daily living and reducing risks of developing chronic medical illnesses, one can maintain independence and improve the quality of life. The potential savings in terms of medical costs, home health assistance costs, and extended care facility costs are also enormous.

Lastly, the psychological benefits of exercise are endless and include improved body image and self-esteem. Much of the time the physically challenged are viewed as being dependent and vulnerable, or as objects of pity. The ability to exercise and compete can help in overcoming these stereotypes. The social value of exercise and the feeling of being mainstreamed into society are important.[26] Athletic participation tends to "level the playing field" in society's evaluation of individuals with physical impairments. Dispelling misperceptions of "disability" in the physically challenged is being achieved again and again in the athletic arena.

OBSTACLES TO EXERCISE FACING THE PHYSICALLY CHALLENGED FEMALE ATHLETE

Major barriers to exercise include inaccessibility of facilities and exercise equipment, high costs of specialized equipment such as lightweight wheelchairs, and the lack of opportunities and events to train and compete. The passage of the ADA created a greater awareness of the needs of people with disabilities, and forced these issues of accessibility and lifestyle to the forefront.

Fortunately for the physically challenged, businesses are beginning to recognize that they are an important consumer spending group, and are developing new products with more sophisticated technology that are specifically designed for their use.[23] These products have often become popular with the able-bodied population. For example, vibrating pagers initially developed for the hearing impaired are now standard for the general population.

Besides the ADA, another force behind this drive is the aging baby-boomer population. As their vision becomes impaired and their function and mobility become limited, they will be requiring more large-type periodicals, easier-to-grip modified free weights, and customized vans. This can only mean that such equipment is likely to be more accessible to the physically challenged population through increased convenience and decreased costs. For example, Cannondale's lightweight racing wheelchairs are being sold in bicycle shops rather than the traditional medical equipment stores.[23] More recreational opportunities are becoming available, such as wheelchair-accessible golf courses and vacation resorts that encourage SCI scuba divers.

Lastly, some of the greatest obstacles to consider may be the societal, cultural, and individual attitudes and values placed on exercise and physical activity. If a physically challenged female perceives that she lacks the ability, or faces a risk of injury, she will not pursue it. If there are no personnel available at the local health club to instruct her in a weight-training program, no matter how accessible the facility or equipment may be, she will not return. It has been suggested that girls with disabilities are protected from failure, while boys are encouraged to challenge those barriers that get in their way.[26] Thus, girls with disabilities may not be encouraged to challenge themselves through sports activity, for fear of failure.

OTHER IMPORTANT ISSUES FACING THE PHYSICALLY CHALLENGED FEMALE

The intention of this section is to familiarize the health care professional with other pertinent medical and psychosocial issues specific to the physically challenged female, whether active or sedentary. It is important to be aware of, counsel, and perhaps treat these issues if one is responsible also for the primary health care of these female athletes.

Obstetric and Gynecologic Issues

Women with disabilities tend to be less likely than women without disabilities to receive pelvic examinations on a regular basis, placing them at a higher risk for delayed diagnosis of breast and cervical cancer.[47] Amenorrhea can occur in 60% of women with SCI; however, within 1 year of injury 90% will resume normal menses.[15] Sexual functioning among women with physical disabilities has been researched, with psychological and social factors such as work status, age, household income, and living with a significant other exerting a strong impact on variables such as sexual desire and activity.[48] More than 50% of women with SCI report weekly sexual activity, 20% use contraception, and 30% have undergone surgical sterilization.[15]

Although pregnancy can result in life-threatening circumstances for women with SCI, such as unrecognized autonomic hyperreflexia from uterine contractions, it is very important to realize that with coordinated prenatal health care services, women with paraplegia and even quadriplegia can safely carry and deliver healthy babies. Often an epidural anesthetic is all that is needed to treat autonomic hyperreflexia and to allow labor to progress.[73] Despite popular belief, women with SCI are not more likely to have miscarriages or long, difficult labors, and by itself SCI is not an indication for a caesarean section.[49] There is no research available on the effects of exercise on the physically challenged pregnant woman.

Certain medical complications of pregnancy, such as urinary tract infection, decubitus ulcers, thrombophlebitis, bowel impactions, and respiratory difficulties, are more likely in the physically challenged female.[4] Adaptations to pregnancy may be needed, such as switching from intermittent catheterization to an indwelling catheter to maintain continence, or changing from a manual to an electric wheelchair.

Childcare issues should initially be addressed at the antepartum visits. Adaptive techniques and devices such as a harness to lift the baby from the floor, changes in the home environment to include crib and changing table adjustments for wheelchair access, and identifying a support network should best be explored before the pregnancy commences. As breastfeeding is the preferred method for feeding infants, the physically challenged mother needs to be given the opportunity and support to breastfeed. An excellent review of the complex interaction that occurs between the sympathetic nervous system and neuroendocrine system during breastfeeding is recommended.[24] The breasts are innervated by the 4th, 5th and 6th intercostal nerves (T4-6). If the lesion is below T6, breastfeeding should be effective, as long as there is adequate nipple simulation from the baby. If the lesion is at T6 and above, there may be a decrease in milk production after 6 weeks postpartum by the lack of the sympathetic nervous system feedback, and thus the inability of the myoepithelial cells to contract.

Domestic Violence and Abuse

Women with disabilities, regardless of age, race, ethnicity, sexual orientation, or class, are assaulted, raped, and abused at a rate 2 times greater than for nondisabled women.[63,64] Eighty-three percent of women with disabilities will be sexually assaulted during their lifetime.[64] The greater the disability, the greater the risk of being assaulted.

Violence can create more disabilities, such as chronic pain, head injury, paralysis, and memory loss. However, health care professionals need to be aware that it is often difficult for physically challenged women to leave abusive situations, both physically and emotionally. They are often financially dependent on their abuser or the physical means of fleeing may be lacking, and few women's shelters are accessible and provide attendant care. Women with children may run the risk of losing custody of their children because authorities may question their ability to care for them alone.

Risk-Taking Behaviors

Nattiv found that able-bodied intercollegiate athletes demonstrated significantly higher risk-taking behaviors than their nonathlete peers, and athletes with 1 risk-taking behavior were at risk for multiple risk-taking behaviors.[43] Risk-taking behaviors also appear to be common in physically challenged athletes. Some of these athletes, such as the SCI athlete who survived a motor vehicle accident, or an amputee athlete who lost her leg to osteosarcoma, have already "faced death" once. Therefore, experimenting with drugs or sex may seem only a minimal risk to them.

People with disabilities show higher rates of illicit drug use than the general population.[41] Problems with adjustment to their disability, social isolation, and chronic medical or health problems can encourage the illicit drug use. Moore and Li's study found that 3 psychosocial variables—negative self-esteem, hostility, and risk-taking—were significantly correlated with illicit drug use.[41]

Suris and coworkers' study of adolescents with chronic diseases and disability found that despite popular belief, even the individuals with "visible" disabilities were at least as sexually active as their healthy peers.[66] Overall, this population also reported a greater history of sexually transmitted diseases, and in addition, 1 in 4 females had sustained sexual abuse.[66] Adolescents will avoid prolonged social contact with a child with a disability if this will jeopardize their social standing with their peers.[75] Thus, physically challenged females may look to sexual activity as a means of gaining acceptance, and demonstrating their "normality."[66]

CONCLUDING REMARKS

This chapter has attempted to provide an overview of issues pertinent to being a sports medicine physician for the physically challenged female athlete. As a sports medicine physician for the physically challenged female athlete, one should work with other professionals as a team to address her many needs. Identifying potential medical issues that could affect performance, educating in preventative strategies, and providing information for local recreation or competitive activities are also roles of the sports medicine physician. Soft-tissue injuries develop in the physically challenged female athlete as readily as in the able-bodied female athlete. It is important to be preventive and address these issues before a training program is commenced. Also it must be remembered that the physically challenged female is first a female. Medical and psychosocial issues pertinent to the female population are just as important to this unique group as to their nondisabled counterparts.

Given the number and variety of physical impairments in this population, sports-specific adaptive equipment and specific sports for each of the physical impairments could not be covered.[50] Although research is ongoing in the area

of physically challenged athletes, most of the research studying the effects of exercise is done in the athletic and nonathletic wheelchair population, and primarily in the male subset.[20,38,59,72] More research is needed to continue to advance physically challenged female athletes and to optimize their athletic performance.

References

1. Adams RC, McCubbin JA: Games, Sports, and Exercises for the Physically Disabled, 4th edition. Pennsylvania, Lea & Febiger, 1990.
2. Armstrong LE, Maresh CM, Riebe D, et al: Local cooling in wheelchair athletes during exercise-heat stress. Med Sci Sports Exerc 27(2):211–6, 1995.
3. Ashworth B: Carisoprodol in multiple sclerosis. Practitioner 192:540–2, 1964.
4. Atterbury JL, Groome LJ: Pregnancy in women with spinal cord injuries. Nurs Clin North Am 33(4):603–13, 1998.
5. Backman E, Johansson V, Hager B, et al: Isometric muscle strength and muscular endurance in normal persons aged between 17 and 70 years. Scand J Rehabil Med 27(2):109–17, 1995.
6. Bednarczyk JH, Sanderson DJ: Comparison of functional and medical assessment in the classification of persons with spinal cord injury. J Rehabil Res Dev 30(4):405–11, 1993.
7. Bloomquist LE: Injuries to athletes with physical disabilities: prevention implications. Phys Sports Med 14(9):97–105, 1986.
8. Braddom RL, Rocco JF. Autonomic dysreflexia: a survey of current treatment. Am J Phys Med Rehabil 70:234–41, 1991.
9. Burnham RS, May L, Nelson E, et al: Shoulder pain in wheelchair athletes. The role of muscle imbalance. Am J Sports Med 21(2):238–42, 1993.
10. Burnham R, Newell E, Steadward R: Sports medicine for the physically disabled: The Canadian team experience at the 1988 Seoul Paralympic Games. Clin J Sports Med 1:193–6, 1991.
11. Burnham R, Wheeler G, Bhambhani Y, et al: Intentional induction of autonomic dysreflexia among quadriplegic athletes for performance enhancement: efficacy, safety, and mechanism of action. Clin J Sport Med 4(1):1–10, 1994.
12. Butler RN, Davis R, Lewis CB, et al: Physical fitness: how to help older patients live stronger and longer. Geriatrics 53(9):26–8, 31–2, 39–40, 1998.
13. Canaday BR, Stanford RH: Propantheline bromide in the management of hyperhidrosis associated with spinal cord injury. Ann Pharmacother 29(5):489–92, 1995.
14. Chandler JM, Duncan PW, Kochersberger G, et al: Is lower extremity strength gain associated with improvement in physical performance and disability in frail, community-dwelling elders? Arch Phys Med Rehabil 79(1):24–30, 1998.
15. Charlifue SW, Gerhart KA, Menter RR, et al: Sexual issues of women with spinal cord injuries. Paraplegia 30:192, 1992.
16. Clark MW: The physically challenged athlete. Adoles Med 9(3):491–9, 1998.
17. Clark MW, Eilert RE (eds): Sports and recreational programs for the child and young adult with physical disability: Proceedings of the Winter Park Seminar. Chicago, American Academy of Orthopaedic Surgeons, 1983, pp 38–9.

18. Corcoran PJ, Goldman RF, Hoerner EF, et al: Sports medicine and the physiology of wheelchair marathon racing. Orthop Clin North Am 11(4): 697–716, 1980.

19. Crespo CJ, Keteyian SJ, Heath GW, et al: Leisure-time physical activity among U.S. adults. Arch Intern Med 156:93–8, 1996.

20. Dallmeijer AJ, Kappe YJ, Veeger D.HEJ, et al: Anaerobic power output and propulsion technique in spinal cord injured subjects during wheelchair ergometry. J Rehabil Res Dev 31(2):120–8, 1994.

21. Ferrara MS, Buckley WE, McCann BC, et al: The injury experience of the competitive athlete with a disability: prevention implications. Med Sci Sports Exerc 24(2): 184–8, 1992.

22. Ferrara MS, Buckley WE, Messner DG, et al: The injury experience and training history of the competitive skier with a disability. Am J Sports Med 20(1):55–60, 1992.

23. Fost D: The fun factor: marketing recreation to the disabled. Am Demograph Feb:54–8, 1998.

24. Halbert LA: Breastfeeding in the woman with a compromised nervous system. J Hum Lact 14(4):327–31, 1998.

25. Hardcastle P, Bedbrook G, Curtis K: Long-term results of conservative and operative management in complete paraplegics with spinal cord injuries between T10 and L2 with respect to function. Clin Orthop 224:88–96, 1987.

26. Henderson KA, Bedini LA: "I have a soul that dances like Tina Turner, but my body can't": physical activity and women with mobility impairments. Res Q Exerc Sport 66(2):151–61, 1995.

27. Hjeltnes N, Wallberg-Henriksson H: Improved work capacity but unchanged peak oxygen uptake during primary rehabilitation in tetraplegic patients. Spinal Cord 36(10):691–8, 1998.

28. Hosking D, Chilvers CED, Christiansen C, et al: Prevention of bone loss with alendronate in postmenopausal women under 60 years of age. N Engl J Med 338:485–92, 1998.

29. Huang Y; Macera CA; Blair SN; et al: Physical fitness, physical activity, and functional limitation in adults aged 40 and older. Med Sci Sports Exerc 30(9):1430–5, 1998.

30. International Paralympic Committee, Bonn, Germany.

31. Jackson RW, Fredrickson A: Sports for the physically disabled. The 1976 Olympiad (Toronto). Am J Sports Med 7(5):293–6, 1979.

32. Jokl E: Sudden Death of Athletes. Springfield, Ill, Charles C Thomas, 1985.

33. Kannisto M, Alaranta H, Merikanto J, et al: Bone mineral status after pediatric spinal cord injury. Spinal Cord 36(9):641–6, 1998.

34. Kerk JK, Clifford PS, Snyder AC, et al: Effect of an abdominal binder during wheelchair exercise. Med Sci Sports Exerc 27(6):913–9, 1995.

35. Kocina P: Body composition of spinal cord injured adults. Sports Med 23(1):48–60, 1997.

36. La Croix AZ, Newton KM, Leveille SG, et al: Healthy aging. A women's issue. Western J Med 167(4):220–32, 1997.

37. Magnusson SP, Constantini NW, McHugh MP, et al: Strength profiles and performance in Masters' level swimmers. Am J Sports Med 23(5):626–31, 1995.

38. Maki KC, Langbein WE, Reid-Lokos C: Energy cost and locomotive economy of handbike and rowcycle propulsion by persons with spinal cord injury. J Rehabil Res Dev 32(2):170–78, 1995.

39. Middleton JW, Siddall PJ, Walker S, et al: Intrathecal clonidine and baclofen in the management of spasticity and neuropathic pain following spinal cord injury:

a case study. Arch Phys Med Rehabil 77(8):824–6, 1996.

40. Mitten MJ: Amateur athletes with handicaps or physical abnormalities: who makes the participation decision? Nebraska Law Rev 71:987–1032, 1992.

41. Moore D, Li L: Prevalence and risk factors of illicit drug use by people with disabilities. Am J Addict 7(2):93–102, 1998.

42. Mutton DL, Scremin AM, Barstow TJ, et al: Physiologic responses during functional electrical stimulation leg cycling and hybrid exercise in spinal cord injured subjects. Arch Phys Med Rehabil 78(7):712–8, 1997.

43. Nattiv A, Puffer JC, Green GA: Lifestyles and health risks of collegiate athletes: a multi-center study. Clin J Sport Med 7(4):262–72, 1997.

44. Needham-Shropshire BM, Broton JG, Klose KJ, et al: Evaluation of a training program for persons with SCI paraplegia using the Parastep 1 ambulation system: part 3. Lack of effect on bone mineral density. Arch Phys Med Rehabil 78(8):799–803, 1997.

45. IX Paralympic Games. General and functional classification guide. Barcelona, 1992.

46. Noreau L, Shephard RJ: Spinal cord injury, exercise and quality of life. Sports Med 20(4):226–50, 1995.

47. Nosek MA, Howland CA: Breast and cervical cancer screening among women with physical disabilities. Arch Phys Med Rehabil 78(12 Suppl 5):S39–44, 1997.

48. Nosek MA, Rintala DH, Young ME, et al: Sexual functioning among women with physical disabilities. Arch Phys Med Rehabil 77(2):107–15, 1996.

49. Oshima S, Kirschner KL, Heinemann A, et al: Assessing the knowledge of future internists and gynecologists in caring for a woman with tetraplegia. Arch Phys Med Rehabil 79(10):1270–6, 1998.

50. Paciorek MJ, Jones JA: Sports and Recreation for the Disabled, 2nd edition. New York, McGraw-Hill/Carmel, IN Cooper Publishing Group, 1994.

51. Park HW, Jahng JS, Hahn SB, et al: Lengthening of an amputation stump by the Ilizarov technique. A case report. Int Orthopaed 21(4):274–6, 1997.

52. Pearson EG, Nance PW, Leslie WD, et al: Cyclical etidronate: its effect on bone density in patients with acute spinal cord injury. Arch Phys Med Rehabil 78(3):269–72, 1997.

53. Perloff JK: The Clinical Recognition of Congenital Heart Disease, 4th edition. Philadelphia, WB Saunders, 1994.

54. Phillips WT, Kiratli BJ, Sarkarati M, et al: Effect of spinal cord injury on the heart and cardiovascular fitness. Curr Probl Cardiol 23(11):641–716, 1998.

55. Pitetti KH, Barrett PJ, Campbell KD, Malzahn DE: The effect of lower body positive pressure on the exercise capacity of individuals with spinal cord injury. Med Sci Sports Exerc 26(4):463–8, 1994.

56. Rantanen T, Guralnik JM, Sakari-Rantala R, et al: Disability, physical activity, and muscle strength in older women: the Women's Health and Aging Study. Arch Phys Med Rehabil 80(2):130–5, 1999.

57. Raymond J, Davis FM, Climstein M, et al: Cardiorespiratory responses to arm cranking and electrical stimulation leg cycling in people with paraplegia. Med Sci Sports Exerc 31:822–8, 1999.

58. Reynolds J, Stirk A, Thomas A, et al: Paralympics-Barcelona 1992. Br J Sports Med 28(1):14–7, 1994.

59. Rodgers MM, Gayle W, Figoni SF, et al: Biomechanics of wheelchair propulsion. Arch Phys Med Rehabil 75(1):85–93, 1994.

60. Sawka MN, Latzka WA, Pandolf KB: Temperature regulation during upper body exercise: able-bodied and

spinal cord injured. Med Sci Sports Exerc 21:S132–40, 1989.

61. Schmid A, Huonker M, Stober P, et al: Physical performance and cardiovascular and metabolic adaptation of elite female wheelchair basketball players in wheelchair ergometry and in competition. Am J Phys Med Rehabil 77(6):527–33, 1998.
62. Scrooten J: Stoke Mandeville: Road to the Paralympics. Aylesbury Buckinghamshire Peterhouse Press, 1998.
63. Sobsey D: Sexual offenses and disabled victims: research and practical implications. Vis-a-Vis 6(4), 1988.
64. Sobsey D: Violence and Abuse in the Lives of People with Disabilities. Baltimore, P. H. Brook Pub. Co. 1994.
65. Stoke Mandeville Games Federation: International Stoke Mandeville Games Federation guide for doctors. International Stoke Mandeville Games Federation guide for doctors. Aylesburg, Stroke Mandeville Games Federation, 1982.
66. Suris JC, Resnick MD, Cassuto N, et al: Sexual behavior of adolescents with chronic disease and disability. J Adolesc Health 19(2):124–31, 1996.
67. Thomas AJ, Davis GM, Sutton JR: Cardiovascular and metabolic responses to electrical stimulation-induced leg exercise in spinal cord injury. Methods Inf Med 36(4–5):372–5, 1997.
68. Thoumie P, Le Claire G, Beillot J, et al: Restoration of functional gait in paraplegic patients with the RGO-II hybrid orthosis. A multicenter controlled study. II: Physiological evaluation. Paraplegia 33(11):654–9, 1995.
69. Uebelhart D, Demiaux-Domenech B, Roth M, et al: Bone metabolism in spinal cord injured individuals and in others who have prolonged immobilisation. A review. Paraplegia 33(11):669–73, 1995.
70. United States Olympic Committee (USOC) Disabled Sports Services, Colorado Springs, Colo.
71. USOC Information Resource Center, Colorado Springs, Colo.
72. van der Woude LHV, Drexhage D, et al: Peak power production in wheelchair propulsion. Clin J Sport Med 4(1):14–24, 1994.
73. Verduyn WH. Pregnancy and delivery in tetraplegic women. J Spinal Cord Med 20(3):371–4, 1997.
74. Warms CA: Health promotion services in post-rehabilitation spinal cord injury health care. Rehabil Nurs 12(6):304–8, 1987.
75. Weiserbs B, Gottlieb J: The perception of risk over time as a factor influencing attitudes toward children with physical disabilities. J Psychol 129(6):689–99, 1995.
76. Wilson PE, Washington RL: Pediatric wheelchair athletics: sports injuries and prevention. Paraplegia 31: 330–7, 1993.

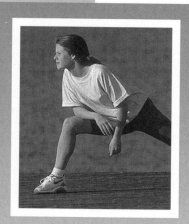

Section VI

Orthopaedic Conditions

Chapter 30

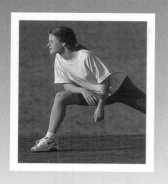

Stress Fractures

Angus M. McBryde Jr., M.D.
William R. Barfield, Ph.D.

Stress fractures are partial or complete breaks in the continuity of bone that result from rhythmic, repeated, subthreshhold tensile or compressive loads. They comprise 6% to 20% of repetitive stress injuries in athletes and 2.3% to 21% of injuries in women in military basic training.[9,12,16,17,35,45,47,54,77,94,105,170] When increased mechanical demands on the skeletal system overwhelm that system's ability to biologically repair the produced wear and tear, the probability of stress fractures increases.[20,58,81,128,171] Injury results from repetitive microtrauma overwhelming the capacity of bone to repair itself. Stress fractures are not due to a single excessive load, but rather result from a series of low repetitive loads. In vivo, the number of cycles that lead to bone microfailure is infinite owing to adaptation occurring as a result of frequency and duration of loading.

Causes are commonly divided into 2 types: (1) abnormal stresses exerted on normal bone, and (2) normal stresses placed on abnormal bone.[156] Bone, like many other body tissues, is a viscoelastic, anisotropic material whose properties depend on the direction and rate of loading.[13,71,154] Adaptation of bone is a function of the number and frequency of loading cycles, strain rate, and duration of strain per cycle.[111]

Although case reports describe stress fractures in virtually every bone in the body, the most common area remains the leg, specifically the tibia, foot, and ankle.[33,109] Data from a recent in-vivo investigation demonstrated differing local tibial deformations, with posteromedial deformation being larger than previously reported from other parts of the tibia and mid-diaphysial findings being consistent with prior findings. These findings support the clinical suspicion of different causes for stress fractures of the tibia based on location.[49] During movement, as the muscle envelope fatigues and becomes less able to attenuate forces, bone may be exposed to abnormally high loads. Therefore, stress fractures may result from repetitive impact loads or may be caused by the decreased ability of a muscle to neutralize forces.[118] It has not been demonstrated conclusively whether compressive loads associated with gravitational pull or stresses associated with muscle contraction put bone at greatest risk for stress fracture.[101] However, Stanitski and coworkers found that relentless eccentric and concentric muscle forces provide sufficient, unresolved submaximal insults to establish an environment in which stress fractures can occur.[155] This submaximal trauma causes focal circumferential periosteal resorption. Lower and more widely distributed magnitudes of force provide a stimulus for bone accretion. However, at higher levels net periosteal resorption occurs. This weakens the cortex, thereby increasing the chance of stress fractures.[155] The process of stress reactions can be altered by numerous confounding variables (eg, poor nutritional habits) that reduce the body's ability to provide concurrent repair of the microscopic "wear and tear" of daily activity. Disorders associated with collagen formation also have been implicated in this problem.[103] What does seem clear is that most stress reactions and fractures occur in the lower extremities of young, otherwise healthy populations involved in vigorous exercise.[82,108,111]

In 1855, Breithaupt was the first to be credited with identifying a stress reaction through his observations of Prussian Army soldiers who developed swollen, painful feet associated with marching.[23] These, stress fractures, first reported in the feet of soldiers, are also known as "march fractures." Reports of march fractures in the early 20th century described injuries primarily to the metatarsals.[15,16,32] By the 1960s greater numbers of fractures in the lower extremity were observed.[171] By the 1980s approximately 35% involved the lower leg (below the knee) and a smaller percentage involved the femur.[25,31,63] Giladi and coworkers speculated that these changes were due to modifications in the nature of training, from marching to running, use of better equipment, and more appropriate selection of personnel.[58] Soldiers with low-arched feet were found to have fewer stress fractures than those with average and high arches. That this functional anatomic characteristic is more common in African American military recruits, in addition to genetic or other as-yet unknown factors, may help explain why this segment of the population incurs fewer stress fractures than their Caucasian counterparts when undergoing the same types of training.[60]

Military experiences, primarily involving men, have contributed much to our understanding of the etiology and epidemiology of stress fractures.[135] Because the military is a controlled setting, however, the military experience cannot easily be applied to an individual male or female athlete presenting with a repetitive stress injury that might be a stress fracture. Stress fractures among athletes result from isolated and varied activities, while military stress fractures frequently occur as a result of group activities.[55,77,80,81,117,159,169,171]

The incidence of stress fractures among females, particularly those in a military environment, is higher than among males in most, but not all studies. Gender differences are not as great among athletic populations. It is suspected that this lack of difference among athletic populations may be a function of the compensatory methods that females employ to modify their activity levels[11,12,29,62,81,130] or may be related to nutritional and hormonal factors.

Research provides evidence that "new" loading regimens must be in effect for 2 weeks before bone can respond physiologically and biomechanically with increased mineral content, and thereby increased bone strength. The results of a study of 440 military recruits found that recruits who altered their activity patterns (less running, jumping, and double-timing) during the third week of basic training suffered one third the number of lower-extremity stress fractures of those who failed to modify training.[148]

Research with regard to prior activity among military recruits is inconclusive, with contradictory findings reported among several different populations. Several authors[36,61,63,172] found retrospectively that prior physical activity can help prevent stress fractures; however, 2 prospective studies, 1 involving military recruits, contradicted these earlier findings, showing that prior participation in sports and aerobic activities did not reduce likelihood of stress fracture.[112,157] Stress fractures occur frequently in untrained populations during the initial weeks of training.[16,19,29,31,61,62,65,66] In studies of women in military training environments, the relative risk for women is 1.2 to 10 times that of men for similar training volume. In athletic populations, gender differences in stress fracture occurrence is not as evident, which may be a function of initial fitness levels[28] or be due to the effects of nutritional and menstrual patterns on bone, as well as other factors.[11]

In 1976, the first year female recruits were admitted to the United States Military Academy, physiologic factors that influenced performance were measured during the first 8-week training period. Short-term findings concluded that women and men placed in an environment where equal physical training was expected demonstrated measurably different performance standards. Protzman[133] reported that 10 of 102 women cadets (9.8%) and 12 of 1228 men (1%) developed stress fractures. Men were injured less, and females sustained 10 times the number of stress fractures, although women were equal in areas such as aerobic metabolism.[133,134]

EPIDEMIOLOGY

Injury risk in population-based studies is a function of the dose–response relationship.[18,81,165] Although a number of previous military reports of stress fracture epidemiology described male recruits primarily,[59,148] there have been a number of military studies including both genders that have found an increased incidence of stress fractures in women compared to men.[25,81,82,130,134,140] In the athletic population, there are fewer epidemiologic studies assessing gender differences in stress fracture rates.[12,29,62,80,116] These athlete studies show either a modest increased risk or no increase in risk of stress fractures in women. As noted above, the reasons for these gender differences in the athletic and military studies are not clear. Although some of the epidemiologic studies in athletes are also not gender specific,[100,104] there are reported series[90] and case reports[7,21,25,34,67,69,73,83,131,149,158,174,175] that describe the occurrence of stress fractures in female athletes,[93,127,132] especially female athletes with menstrual dysfunction.[6,11,98]

Mechanical forces, an inherent aspect of locomotion, have been examined in several studies.[2,38,39,41,59,152,166] However, time frames, definitions of what qualifies as an overuse injury, and measurement techniques vary widely.

Stress fractures occur in athletes who run, jump, throw,[113] and perform combinations of these movements, such as rowers[73]; however, primarily lower extremities activities, soldiers, distance runners, and professional dancers are at increased risk for repetitive stress injuries, including stress fractures.[11,12,36,51,55,78,80,89,138,164] Initiating an exercise program that includes weight bearing and other forms of resistance training increases bone mass. While non-weight-bearing activities such as swimming and cycling have no appreciable effect on bone mass,[71,141–143] stress fractures have been shown to occur in non-weight-bearing bones of the skeleton.[8,66,69,73] Various forms of weight training have been shown to be more effective for stimulating bone formation than cyclic, repetitive activities such as distance running.[37,143]

GENDER-SPECIFIC FACTORS RELATING TO STRESS FRACTURES

Females may be at greater risk than males for stress fractures for a number of reasons. Some of these factors appear to be associated with alteration of endocrine function, surfacing as abnormal menstrual patterns. Up to 50% of female runners have irregular menses, which is a risk factor for stress fractures.[5,11,21,98] In a recent study, bone mineral density (BMD), when measured at 3 different anatomic sites, revealed that menstrual dysfunction was linearly associated with declining BMD. Even moderate menstrual irregularities may have a negative impact on BMD. Women in the marines with fewer than 10 menstrual cycles per year demonstrated a higher incidence of stress reactions.[172] Furthermore, greater observed BMD differences between females who were oligomenorrheic and those who were eumenorrheic were observed in weight-bearing bones of the lower extremity. This may indicate that females with menstrual abnormalities do not adapt to increasing mechanical loading associated with exercise.[25,54,80,161,169] Weight-bearing exercise is a stimulus for growth and bone remodeling. Whether increased BMD or stress fracture results is based on several factors, including a history of amenorrhea.[54]

Underlying the stress fracture picture is the "female athlete triad," also known as the "unhappy triad,"[115,125] which includes the following:

1. Disordered eating, which may include restricting food intake as well as bingeing and purging, and use of diet pills, diuretics, and laxatives, which can lead to other negative consequences such as infertility, depression, immune system dysfunction, and extended healing time following injury in addition to stress fractures.[5,92,147,168]
2. Amenorrhea (lack of menses for longer than 3 months) or menstrual irregularities.
3. Osteoporosis (BMD values greater than 2.5 standard deviations below mean peak bone mass for young women) or osteopenia (BMD values between 1 and 2.5 standard deviations below mean peak bone mass for young women).[5,124]

Onset of stress fracture pain is frequently insidious and activity related. Even when applied loads are increased to reasonable levels gradually, females may be at increased risk because of reduced BMD associated with secondary amenorrhea.[25,27,82,87,130,134,140]

Acute injuries resulting from the "female athlete triad" have been reported. For example, a 15-year-old avid female runner presented with acute right hip and thigh pain that developed while jogging. Initial treatment included analgesics and physiotherapy; however, pain did not subside. Subsequent non-weight-bearing activity (swimming) resulted in a "crack" in the right groin. Radiographic examination revealed an acutely displaced stress fracture of the right femoral neck. Clinical questioning revealed a 2-year history of a vegan diet, weight loss totaling 17 pounds, and amenorrhea. Injury did not appear to result from increased mileage. Repair with a 6.5mm cancellous screw and an autograft decreased pain, rigidly fixed the femoral neck, and led to eventual union.[68]

Amenorrhea is based on such factors as family history,[150] race,[50] low body weight,[137] energy deficit,[99] exercise,[19,46] smoking, and reduced estrogen levels.[1] Evidence that race may be a positive risk factor for stress fractures was shown by Bernstein and Stone[16] and Leabhart,[96] and later by Brudvig and coworkers[25] and Gardner and colleagues.[56] African Americans have a greater BMD than Caucasians, which may serve as a primary protective factor against stress fractures, although recent studies revealed no significant relationships when race, age, and height among female army recruits were considered.[36,79,163] Use of oral contraceptives also has been demonstrated to ameliorate the impact of stress fractures among an active female population,[5] although this has not been demonstrated consistently. Myburgh and coworkers[114] and Drinkwater and coworkers[46] demonstrated that hypoestrogenic athletes have a lower BMD, a lower calcium intake, a negative calcium balance, menstrual irregularities, and lower rate of oral contraceptive use.

Another less common factor that predisposes to and/or correlates with stress fractures in older women is the use of fluoride etidronate to treat osteoporosis.[64] Middle-aged (mid-career) or elderly osteopenic women with "insufficiency fractures" who endeavor to run certainly are at risk for complications.

There are numerous variables that may explain the predisposition of female athletes to stress fractures. Anatomic and physiologic male/female differences are documented and are pertinent to many performance elements, not just to injury {including stress fractures}.[75] Suspected causes for stress fractures among females include (1) lower BMD, (2) static and dynamic biomechanical differences (gait, coxa vara, genu valgum), (3) bone geometry differences, (4) higher levels of adipose tissue compared with lean body mass, (5) menstrual factors,(6) nutritional factors, and (7) lower initial levels of physical fitness.[12,29,62,80]

Winfield and colleagues examined a variety of anatomic and biomechanical characteristics possibly associated with stress fractures, including pelvic width and subtalar joint range of motion. No remarkable findings were observed.[172] Despite conflicting results, current research findings do not unequivocally support the often-held view that varus knee alignment and a low foot arch contribute to an increased risk of overuse injuries, particularly stress fractures.[76] Other possible factors include the following:

1. *Genetic factors:* Inherent anatomic factors that are not well correlated, including a broader pelvis and genu valgus with a slightly altered foot plant in the female. Biomechanical studies do not show male/female differences in selected stress fractures based on these variables.[160]

2. *Developmental factors:* Many anatomic changes reflect participation in sports in which traditionally the majority of participants are female.[64] For instance, metatarsal hypertrophy is commonly found in ballet dancers. In ballet, *demi-pointe* and *full pointe* require supporting 3 to 4 times body weight through the metatarsophalangeal joint. Great-toe changes in ballet performers as young as 6 years have been documented.[51,164] The most common site for stress fractures in female dancers is at the base of the second metatarsal. The patient frequently presents with insidious onset of midfoot pain prior to medical intervention; most can be treated symptomatically with conservative care.[122] In a retrospective study of female track and field athletes, a high incidence of navicular stress fractures was seen. Those with a prior history of stress fractures,

delayed commencement of menarche, and self-imposed restricted eating patterns appeared to be at greatest risk. BMD, body composition, and current training load did not differ between females with and without a stress fracture history. This latter finding may be a function of analyzing females in all track and field events as a single group rather than by event. Most studies have found that distance running and marching present the greatest risk of stress fractures.[11,116]

3. *Training discrepancies*
   a. Womens' team coaches traditionally have been less skilled than coaches of men's teams; this implies that different demands are placed on female athletes (eg, female athletes are not pushed as hard in training and competition as are men).[70]
   b. Patterns for males differ from those for females (eg, males are predominant in the military; organized "playing" of sports in preschool and primary grades traditionally has involved primarily male participants).
   c. Sociocultural/parenting patterns. Generations of sedentary and nonathletic lifestyles have imbued a lower tolerance for repetitive stress into females. Male parents tend to push boys more than girls to early sports competition and to push harder than mothers.[57] Overuse injuries, including stress fractures, have become increasingly troublesome in the sports medicine field during the last quarter of the 20th century. As trends in the 21st century, especially among the aging female population, continue toward greater quality and quantity of training, overuse injuries are likely to increase in number. In a recent 12-month survey, overuse injuries outnumbered acute injuries by a ratio of 2:1.[4]
   d. Athletic shoe characteristics, including foot patterns and sizing, traditionally have reflected male needs. This inherently offers less protection to the female foot and ankle.

PATHOGENESIS

A stress fracture results from a distinct series of events; it is a process, not an event.[40,105,106] The number of ongoing investigations related to the pathoanatomy of stress fracture is considerable, with numerous flow charts and algorithms having been devised.[74,82] On a basic level, stress fractures occur with decreased cellular repair and inadequate or insufficient remodeling of strained bone (Fig. 30–1).[30]

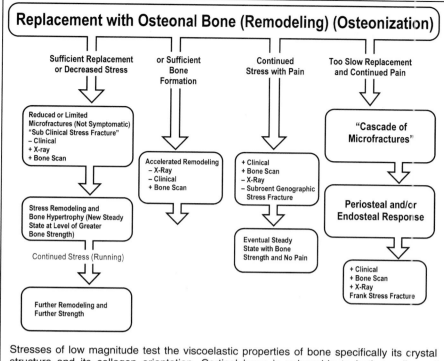

Replacement with Osteonal Bone (Remodeling) (Osteonization)

Sufficient Replacement or Decreased Stress

or Sufficient Bone Formation

Continued Stress with Pain

Too Slow Replacement and Continued Pain

Reduced or Limited Microfractures (Not Symptomatic) "Sub Clinical Stress Fracture"
– Clinical
+ X-ray
+ Bone Scan

Accelerated Remodeling
– X-Ray
– Clinical
+ Bone Scan

+ Clinical
+ Bone Scan
– X-Ray
– Subroent Genographic Stress Fracture

"Cascade of Microfractures"

Stress Remodeling and Bone Hypertrophy (New Steady State at Level of Greater Bone Strength)

Periosteal and/or Endosteal Response

Continued Stress (Running)

Eventual Steady State with Bone Strength and No Pain

+ Clinical
+ Bone Scan
+ X-Ray
Frank Stress Fracture

Further Remodeling and Further Strength

Stresses of low magnitude test the viscoelastic properties of bone specifically its crystal structure and its collagen orientation. Cortical bone is vulnerable to both tensile and compressive fluctuating stresses. Microscopic cracks along the cement lines permit the loss of strain energy and can lead to progressive accumulation of micro damage in cortical bone. Continuation of the stress can cause eventual failure through fracture crack propagation. Living bone with periosteal callus and new bone near the microscopic cracks can arrest the crack propagation by reducing the high stresses at the tip of the crack. The above figure describes a flow pattern of stress fracture seen from the clinician's point of view.

Figure 30-1. Bone dynamics.

Knapp and Mandelbaum proposed that for every change in the form and function of bone, there is a change in the internal architecture, and that stress fracture ultimately results from mal-adaptation to abnormal doses of stress. Adequate adaptive response dictates that stress be cyclic with periodic rest, which is dictated by the host bone. When periosteal resorption overwhelms remodeling of bone, a weakened cortex results in increased probability of stress fractures.[91] In a 12-month prospective study examining bone remodeling and pathogenesis of stress fractures among male and female track and field athletes in which the serum osteocalcin level was used to assess bone formation and urinary excretion of pyrvinium cross-links and N-telopeptides of type-1 collagen was used to assess bone resorption. No differences in bone turnover levels prior to or following onset of bony pain were found.[10] This indicates that the variables examined were not useful as single and/or multiple measures of bone turnover and were not clinically useful in predicting the likelihood of stress fractures in male or female athletes.

Animal models provide information about fatigue properties of cortical bone.[119] Li and colleagues,[97] when examining an animal model, found that vascular changes were the first pathologic sign in tibial stress fractures. Disturbances in haversian circulation, cracks, and vasodilation were observed initially. Subsequent acceleration of osteoclastic activity created cavities originally caused by ischemia and anoxia. More recently, comparison of specimens harvested from the right third metacarpal of exercised horses with specimens from controls showed that exercised horses demonstrated higher bone toughness. There were remarkable impact strength differences (impact strength and work, measured as the area under the load–deformation curve related to a material's intrinsic energy absorption capacity) in cortical bone between the 2 groups, with exercised horses showing greater strength. Young's modulus and inner bone strength were greater in exercised animals compared with controls, but outer bone strength, indicative of rapid circumferential growth associated with exercise, was even greater than inner bone strength. Study results suggest that exercise improves bone stock through improved mechanical properties, thereby lessening fracture risk.[139]

Resorption of bone and increased osteoblastic activity are common responses to physical stress, however, there may be a time window during the resorption phase when osteoclastic response to stress overwhelms formation of new bone, thereby temporarily weakening the bone.[97] That weakness in certain women who present with menstrual disturbances, and who develop osteopenia as a result of menstrual disturbances, appears to be most pronounced at the lumbar spine. Magnitude of loss is not as apparent at appendicular sites. These findings suggest that trabecular bone is more sensitive to endocrine changes and may be less responsive to mechanical loading when compared to cortical bone.[13]

Initial healing of a fracture requires an inflammatory response involving disruption of blood supply, hemorrhage, clotting, and an influx of inflammatory cells, followed by repair and remodeling. Following necrosis at the fractured bone ends and the phagocytic response, osteocytes die. Within days a 1- to 2-mm radiolucent space can be observed at the fractured ends. The callus formed by a proliferation of capillaries, fibroblasts, collagen, and osteoid serves as a form of internal fixation at the fractured ends. When movement at the fracture site occurs, predominant cartilage forms. In that case new bone formation follows the process of endochondral sequencing.[24,159] If stress fractures fail to heal, location, inadequate immobilization, distraction, or damage to blood supply may be the causative factor, as described for acute fracture.[24]

Decreased electrical activity and the piezoelectric phenomenon play a definite role in stress fracture risk.[153] The piezoelectric phenomenon is related to (1) tensile and rotational forces that reflect electropositivity, osteoclastic activity, and bone resorption; and (2) compressive forces reflecting electronegativity, osteoblastic activity, and bone accretion.[111]

Analysis of female gait and other correlative studies will help target training modifications and other preventive methods that may reduce the female tendency for stress fractures.[153]

DIAGNOSIS

Diagnosis of stress fractures relies on the amalgamation of history, physical examination, predisposing factors,[27] a high index of suspicion, and imaging studies. Certain stress fractures are clinically obvious; others may present symptoms and produce findings that have not yet manifested clear characteristic stress fracture findings. Symptoms and findings can be vague, referred, noncorrelative, subtle, and misleading, contributing to misdiagnosis (eg, ankle sprain with distal tibial stress fracture or plantar fasciitis with an os calcis stress fracture; or with upper rib stress fractures a misdiagnosis of neck strain, cervical radiculopathy, or rotator cuff pathology).[73] If the stress fracture is located in the lower extremity, a patient may present with antalgic gait, particularly if the fracture site is located in the fibula.[126] When a female runner presents with low-back and buttock pain a sacral stress fracture should be suspected. Most will respond favorably to rest and/or modification of activity.[110] Patients with these undiagnosed fractures can be considered "at risk" or "not at risk" for increased morbidity with continued stress.

High-risk fractures occur when there are excessive tensile forces and relative reduced vascularity.[22] The at-risk fractures include the superior aspect of the femoral neck, patella, anterior cortex of the tibia, medial malleolus, talus, tarsal navicular, fifth metatarsal, metaphyseal Jones' type, and great toe sesamoids.

The female basketball athlete depicted in Figure 30–2 complained of anterior calf pain. Radiographs demonstrated radiolucency in the anterior cortex, the dreaded "black line."

The first step in successful prevention is to diagnose, understand, and analyze, early on, the factors associated with stress fractures in women, and then to modify those factors found to be most egregious. Extrinsic and intrinsic factors have been cited as possible culprits. These previously documented factors include errors in training; surface changes; ill-fitted and/or inappropriate footwear; hormonal, psychological, and nutritional factors; late onset of menarche; amenorrhea or oligomenorrhea; low BMD; malalignment of the lower extremity; a wide pelvis; poor flexibility; and muscle imbalances.[12,26,172]

With the diagnosis of stress fractures, 3 questions need to be addressed:

1. Does the pain have a bony origin?
2. Which bone(s) is/are involved?
3. Where on the continuum of bone stress is the injury located (since stress fracture is a process and not the result of a single acute event)?

Assessment can include a detailed history encompassing time and onset of symptoms; training and activity history, including quantity

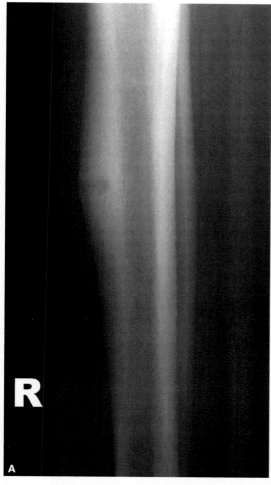
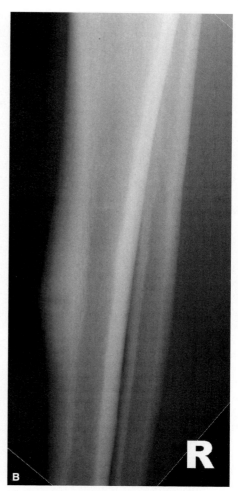

Figure 30-2. This female basketball athlete with physiologic anterior bowing of the tibia developed a stress fracture. **A.** Healing occurred after 3 months' rest. **B.** In nonunion the tibia requires intramedullary rodding. (Courtesy of Mary Lloyd Ireland.)

and quality of training; training surfaces; shoe type; biomechanical ambulation technique, particularly foot placement (anterior/posterior, medial/lateral, and whether subject is a heel striker, midfoot striker, or forefoot striker); nutritional history; age at menarche; menstrual history; general health; medications; occupation; and level of commitment to their activity.[27]

Mid-foot plantar and dorsal pain of 2 months duration was the complaint of a female basketball athlete, whose radiographs (Fig. 30–3) show the typical orientation of a tarsonavicular stress fracture. Technetium bone scanning and computed tomography (CT) confirmed the fracture.

Physical examination should locate the site of bony tenderness (whether superficial or deep) and the presence of palpable periosteal thickening, which may indicate initial bony inflammation. Imaging with plain roentgenography has high specificity, but low sensitivity. Radiographic

abnormalities may not be present for 2 to 3 weeks following injury. If suspicion for stress fracture is high and the radiograph is negative, a triple-phase bone scan will provide nearly 100% sensitivity, with changes seen as early as 48 to 72 hours after presentation of symptoms. The radionuclide may actually detect accelerated remodeling prior to the onset of symptoms.[27,144] Bone scintigraphy lacks specificity and reflects osteoblastic response of bone to insult without regard to actual etiology.[86] The lack of specificity with nuclear imaging does not permit differentiation of nontraumatic lesions such as osteomyelitis and other bony dysplasias. CT and magnetic resonance imaging (MRI) lend improved specificity for diagnosing bone stress injury.[14] CT and MRI can differentiate between stress reactions and stress fractures, and MRI can distinguish between stress fracture and bone tumor or infectious conditions.[27,53]

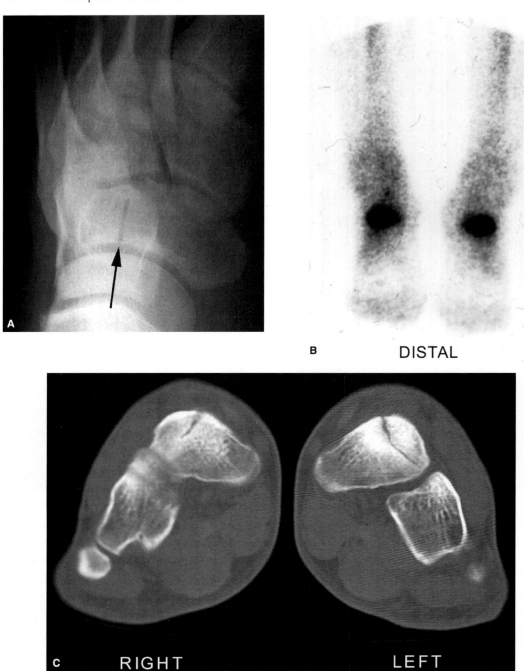

Figure 30-3. This at-risk tarsonavicular stress fracture occurred in an 18-year-old female basketball athlete with a history of 2 months of pain in her left foot. She denied pain in her right foot. Radiographs initially were normal but repeat films in another 2 months showed fracture. **A.** *(arrow)* The pattern of lateral third longitudinal is common. Bone scan was performed that showed increased activities in both tarsonavicular. **B.** CT scan showed the fracture on the left had propagated toward the plantar aspect. **C.** The asymptomatic right tarsonavicular began, as is typical, on the proximal dorsal articular side and had not yet propagated through the distal plantar cortex. Patient underwent open reduction internal fixation and local bone grafting of the left tarsonavicular. Follow-up radiographs revealed healed navicular fracture.

T_2-weighted MRI was used to confirm the medial femoral stress fracture depicted in Figure 30–6.

Radiologic grading systems for stress fractures have been developed.[3] Using MRI, stress fractures have been graded 1 to 4, with 1 being positive short-tau inversion sequence (STIR); 2, positive STIR and T_2-weighted images; 3, no definite cortical break and positive T_1- and

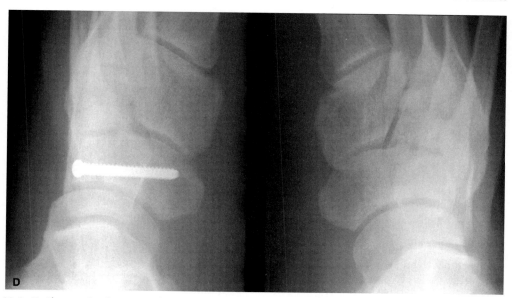

Figure 30-3. D. She remained symptom-free on the right side throughout her 4-year collegiate career. (Courtesy Mary Lloyd Ireland.)

T_2-weighted images; and 4, fracture line–positive T_1- and T_2-weighted images (Table 30–1).

MRI can detect areas in which bone marrow is overwhelmingly fatty, thus providing a distinct advantage in the lower extremity and foot, areas that, except in young individuals, are primarily fatty marrow.[43]

The nonbony aspect of the differential diagnosis should include muscle or other soft-tissue injury, muscle soreness and/or inflammation, strain (ie, post-tibial stress syndrome), and degenerative changes. Periostitis, compartment syndrome, tumor, and infection can all mimic stress fracture.[27]

TREATMENT

Algorithms for treatment of overuse injuries, particularly stress fractures, involve (1) identifying, isolating, and nullifying exacerbating factors, and (2) encouraging the patient to reduce the frequency, intensity, and duration of initiating activities. Cessation or change of stress will allow repair to dominate resorption, with 6 to 8 weeks needed for most fractures, although pubic rami fractures may require 2 to 5 months to heal completely.[103] Conservative training that involves a 10% increase in intensity per week combined with a modified periodization

Table 30-1. Radiologic Grading System for Stress Fractures

GRADE	RADIOGRAPHY	BONE SCANING	MRI	TREATMENT
1	Normal	Mild uptake confined to 1 cortex	Positive STIR image	Rest for 3 weeks
2	Normal	Moderate activity; larger lesion confined to unicortical area	Positive STIR and T_2-weighted images	Rest for 3–6 weeks
3	Discrete line (+/–), periosteal reaction (+/–)	Increased activity (>50% width of bone)	No definite cortical break; positive T_1-and T_2-weighted images	Rest for 12–16 weeks
4	Fracture or periosteal reaction	More intense bicortical uptake	Fracture line; positive T_1- and T_2-weighted images	Rest for 16+ weeks

Adapted from Arendt EA, Griffiths HJ: The use of MR imaging in the assessment and clinical management of stress reactions of bone in high-performance athletes. Clin Sports Med 16:291–306, with permission.
STIR, short-tau inversion sequence.

schedule and a variety of substitute activities seem to work best.[77,145] Any specific stress fracture may be at risk and, if so, needs special and aggressive attention. Those fractures not at risk require continued stimulation with a balanced program that keeps the activity level below that which causes pain. It is necessary that the patient understand the importance of stimulating his or her involved bone in a way so as not to cause pain. Sports activity substitution (ie, swimming for soccer or avoiding impact by using a Stairmaster), taping, and/or orthoses and other forms of bracing and changed mechanics are effective means of treatment. Care must be taken so that forces do not cause other bony areas to become symptomatic.[103] In short, stress must be reduced to a subalgic level in all sports activities, not only that thought to cause the injury.[44] Even with such a regimen, routine stress fractures can cause problems.[120] Stress fractures of the medial malleolus, primarily low-risk running injuries, usually unite in 3 to 4 months with nonoperative therapy. However, use of a pneumatic brace or early screw fixation may be necessary in an elite female athlete who needs a timely return to training and competition.[121,122] Unique treatment as described should be applied on an individual basis.

More proximal stress fractures are common in females.[75,129] Femoral neck stress fractures are 4 times as common in female runners as in males, although they are less common than tibial and fibular injuries in both populations.[48,106]

If the fracture is on the superior tensile side, pinning in situ is recommended; if on the compression side, as in the recreational runner depicted in Figure 30–4, observation and foot-flat weight bearing will be sufficient to allow healing.

When males and females participate in integrated military training, increased stride length by females, especially when in formation marching and/or running, can place them at a mechanical disadvantage, with stresses focused more proximally. Of 12 reported stress fractures of the inferior pubic ramus, 11 occurred in females undergoing training. This finding was attributed to integrated training of males and females, whereby female stride length, when marching, was dictated by men, most of whom by nature of stature take longer strides.[72] Femoral neck stress fracture can have compressive and tensile components. Excursion across the femoral neck is related primarily to continuation of the inciting activity.[102] Femoral neck stress fracture is an at-risk injury and must be treated as follows:

1. Immediate discontinuation of weight-bearing or equivalent rest to eliminate pain.
2. Avoidance of any activity that causes discomfort.

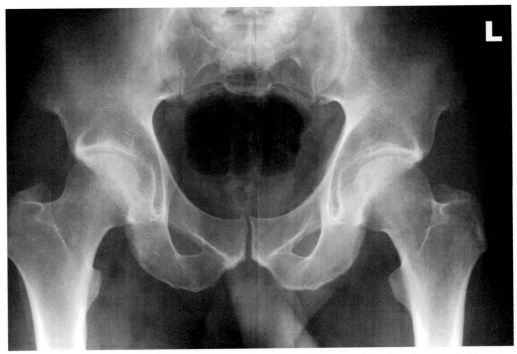

A

Figure 30-4. This 45-year-old recreational runner was preparing for a summer 10K run and developed groin pain. The anteroposterior pelvis was negative. **A.** The bone scan was positive.

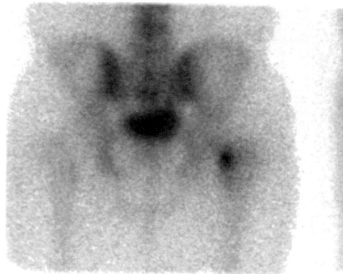
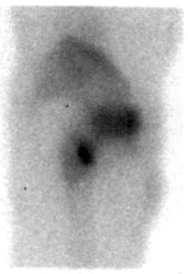

B   POSTERIOR   RT LAT

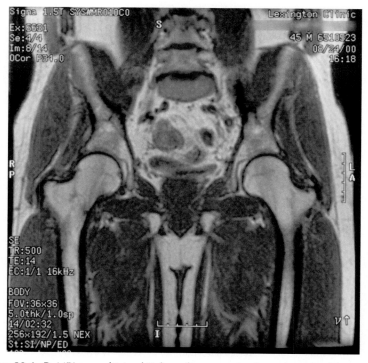

C

Figure 30-4. B. MRI scan obtained 5 days after onset of pain was positive for a compression inferior femoral neck fracture seen on T_1. **(C)** and T_2.

3. Hip pinning in 7 to 10 days if pain is not under control (pinning is indicated if there is radiographic evidence of stress fracture excursion across the femoral neck).[48,95,156]

Return to full or partial weight bearing must be dictated by the patient's clinical symptoms, the physical examination, and the findings from imag-

ing studies. Upper- or lower-extremity complete or extra-articular displaced fractures and nonunions are treated with immobilization in a plaster cast. These may require immobilization and non-weight bearing for 6 to 8 weeks. Weight-bearing devices may be especially necessary for intra-articular fractures. Delayed union or nonunion may require bone stimulation or

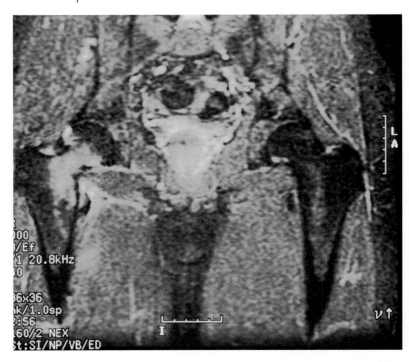

Figure 30-4. (D) weighted images. Follow-up radiographs at 3 months after fracture diagnosis shows healing medially.

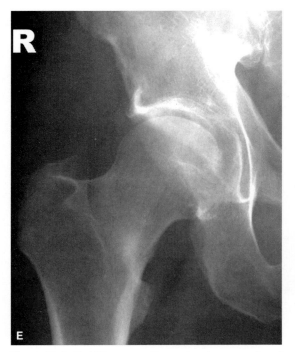

Figure 30-4. E. MRI scan at 3 months shows continued edema in T_1.

curettage and bone grafting assuming a fibrous union has not occurred; open reduction and internal fixation should not be attempted since this may further disrupt the healing process.[91] Length of relative rest depends on the fracture site, spectrum of injury, and duration of symptoms.[27]

As discussed, the increased incidence of stress fractures in females in the military is more apparent when compared with males in an equal training environment. In the female athletic setting, the training environment may not be as uniform; assessment of training in this setting presents a further opportunity for study.[5,108]

CONSIDERATIONS FOR RETURN TO ACTIVITY

Not-at-risk lower-extremity stress fractures usually heal in a straightforward way, with return to activity in 4 to 6 weeks with 1 to 2 weeks rest often sufficient.[86] Initial management includes relief of pain with mild analgesics and relative rest.[111] If normal daily activities cause pain, non-weight bearing or splinting is indicated for 7 to 10 days.

Resumption of activity with any lower-extremity stress fracture is a function of pain, symptoms, physical findings, and fracture location. Management of lower-limb stress fractures follows a periodized approach involving walking to running with eventual return to full activity. Interim maintenance of fitness can be achieved through cross-training, including cycling, water

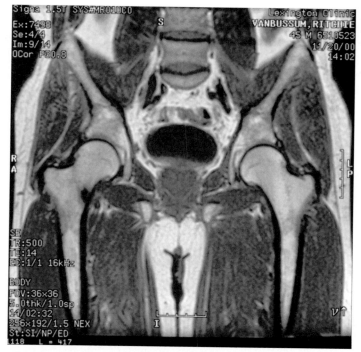

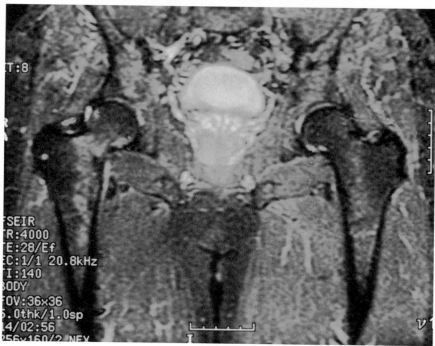

Figure 30-4. **(F)** and T_2 **(G)** views. Grade I fractures have periosteal edema on fat suppressed (T_2 weighted) image and grade II have increased periosteal signal intensity. Correlation with plain films and MRI is interesting in that the MRI scan appears to show the healing fracture more clearly, propagating toward the tensile superior aspect of the femoral neck. The patient was treated with foot-flat weight bearing for 6 weeks and at 4 months follow-up is clinically healed.

activities, appropriate weight training, and flexibility exercises.[27]

In women who have menstrual dysfunction, establishment of an appropriate cyclic menstrual period is beneficial in the attempt to preserve BMD. Immobilization is seldom necessary although casts and/or bracing may be considered.[111] Tarsonavicular and femoral neck fractures require extra caution because of the risk of intra-articular involvement and avascular necrosis.[35,89] For navicular stress fractures the average time between onset of symptoms and eventual diagnosis is 7 months. This poses a difficult diagnostic and treatment dilemma for the practitioner.[162]

SUGGESTIONS FOR PREVENTION

Some females who are actively involved in athletic activities follow severe dietary restrictions that subsequently deprive their bodies of essential nutrients, including calcium. Diets with little or no calcium are associated with an increased incidence of stress fractures. When the effect of calcium supplementation on BMD was examined, it was found that there were no statistical differences between a control group and a calcium supplementation group (1000 mg/day). Data suggest that the experimental group was noncompliant yet there was some benefit on BMD, although not a statistically significant benefit.[146]

Cost of patient care and the subsequent impact on the lives of active young women makes the primary goal for all sports medicine practitioners one of reducing the incidence of repetitive stress injury, particularly stress fracture. This involves identification of risk factors and instructing athlete-patients to reduce the frequency, intensity, and duration of activities that lead to stress fractures. Conservative training with a variety of activities, including cross-training, seems to work best.[27,159]

Studies of female athletes with delayed onset of menarche have yielded conflicting data concerning stress fracture incidence. Several studies found that delayed menarche increased the incidence of stress fractures, with one study indicating a 4-fold increase for every additional year of age at menarche.[11,12,31,167,168] Others found no differences in age at menarche and the effect on stress fracture incidence.[55,84,114,116]

Menstrual abnormalities that lead to decreased BMD also have been credited with contributing to a higher incidence of stress fractures,[11] however, study subjects demonstrated confounding risk factors such as greater training loads,[65] lower calcium intake,[42,85] and differences in soft-tissue structure and composition.[88,173]

Biomechanical factors such as abnormally high levels of pronation and supination also have been proposed to contribute to increased incidence of stress fractures.[27] There is some evidence, though in males, that nonrigid orthoses may be warranted to reduce the incidence of stress fracture in the military environment.[52]

Attention to all of these factors prior to athletic participation is important.

CONCLUDING REMARKS

Whether the athletic program is recreational, competitive, or occupational (eg, school environment), the requirement for uniform medical attention—diagnosis, treatment, and rehabilitation—in females parallels that in males. The overall incidence of stress fracture appears to be greater in females, but this is more apparent in military studies than in athletic studies. Parity with men in terms of conditioning, quality and quantity of training, access to knowledgeable and quality sports medicine resources, and coverage are necessary but still inadequately provided at the outset of the 21st century. As parity is reached at all levels, it is hoped that injury incidence, including stress fractures, of females will decline to that of males. The following general guidelines will assist in this endeavor:

1. Educate young females and parents with regard to appropriate levels of calcium intake through the diet or with supplementation so that the female athlete receives 1000 to 1500 mg of calcium per day.
2. Train coaches, parents, and sports medicine personnel concerning age- and gender-appropriate athletic training such that the dose–response adaptation can occur gradually.
3. Closely examine training and competition shoes, as well as the training grounds.
4. Be observant of disordered eating.
5. Educate young females regarding the importance of normal menses and the consequences of ignoring irregular and/or amenorrheic conditions.
6. Finally, understand that men and women cannot be trained under the same circumstances without some negative consequences, especially in females.[89]

Stress fractures in females need practitioners who have a high index of suspicion, who understand the treatment principles for repetitive stress injuries, and who realize the importance of prevention as well as techniques for complete patient rehabilitation.

References

1. Aloia JF, Cohn SH, Vaswani A, et al: Risk factors for postmenopausal osteoporosis. Am J Med 78:95–100, 1985.

2. Arangio GA, Xiao D, Salathe EP: Biomechanical study of stress in the fifth metatarsal. Clin Biomech 12(3):160–4, 1997.

3. Arendt EA, Griffiths HJ: The use of MR imaging in the assessment and clinical management of stress reactions of bone in high-performance athletes. Clin Sports Med 16:291–306, 1997.

4. Baquie P, Brukner PD: Injuries in presenting to an Australian sports medicine clinic. Clin J Sports Med 7(1):28–31, 1997.

5. Barfield WR, McBryde AM, Otteni JF, et al: Evaluation of factors associated with increased risk of stress fracture among a group of female freshmen cadets and a female control group–an initiated study. MUSC Orthop J 2:68–74, 1999.

6. Barrow GW, Saha S: Menstrual iregularity and stress fractures in collegiate female distance runners. Am J Sports Med 16:209–16, 1988.

7. Beaman DN, Roeser WM, Holmes JR, Saltzman CL: Cuboid stress fractures: A report of two cases. Foot Ankle 14:525–8, 1993.

8. Belkin SC: Stress fractures in athletes. Orthop Clin North Am 11:735–41, 1980.

9. Bell NS, Jones BH: Injury risk factors among male and female trainees. Abstract from 121st Annual Meeting of the American Public Health Association, 1993, p 95.

10. Bennell KL, Malcolm SA, Brukner PD, et al: A 12-month prospective study of the relationship between stress fractures and bone turnover in athletes. Calcif Tissue Int 63(1):80–5, 1998.

11. Bennell KL, Malcolm SA, Thomas SA, et al: Risk factors for stress fractures in track-and-field athletes: a twelve month prospective study. Am J Sports Med 24:810–8, 1996.

12. Bennell KL, Malcolm SA, Thomas SA, et al: The incidence and distribution of stress fractures in competitive track and field athletes. A twelve-month prospective study. Am J Sports Med 24(2):211–7, 1996.

13. Bennell KL, Malcolm SA, Wark JD, Brukner PD: Skeletal effects of menstrual disturbances in athletes. Scand J Med Sci Sports 7:261–73, 1997.

14. Bergman AG, Fredericson M: MR imaging of stress reactions, muscle injuries, and other overuse injuries in runners. MRI Clin North Am 7(1):151–76, 1999.

15. Bernstein A, Childers MA, Fox KW, et al: March fractures of the foot: care and management of 692 patients. Am J Surg 71:355–62, 1946.

16. Bernstein A, Stone JR: March fracture: a report of 307 cases and a new method of treatment. J Bone Joint Surg 26:743–50, 1944.

17. Bijur PE, Horodyski M, Egerton W, et al: Comparison of injury during cadet basic training by gender. Arch Pediatr Adolesc Med 151(5):456–61, 1997.

18. Blair SN, Kohl HW, Goodyear NN: Rates and risks for running and exercise injuries: studies in three populations. Res Q Exerc Sport 58:221–28,1987.

19. Block JE, Smith R, Black D, Genant HK: Does exercise prevent osteoporosis? JAMA 257:3115–7, 1987.

20. Bollen SR, Robinson DG, Critchton KJ, Cross MJ: Stress fractures of the ulna in tennis players using a double-handed backhand stroke. Am J Sports Med 32:751–2, 1993.

21. Bottomley MB: Sacral stress fracture in a runner. Br J Sports Med 24:243–4, 1990.

22. Boden BP, Osbabr DC: High-risk stress fractures: Evaluation and treatment. J Am Acad Orthop Surg 8(6):344–53, 2000.

23. Breithaupt M: Zur Pathologie des mensch lichen fusses. Med Z 24:169–71, 175–7, 1855.

24. Brighton CT: Principles of fracture healing. In Instructional Course Lectures. St. Louis, CV Mosby, 1984.

25. Brudvig TJS, Gudger TD, Obermeyer L: Stress fractures in 295 trainees: a one-year study of incidence as related to age, sex, and race. Mil Med 148:666–7, 1983.

26. Brukner P: Overuse injuries: where to now? Br J Sports Med 31:2, 1997.

27. Brukner P, Bennell K: Stress fractures in female athletes. Diagnosis, management and rehabilitation. Sports Med 24(6):419–29, 1997.

28. Brukner P, Bradshaw C, Bennell K: Managing common stress fractures:let risk level guide treatment. Physician Sports Med 26(8):39–47, 1998.

29. Brunet ME, Cook SD, Brinker MR, Dickinson JA: A survey of running injuries in 1505 competitive and recreational runners. J Sports Med Phys Fitness 30(3):307–15, 1990.

30. Burr DB, Martin RB, Schaffler MB, Radin EL: Bone remodeling in response to in-vivo fatigue microdamage. J Biomech 18:189–200, 1985.

31. Carbon R, Sambrook PN, Deakin V, et al: Bone density of elite female athletes with stress fractures. Med J Aust 153(7):373–6, 1990.

32. Carlson GD, Wertz RF: March fractures including others than those of the foot. Radiology 43:45–53, 1944.

33. Chen JB: Cuboid stress fracture: a case report. J Am Podiatr Med Assoc 83:153–5, 1993.

34. Chowchuen P, Resnick D: Stress fractures of the metatarsal heads. Skeletal Radiol 27(1):22–5, 1998.

35. Clement DB, Ammann W, Taunton JE, et al: Exercise-induced stress injuries to the femur. Int J Sports Med 14(6):347–52, 1993.

36. Cline AD, Jansen GR, Melby CL: Stress fractures in female army recruits: implications of bone density, calcium intake, and exercise. J Am Coll Nutr 17(2):128–35, 1998.

37. Conroy BP, Kraemer WJ, Maresh CM, et al: Bone mineral density in elite junior olympic weightlifters. Med Sci Sports Exerc 25(10):1103–9, 1993.

38. Cowan DN, Jones BH, Frykman PN, et al: Lower limb morphology and risk of overuse injury among male infantry trainees. Med Sci Sports Exerc 28(8):945–52, 1996.

39. Cowan DN, Jones BH, Robinson JR: Foot morphologic characteristics and risk of exercise-related injury. Arch Fam Med 2:773–7, 1996.

40. Daffner RH, Pavlov H: Stress fractures: current concepts. Am J Radiol 159:245–52, 1992.

41. Dahle LK, Mueller M, Delitto A, Diamond JE: Visual assessment of foot type and relationship of foot type to lower extremity injury. J Orthop Sports Phys Ther 14:70–4, 1991.

42. Dalen N, Olsson KE: Bone mineral content and physical activity. Acta Orthop Scand 45:170, 1974.

43. Deutsch AL, Mink JH, Kerr R: MRI of the Foot and Ankle. New York, Raven Press, 1992.

44. Dickson TB, Kichline PD: Functional management of stress fractures in female athletes using a pneumatic leg brace. J Sports Med 15:86–9, 1987.

45. Dishman RD, Steinhardt M: Reliability and concurrent validity for a 7-d re-call of physical activity in college students. Med Sci Sports Exerc 20:14–25, 1988.

46. Drinkwater BL, Nilson KN, Chestnut CH, et al: Bone mineral content of amenorrheic and eumenorrheic athletes. N Engl J Med 311:277–80, 1984.

47. Duester PA, Jones BH, Moore J: Patterns and risk factors for exercise-related injuries in women: a military perspective, Mil Med 162(10):649–55, 1997.

48. Egol KA, Koval KJ, Kummer F, Frankel VH: Stress fractures of the femoral neck. Clin Orthop Rel Res 348:72–8, 1998.

49. Ekenman I, Halvorsen K, Westblad P, et al: Local bone deformation at two predominant sites for stress fractures of the tibia–an in-vivo study. Foot Ankle Int 19(7):479–84, 1998.

50. Farmer ME, White LR, Brody JA, Bailey KR. Race and sex differences in hip fracture incidence. Am J Public Health 74:1374–9, 1984.

51. Fehlandt AF Jr, Micheli LF: Lumbar facet stress fracture in a ballet dancer. Spine 18:2537–9, 1993.

52. Finestone, A, Giladi M, Elad H, et al: Prevention of stress fractures using custom biomechanical shoe orthoses. Clin Orthop Rel Res 360:182–90, 1999.

53. Fredericson M, Bergman AG, Hoffman KL, et al: Tibial stress reaction in runners: correlation of clinical symptoms and scintigraphy with a new magnetic imaging grading system. Am J Sports Med 23:472–81, 1995.

54. Friedl KE, Nuovo JA, Patience TH, Dettori JR. Factors associated with stress fracture in young army women: indications for further research. Mil Med 157:334–8, 1992.

55. Frusztager NT, Dhuper S, Warren MP, et al: Nutrition and the incidence of stress fractures in ballet dancers. Am J Clin Nutr 51(5):779–83, 1990.

56. Gardner L, Dziados JE, Jones BH, et al: Prevention of lower extremity stress fractures: a controlled trial of a shock absorbent insole. Am J Public Health 78:1563–7, 1988.

57. Garrick JG, Requa RK. Girls' sports injuries in high school athletics. JAMA 239:2245–8, 1978.

58. Giladi M, Ahronson Z, Stein M, et al: Unusual distribution and onset of stress fractures in soldiers. Clin Orthop Rel Res 192:142–6, 1985.

59. Giladi M, Milgrom C, Simkin A, et al: Stress fractures and tibial bone width: a risk factor. J Bone Joint Surg 69B:326–9, 1987.

60. Giladi M, Miligrom C, Stein M, et al: The low arch, a prospective factor in stress fracture: a prospective study of 295 military recruits. Orthop Rev 14:81–4, 1985.

61. Gilbert RS, Johnson HA: Stress fractures in military recruits—a review of twelve years' experience. Mil Med 131:716–21, 1996.

62. Goldberg B, Pecora C: Stress fractures: a risk of increased training in freshmen. Phys Sports Med 22:68–78, 1994.

63. Greaney RB, Gerber FH, Laughlin RL, et al: Distribution and natural history of stress fractures in U.S. marine recruits. Radiology 146:339, 1983.

64. Guanabens N, Peris P, Monegal A, et al: Lower extremity stress fractures during intermittent cyclical etidronate treatment for osteoporosis. Calcif Tissue Int 54:431–4, 1994.

65. Guler F, Hascelik Z: Menstrual dysfunction rate and delayed menarche in top athletes of team games. Sports Med Train Rehabil 4:99–106, 1993.

66. Haapasalo H, Kannus P, Sievanen H, et al: Long-term unilateral loading and bone mineral density and content in female squash players. Calcif Tissue Int 54(4):249–55, 1994.

67. Haasbeek JF, Green NE: Adolescent stress fractures of the sacrum: two case reports. J Pediatr Orthop 14:336–8, 1994.

68. Haddad FS, Bann S, Hill RA, Jones DH: A displaced stress fracture of the femoral neck in an active amenorrhoeic adolescent. Br J Sports Med 31:70–5, 1997.

69. Hall RJ, Calvert PT: Stress fractures of the acromion. an unusual mechanism and review of the literature. J Bone Joint Surg, 77B:153–4, 1995.

70. Haycock CE, Gillette JV: Susceptibility of women athletes to injury; myths vs reality. JAMA 236:163–5, 1976.

71. Heinonen A, Oja P, Kannus P, et al: Bone mineral density of female athletes in different sports. Bone Min 23:1–14, 1993.

72. Hill PF, Chatterji S, Chambers D, Keeling JD: Stress fracture of the pubic ramus in female recruits. J Bone Joint Surg 78:383–6, 1996.

73. Holden DL, Jackson DW: Stress fractures of the ribs in female rowers. Am J Sports Med 18:242–9, 1985.

74. Horn TS: The identification of cortical microdamage in fatigue-loaded bone using a non-invasive impulse response vibration testing technique. Bone 14:259–64, 1993.

75. Hunter LY, Andrews JR, Clancy WG, Funk FJ: Common orthopaedic problems of female athletes. In Frankel VH (ed): Instructional Course Lectures, vol XXXI. St. Louis, CV Mosby, 1982, 126–51.

76. Ilahi OA, Kohl HW: Lower extremity morphology and alignment and risk of overuse injury. Clin J Sports Med 8:38–42, 1998.

77. James SL, Bates BT, Osternig LR: Injuries to runners. Am J Sports Med 6:40–50, 1978.

78. Jensen JE: Stress fracture in a world class athlete: a case study. Med Sci Sports Exerc 30(6):783–7, 1998.

79. Johnson CC, Smith DM, Yu P, Deiss WP: In-vivo measurements of bone mass in the radius. Metabolism 17:1140–53, 1968.

80. Johnson AW, Weiss CB, Wheeler DL: Stress fractures of the femoral shaft in athletes—more common than expected: a new clinical test. Am J Sports Med 22:248–56, 1994.

81. Jones BH, Bovee MW, Harris J McA, Cowan DN: Intrinsic risk factors for exercise-related injuries among male and female army trainees. Am J Sports Med 21:705–10, 1993.

82. Jones BH, Harris JM, Vinh TN, Rubin C: Exercise-induced stress fractures and stress reactions of bone: epidemiology, etiology, and classification. Exerc Sport Sci Rev 17:379–422, 1989.

83. Jowett AD, Brukner PD: Fifth metacarpal stress fracture in a female softball pitcher. Clin J Sports Med 7(3):220–1, 1997.

84. Kadel NJ, Teitz CC, Kronmal RA: Stress fractures in ballet dancers. Am J Sports Med 20:445–9, 1992.

85. Kaiserauer S, Snyder AC, Sleeper M, Zierath J: Nutritional, physiological and menstrual status of distance runners. Med Sci Sports Exerc 21:120–5, 1989.

86. Kanstrup IL: Bone scintigraphy in sports medicine: a review. Scand J Med Sci Sports 7:322–30, 1997.

87. Keating TW: Stress fracture in the sternum of a wrestler. Am J Sports Med 15:92–3, 1987.

88. Keay N, Fogelman I., Blake G: Bone mineral density in professional female dancers. Br J Sports Med 31:143–7, 1997.

89. Khan KM, Fuller PJ, Brukner OD, et al: Outcome of conservative and surgical management of navicular stress fracture in athletes. Am J Sports Med 20(6):657–66, 1992.

90. Kiss ZX, Khan KM, Fuller PJ: Stress fractures of the tarsal navicular bone: CT findings in 55 cases. Am J Radiol 160:111–5, 1993.

91. Knapp TP, Mandelbaum BR: Stress fractures. In Garrett WE, Kirkendall, DT, Contiguglia SR (eds): The US Soccer Sports Medicine Book. Baltimore, Williams & Wilkins, 1996.

92. Knapp TP, Mandelbaum BR, Garrett WE: Why are stress injuries so common in the soccer player? Clin Sports Med 17:835–53, 1998.

93. Koskinen SK, Mattila KT, Alanen AM, Aro HT: Stress fracture of the ulnar diaphysis in a recreational golfer. Clin J Sport Med 7(1):63–5,1997.

94. Kowal DM: Nature and causes of injuries in women resulting from an endurance training program. Am J Sports Med 8:265–9, 1980.

95. Kupke MJ, Kahler DM, Lorenzoni MH, Edlich RF: Stress fracture of the femoral neck in a long distance runner: biomechanical aspects. J Emerg Med 11 587–91, 1993.

96. Leabhart JW: Stress fractures of the calcaneus. J Bone Joint Surg 41:1285–90, 1959.

97. Li G, Zhang SD, Chen G, et al: Radiographic and histologic analyses of stress fracture in rabbit tibias. Am J Sports Med 13:285–94, 1985.

98. Lloyd T, Triantafyllou SJ, Baker ER, et al: Women athletes with menstrual irregularity have increased musculoskeletal injuries. Med Sci Sports Exerc 18:374–9, 1986.

99. Loucks AB, Verdun M, Heath EM, et al: Low energy availability, not the stress of exercise, alters LH pulsatility in exercising women. J Appl Physiol 84(1):37–46, 1998.

100. Lysholm J, Winklander J: Injuries in runners. Am J Sports Med 15:168–71, 1987.

101. Major NM, Helms CA: Pelvic stress injuries: the relationship between osteitis (symphysis pubis stress injury) and sacroiliac abnormalities in athletes. Skeletal Radiol 26:711–7, 1997.

102. Maquet P: Letter to the editor concerning stress fracture. Clin Orthop Rel Res 360:269–70, 1999.

103. Markey KL: Stress fractures. Clin Sports Med 6:405–25, 987.

104. Marti B, Vader JP, Minder CE, Abelin T: On the epidemiology of running injuries: The 1984 Bern Grand-Prix study. Am J Sports Med 16:285–94, 1988.

105. McBryde A: Stress fractures of the foot and ankle. In DeLee JC, Drez D (eds): Orthopaedic Sports Medicine: Principles and Practice, Vol 2. Philadelphia, WB Saunders, 1994, pp 1970–1981.

106. McBryde AM Jr: Stress fractures in athletes. J Sports Med 3:212–7, 1976.

107. McBryde AM Jr: Stress fractures in runners. In Prevention and Treatment of Running Injuries. Thorofare, NJ, Charles B. Slack, 1982, pp 23–42.

108. McBryde AM, Barfield WR: Stress fractures of the foot and ankle. Foot Ankle Clin. 4(4):881–909, 1999.

109. McBryde AM, Bassett FH III: Stress fracture of the fibula. Gen Pract 38:120, 1968.

110. McFarland EG, Giangarra C: Sacral stress fractures in athletes. Clin Orthop Rel Res 329:240–3:1996.

111. Monteleone GP: Stress factures in the athlete. Orthop Clin North Am 26(3):423–32, 1995.

112. Mustajoki P, Laapio H, Muerman K: Calcium metabolism, physical activity and stress fractures. Lancet 2:797, 1983.

113. Mutoh Y, Mori T, Suzuki Y, Sugiura Y: Stress fractures of the ulna in athletes. Am J Sports Med 10:365–7, 1982.

114. Myburgh KH, Hutchins J, Fataar AB, et al: Low bone density is an etiologic factor for stress fractures in athletes. Ann Int Med 113(10):754–9, 1990.

115. Nattiv A, Agostini R, Drinkwater BL, Yeager KK: The female athlete triad: The interrelatedness of disordered eating, amenorrhea, and osteoporosis. Clin Sports Med 13(2):405–18, 1994.

116. Nattiv A, Puffer JC, Casper J, et al: Stress fracture risk factors incidence and distribution: A three year prospective study in collegiate runners. Med Sci Sports Exerc (suppl 5):S347, 2000.

117. Nickerson SH: March fractures or insufficiency fractures. Am J Surg 62:154–64, 1943.

118. Nordin M, Frankel VH: Biomechanics of whole bones and bone tissue. In Frankel VH, Nordin M (eds): Basic Biomechanics of the Skeletal System. Philadelphia, Lea & Febiger, 1980, pp 15–60.

119. Nunamaker DM, Butterweck DM, Provost MT: Fatigue fractures in thoroughbred racehorses: relationships with age, peak bone strain, and training. J Orthop Res 8:604–11, 1990.

120. O'Brien T, Wilcox N, Kersch T: Refractory pelvic stress fracture in a female long-distance runner. Am J Orthop 24:710–6, 1995.

121. Okada K, Senma S, Sato K, Minato S: Stress fractures of the medial malleolus: a case report. Foot Ankle 16:49–52, 1995.

122. O'Malley MJ, Hamilton WG, Munyak J, Defranco MJ: Stress fractures at the base of the second metatarsal in ballet dancers. Foot Ankle Int 17(2):89–94, 1996.

123. Orava S, Karpakka J, Taimela S, et al: Stress fractures of the medial malleolus. J Bone Joint Surg 77A:362–5, 1995.

124. Otis CL: Exercise-associated amenorrhea. Clin Sports Med 11:351–62, 1992.

125. Otis CL, Drinkwater BL, Johnson M, et al: American College of Sports Medicine position stand on the female athlete triad. Med Sci Sports Exerc 29(5):i-ix, 1997.

126. Palamarchuk HJ, Sabo M: Fibular stress fracture in a female runner. J Am Podiatr Med Assoc 88(1):34–6, 1998.

127. Pecina M, Bojanic I, Dubravcic S: Stress fractures in figure skaters. Am J Sports Med 18:277–9, 1990.

128. Penix AR: Stress fractures. In Baker CL (ed): The Hughston Clinic Sports Medicine Book. Baltimore, Williams & Wilkins, 1995.

129. Peris P, Guanabens N, Pons F, et al: Clinical evolution of sacral stress fractures: influence of additional pelvic fractures. Ann Rheum Dis 52:545–7, 1993.

130. Pester S, Smith PC: Stress fractures in the lower extremities of soldiers in basic training. Orthop Rev 21:297–303, 1992.

131. Petschnig R, Wurnig C, Rosen A, Baron R: Stress fracture of the ulna in a female table tennis tournament player. J Sports Med Phys Fitness 37(3):225–7, 1997.

132. Powell KE, Kohl HW, Capersen CJ, Blair SN: An epidemiological perspective on the causes of running injuries. Physician Sports Med 14:100–14, 1986.

133. Protzman RR: Physiologic performance of women compared to men. Observations of cadets at the United States Military Academy. Am J Sports Med 7:191–4, 1979.

134. Protzman RR, Griffis CC: Comparative stress fracture incidence in males and females in an equal training environment. Athletic Training 12:126–30, 1977.

135. Protzman RR, Griffis CC: Stress fractures in men and women undergoing military training. J Bone Joint Surg 59A(6):825, 1977.

136. Provost RA, Morris JM: Fatigue fracture of the femoral shaft. J Bone Joint Surg 51:487–91, 1969.

137. Pruzansky ME, Turano M, Luckey M, Senie R: Low body weight as a risk factor for hip fracture in both black and white women. J Orthop Res 7:192–7, 1989.

138. Reeder MT, Dick BH, Atkins JK, et al: Stress fractures—current concepts of diagnosis and treatment. Sports Med 22(3):198–212, 1996.

139. Reilly GC, Currey JD, Goodship AE: Exercise of young thoroughbred horses increases impact strength of the third metacarpal bone. J Orthop Res 15(6):862–8, 1997.

140. Reinker KA, Ozburne S: A comparison of male and female orthopaedic pathology in basic training. Mil Med 144:532–6, 1979.

141. Rico H, Revilla M, Hernandez ER, et al: Bone mineral content and body composition in postpubertal cyclist boys. Bone 14(2):93–5, 1993.

142. Risser WL, Lee EJ, LeBlanc A, et al: Bone density in eumenorrheic female college athletes. Med Science Sports Exerc 22(5):570–4, 1990.

143. Robinson TL, Snow-Harter C, Taaffe DR, et al: Gymnasts exhibit higher bone mass than runners despite similar prevalence of amennorrhea and oligomenorrhea. J Bone Miner Res 10(1):26–35, 1995.

144. Rosenthall L, Hill RO, Chuang S: Observation of the use of 99mTC-phosphate imaging in peripheral bone trauma. Radiology 119(3):637, 1976.

145. Roub LW, Gumerman LW, Hanley EN Jr, et al: Bone stress: a radionuclide imaging perspective. Radiology 132:431–8, 1979.

146. Rourke K, Bowering J, Turkki P, et al: Effect of calcium supplementation on bone mineral density in female athletes. Nutr Res 18(5):775–83, 1998.

147. Sanborn CF, Albrecth BH, Wagner WW: Athletic amenorrhea: lack of association with body fat. Med Sci Sports Exerc 19:207–12, 1987.

148. Scully TJ, Besterman G: Stress fracture: a preventable training injury. Mil Med 147:285–7, 1982.

149. Shiraishi M, Muzuta H, Kubota K, et al: Stress fracture of the proximal phalanx of the great toe. Foot Ankle 14:28–34, 1993.

150. Silverberg SJ, Lindsay R: Postmenopausal osteoporosis. Med Clin North Am 71:41–57, 1987.

151. Slawson SH, Arendt E, Engebretsen L, et al: Fibular stress fracture in a 20-year old woman. Orthopaedics 17(4):375, 378–9, 1994.

152. Sommer HW, Vallentyne SW: Effect of foot posture on the incidence of medial tibial stress syndrome. Med Sci Sports Exerc 27:800–4, 1995.

153. Soutas-Little P, Fredericksen R, Schwartz M, et al: Dynamic profile of female gait. Biomechanics 84:153–6, 1987.

154. Stanitski CL: Overuse injuries. In Stanitski CL, DeLee JC, Drez D (eds): Pediatric and Adolescent Sports Medicine. Philadelphia, WB Saunders, 1994.

155. Stanitski CL, McMaster JH, Scranton PE: On the nature of stress fractures. Am J Sports Med 6:391–6, 1978.

156. Sterling JC, Webb RF, Meyers MC, Calvo RD: False negative bone scan in a female runner. Med Sci Sports Exerc 25:179–85, 1993.

157. Swissa A, Milgrom C, Gilardi M, et al: The effect of pretraining sports activity on the incidence of stress fractures among military recruits: a prospective study. Clin Orthop Rel Res 245:256–60, 1989.

158. Taimela S, Kujala UM, Orava S: Two consecutive rib stress fractures in a female competitive swimmer, Clin J Sports Med 5(4):254–7, 1995.

159. Teitz CC: Scientific Foundations of Sports Medicine. Philadelphia, BC Decker, 1989.

160. Ting A, King W, Yocum L, et al: Stress fractures of the tarsal navicular in long-distance runners. Clin Sports Med 7:89–101, 1988.

161. Tomten SE, Falch JA, Birkeland KI, et al: Bone mineral density and menstrual irregularities: a comparative study on cortical and trabecular bone structures in runners with alleged normal eating behavior. Int J Sports Med 19:92–7, 1998.

162. Torg JS, Pavlov H, Cooley LH, et al: Stress fractures of the tarsal navicular: a retrospective review of twenty-one cases. J Bone Joint Surg 64(5):700–12, 1982.

163. Trutter M, Broman GE, Peterson RR: Densities of white and Negro skeletons. J Bone Joint Surg 42A:50–8, 1960.

164. van de Muslebroucks B, Dereymaeker G: Stress lesions of the forefoot in ballet dancers. Acta Orthop Belg 60 Suppl 1:47–9, 1994.

165. van Mechelen W: Running injuries: a review of the epidemiological literature. Sports Med 14:320–5, 1992.

166. Vitasalo JT, Kvist M: Some biomechanical aspects of the foot and ankle in athletes with and without shin splints. Am J Sports Med 11:125–30, 1983.

167. Warren MP, Brooks-Gunn J, Fox RP, et al: Lack of bone accretion and amenorrhea: evidence for relative osteopenia in weight-bearing bones. J Clin Endocrinol Metab 72(4):847–53, 1991.

168. Warren MP, Brooks-Gunn J, Hamilton LH, et al: Scoliosis and fractures in young ballet dancers. Relation to delayed menarche and secondary amenorrhea. N Engl J Med 314(21):1348–53, 1986.

169. Wendenberg B: Mineral metabolism of fractures of the tibia in man studied with external counting of Sr 85. Acta Orthop Scand (Suppl) 52:1–79, 1961.

170. Westphal KA, Friedl KE, Sharp MA, et al: Health, performance, and nutritional status of US Army women during basic combat training. Technical Report No. T96–2. Natick, Mass, US Army Research Institute of Environmental Medicine, 1996.

171. Wilson ES, Katz FN: Stress fractures: an analysis of 250 conservative cases. Radiology 92:481–6, 1969.

172. Winfield AC, Moore J, Bracker M, Johnson CW: Risk factors associated with stress reactions in female marines. Mil Med 162(10):698–702, 1997.

173. Wolman RL, Harries MG: Menstrual abnormalities in elite athletes. Clin Sports Med 1:95–100, 1989.

174. Yokoe K, Mannoji T: Stress fracture of the proximal phalanx of the great toe: a report of three cases. Am J Sports Med 14:240–2, 1986.

175. Young CC, Raasch WG, Geiser C: Ulnar stress fracture of the nondominant arm in a tennis player using a two-handed backhand. Clin J Sports Med 5(4):262–4, 1995.

Chapter 31

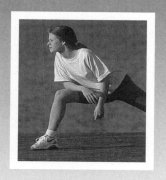

Total Hip and Knee Arthroplasty

David A. Mattingly, M.D.
Geoffrey J. Van Flandern, M.D.

Women of all ages have been introduced to the understanding that staying active and athletic may be a way to maintain and improve overall physical and mental health. At the same time, physical activity can prevent bone stock loss, control weight, and improve the quality of life.

This chapter will deal with those physically active women who have already undergone, or who plan to undergo, a total hip or total knee arthroplasty. In these patients, the need to exercise—to maintain their weight, bone stock, and physical and mental wellness—is no less than that in other athletes. The drive to maintain physical wellness must be moderated by the fact that the components in total joint arthroplasties are "artificial" man-made parts and therefore have a predictable natural history for wear and durability. When loaded repetitively, these implants will wear. In the same way, when loads are reduced, wear slows. For this reason, the key to implant longevity is activity modification and force control. Total joint arthroplasty in active women should only be considered after conservative medical and surgical management has failed to relieve pain or improve function.

THE HIP

Hip Pathology

Arthritic conditions necessitating total hip arthroplasty are of 2 basic types: noninflammatory and inflammatory arthritis. Noninflammatory entities occur more frequently than inflammatory conditions. Noninflammatory conditions include primary or secondary osteoarthritis (degenerative joint disease). Primary osteoarthritis involves degeneration of the joint cartilaginous tissues themselves. Related to the aging process, cartilage can undergo structural changes with time. Cartilage integrity can be lost over time, leading to joint irregularity and deformity

(Fig. 31-1A). Secondary osteoarthritis includes degeneration as a result of other etiologies: trauma, childhood and adolescent hip abnormalities, and avascular necrosis. Trauma can initiate deformity, change weight-bearing dynamics, and eventually lead to degeneration. Childhood and adolescent hip diseases include hip dysplasia, Legg—Calvé–Perthes disease, slipped capital femoral epiphysis, and hip sepsis during youth. All can lead to anatomic irregularities of the hip during development, causing a substantial change in the weight-bearing distribution across the hip joint and leading to early degeneration. Finally, avascular necrosis results from an alteration to the normal vasculature to the femoral head. This can lead to ischemia and even large-scale cellular death in the femoral head. The death of the femoral head and the subsequent repair process greatly decrease the strength of the bone superstructure. Collapse of the bone may follow. Collapse leads to deformity, changed weight-bearing dynamics, and, often times, rapid degeneration.

Inflammatory arthritides combine all of the hip pathologies that begin as a primary inflammatory process, including rheumatoid arthritis. Rheumatoid arthritis describes a process in which the joint lining (synovium) mounts an autoimmune inflammatory response to cartilage itself. In this process, cartilage is degraded and the joint is degenerated. Other inflammatory etiologies include psoriatic arthritis and systemic lupus erythematosus.

Alternatives to Total Hip Arthroplasty

In the years prior to the advent of successful total joint arthroplasty (late 1960s), hip disease was treated in many different ways. It is important to note that many of these techniques are still used today as alternatives to total joint arthroplasty. Generally speaking, these alternatives are technically demanding and provide less

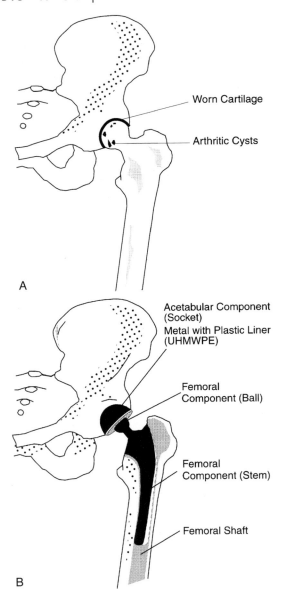

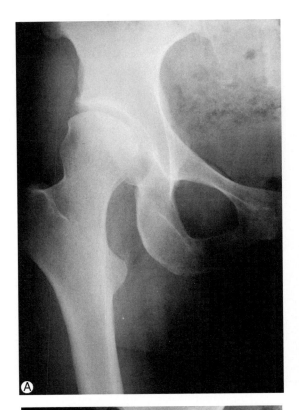

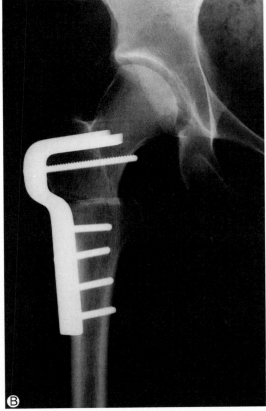

Figure 31-1. Artist's depiction of an arthritic hip with cartilage loss (**A**) and following total hip arthroplasty (**B**).

predictable pain relief and functional return than total hip arthroplasty.

For the carefully selected patient, proximal femoral (Fig. 31-2) or acetabular (Fig. 31-3) osteotomies may be an alternative to total joint arthroplasty.[7,13,16,19,29] The selected patient must fulfill strict criteria. The patients are typically younger and have a higher demand, with an excellent range of motion and either mild or isolated degeneration in the face of worsening anatomic/biomechanical function that can be remedied by a bony realignment.[4,23,26,46] Osteotomies, when correctly performed, allow the patient to resume impact-loading activities with few restrictions. An

Figure 31-2. Valgus hip deformity (**A**) treated by varus osteotomy of the proximal femur (**B**) to improve containment of the femoral head.

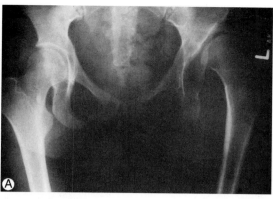 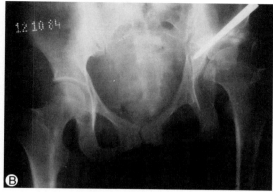

Figure 31-3. Dysplastic acetabulum **(A)** treated by acetabular osteotomy **(B)** to improve containment of the femoral head.

added advantage to acetabular osteotomy is that it usually improves hip bone stock. This may make total hip arthroplasty easier to perform at a later date. However, osteotomy techniques can be extremely technically demanding, making results difficult to reproduce. In addition, particularly with femoral osteotomies, later joint reconstruction can be more difficult. The selection criteria are very strict and the rehabilitation time may be substantially longer than a joint arthroplasty. Crutch ambulation may be required for 6 months or longer.

Another alternative for the very high-demand user is hip fusion (arthrodesis) (Fig. 31-4).[31,38,39] Typically used in the younger, higher-demand patient, arthrodesis trades motion for comfort and stability. Fusion, when healed, allows heavy, high-demand, dependable func-

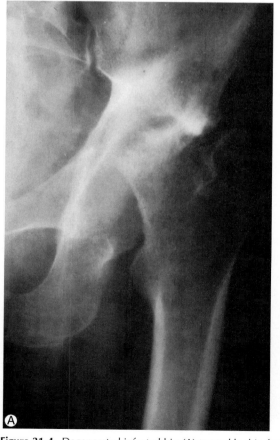 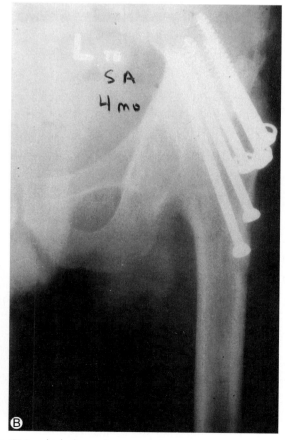

Figure 31-4. Degenerated infected hip **(A)** treated by hip fusion **(B)** in a high-demand, young patient.

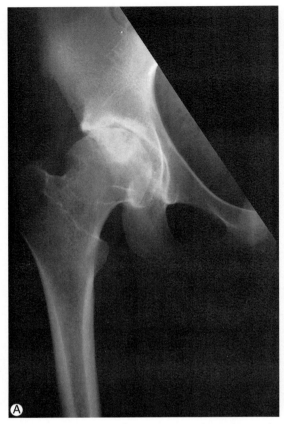
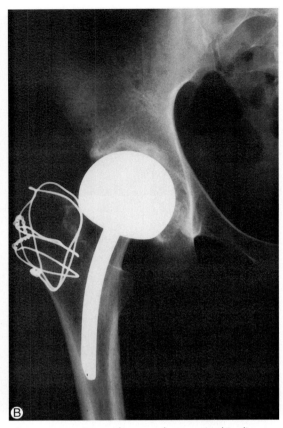

Figure 31-5. Pre- **(A)** and post- **(B)** operative surface replacement in a young patient with severe degenerative hip disease.

tion with no further hip wear. Durability is high but hip motion is totally eliminated; prolonged sitting, especially in cars, planes, and theaters, may be difficult or awkward. With hip motion eliminated, additional functional and anatomic demands are placed on the surrounding joints, particularly the lumbar spine, the ipsilateral knee, and the contralateral hip. Later-life function may be limited by progressive wear and degeneration in these locations.

In addition to total hip arthroplasty, surface replacement (Fig. 31-5) may provide substantial return of function with limited rehabilitation.[1,5,6,41–43,45] As with previous procedures, patient selection is the key to success. Resurfacing may function best in younger patients with good bone stock, noninflammatory arthritis, and head involvement severe enough to deter osteotomy. These criteria are combined with demands low enough to discourage fusion. As opposed to osteotomy, bone healing is not required and rehabilitation is usually rapid. In contradistinction to fusion, this procedure preserves bone stock and musculature, allowing predictable conversion to total hip arthroplasty at a later date.

Total Hip Arthroplasty

When all other options have failed or are inappropriate, total hip arthroplasty (Fig. 31-1B) can provide pain-free function and satisfactory durability. The best long-term results in active patients occur when ideal weight is maintained and activities are moderated. For example, running and high-impact loading are to be avoided.

Technical considerations can be complex for total hip arthroplasty. Since the mid 1980s, cementless ingrowth sockets have been performed over cemented sockets for acetabular fixation in high-demand patients.[2,15,47] The choice for femoral fixation, however, is still controversial. Cementless stems (Fig. 31-6A) require superior bone stock and necessitate longer rehabilitation with possibly less-predictable pain relief.[10,11] Cemented stems (Fig. 31-6B), on the other hand, may provide more rapid, solid fixation but at the expense of later durability.[8,9,25] Although the literature can be conflicting, an ingrowth stem may provide longer life, whereas a cemented interface lends more immediate return to function.

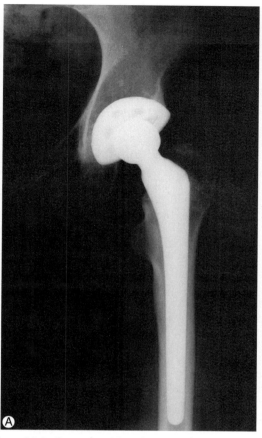

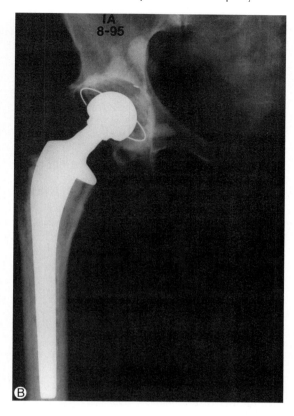

Figure 31-6. Cementless (**A**) and cemented (**B**) total hip arthroplasty.

With all of the theories of stem and socket aside, the longevity-limiting component is ultra-high-molecular-weight polyethylene (UHMW-PE). Polyethylene wear at the bearing surface is now recognized as the major cause of failure of a previously well-functioning total hip arthroplasty.[17,33] Implants should be selected to help to decrease wear. Possibilities include optimizing polyethylene thickness (minimum 6 mm), head size (26 to 28 mm), and head bearing surface materials. Newly "perfected" ceramic materials actually provide decreased friction but may be subject to breakage because of their brittle property. The drive to optimize the bearing surface is one of the most studied and controversial facets of total joint arthroplasty. This topic is revisited in the final portion of this chapter.

What about failure of the previously successful arthroplasty? There are 2 distinct types of failure: mechanical and biologic.

Mechanical wear and failure are difficult to avoid in any joint arthroplasty. Although metal–polyethylene articulations have the best function and durability for the bearing surface at this time, the days of function for a bearing surface with polyethylene are always numbered. Unlike the native joint, which responds to loading with nutrient production and collagen distribution, polyethylene's only response to repetitive demand is wear. As with the brake linings on an automobile, wear can be a gradual, slow process or it can be rapid and precipitous. Repetitive loading—especially when associated with high impact—can increase wear rates by increasing bearing surface loads to 4 to 5 times normal body weight. The debris generated by the wear process is addressed in the next few paragraphs.

The other obvious mechanical failure pattern is dislocation. For the posterior approach, the dislocation rate can approach 3%.[14,29,44] Most commonly, the components dislocate with the femur directed posteriorly. Activities such as excessive flexion at the hip—especially when combined with internal rotation—can precipitate posterior dislocation of the prosthesis. A recurrent dislocation problem forces restriction of motion and limited function. Potentially caused by malpositioned components, recurrent dislocations can often be corrected by revision surgery.

Biologic causes of failure include the devastating problems of osteolysis and infection. Osteolysis (Fig. 31-7) is the bone loss and consequent interface failure and loosening resulting from the foreign-body reaction to particles of UHMWPE as they are shed with bearing surface wear.[22] Not only does the bearing surface thin to failure, but debris shed along the way incites a biologic response—osteolysis. The foreign-body response to particles of UHMWPE was initially thought to be a response to cement particles—so-called cement disease. It is now known that the debris shed by wear of UHMWPE is of the correct size to cause the impressive osteolytic reactions. Osteolysis causes surrounding bone loss leading to stem and socket interface breakdown and loosening.

The other, more devastating, mode of biologic failure is infection (sepsis). Having many origins, sepsis can arise early or late in the life of a joint arthroplasty.[21,34] In the 1960s, sepsis was seen in 5% to 10% of arthroplasties. With the advent of perioperative antibiotics and improved operating room conditions, (laminar flow, ultra-violet lights, body exhaust systems), present perioperative infection rates are 0.5% to 1%. Late infection results almost universally from hematogenous seeding. Dental visits, operative procedures, and urinary tract or other bacterial infections can produce transient bacteremia, possibly leading to hematogenous seeding of the joint. Since the 1990s, the American Heart Association protocols are followed, which recommend giving broad-spectrum oral antibiotic coverage during times of potential bacteremia. After bacterial seeding, joint sepsis can proceed at different rates and fulminance depending on the organism involved as well as the susceptibility of the host. Bacterial sepsis proceeds most commonly in an accelerated form of bone loss. Joint effusion and inflammation cause new pain, often at rest. As sepsis passes through the acute phase, surrounding bone may become infected (osteomyelitis). The combination of joint infection/inflammation, bone loss, and surrounding osteomyelitis will eventually break down any implant/bone interface, with resulting component loosening. Usually diagnosed earlier than the implant failure stage, most forms of joint sepsis require temporary or permanent implant removal for eradication.

Return to Activity

Total hip arthroplasty is performed to return patients to their desired activities. At the same time, moderation of activities is suggested to help slow wear. Restricting or slowing wear can be accomplished in 2 ways: reduce the load or reduce the demand. Load reduction—as common sense might dictate—refers to weight reduction. In activities of daily living, forces up to 3 to 4 times body weight can be transmitted across the hip joint. Decreasing body weight will markedly reduce the loads seen on the bearing surface. Demand reduction can come from modification of activity and/or increased efficiency of joint reactive forces. High-impact or repetitive-impact activities (singles tennis, basketball, running, racquetball) can cause accelerated wear. Activities that involve running or jumping should be avoided. However, strengthening of the hip extensors (gluteus maximus) and hip abductors (gluteus medius and minimus) can improve hip motion and efficiency by distributing load to multiple areas of the bearing surface and reducing isolated wear areas.

Total hip arthroplasty provides rapid return of function to the low-demand female athlete. Total hip arthroplasty often gives the female athlete nearly complete return of activities previ-

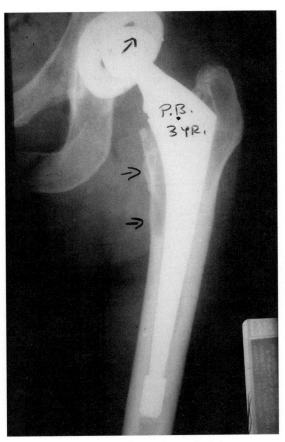

Figure 31-7. Osteolysis (bone destruction) in a young, active patient with significant polyethylene wear debris.

ously impossible in the arthritic extremity. Sports such as low-impact aerobics, cross-country skiing, bicycling, brisk walking, golf, swimming, unloaded hiking, and recreational horseback riding all improve strength, flexibility, and coordination of the hip while providing endurance challenges for the athlete. Activities such as these can be experienced safely by the postoperative arthroplasty patient. These activities, when performed in moderation, help endurance, deter osteoporosis, and provide the feeling of wellness sought by the mature physically active female.

However, certain sports are not recommended. High-impact sports or those with significant fall/injury risk are ill-advised. Downhill skiing, for example, provides a challenging workout for both the cardiovascular system and the hip. At the same time, a high-impact/low-control fall during skiing can cause a catastrophic fracture and/or dislocation. Resistance exercises should be limited to 3 to 5 pounds of weight. Singles tennis and racquetball provide too extreme a repetitive loading environment. All allowable activities should be done in moderation. Aggressive exercise (except golf) should be limited to 30 minutes per day.

After total hip arthroplasty, function can be maintained/improved through long-term exercise. Walking (outdoor or treadmill) each day should allow progressive endurance improvement as well as continued confidence in hip function. Muscle strengthening about the hip joint, especially the hip extensors (gluteus maximus) and the hip abductors (gluteus medius and minimus), will correct the muscular atrophy and contraction seen with the long-term loss of motion and function that correspond with

joint deterioration. Restoration of muscle strength is the way to eliminate surgical limp resulting from the hip disease. Other exercise outlets are bicycling, cross-country ski machine use, swimming, and even use of the StairMaster in moderation.

THE KNEE

As with the hip, end-stage knee wear and degeneration can severely limit the mature active female with pain and compromised motion. In order to pursue activities related to ambulating, an extremity must provide stable, strong, preferably pain-free function. Prior to the development of total knee arthroplasty, end-stage disease of the knee, like that of the the hip, has been treated in many ways. In the same way, end-stage knee disease has many causes.

Knee Pathology

As in the hip, causes of end-stage arthritis can be divided into noninflammatory and inflammatory causes. Noninflammatory causes can then be further subdivided into primary and secondary arthritis. Primary causes are a function of structural changes in the cartilage coincidental with the aging process. Primary breakdown of the joint cartilage leads eventually to end-stage degeneration (Fig. 31-8A). Secondary causes of knee degeneration usually involve trauma. Mild to moderate trauma can cause meniscal injury. Loss of effective meniscal force distribution leaves knee condylar surfaces to endure overwhelming forces in repetitive point loading with daily activities. These point

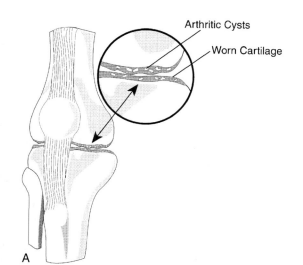

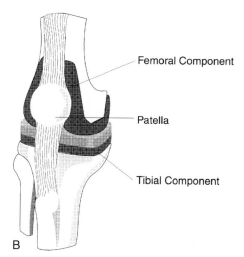

Figure 31-8. Artist's depiction of an arthritic knee with cartilage loss (**A**) and following total knee arthroplasty (**B**).

forces will, over time, lead to degeneration. More significant trauma to the knee can compromise ligamentous integrity. The anterior cruciate ligament (ACL) and posterior cruciate ligament (PCL) provide anterior and posterior translational stability, respectively, therein protecting the menisci. Injury to one or both of the cruciates—especially in combination with injury to secondary knee stabilizers—results in significant translational and rotational instability. The resulting instability allows knee motion beyond physiologic limits, giving opportunity for further meniscal/ligamentous injury. Instability allows wear patterns outside of the normal condylar glide and degeneration can ensue. Fractures about the knee can alter alignment, damage joint cartilage, and change force distribution in the knee. This also accelerates wear by isolating forces in a nonphysiologic manner. Inflammatory disease processes involve the knee similar to the hip. Diseases such as rheumatoid arthritis and systemic lupus erythematosus can lead to rapid total joint arthritic destruction.

Alternatives to Total Knee Arthroplasty

Prior to and in the years of the development of total knee arthroplasty, many treatment alternatives had been developed. Many of these are used today in selected patient populations.

Still performed in substantial numbers, a high tibial osteotomy (Fig. 31-9) can improve alignment of the mechanical forces across the knee.[3] Change of alignment produces redistribution of forces from areas of isolated degeneration to sections of the joint surface better preserved. High tibial osteotomy, along with the somewhat less frequently performed distal femoral osteotomy, can give 8 to 10 years of improved comfort and function in selected patients.[24,28,30] Conversion to total knee arthroplasty, though, has been reported to have complication rates rivaling those of revision total knee arthroplasty.[48] High tibial osteotomy requires strict selection criteria: good to excellent range of motion, ligamentous stability (including the ACL), weight-bearing pain without rest pain, and noninflammatory etiology. Assuming these criteria, the best candi-

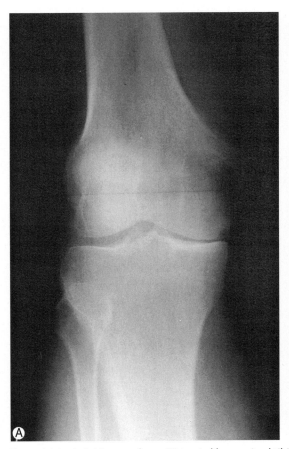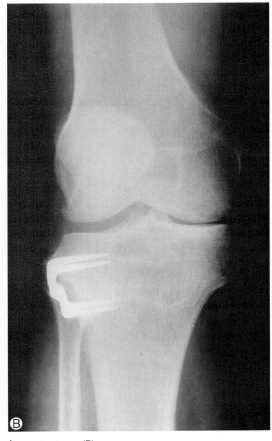

Figure 31-9. Arthritic varus knee **(A)** treated by proximal tibial valgus osteotomy **(B)**.

date is young (below 55) with a high demand, and must have unicompartmental disease (preserved medial or lateral compartment and patellofemoral articulation). The patient with activity-related weight-bearing pain and no rest pain may have the most predictably positive outcome. Osteotomy allows eventual full activity return and high-demand durability but an almost certainly limited life span. Osteotomies can be technically challenging, may not provide as much pain relief as total knee arthroplasty, and have been known to complicate a conversion to total knee arthroplasty.

Resurfacing procedures for the knee also function well in the selected patient. Although total knee arthroplasty is a version of resurfacing, more conservative bone-sparing options are still available. An example is the McKeever hemiarthroplasty resurfacing prosthesis (Fig. 31-10A). This prosthesis provides resurfacing for unicompartmental disease— medial or lateral. The resurfacing provides a metal-on-bone bearing surface with no intervening polyethylene.[36,40] The McKeever has been most often used in the young, very active and/or heavy

patient. The patient must have full ligamentous stability, including the ACL, PCL, and collaterals. The advantage to this procedure, in addition to its bone-sparing qualities, is elimination of intervening polyethylene and the problems of plastic wear and osteolysis. Although the metal-on-bone bearing surface is subject to wear, eliminating the polyethylene markedly increases the durability of the surface, allowing the patient to return to full impact loading as tolerated. The downside is that the prosthesis can loosen—especially with repetitive impact loading. Also, pain relief can be incomplete. Pain relief is not as predictable as with total knee arthroplasty or even with unicompartmental knee replacement. Conversion to total knee arthroplasty, however, is not difficult.

Realizing the limitations of the McKeever-type resurfacing and high tibial osteotomy, more complete unicompartmental arthroplasties were developed to resurface both sides of the tibiofemoral joint.[18,35] These unicompartmental arthroplasties (Fig. 31-10B) still allow limited bone resection and ligamentous preser-

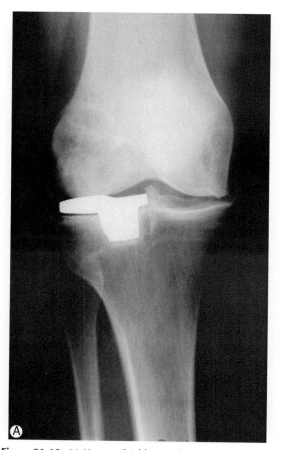 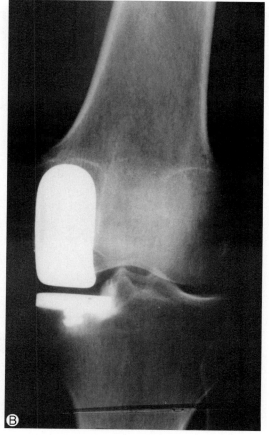

Figure 31-10. McKeever tibial hemiarthroplasty **(A)** and medial unicompartmental knee arthroplasty **(B)** for arthritis limited to only a portion of the knee joint.

vation, but UHMWPE now is introduced as the bearing surface. Indications for unicompartment replacement include relative youth (50 to 60 years), rest pain, ligamentous integrity, and unicompartmental disease (excluding severe patellofemoral disease). Inflammatory arthritides are a contraindication to unicompartmental replacement. Because of the UHMWPE bearing surface, additional guidelines for patient selection might include moderate to low activity (for a younger person) and body weight under control. By maintaining both cruciates, patients may feel as though it is more like "their own knee." The introduction of UHMWPE makes pain relief more predictable, but adds the component of polyethylene wear. Because of the polyethylene, activity restrictions postoperatively will be somewhat the same as those following total knee arthroplasty.

Total Knee Arthroplasty

Total knee arthroplasty (Fig. 31-8B) still provides the most predictable pain relief in end-

stage knee disease. Total knee arthroplasty is best indicated in end-stage disease of more than one compartment—or for any end-stage inflammatory arthritis. Total knee arthroplasty can provide correction of deformity not achieved by other treatments. With total knee arthroplasty, the distal femur and the proximal tibia are resurfaced. Usually, the patella is also resurfaced.

As total knee arthroplasty has become more prevalent, and reproducible, the desire came to provide this for younger, more active patients. In the interest of longevity of the interface, cementless technology has been applied to the total knee arthroplasty. Cementless, ingrowth femurs (Fig. 31-11) have been found successful at intermediate follow-up. The primary indication is the high-demand, younger patient. Even with short and intermediate results for the cementless femurs very similar to those of the cemented components, it has been theorized that cementless femurs may better maintain bone stock into the second decade. Cementless tibial components have not, to this date, performed as well as their cemented counterparts. Although still used in many centers, cementless tibial components are less commonly used.

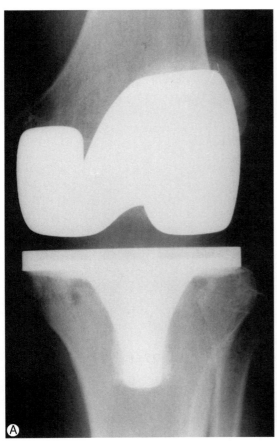
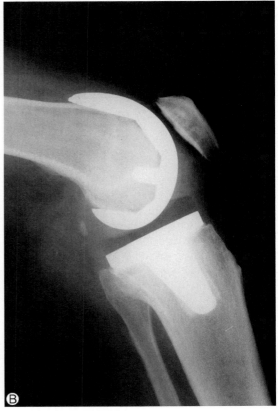

Figure 31-11. Anteroposterior (**A**) and lateral (**B**) roentgenograms of a hybrid total knee arthroplasty: cemented tibial and patellar components and cementless femoral component.

Cementless patellar resurfacing requires a metal backing for ingrowth surface. Metal backing of the patella, with a few exceptions, has been abandoned because of insufficient thickness of the overlying polyethylene.

Two final considerations involve the patella and the posterior cruciate ligament. Patellar resurfacing is not mandatory in total knee arthroplasty performed for osteoarthritis.[12,27] Native patellae, with limited disease, can articulate well with properly selected femoral components. Patellar bone stock is preserved and complications resulting from patellar resurfacing are avoided. Pain relief may not be complete. Predicting patellofemoral pain relief is difficult. For that reason patellae are largely being resurfaced. The ACL must be sacrificed in total knee arthroplasty. The PCL, however, can be preserved or sacrificed. The 2 options have largely the same results with similar follow-up (slightly longer with the PCL sacrificing). PCL-preserving total knee arthroplasty is more technically demanding, but may preserve bone and provide better knee kinematics on stairs.[37,49]

Modes of failure with total knee arthroplasty are in many ways similar to those of the total hip arthroplasty. Except for dislocation, very rare in total knee arthroplasty, the same mechanical and biologic concerns exist for the knee. Mechanical wear, osteolysis, and sepsis impact life of the total knee in almost the exact fashion that they do the hip.

Return to Activity

In many ways, because UHMWPE still provides the bearing surface, activity restrictions are also quite similar to those of total hip arthroplasty. In order to regain motion and function, strength in the lower extremity is critical. To a large extent, bony anatomy and component position provide stability in the hip. This is not true in the knee. The knee depends on ligaments for static and dynamic stability with extensor/flexor musculature for added dynamic stability. Quadriceps and hamstring strengthening provide the final ingredient for confident use of the new total knee arthroplasty.

Sports that are recommended for the mature, active female with a total knee arthroplasty include bicycling, walking, cross-country ski machine use, golfing, unloaded hiking, swimming, and horseback riding. As with the total hip arthroplasty, UHMWPE governs the life of the total knee arthroplasty. Wear prevention is an important component of postoperative total knee arthroplasty considerations. In order to

preserve the bearing surface, activities that involve high-impact, repetitive loading should be avoided. Activities such as prolonged running, jogging, or high-impact aerobics cause the arthroplasty excessive wear risk. The replaced knee is by definition ACL deficient, with a good deal of proprioception lost. This eliminates fast starts and predictable cutting motions with the knee. StairMaster and LifeStep use, step aerobics, squatting, and kneeling all may place undue stress on the component bearing surface as well as the ligamentous integrity.

Isolated strengthening of the total knee does add stability and function. Quadriceps musculature does respond well to quadriceps setting extension exercises. Performed from $0°$ to $30°$ of flexion, a few pounds of weight (3 to 5 pounds) can be added for advanced strengthening. Quadriceps setting provides strength that improves confident use as well as patellar tracking. Flexion exercises, such as leg curls, strengthen the hamstrings. Together with flexibility exercises, quadriceps and hamstring strengthening will improve endurance while easing stiffness in the total knee arthroplasty.

THE FUTURE

Total hip and total knee arthroplasty classically depend upon metal–polyethylene bearing surfaces. This combination has been effective since 1961. Unfortunately, as repetitive loading proceeds, polyethylene can wear and shed debris.

Research and clinical trials are proceeding for alternative bearing surfaces. Ceramic against ceramic and metal on metal surfaces are both being examined. Both show tremendous promise in decreasing wear debris generation and the bone reaction. Trials are ongoing to examine the ability of these materials to withstand the repetitive forces of joint arthroplasty. If successful, these alternative bearing surfaces could greatly slow the major cause of present hip and knee failure.

CONCLUDING REMARKS

While total hip arthroplasty and total knee arthroplasty relieve pain and return function to most active women with hip and/or knee arthritis, long-term survivorship and function of these artificial joints is best seen in lower-weight, lower-demand patients. Motion and activity are encouraged, whereas running, jumping, twisting, and excessive repetitive loading (overuse) are discouraged. Though joint replacements may not withstand excessive demand, total joint arthroplasty has been very successful in allowing pain-free activities of daily living and enthusiastic return to moderate-demand athletics.

References

1. Amstutz HC, Thomas BJ, Jimak R: Treatment of primary osteoarthritis of the hip: a comparison of total joint and surface replacement arthroplasty. J Bone Joint Surg 66A(2):228, 1984.
2. Amstutz HC, Yao J, Dorey FJ, et al: Survival analysis of T-28 hip arthroplasty with clinical implications. Orthop Clin North Am 19(3):491–503, 1988.
3. Berman AT, Bosacco SJ, Kirsher S, et al: Factors influencing long-term results in high tibial osteotomy. Clin Orthop 272:192–8, 1991.
4. Bombelli R, Santore RF, Poss R: Mechanics of normal and osteoarthritic hips: a new perspective. Clin Orthop 182:69–78, 1984.
5. Capello WN, Misamore GW, Trancik TM: Conservative total hip arthroplasty. Orthop Clin North Am 13:833, 1982.
6. Chandler HP, Remech RL, Wixson RL, McCarthy JC: Total hip replacement in patients younger than 30 years old. J Bone Joint Surg 63A:1426, 1981.
7. Chiari K: Medial displacement osteotomy of the pelvis. Clin Orthop 55:98, 1974.
8. Dorey FJ, Kilgus DJ, Amstutz HC: The effect of patient activity, sports participation and impact loading on the durability of cemented total hip arthroplasty. Presented at the AAOS Annual Meeting, Atlanta, 1988.
9. Dorr LD, Luchett M, Conaty JP: Total hip arthroplasties in patients younger than 45 years: a 9 to 10 year follow-up study. Clin Orthop 260:215–9, 1990.
10. Engh CA, Bobyn JD, Glassmen AH: Porous coated hip replacements. J Bone Joint Surg 69B:45–55, 1987.
11. Engh CA, Massini P: Cementless total hip arthroplasty using the AML. Clin Orthop 249:141–58, 1989.
12. Enis JE, Gardner R, Robledo MA, et al: Comparison of patellar resurfacing vs nonresurfacing in bilateral total knee arthroplasty. Clin Orthop 260:38–42, 1990.
13. Eppright RH: Dial osteotomy of the acetabulum. J Bone Joint Surg 58A:283, 1976.
14. Fackler CD, Poss R: Dislocation in total hip arthroplasty. Clin Orthop 151:169–78, 1980.
15. Harris WH, Maloney WJ: Hybrid total hip arthroplasty. Clin Orthop 249:21–9, 1989.
16. Hirohata K, Shiba R, Shimizu T: Follow-up results of Chiari pelvis osteotomy for patients with acetabular dysplasia. In: Hirohata K (ed): Joint Surgery Up-To-Date. New York, Springer-Verlag, 1989.
17. Huddleston HD: Femoral lysis after cemented hip arthroplasty. J Arthroplasty 3:285–97, 1988.
18. Kozinn SC, Scott RD: Unicondylar knee arthroplasty. J Bone Joint Surg 71A:145–50, 1989.
19. Lach W, Windhager R, Kutschera HP: Chiari pelvic osteotomy for osteoarthritis secondary to hip dysplasia: indications and long-term results. J Bone Joint Surg 73B:229–34, 1991.
20. Lidwell OM: Clean air at operation and subsequent sepsis in the joint. Clin Orthop 211:91, 1986.
21. Lidwell OM, Lowbury EJ, Whyte W, et al: Infection and sepsis after operation for total hip or total knee replacements—influence of ultra clean air, prophylactic antibiotics and other factors. J Hyg London 93:505–29, 1984.
22. Livermore J, Ilstrip D, Money B: Effective femoral head size on wear of the polyethylene acetabular component. J Bone Joint Surg 72A:518–28, 1990.
23. Maquet PGJ: Biomechanics of the Hip. Berlin, Springer-Verlag, 1985.
24. McDermott AG, Finklestein JA, Farine I, et al: Distal femoral varus osteotomy for valgus deformity of the knee. J Bone Joint Surg 70A:110–6, 1988.
25. Michelson JA, Riles LH Jr: Considerations in the comparison of cemented and cementless total hip arthroplasty. J Arthroplasty 4:327–34, 1989.
26. Petty W: Total Joint Replacement. Philadelphia, WB Saunders, 1991.
27. Picette GD III, McGann WA, Welch RB: The patellofemoral joint after total knee arthroplasty without patellar resurfacing. J Bone Joint Surg 72A:1379–82, 1990.
28. Ritter MA, Fechtman RA: Proximal tibial osteotomy: a survivorship analysis. J Arthroplasty 3(4):309–11, 1988.
29. Roberts JM, Fu FH, McClaine EJ, Ferguson AB: A comparison of posterolateral and anterolateral approaches to total hip arthroplasty. Clin Orthop 187:205–10, 1984.
30. Rudan JF, Simuda MA: High tibial osteotomy: a prospective clinical and x-ray review. Clin Orthop, 255:251–6, 1990.
31. Russell TA: Arthrodesis of lower extremity and hip. In: Campbell's Operative Orthopedics. St Louis, CV Mosby, 1987.
32. Salter RB, Harrisson G, Thompson GH: Innominate osteotomy in the management of congenital subluxation of the young adult. Clin Orthop 182:53–68, 1984.
33. Santavirta S, Hoikka V, Eskola A, et al: Aggressive granulomatous lesions in cementless total hip arthroplasty. J Bone Joint Surg 72B:980–4, 1990.
34. Schutzer SF, Harris WH: Deep wound infection after total hip arthroplasty under contemporary aseptic conditions. J Bone Joint Surg 70A:724–7, 1988.
35. Scott RD, Cobb A, McQueary F, et al: Unicompartmental knee arthroplasty: 8–12 year follow-up evaluation with survivorship analysis. Clin Orthop 271:96–100, 1991.
36. Scott RD, Joyce MJ, Ewald FC, et al: McKeever metallic hemiarthroplasty of the knee in unicompartmental degenerative arthritis: long-term clinical follow-up and current indications. J Bone Joint Surg 67A:203–7, 1985.
37. Scuderi GR, Insall JN, Windsor RE, et al: Survivorship of cemented knee replacements. J Bone Joint Surg 71B:798–803, 1989.
38. Sofue M, Kono S, Kawaji W, et al: Long-term results of arthrodesis in the hip in young adults. Int Orthop 13:129–33, 1989.
39. Strathy GM, Fitzgerald RH Jr: Total hip arthroplasty in the ankylosed hip: a ten year follow-up. J Bone Joint Surg 70A:963, 1988.
40. Swanson AB, Swanson GDE, Powers T, et al: Unicompartmental and bicompartmental arthroplasty of the knee with a thin metal-tibial implant. J Bone Joint Surg 67A:1175–82, 1985.
41. Tanaka S: Surface replacement of the hip joint. Clin Orthop 134:75, 1978.
42. Townley CO: Conservative total articular replacement arthroplasty (tara) with fixed femoral cup. Orthop Trans 5:463, 1981.
43. Turner RH, Scheller AD: Revision Total Hip Arthroplasty. New York, Grune & Stratton, 1982.

44. Vicar AJ, Coleman CR: A comparison of the anterolateral, transtrochanteric and posterior surgical approaches in primary total hip arthroplasty. Clin Orthop 188:152–9, 1984.
45. Wagner H: Surface replacement arthroplasty of the hip. Clin Orthop 134:102–30, 1978.
46. Watillon M, Maquet P: Indications for femoral intertrochanteric osteotomy for arthritic sequelae of hip dysplasia. Acta Orthop Belg 56:371–7, 1990.
47. White SH: The fate of cemented total hip arthroplasty in young patients. Clin Orthop 231:29–34, 1988.
48. Windsor RE, Insall JN, Vince KG: Technical considerations of total knee arthroplasty after proximal tibial osteotomy. J Bone Joint Surg 70A:547–55, 1988.
49. Wright J, Ewald FC, Walker PS: Total knee arthroplasty with the kinematic prosthesis: results after 5–9 years: a follow-up note. J Bone Joint Surg 72A(7):1003–9, 1990.

Chapter 32

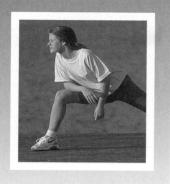

Biomechanical Considerations

Cheryl Riegger-Krugh, Sc.D., P.T.
Barney F. LeVeau, Ph.D., P.T.

Many disciplines contribute to competitiveness and the ability to excel in physical performance in sports. These disciplines include biomechanics, motor control/motor learning, physiology, and psychology, whether known under these or other names. These disciplines as well as issues related to hormones and nutrition affect the physical performance of the female athlete. This chapter will address the biomechanical aspects of physical performance as related to the female athlete.

TERMINOLOGY

Rigid-Body Biomechanics

Biomechanics is the application of forces and their effects on living systems, including the human body. In the simplest form, a *force* is a push or a pull. When motion is involved, *force* can be defined as the entity that causes a mass to accelerate or decelerate. All forces are fully characterized by indicating their line of action, direction, point of application, and magnitude. If the objects involved are completely stationary or moving at a constant velocity, the field of statics is considered. The field of dynamics is considered when change in motion occurs. Within the broad field of biomechanics, *kinematics* involves the description of motion of body segments or the body as a whole and *kinetics* involves the forces involved in either a static posture or a motion. Body segments are considered as rigid bodies when movement of body segments is analyzed, therefore, this area of biomechanics may be called *rigid-body biomechanics*.

Deformable-Body Biomechanics

Biomechanics involves the response of the musculoskeletal system structures inside the body to forces external to the body. This area of study is called *deformable-body biomechanics* because these structures can deform, or undergo mechanical strain, under loading. Five different strains exist:

1. Tensile forces tend to pull structures apart, producing tensile strain.
2. Compressive forces tend to push together, producing compressive strain.
3. Shear forces tend to cause sliding, producing shear strain.
4. A combination of the above forces can tend to cause bending, with bending strain, if the forces are not collinear or in the same straight line.
5. Torsional forces tend to cause twisting within a structure, producing torsional strain.

Relevant aspects of each of these areas will be introduced and discussed in the context of female participation in sports. The emphasis of this chapter will be on rigid-body biomechanics, as the concepts of deformable-body biomechanics are more closely linked to sports-related injuries and will be addressed in the chapters related to sport-specific conditions.

GENERAL REQUIREMENTS OF POSTURE AND MOVEMENT DURING PHYSICAL PERFORMANCE IN SPORTS

Physical performance involves an ability to maintain posture and to move. Some non-gender-specific concepts related to physical performance will be reviewed initially within this context and then related to the differences in females and males. These abilities involve requirements for muscle force production in synchrony with other muscles, duration and timing of force production, and application of these abilities in optimal amounts toward the sport skill. To maximize these abilities, external forces, or forces outside the body, must be overcome, matched, or controlled by the internal forces, or forces inside the body. External forces include force produced by gravity's pull on a mass, resisting loads, buoyancy, wind resistance, and friction on the surface of the body. Internal forces are produced by muscle–tendon units (MTUs), ligamentous–joint reactions, and tendon-on-bone friction. External and internal forces cause or tend to cause linear or angular motion.

Static Posture

Maintaining a posture during a sport involves producing the required net linear internal forces and net resultant internal moments to hold the posture.

The ability to maintain static postures involves the body's response to external forces, so that the external forces will not produce angular motion (external moment or torque) or linear motion. The tendency to produce angular motion or rotation in all directions must balance, that is, the Σ (Sum) of moments in any direction must equal 0. Linear forces in all directions must balance, that is, the Σ (Sum) of forces in any direction must equal 0. For example, as a person stands in a squat posture, the knee flexion external moment produced by the pull of gravity must equal the knee extensor internal moment, mostly produced by the quadriceps. If the anterior cruciate ligament is not strong enough, anterior shear of the tibia on the femur will occur.

Since the moment or torque is determined by multiplying the applied force by a distance, called the *moment arm* (the perpendicular distance from the line of action of the force to the axis of motion), a larger force production or a larger moment arm allows a greater moment or torque production. A larger moment arm provides a mechanical advantage for the identified force. The gluteus medius and biceps brachii have relatively large moment arms.

Motion

Producing movement or motion during a sport involves producing the net linear internal forces and net resultant internal moments required for movement. Force production during linear movement involving accelerations and decelerations is determined by the equation: Force = mass $\times$ acceleration (Newton's second law). Linear acceleration is directly proportional to the force applied. The acceleration is inversely proportion-

al to the magnitude of the mass. Therefore, the mass tends to resist any change in linear motion.

Moments involving angular motion are analyzed by the equation: Σ Moments = Moment of inertia (I) $\times$ angular acceleration (α). This equation means that opposite moments do not balance. The general equation for the moment of inertia is $I = mr^2$. This equation illustrates that the important factors involving the direction of movement of the object include the object's mass, the location of the object's mass along the segment, and the relationship of the mass to the axis of rotation. The moment of inertia tends to resist the change in angular motion. Therefore, the angular acceleration is inversely proportional to the moment of inertia. The positive or negative aspect of the summed equation indicates the direction of motion and muscle moment required.

While maintaining postures involves isometric MTU actions, active movement usually involves either concentric or eccentric muscle actions.

- Concentric MTU activity: force production while the MTU is shortening.
- Eccentric MTU activity: force production while the MTU is lengthening.

Concentric action occurs when a muscle group overcomes external forces or moments to produce linear motion or angular motion in the direction opposite the tendency of the external forces or moments. For example, in a jumping up task, net knee extensor concentric MTU force production would be required to extend the knees. Concentric action also is needed to produce motion in the same direction as the external force or moment, if the desired movement is faster and/or more forceful than would be produced with the external force or moment alone. For example, elbow extensors are needed to produce a forceful planting of a ski pole into the snow even though the pull of gravity on the forearm, hand, and ski pole would tend to produce elbow extension motion, although not as quickly or forcefully as needed.

Eccentric action occurs when a muscle group controls external forces or moments to produce smooth coordinated linear motion or joint motion in the same direction as the tendency of the external forces or moments. In landing from a jump, knee extensor eccentric MTU force production would be required to allow smoothly controlled movement into knee flexion.

Movement produced during a sport requires a coordinated sequence of concentric and eccentric muscle actions, as well as optimal active stabilization from muscle groups and passive stabilization from ligaments, fascia, bone, and articular surface geometry. Muscle force is produced by a combination of force from the active contractile portion of muscle (ie, muscle tissue) as well as the tension produced in the connective tissue components of a muscle. The connective tissue components include the tendon and the connective tissue that wraps around the muscle bundles from fibers to fascicles to the entire muscle. Maximum force production from the active contractile part of a MTU is available during concentric and eccentric contractions. However, maximum force production from stretching connective tissue components is limited during concentric contractions. There is greater ability to stretch connective tissue during eccentric contractions. Several implications result:

1. Eccentric contractions offer maximum MTU force production.
2. Greater MTU force can occur concentrically during slow muscle action as compared to fast motions.
3. During a movement task, which alternates between concentric and eccentric phases at the same speed, the eccentric phase may seem easier. However, the eccentric portion may be associated with less fine motor control, because more of the total force production is from the passive stretch of connective tissue.
4. Muscle activity (monitored by electromyography [EMG]) will be less during the eccentric than concentric phase of a task of the same speed. EMG monitors only the muscle activity and not force production from the stretching of connective tissue.

Force production during movement also occurs as a result of inertial effects. Inertial effects involve the ongoing motion effect of an object or body segment. In many ballistic or burst-type movements in sports, a body segment is accelerated with concentric action, carried through passively with the inertial effect, and slowed by activation of the antagonist muscles. For example, in a tennis serve, glenohumeral adductors, horizontal adductors, and medial rotators likely initiate the forward motion of the serve, the inertial effect of momentum continues the forward upper limb motion, and control or slowing occurs with eccentric activation of the glenohumeral horizontal abductors and lateral rotators. Momentum can be quantified by multiplying mass by velocity for momentum in a linear path and by multiplying moment of inertia (I) (a mass equivalent for angular movement) $\times$ angular velocity (ω) for momentum in an angular or rotational path. The baseball batter who maximally horizontally adducts the gleno-

humeral joint allows more angular velocity and therefore more momentum to occur before the ball is hit.

Angular momentum also can be used to increase the speed of rotation. The angular term of $I\omega$ is equivalent to $mr^2\omega$, since $mr^2 = I$. In conditions with angular momentum, the location of the mass is important. Divers, ice skaters, and gymnasts control their spins and turns by changing positions of their limbs and trunk. For example, in the trunk-tucked position, the spin will be faster, because I is decreased and provides less resistance to change in angular velocity. The sprinter flexes the lower limb joints to decrease moment of inertia during the swing phase, allowing a quicker swing phase to occur.

Since the momentum (mass $\times$ velocity) of an object equals the impulse of the force at contact (force magnitude $\times$ time interval), the force at contact can be decreased if the time interval is increased. During a bunt in baseball, the batter skillfully draws back, reducing the force imposed on the ball, and therefore causes the ball to drop close to the batter.

Shock absorption is important to prevent injury in sports. Passive shock absorption is provided by nonmuscular structures, such as wood surfaces (as opposed to concrete) and shock-absorbing shoewear and shoe inserts.[121] Well-timed eccentric muscle actions provide the active component of shock absorption needed to dampen forces imposed by ground reaction forces, body contact hits during contact sports, and so forth. These muscle actions require strength and coordination of muscle force production.[94]

Components of Physical Performance Competitiveness

There are many components to achieving competitiveness in physical performance. Many of these components are included in preseason physical examinations for athletes.[5,19,57] Each of the components, such as strength and flexibility, will be explained briefly relative to the female athlete. Some equalization of training resources for men and women has occurred through Title IX of the 1972 Education Amendments Act[73] and the Civil Rights Restoration,[126] the realization of the athletic competitiveness of women,[8,75,88] and the encouragement of physical activity for health benefits.[48,73,133] The boldfaced first sentence under each topical component is a summary statement relative to the female athlete and that component.

With physical performance competitiveness comes injuries and the risk for injuries.[116] While most injuries are sport specific rather than gender specific,[4,5,10,57,104] some injuries and incidence of other injuries are distinctive for females.[5,9,63,104,127] The biomechanical basis for injury risk is addressed in this chapter. Risk and injury status related to specific sports are addressed in individual chapters of this book.

Muscle Strength

While absolute strength is less for adult females than adult males, relative strength generally is the same. An adequate magnitude of muscle strength is required for physical performance, including moving body segments against the pull of gravity, appropriate accelerations and decelerations of body segments, and static and dynamic postural control. Often equally critical issues are balanced agonist/antagonist muscle strength,[49,58] avoidance of excessive strength in overused muscle groups, and avoidance of muscle force production at a disadvantageous muscle length. An example of agonist overuse would be stronger glenohumeral medial rotator than lateral rotator muscles for swimmers. Of the 4 main strokes used in swimming (freestyle, butterfly, breaststroke, and backstroke), 3 use glenohumeral medial rotators during the pull-through phase of the arm stroke.[59] Speed of muscle contraction is important for producing quick movements in sporting activities and for protecting joints from injury. The ability of an athlete to maintain a muscular contraction or to perform many repeated contractions at a high level of strength is required in many sports.

There are different types of muscle strength, which relate to different types of sport skills:

- Static muscle moment or torque: strength related to holding postures.
- Dynamic muscle moment or torque: strength related to producing movement with concentric MTU action or controlling movement with eccentric MTU action.
- Muscle force: strength related to producing gliding or linear motions (such as scapular depression) and the force component of muscle moment or torque.
- Muscle power: strength within a given time period, usually a short time period.
- Strength in endurance: ability to maintain a level of muscle moment or force for a given time period (ie, resistance to fatigue).

Since static muscle strength does not correlate well with dynamic strength,[4] the type of strength training needs to be chosen carefully. Great static muscle strength is needed to maintain the challenging postures held by female ballet dancers, for example. Dynamic strength requirements involving muscle power and strength in endurance would be greater for tennis players, soccer players, and basketball players. Most sports involve both static and dynamic strength requirements.

Strength correlates well with physical performance related to daily functional mobility tasks *if* strength is the limiter of the physical performance achievement.[12,56] This same correlation exists relative to sports.[7,13,39,45,120]

In general, adult males have absolute greater muscle moment or torque capacity than adult females,[3,11,23,60,61,67,85] and this difference is greater for upper body than lower body muscle groups.[20,106] Fuster and coworkers reported 53% greater maximum strength in men than women in pulling activities and hand-grip strength.[32] In the first decade of life, however, absolute strength is similar in girls and boys.[86] By late adolescence, females reach an average of two thirds of lean body mass (mass of a body less all but essential fat) and total muscle mass of males.[76] This strength development difference in adults is apparent in 100- and 200-meter sprints, which require great force development in muscles of the upper as well as lower limb muscles and result in a 9% to 10% advantage for men.[20] Neder and colleagues reported absolute greater strength in knee extensors and flexors in nonathletic men as compared to women from 20 to 80 years old.[85] Gibbs reported on female versus male Alpine and Nordic skier power.[33] From best to least power capacity were male Alpine skiers, male Nordic skiers, female Alpine skiers, and female Nordic skiers. From best to least agility, with agility being undefined, were male Alpine skiers, female Alpine skiers, male Nordic skiers, and female Nordic skiers. Hakkinen reported shorter time to absolute and relative force level of muscle contraction in knee extensors, trunk flexors, and trunk extensors for male versus female basketball players.[39] He explained that the differences involved gender differences as well as training. Holloway and Baechle[46] reported overall absolute strength and power for women as two thirds of that for men. Muscle fiber and muscle cross-sectional area, both of which relate to strength capacity for different tasks, for females are 60% to 85% of that for males.[105]

The number of muscle fibers correlates to strength, but there is no evidence that men and women differ in number of fibers.[20] Relative proportion of fast-twitch to slow-twitch fibers, which relates to speed and power, does not appear different for men and women,[1,20,21,108] however, some studies indicate that males have larger fibers than females.[1] In the general population, muscle fiber composition is approximately 52% slow-twitch and 48% fast-twitch fibers in women.[20] The percentage of fiber type may change with age for females.[35,36]

Relative strength between men and women has been compared by normalizing values to body weight,[3,11,39,49,100] fat-free weight,[105] limb-length volume,[23] and bone-free lean mass,[85] or by normalizing strength measured by dynamometer to limb or segment length. An isokinetic strength comparison of elite female athletes with male college football players showed females to have statistically weaker quadriceps and hamstring muscle strength at 60°/sec. This difference also was apparent when values were normalized to body weight. Hakkinen evaluated the isometric force production of the knee extensor, trunk flexor, and trunk extensor muscles in male and female basketball players.[39] Male players had greater absolute maximal strength in all 3 muscle groups than the females. When strength per body weight was determined, the knee extensor muscles showed no significant difference. However, significant differences remained for the trunk muscles. Ramos and coworkers[100] studied gender differences in strength at 3 different age levels. The younger groups (11 to 12 and 13 to 14 years old) had no difference in either absolute or relative strength to body weight. In the oldest group (17 to 18 years old), boys were stronger than girls of the same age in absolute (65%) and relative to body weight (74%) strength. Gibbs[33] reported on female versus male Alpine and cross-country skier strength adjusted for weight. From most to least strength were male Alpine skiers strongest, with female Alpine skiers, male cross-country skiers, and female cross-country skiers having equal strength. Davies and colleagues[23] tested 79 young adult males and females using the handgrip and standing long jump. They determined that males had greater absolute strength than the females. When they normalized the results using lean limb volume, the differences were less, but still significant. While Neder and coworkers[85] reported absolute greater strength in knee extensors and flexors in nonathletic men and women from 20 to 80 years old, they found no consistent significant difference in isokinetic strength, power, or ratio of knee flexor:extensor strength when values were normalized. In contrast to Neder's finding for the knee in nonathletic women, imbalance in strength of agonist and antagonist knee muscles in soccer players has been considered as one reason for injuries to

be twice as high in girls as in boys.[94] Since training results in similar relative gains in strength for females and males at all ages,[21,69,70] Sanborn[105] interpreted the differences in muscle strength between trained men and women as a factor of muscle mass size.

MTUs produce the internal muscle moment required by the sport. Since muscles do not produce the same force and moment throughout the entire joint range of motion,[37,42,51,128,130] physical performance strength ability should be optimized by having muscles produce the greatest moment during a sport skill at a point in the joint range where maximum muscle moment is possible. For most muscle groups, maximum muscle moment capacity occurs at a muscle length that is slightly elongated from the resting position. However, the elbow flexors and extensors have maximum muscle capacity near 100° of elbow flexion with the shoulder neutral, where the moment arms of the muscles are greatest. The ankle plantarflexors have maximum muscle capacity in slight plantar flexion, when the muscle length and moment arms are equally advantageous.[51,130] When isometric, isotonic, and isokinetic torque curves for knee extensor, knee flexor, elbow extensor, and elbow flexor muscles were determined by Knapik and colleagues,[61] the shapes of these curves for males and females were similar. The curves were generally an inverted-U shape that tended to follow the mechanical requirements of the joint position or muscle length.

Muscle contraction time can determine whether an athlete will succeed in an event, or, in some instances, whether an injury will result. Females may require more time to generate maximum force than males.[10,39,49,52,61,62,66] In their torque curve study, Knapik and coworkers[61] found that males demonstrated peak torque earlier in the isometric contraction, and earlier in the range of motion, than females. The rate of force development to maximum was shown to be greater for male than female basketball players. The males took less time to reach a higher force level. This rate remained statistically significant when calculated to a relative force scale. The males also demonstrated a faster muscle relaxation time than the females. This neuromuscular efficiency was evaluated by Huston and Wojtys.[49] They found no significant differences in time to peak torque for knee extension among female or male athletes or controls. However, they did find that the female athletes were much slower than the male athletes for knee flexion time to peak torque. This slower generation of torque in hamstring muscles for females may have implications related to anterior cruciate ligament injuries in female athletes.

Muscular Endurance

Comparisons of muscular endurance of females and males are inconclusive. Muscular endurance, the ability to perform many repetitions at submaximal load, is an important component in many sports. Adequate endurance is required for many aspects of physical performance, including maintaining prolonged postures, stamina for the length of the competition, and requirements for specific skills, such as strength or precision, well into the event. These skills involve training to acquire necessary resistance to fatigue.

Gender comparisons of muscular endurance are inconclusive. Muscular endurance of the quadriceps, as measured by the number of knee extension efforts before 50% reduction in peak torque on a Cybex machine, has been positively correlated with ability in the slalom event,[33] but no female–male differences were found on this measure of muscular endurance. However, muscular endurance as measured by the Biodex was found by Huston and Wojtys[49] to be greater in male athletes than female athletes. This significant difference remained when the results were normalized to body weight. Three separate studies comparing gender differences in fatigue found that females were less fatigable than males.[18,45,80] Muscular endurance should be affected by the percentage of fast- or slow-twitch fibers in a muscle, but, as mentioned, the relative proportion of fast-twitch to slow-twitch fibers does not appear to differ by gender.

Strength of Musculoskeletal Structures

A "Wolff's Law" concept applies to bone, and also to other musculoskeletal structures. Each musculoskeletal structure must have adequate strength to avoid injury during a sport. Strength of structures such as bone, tendon, ligament, cartilage, and fascia can be indicated by maximum stress, strain, or stiffness as defined by a stress–strain curve.[30] While adequate strength of tissue is required, adequate strength of junctions, such as the muscle–tendon or ligament–bone junctions, also is required. Wolff's Law relates to bone's ability to remodel to the stress placed on it.[101,132] Wolff's Law paraphrased states that bone is in a constant state of remodeling, with deposition occurring if appropriate stress is imposed on it and resorption occurring if either too much or too little stress is imposed. While this law relates to bone, the other structures appear to follow the same pattern of remodeling, although with different types and degrees of stresses serving as stimuli for building and breaking down and with different rates of adaptation. To very briefly summarize the main stresses and remodeling patterns:

- Long bones require intermittent compressive forces to remodel. Growth at muscle attachment sites is due to tensile forces. Remodeling factors are numerous.[101]
- Tendon remodeling occurs with tensile forces in the direction of collagen fibers.[38]
- Ligament remodeling occurs with tensile forces in the direction of collagen fibers.[15]
- Articular cartilage responds very slowly to intermittent compressive forces.[122] Cartilage degeneration occurs with excessive pressure and too little pressure, such as with immobilization.[122] Epiphyseal or growth plates of hyaline cartilage within bone adapt to the alignment of forces on the bone, such that the plate orients perpendicular to the resultant compressive force on the bone. This has great implication for orientation of forces imposed on bone and resulting skeletal alignment in the bone or at the joint.[103]

Application of these concepts relates to implications of stresses on structures by different sports and the ability of structures to either adapt to these stresses or be injured by them.

Many examples of application of these concepts occur within sports. Intermittent compressive forces within optimal physiologic limits on long bones will maintain bone density or cause bone deposition.[27] For example, gymnasts have significantly greater bone mineral density in upper limb sites than many other athletes. Gymnasts have greater bone mineral density in the lower limb bones and pelvis than swimmers and greater bone mineral density in the torso than other athletes. Weight training, which provides greater impact loading than endurance training, resulted in a greater osteogenic stimulus than did endurance training.[43] During weight training, bone mineral density increase was specific to loaded bony sites. Higher bone mineral density has been reported in females who participate in high-impact physical activity as compared to female nonathletes.[24]

Loading outside optimal physiologic limits leads to bone resorption. Excessive compressive and repetitive forces can result in stress fractures. Female ballet dancers who do pointe work have a high incidence of stress fractures of the second metatarsal bone.[107] Relative to the spine, spondylolysis in female gymnasts has been linked to repetitive forces related to trunk hyperextension, hyperflexion, and compression and repetitive torques.[40,127] Too little bone compressive force results in loss of bone mass and strength. Imposing compressive loads on bone with a bowed shaft, such as the tibia, may cause the bone to bow even more. Bone that is resistant to bending and fracture has adequate bone mass and adequate distance of bone mass from the bending axis. Biomechanically, these 2 characteristics result in area or bending moment of inertia (I), determined by the summation of each mass (m) times the distance (d) squared of the mass from the bending axis ($I = \Sigma$ mass $\times$ d^2). While tibial area moment of inertia has been reported to predict the risk for stress fractures during the first year of military training for men,[79] this relationship has not been supported for women.[134]

During growth, tendon and ligament insertions migrate through a process of bone resorption and deposition. Tendons and ligaments often are attached to bone on the side of the epiphyseal plate that is distant from the joint surface. Migration of tendon/ligament insertion site occurs, so that excessive length of the structure is prevented during growth. This occurs for the patellar ligament during growth.[87] Stimuli such as excessive physical activity during a growth period or excessive tightness of an MTU or ligament may not allow controlled migration but instead may lead to an inflammatory process.[57] Examples of such processes are apophysitis of the tibial tuberosity (Osgood–Schlatter disease), apophysitis of the distal pole of the patella (Siding—Larson–Johansson syndrome), and calcaneal apophysitis (Sever's disease).

Excessively forceful intermittent compressive forces at an epiphyseal plate may result in damage or premature closure of growth plates, exemplified by changes that occur in the distal radial plate in young gymnasts.[57] Medial epicondylitis of the elbow has been characterized by hyperplasia and degeneration of collagen occurring from overuse of the tendons that attach to the medial epicondyle of the humerus,[41] whereas gradually increasing use of the tendons may result in strengthening without the damaging response.

Frictional forces of soft tissue on bone can lead to pathology, and one example is the tendency for the iliotibial band to shear on the lateral femoral epicondyle at approximately 30° of knee flexion. This condition is worsened when the friction is increased, as it can be in someone with a genu varus deformity or with excessively pronated feet.[20,63]

Flexibility

There are many aspects to flexibility, and each must be discussed separately. Adequate flexibility is required for many aspects of physical performance, including attaining specific joint range,[89] moving through joint range with specific speed by minimizing soft tissue stiffness, and preventing excessive tissue or joint flexibility while reaching desired end-point joint range.

In one study of 2000 secondary school and college athletes, females were more flexible than males in all measures of a preparticipation physical examination.[60] The knees of women have been reported to have greater laxity than the knees of men,[49] and this may give women an overall advantage in attaining greater end-point range of motion. Ballet dancers are exemplary in this aspect of flexibility.

Stiffness in muscles, other soft tissues, and joints can be a mechanism to prevent quick joint movement, which often is needed to compete athletically. *Stiffness* can be defined as resistance to stretch, especially quick stretch in muscles and soft tissues opposing motion.[47] Stiffness has been categorized as skeletal stiffness, muscle stiffness, and joint stiffness.[47,54] Muscle stiffness can be separated into passive (connective tissue), contractile apparatus or muscle fiber, and reflex action[54,111] or dynamic-passive (stiffness and the inverse, compliance while muscles are inactive) and dynamic-active (stiffness/compliance while muscles are active).[34] While optimal skeletal stiffness is high, optimal joint stiffness is low, and optimal muscular stiffness changes based on the requirement for the sport surfaces.[47]

Stiffness in some circumstances can enhance physical performance. Increased stiffness in the MTU may enhance physical performance by increasing force production capacity in the contractile component.[34,131] Jahnke and coworkers[54] noted that muscle stiffness changes were accompanied by changes in electromyographic and muscle spindle response. Increased muscle responsiveness can enhance physical performance requiring rebound activity from eccentric muscle action,[34] or quick reactiveness in the MTU. Force resulting from passive stretching of tight soft tissues can be considerable in magnitude and may be mistakenly overlooked as a source of stiffness.[78] Quick reactiveness in sports could involve training to decrease force production in the antagonist quickly enough. Female volleyball players have been reported to have a quadriceps muscle recruitment order different from that of male volleyball players in response to anterior tibial translation.[49] The authors hint that this phenomenon could result from different training programs or from the fact that women may require different training programs than men.[36]

Interestingly, some detriments of stiffness have been noted during physical performance. Damped oscillations during brief perturbations in supine leg presses were used to classify MTU stiffness in 20 trained men. When subjects performed a series of jump maneuvers, the stiffer subjects demonstrated poorer eccentric performance during landings from the jumps; that is, they were less able to dampen the high eccentric loads.[123]

Prevention of excessive joint or muscle flexibility during movement involves adequate and well-timed eccentric muscle action. An example would be injury from excessive glenohumeral lateral rotation from inadequate restraint by the subscapularis and pectoralis major just prior to the initiation of the acceleration phase of a tennis serve. Warmth does appear to decrease muscle stiffness,[26] through appropriate warm-up activity or with superficially applied heat.

Skeletal Alignment

Skeletal alignment affects movement efficiency and risk for pathology. Skeletal alignment has been defined as either the alignment of 2 bones at the joint or the alignment of different areas, such as proximal and distal ends, within a bone. *Skeletal malalignment* is defined as either abnormal joint alignment, such as genu varus or valgus, or deformity within a bone, such as excessive tibial torsion.[103]

Weight-bearing on skeletally malaligned joints can result in many problems for the athlete. Muscles designed to provide force along an established line of action now pull nonoptimally. Excessive joint motion can occur at the site of the skeletal malalignment or as a result of correlated or compensatory motions or postures,[103] causing time loss and/or muscle imbalance in a sport skill. Correlated motions/postures are ones that normally occur with closed kinetic chain relationships. Compensatory motions/postures occur as an adjustment for problematic closed kinetic chain relationships to improve neuromusculoskeletal function or foot contact with some external surface or cosmetic appearance. Compensatory motions or postures do not occur in a predictable manner during closed kinetic chain activities. For example, a person with a genu varus, or bow-legged, knee posture would demonstrate the correlated posture of standing on the lateral aspects of the feet if normal tibial to rearfoot alignment were maintained with the genu varus posture. During

weight-bearing, this could result in risk for lateral ankle sprains, a risk that is higher for females than males.[57] When weight-bearing, however, this person may demonstrate a compensatory posture of excessive subtalar pronation to allow the medial calcaneus and medial forefoot to contact the floor to increase the base of support and stability of the foot on the ground. A person with genu varus and this compensatory subtalar motion may increase time to weight-bear on this lower limb because of the excessive time to move into and out of the compensatory motions.

In general, the athlete with excellent skeletal alignment appears to be at a distinct advantage relative to physical performance and decreased risk for injury. Perfect skeletal alignment is not currently established, but there are few competitive athletes with marked observable skeletal malalignment. Optimal skeletal alignment may change by specific sport. For example, in weight-bearing sports such as basketball and baseball, athletes with in-toed lower limb posture can be competitive. This in-toed posture may allow optimal force production in the gastrocnemius and soleus for jumping or running, as these muscles produce both ankle plantar flexion and subtalar inversion needed in running and jumping. In addition, this in-toed posture could decrease the mediolateral distance through which the body center of mass (CoM) has to displace during right-to-left weight shifts. In these same sports, some athletes, and often the same athletes, appear to have a genu varus posture. People with these skeletal malalignments may be able to compete athletically, but also may have a higher-than-normal risk for pathology, such as medial knee osteoarthritis.

Some skeletal alignment differences exist between females and males. Females tend to have more genu valgus, excessive femoral antetorsion or anteversion, and foot pronation than men.[50,57] Males have a femoral neck-to-shaft angle of 125°, whereas females have an angle of less than 125°.[126] The neck-to-shaft angle, a wider pelvis, and shorter femur often lead to the genu valgus, so that the feet are normally spaced in relation to each other. A combination of skeletal alignments, including hip coxa vara, excessive femoral antetorsion or anteversion, genu valgus, lateral placement of the tibial tuberosity, and valgus posture of the calcanei has been termed the "miserable malalignment syndrome."[5,17] Women have a wider pelvis and a greater Q angle than men,[20] which, together with excessive femoral antetorsion, puts stress on the medial compartment of the tibiofemoral joint, the lateral patellofemoral joint, and medial aspect of the ankle.[20] Genu valgus posture, increased Q angle, and the wider pelvis can lead to patellofemoral problems in female equestrians, who increase the malalignments when pressing the knees against the horse.[28] Lower limb alignment has been implicated in the high incidence of soccer injuries in females.[94]

Weight-bearing on skeletally malaligned joints can increase the risk for arthritis pathology. Weight-bearing on a skeletally malaligned joint involves joint loading on reduced joint contact surface and may produce a tendency to increase the skeletal malalignment. Joint degeneration in arthritis can occur from excessive joint contact pressure with loading on reduced contact area.[71,98,118,122] Patellofemoral arthritis is linked to genu valgus, excessive femoral antetorsion or anteversion, and excessive lateral tibial rotation.[84] Less often joint degeneration occurs from too little weight-bearing on articular cartilage that is unloaded by skeletal malalignment.[14,31,109,122] Sites that are inadequately loaded receive too little nutrition to maintain healthy articular cartilage,[14] however, joint degeneration from too little loading is less progressive than joint degeneration caused by too much joint contact pressure.[109,124] Interestingly, running does not result in greater incidence of arthritis or joint degeneration in people who are "biomechanically elite," that is, those who have excellent skeletal alignment, strength and muscle balance, flexibility, and movement performance during running. Running, however, can lead to arthritis in those who have skeletal malalignment or poor movement performance.[90,91]

Weight-bearing on skeletally malaligned joints can result in risk for soft-tissue pathology. Weight-bearing on a skeletally malaligned joint can produce a moment that tends to increase the skeletal malalignment, and this increase in skeletal malalignment usually is prevented by soft tissue. For example, excessive subtalar pronation in weight-bearing produces the correlated motion of excessive medial tibial rotation, which can lead to excessive stress and strain on the anterior cruciate ligament.[117] Friction syndromes and the pathologies of association are correlated with skeletal malalignment. Genu varum posture may increase friction of the iliotibial band on the lateral femoral epicondyle,[118] which can be problematic in sports such as rowing and running.[84]

Symmetry

Implications of symmetry and asymmetry are specific to a sport skill. Symmetry in skeletal alignment, strength, flexibility, and so forth may be an issue related to physical performance for the athlete. Symmetry is important for symmetrical sports, such as swimming, diving, and running. Asymmetry may result from repetitive performance of a unilateral task, such as baseball pitching, and may not be problematic. Some aspects of asymmetry, such as asymmetrical bone density, may be a response to skill-related stresses imposed as necessary adaptation. Asymmetry in skeletal alignment may result in imbalance in timing, right-to-left muscle group strength, or agonist-to-antagonist muscle group strength,[61,125] and may be problematic. Asymmetry in joint range of motion or adequate control throughout the joint range can complicate physical performance ability, especially for a bilaterally symmetrical sport.

Anthropometrics

Athletes have an easier and better chance to excel in a specific sport if body dimensions closely match the mechanical requirements of the sport. Most postural or movement tasks, including physical performance in sports, are more or less challenging based on a person's anthropometrics. Anthropometrics incorporates measures of body dimension, such as body shape, height and width of segments, relative length of body segments, segmental weight, location of body center of mass, and percentage of body fat versus muscle. For example, swimming speed is positively correlated with broader shoulder width, larger chest circumference, and greater fat-free weight.[44] Some predictive gender-related anthropometric differences have been reported.[32] Fuster and colleagues[32] reported that the vertical jump height was more dependent on trunk length than body height or size for women, whereas this skill was more dependent on all longitudinal dimensions for men. While the morphologic or structural differences of females and males can be contrasted, often variations within gender are greater than variations between genders,[126] or among races.[16] Racial differences between Japanese and American male gymnasts were reported by LeVeau and colleagues.[68] As an example of relative task difficulty, standing at self-selected speed after being seated in a standard height chair is easier for a person with normal thigh and leg length than for a person with very long thighs and legs (as long as both feet reach the floor). The long-legged person has to achieve more knee joint flexion to sit, probably generate more knee extensor strength to do the same task, and possibly generate maximum knee extensor strength in a less advantageous point in the joint range than does the person with normal segment lengths.

Relative difficulty of functional movement tasks has been studied in the context of constrained and unconstrained tasks. Unconstrained tasks are set as absolute tasks in an attempt to maintain conformity of the task. In the example of rising from the chair, the chair height might be set at the usual height of chairs in the community to learn how many in the community could use a certain type of chair. Constrained tasks, however, are relatively difficult for all participants and indicate that some restriction of normal motion has been imposed. In the example of rising from the chair, chair height might be altered to popliteal height for each individual. Athletic events are a combination of constrained and unconstrained tasks. Some historical opinion that females were not competitive athletically may be due to the development of sports as unconstrained tasks, based on ability of male athletes. Some unconstraint persists, such as the 10-foot height of basketball hoops for men and women. Some constraint has been developed, such as a smaller-diameter basketball for women's basketball than for men's basketball.[93]

There are a number of anthropometric differences between females and males. These anthropometric differences affect different sports in different ways. Theories have been proposed regarding anthropometric risks for injury.[88] An example of such a theory includes shorter people being at risk for stress fractures, because shorter step lengths result in more foot contacts per distance run. If the athlete has an impulsive landing foot contact pattern, then risk might be increased for this reason. Christine Wells[126] has compiled a great deal of information on profiles for female athletes competing in different sports. Each difference will be discussed below.

Length Dimensions. Average body height, limb segment length, and trunk length for females are less than for males.[25,64,72,126] Adult height is reached by 17 to 19 years for females and by the early 20s for males.[74] Females have shorter limbs relative to body height.[126] After adolescence, leg length is approximately 52% of a male's height and 51.2% of a female's height, with most of this difference existing in the knee-to-ankle length.[126] Males have longer and wider feet, and longer arms and forearms on average.[126] Peak height velocity occurs during years 10.5 to 13 for females and 12.5 to 15 for males.[64,115] Atwater reviewed the literature regarding height of the CoM and athletic achievement in jumping and running and concluded that people do not appear to be disadvantaged in these activities based on this parameter.[6]

Sports that have absolute height-related goals for achievement will be relatively more difficult for females. In basketball, the rim height for men's and women's basketball is 10 feet (120 inches). In this case, the athlete who is taller and has a longer upper limb length will be much closer to the rim before initiating the jump for the rim. In 1983, Krugh and LeVeau[65] measured a standing vertical reach of 93.67 inches, a vertical reach displacement during a jump from standing of 35.93 inches, and a vertical reach displacement during a jump from running of 45.76 inches for Michael Jordan. During the standing vertical reach, Michael Jordan already had 78% of the height needed to reach the rim.

Sports that have absolute length-related goals for achievement will be relatively more difficult for females. The athlete with the longer upper limb length, which males generally have, has an advantage in contacting a tennis ball, squash ball, or racquetball. Length-related components of sports that are normalized by anthropometrics are relatively the same difficulty in that component for females and males. The average size of the female hand was used in making a smaller-diameter standard-size ball for women's basketball compared to that used in men's basketball.

Some gender differences in anthropometrics have implications for sport success. Adult females have a wider pelvis and greater tibiofemoral valgus angle[25,64,72] than males, which could result in differences in time from right to left weight shifts for females. Morris and Underwood[83] summarized that the athletes from various sport groups had distinctive anthropometric characteristics. Relatively, basketball players had longer hands, forearms, arms, total upper limb length, feet, legs, thighs, total lower limb and trunk lengths, and wider shoulders. Softball players had shorter hands, forearms, feet, and legs, and longer trunks, which gave them a low leg length:trunk length ratio. Body-segment ratios varied, with softball players having a low shoulder:hip width ratio, field hockey players having a low leg length:trunk length ratio, and track and gymnastic athletes having a high leg length:trunk length ratio. Track athletes had a higher shoulder:hip width ratio. Athletes in track and gymnastics had many anthropometric similarities. Divers and basketball players had very different anthropometrics. Swimmers were not extreme in any of the anthropometric measures.

Weight. Average body weight is less for females than for males. However, muscle mass is less and fat is more of the total percentage of body weight for females than for males.[72] Overall, adult women have 8% to 10% more body fat than men.[105]

For the same muscle mass, the same strength exists for men and women. Relative strength measures are comparable, as discussed earlier. However, the greater percentage of body fat is not a force-producing substance. For land-based sports, females may be at a disadvantage. However, for water-based sports, females will tend to be more buoyant.[126]

Shape and Size. Overall, females tend to be pear shaped and males tend to be triangular or rectangular.[25] The body CoM is lower in females (at the level of the S2 vertebra) than males (at the level of the S1 vertebra) to reflect this body-shape difference. However, CoM is determined more by a person's body type and height than gender.[126] This general shape difference incorporates the wider pelvis in females[64] and less upper body muscle mass. Coordination of efforts to maintain balance during a postural hold involves control of the body CoM. The higher the body CoM, the more challenge to balance control tasks.

Body shape may be sport specific for females.[25,119] Female runners, compared to the average female, may be slightly taller; have a higher ponderal index (ie, height/weight ratio, meaning that the taller person is at an advantage) and may be more ectomorphic; have a narrower pelvis and smaller feet; and have a lower percentage[2] of body fat.[2] Williams and colleagues[129] reported that elite female distance runners had a narrower pelvis and less body fat than the typical female in the population.[129] However, their elite female distance runners were shorter and had shorter lower limbs than the average female. Female track and field athletes, jumpers, discus/javelin throwers, and shot-putters were reported to have anthropometric body proportions similar to those for college-age males.[77] Young swimmers, 39 males and 54 females, have been reported as being taller and heavier, and having wider shoulders than same-aged nonswimmers.[44] In these swimmers, swimming speed was positively correlated with shoulder width, chest circumference, hand and foot size, and fat-free weight. Female speed skaters had a lower amount of body fat and greater total muscle mass than female controls,[112] and had more fat on their thighs than the male speed skaters and male controls but less than female controls. Female speed skaters had greater thigh mass than female 400-meter

sprinters, marathon runners, cross-country skiers, and figure skaters.

Surface Area:Mass Ratio. Females have a larger body surface area:mass ratio than males.[126] While this larger body surface area is advantageous for cooling in dry heat, there is no advantage in humid heat.[105] Larger body surface area could lead to hypothermia in females,[29,105] although this tendency may be offset if the female had the characteristically thicker layer of subcutaneous fat.[105]

Clothing, Sports Equipment, and Playing Surfaces. Clothing, sports equipment, and even playing surfaces have relevance to anthropometrics. In the past, women wore men's athletic clothing, because it was the only sport clothing available.[113] Initial attempts to adapt clothing mainly consisted of making men's clothing in a variety of pastel colors and calling the skis, snowboards, and so forth "women-specific" equipment.[92] In recent years, clothing has become "anthropometrically correct" for a variety of sports.[113] Shoes have been redesigned for the female foot.[114]

Sports equipment likewise has been adapted for females.[113] Components of bicycles, skis, and wind-surfing equipment are examples of sport equipment adapted for women. Shorter bicycles with narrower handlebars and wider saddle designs are available for women.

A stiff playing surface of concrete can increase risk of injury for all athletes, especially those landing with high impact. Athletes who have insufficient shock absorption from well-timed eccentric MTU actions after landing would be at greater risk of injury if they were playing their sport on a very stiff surface, such as concrete.[22]

Movement Performance

Appropriate movement performance is required for many aspects of physical performance, including timing parameters and the optimum use of movement strategies. Movement performance is the quality of a movement; it involves aspects such as coordination, forcefulness, and speed. Some would include balance, while others would see balance as a separate entity. Each aspect incorporates biomechanical, neurologic, motor control/motor learning, and behavioral (such as motivational) aspects of movement. Timing parameters include appropriate bursting of muscle activity (power), release and initiation of muscle activity, and smooth coordination. Eccentric muscle actions precede concentric actions of the same muscles, as exemplified in diving when the diver allows the ankle to dorsiflex under eccentric control of the plantarflexors and then forcefully plantarflex by concentric plantarflexor action to propel the diver into the air. If the concentric muscle action is too late, the MTU force from the rebound of the eccentric stretch of the plantarflexors is lost.

Optimum movement strategies involve adequate use of muscle and soft-tissue properties, minimization of extraneous movements, and adequate shock absorption for the sport skill. Repetitive impulsive loading (RIL) is an example of movement performance characterized by insufficient shock absorption.[97] RIL has been identified mostly in human gait and involves hard and fast heel landings and insufficient shock absorption in subtalar eversion and knee flexion from subtalar invertor and knee extensor eccentric muscle activity, respectively, following initial contact.[96,99] Ability to use well-timed eccentric muscle activity is very important in sport skill. The high incidence of anterior cruciate injuries in female soccer players landing with extended knees, which limits shock absorption, points out the need for shock absorption in sports.[94] Contrary to what was once thought, articular cartilage and synovial fluid have little inherent shock-absorbing capacity.[95]

Parameters of movement performance require valid analysis of the sport skill and determination of meaningfulness. For some sports, especially fast moving sports, videotaping can be very helpful in allowing slow-motion playback of the movement strategy. For some sports, 3 dimensional motion analysis can assist analysis significantly. The hard heel landings have been documented as the large magnitude slope of the vertical component of the ground reaction force as measured on a force plate at initial contact and beginning loading response of the gait cycle. Validation of a movement performance characteristic or subtle movement with videotaping, 3-dimensional analysis, or force plate analysis might be learned as an observational skill.[102] Monitoring muscle action patterns with surface or fine-wire electromyography offers insight into magnitudes of muscle firing and timing of muscle firing. Since movement can be performed with a variety of muscle-action combinations, ability to complete a movement does not allow prediction of specific muscles or magnitudes of muscle actions used to accomplish the task.[12] The next step is determining whether the analysis gained by these procedures is meaningful (ie, makes a difference for the athletic physical performance). Often these analyses do make a difference, both to the trainer and to the athlete who needs to understand how to alter movement strategies. The coach, trainer, or athlete may use electromyography, videotaping, or other feedback to help improve performance. Such analysis is common in baseball for pitchers and batters. Analysis with feedback has been shown to be effective in enhancing rapid walking on a treadmill,[53] playing a stringed instrument,[82] and playing the piano.[81] Video analysis has helped improve skills on the balance beam,[110] and with throwing a ball.[55]

CONCLUDING REMARKS

In summary, each variation within athletic events adds complexity to the picture of competitive physical performance. The addition of gender difference from athletic events that were originally competitive events for males adds one more variation. For some aspects of physical performance, biomechanical differences between females and males are significant, whereas for other aspects, intragender differences are as great or greater than intergender differences.

Acknowledgments

I am grateful for the review and comments by Mary Christenson, MS, PT; Alexander Benson, BS; and Celeste Hancock, BS in Biology, PT.

Suggested Readings

Cerny K: Pathomechanics of stance, Phys Ther 64(12):1851–95, 1984.

Craik RL, Oatis CA: Gait Analysis—Theory and Application. St. Louis, CV Mosby, 1995.

Enoka RM: Neuromechanical Basis of Kinesiology. Champaign, Ill, Human Kinetics Books, 1988.

Frankel V, Nordin M: Basic Biomechanics of the Musculoskeletal System. Philadelphia, Lea & Febiger, 1990.

Hamill J, Knutzen KM: Biomechanical Basis of Movement. Baltimore, Williams & Wilkins, 1995.

LeVeau B: Williams and Lissner's Biomechanics of Human Motion, 3rd edition. Philadelphia, WB Saunders, 1992.

Perry J: Gait Analysis, Normal and Pathological Function. Thorofare, NJ, Slack, 1992.

Physical Therapy—December 1984 issue on Biomechanics

Root ML, Orien WP, Weed JH: Normal and Abnormal Function of the Foot. Los Angeles, Clinical Biomechanics Corporation, 1977.

Rose J, Gamble JG: Human Walking. Baltimore, Williams & Wilkins, 1994.

Soderberg GL: Kinesiology: Application to Pathological Motion. Baltimore, Williams & Wilkins, 1986 and 1997.

Winter DA: The Biomechanics and Motor Control of Human Movement, New York, John Wiley & Sons, 1990.

References

1. Alway SE, Grumbt WH, Gonyea WJ, Stray-Gunderson J: Contrasts in muscle and myofibers of elite male and female bodybuilders. J Appl Physiol 67:24–31, 1989.

2. Anderson T: Biomechanics and running economy. Sports Med 22:76–89, 1996.

3. Andrews AW, Thomas MW, Bohannon RW: Normative values for isometric muscle force measurements obtained with hand-held dynamometers. Phys Ther 76(3):248–59, 1996.

4. Aniansson A, Gustafsson E: Physical training in elderly men with special reference to quadriceps muscle strength and morphology. Clin Physiol 1:87–98, 1981.

5. Arendt EA: Knee injuries. In: Agostini R (ed): Medical and Orthopedic Issues of Active and Athletic Women. St Louis, CV Mosby, 1994, p 307.

6. Atwater AE: Biomechanics and the female athlete. In: Puhl J, Brown CH, Voy R (eds): Sport Science Perspectives for Women, Champaign, Ill, Human Kinetics Publishers, 1988, pp 1–12.

7. Bale P, McNaught-Davis P: The physiques, fitness and strength of top class women hockey players. J Sports Med Phys Fit 23:80–8, 1983.

8. Barnett NP, Wright P: Psychosocial factors and the developing female athlete. In: Agostini R (ed): Medical and Orthopedic Issues of Active and Athletic Women. St Louis, CV Mosby, 1994, p 92.

9. Beim G, Stone DA: Issues in the female athlete. Orthop Clin North Am 26:443–51, 1995.

10. Bell DG, Jacobs I: Electro-mechanical response times and rate of force development in males and females. Med Sci Sports Excerc 18:31–6, 1986.

11. Bohannon RW:Reference values for extremity muscle strength obtained by hand-held dynamometry from adults aged 20–79 years. Arch Phys Med Rehabil 78:26–32, 1997

12. Bohannon RW, Andrews AW, Thomas MW: Walking speed: reference values and correlates for older adults. J Orthop Sports Phys Ther 24(2):86–90, 1996.

13. Bowerie W, Cummings GR: Sustained handgrip in boys and girls: variation and correlation with performance and motivation to train. Res Q 43:131–41, 1972.

14. Bullough P, Goodfellow J, O'Connor J: The relationship between degenerative changes and load-bearing in the human hip. J Bone Joint Surg 55B(4):746–58, 1973.

15. Butler DL, Grood ES, Noyes FR, Zernicke RF: Biomechanics of ligaments and tendons. Exerc Sport Sci Rev 6:125–81, 1978.

16. Cheng JC, Leung SS, Lau J: Anthropometric measurements and body proportions among Chinese children. Clin Orthop 323:22–30, 1996.

17. Ciullo JV: Lower extremity injuries. In: Pearl AJ (ed): The Athletic Female. Champaign, Ill, Human Kinetics Publishers, 1990, pp 267–98.

18. Clarke DH: Sex differences in strength and flexibility. Res Q Exer Sport 57:144–9, 1986.

19. Claypoole C, Agassiz S: Physical therapy approaches to patellofemoral stress syndrome. In: Agostini R (ed): Medical and Orthopedic Issues of Active and Athletic Women. St Louis, CV Mosby, 1994, p 316.

20. Colliton JW: Personal safety and exercise. In: Agostini R (ed): Medical and Orthopedic Issues of Active and Athletic Women. St Louis, CV Mosby, 1994, p 123.

21. Cureton KJ, Collins MA, Hill DW, McElhannon FM: Muscle hypertropy in men and women. Med Sci Sports Exerc 20, 338–44, 1988.

22. Davidson CJ, Harty DJ: Volleyball. In: Agostini R (ed): Medical and Orthopedic Issues of Active and Athletic Women. St Louis,CV Mosby, 1994, p 489.

23. Davies BN, Greenwood EJ, Jones SR: Gender difference in the relationship of performance in the handgrip and standing long jump tests to lean limb volume in young adults. Eur J Appl Physiol 58:315–20.

24. Dook JE, James C, Henderson NK, Price RI: Exercise and bone mineral density in mature female athletes. Med Sci Sports Exerc 29:291–6, 1997.

25. Espenschade AS, Eckert HM: Motor Development. Columbus, Ohio, Charles E Merrill Books, 1967.

26. Ettema GJ, Huijing PA: Skeletal muscle stiffness in static and dynamic contractions. J Biomech 27(11):1361–8, 1994.

27. Fehling PC, Alekel L, Clasey J, et al: A comparison of bone mineral densities among female athletes in impact loading and active loading sports. Bone 17:205–10, 1995.

28. Finnegan MA: Equestrian events. In: Agostini R (ed): Medical and Orthopedic Issues of Active and Athletic Women. St Louis, CV Mosby, 1994, p 439.

29. Foyster P: Heat and cold. In: Agostini R (ed): Medical and Orthopedic Issues of Active and Athletic Women. St Louis, CV Mosby, 1994, p 333.

30. Frankel V, Nordin M: Basic Biomechanics of the Musculoskeletal System. Philadelphia, Lea & Febiger, 1990.

31. Freund E, Goodfellow JW, Bullough TP: The pattern of ageing of the articular cartilage of the elbow joint. J Bone Joint Surg 49B(1):175–81, 1967.

32. Fuster V, Jerez A, Ortega A: Anthropometry and strength relationship: male-female differences. Anthropol Anz 56(1):49–56, 1998.

33. Gibbs P: Skiing. In: Agostini R (ed): Medical and Orthopedic Issues of Active and Athletic Women. St Louis, CV Mosby, 1994, p 347.

34. Gleim GW, McHugh MP: Flexibility and its effects on sports injury and performance. Sports Med 24(5): 289–99, 1997.

35. Glenmark B, Hedberg G, Jansson E: Changes in muscle fiber type from adolescence to adulthood in women and men. Acta Physiol Scand 146:251–9, 1992.

36. Glenmark B, Hedberg G, Kaijser L, Jansson E: Muscle strength from adolescence to adulthood-relationship to muscle fiber types. Eur J Appl Physiol 68:9–19, 1994.

37. Gravel D, Richards CL, Filion M: Angle dependency in strength measurements of the ankle plantar flexors. Eur J Appl Physiol 61:182–7, 1990.

38. Gross MT: Chronic tendinitis: pathomechanics of injury, factors affecting the healing response and treatment. J Orthop Sport Phys Ther 16(6):248–60, 1992.

39. Hakkinen K: Force production characteristics of leg extensor, trunk flexor and extensor muscles in male & female basketball players. J Sports Med Phys Fitness 31(3):325–31, 1991.

40. Hall SJ: Mechanical contribution to lumbar stress injuries in female gymnastics. Med Sci Sports Exerc 18:599–602, 1986.

41. Hannafin JA: Upper extremity injuries. In: Agostini R (ed): Medical and Orthopedic Issues of Active and Athletic Women. St Louis, CV Mosby, 1994, p 294.

42. Harms-Ringdahl K, Ekholm J: Biomechanical aspects of exercise. In: Harms-Ringdahl K (ed): Muscle Strength. New York, Churchill Livingstone, 1993.

43. Heinonen A, Oja P, Kannus P, et al: Bone mineral density of female athletes in different sports. Bone Miner 23:1–14, 1993.

44. Helmuth HS: Anthropometric survey of young swimmers. Anthropol Anz 38(1):17–34, 1980.

45. Heyward V, McCreary L: Analysis of static strength and relative endurance in women athletes. Res Q 48:703–10, 1977.

46. Holloway JB, Baechle TR: Strength training for female athletes. A review of selected aspects. Sports Med 9(4):216–28, 1990.

47. Hortobagyi T, DeVita P: Altered movement strategy increases lower extremity stiffness during stepping down in the aged. J Gerontol 54:B63–70, 1999.
48. Huang Y, Macera C, Blair SN, et al: Physical fitness, physical activity, and functional limitation in adults aged 40 and older. Med Sci Sports Exerc 30(9):1430–5, 1998.
49. Huston LJ, Wojtys EM: Neuromuscular performance characteristics in elite female athletes. Am J Sports Med 24:427–36, 1996.
50. Hutchinson MR, Ireland ML: Knee injuries in female athletes. Sports Med 19:288–302, 1995.
51. Inman VT, Ralston HJ, Todd F: Human Walking. Baltimore, Williams & Wilkins, 1981.
52. Ives JC, Kroll WP, Bultman LL: Rapid movement kinematic and electromyographic control characteristics in males and females. Res Q Exerc Sport 64:274–83, 1993.
53. Jaeger BJ, Olivares SA, Wetzel MC: Operant conditioning in relation to natural EMG during rapid treadmill walking. Am Phys Med 66:59–76, 1987.
54. Jahnke MT, Proske U, Struppler A: Measurements of muscle stiffness, the electromyogram, and activity in single muscle spindles of human flexor muscles following conditioning by passive stretch or contraction. Brain Res 24:493(1):103–12, 1989.
55. Janelle CM, Barba DA, Frehlich SG, et al: Maximizing performance feedback effectiveness through videotape replay and a self-controlled learning environment. Res Q Exerc Sport 68:269–79, 1997.
56. Jette AM: Outcomes research: shifting the dominant research paradigm in physical therapy. Phys Ther 75(11):965–70, 1995.
57. Johnson MD: Preseason sports examination for women. In: Agostini R (ed): Medical and Orthopedic Issues of Active and Athletic Women. St Louis, CV Mosby, 1994, p 35.
58. Kellis E, Baltzopoulos V: The effects of the antagonist muscle force on intersegmental loading during isokinetic efforts of the knee extensors. J Biomech 32:19–25, 1999.
59. Kenal K: Swimming and water polo. In: Agostini R (ed): Medical and Orthopedic Issues of Active and Athletic Women. St Louis, CV Mosby, 1994, p 363.
60. Kibler WB, Chandler TJ, Uhl T, Maddux RE: A musculoskeletal approach to the preparticipation physical examination. Am J Sports Med 17:525–31, 1989.
61. Knapik JJ, Wright JE, Mawdsley R, Braun J: Isometric, isotonic, and isokinetic torque variations in four muscle groups through the range of joint motion Phys Ther 63:938–47, 1983.
62. Komi PV, Karlsson J: Skeletal muscle fiber types, enzyme activities and physical performance in young males and females. Acta Physiol Scand 103:210–8, 1978.
63. Krivickas LS: Basketball. In: Agostini R (ed): Medical and Orthopedic Issues of Active and Athletic Women. St Louis, CV Mosby, 1994, p 465.
64. Krogman WM: Child Growth. Ann Arbor, Mich, The University of Michigan, 1972, p 231.
65. Krugh J, LeVeau B: Michael Jordan's vertical jump. J Orthop Sports Phys Ther 29(1):A–10, 1999.
66. Lennmarken C, Bergman T, Larsson J, Larsson LE: Skeletal muscle function in man: force, relaxation rate, endurance and contraction time-dependence on sex and age. Clin Physiol 5:243–55, 1985.
67. LeVeau B: Sports for women. In: Harris DV (ed): DGWS Research Reports. Washington DC, AAHPER, 1971, pp 3–13.
68. LeVeau BF, Ward T, Nelson RC: Body dimensions of Japanese and American gymnasts. Med Sci Sports Exerc 6:146–50, 1974.

69. Lexell J, Downham DY, Larsson Y, et al: Heavy-resistance training in older Scandinavian men and women: short- and long-term effects on the arm and leg muscles. Scand J Med Sci Sports 5:329–41, 1995.
70. Lillegard WA, Brown EW, Wilson DJ, et al: Efficacy of strength training in prepubescent to early postpubescent males and females: effects of gender and maturity. Pediatr Rehabil 1:147–57, 1997.
71. Lindgren U, Seireg A. The influence of mediolateral deformity, tibial torsion, and foot position on femorotibial load. Arch Orthop Trauma Surg 108:22–6, 1989.
72. Lohman TG, Roche AF, Martorell R (eds): Anthropometric Standardization Reference Manual. Champaign, Ill, Human Kinetics Publishers, 1988.
73. Lopiano DA: Gender equity in sports. In: Agostini R (ed): Medical and Orthopedic Issues of Active and Athletic Women. St Louis, CV Mosby, 1994, p 13.
74. Lowry GH: Growth and Development of Children, 6th edition. Chicago, Year Book Medical Publishers, 1973.
75. Mahle Lutter J: Sociologic considerations on women and sports. In: Agostini R (ed): Medical and Orthopedic Issues of Active and Athletic Women. St Louis, CV Mosby, 1994, p 6.
76. Malina RM: Growth, performance, activity, and training during adolescence. In: Shangold M, Mirkin G, (eds): Women and Exercise Physiology and Sports Medicine, Philadelphia, FA Davis, 1988.
77. Malina RM, Zavaleta AN: Androgeny of physique in female track and field athletes. Ann Hum Biol 3:441–6, 1976.
78. Mansour JM, Audu ML: The passive elastic moment at the knee and its influence in gait. J Biomech 19(5):369–73, 1986.
79. Milgrom C, Giladi M, Simkin A, et al: The area moment of inertia of the tibia: a risk factor for stress fractures. J Biomech 22:1243–8, 1989.
80. Misner JE, Massey BH: Sex differences in static strength and variability in three different muscle groups. Res Q Exer Sport 61:238–42, 1991.
81. Montes R, Bedmar M, Sol Marin M: EMG biofeedback of the abductor pollicis brevis in piano performance. Biofeedback Self Regul 18:67–77, 1993.
82. Morasky RL, Reynolds C, Clarke C: Using biofeedback to reduce left arm extensor EMG of string players during musical performance. Biofeedback Self Regul 6:565–72, 1981.
83. Morris PC, Underwood CS: The woman athlete structurally speaking. In: Harris DV (ed): DGWS Research Reports: Women in Sports. Washington DC, AAHPER, 1973, pp 101–37.
84. Musnick DJ: Rowing. In: Agostini R (ed): Medical and Orthopedic Issues of Active and Athletic Women. St Louis, CV Mosby, 1994, p 373.
85. Neder JA, Nery LE, Shinzato GT, et al: Reference values for concentric knee isokinetic strength and poser in nonathletic men and women from 20–80 years old. J Orthop Sports Phys Ther 29(2):116–26, 1999.
86. Oded Bar-Or: The prepubescent female. In: Shangold M, Mirkin G (eds): Women and Exercise Physiology and Sports Medicine. Philadelphia, FA Davis, 1988.
87. Ogden JA, Grogan DP: Prenatal development and growth of the musculoskeletal system. In: Albright J, Brand R (eds): The Scientific Basis of Orthopaedics, 2nd edition. Norwalk, Conn, Appleton & Lange, 1987.
88. Otis CL: Stress fractures in athletes. In: Agostini R (ed): Medical and Orthopedic Issues of Active and Athletic Women. St Louis, CV Mosby, 1994, p 325.

89. O'Toole ML, Douglas PS: Fitness: definition and development. In: Shangold M, Mirkin G (eds): Women and Exercise Physiology and Sports Medicine. Philadelphia, FA Davis, 1988.

90. Panush RS, Lane NE: Exercise and the musculoskeletal system. In: Panush RS, Lane NE (eds): Bailliere's Clinical Rheumatology: Exercise and Rheumatic Disease. Vol 8(1). Philadelphia, Bailliere Tindall, 1994, p 79.

91. Panush RS, Schmidt C, Caldwell JR, et al: Is running associated with degenerative joint disease? JAMA 255(9):1152–4, 1986.

92. Parker P: Volant targets female skiers. The Denver Post Friday, March 12, 1999.

93. Politi S: Wave of the future? UNC women not only ones to jam. The Daily Tar Heel November 12, 1992.

94. Putukian M: Soccer. In: Agostini R (ed): Medical and Orthopedic Issues of Active and Athletic Women. St Louis, CV Mosby, 1994, p 478.

95. Radin EL, Paul IL: Response of joints to impact loading. I. In vitro wear. Arthritis Rheum 14:356–62, 1971.

96. Radin EL: Osteoarthrosis. In: Wright V, Radin EL (ed): Mechanics of Human Joints. New York, Marcel Dekker, 1993.

97. Radin EL, Martin RB, Burr DB, et al: Effects of mechanical loading in the tissues of the rabbit knee. J Orthop Res 2:221–34, 1984.

98. Radin EL, Burr DB, Caterson B, et al: Mechanical determinants of osteoarthrosis. Semin Arthritis Rheum 21(3), Suppl 2:12–21, 1991.

99. Radin EL, Yang KH, Riegger C, et al: Relationship between lower limb dynamics and knee joint pain. J Orthop Res 9:398–405, 1991.

100. Ramos E, Fontera WR, Llopart A, Feliciano D: Muscle strength and hormonal levels in adolescents: gender related differences. Int J Sports Med 19:526–31, 1998.

101. Riegger-Krugh C. Bone. In: Malone TR, McPoil TG, Nitz AJ (eds): Orthopaedic and Sports Physical Therapy, 3rd edition. St Louis, CV Mosby, 1996, pp 3–46.

102. Riegger-Krugh C: Poor shock absorption may contribute to OA. Biomechanics 33–36, June 1999.

103. Riegger-Krugh C, Keysor JJ: Skeletal malalignments of the lower quarter: correlated and compensatory motions and postures. J Orthop Sports Phys Ther 23(2):164–70, 1996.

104. Rubin CJ: Sports injuries in the female. NJ Med 88:643–5, 1991.

105. Sanborn CF, Jankowski CM: Gender-specific physiology In: Agostini R (ed): Medical and Orthopedic Issues of Active and Athletic Women. St Louis, CV Mosby, 1994, p 23–27.

106. Sanborn CF, Janowski CM: Physiological considerations for women in sport. Clin Sports Med 13:315–27, 1994.

107. Schafle MD: The child dancer. In: Agostini R (ed): Medical and Orthopedic Issues of Active and Athletic Women. St Louis, CV Mosby, 1994, p 395.

108. Schantz P, Randall-Fox E, et al: Muscle fiber distribution, muscle cross-sectional area and maximal voluntary strength in humans. Acta Physiol Scand 117:219–26, 1983.

109. Seedhom B, Takeda T, Tsubuku T, Wright V: Mechanical factors and patellofemoral osteoarthritis. Ann Rheum Dis 38:307–16, 1979.

110. Selder DJ, Del Rolan N: Knowledge of performance, skill level and performance on the balance beam. Can J Appl Sport Sci 4:226–9, 1997.

111. Sinkjaer T, Toft E, Andreassen S, Hornemann BC: Muscle stiffness in human ankle dorsiflexors; intrinsic and reflex components. J Neurophysiol 60(3):1110–21, 1988.

112. Sovak D, Hawes MR: Anthropological status of international calibre speed skaters. J Sports Sci 5:287–304, 1987.

113. Stuhr R: Women's sports equipment: is it a marketing ploy? In: Agostini R (ed): Medical and Orthopedic Issues of Active and Athletic Women. St Louis, CV Mosby, 1994, p 134.

114. Sullivan K: Women's athletic shoes. In: Agostini R (ed): Medical and Orthopedic Issues of Active and Athletic Women. St Louis, CV Mosby, 1994, p 138.

115. Tanner JM: Growth at Adolescence, 2nd edition. Oxford, UK, Blackwell Scientific Publishers, 1962.

116. Teitz CC (ed): The Female Athlete. Seattle, Wash, American Academy of Orthopaedic Surgeons, University of Washington, 1997.

117. Tiberio D: Pathomechanics of structural foot deformities. Phys Ther 68(12):1840–9, 1988.

118. Ting AJ, Tarr RR, Sarmiento A, et al: The role of subtalar motion and ankle contact pressure changes from angular deformities of the tibia. Foot Ankle 7(5):290–9, 1987.

119. Tsunawake N, Tahara Y, Yukawa K, et al: Characteristics of body shape of female athletes based on factor analysis. Appl Human Sci 14:55–61, 1995.

120. Vaccar P, Clark DH, Wrenn JP: Physiological profiles of elite women basketball players. J Sports Med 19:45–54, 1979.

121. Voloshin A, Wosk J: Influence of artificial shock absorbers on human gait. Clin Orthop 160:52–6, 1981.

122. Walker JM: Pathomechanics and classification of cartilage lesions, facilitation of repair. J Orthop Sport Phys Ther 28(4):216–31, 1998.

123. Walshe AD, Wilson GJ: The influence of musculotendinous stiffness on drop jump performance. Can J Appl Physiol 22(2):117–32, 1997.

124. Wang H, Olney ST: Relationships between alignment, kinematic and kinetic measures of the knee of normal elderly subjects in level walking. Clin Biomech 9(4):245–52, 1994.

125. Watkins MP, Harris BA: Evaluation of skeletal muscle performance. In: Harms-Ringdahl K (ed): Muscle Strength. New York, Churchill Livingstone, 1993.

126. Wells CL (ed): Women, Sport, and Performance, A Physiological Perspective, 2nd edition. Champaign, Ill, Human Kinetics Publishers, 1991.

127. Wiggins DL, Wiggins ME: The female athlete. Clin Sports Med 16:593–611, 1997.

128. Wilk K: Dynamic muscle strength testing. In: Amundsen LA (ed): Muscle Strength Testing. New York, Churchill Livingstone, 1990.

129. Williams KR, Cavanagh PR, Ziff JL: Biomechanical studies of elite female distance runners. Int J Sports Med 8(Suppl 2);107–18, 1987.

130. Williams M, Stutzman L: Strength variation through the range of joint motion. Phys Ther Rev 39(3):145–52, 1959.

131. Wilson GJ, Murphy AJ, Pryor JF: Musculotendinous stiffness: its relationship to eccentric, isometric, and concentric performance. J Appl Physiol 76(6):2714–9, 1994.

132. Woo SL-Y, Kuei SC, Amiel D, et al: The effect of physical training on the properties of long bone: A study of Wolff's law. J Bone Joint Surg 63A:780–6, 1981.

133. Yeager KK, Macera C. Women, activity, and health profiles and healthy people 2000. In: Agostini R (ed): Medical and Orthopedic Issues of Active and Athletic Women. St Louis, CV Mosby, 1994, p 29.

134. Zernicke RF, McNitt-Gray J, Otis C, et al: Stress fracture risk assessment among elite collegiate women runners (abstract). Presentation at the International Society of Biomechanics, 1993.

Chapter 33

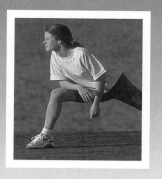

Soft-Tissue Injuries

W. Ben Kibler, M.D.

Soft-tissue injuries, such as tendinitis and acute chronic muscle strains, are very common among female athletes; however, there are very few reports of an increased or decreased incidence of any particular type of injury in female athletes compared to males. This chapter will summarize the known pathophysiology of this class of injuries, and then use this knowledge as a basis for evaluation and prevention of the injuries. Special concerns for the female athlete will be highlighted.

PATHOPHYSIOLOGY

Soft-tissue injuries occur by 2 mechanisms: acute macrotrauma and chronic microtrauma. Each mechanism has unique characteristics that should be identified during evaluation and treatment.

Acute macrotrauma occurs as an *event*. The tissues are normal, and then are instantly abnormal and symptomatic as a result of the physical disruption of the tissues. This event may be a direct-blow injury, such as a muscle contusion. More commonly, the event is an acute tensile overload, such as in an acute hamstring tear. This type of event is an absolute overload, in that the normal tissues are overloaded by a supranormal load (Table 33-1).

Eighty-five to ninety percent of all soft-tissue injuries, however, are due to chronic microtrauma.[10] Chronic microtrauma injuries occur as a result of a *process* that occurs over time. This mechanism results from a failure of homeostasis of the cellular activities and tissue constituents to maintain tissue integrity in the face of continued athletic demand.[23]

Failure of cellular activities can be seen in alteration of the size and shape of mitochondria with a decrease in mitochondrial enzyme levels,[13] alterations in calcium release and uptake,[1] and alterations in fiber formation, kinking, and cross links.[13] The net result of this degenerative process is the loss of normal cell matrix and resultant scar tissue formation as normal reparative mechanisms fail. The abnormal matrix shows fatty vacuoles, hydroxyapatite clefts ("tombstones" of cell injury), and disorganization of fibrils.[22] This abnormal cell matrix fails under load, giving rise to clinical symptoms. Pathologic specimens from many types of soft-tissue injuries, including epicondylitis, plantar fasciitis, patellar tendinitis, and Achilles tendinitis, are similar and show the end result of this degenerative process.[14,22] These specimens show many blood vessels, unorganized fibrotic tissue, and few inflammatory cells. This unorganized tissue cannot respond to normal biologic signals for repair and recovery, collagen orientation, or maturation.[22]

It appears that initiation of these degenerative changes is multifactorial. Tissue aging, humoral factors, and vascular factors ("heart attack" of the tendon) have been proposed as causative factors.[14,22,24,27] It also appears that these may be the cumulative result of mechanical strain on the cells of multiple tensile loads, either by tissue strength or eccentric contraction.[7,25,29,30]

These cellular changes have major effects on tissue function. Alterations in function include inflexibility caused by scar formation, muscle weakness, imbalance of strength between pairs of a force couple, and the inability to absorb loads resulting from weakness of eccentric muscle contraction.[10,14,22] Since this process is gradual, the body can usually adapt to maintain athletic activity by recruiting other muscles from the same

Table 33-1. Comparison of Macrotrauma and Microtrauma Mechanisms

MACROTRAUMA	MICROTRAUMA
Event (normal → abnormal)	Process (normal → adaptation → abnormal)
Crush injury	
Absolute overload (normal tissues, supranormal load)	Relative overload (abnormal tissues, normal load)

area, by using different mechanics, or by decreasing the performance level. These alterations are often present without producing symptoms, but do impose biomechanical and physiological inefficiencies on the athlete, and have been implicated as risk factors in producing injuries in various anatomic areas, including the shoulder,[28] plantar fascia,[19] and lower extremity.[21]

These alterations can be measured objectively as decreases in joint range of motion, muscle flexibility, strength production, or work output. They are present in a large majority of symptomatic athletes with soft-tissue injury. However, they are rarely implicated in a one-to-one cause and effect relationship with specific diagnosis. They act as some of the "intrinsic risk factors" that the athlete brings to the sport (Table 33-2). These may create a predisposition to injury.[26] The predisposed athlete may then interact with "extrinsic" risk factors, such as sport-specific demands, training schedule, or equipment (Table 33-2) in such a way that the tissues become overloaded to the point of clinical symptoms or performance decrement.[16,26] This type of injury may be characterized as a relative overload (Table 33-1), with basically normal loads acting upon abnormal tissues.

In summary, soft-tissue injuries occur as a result of direct trauma, macrotrauma with absolute overload, or chronic microtrauma with relative overload. Chronic microtrauma, with degenerative cellular effects that lead to objective tissue alteration, is the most common mechanism. There is no literature or clinical evidence to support the idea that gender affects the tissue alterations. It appears that males and females have the same cellular and tissue responses to macrotrauma and microtrauma. Females are generally more flexible than males, but appear to respond to chronic tensile load in the same manner and develop inflexibilities in the same fashion as males.[18,19] When an athlete presents with an acute or chronic soft-tissue injury, evaluation should be inclusive, to identify all extrinsic and intrinsic risk factors that may be present, as well as to identify the clinical symptoms.[16,26] It is important to recognize that these injuries are the result of a process and that adaptations are usually present.

SOFT-TISSUE INJURIES IN WOMEN

There are very few studies that break out gender-specific rates of soft-tissue injuries. In a series of U.S. Tennis Association Studies,[15] no statistical difference was found between competitive males and females. Overload injuries predominated, the most common sites being the back, shoulder, and knee, in that order. This corroborates earlier studies that showed no increase in injury rate in conditioned women athletes compared to males.[14] However, the level of conditioning does play a role in the injury rate, and unconditioned women do have a higher injury rate when exposed to athletic activity.[15] It appears that soft-tissue injuries are more sport specific than gender specific in most instances. Exceptions are seen in the knee, where the incidence of "anterior knee pain" is higher in females, and in the shoulder, where injury rates are higher for female swimmers than male swimmers. The exact reasons are not known, but the larger amount of joint flexibility and the relative weakness in strength seen in women are thought to be causative factors.[12]

EVALUATION

Any system of evaluation of soft-tissue injuries should take into account the broad scope of causative and contributing factors that may exist in addition to the clinical symptoms. These include any gender-based differences, such as joint flexibility, any intrinsic risk factors, and any biomechanical deficits that may be present. Our evaluation is based on a framework in which most of the factors are categorized into 5 main areas, called complexes.[16] These complexes interact with each other in the causation of microtrauma injuries, can be present as a result of macrotrauma injuries, and are detectable on a clinical level. These complexes are as follows:

1. *Tissue injury complex*: the group of anatomic structures that have overt pathologic change.
2. *Clinical symptom complex*: the group of overt symptoms and signs that clinically characterize the injury.
3. *Tissue overload complex*: the group of structures that have nonsymptomatic, but clinically detectable changes.

Table 33-2. Intrinsic and Extrinsic Risk Factors in Causation of Tissue Injury

INTRINSIC	EXTRINSIC
Age	Inherent demands of the sport
Inflexibility	Biomechanical demands
Strength weakness	Equipment
Muscle imbalance	Surfaces
Previous injury	Schedule of training or events

4. *Functional biomechanical deficit complex*: alterations in biomechanics due to injury or overload.
5. *Subclinical adaptations*: substitute actions that the athlete uses to compensate for altered mechanics to maintain performance.

These complexes interact in a negative-feedback vicious cycle (Fig. 33-1) to cause or maintain a soft-tissue injury. In microtrauma cases, an athlete may "cycle" as a "susceptible" athlete for some time before overt clinical symptoms appear. Most acute injuries will exhibit fewer overloads and biomechanical deficits, but some may result from treatment, such as immobilization after Achilles tendon surgery. In this model, clinical symptoms are a relatively small part of the entire pathophysiologic picture. They obviously need to be treated, but emphasis should be placed on restoration of function, including all of the alterations, rather than only resolution of symptoms.

DIAGNOSIS USING VICIOUS CYCLE COMPLEXES

The following examples illustrate the use of the vicious cycle complexes to evaluate various soft-tissue injuries. These findings are present in most cases.

Rotator Cuff Tendinitis

- *Tissue Overload*: Posterior capsule, shoulder external rotator muscles, scapular stabilizers.

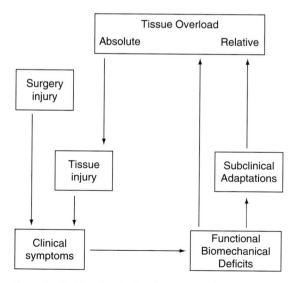

Figure 33-1. Negative-feedback vicious cycle.

- *Tissue Injury*: Rotator cuff impingement or tensile stretch, glenoid labrum, anterior capsule.
- *Clinical Symptoms*: Pain over anterior lateral acromion, impingement on abduction and rotation, glenohumeral subluxation, positive "clunk test" or anterior slide test.
- *Functional Biomechanical Deficit*: Functional lateral scapular slide consisting of inflexibility in internal rotation; muscle-strength deficits in shoulder external rotators and scapular stabilizers; and in later cases, superior or anterior glenohumeral translation.
- *Subclinical Adaptations*: Short-arming the throw; alteration of arm position during throwing or lifting; muscle recruitment from anterior shoulder, forearm, or trunk.

Lateral Epicondylitis

- *Tissue Overload*: Lateral muscle mass, mainly extensor carpi radialis brevis, wrist supinators and extensors, shoulder external rotators.
- *Tissue Injury*: Same as for tissue overload, plus annular ligament and joint capsule.
- *Clinical Symptoms*: Point tenderness over extensor muscle mass, with or without swelling, pain upon hitting backhand, usually in recreational athlete.
- *Functional Biomechanical Deficit*: Extensor inflexibility and muscle weakness, decreased range of motion in pronators and supinators, decreased shoulder external rotation strength.
- *Subclinical Adaptations*: Hitting behind the body, hitting with wrist movement, recruitment of triceps or alteration of position of elbow.

Medial Epicondylitis

- *Tissue Overload*: Forearm flexor mass, biceps, pronator teres, usually absolute overload.
- *Tissue Injury*: Same as for tissue overload, plus medial collateral ligament, ulnar nerve, and/or posterior medial olecranon.
- *Clinical Symptoms*: Point tenderness over flexor muscle mass, medial collateral ligament, posterior medial elbow, with or without ulnar nerve symptoms; usually in competitive athlete.
- *Functional Biomechanical Deficit*: Functional pronation, consisting of elbow

flexion and pronation inflexibility, and tight and weak flexors.

- **Subclinical Adaptations**: Hitting behind the body, more overhead throwing motion, more wrist snap, more use of shoulder in throwing motion.

Mechanical Low Back Pain in the Athlete

- **Tissue Overload**: Hamstring muscles, quadratus lumborum and erector spinae muscles, hip external rotators, obliques.
- **Tissue Injury**: Facet joints, lumbosacral joints, quadratus, obliques.
- **Clinical Symptoms**: Nonradiating back pain upon extension or rotation of low back, stiffness.
- **Functional Biomechanical Deficit**: Abnormal pelvic tilt and hip rotation secondary to tight hamstrings, hip rotators, and quadratus and weak erector spinae and hamstrings.
- **Subclinical Adaptations**: Lack of trunk rotation in throwing, using more arm motion, decreased bending from the waist in defensive position or for low shots.

"Anterior Knee Pain"

- **Tissue Overload**: Patellar retinaculum, quadriceps, iliotibial band.
- **Tissue Injury**: Patellar retinaculum, retropatellar articular cartilage.
- **Clinical Symptoms**: Diffuse pain, patellofemoral crepitus, pain upon sitting or upon getting up.
- **Functional Biomechanical Deficits**: Quadriceps and iliotibial band inflexibility, quadriceps/hamstring force couple imbalance, patella infera.
- **Subclinical Adaptations**: Less knee flexion, jumping or climbing off opposite leg.

Patellar Tendinitis

- **Tissue Overload**: Quadriceps, iliotibial band, patellar tendon.
- **Tissue Injury**: Point tenderness, infrapatellar pain, no joint internal derangement.
- **Clinical Symptoms:** Point tenderness, infrapatellar pain, no joint internal derangement.
- **Functional Biomechanical Deficit**: Quadriceps and iliotibial band inflexibility, hamstring muscle weakness.
- **Subclinical Adaptations**: No terminal knee extension, jumping off opposite leg.

Deep Thigh Muscle Contusion

- **Tissue Overload**: None.
- **Tissue Injury**: Vastus lateralis, with mechanical disruption.
- **Clinical Symptoms**: Localized pain, swelling, and bruising, athletic dysfunction.
- **Functional Biomechanical Deficit**: Muscle imbalance due to muscle weakness.
- **Subclinical Adaptations**: Limp.

Anterior Tibial Shin Splints

- **Tissue Overload**: Anterior compartment muscles at tendon–bone junction, sometimes posterior tibial muscle.
- **Tissue Injury**: Anterior muscle at tendon–bone junction.
- **Clinical Symptoms**: Localized tenderness and swelling, increased compartment pressure.
- **Functional Biomechanical Deficits**: Anterior muscle weakness and inflexibility, posterior muscle weakness.
- **Subclinical Adaptations**: More inversion upon running, shortened stride length and stance time.

Achilles Tendinitis

- **Tissue Overload**: Achilles tendon, plantar flexor muscles.
- **Tissue Injury**: Achilles tendon, paratenon.
- **Clinical Symptoms:** Point tenderness to palpation over tendon, especially with dorsiflexion.
- **Functional Biomechanical Deficits**: Plantar flexor inflexibility, inability of gastrocnemius/soleus complex to absorb loads.
- **Subclinical Adaptations**: Staying on toes, landing on opposite leg, shortened stance phase.

Plantar Fasciitis

- **Tissue Overload**: Plantar flexor muscles, plantar fascial insertion at heel, foot intrinsic muscles.
- **Tissue Injury**: Same, plantar fascial attachment at heel.
- **Clinical Symptoms**: Point tenderness at base of calcaneus, worse at first run or after running.

- *Functional Biomechanical Deficits*: Plantar flexor inflexibility and weakness, creating functional pronation.
- *Subclinical Adaptations*: Running on toes, shortened stride length, foot inversion.

REHABILITATION

Rehabilitation protocols and procedures will be discussed elsewhere in this book. Several principles should guide the process of rehabilitation. Rehabilitation should be an orderly process based on healing of tissue and restoration of functional capability. However, this process should be based on a complete and accurate diagnosis of the entire pathophysiologic process, and definite criteria for proceeding through the phases of rehabilitation should be understood. We use a 3-phase rehabilitation program[16,20] that comprises acute, recovery, and functional phases.

The *acute phase* is concerned with anatomic tissue healing. The focus is on resolving the clinical symptoms and tissue-injury complexes. It is the broadest phase because of the many presentations of soft-tissue injuries.

The *recovery phase* is concerned with restoration of functional capability. It deals with normalizing the tissue overloads and the functional biomechanical deficits. Because these deficits are subtle and of a long-standing nature, this phase is usually the longest. Appropriate loading of the tissue within safe ranges and tolerances will provide the proper stimulus for healing on both the tissue and cellular levels.

The *functional phase* is concerned with normalization of functional ability. Resolution of biomechanical deficits and elimination of subclinical adaptations are central to this phase. Sport- or activity-specific progressions should be employed to prepare the tissues biomechanically and physiologically for the sport or activity demands. Most athletes develop soft-tissue injuries as a result of failure to meet demand, so completion of this phase is important before return to play is allowed.

Return to play can be allowed when clinical symptoms are resolved, the vicious cycle complexes are normalized, and the athlete has completed activity- or sport-specific progressions.

PREVENTION

Soft-tissue injuries usually are fairly minor injuries, but they are often slow to resolve and frustrating to rehabilitate. In this setting, pre-vention would be preferable to treatment. Little can be done to prevent direct-blow macro-trauma, other than use of judicious padding and enforcement of rules. However, since chronic microtrauma injuries represent a process that has identifiable risk factors, preventative efforts may have some efficacy.[22,26]

Close attention should be paid to assessing athletes for inflexibilities, muscle-strength imbalances, and postural abnormalities that may exist. A convenient format for this is the preseason physical examination.[18] Several specific postural areas should be checked in female athletes. Identification of generalized joint laxity by checking elbow hyperextension, knee hyperextension, patellar mobility, thumb to forearm, and pes planus should be done. Spine posture should be evaluated to rule out scoliosis or kyphosis. Patellar tracking and malalignment can be checked. Genu valgum can be evaluated by measurement of the "Q-angle" between the quadriceps and patellar tendon. Hip posture is a key to lower-leg function and must be assessed carefully. Specific tests for hip strength include step up/step down, one-legged stance, one-legged half squat, and one-legged hopping.[11] Identification of the postural abnormalities can suggest treatment, rehabilitation, or bracing to modify the risk factors.

Despite being more flexible in general than males, females respond to chronic tensile load by developing the same type and magnitude of inflexibilities.[18,24] These are most common in the posterior shoulder, low back and hamstrings, and gastrocnemius. Females should be evaluated for these inflexibilities just as closely as males.

Female athletes have less muscle mass per body weight[8] and produce less strength[23] than males. We have also found that a much higher percentage of females (78%) than males (23%) do not achieve normative hamstring/quadriceps ratios on isokinetic testing (Lexington Clinic Sports Medicine Center, unpublished data). Since strength, and especially strength balance, is important in the genesis of soft-tissue injuries, this area should have high priority for evaluation and correction of deficits. These deficits can be largely corrected by proper strengthening, as females can respond in the same manner, but at a lower magnitude, to a strength-training stimulus as males.[27]

Prevention of soft-tissue injuries is largely a matter of matching the athlete's musculoskeletal base to the demands of the sport or activity. This process is termed *prehabilitation*. It starts with the evaluation as described, and then involves a periodized conditioning program[17] to prepare musculoskeletal flexibility, strength, and endurance for the athletic season. This program matches volume of conditioning and type of conditioning exercises to the season (preseason, in-season, off-season) of the particular sport to keep the body from being overloaded during conditioning or play. Although prevention has not been studied extensively in female athletes, this approach has shown success in athletes in several sports and activities.[6,9,17]

CONCLUDING REMARKS

Soft-tissue injuries are quite common in female athletes. These injuries largely occur as a failure of homeostasis or body repair in the face of a chronic tensile overload. This process of injury is often associated with alterations in tissues other than those responsible for the clinical symptoms. These alterations may cause or exacerbate the clinical symptoms, or prolong rehabilitation efforts. In the female athlete, special attention should be placed on evaluation, correction, or bracing of postural deficits, joint hyperlaxity, muscle inflexibility, and muscle weakness and imbalance, as these are the most common risk factors in these types of injuries.

References

1. Armstrong RB: Initial events in exercise induced muscle injury. Med Sci Sports Exerc 22:429–35, 1990.
2. Chandler TJ, Kibler WB: Muscle training in injury prevention. In Renstrom P (ed): Sports Injuries—Basic Principles of Prevention and Care. London, Blackwell, 1993, pp 252–61.
3. Chandler TJ, Kibler WB, Kiser AM, et al: Shoulder strength, power, and endurance in college tennis players. Am J Sports Med 20(4):455–7, 1992.
4. Chandler TJ, Kibler WB, Uhl TL, et al: Flexibility comparisons of junior elite tennis players to other athletes. Am J Sports Med 18:134–6, 1990.
5. Clark KS, Buckley WE: Women's injuries in collegiate sports. Am J Sports Med 8:187–91, 1980.
6. Ekstrand J, Gillquist J: The avoidability of soccer injuries. Int J Sports Med 4:124–8, 1983.
7. Garrett WE, Tidball JG: Myotendinous junction: Structure, function, and failure. In Woo, SL-Y, Buckwalter JS, et al (eds): Injury and Repair of Musculoskeletal Soft Tissues. Park Ridge, Ill, American Academy of Orthopaedic Surgeons, 1988, pp 171–205.
8. Griffin LY: The female athlete. In Renstrom P (ed): Sports Injuries—Basic Principles of Prevention and Care. London, Blackwell, 1993, pp 194–202.
9. Heiser TM, Weber T, Sullivan G, et al: Prophylaxis and management of hamstring muscle injuries in intercollegiate football. Am J Sports Med 12:368–70, 1984.
10. Herring SA, Nilson KL: Introduction to overuse injuries. Clin Sports Med 6(2):225–39, 1987.
11. Host JV, Craig R, Lehman RC: Patellofemoral dysfunction in tennis players—a dynamic problem. Clin Sports Med 14:177–205, 1995.
12. Hunter LY: Women's athletics: The orthopedic viewpoint. Clin Sports Med 3(4):809–27, 1984.
13. Kannus P, Jozsa L: Histopathologic changes preceding spontaneous rupture of a tendon. J Bone Joint Surg 73A:1715–25, 1991.
14. Kibler WB: Pathophysiology of overload injuries around the elbow. Clin Sports Med 14(2):447–57, 1995.
15. Kibler WB, Chandler TJ: Racquet sports. In Fu F, Stone R (eds): Sports Injuries: Mechanisms, Prevention, and Treatment. Baltimore, Williams & Wilkins, 1994, pp 531–50.
16. Kibler WB, Chandler TJ, Pace BK: Principles of rehabilitation after chronic tendon injuries. Clin Sports Med 11(3):666–71, 1992.
17. Kibler WB, Chandler TJ, Reuter BH: Advances in Conditioning. Orthopedic Knowledge Update—Sports Medicine. Rosemont, Ill, American Academy of Orthopaedic Surgeons, 1994, pp 65–73.
18. Kibler WB, Chandler TJ, Uhl TL, et al: A musculoskeletal approach to the preparticipation physical examination. Preventing injury and improving performance. Am J Sports Med 17:525, 531, 1989.
19. Kibler WB, Goldberg C, Chandler TJ: Functional biomechanical deficits in running athletes with plantar fasciitis. Am J Sports Med 19:66–71, 1991.
20. Kibler WB, Herring SA, Press JM: Functional Rehabilitation of Sports and Musculoskeletal Injuries. Gaithersburg, Md, Aspen, 1998.
21. Knapik JJ, Bauman CL, Jones BA, et al: Preseason strength and flexibility imbalances associated with athletic injuries in female collegiate athletes. Am J Sports Med 19:76–81, 1991.
22. Leadbetter WB: Cell matrix response in tendon injury. Clin Sports Med 11:533–79, 1992.
23. Leadbetter WB. Physiology of tissue repair. In Athletic Training and Sports Medicine, Park Ridge, Ill, American Academy of Orthopaedic Surgeons, 1991, pp 45–55.
24. Leadbetter WB, Mooar PA, Lane GJ, et al: The surgical treatment of tendinitis. Clin Sports Med 11:679–711, 1992.
25. Lieber RL, Friden J: Muscle damage is not a function of muscle force but active muscle strain. J Appl Physiol 74:520–6, 1993.
26. Meeuwisse WH: Assessing causation in sport injury: a multifactorial model. Clin J. Sports Med 4:166–70, 1994.
27. Nirschl RP: Elbow tendinitis/tennis elbow. Clin Sports Med 11:851–69, 1992.
28. Silliman JF, Hawkins RJ: Current concepts and recent advances in the athlete's shoulder. Clin Sports Med 4:693–706, 1991.
29. Teague BN, Schwane JA: Effect of intermittent eccentric contraction on symptoms of muscle microinjury. Med Sci Sports Exerc 27:1378–84, 1995.
30. Warren GL, Hayes DA, Lowe DA, et al: Materials fatigue initiates eccentric contraction-induced injury in rat soleus muscle. J. Physiol (Lond) 464:477–89, 1993.

Chapter 34

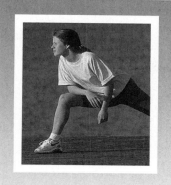

Thoracic and Lumbar Injuries

Peter G. Gerbino, II, M.D.
Lyle J. Micheli, M.D.

Back injury and back pain are extremely common, and athletes are particularly at risk. Understanding the risk factors inherent in athletic activities is the key to successful management.

Risk factors arise from the host (eg, from a pre-existing medical condition) or the environment (eg, from a training error) (Table 34-1). Most risk factors may be present in both female and male athletes. The relative weight given to a risk factor varies according to the athlete's age, the level of intensity, the location of back injury, and the chronicity of symptoms, as well as gender. Female-specific risk factors are only now being actively studied. The two most important risk factors in the etiology of the female athlete's back pain is a prior history of back injury and the sport in which she is engaged. Sports in which repetitive lumbar hyperextension is common (eg, gymnastics,[22,25] figure skating,[43] ballet[44]) produce the greatest number of back problems in women. Whether women have a greater or lesser number of back injuries than men is open to debate.[23,82] As a group, women do not seem to have more back pain than men, but 1 study has found that 1 year after reporting low back pain symptoms, women were 1.5 times more likely to have a poor outcome than men.[77]

ANATOMY

Sources of pain in the lumbar spine include the vertebral bones, intervertebral discs, spinal nerves, facet joints, sacroiliac joints, paraspinal muscles, and tendons and ligaments; in addition, pain may be referred from the viscera or be psychogenic. Figure 34-1 depicts a spinal motion segment and the associated structures most often associated with pain. The close proximity of the various pain sources can make definitive diagnosis difficult, but a carefully obtained history and physical examination can lead to the source of injury.

Table 34-1. Risk Factors for Overuse Injury

HOST	ENVIRONMENTAL
Growth process	Training or technique error
Anatomic malalignment	Improper equipment
Muscle–tendon imbalance	Playing surface
Associated disease state	Nutrition
Psychological factors	Cultural deconditioning
Gender	Drugs

ACUTE TRAUMATIC SOURCES OF THORACIC AND LUMBAR BACK PAIN

The female spine subjected to trauma sustains the same injuries as the male spine. For athletes of a given size, there is no evidence that the female spine is at greater risk for traumatic injury than the male spine. The spectrum of spinal trauma ranges from minimal contusions to catastrophic fractures.

Contusions, Strains, and Sprains

Contusions and tears of the muscles, tendons, and ligaments of the back are common. Most athletes will effectively self-diagnose and treat. The etiology of a ligament *sprain* is a stretch beyond the elastic limit of that ligament. Muscle and tendon *strains* occur as a result of excessive stretching or overexertion during a concentric or eccentric contraction.

The greatest risk factor for strain or sprain is inadequate warming up and stretching. The viscoelastic properties of tendon, ligament, and muscle are greatly improved with warming,[64] and the neurophysiologically governed length and coordination of muscle is enhanced by both warming up and gently stretching.[69] Women with tight thoracolumbar soft tissues from constitutional factors, following injury, or during the adolescent growth spurt are at increased risk.[39]

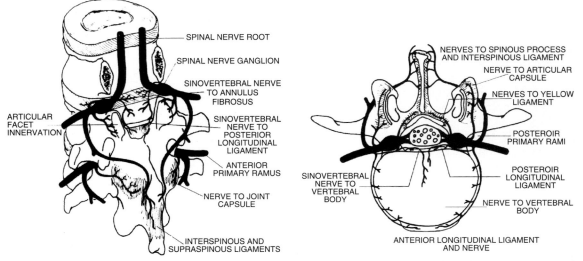

Figure 34-1. A spinal motion segment comprises two adjacent vertebrae, the intervertebral disc, facet joints, and interconnecting tendons and ligaments. Sensory nerve endings are present at every structure. (From White AA, Panjabi MM: Clinical Biomechanics of the Spine, 2nd edition. Philadelphia, JB Lippincott, 1990, pp 1–19, with permission.)

The history frequently will uncover the causative event, but since muscular hypertonicity and pain is common with most types of back injury, this physical finding alone is not diagnostic. The physical examination is more useful in *excluding* other possible injuries, such as a herniated disc or fracture, than confirming strain or sprain. Likewise, diagnostic imaging is better at detecting other causes than confirming soft tissue tear.

Treatment of strains and sprains of the back is similar to that of contusion, with 48 to 72 hours of icing, relative rest, and early mobilization and stretching to minimize scarring. Achieving relative rest is difficult in the spine, so a soft corset may be employed to decrease demands on the injured tissues. Stretching and strengthening must be maintained to prevent atrophy and maintain length. Evidence exists that spinal manipulation can have a beneficial effect in some patients.[20] Prevention requires low back and abdominal strengthening, adequate warming up, stretching of the hamstrings and dorsal back, and avoidance of sudden, strenuous maneuvers.

Acute Disc Herniation

Herniation of the nucleus pulposus (HNP) is common. It is estimated that 2% of the general population will have a clinically significant HNP at some time.[21]

Etiology

Intradisc pressures are greatest during sitting.[49] A disc under pressure will herniate when the annulus tears. These tears are most common just lateral to the midline posteriorly in the area where the posterior longitudinal ligament is weakest.[46] The mean age for HNP is 35,[31] but herniation can occur in childhood and late adulthood as well. Simultaneous spinal extension and rotation after sitting is thought to be particularly risky.[81]

Risk Factors

There are no reported gender differences in the etiology or incidence of HNP. A recent study of male and female athletes looked at the epidemiology of HNP. Neither gender nor amount of weight lifting was related to the incidence of HNP. Of several sports studied, only *bowling* had a positive correlation to the occurrence of HNP.[47]

History

An inciting event may or may not be recalled. Only 35% of patients with HNP develop sciatica,[46] but most will have low back pain. Pain is typically worse with sitting or activities such as coughing, sneezing, or straining. Inability to urinate and perineal sensory changes suggest a cauda equina syndrome[63] and warrant emergent evaluation and treatment.

Physical Examination

In acute HNP, the patient may be unable to move without severe pain. The athlete with acute HNP will more commonly have restricted lumbar flexibility with varying amounts of back and leg pain. Once cauda equina syndrome is ruled out, a detailed motor, sensory, and reflex evaluation is performed on the lower extremities. Single-leg toe raises to the point of fatigue may be necessary to demonstrate subtle S_1 weakness on the affected side. Neurotension tests are done with the patient supine (sciatic nerve) and prone (femoral nerve) and bilaterally. Pain or paresthesias radiating past the knee with supine straight-leg raising indicates sciatic irritation. Hamstring or back pain with straight-leg raising does not necessarily indicate disc-related neuropathy. Any evidence of neuritis warrants a further search for herniated disc at the involved level.

Imaging

Plain radiographs of an athlete with HNP will usually be negative. In an older athlete, disc-space narrowing or early degenerative changes may be seen. Computed tomography (CT) or magnetic resonance imaging (MRI) of the lumbosacral spine will demonstrate the herniation. Studies such as CT-myelography, discography, electromyography, and sensory evoked potentials are reserved for special circumstances and have no place in the initial evaluation of an athlete with back pain.

Treatment

Bed rest is no longer used to treat acute HNP.[21] A day or 2 of bedrest may be required for patient comfort, but bed rest does not expedite healing and, in fact, frequently leads to increased back and hamstring tightness. As long as there are no cauda equina symptoms or no progressive neuropathy, the athlete is encouraged to perform as much as she can within the limits of pain. Activities such as prolonged sitting, jumping, spine hyperflexion or extension, and straining as in weight lifting are contraindicated.

A large body of research shows that up to 90% of all adult cases of HNP will resolve within 12 weeks without surgery.[12,16] We strongly believe that in the young athlete, even fewer will require operative excision, but there are published data indicating high operative rates for children.[17]

Therapeutic nonoperative interventions with a proven benefit include relative rest, nonsteroidal anti-inflammatory drugs (NSAIDs), aerobic exercise, lumbar and hamstring flexibility training, avoiding stressful postures (sitting, lordosis) and utilizing the semi-Fowler position to relieve disc stresses. Utilizing the Boston overlap brace in 15° lordosis to decrease terminal flexion and extension has proved extremely successful for relieving symptoms and avoiding surgery in our young patients. Studies at our institution are ongoing to document this effect and demonstrate how bracing restricts motion. Lumbar epidural steroid therapy can provide dramatic relief and resolution of symptoms in a subset of patients with acute HNP.[18] Unfortunately, this subset has not been well defined and some patients with acute HNP receive no benefit from lumbar epidural steroid therapy. Muscle relaxants have a limited role in the acute setting, but are usually of little long-term value.

Treatment mainstays remain relative rest, NSAIDs, and maintenance of flexibility. If this regimen has failed after 6 weeks, referral to a spine surgeon is made for consideration of lumbar epidural steroid therapy and, if the injections fail, discectomy.

Acute Apophyseal Avulsion

In the immature athlete, physeal and apophyseal cartilage is present at the vertebral end plates and in other locations about the spine. Macrotrauma in this age group can result in apophyseal avulsion, and microtrauma can lead to apophysitis.

Etiology

The two most common traumatic apophyseal injuries about the spine are lumbar vertebral end-plate avulsions and posterior iliac crest apophyseal avulsions.[61] The pathomechanics of both are thought to be either a sudden large traction force or a relatively minor traction force following fatigue fracture (apophysitis) of the growth cartilage in an athlete with growth-related tightness.

Spine extension can cause anterior vertebral end-plate apophyseal avulsion and spine flexion can avulse a portion of the posterior end plate. Ikata and coworkers have published a review of MR analyses of these injuries. They found that these were true osteochondroses with a risk of nonunion and, in the case of posterior avulsions, canal compromise. Their work showed that only two thirds of end-plate fragments had interposed herniated disc material (limbus-vertebra). The remaining third did not have interposed disc demonstrating that a subset of these lesions are primary apophyseal/epiphyseal fractures.[28] Posterior end-plate injuries usually occur in conjunction with other spinal trauma and can result in canal stenosis.[15,61,79]

History

Traumatic avulsions present as severe strain-type injuries with focal pain. *Overuse* anterior end-plate apophyseal avulsion presents with non-specific aching low back pain. There may be some buttock pain, but not sciatica. A history of trauma or a known onset of symptoms is uncommon. Traumatic posterior end-plate fractures that result in spinal canal compromise will have associated neurologic complaints.

Physical Examination

Discrete point tenderness is unusual in vertebral avulsions, but common with iliac crest avulsions. There is increased paraspinal muscle tone with both. Anterior vertebral end-plate injuries are exacerbated by extension. Physical findings of posterior fractures with associated canal compromise can mimic those of HNP or spinal stenosis.[79]

Imaging

Plain radiographs will show what has been called a "limbus" vertebra.[79] MRI is the only way to know whether there is herniated disc material within the fracture,[28] but the usefulness of such knowledge is unknown. For posterior end-plate fractures, knowing whether there is canal compromise by the disc is important and MRI is indicated. CT is the test of choice to study the relationship of multiple fracture fragments.

Treatment

Relative immobilization is the most appropriate treatment for overuse apophyseal avulsion. If the painless state can be achieved by decreased activity or using a soft lumbar support, bracing is not necessary. More often, a rigid lumbosacral orthosis such as the Boston overlap brace[42] is necessary. The advantage to bracing is that the sport frequently can be continued without pain in the brace. In the case of posterior end-plate injuries associated with trauma, treatment of the associated fractures or herniated disc takes precedence.

Fractures

Etiology

Acute spine fracture in sports is uncommon. Athletes fracture their spines as a result of severe trauma. Excessive force in flexion, extension, axial compression, horizontal shear, or any combination of these motions can lead to failure of the spinal elements. Bony failure (fracture) is most common, but purely ligamentous and/or disc failure can occur.

Risk Factors

Collision with a restraining device, an immovable object, or another athlete provides the forces required to fracture the spine. Equestrians who are thrown or trampled may fracture the spine.[34] Falls from a trampoline,[65] while skiing[48] and while tobogganing[55] are associated with thoracolumbar fractures as well as with cervical spine injury. Women are not known to be at greater risk for these injuries than men.

History

Trauma severe enough to cause spine fracture is frequently a witnessed event where the mechanism is obvious. It is important to perform a full trauma assessment in these individuals. If they are alert and communicative, it is necessary to ask questions pertaining to mental and neurologic status.

Physical Examination

Strict spinal precautions must be employed without moving the athlete. In all cases, the Advanced Trauma Life Support (ATLS) protocol is strictly followed.[14] *A*irway, *b*reathing, *c*irculation, and neurologic *d*isability (ABCD) are assessed. The athlete can be logrolled onto a spine board where the assessment can be continued.[56]

Treatment

If an on-field diagnosis of spinal fracture with neurologic deficit is made, intravenous methylprednisolone (30 mg/kg bolus, 5.4 mg/kg/hr maintenance) should be started within 8 hours and continued for 24 hours. This regimen has been shown to mitigate neurologic damage.[10] Assessment and stabilization on a spine board with or without steroid administration is immediate care. The athlete is then transported by ambulance to a trauma center for definitive management.

Other Traumatic Injuries

There are many other acute injuries that can occur around the thoracolumbar spine and present as back pain. Trauma to the abdominal or pelvic organs can present as back pain. The liver, spleen, and abdomen should be carefully palpated. Pelvic tenderness or vaginal bleeding warrants immediate transfer to a facility where a complete pelvic examination can be performed.

Costovertebral fractures, subluxations, and dislocations present as thoracic back pain.[54] An acutely subluxated rib can sometimes be manually reduced[72] resulting in dramatic pain relief. Other times, gentle massage, pain-relieving medicines, and occasional steroid injections may be required for several weeks.[40]

OVERUSE INJURIES TO THE THORACIC AND LUMBAR SPINE

Spondylolysis

Spondylolysis encompasses a progression of events from "prespondylolytic stress reaction" of the pars interarticularis to "lysis" and sometimes on to displacement (spondylolisthesis). In athletes, understanding this process is essential to making the diagnosis and effectively managing the condition.

Etiology

Spondylolysis in the athlete must be differentiated from that occurring in the nonathlete. All spondylolysis occurs as a result of mechanical forces on the posterior elements of the lumbosacral spine. In a classic study, Rosenberg and coworkers demonstrated that pars interarticularis fracture did not exist in nonambulators.[56] Several studies have conclusively shown that repetitive hyperextension of the lumbar spine leads to fatigue and ultimately fracture of the pars interarticularis.[29,33,74,78] The difference between athletes and nonathletes is that the nonathletes are predisposed to develop these fractures with minimal stresses and the athletes require higher and more repetitive forces. The pain associated with athletes' spondylolysis is more severe than that found in the nonathletes, who are frequently asymptomatic.

Risk Factors

Two absolute risk factors for developing spondylolysis in the *nonathlete* are Alaskan Native American heritage and a first-degree relative already having spondylolysis. Both circumstances carry a 50% risk of developing spondylolysis.[32,85]

In the athlete, repetitive hyperextension is the major risk factor for developing spondylolysis. This information is derived from the sports with the highest incidences of spondylolysis and from

the maneuvers that produce symptoms. The incidence of spondylolysis in diving is 63% and in gymnastics is 32%.[57] Other activities such as dancing[44] and figure skating[43] have an increased incidence of spondylolysis (Fig. 34-2). The young athlete is particularly at risk for this process. In an epidemiologic study looking at all causes of back pain in adolescent and adult athletes, 47% of adolescent back pain was related to the spondylolytic process (Table 34-2).[45] Risk factors for progression from spondylolysis to spondylolisthesis are unknown.

History

The female athlete with spondylolytic low back pain will complain of aching pain with hyperextension of the spine. Sciatica can occur, but is rare. The pain is focally located to the bony posterior spine, usually at L4 or L5. The athlete may also complain about back and hamstring tightness. NSAIDs, rest, and heat have been found to decrease symptoms.

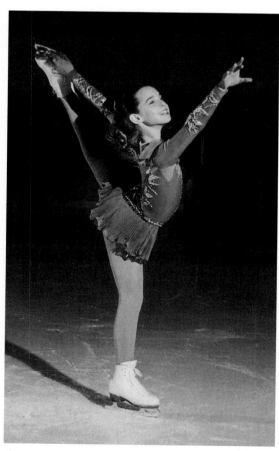

Figure 34-2. Spine hyperextension, a common maneuver in many sports.

Table 34-2. Epidemiology of Low Back Pain in Athletes[a]

LESION	YOUTH	ADULT
Discogenic	11	48
Herniated	9	24
Degenerated	1	22
Both	1	2
Spondylolysis/spondylolisthesis	47	5
Hyperlordotic mechanical back pain	26	0
Lumbosacral strain	6	27
Scoliosis	8	7
Osteoarthritis	0	4
Spinal stenosis	0	6
Neoplasm	0	2
Hamstring strain	1	0
Trochanteric bursitis	1	0
Ankylosing spondylitis	0	1
Total	*100*	*100*

[a]Evaluation of 100 adults and 100 adolescents with sports-related low back pain. The majority of adult back pain was discogenic, while in adolescents the spondylolytic process was dominant. (From Micheli LJ, Wood R: Back pain in young athletes: Significant differences from adults in causes and patterns. Arch Pediatr Adolesc Med 149: 15–8, 1995, with permission.)

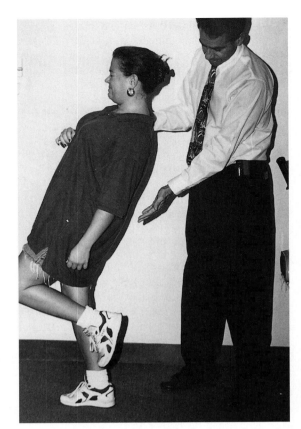

Figure 34-3. Hyperextension of the lumbar spine putting focused stresses on left posterior elements.

Physical Examination

It must be borne in mind that the female athletes who develop spondylolysis are usually involved in sports demanding increased ranges of motion. An injured athlete's flexibility *must be compared to her preinjury flexibility.* Specifically, in evaluation of low back pain, forward flexion (fingertips to the toes) is assessed. Hamstring tightness is always present with low back pain. Hyperlordosis is common. Gymnasts or dancers with spondylolysis may have relative low back and hamstring tightness, but appear to have normal flexibility on examination. Only if a preparticipation screening examination has been done will the examiner know the change from the athlete's preinjury spine flexibility.

Lumbar and hamstring tightness is present in most cases of low back pain and is not isolated to spondylolysis. Once the general low back pain examination has been performed and all dermatomes, myotomes, and reflexes cleared, specific tests are performed. Spondylolytic pain is elicited with hyperextension of the spine in the standing patient. Since spondylolysis is frequently unilateral, the symptomatic side can usually be identified by having the athlete stand on alternate legs while hyperextending the spine. The painful injured side will be found to correspond to the weight-bearing side (Fig. 34-3). Forward flexion should not increase symptoms.

Imaging

Plain radiographs of the lumbar spine in an athlete should include anteroposterior, lateral, and oblique views. Flexion-extension lateral views can be obtained if spondylolisthesis is present or stability is in question. The anteroposterior view is usually normal, although in athletes with familial spondylolysis, other associated spinal irregularities such as scoliosis, spina bifida occulta, and transitional vertebrae may be present.[62] The lateral film will show the spondylolysis if fracture has occurred and will demonstrate the degree of slip and slip angle in spondylolisthesis (Fig. 34-4). Oblique films can pick up a more subtle unilateral spondylolysis.

There are many schemes for classifying spondylolisthesis based on radiographic appearance. The grading system of Wiltse describes the various morphologic types of spondylolisthesis.[84] A percent slip grading system indicates the slip severity (Fig. 34-5).[37] An athlete with hyperextension low back pain in an at-risk sport with normal plain films requires further studies. A technetium 99m bone scan will identify many pars stress fractures otherwise missed by oblique

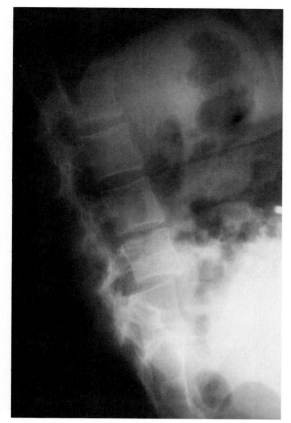

Figure 34-4. Lateral radiograph demonstrating L4 spondylolisthesis.

plain films. Several studies have further shown that a standard bone scan is inadequate. A single photon emission computed tomographic (SPECT) bone scan is necessary to identify the more subtle (and common) prespondylolytic stress reactions (Fig. 34-6).[2,13,50,51]

The SPECT bone scan is also useful as a management tool. The physical examination might indicate a right-sided painful pars, but plain-film oblique views could show fracture or sclerosis on the left and a normal-appearing right pars. The SPECT scan will show increased metabolism on the nonfractured, symptomatic right. This situation is fairly common as the process is thought to be a progression of stresses to both sides. The athlete in this circumstance can be treated to prevent the right pars from fracturing.

Other studies can be used to obtain specific information. A CT scan through the fracture gives excellent bony detail (Fig. 34-7) and may be obtained if surgery is contemplated or to document healing.

Treatment

The notion persists that spondylolysis is an asymptomatic or minimally symptomatic condition for which there is no treatment. This attitude probably stems from the experience of orthopaedists treating familial spondylolysis, which is far less often symptomatic. It is also the result of treating radiographically obvious or long-standing spondylolysis and spondylolisthesis. These fractures rarely heal and aggressive treatment is thought by some to be unrewarding.[68]

Fortunately, earlier detection with SPECT or CT allows earlier intervention and frequent healing before overt fracture occurs. The most successful therapy has been antilordotic bracing in a thoracolumbosacral orthosis such as the Boston overlap brace.[4,67] The brace is molded

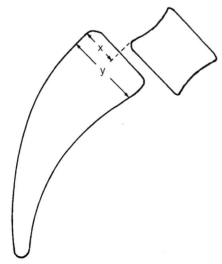

Figure 34-5. Classification of spondylolisthesis by percent displacement. X/Y = % slip.

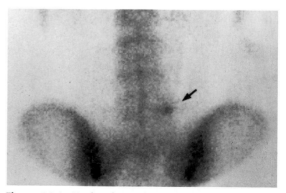

Figure 34-6. Single photon emission computed tomography (SPECT) bone scan showing prespondylolytic stress reaction. Plain films were normal.

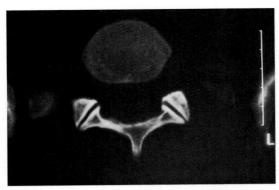

Figure 34-7. CT scan through L5 spondylolysis. Note sclerosis of a healed, asymptomatic stress fracture of the right pars and a normal-appearing left side. The SPECT scan showed uptake on the nonsclerotic side.

in 0° of lordosis to help unload the posterior elements. Over 2 to 3 weeks, the athlete gets used to wearing the brace until the brace is on for 23 hours per day. Initial therapy emphasizes hamstring stretching in the brace. As symptoms subside, lumbar flexion exercises (Williams) are begun out of the brace.[83] Activity in the brace, including most aspects of the athlete's sport, is progressively increased as long as there is no back pain. When the athlete has no back pain with full sports activity in the brace, weaning from the brace is begun. First, sleeping is permitted out of the brace. If pain does not return, more and more time is spent out of the brace. The sporting activity itself is the final activity for which the brace is used. It may take 6 to 9 months before all bracing can be stopped.

A complete cure can be routinely expected for prespondylolytic stress reaction and very early spondylolysis that is metabolically active by bone scan. Long-standing spondylolysis and all spondylolisthesis lesions are unlikely to heal with bony union. The pain-free state can be achieved in these cases, but with a fibrous union. Using bone stimulators to enhance healing of all stages of this process holds tremendous promise. Electromagnetic field treatment has been used[71] and studies are now underway at our institution using ultrasonic and electromagnetic bone stimulation.[52]

Painful spondylolysis nonunion and spondylolisthesis that continues to slip require operative intervention. The pars defect may be repaired[26,30] or more commonly a limited posterior fusion is performed. Historically, in situ fusion with bone graft has been the standard operation.[8,9,24] More recently, limited fusion with bone graft and hardware fixation is being used to minimize the number of vertebrae fused and obtain reduction of the slip.[19]

Degenerative Disc Disease

Etiology

Intermittent aching low back pain can be caused by one or more degenerative discs. In the majority of patients with pain resulting from degenerative disc disease (DDD), the pain is thought to arise initially in the annulus fibrosis, but frequently these patients have facet degenerative changes or spinal stenosis as well.[76] Of all adult athletes' low back pain, 48% is from DDD, whereas only 11% of adolescents' low back pain will be discogenic.[45] MRI studies have confirmed DDD in gymnasts as young as 10 years.[71]

Risk Factors

Sports such as gymnastics carry an increased risk of DDD, but the reasons are unclear. Women do not seem to be at increased risk as compared with men. Known risk factors for DDD include aging, heavy labor, and a family history of disc problems. Males have more mechanical back pain than females in the general population.[7] Disc degeneration has been documented by MRI in gymnastics[38,70,71] and several other sports. The at-risk sports place increased axial loads and flexion loads on the spine. The most likely conclusion is that in any sport in which there is increased stress on the annulus, whether from increased intradisc pressures, or external strain in flexion or rotation, the disc is at risk for premature degeneration. The athlete's age and family history must also be considered.

History

Unlike an acute disc herniation, DDD presents with waxing and waning low back pain. In the early stages of the process, there is no associated degenerative spondylolysis, facet arthropathy, or degenerative stenosis. Pain is dull and aching and comes on with increased activity. There is no morning stiffness, but the low back and hamstrings are always tightest in the morning. A history of radicular symptoms should make the examiner suspicious for a disc herniation. In long-standing DDD, neurologic symptoms after exercise (claudication) indicate degenerative stenosis.

Physical Examination

The standard low back pain examination is performed. Gait, flexibility, and complete neurologic testing is done to rule out radiculopathy. Hyperflexion or hyperextension will increase back pain. Hyperextension causing radicular symptoms points to foraminal or central stenosis and facet hypertrophy. Most commonly, the low back examination is nonspecific, showing no neurologic deficits, diffuse lower lumbar tenderness, and a vague ache with provocative flexion or extension. Paraspinal and hamstring muscles are invariably tight.

Imaging

For most athletes, the plain radiographs are normal early in the disease. Only with advanced DDD is disc space narrowing or traction osteophyte formation seen. As the process progresses further, facet hypertrophy and degeneration occur and can be seen on plain radiographs.

MRI gives excellent documentation of disc dehydration and degeneration. MRI also has the advantage of identifying herniated disc material and allowing measurements of stenosis to be made. Unfortunately, it is common to see MR evidence of disc degeneration in a completely asymptomatic adult patient.[6] It is unknown whether adolescents have a similar rate of false-positive MR findings. CT with multiplanar reformation can give similar evidence of disc degeneration without being able to identify the symptomatic from the asymptomatic. A secondary advantage of CT is that central and foraminal stenosis is easily seen if present.

The only known technique for identifying *symptomatic* degenerative discs is discography. A small amount of saline or contrast medium is injected into the suspect disc under fluoroscopy. If the patient's *usual* low back pain symptoms are duplicated by the injection, the test is positive and that disc is said to be the source of the low back pain.[66]

Treatment

The vast majority of athletes with DDD will respond to nonoperative treatment. NSAIDs help relieve pain. Decreasing axial loads and flexion moments by activity modification may be all that is necessary to relieve pain at rest. Unfortunately, getting an athlete back to full sports without recurrence can be difficult. Using a soft lumbosacral corset will help, but more commonly, a polypropylene thoracolumbosacral orthosis in 10° to 15° of lordosis is required to relieve symptoms and permit sports. The athlete is weaned from the brace as symptoms permit, which takes 4 to 6 months in most cases.

Operative intervention is rarely required. In the most severe cases, discography would be performed and if positive, the athlete would receive anterior and/or posterior fusion of that motion segment.[80]

Atypical Scheuermann's Thoracolumbar Kyphosis

Etiology

Atypical Scheuermann's kyphosis is manifested by anterior intravertebral disc herniation and Schmorl's node formation.[5] Increased axial loads in flexion are thought to be causative, but how and why the herniations occur is unclear.

Risk Factors

At-risk sports for atypical Scheuermann's kyphosis are thought to be diving and gymnastics, in which athletes are subject to increased axial loads, especially when combined with forward flexion. Tight lumbosacral soft tissues put increased demands on the thoracolumbar kyphosis. There are no known gender, heredity, or other host or environmental risk factors associated with this condition.

History

The athlete's back pain is associated with lifting and forward flexion. There may be some low back pain at rest.

Physical Examination

The back examination is nonspecific, with the exception of the inability to reverse the lumbar lordosis. Tenderness is midline and diffuse. Forward flexion may increase symptoms and the lumbosacral soft tissues are tight. No pain is found with spine extension. The neurologic examination is normal.

Imaging

Anterior end-plate changes are seen in the lateral plain films (Fig. 34-8). MRI shows disc material herniated into the adjacent vertebrae (Schmorl's nodes) (Fig. 34-9). Technetium 99m bone scanning, CT, and other studies are of little additive value.

Treatment

Relative rest is prescribed, especially from the etiologic activity within the sport. Hyperextension bracing in a 15° lordosis Boston overlap brace relieves the pain. Pain relief in the brace is so dramatic that whether the brace leads to "healing" is secondary. Patients, even adolescents highly

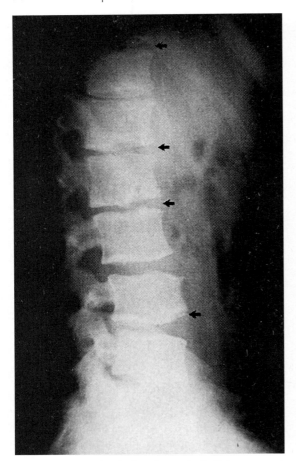

Figure 34-8. Radiograph of atypical Scheuermann's thoracolumbar kyphosis. Note multiple anterior vertebral end-plate changes without avulsion.

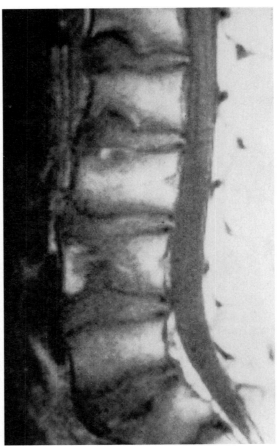

Figure 34-9. MR image of atypical Scheuermann's kyphosis demonstrating the intravertebral disc herniations of the anterior spinal column.

resistant to a plastic brace, will gratefully wear the brace 23 hours a day to remain pain free. Physical therapy stresses McKenzie-type extension exercises[36] for the thoracolumbar region and flexion stretching of the lumbosacral region and hamstrings. Weaning from the brace is begun after the patient has been symptom free for 1 month.

Vertebral End-Plate Apophysitis

Etiology

Closely related to atypical Scheuermann's thoracolumbar kyphosis is vertebral end-plate apophysitis. The ring apophysis of the immature vertebra is the attachment site of the annulus fibrosis and longitudinal ligaments as well as being the growth center. Repetitive traction, compression, and shear can lead to fatigue fracture of growing cartilage, but how these mechanisms lead to failure in the ring apophysis is

unknown. Ikata and coworkers have shown that there are several variations of vertebral apophysis failure.[28] Apophyseal widening with interposed disc material, for example, could be a variant of atypical Scheuermann's in which the disc forces its way into the apophysis. Conversely, disc herniation could occur after stress fracture or avulsion of the ring apophysis. Anterior apophyseal fractures without interposed disc are also found. These must result from acute or stress fracture of the apophysis and, therefore, represent a distinct entity as a source of low back pain.

Risk Factors

Like other apophyseal cartilages, vertebral apophyses are most likely damaged by repetitive stress in tension. For the anterior portion to fail in tension, repetitive hyperextension with or without rotation would be implicated. Precise risk factors remain theoretical.

History

The classic complaint is that of aching low back pain with activity. All forms of increased motion seem to induce symptoms.

Physical Examination

Localized tenderness may be present, but is unusual. Hyperflexion, hyperextension, and extreme lateral bending may duplicate symptoms. All the athletes have tight hamstrings, but only some have tight lumbar fascia and "flat back." This group may, in fact, be the same population at risk for atypical Scheuermann's kyphosis. The neurologic examination is normal.

Imaging

Plain radiographs are usually diagnostic. On the lumbosacral spine lateral view, widening of the ring apophysis is seen. This may occur at one or more vertebrae. Multiple levels with or without Schmorl's node formation is more typical of thoracolumbar Scheuermann's than apophysitis. MRI will show whether there is disc material in the defect. This information is helpful in determining etiology, but is not useful for treatment at this time.

Treatment

Relative rest is prescribed to alleviate the apophysitis. Although the term *apophysitis* implies inflammation, the process is more likely a stress fracture of growth cartilage. Hamstring and gentle lumbar flexibility is begun. If symptoms persist, bracing in the Boston overlap brace is required. Healing is usually complete in 6 to 8 weeks, but occasionally pain will persist for 3 to 4 months. As with the other overuse conditions of the low back, sport participation is permitted in the brace as long as there is no pain.

Chronic Mechanical Low Back Pain

Mechanical low back pain in the female athlete can occur when a simple muscular strain is not adequately rehabilitated. Flexibility and strength must be restored to normal values or repeated injury can occur.

Lordotic Low Back Pain

In the adolescent, the growth spurt may lead to a temporary state of pathologic soft-tissue tightness. Manifestations in the low back include hyperlordosis, "flat back" and compensatory hyperkyphosis of the thoracic spine. This is the functional equivalent of adult chronic strain. Treatment is exactly the same, with even greater emphasis on hamstring and low back stretching.

Other Causes of Overuse Low Back Pain

Transitional Vertebra

When a transitional vertebra forms a pseudarthrosis with the iliac wing or sacrum, the pain can be debilitating.[3] This is readily seen on plain radiographs (Fig. 34-10), but may require bone scanning or CT for clarification. The goal is to achieve a painless pseudarthrosis at the impingement. Rest and NSAIDs may work, but occasionally a corticosteroid injection to the space is necessary. Persistent pain requires spinal fusion or resection of the offending bone.[59]

Facet Syndrome

Repetitive flexion and extension can lead to facet pain and eventual degeneration. This process may be the result of increased motion segment excursion because of disc degeneration. If the pain source is the facet joints, symptoms can be relieved with rest and motion limitation (with a brace if necessary), and by injecting the facets with corticosteroid when necessary. Only in the older athlete who develops spinal stenosis and facet hypertrophy is operative decompression considered.

Sacroiliitis

Whether following trauma or as a result of an arthritic process,[35] the sacroiliac joint can de-

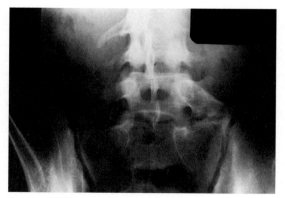

Figure 34-10. Transitional vertebra at L5-S1, with pseudarthrosis of the transverse process of L5 upon the sacral ala.

velop painful degenerative arthritis. As in facet arthropathy, the goal is to decrease excessive motion and inflammation with rest, heat, and NSAIDs if possible. Similarly, corticosteroid injection of the sacroiliac joint occasionally is necessary.

Rib Stress Fracture

An overuse injury that occasionally occurs in female rowers is rib stress fracture. As reported by Holden and Jackson, this develops from the specific demands of rowing.[27] As in other stress fractures, treatment requires relative rest until symptoms resolve and the bone is healed.

ATRAUMATIC SOURCES OF BACK PAIN IN WOMEN

While acute trauma is rarely missed, microtrauma can be insidious. When microtrauma is suspected, it is always necessary to rule out atraumatic sources of back pain.

A wide variety of atraumatic conditions can present as thoracic or lumbar pain in a female athlete. These include infection, arthritis, congenital or developmental problems, neoplasm, and referred pain. Exhaustive lists of known causes of back pain have been developed, but it is more important to understand the broad categories of atraumatic back pain and to then know the more common diagnoses from each group.

Scoliosis

Back pain is so prevalent in the general population that demonstrating whether or not scoliosis directly causes back pain is extremely difficult. We believe it cannot be said that scoliosis, per se, is a cause of back pain. Mechanical and discogenic back pain are more likely to occur in someone with moderate to severe curvature.

Females are affected by significant adolescent idiopathic scoliosis nearly 10 times as frequently as males, making scoliosis probably the second most common back condition encountered in the adolescent athlete behind spondylolysis and overuse injuries.

Etiology

Adolescent idiopathic scoliosis (AIS) has no definite cause, but a multifactorial etiology is postulated with variable contributions from genetics, neuromuscular status, and growth. Although poorly defined, the genetic associations are definite. Numerous experimental and prevalence studies point toward a subtle neuropathic etiology in AIS. Compared with their peers, adolescents with progressive AIS are taller than and grow later than average.[1]

Juvenile idiopathic scoliosis presents in childhood and may be rapidly progressive. Significant juvenile scoliosis may have a definite neuropathic etiology and should be screened for Chiari I malformation and syringomyelia by MRI.[60] Adolescent idiopathic scoliosis is usually first detected in late childhood or early puberty and has a variable natural history. Some cases progress but then spontaneously stabilize; some progress further during the puberty growth spurt but stabilize and some progress rapidly during the puberty growth spurt and are troublesome. The risk of progression generally correlates with the amount of growth remaining and the severity of the curve. School screening of fifth to ninth graders for adolescent idiopathic scoliosis has been advocated but is imperfect. The United States Public Health Service task force on screening was neutral in its recommendation of school screening.[75] Physician screening of the same population group is probably more effective and is advocated. The rationale for screening is straightforward: earlier detection of progressive curves allows nonoperative brace treatment and can potentially diminish the incidence of surgery and the incidence of larger curves at the end of growth. Standard screening examination includes a search for asymmetry of the shoulders, scapulae, iliac crest heights, and distance between the trunk and arms. The forward bend test in which the examiner sights down the spine searching for asymmetries is performed. The scoliometer or "inclinometer" popularized by Bunnell is a modified spirit level used to quantify the amount of rib or lumbar paraspinal muscle hump.[11] The device is centered on the spine at the point of maximum deviation and the degree of inclination recorded. Radiographic investigation of curves with scoliometer or inclinometer readings in excess of 5° is generally recommended. Curves with inclinometer readings of less than 5° are unlikely to be large curves at the time of screening and although follow-up may be appropriate, radiographs are probably not needed unless there is associated pain or other abnormalities. Curves with inclinometer readings less than 5° probably can be followed periodically through growth by primary care physicians. Patients with curves with inclinometer readings greater than 5° generally should be either referred for radiography and, if the curve is in excess of 20°, referred to an orthopaedist for follow-up or simply referred on to an orthopaedist for follow-up. The frequency of follow-up and follow-up radiography depends on the risk of curve progression, which in turn hinges upon growth remaining and severity of the curvature.

The only nonoperative treatment with statistical support is full-time or nearly full-time brace treatment.[58] Although juvenile idiopathic scoliosis is braced earlier, bracing of adolescent idiopathic scoliosis is generally reserved for progressive curves between 20° and 30° or any curve between 30° and 45° Cobb with growth remaining. After 45° to 50° of curvature braces are generally less effective and a zone where primary surgical treatment may be preferable is entered. If adolescents have a large curve that has failed to respond to bracing or have a curve in excess of 45° to 50°, surgical fusion and instrumentation may be advocated.[53,73] Since on average bracing only stops progressive curvatures, it is important to initiate bracing early in the course of progressive curves.

When a female athlete complains of back pain and is found to have scoliosis, a thorough search must be made for the common sources of back pain such as spondylolysis and lordotic back pain. Muscle and soft-tissue tightness found with significant scoliosis may cause recurrent strains if not adequately stretched.

Referred Back Pain

Within the context of atraumatic back pain, pain referred to the spine from other areas must be considered. Trauma or disease in almost every organ has been reported to present as back pain. Most often, referred thoracic or lumbar back pain originates in the kidney, lung, liver, spleen, aorta, bowel, or uterus.

CONCLUDING REMARKS

Back pain is one of the most common and vexing problems that human beings must endure. Most injuries result from the overuse of the skeletal support system that is the thoracolumbar spine. In terms of types of injuries, there is really no difference between females and males. Different age groups and different sports are at risk for specific problems. Knowing the risk factors permits precise diagnosis and appropriate management. Overuse injuries, and the spondylolytic process in particular, demand persistent diagnostic efforts and aggressive use of bracing

and physical therapy to maximize function and minimize recurrence. Pain is the variable that determines level of permissible activity. When pain has been eliminated by healing, bracing or even fusion,[41] full return to athletic activity is possible.

References

1. Archer IA, Dickson RA. Stature and idiopathic scoliosis. A prospective study. J Bone Joint Surg 67B:185–8, 1985.
2. Bellah RD, Summerville DA, Treves ST, et al: Low-back pain in adolescent athletes: Detection of stress injury to the pars interarticularis with SPECT. Radiology 180:509–12, 1991.
3. Bertolotti M: Contributo alla conoscenza dei vizi di differenzazione regionale del rachide con speciale riguardo alla assimilazione sacrale della V lombare. Radiol Med (Torino) 4:113–44, 1917.
4. Blanda J, Bethem D, Moats W, Lew M: Defects of pars interarticularis in athletes: a protocol for nonoperative treatment. J Spinal Disorders 6(5):406–11, 1993.
5. Blumenthal SL, Roach J, Herring JA, et al: Lumbar Scheuermann's: a clinical series and classification. Spine 12:929–32, 1987.
6. Boden SD, David DO, Dina TS, et al: Abnormal magnetic-resonance scans of the lumbar spine in asymptomatic subjects: A prospective investigation. J Bone Joint Surg 72A:403–8, 1990.
7. Borenstein DG, Wiesel SW: Low Back Pain. Medical Diagnosis and Comprehensive Management. Philadelphia, WB Saunders, 1989, pp 51–4.
8. Bosworth D, Fielding J, Demarest L, et al: Spondylolisthesis: A critical review of a consecutive series of cases treated by arthrodesis. J Bone Joint Surg 37A:767–86, 1955.
9. Boxall D, Bradford D, Winter R, Moe J: Management of severe spondylolisthesis in children and adolescents. J Bone Joint Surg 61A:479–95, 1979.
10. Bracken MB, Shepard MJ, Collins WF, et al: A randomized, controlled trial of methylprednisolone or naloxone in the treatment of acute spinal-cord injury: Results of the Second National Acute Spinal Cord Injury Study. N Engl J Med 322:1405–11, 1990.
11. Bunnell WP: Outcome of spinal screening. Spine 18:1572–80, 1993.
12. Cherkin DC, Deyo RA, Loeser JD, et al: An international comparison of back surgery rates. Spine 19:1201–6, 1994.
13. Collier BD, Johnson RP, Carrera GF, et al: Painful spondylolysis or spondylolisthesis studied by radiography and single photon emission computed tomography. Radiology 154:207–11, 1985.
14. Committee on Trauma (eds). Advanced Trauma Life Support for Doctors, 6th edition, Chicago, American College of Surgeons, 1997.
15. Crawford AH: Operative treatment of spine fractures in children. Orthop Clin North Am 21:325–39, 1990.
16. Davis H: Increasing rates of cervical and lumbar spine surgery in the United States, 1979–1990. Spine 19:1117–23, 1994.
17. DeOrio JK, Bianco AJ: Lumbar disc excision in children and adolescents. J Bone Joint Surg 64A(7):991–5, 1982.
18. Dilke T&W, Burry HC, Grahame R: Extradural corticosteroid injection management of lumbar nerve root compression. Br Med J 2:635–9, 1973.

19. Edwards C: Reduction of spondylolisthesis. In Bridwell K, DeWald R (eds): Textbook of Spinal Surgery. Philadelphia, JB Lippincott, 1991.
20. Erhard RE, Delitto A, Cibulka M: Relative effectiveness of an extension program and a combined program of manipulation and flexion and extension exercises in patients with acute low back syndrome. Phys Ther 74(12):1093–100, 1994.
21. Frymoyer JW: Back pain and sciatica. N Engl J Med 318:291–300, 1988.
22. Garrick JG, Requa RK: The epidemiology of woman's gymnastics injuries. Am J Sports Med 8:261–4, 1980.
23. Germanaud J, Bardet M: Is the female sex a risk factor for acute low back pain? (letter) Rev Rhum 60(11):850–1, 1993.
24. Gill G, Manning J, White H: Surgical treatment of spondylolisthesis treated by arthrodesis. JAMA 163:175–9, 1957.
25. Goldberg MJ. Gymnastics injuries. Orthop Clin North Am 11:717–26, 1980.
26. Hardcastle PH: Repair of spondylolysis in young fast bowlers. J Bone Joint Surg 75B:398–402, 1993.
27. Holden DL, Jackson DW: Stress fractures of the ribs in female rowers. Am J Sports Med 13:342–5, 1985.
28. Ikata T, Morita T, Katoh S, et al: Lesions of the lumbar posterior end plate in children and adolescents. J Bone Joint Surg 77B:951–5, 1995.
29. Jackson DW, Wiltse LL, Dingeman RD, et al: Stress reactions involving the pars interarticularis in young athletes. Am J Sports Med 9:304–12, 1981.
30. Johnson GV, Thompson AG: The Scott wiring technique for direct repair of lumbar spondylolysis. J Bone Joint Surg 74B:426–30, 1992.
31. Kelsey JL: An epidemiological study of acute herniated lumbar intervertebral disc. Rheumatol Rehabil 14:144–59, 1975.
32. Kettlekamp DB, Wright GD: Spondylolysis in the Alaskan Eskimo. J Bone Joint Surg 53A:563–6, 1971.
33. Letts M, Smallman T, Afanasen R, et al: Fracture of the pars interarticularis in adolescent athletes: a clinical biomechanical analysis. J Pediatr Orthop 6:40–6, 1986.
34. Lloyd RG: Riding and other equestrian injuries: Considerable severity. Br J Sports Med 21:22–4, 1987.
35. Marymount JV, Lynch MA, Henning CE: Exercise-related stress reaction of the sacroiliac joint. An unusual cause of low back pain in athletes. Am J Sports Med 14:320–3, 1986.
36. McKenzie RA: The Lumbar Spine. Mechanical Diagnosis and Therapy. Lower Hutt, New Zealand, Spinal Publications, 1981.
37. Meyerding HW: Low backache and sciatic pain associated with spondylolisthesis and protruded intervertebral disc. J Bone Joint Surg 23A:461–70, 1941.
38. Micheli LJ: Back injuries in gymnastics. Clin Sports Med 4:85–93, 1985.
39. Micheli LJ: Spinal deformities and the athlete. In Welch RP, Shephard RJ (eds): Current Therapy in Sports Medicine. Philadelphia, BC Decker, 1985, pp 158–64.
40. Micheli LJ: The spine and chest wall. In Johnson RL, Lombardo J (eds): Current Review of Sports Medicine. Philadelphia, Current Medicine, 1994, pp 1–16.
41. Micheli LJ: Sports following spinal surgery in the young athlete. Clin Orthop 198:152–7, 1985.
42. Micheli LJ, Hall JE, Miller ME: Use of modified Boston brace for back injuries in athletes. Am J Sports Med 8:351–6, 1980.
43. Micheli LJ, McCarthy C: Figure skating. In Watkins RG (ed): The Spine in Sports. St. Louis, Mosby-Year Book, 1996.
44. Micheli LJ, Micheli ER: Back injuries in dancers. In Shell CG (ed): The 1984 Olympic Scientific Congress

Proceedings, vol 8: The Dancer as Athlete. Champaign, Ill, Human Kinetics Publishers, 1986, pp 91–4.
45. Micheli LJ, Wood R: Back pain in young athletes: Significant differences from adults in causes and patterns. Arch Pediatr Adolesc Med 149:15–8, 1995.
46. Mixter WJ, Barr JS: Rupture of the intervertebral disc with involvement of the spinal canal. N Engl J Med 211:210–1, 1934.
47. Mundt DJ, Kelsey JL, Golden AL, et al: Northeast Collaborative Group on Low Back Pain. An epidemiologic study of sports and weight lifting as possible risk factors for herniated lumbar and cervical discs. Am J Sports Med 21(6):854–60, 1993.
48. Myles St, Mohtadi NG, Schnittker J: Injuries to the nervous system and spine in downhill skiing. Can J Surg 35:643–8, 1992.
49. Nachemson A, Morris JM: In vivo measurements of intradiscal pressure. J Bone Joint Surg 46:1077–84, 1964.
50. Papanicolaou N, Wilkinson RH, Emans JB, et al: Bone scintigraphy and radiography in young athletes with low back pain. AJR 145:1039–44, 1985.
51. Pennell, RG, Maurer AH, Bonakdarpour A: Stress injuries of the pars interarticularis: Radiologic classification and indications for scintigraphy. AJR 145:763–6, 1985.
52. Pettine KA, Salib RN, Walker SG: External electrical stimulation and bracing for treatment of spondylolysis. A case report. Spine 18(4):436–9, 1993.
53. Pizzutillo PD: Idiopathic scoliosis and kyphosis. Instr Course Lect 43:185–91, 1994.
54. Porter GE: Slipping rib syndrome: An infrequently recognized entity in children: A report of 3 cases and review of the literature. Pediatrics 76:810–3, 1985.
55. Reid DC, Saboe L: Spine fractures in winter sports. Sports Med 7(6):393–9, 1989.
56. Rosenberg NJU, Bargar WL, Friedman B: The incidence of spondylolysis and spondylolisthesis in nonambulatory patients. Spine 6:35–8, 1981.
57. Rossi F: Spondylolysis, spondylolisthesis and sports. J Sports Med Phys Fitness 18(4):317–40, 1988.
58. Rowe DE, Bernstein SM, Riddick MF, et al: A meta-analysis of the efficacy of non-operative treatments for idiopathic scoliosis (see comments). J Bone Joint Surg 79A:664–74, 1997.
59. Santavirta S, Tallroth K, Ylinen P, et al: Surgical treatment of Bertolotti's syndrome. Follow-up of 16 patients. Arch Orthop Trauma Surg 112:82–7, 1993.
60. Schwend RM, Hennrikus WL, Hall JE, Emans JB: Childhood scoliosis: Clinical indications for magnetic resonance imaging. J Bone Joint Surg 77A:46–53, 1995.
61. Schwobel MG. Apophyseal fractures in adolescents. Chirurg 56:699–704, 1985.
62. Shands AR, Bundens WD: Congenital deformities of the spine. Analysis of the roentgenograms of 700 children. Bull Hosp Jt Dis 17:110–33, 1956.
63. Shapiro S: Cauda equina syndrome secondary to lumbar disc herniation. Neurosurgery 32:743–6, 1993.
64. Shellock FG, Prentice WE. Warming up and stretching for improved physical performance and prevention of sports-related injuries. Sports Med 2:267–78, 1985.
65. Silver JR, Silver D, Godfrey JJ: Trampolining injuries of the spine. Injury 17:117–24, 1986.
66. Simmons EH, Segil CM: An evaluation of discography in the localization of symptomatic levels in discogenic disease of the spine. Clin Orthop 108:57–62, 1975.
67. Steiner ME, Micheli LJ: Treatment of symptomatic spondylolysis and spondylolisthesis with the modified Boston brace. Spine 10:937–43, 1985.

68. Stinson JT: Spondylolysis and spondylolisthesis in the athlete. Clin Sports Med 3:517–28, 1993.

69. Svendsen DA, Matyas TA: Facilitation of the isometric maximum voluntary contraction with traction. A test of PNF predictions. Am J Phys Med 62(1):27–37, 1983.

70. Sward L, Hellstrom M, Jacobsson B, et al: Disc degeneration and associated abnormalities of the spine in elite gymnasts: a magnetic resonance imaging study. Spine 16:437–43, 1991.

71. Tertti M, Paajanen H, Kujala UM, et al: Disc degeneration in young gymnasts: a magnetic resonance imaging study. Am J Sports Med 18:206–8, 1991.

72. Thomas PL: Thoracic back pain in rowers and butterfly swimmers—Costovertebral subluxation. Br J Sports Med 22:81–8,1988.

73. Tolo VT: Surgical treatment of adolescent idiopathic scoliosis. AAOS Instr Course Lect 38:143–56. 1989.

74. Troup JDG: Mechanical factors in spondylolisthesis and spondylolysis. Clin Orthop 147:59–67, 1976.

75. USPHS: United States Preventive Services Task Force: Screening for adolescent idiopathic scoliosis. Review article. JAMA 269:2667–72,1993.

76. Verbiest H: Pathomorphologic aspects of developmental lumbar stenosis. Orthop Clin North Am 6:177–96, 1975.

77. Von Korff M, Deyo RA, Cherkin D, Barlow W: Back pain in primary care. Outcomes at one year. Spine 18(7):855–62, 1993.

78. Weir MR, Smith DS: Stress reaction of the pars interarticularis leading to spondylolysis. A cause of adolescent low back pain. J Adolesc Health Care 10:573–7, 1989.

79. Weissman B, Sledge C: The lumbar spine. In Orthopaedic Radiology. WB Saunders, Philadelphia, 1986, p 285.

80. Wetzel FT, LaRoca HS, Lowery GL, et al: The treatment of lumbar spinal pain syndromes diagnosed by discography: lumbar arthrodesis. Spine 19:792–800, 1994.

81. White AA, Panjabi MM: Clinical Biomechanics of the Spine, 2nd edition. Philadelphia, JB Lippincott, 1990, pp 1–19.

82. Whiteside P: Men's and women's injuries in comparable sports. Phys Sportsmed 8:130–40, 1980.

83. Williams PC: The conservative management of lesions of the lumbosacral spine. AAOS Instruct Course Lect 10:80–102, 1953.

84. Wiltse LL, Neuman PH, MacNab I. Classification of spondylolysis and spondylolisthesis. J Bone Joint Surg 65A:768–72, 1983.

85. Wynne-Davies R, Scott J: Inheritance and spondylolisthesis. J Bone Joint Surg 61B:301–5, 1979.

Chapter 35

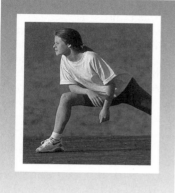

Pelvis and Hip Injuries

Sharon L. Hame, M.D.
Gerald A. M. Finerman, M.D.

Injuries to the hip and pelvis can occur in any sporting activity and are relatively common. The complexity of the anatomy in and around the pelvis and hip often makes diagnosis difficult. Approximately 5% to 6% of all injuries sustained by adult athletes involve the hip and pelvis.[13] Although hip and pelvis injuries can occur in any sport, runners and soccer players are at increased risk.

There is no evidence that female athletes sustain more pelvic and hip injuries than male athletes, however, it appears that female athletes are more susceptible to pelvic stress fractures.[9,47] Other hip and pelvic injuries that are common to the athlete include soft tissue contusions, bursitis, and muscle injuries. Common bony injuries include osteitis pubis, pelvic fractures, and hip avulsion fractures. Acute hip and pelvic fractures are unusual in athletes.

When examining a female athlete with hip or pelvic injury, many sources of pain must be considered. Organ systems to include in the differential diagnosis are the musculoskeletal system and the gynecologic and genitourinary tracts; pregnancy is also a consideration. Several other medical conditions brought on by sporting activities may present as hip or pelvic pain. These include infections, tumors, metabolic bone diseases, and inflammatory conditions such as rheumatoid arthritis, juvenile arthritis, and ankylosing spondylitis. The treating physician must be aware of the wide variety of medical problems that may affect the hip and pelvis, form a differential diagnosis, order the appropriate diagnostic tests, and prescribe the appropriate treatment plan. Knowledge of anatomy and careful review of plain radiographs and magnetic resonance imaging (MRI) scans enable the practitioner to make the specific diagnosis and implement appropriate treatment.[6] Consideration of the sport in which the female athlete participates and the type of injury sustained will influence the treatment plan and safe return to sport.

ANATOMY AND BIOMECHANICS OF THE PELVIS AND HIP

The anatomy of the hip and pelvis is complex. The pelvis is the site of many large muscle and ligament attachments, from the torso as well as from the lower extremities. As a result, the pelvis and hip are the major contributors to gait and overall lower extremity alignment. In addition, the pelvis also supports and protects the pelvic viscera.

The bony pelvis is composed of 2 paired innominate bones, the sacrum, and the coccyx. Together, the sacrum and the innominate bones make up the pelvic ring and are joined posteriorly at the sacroiliac joints and anteriorly at the pubic symphysis. The innominate bones themselves are formed by 3 separate parts, the ilium, ischium, and pubis, which fuse during development at the tri-irradiate cartilage and help form the acetabulum. Femoral anteversion develops during the second half of pregnancy and reaches 35° by birth.[97,102] The sacrum, which articulates with the 2 innominate bones, is formed by the fusion of 5 distal vertebrae, and the coccyx is formed by the union of the terminal 3 to 5 rudimentary vertebral bodies.

The sacroiliac joints are irregular in nature and are covered with hyaline cartilage. Differences in the male and female articular cartilage have been noted and may be related to childbearing or differences in center of gravity.[99] Despite these differences, there is relatively little motion across the sacroiliac joints and no muscle action in either gender. Forward and backward tilting of the sacrum relative to the iliac bones is the sacrum's main motion.[99] Although the configuration of the joints provides some stability, the sacroiliac joints are primarily stabilized by the posterior interosseous sacroiliac ligaments, which resist downward migration and forward rotation of the sacrum. In contrast to the posterior interosseous ligaments, the anterior interosseous sacroiliac ligaments are thin and contribute little to the stability of the joint. Additional support is provided by the sacrotuberous and sacrospinous ligaments, which originate from the sacrum and attach to the ischial tuberosity and ischial spine, respectively. They contribute to rotatory stability of the sacroiliac joints by helping to control forward tilting of the pelvis.[99] Further reinforcement is provided by the sturdy dorsal sacroiliac ligament, which unites with the interosseous sacroiliac ligament to support the downward force produced by body weight on the pelvis and assists in controlling backward tilting of the pelvis.[99]

Like the sacroiliac joints, the pubic symphysis is supported by strong ligaments and is covered with hyaline cartilage. In contrast to the sacroiliac joints, the pubic symphysis has a fibrocartilaginous disc that lies between the 2 innominate bones. Superiorly, the pubic symphysis is stabilized by the suprapubic ligament; inferiorly, it is supported by the arcuate portion of the pubic ligament. Additional support is provided by the anterior interpubic ligament.

Differences between the male and female pelvis have been reported. Females are smaller and have a lower body mass, and have pelvic anatomy that reflects these features. The female bones and joints are smaller and the markings for ligament and tendon attachments are less pronounced.[7] The true pelvis in the female is larger than that of the male (Fig. 35-1). The female pelvic inlet is 1/4 inch larger and the pelvic outlet 1 inch larger in diameter as compared to the male pelvis.[17] The ischial tuberosities of the female pelvis are more everted and the pubic arch is almost 90° as compared to the acutely angled male pubic arch.[7] The acetabular anteversion also

appears to be increased in females. In addition, the pubic symphysis in the female is shorter and has a wider fibrocartilage disc.[7] These anatomic differences reflect the functional differences between the male and the female pelvis and may contribute to the increase in injury to the lower extremities in the female athlete.

A large number of important muscular groups originate and insert onto the pelvis (Fig. 35-2). The semimembranosus, semitendinosus, and biceps femoris muscles comprise the hamstring muscles, which originate from the ischial tuberosity and attach to the proximal tibia and fibula. These muscles span 2 joints and are involved in knee flexion and hip extension. The hip adductors originate on the pubis and insert onto the medial femur (Fig. 35-3). The adductor brevis and adductor longus have a lateral and midline origin, respectively; the gracilis, a hamstring muscle, originates most medially and spans to insert on the medial tibia. Anteriorly, the rectus femoris and the sartorius originate from the anterior inferior iliac spine and anterior superior iliac spine, respectively. The tensor fascia lata also takes its origin from the pelvis and inserts into the iliotibial tract. The iliopsoas muscle and the abdominal musculature also have attachment sites on the pelvis. Posteriorly, the large muscles of the back attach to the iliac crest. In addition to the large muscles, which affect hip and pelvic motion, there are smaller, deeper muscles that originate on the pelvis and control internal and external rotation of the hip. These include the piriformis muscle, the gemellus, the quadratus femoris, and the obturator internus and externus.

In addition to providing protection for the pelvic viscera, the bony pelvis is responsible for transferring weight from the trunk to the lower

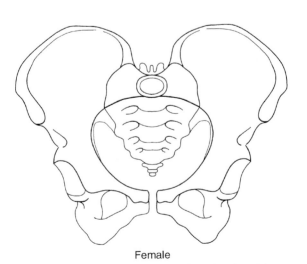

Female

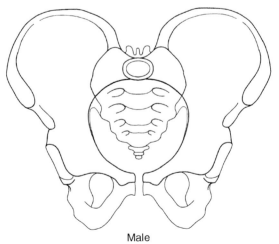

Male

Figure 35-1. Comparison of the female and male pelvis.

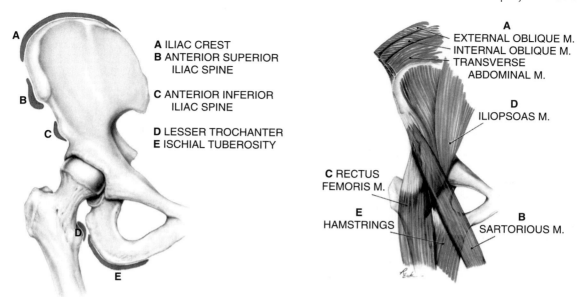

A ILIAC CREST
B ANTERIOR SUPERIOR
    ILIAC SPINE

C ANTERIOR INFERIOR
    ILIAC SPINE

D LESSER TROCHANTER
E ISCHIAL TUBEROSITY

A
EXTERNAL OBLIQUE M.
INTERNAL OBLIQUE M.
TRANSVERSE
ABDOMINAL M.

D
ILIOPSOAS M.

C RECTUS
FEMORIS M.

E
HAMSTRINGS

B
SARTORIOUS M.

Figure 35-2. The origins and insertions of muscles about the pelvis. Muscles with origins on the iliac crest (**A**) are the external oblique, internal oblique, and transverse abdominal muscles. The sartorius muscle has its origin on the anterior superior iliac spine (**B**). The rectus femoris muscle has its origin on the anterior inferior iliac spine (**C**). The iliopsoas muscle has its origin on the lesser trochanter (**D**). The hamstrings have their origin on the ischial tuberosity (**E**). (From Keats TE: Radiology of Musculoskeletal Stress Injury. Chicago, Year Book Medical Publishers, 1990, p 53, with permission.)

extremities. While standing, the force is transmitted through the fifth lumbar vertebra to the sacrum, through the sacroiliac joints and ileum to the acetabulum and hip. When sitting, the force is transmitted to the ischial tuberosities (Fig. 35-4).

Motion of the pelvis is distinct but results from a complex interaction of musculature. Anteroposterior tilting, lateral tilting, and rotation all occur about the pelvis. Anterior tilting occurs in the sagittal plane and is the result of

contraction of the hip flexors, including the iliopsoas and the extensors of the lumbar spine. The female is more likely to have an anteriorly tilted pelvis and in some instances this may lead to an increased risk of lower extremity injury. The combined actions of the rectus abdominis, abdominal oblique, gluteus maximus, and hamstring muscles create posterior tilting of the pelvis. The hip joint serves as the axis of rotation for lateral tilting of the pelvis; therefore, motion in this plane produces abduction or adduction

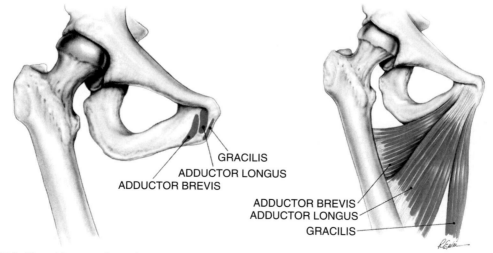

GRACILIS
ADDUCTOR LONGUS
ADDUCTOR BREVIS

ADDUCTOR BREVIS
ADDUCTOR LONGUS
GRACILIS

Figure 35-3. The adductor and gracilis origins from the pubis. (From Keats TE: Radiology of Musculoskeletal Stress Injury. Chicago, Year Book Medical Publishers, 1990, p 60, with permission.)

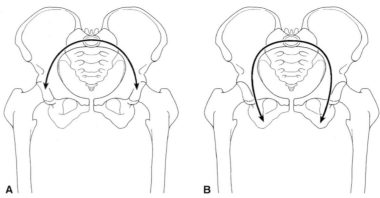

Figure 35-4. A. The force is transmitted to the acetabulum and hip when standing. **B.** The force is transmitted to the ischium when sitting.

of the hip. The abductors of the hip control pelvic tilting through eccentric contraction. Pelvic rotation occurs in the transverse plane and is controlled by a complex interaction of pelvic musculature.

The acetabulum of the pelvis and the head of the femur join to form the hip joint. Stability of the hip joint during motion is maintained by its ball-and-socket configuration.

The femoral head forms two thirds of a sphere and is covered with hyaline cartilage. Kersnic[52] noted that females have a smaller femoral head radius and a larger distance between the inner acetabular rims than males. Therefore, females may be subject to greater contact stresses in the hip joint articular surface than males. The acetabulum is also covered with hyaline cartilage. The rim of the acetabulum is increased by the surrounding labrum. Additional stability is provided by several intracapsular ligaments that originate on the pelvis and attach to the greater and lesser trochanters of the femur.

The bony configuration and blood supply of the proximal femur have been well studied. The neck–shaft angle of the femur ranges from 125° to 135°. Femoral anteversion measures approximately 15° in adults.[37] Staheli and coworkers[92] reported greater femoral anteversion in girls compared to boys. Differences in female anteversion have been associated with increased hip abnormalities[97] and may lead to increased risk of injury to the hip. The ligamentum teres lies within the hip joint and inserts into the fovea capitis of the femoral head. It provides a small portion of the blood supply to the femoral head through a branch of the obturator artery. Additional blood supply to the femoral head is provided by the extracapsular ring of vessels at the base of the femoral neck and its ascending branches.

The internal architecture of the femoral neck is important because it is related to the stress placed on the femoral neck. No gender differences in the internal architecture of the femoral, neck have been reported. In the femoral neck cancellous bone is arranged in a trabecular pattern along the principal lines of stress. Two primary systems exist: a medial or compression trabecula and a lateral or tension trabecula. The medial system arises from the cortical bone of the medial femoral shaft and extends to the superior femoral head. The subchondral layers of this system support the joint reaction force of the hip and are often referred to as the *calcar*. The lateral system, which forms in response to the forces produced by the abductor muscles and the fascia lata,[66,70] begins at the lateral cortical surface inferior to the greater trochanter, passes in a curved fashion through the medial system, and ends at the inferomedial portion of the femoral head. Secondary compressive and tensile systems also exist.

In addition to being quite stable, the hip joint is very mobile. The large muscle groups that originate on the pelvis and insert on the femur, such as the gluteals, the adductors, the abductors, the hip flexors, and the hamstrings, control hip motion in sagittal, transverse, and frontal planes. The greatest motion occurs in the sagittal plane. During gait motion occurs in all 3 planes. Although during normal activities of daily living a limited range of motion of the hip is necessary, during athletics large ranges of motion are required.

Forces about the hip also increase during athletic participation. During one-legged stance the force transmitted across the hip is 2.6 times body weight.[66] During slow walking the force on the hip is 1.6 times body weight and this increases as speed is increased. Running further increases the force across the hip to 5 times body weight in the stance phase and 3 times body weight in the swing phase.[66] Since it has been reported that females have higher contact stresses within the hip joint,[52] the large forces across the hip during athletic participation may significantly increase the risk of injury to the hip of a female athlete.

Skeletally Immature Athletes

In the young female athlete who is skeletally mature, disorders such as slipped capital femoral epiphysis (SCFE), transient synovitis, and Legg–Calvé–Perthes syndrome must be considered. In a young athlete with knee pain, careful examination of the hip should be performed. In cases of SCFE the hip will externally rotate with flexion and pain occurs with internal rotation.

Avulsion injuries will occur at the attachments of the large muscle groups, usually at the ilium or pelvis, or of the insertion of the iliopsoas onto the lesser trochanter. The exact locations of the apophyses are shown in Figures 35-2 and 35-3. Pain on palpation and radiographically demonstrated asymmetry will allow the practitioner to make the correct diagnosis. The basketball athlete shown in Figure 35-5 complained of pain over the iliac crest of several months' duration. The pain could be reproduced on hip abduction and flexion. An MRI scan (Fig. 35-5A) showed abnormal signal over the iliac crest apophysitis. Plain radiographs (Fig. 35-5B) confirmed iliac apophysitis. Apophyseal injuries at the heel or calcaneal apophysitis and tibial tubercle apophysitis (Osgood–Schlatter disease) are less common in female compared to male athletes. There are no comparable repetitive overuse conditions to those mentioned above. Apophyseal inflammatory conditions about the pelvis are usually due to one specific incident, but iliac apophysitis can occur in a repetitive running and cutting sport such as soccer.

SOFT-TISSUE INJURIES OF THE PELVIS AND HIP

Contusions

Soft-tissue contusions are very common among all athletes, male and female. Treatment is the standard rest, ice, and compression. Aspiration of a hemarthrosis is rarely necessary. The timing and intensity of stretching and strengthening depends on the severity of the injury. Local modalities and nonsteroidal anti-inflammatory drugs (NSAIDs), which affect platelet function, should be avoided if the hematoma is large.

Pelvic and hip contusions may be superficial or deep, depending on the injured site and force of

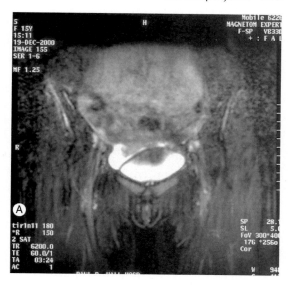

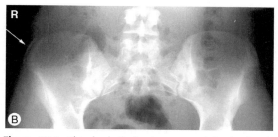

Figure 35-5. This basketball player complained of right iliac crest pain. **A.** The MRI showed abnormal signal over iliac apophysis. **B.** Plain roentgenograms showed widening asymmetry from normal left iliac crest.

the impact. Frequently, contusions occur over bony prominences, such as the greater trochanter and iliac crest. Subperiosteal hemorrhage and hematoma formation occur at the iliac crest. This injury, termed a "hip pointer,"[4,54,71] can be quite painful and should be differentiated from an avulsion injury or fracture.

Care must be taken not to allow return to athletic participation too soon to avoid reinjury. Injection of a local anesthetic and corticosteroid may be beneficial and allow for earlier return to sport.

Deep contusions within large muscles such as the gluteus maximus may cause significant hemorrhage, resulting in chronic bursitis, myositis ossificans, sciatic nerve injury, compartment syndrome, and infection. Chronic bursitis occurs frequently over the ischial tuberosity and greater trochanter and will usually resolve. Myositis ossificans should be suspected in a severe contusion of the quadriceps or adductor muscle groups that is not improving. Radiographs may not show calcification of the soft tissue. Initial treatment includes rest, active stretching, NSAIDs (indomethacin), and avoidance of local modalities. In addition to myositis ossificans, a severe blow to the buttock can result in sciatic nerve contusion. The pain frequently involves the entire distribution of the sciatic nerve, from the buttock to the foot. Gluteal compartment syndrome is rare but should be considered if the injury, pain, and swelling are severe.

Muscle and Tendon Injuries

Muscle and musculotendinous injuries are quite common around the pelvis and hip of the female athlete. Muscle strains and pulls about the pelvis compose most of these injuries. Strains or tears (partial or complete) of muscles or muscle–tendon units result from violent muscular contraction.[38] Any muscles that originate and insert on the pelvis or hip may be injured, causing significant disability. In the skeletally immature, an apophyseal injury at the bony origin must be considered. Knowledge of muscular origins and insertions aids in diagnosis (see Figs. 35-2 and 35-3). Muscles typically involved include the abdominal, iliopsoas, adductor, gluteal, iliac, sartorius, and rectus femoris muscles. Pain with isolated strength testing of the injured muscle will help clarify the diagnosis.

The frequency of muscle injury has resulted in the development of specific treatment protocols. Gross and coworkers[42] outlined a 5-phase treatment protocol based on the 4-stage plan presented by Sim and Scott.[91] The first phase involves rest, ice, compression, and protection, followed by a second phase that emphasizes regaining range of motion. Phase 3 is begun when the athlete is pain free, and the emphasis is on increasing strength, flexibility, and endurance. Dynamic-resistance exercises are initiated in phase 4. Phase 5 emphasizes coordination and proprioception. Sport-specific exercises are also started and return to full participation is allowed when all aspects of phase 5 are mastered by the athlete.

Groin Pull

Injuries to the adductor muscles are quite common, particularly in hockey players and soccer players, and are often referred to as "groin pulls." Adductor injury is caused by forced external rotation of an abducted leg. Weakness of the adductor muscles may predispose an athlete to this injury.[63] Further, muscles that span 2 joints, such as the gracilis, are susceptible to this type of injury. When injury does occur, pain is immediate and the athlete is unable to return to the activity. Tenderness can be palpated at the groin and pain increases with passive abduction and resisted adduction. Treatment follows the 5-phase protocol as described for muscle and tendon injuries. Stretching and strengthening of the adductor musculature has been advocated by some authors for prevention of groin pulls.[18,38,63,83] Reinjury is common.

Bursitis

A bursa is a sac-like structure filled with viscous fluid found in areas of the body that produce friction, such as over bony prominences and between tendons. The most commonly inflamed bursae are the trochanteric, iliopectineal, and ischial bursae. Sports that require repetitive hip motion result in pain and tenderness over the area of the bursa. Treatment generally involves anti-inflammatory medication, rest, and icing. Corticosteroid injection may also be beneficial.

Trochanteric bursitis must be considered in a female athlete with hip pain. Three bursae are associated with the greater trochanter of the hip, the largest being the gluteus maximus bursa, which lies just deep to gluteus maximus tendon fibers. The other, smaller bursae help protect the gluteus medius and minimus, respectively. Trochanteric bursitis can be an isolated or combined with other hip or pelvic pathology. Oftentimes the patient has had local trauma or repetitive activity, or has changed her running surface. On physical examination, the tenderness is localized over the greater trochanter and increases with external rotation and adduction of the hip. Athletes may describe a snapping sensation at the greater trochanter, which is a result of the iliotibial band passing over the greater trochanter.

Rest, anti-inflammatory medication, and stretching of the gluteal muscles and iliotibial band is initiated. Local injection of corticosteroids has been shown to be both diagnostic and therapeutic.[31,85,89] In rare instances, refractory cases have been found to respond to excision of a portion of the iliotibial band and débridement of the underlying bursae[109] or z-plasty.[15]

The "Snapping Hip"

"Snapping hip" refers to a constellation of problems that occur around and in the hip joint that cause a snapping sensation.[3,84] It may be the result of a wide variety of extra-articular as well as intra-articular pathologies. Most commonly it is associated with trochanteric bursitis, which causes the iliotibial band to snap over the greater trochanter. Other extra-articular causes include stenosing tenosynovitis of the iliopsoas tendon sheath, subluxation of the iliopsoas tendon over the iliopectineal eminence of the pelvis, iliofemoral ligaments over the femoral head, and tendinous origin of the long head of the biceps femoris muscle over the ischial tuberosity. Iliopsoas bursography may be helpful in confirming the diagnosis.[3,84]

HIP INTRA-ARTICULAR CONDITIONS

If an extra-articular entity is ruled out, intra-articular pathologies should be considered. These include loose bodies, synovial chondromatosis, subluxation of the hip, osteocartilaginous exostosis, and labral tears (Fig. 35-6).

Labral tears can occur as a result of a minor injury usually involving slipping or twisting. Often the athlete does not recall a particular incident. The athlete may present with a hip "click" and groin pain. These symptoms may be audible or palpable during the physical examina-

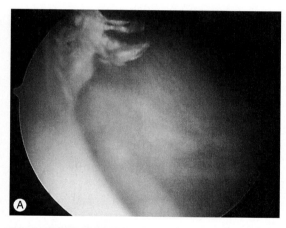

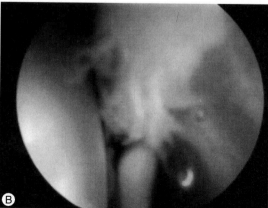

Figure 35-6. A. Posterosuperior acetabular labral tear. **B.** Superior labral tear displaced into the joint.

tion. An anterior labral tear may be identified with hip flexion, external rotation, and abduction followed by extension with internal rotation and adduction.[6] Radiographically, diagnosis of labral tears includes arthrography, MRI, high-resolution MRI, and MR arthrography. Initial treatment should include a brief period of rest followed by hip strengthening exercises. If conservative treatment fails, arthroscopic débridement of the labrum has been shown to be successful.[20,34] Return to sport following hip arthroscopy and labral débridement is allowed in 4 to 6 weeks if the athlete is symptom free.

OSTEITIS PUBIS

The pubic symphysis is a complex structure involving the interaction of fibrocartilage, muscle attachments, and ligaments. In the female, abnormalities at the pubic symphysis can be the result of congenital, metabolic, degenerative, traumatic, infectious, and inflammatory disorders. The female pubic symphysis is vertically shorter and the interposed fibrocartilage is wider.[7] Osteitis pubis should be considered in the female athlete who complains of groin or hip pain.

Osteitis pubis was first described by Beer[8] in 1924 in association with urologic procedures. It is a self-limiting inflammation of the pubic symphysis reported in runners, football players, soccer players, and weight lifters. There is no reported difference in incidence between genders. The constellation of symptoms includes most commonly gradual onset of pubic pain with radiation into the groin, medial aspect of the thigh, or abdomen. Other symptoms may include groin discomfort when climbing stairs, coughing, or sneezing. Physical examination often demonstrates symphysis tenderness, adductor muscle spasm with restricted abduction, pain on pelvic compression, and an antalgic gait. Radiographic evidence of osteitis pubis may not become evident until several weeks after the onset of pain. Depending on the severity of the case, radiographic findings may range from reactive sclerosis to superficial bone destruction (Fig. 35-7).

Bone scans are usually positive in athletes with osteitis pubis and will be positive earlier in the course of the problem than a radiograph. MRI findings demonstrate a high signal within the pubic symphysis and marrow edema in the surrounding bone early in its course.[98] Later, low signal is seen in both T_1- and T_2-weighted

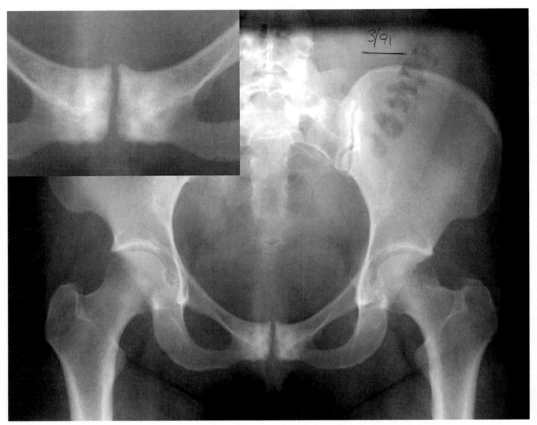

Figure 35-7. Osteitis pubis. This runner complained of pain centrally over her pubis. Acute roentgenograms showed sclerosis. After 12 months of conservative management, she was pain free.

images.[98] Biopsies of the affected area reveal fibrosis with minimal inflammation.[68]

The etiology of osteitis pubis is unknown at this time. However, in the female athlete it appears that repetitive trauma to the area is the source of the inflammation. Differential diagnosis in the athlete includes pubic or femoral stress fracture, inguinal hernia, isolated muscle tear, apophysitis, bony avulsion, genitourinary problem, nerve entrapment and osteomyelitis.

Treatment of osteitis pubis consists of rest, oral anti-inflammatory medication, and a functional rehabilitation program that should include pelvic and lower extremity stretching. Recovery may require many months. Athletes should not return to their sport until pain free. To decrease time away from sport, Holt and coworkers[45] suggest the use of corticosteroid injections into the affected area. A decrease in recovery time has been reported. Refractory cases should be treated with pubic symphysis débridement, excision, or fusion.[45] Surgery is rarely indicated and return to previous activity not predictable following surgery.

FRACTURES OF THE PELVIS AND HIP

Avulsion Fractures

Avulsion fractures of the hip and pelvis are more common in male athletes[35,94]; however, there is some evidence that this type of injury is increasing in women.[94] Generally, avulsion fractures of the hip and pelvis occur as a result of a sudden forceful stress across an open apophysis, therefore, they occur more often in adolescents. The incidence ranges from 4% to 13%.[22,80] Football players, soccer players, sprinters, and jumpers appear to be at greater risk for this injury.[64,103]

Athletes will report a sudden onset of pain and have tenderness and swelling in the affected area. Some may report previous symptoms in the area. A displaced fragment may be palpable on physical examination. Radiographs of the pelvis and hip may show the avulsed fragment and should be analyzed for fragment displacement. Comparison films of the contralateral side may be necessary to identify fractures and to assess the level of skeletal maturity. Chronic avulsion fractures may have abundant callus formation and should not be confused with tumor formation.

Generally, the current literature supports nonoperative treatment of avulsion fractures.[35,64,94] Metzmaker and Pappas[64] successfully treated 27 patients with avulsion fractures of the pelvis with a directed nonoperative program. Surgical open reduction and internal fixation has been described but is not widely advocated.[22] Athletes typically tolerate partial weight bearing and advance to athletic participation within 6 to 8 weeks if symptoms allow. Late or refractory cases may require surgical excision of the displaced fragment.

Avulsion fractures in the hip and pelvis occur at the ischial tuberosity, anterior superior iliac spine, anterior inferior iliac spine, iliac crest, and lesser and greater trochanters of the femur. Avulsion fractures of the ischial tuberosity are the most common and are caused by a forceful contraction of the hamstrings with the hip flexed and the knee extended (Fig. 35-8).[1,10,60,65] This type of injury is common in hurdlers and gymnasts.[86] Successful return to sport has been reported by most investiga-

tors[35,64,105]; however, Sundar and Carty[94] described 8 patients with ischial tuberosity avulsions who reported a reduction in athletic ability. Additionally, Schlonsky and Olix[86] reported on 2 sprinters who did not completely recover from their injury. Surgical intervention is uncommon but may be required in cases wide fracture separations[86] and of symptomatic excess callus formation at the avulsion site. In these avulsion injuries, treatment is similar, consisting of relative rest, ice, stretching, and functional rehabilitation program. Predictable return to sport is the rule.

Avulsions of the anterior superior iliac spine occur as a result of a forceful contraction of the sartorius muscle during jumping or running. Commonly, this occurs when the hip is extended and the knee is flexed.[22,81] Displacement of the bony fragment rarely occurs and is prevented by the fascia lata and the lateral aspect of the inguinal ligament.[81,82]

Avulsions of the anterior inferior iliac spine are less common. Earlier ossification of the anterior inferior iliac spine may contribute to the stability of this apophysis.[80,104,106] The mechanism of injury classically involves kicking, however, any activity that may cause forceful contraction of the straight head of the rectus femoris muscle

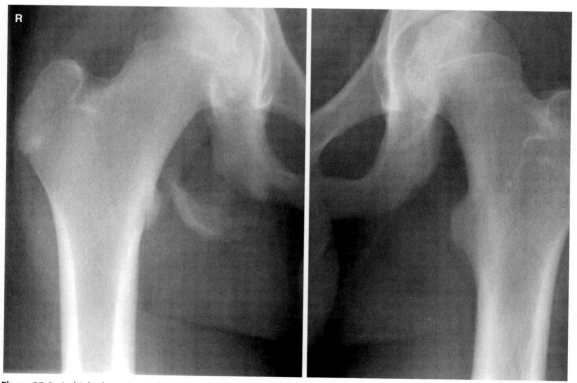

Figure 35-8. Ischial tuberosity avulsion fracture. This basketball player was running the court at end of practice and felt a pop and pain in her right buttock. Roentgenograms showed an avulsion fracture of ischial tuberosity. Treatment was use of crutches for 2 weeks, followed by gradual resumption of activities. She returned to full activity 9 months after sustaining this fracture.

may lead to this injury. Bilateral avulsions can occur and have been reported in a runner.[40] Displacement of the fragment is prevented by the intact reflected head of the rectus femoris and its insertion through the conjoined tendon.[22]

Iliac crest avulsion fractures have been reported to occur as a result of forceful contraction of the abdominal muscles and as a result of a direct blow.[19,41] Symptoms include pain and tenderness at the iliac crest. Bending at the torso and contraction of the abdominal muscles may cause pain. True avulsions may be confused with apophysitis or contusion. Radiographs including oblique views and comparison films of the unaffected side may be necessary to make the diagnosis.[41]

Avulsion fractures of the lesser and greater trochanter of the proximal femur can occur in the athlete. The lesser trochanter is the insertion site for the powerful iliopsoas muscle. Avulsions of the lesser trochanter occur as a result of forceful contraction of this muscle. Athletes who experience sudden and severe pain in the anteromedial thigh while running, jumping, or kicking should be evaluated for an avulsion fracture (Fig. 35-9). Athletes will have increased pain with resisted hip flexion. Radiographs will show the avulsed fragment. As with most avulsion fractures, treatment consists of rest, protective weight bearing, and rehabilitation.[28,30,74,77,95] At this time there are no indications for operative treatment. Return to sport is allowed at 6 to 8 weeks but up to 12 weeks may be required before full participation.[30,42]

The greater trochanter is the insertion site of the gluteus medius and minimus, and external rotators of the hip. Avulsion fractures of the greater trochanter are rare[5,62] but can occur with vigorous contraction of the abductor muscles.[25] Symptoms include pain over the greater trochanter and difficulty walking. In thin athletes a fracture fragment may be palpable. Radiographs of the hip will demonstrate the avulsed fragment. Treatment of greater trochanter avulsion is controversial. Several investigators recommend operative intervention, particularly if the fragment is displaced more than 1 cm.[5,28] Others recommend rest, protective weight bearing, and rehabilitation.[61] Regardless of treatment, full athletic participation is not allowed until the athlete is symptom free.

Stress Fractures

Stress fractures were first diagnosed clinically by the Prussian surgeon Breithraupt in 1855.[14] The definition of a stress fracture has evolved along

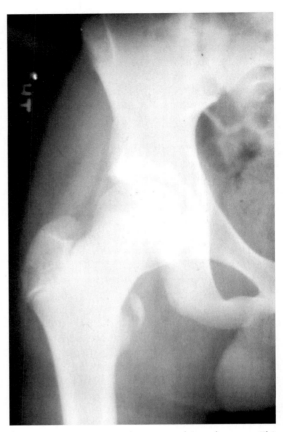

Figure 35-9. Lesser trochanter avulsion fracture. This softball player felt a rip and pain in her groin while running bases. Roentgenography confirmed lesser trochanter avulsion fracture.

with the advances in radiologic imaging of bone. Today, stress injury to the bone is thought to lie on a continuum ranging from normal bone remodeling to cortical disruption.[51] A stress fracture can, therefore, be defined as a partial or completed fracture of the bone resulting from the bone's inability to withstand non-violent stress that is applied in a rhythmic, repeated, subthreshold manner.[59]

Female athletes appear to be more susceptible to stress fractures than their male counterparts. They have been reported to have an increased risk of 1.5 to 3.5 times that of male athletes.[16,39,72,108] Military studies have also shown that females have a greater incidence of stress fractures when compared to men.[43,44,78,107] In addition, studies suggest that pelvic,[9,47] femoral,[9] and metatarsal[9,47,73] stress fractures are more common in women. It is not well understood whether these results are due to gender inherently or simply to sex-related factors. However, if a pelvic or hip stress fracture occurs in a female athlete, contributing factors such as levels of hormones, bone density, diet, training program, and fitness level must be evaluated by the clinician.

Pelvic Stress Fractures

Stress fractures of the pelvis are very rare and are reported to account for 1% to 5% of all stress fractures that occur as a result of running or track and field.[9,73,93] Most pelvic stress fractures occur in joggers and runners, however, they have also been reported in bowling and during gymnastic activities.[27] Within the pelvis, stress fractures occur most often in the inferior pubic ramus medially close to the pubic symphysis.[44,75,93] They have also been reported in the superior pubic ramus[73,88] and even more rarely in the sacrum.[61,100]

As reported in the literature, women appear to be more susceptible to pelvic stress fractures than men. Anatomic differences in the female pelvis such as smaller bones and a wider pelvis do not account for the high tensile stresses in the pelvis that would lead to a stress reaction or fracture. Pavlov and coworkers[75] suggest that differences in gait between men and women may account for the increase in tension in the pubic rami. She states that the female runner relies on hip-extension forces more than the male runner. In doing so, the female pelvis would potentially be presented with an increase in tensile stresses leading to a stress fracture. Latshaw and coworkers[55] suggest that during the alternating phases of running, the ischial pubic ramus is stressed by the forces produced by the external rotators and adductor muscles of the hip joint during the swing phase and stance phase of running. Thus, the repetitive insult to the pubic arch would lead to stress fracture or reaction. Differences in female anatomy and running style may increase the risk for development of a stress fracture, however, to date, there is no scientific support for these hypotheses. Additional research in this area is necessary and may potentially impact female running styles and training regimens.

Athletes with pelvic stress fractures usually complain of pain in the inguinal, peroneal, or adductor regions. As with most stress fractures, the pain increases with continued activity and decreases with periods of rest. On physical examination athletes may have a limp, pain with palpation of the hip or groin, and pain with hip rotation. It may be difficult to differentiate the athlete's diagnosis from referred pain from the lumbar spine, adductor tendinitis, trochanteric bursitis, osteitis pubis, or visceral pain. Noakes and coworkers[69] suggested that the presence of a "positive standing sign" in which a patient has difficulty standing unsupported on the affected side. In addition, he suggested that the positive standing sign, groin pain sufficient enough to prevent running, and exquisite tenderness localized only to the affected inferior pubic ramus were diagnostic of an inferior pubic ramus stress fracture. Regardless of other diagnostic signs, a pelvic stress fracture should be considered in a female athlete with groin pain, an intense workout schedule, an abnormal menstrual history, or disordered eating.

After a careful history and physical examination, an anteroposterior pelvic roentgenogram should be taken. If a sacral stress fracture is suspected, sacral views should also be evaluated. If the onset of symptoms is recent, initial roentgenograms are normal. Long-standing problems may show callus formation at the fracture site. A bone scan should be ordered early. MRI has now become another diagnostic tool for early diagnosis of a stress reaction or stress fracture.

Treatment includes cessation of any symptom causing activity. Training in other activities to maintain aerobic health such as bicycle riding and swimming may continue if the athlete is pain free. Other issues, including intrinsic and extrinsic mechanical factors, amenorrhea, oligomenorrhea, and nutritional problems, must be adequately addressed by the appropriate caregiver. Unfortunately for the athlete, pelvic stress fractures may require longer periods of rest than other lower extremity stress fractures. Pavlov and coworkers,[75] in their series of 12 runners with inferior pubic ramus stress fractures, found 10 runners who were clinically asymptomatic 2 to 5 months after cessation of running. Two runners continued to run and had symptoms for 13 and 27 months, respectively. Therefore, athletes must be counseled on the severity of their injury and given realistic goals for returning to their sport. Return to sport should be gradual and full participation is allowed when the athlete is pain free.

Sacral Stress Fractures

Sacral stress fractures are more common in the elderly and in those with predisposing factors such as idiopathic osteoporosis and osteoporosis associated with radiation, steroids, or malignancy.[2,23,26,57] A small number of cases have been reported in female athletes[61] and military recruits.[100] Sacral stress fractures most commonly occur in runners or those involved in running sports.[61] In runners, sacral stress fractures are believed to be the result of cyclic loading of the sacrum.[46]

Sacral stress fracture should be considered if complaints include low back pain, or pain radiating into the buttock or groin or down the leg. The vast array of symptoms may be caused by irritation of the cauda equina or sacral nerve roots, and diagnosis based on physical examination may be difficult. There may be only localized tenderness over the sacrum and sacroiliac joint. Radiographs of the pelvis and sacrum are typically normal. Additional radiographic studies including bone scan and MRI may be necessary to confirm the diagnosis (Fig. 35-10). Treatment involves rest and gradual return to sport if pain free. Cycling or pool running is allowed during the rest period to maintain strength and aerobic capacity. As with other stress fractures in the female athlete, a multidisciplinary approach may be necessary. Fortunately, most athletes fully recover from this injury without sequelae.

Femoral Stress Fractures

As with stress fractures of the pelvis, stress fractures of the femur are rare.[56] The reported incidence ranges from 7% to 20%.[49,58] However, if missed, femoral stress fractures have a high complication rate. They can occur in the femoral neck, shaft, and condyles. As with other pelvic stress fractures, a femoral neck stress fracture should be considered in an athlete with groin pain.

Clinically, athletes will complain of groin or hip pain that is increased with activity. They may limp. Hip range of motion may be painful and limited, especially in internal rotation. Overlying soft tissue may make bony tenderness difficult to elicit on physical examination. Athletes may present with bilateral symptoms, therefore, roentgenograms should be taken of both hips and the pelvis. If roentgenograms do not demonstrate a fracture and one is suspected, a bone scan may also be performed to rule out a stress fracture. Despite being more expensive, MRI is becoming the standard for diagnosing hip pain in athletes. It has been shown to be more accurate and can demonstrate a fracture earlier without exposing the athlete to radiation. Shin and coworkers[90] reported 100% accuracy in diagnosing femoral neck fractures with MRI and only 68% accuracy with radionucleotide bone scanning.

To date, the biomechanics of femoral neck stress fractures are not fully understood. During walking or running loads on the femoral head can exceed 3 to 5 times body weight. During prolonged or repetitive activity hip musculature becomes weakened and fatigued and no longer can provide a protective shock absorbing effect. This may lead to increased stress on the femoral neck. Additional factors such as a congenital hip deformity may predispose an athlete to femoral neck stress fracture. As with pelvic stress fractures, training regimen, shoe wear, training facility, menstrual irregularities, osteopenia, and eating or nutritional disorders play a role in the development of the fracture.

Devas[29] first classified femoral neck fractures into 2 different types: tension and compression (Figs. 35-11 and 35-12). A tension femoral neck fracture occurs on the superolateral aspect of the neck and is at increased risk for fracture displacement. A compression femoral neck fracture occurs on the inferomedial aspect of the femoral neck and is thought to be mechanically stable. In 1966, Blickenstaff and Morris[11] classified femoral neck fractures by the appearance of a fracture line and fracture displacement. Type 1 had periosteal reaction or callus formation along the inferior neck and no evidence of a fracture line; type 2 was a nondisplaced fracture across the femoral neck or calcar; and type 3 was a displaced fracture. They did not take into account

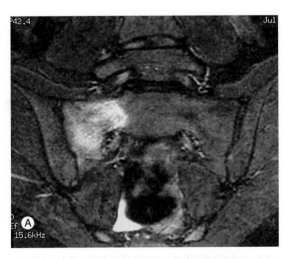

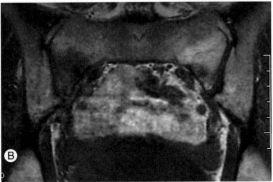

Figure 35-10. Sacral stress fracture. **A.** MRI scan of the sacrum of a 20-year-old female distance runner. **B.** MRI scan of the sacrum of a 22-year-old female distance runner.

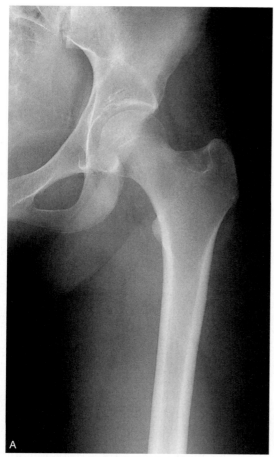

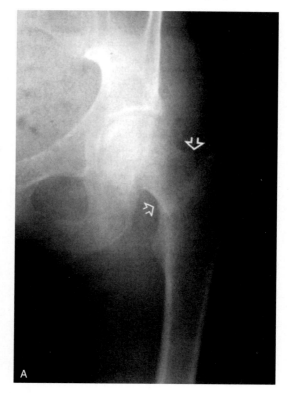

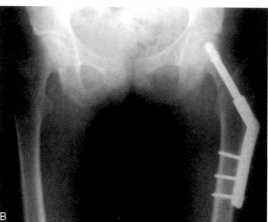

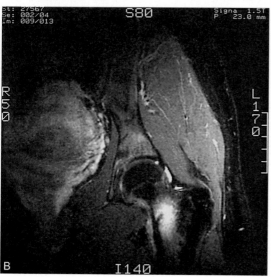

Figure 35-11. Femoral neck stress fracture in a female distance runner. **A.** Normal roentgenogram of hip. **B.** MRI scan of a compression femoral neck fracture.

Figure 35-12. Femoral neck stress fracture in a female distance runner. **A.** Displaced tension-sided femoral neck stress fracture. **B.** Fracture treated with internal fixation. (From Anderson K, Strickland SM, Warren R: Hip and groin injuries in athletes. Am J Sports Med 29:521–33, 2001, with permission.)

the position of the fracture line within the femoral neck. More recently, Fullerton and Snowdy[36] have modified Devas' classification to include a third type of stress fracture—the displaced femoral neck fracture.

Treatment of femoral neck stress fractures depends on the type of stress fracture. Compression (medial side) stress fractures are stable. The treatment is a period of rest and non-weight bearing for several months until the athlete is pain free. Radiographs should be taken at regular intervals to ensure no change of position and to monitor fracture healing. If healing does not occur or refracture occurs, internal fixation is required. Tension (superior side) femoral neck stress fractures are inherently unstable and require immediate internal fixation with multiple hip pins or screws (Fig. 35-12).[12,32] Nonoperative treatment may lead to fracture displacement. Complications of displaced femoral neck fractures can be career ending and include nonunion, delayed union, varus deformity, and avascular necrosis. Displaced femoral neck stress fractures require immediate open reduction and internal fixation. Return to sport after internal fixation of the hip should be gradual and depend on the symptoms and radiologic findings.

FRACTURES OF THE PELVIS

Fortunately, other than avulsion fractures and stress fractures, fractures of the pelvic ring are rare[103] in athletes. They have, however, been reported in cycling[50] and hang gliding.[53] Female athletes who participate in contact sports are also at risk for pelvic fracture. Athletes who sustain pelvic fractures must be resuscitated, stabilized, and transferred to a medical facility for appropriate evaluation.[17] Careful evaluation of the athlete for other long bone injuries and visceral injuries is important.[17] Although minor pelvic fractures may only require non-weight-bearing treatment, severe injury may require external fixation, open reduction and internal fixation, or both.[17] Time to return to sport will depend on the severity of the injury. Severe pelvic trauma will require a long period of rehabilitation. Athletes with this type of injury may be unable to successfully return to their sport. Further discussion of the classification and surgical management of pelvic fractures is beyond the scope of this chapter.

Coccyx Fractures

The coccyx is composed of the last 4 or 5 rudimentary vertebrae. Its position makes it susceptible to injury from a backward fall or kick to the area. The athlete will report pain and tenderness in the region. Local swelling and ecchymosis may be evident. Roentgenograms will confirm the diagnosis. Treatment should include ice, rest, and pain medication. Cessation of athletic activity is advised until pain has decreased. A doughnut cushion will provide some comfort while sitting. Athletes may return to sport as tolerated with appropriate padding. Although rare, cases of painful nonunion and disability may require excision of the fracture fragment.

Hip Fractures

Hip fractures require a great deal of force and are, therefore, not common on the athletic field. At this time there are no reported gender differences with respect to hip fractures that occur in athletic participation. Although rare, fractures of the hip must be considered if the athlete has an inability to move and a shortened and externally rotated leg. After careful neurovascular examination, the athlete should be immobilized, not allowed to move, and transported to a hospital emergency department for further evaluation and radiography.

Femoral neck and subcapital hip fractures are classified by fracture pattern and the amount of displacement.[28] Intertrochanteric fractures are rare in this population. Surgery is required. A wide variety of internal fixation devices are available and include multiple parallel pins or screws, sliding hip screws, and hemiarthroplasty.

An acute femoral neck fracture in the young adult is very rare, but when it occurs it is an orthopaedic emergency because of the risk of avascular necrosis of the femoral head. Pediatric hip fractures, as described by Delbert and reported by Colonna,[24] are classified as transepiphyseal, transcervical, cervicotrochanteric, and trochanteric. Transepiphyseal fractures cross the growth plate and, therefore, rates of avascular necrosis reach 100% with this type of injury. Treatment ranges from closed reduction with spica casting to transphyseal pinning.[21,48,79] Regardless of treatment results are generally poor. Transcervical fractures are generally treated with closed reduction and internal fixation with pins. Care must be taken to use smooth pins when crossing the physis with fixation. The rates of osteonecrosis from this injury range from 15% to 50%. Cervicotrochanteric fractures result in avascular necrosis 30% to 40% of the time. Intertrochanteric fractures are the least complicated of pediatric hip fractures and are treated with internal fixation. The incidence of avascular necrosis in this type of fracture is the lowest. Return to sport is dependent on fracture type, treatment, and healing.

DISLOCATION OF THE HIP

Dislocations of the hip require very large forces and are rare in the athletic population. However, a dislocation of the hip is a true orthopaedic emergency. When the hip is dislocated the blood supply to the femoral head and the sciatic nerve is compromised. Therefore, prompt intervention is required.

Hip dislocations can be anterior, posterior, and central. Posterior dislocations of the hip are the most common.[101] Thompson and Epstein[96] classified them into 5 different types taking into account associated fractures of the acetabulum and femoral head. Type V posterior dislocations of the hip have been further classified by Pipkin[76] into 4 different types depending on the type of femoral head fracture and whether or not there is an associated acetabular fracture. Anterior hip dislocations have been classified by Epstein[33] into superior and inferior dislocations with or without associated fractures of the femoral head, neck, or acetabulum. They account for 8% to 15% of hip dislocations.[87] Central hip dislocations require severe disruption of the acetabulum and are rare.

Athletes with hip dislocation complain of intense pain and inability to move the affected hip. On inspection of the leg, deformity will be apparent. In a posterior hip dislocation, the leg will be in a position of flexion, adduction, and internal rotation. Anterior dislocations will present with the limb extended, abducted, and externally rotated. Neurovascular status of the limb must be determined immediately. The athlete should be transferred to an appropriate medical facility and roentgenograms of the hip and pelvis obtained. Care must be taken to assess surrounding joints, including the knee, for any associated fracture or ligament damage. Closed reduction with adequate sedation is performed emergently. Due to the speed at which reduction must be completed, computed tomography is not usually recommended prior to reduction maneuvers.

Postreduction roentgenograms and computed tomography should be obtained to determine adequacy of reduction, to rule out any intra-articular bony fragments and to assess the acetabulum. Postreduction stability testing is performed. If the hip is stable and there is no other bony pathology, 48 hours of gentle traction followed by range of motion and ambulation with crutches is initiated. This generally involves advancement to full weight bearing over 3 to 4 weeks. Follow-up roentgenograms are essential to assess the hip for signs of avascular necrosis. Epstein[33] recommends follow-up roentgenograms every 3 months for the first year and every 6 months for the following 2 years. MRI may lead to earlier diagnosis of avascular necrosis. For patients with loose bodies in the joint after reduction of the hip, arthroscopic surgery or open removal of the fragments is indicated. Athletes with hip instability due to associated acetabular or femoral head fractures will require open reduction and internal fixation.

Complications of hip dislocation include avascular necrosis of the femoral head and neurologic injury. The incidence of avascular necrosis is directly related to amount of time the hip remained dislocated. Additionally, sciatic nerve injury may occur with posterior dislocations and femoral nerve injury may occur with anterior dislocations. Return to sport after this injury depends on the severity of the injury and the athlete's progress in a rehabilitation program. Recurrence of the instability is rare but if it does occur would require an open capsular repair of the hip.[67,87]

CONCLUDING REMARKS

To prevent injuries about the hip and pelvis from becoming recurrent and chronic, it is very important to make a precise and early diagnosis when an athlete presents. A bone scan is indicated early on if there is groin pain in a runner to rule out stress fracture. Fortunately, more significant fractures of the femoral neck in a trochanteric level are unusual in sport but are being seen earlier in female athletes because of osteoporosis or insufficiency origin. Institution of a core strengthening program that emphasizes abdominal lumbosacral pelvic position and strength is critical in the female athlete. With a stable core and preprogram position, with pelvis position backward, rotated, the stage is set for healthy participation in sports. Prevention of lower extremity injuries starts at the pelvis with strengthening and proper position of the pelvis and sacrum.

References

1. Abbate CC: Avulsion fracture of the ischial tuberosity: A case report. J Bone Joint Surg 27:716, 1945.
2. Abe H, Nakamura M, Takahashi S, et al: Radiation-induced insufficiency fractures of the pelvis: Evaluation with Tc-methylene diphosphonate scintigraphy. Am J Radiol 158:599–602, 1992.
3. Allen WC, Cope R: Coxa saltans: The snapping hip revisited. J Am Acad Orthop Surg 3:303–8, 1995.
4. American Medical Association, Subcommittee on Classification of Sports Injuries: Standard Nomenclature of Athletic Injuries. Chicago, American Medical Association, 1966.
5. Armstrong GE: Isolated fracture of the greater trochanter. Ann Surg 46:292–7, 1907.
6. Anderson K, Strickland SM, Warren R: Hip and groin injuries in athletes. Am J Sports Med 29(4):521–33, 2001.
7. Basmajian JV: Female pelvis. In Grant's Method of Anatomy. By Regions Descriptive and Deductive, 10th edition. Baltimore, Williams & Wilkins, 1980, pp 227–37.
8. Beer E: Periostitis and osteitis of the symphysis pubis following suprapubic cystotomies. J Urol 20:233, 1928.

9. Bennell KL, Malcolm SA, Thomas SA, et al: The incidence and distribution of stress fractures in competitive track and field athletes: A twelve month prospective. Am J Sports Med 24:211–7, 1996.
10. Berry JM: Fracture of the tuberosity of the ischium due to muscular action. JAMA 59:1450, 1912.
11. Blickenstaff LD, Morris JM: Fatigue fractures of the femoral neck. J Bone Joint Surgery 48A:103–4, 1966.
12. Boden BP, Speer KP: Femoral stress fractures. Clin Sports Med 16: 307–17, 1997.
13. Boyd KT, Pierce NS, Batt ME: Common hip injuries in sport. Sports Med 24:273–88, 1997.
14. Breithaupt MD: Zur pathologie des menschlichen fusses. Med Z 24:169, 1855.
15. Brignall CG, Stainsby GD: The snapping hip. Treatment by Z-plasty. J Bone Joint Surg 73B(2):253–4, 1991.
16. Brunet ME, Cook SD, Brinker MR, Dickinson JA: A survey of running injuries in 1505 competitive and recreational runners. J Sports Med Phys Fitness 30:307–15, 1990.
17. Burgess AR, Tile M: Fractures of the pelvis. In Rockwood CA Jr, Green DP, Bucholz RW (Eds): Fractures in Adults. Philadelphia, JB Lippincott, 1991, pp 1399–1479.
18. Burkett LN: Causative factors in hamstring strains. Med Sci Sports 2:39–42, 1970.
19. Butler JE, Eggert AW: Fracture of the iliac crest apophysis: An unusual hip pointer. Am J Sports Med 3:192–3, 1975.
20. Byrd JW, Jones KS: Prospective analysis of hip arthroscopy with 2 year follow-up. Arthroscopy 16(6):578–87, 2000.
21. Canale ST, Bourland WL: Fractures of the neck and intertrochanteric region of the femur in children. J Bone Joint Surg 59A:431–43, 1977.
22. Canale ST, King RE: Pelvic and hip fractures. In Rockwood C A Jr, Wilkins KE, King RE (eds): Fractures of Children. Philadelphia, JB Lippincott, 1991.
23. Carter SR: Stress fracture of the sacrum: A brief report. J Bone Joint Surg 69B:843–4, 1987.
24. Colonna PC: Fractures of the neck of the femur in children. Am J Surg 6:793, 1929.
25. Combs JA: Hip and pelvis avulsion fractures in adolescents. Physician Sportsmed 22(7):41–9, 1994.
26. Cooper KL, Beabout JW, Swee RG: Insufficiency fractures of the sacrum. Radiology 156:15–20, 1985.
27. Daffner RH, Pavlov H: Stress fractures: Current concepts. Am J Roentgenol 159:245–52, 1992.
28. Delee JC: Fractures and dislocations of the hip. In Rockwood CA Jr, Green DP, Bucholz RW (Eds): Fractures in Adults. Philadelphia, JB Lippincott, 1991.
29. Devas MB: Stress fractures of the femoral neck. J Bone Joint Surg 47B:728, 1965.
30. Dimon JH III: Isolated fractures of the lesser trochanter of the femur. Clin Orthop 82:144–8, 1972.
31. Ege Rasmussen KJ, Fan N: Trochanteric bursitis: Treatment with corticosteroid injection. Scand J Rheumatol 14:417–20, 1985.
32. Egol KA, Koval KJ, Kummer F, Frankel VH: Stress fracture of the femoral neck. Clin Orthop 348:72–8, 1998.
33. Epstein HC: Traumatic dislocations of the hip. Clin Orthop 91:116, 1973.
34. Farjo LA, Glick JM, Sampson TG: Hip arthroscopy for acetabular labral tears. Arthroscopy 15(2):132–7, 1999.
35. Fernbach SK, Wilkinson RH: Avulsion injuries of the pelvis and proximal femur. Am J Roentgenol 137:581–4, 1984.
36. Fullerton LR, Snowdy HA: Femoral neck stress fractures. Am J Sports Med 16:365–77, 1988.
37. Gardener E, Gray DJ, O'Rahilly R: Anatomy, A Regional Study of Human Structure. Philadelphia, WB Saunders, 1975.
38. Garrett WE, Safran MR, Seaber AV, et al: Biomechanical comparison of stimulated and nonstimulated muscle pulled to failure. Am J Sports Med 15:448–54, 1987.
39. Goldberg B, Pecora C: Stress fractures: A risk of increased training in freshman. Physician Sportsmed 22:68–78, 1994.
40. Gomez JE: Bilateral anterior inferior iliac spine avulsion fractures. Med Sci Sports Exerc 28:161–4, 1996.
41. Goodshall RW, Hansen CA: Incomplete avulsion of a portion of the iliac epiphysis: An injury of young athletes. J Bone Joint Surg 55A:1301–2, 1973.
42. Gross ML, Nassar S, Finerman GAM: Hip and pelvis. In Delee JC, Drez D (Eds): Orthopaedic Sports Medicine: Principles and Practice. Philadelphia, WB Saunders, 1994.
43. Ha KI, Hahn SH, Chung M, et al: A clinical study of stress fractures in sports activities. Orthopaedics 14:1089–95, 1991.
44. Hill PF, Chatterji S, Chambers D, Keeling JD: Stress fracture of the pubic ramus in female recruits. J Bone Joint Surg 78B:383–6, 1996.
45. Holt MA, Keene JS, Graf BK, Helwig DC: Treatment of osteitis pubis in athletes: Results of corticosteroid injections. Am J Sports Med 23:601–6, 1995.
46. Holtzhausen LM, Noakes TD: Stress fracture of the sacrum in two distance runners. Clin J Sports Med 2:139–42, 1992.
47. Hulkko A, Orava S: Stress fractures in athletes. Int J Sports Med 8:221–6, 1987.
48. Ingram AJ, Bachynski B: Fractures of the hip in children. Treatment and results. J Bone Joint Surg 35A:867, 1953.
49. Johnson AW, Weiss CB, Wheeler DL: Stress fractures of the femoral shaft in athletes—more common than expected. Am J Sports Med 22:248–56, 1994.
50. Judet R, Judet J, Letournel E: Fractures of the acetabulum: Classification and surgical approaches for open reduction. J Bone Joint Surg 46A:1615–46, 1964.
51. Keats TE: Radiology of Musculoskeletal Stress Injury. Chicago, Year Book Medical Publishers, 1990.
52. Kersnic B, Iglic A, Kralj-Iglic V, et al: Increased incidence of arthrosis in women could be related to femoral and pelvic shape. Arch Orthop Trauma Surg 116:345–7, 1997.
53. Krissoff WB: Follow-up on hang gliding injuries in Colorado. Am J Sports Med 4:222–9, 1976.
54. Kulund DN: The Injured Athlete. Philadelphia, JB Lippincott, 1982.
55. Latshaw RF, Kantner TR, Kalenak A, et al: A pelvic stress fracture in a female jogger. Am J Sports Med 9:54–6, 1981.
56. Lombardo SJ, Benson DW: Stress fractures of the femur in runners. Am J Sports Med 10:219–27, 1982.
57. Lourie H: Spontaneous osteoporotic fracture of the sacrum. JAMA 248:715–7, 1982.
58. Matheson GO, Clement DM, McKenzie DC, et al: Stress fractures in athletes: A study of 320 cases. Am J Sports Med 15:46–58, 1987.
59. McBryde AM: Stress fractures in athletes. Am J Sports Med 5:212, 1976.
60. McCleod SB, Lewin P: Avulsion of the epiphysis of the tuberosity of the ischium. JAMA 92:1957, 1929.
61. McFarland EG, Giangarra C: Sacral stress fractures in athletes. Clin Orthop 329:240–3, 1996.
62. Merlino AF, Nixon JE: Isolated fractures of the greater trochanter: Report of twelve cases. Int Surg 52:117–24, 1969.

63. Merrifield HH, Cowan RF: Groin strain injuries in ice hockey. J Sports Med 1:41–2, 1973.
64. Metzmaker JN, Pappas AM: Avulsion fractures of the pelvis. Am J Sports Med 13:349–58, 1985.
65. Milch H: Avulsion fracture of the tuberosity of the ischium. J Bone Joint Surg 8:832, 1926.
66. Morris JM: Biomechanical aspects of the hip joint. Orthop Clin North Am 2:33–54, 1971.
67. Nelson CL: Traumatic redislocation of the hip. J Bone Joint Surg 52A:128–30, 1970.
68. Nicholas JA, Hershman EB: The Lower Extremity and Spine in Sports Medicine. St Louis, Mosby, 1986, pp 1151–2.
69. Noakes TD, Smith JA, Lindenberg G: Pelvis stress fractures in long distance runners. Am J Sports Med 13:120–3, 1985.
70. Nordin M, Frankel VH: Biomechanics of the hip. In Frankel V. H, Burstein AH (Eds): Orthopaedic Biomechanics. Philadelphia, Lea & Febiger, 1970.
71. O'Donoghe DH: Treatment of Injuries to Athletes. Philadelphia, WB Saunders, 1970.
72. O'Toole ML: Prevention and treatment of injuries to runners. Med Sci Sports Exerc 24:360–3, 1992.
73. Orava S, Puranen J, Ala-Ketola L: Stress fractures caused by physical exercise. Acta Orthop Scand 9:19, 1978.
74. Paletta GA, Andrish JT: Injuries about the hip and pelvis in the young athlete. Clin Sports Med 14:591–628, 1995.
75. Pavlov H, Nelson TL, Warren RF, et al: Stress fractures of the pubic ramus. J Bone Joint Surg 64A:1020–5, 1982.
76. Pipkin G: Treatment of grade IV fracture—dislocation of the hip, J Bone Joint Surg 39:1027–42, 1957.
77. Poston H: Traction fracture of the lesser trochanter of the femur. Br J Surg 9:256, 1921.
78. Protzman RR, Griffis CC: Comparative stress fracture incidence in males and females in equal training environment. Athletic Training 12:126–30, 1997.
79. Ratliff AHC: Fractures of the neck of the femur in children. J Bone Joint Surg 44B:528–42, 1962.
80. Reed MH: Pelvic fractures in children. J Can Assoc Radiol 27:255–61, 1976.
81. Robertson RC: Fracture of the anterior superior iliac spine of the ilium. J Bone Joint Surg 17:1045, 1935.
82. Russ LV, Rush HL: Avulsion of the anterior superior spine of the ilium. J Bone Joint Surg 21:206, 1939.
83. Safran MR, Garrett WE, Seaber AV, et al: The role of warm-up in muscular injury and prevention, Am J Sports Med 16:126–9,1988.
84. Schaberg JE, Harper MC, Allen WC: The snapping hip syndrome. Am J Sports Med 12 (5):361–5, 1984.
85. Schapira D, Menachem N, Scharf Y: Trochanteric bursitis: A common clinical problem. Arch Phys Med Rehabil 67:815–7, 1986.
86. Schlonsky J, Olix ML: Functional disability following avulsion fracture of the ischial epiphysis. J Bone Joint Surg 54A:641–4, 1972.
87. Scudese VA: Traumatic anterior hip redislocation. Clin Orthop 88:60–3, 1972.
88. Selakovich W, Love L: Stress fractures of the pubis ramus. J Bone Joint Surg 36A:573–6, 1954.

89. Shbeeb MI, O'Duffy JD, Michet Jr, et al: Evaluation of glucocorticoid injection for the treatment of trochanteric bursitis J Rheumatol 23:2104–6, 1996.
90. Shin AY, Morin WD, Gorman JD, et al: The superiority of magnetic resonance imaging in differentiating the cause of hip pain in endurance athletes. Am J Sports Med 24:168–76, 1996.
91. Sim FH, Scott HG: Injuries of the pelvis and hip in athletes. In Nicholas JA, Hershmann EB (Eds): The Lower Extremity and Spine in Sports Medicine. St Louis, CV Mosby, 1986.
92. Staheli LT, Corbett M, Wyss C, King H: Lower extremity rotation problems in children: Normal values to guide management. J Bone Joint Surg 67-A:39–47, 1985.
93. Sullivan D, Warren R, Pavlov H, Kelman G: Stress fractures in 51 runners. Clin Orthop 187:188–92, 1984.
94. Sundar M, Carty H: Avulsion fracture of the pelvis in children: A report of 32 fractures and their outcome. Skeletal Radiology 23(2):85–90, 1994.
95. Sweetman RJ: Avulsion fracture of the lesser trochanter. Nursing Times 68:122–3, 1973.
96. Thompson VP, Epstein HC: Traumatic dislocation of the hip. J Bone Joint Surg 33A:746–78, 1951.
97. Tonnis D, Heinecke A: Acetabular and femoral anteversion: Relationship with osteoarthritis of the hip. J Bone Joint Surg 81A(12):1747–70, 1999.
98. Tuite MJ, De Smet AA: MRI of selected sports injuries; Muscle tears, groin pain and osteochondritis dessicans Semin Ultrasound CT MR 15:318–40, 1994.
99. Vleeming A, Snijders SF, Stoeckart R, Mens JMA: The role of the sacroiliac joints in coupling between spine, pelvis, legs and arms. In Vleeming A, Mooney V, Snijders CJ, et al: Movement, Stability and Low Back Pain: The Essential Role of the Pelvis. New York, Churchill Livingstone, 1997, pp 53–71.
100. Volpin G, Milgrom C, Goldsher D, et al: Stress fractures of the sacrum following strenuous activity. Clin Orthop 243:184–8, 1989.
101. Walsh ZT, Micheli LJ: Hip dislocation in a high school football player. Physician Sportsmed 17:112, 1989.
102. Watanabe RS: Embryology of the human hip. Clin Orthop 98:8–26, 1974.
103. Waters PM, Millis MB: Hip and pelvic injuries in the young athlete. Clin Sports Med 7:513–26, 1988.
104. Watson-Jones R: Dislocations and fracture dislocations of the pelvis. Br J Surg 25:773, 1938.
105. Watts HG: Fractures of the pelvis in children. Orthop Clin North Am 7:615, 176.
106. Weitzner I: Fractures of the anterior superior spine of the ilium in one case and anterior inferior in another case. Am J Roentgenol 33:39, 1935.
107. Winfield AC, Moore J, Bracker M, Johnson CW: Risk factors associated with stress reactions in female marines. Mil Med 162:698, 1997.
108. Zernicke R, McNitt-Gray J, Otis C, et al: Stress fracture risk assessment among elite collegiate women runners. International Society of Biomechanics XIVth Congress, 1993, pp 1506–1507.
109. Zoltan DJ, Clancy WG, Keene JS: A new operative approach to snapping hip and refractory trochanteric bursitis in athletes. Am J Sports Med 14:201–4, 1986.

Chapter 36

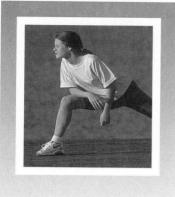

Knee Injuries

Mark R. Hutchinson, M.D.
Richard I. Williams, M.D.
Mary Lloyd Ireland, M.D.

The knee accounts for a significant portion of injuries in most sports for both genders. The knee is the largest joint in the body. It is a complex interaction of ligament restraints, active muscle motors, and mobile and immobile articulating surfaces that allow the athlete to flex, extend, twist, cut, run, jump, and squat. The functional demands upon the knee are specific for each sport and not specific to each gender. A female basketball player needs to run, jump, stop, twist, and cut just like a male basketball player. A female swimmer performs the same breaststroke whip kick as her male counterpart. Nonetheless, knee injury patterns are different between males and females. These differences may be related to variations in levels of conditioning, variations in the performance of proper techniques, differences in style, and differences in anatomic structure. The purpose of this chapter is to discuss knee injuries in the female athlete.

EPIDEMIOLOGY

With added accessibility, encouragement, and an increased focus on fitness over the past few decades, women's participation in organized and recreational sports has increased drastically. A proportional increase in the incidence of sport-related injuries in women has also been noted.[26,33,69,87] However, the increase in total number of injuries can't be explained only by the increasing number of participants. Compared to males, females have increased risk for certain types of injuries and specifically certain types of injuries about the knee.[5,36]

The increased incidence of noncontact anterior cruciate ligament (ACL) injuries in females compared to males has been reported in basketball,[2,3,8,29,51,75,102,103] soccer,[2,3,7,62,75] skiing,[77,95] team handball,[73] and netball.[38,67]

Epidemiology studies must have enough numbers—athletes with ACL tears—over several seasons to develop the power to determine ACL injury rate. The incidence of injury is reported as the number of ACL injuries (numerator) divided by a denominator that represents the number of "athlete exposures" (hours of sport, number of participants, games/practices, etc.).

Studies comparing knee injuries in males and females at the high school, college, Olympic, and professional levels have been published. A summary of those studies was recently published.[48] In studies reported from the San Antonio, Texas, high school system, girls' basketball athletes sustained more knee injuries that required surgery than boys' basketball and football athletes.[19,29] Comparing 3 high school sports, there was a greater need for knee surgery in girls' basketball than boys' football (1.3 times) and boys' basketball (3 times).[19,68,73] In an Iowa high school study, comparing basketball athletes, girls were more likely to be hurt in a game and to have a serious knee injury than boys.[103]

Clarke and Buckley presented data from the National Injury/Illness Reporting System from 1975 to 1978 that showed that knee injuries make up a greater proportion of significant injuries for females in most gender comparable sports.[12] For example, 27% of all injuries in women's gymnastics related to the knee compared to only 14% for men. More specifically, the incidence of knee injuries per 1000 athletic exposures was higher for females in the gender-comparable sports of gymnastics, basketball, softball/baseball, and track and field.

The National Collegiate Athletic Association (NCAA) receives injury reports from representative colleges in 16 sports reported as the Injury Surveillance System[76] (Table 36-1). The incidence is reported as number of injuries divided by 1000 athletic exposures. Survey of

Table 36-1. NCAA Injury Rates for Knee and Knee Structures, 1999–2000

	KNEE		PATELLA		COLLATERAL		ANTERIOR CRUCIATE		POSTERIOR CRUCIATE		TORN MENISCUS		PATELLA/ TENDON		KNEE OTHER	
	Practices	*Games*	P	G	P	G	P	G	P	G	P	G	P	G	P	G
Gymnastics-W	1.01	4.32	0.15	0.00	0.55	1.44	0.35	1.44	0.00	0.48	0.30	0.48	0.20	0.00	0.30	0.96
Gymnastics-M	0.41	1.70	0.00	0.00	0.00	0.85	0.10	0.85	0.00	0.00	0.10	0.85	0.10	0.00	0.20	0.00
Basketball-W	0.68	1.97	0.11	0.17	0.13	0.62	0.12	0.52	0.03	0.07	0.15	0.48	0.20	0.34	0.18	0.31
Basketball-M	0.48	1.13	0.08	0.15	0.14	0.30	0.05	0.12	0.01	0.00	0.09	0.30	0.18	0.18	0.07	0.27
Soccer-W	0.68	3.98	0.06	0.15	0.15	1.80	0.09	1.33	0.01	0.04	0.08	0.99	0.13	0.22	0.24	0.52
Soccer-M	0.55	3.24	0.07	0.16	0.18	1.56	0.05	0.23	0.01	0.08	0.12	0.62	0.08	0.39	0.15	0.39
Lacrosse-W	0.37	1.88	0.05	0.00	0.05	0.70	0.08	0.70	0.00	0.00	0.08	0.23	0.11	0.23	0.05	0.12
Lacrosse-M	0.42	1.23	0.00	0.08	0.07	0.08	0.08	0.33	0.00	0.00	0.09	0.16	0.07	0.25	0.05	0.08
Field Hockey-W	0.45	0.98	0.07	0.09	0.14	0.18	0.05	0.18	0.00	0.00	0.05	0.27	0.14	0.27	0.10	0.27
Volleyball-W	0.44	0.54	0.10	0.06	0.07	0.26	0.02	0.17	0.00	0.00	0.09	0.11	0.21	0.06	0.17	0.11
Softball-W	0.18	0.68	0.09	0.08	0.04	0.20	0.05	0.11	0.00	0.01	0.05	0.09	0.09	0.16	0.06	0.21
Spring Football-M	1.85	0.00	0.12	0.00	0.98	0.00	0.27	0.00	0.07	0.00	0.34	0.00	0.21	0.00	0.26	0.00
Wrestling-M	1.29	8.06	0.07	0.20	0.58	5.30	0.07	1.22	0.01	0.20	0.43	1.84	0.23	0.20	0.12	0.71
Football-M	0.69	9.41	0.05	0.36	0.34	5.58	0.12	1.50	0.02	0.45	0.13	1.39	0.12	0.95	0.11	1.04
Ice Hockey-M	0.29	2.75	0.01	0.09	0.20	2.05	0.01	0.33	0.00	0.00	0.05	0.23	0.00	0.14	0.05	0.23
Baseball-M	0.11	0.47	0.03	0.07	0.04	0.07	0.02	0.10	0.00	0.04	0.03	0.14	0.04	0.15	0.04	0.12

All data are shown as rate per 1000 athletic exposures for 1999–2000.
From NCAA Injury Surveillance System, 1999–2000, with permission.

16% of member institutions are evaluated and reported. Practice and game rate are listed for injuries in the categories of knee, including patella, ligaments (collateral, anterior cruciate, posterior cruciate), torn meniscus, patella/tendon, and knee/other. For 1999 to 2000, injury rates in 16 sports are listed. Comparing the NCAA college divisions and skill levels, there was no statistically significant difference in ACL injury rate comparing the larger and smaller division (I, II, or III) schools.[34]

At the United States Naval Academy, the incidence of ACL injuries was recorded during military training, intercollegiate and intramural athletics from 1991 to 1997.[32] The midshipmen at the United States Naval Academy provide a population base that can be studied with injury reports expressed as rates of number per 1000 athletic exposures. At the intramural level of athletics, which included soccer, basketball, softball, and volleyball, there was no statistically significant increase in the ACL injury rate, male versus female. However, in military training during the timed agility tests, the relative ACL injury risk was 9.74 in women, and in intercollegiate soccer, basketball, and rugby, women had a relative ACL injury risk of 3.96 compared with men midshipmen.

SPECIFIC SPORTS

Basketball

The knee structure injury rates in games and practices for males and females are shown in Figure 36-1.[76] Ratios above compare males to females. Of note is higher injury rates in games

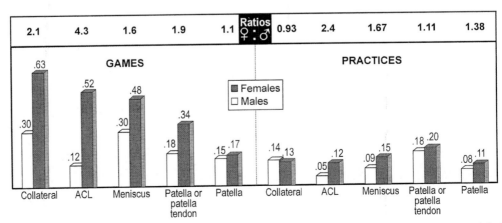

Figure 36-1. Knee structure injury rates in basketball games and practices, 1999–2000. Injury rates represent injuries/1000 athlete-exposures. (Data from the NCAA Injury Surveillance System, 1999–2000.)

and females for all structures except the patella or patellar tendon. In 1999–2000 season, ratios comparing males and females for ACL tears in games were 4.3 and in practice were 2.4. Over a 10-year period, collegiate female basketball players tore their ACL at a 3.5 times greater rate than males. From 1989 to 1993, in basketball, the women's ACL injury rate per 1000 athlete exposures was 0.29 and men's was 0.07 (4 times higher in women).[3] From 1994 until 1998, the rates remained 3 times higher in the female (0.30 versus 0.10).[1] Summary over a 10-year period is shown in Figure 36-2. The Atlantic Coast, Big Ten, and Pacific 10 Collegiate Conference data showed that females were 8 times more likely to sustain an ACL injury than males. In 44 professional male and female basketball players, females sustained an ACL injury at 10 times the rate of the male athletes.[30]

At the professional and Olympic level rates remain significantly higher in the female. In 1982, female professional basketball players were reported at increased risk for knee injuries.[102] At the elite level, males and females selected for the 1988 US Olympic basketball trials were evaluated by questionnaire. The females sustained significantly more knee injuries and required surgery more often than the males. This was prior to the professional male basketball athletes being selected for the

Olympic team. Of 64 female athletes, 13 had ACL injuries and of 80 male athletes, 3 had ACL injuries.[51] Many of the female athletes from the 1988 Olympic study are now playing basketball professionally in the United States.

Soccer

In soccer at the college level, the NCAA statistics were analyzed over two 5-year periods. From 1989 to 1993, women's ACL injury rate per 1000 athlete exposures was 0.31 compared to the men's of 0.13 (2.4 times greater in females than males).[2] The average ACL tear rate from 1994 to 1998 in soccer was 0.33 in women and 0.12 in men (2.3 greater in females than males). Summary over the 10-year period is shown in Figure 36-3. In soccer, the NCAA Injury Surveillance data for 1997 to 1998 reveals the game incidence for males was 0.45 ACL injuries and practice 0.06 (7.5 times greater in games). In the females, the game incidence was 1.12 ACL injuries and practice 0.09 (12.4 times greater).[75]

In a study of recreation league local indoor soccer, Lindenfeld reported on injury rates per 100 player-hours.[62] He found that the overall rate of knee ligament injuries for females was significantly higher at 0.87 for females and 0.29 for males. There were 10 diagnosed ACL tears, with 8 occurring in female athletes.

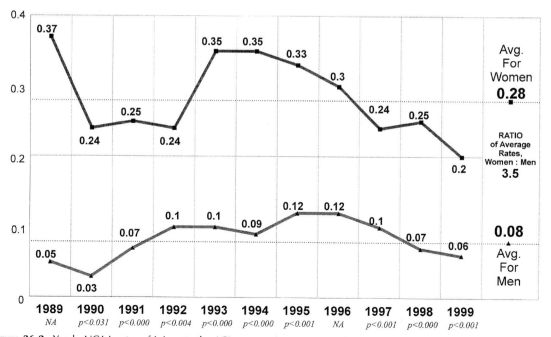

Figure 36-2. Yearly NCAA rates of injury to the ACL, comparing women and men. Basketball, 1989–1990 season through 1999–2000 season. Injury rates represent injuries/1000 athlete-exposures. (Copyright 2002, ML Ireland. Data from NCAA Injury Surveillance System and adapted from Arendt EA, Agel J, Dick R: Anterior cruciate ligament injury patterns among collegiate men and women. J Athletic Training 34(2):86–92, 1999.)

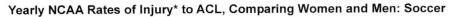

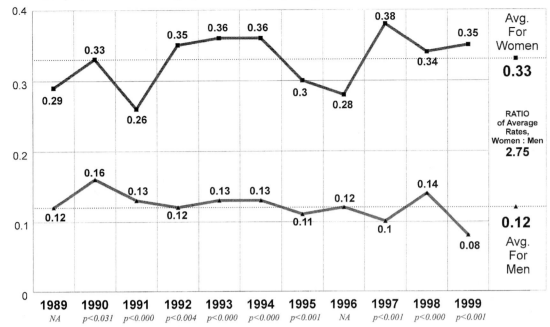

Figure 36-3. Yearly NCAA rates of injury to the ACL, comparing women and men: Soccer. (Copyright 2002, ML Ireland.* Data from NCAA Injury Surveillance System and adapted from Arendt EA, Agel J, Dick R: Anterior cruciate ligament injury patterns among collegiate men and women. J Athletic Training 34(2):86–92, 1999.)

In Norway, soccer injuries were retrospectively reviewed. Females were injured twice as often, based on 1000 game-hours as the denominator, 0.1 for females versus 0.057 for males.[5] Injuries in both sexes occurred more often during games. Average age of injury in the female was 19 and in the males was 26. The rate of injury was greater in the offensive position and in higher-skilled players.[7] In the United States, the indoor recreational soccer knee injury rate was 3 times greater in the female.[62]

Skiing

In the sport of skiing, injury statistics are harder to obtain. Of 450 patients with acute ACL rupture treated in Finland, the number of ACL tears increased by 247% over a 10-year period, from 1980 to 1989. The ACL injuries sustained in cross-country skiing decreased by 2 times and increased by 30 times in downhill skiing. The breakdown of common sports causing ACL injury were soccer 29%, downhill skiing 20%, cross-country skiing 12%, volleyball 12% in this study.[77]

In 1995, a questionnaire was sent to skiers in the New England area.[95] Of the 404 responses received, 25% of the respondents had sustained a new injury. Female racers were 2.3 times more likely to sustain a knee injury than male racers and 3.1 times more likely to sustain ACL injuries

compared to males. For those undergoing ACL surgery, 1 in 5 of the ACL reconstructions failed in female skiers. Although the females had a higher reinjury rate than males (27% to 13%), it was not statistically significant.[95]

Rugby

In women's collegiate and club rugby, 810 athletes from 42 clubs responded to questionnaires regarding knee injuries. The ACL injury rate was 0.36 per 1000 athletic exposures. Sixty-seven percent of ACL tears occurred in rugby backs.[61] No direct comparison was made with male rugby players.

Team Handball

Over three seasons, in Norwegian team handball athletes, a registry of ACL injuries was reported. ACL tears occurred in 23 women and 5 men.[55] The rate per 1000 player-hours was 0.31 in women and 0.06 in men.[74] Over a 2-year period all ACL injuries were registered in 3 upper divisions in Norway. Ninety-three ACL injuries occurred, and 1.4% of the players suffered ACL injuries—1.8% of the females compared to 1.0% of the males. There were 3 divisions, with 4.5% of first-division female players sustaining an ACL injury. Seventy-five percent of the injuries occurred during games and

95% were noncontact. Fifty-five percent of the injuries involved activities in which friction between the shoe and floor was a statistically significant factor.[72]

Netball

In Commonwealth countries, netball is a very popular sport, particularly among women. Female basketball and netball player injury rates were compared.[67] Six thousand nine hundred and seventy-two basketball athletes and 9190 netball athletes were followed for injury. Rates were calculated by injury number per 1000 participants. Netball players sustained severe knee injuries at a rate 3.3 times that of female basketball players. The rates of major and severe injuries occurred in 1:625 games in basketball and 1:250 games in netball.[67] Another study compared the kinanthropometric and performance variables to predict injury. The higher-risk netball athlete was thinner, fitter, and more powerful.[38]

GENDER DIFFERENCES IN STRUCTURE AND PHYSIOLOGY

Anatomic and structural differences between men and women play a significant role in the incidence and type of knee injuries. The increased rate of ACL tears and patellofemoral disorders is due to static and dynamic factors. Underlying structural differences exist.

Extrinsic structural factors, particularly alignment, are also different between men and women. Lower extremity alignment contributes directly to the forces and strain on the knee compartments, ligaments, and musculotendinous structures (Fig. 36-4).

Structurally, in addition, females often have increased femoral anteversion and less development of the vastus medialis obliquus (VMO) compared to males. Genu valgum, VMO hypoplasia, and femoral anteversion increase the laterally directed forces on the patellofemoral joint.[42] Another way to consider this problem is to compare 2 girls, one with mild and one with significant knocked knees (genu valgum). Biomechanics predict that the girl with more significantly angulated knees would be at greater risk of patellar subluxation and dislocation. Since females, in general, have 4° greater increased genu valgum compared to their male counterparts, it is not surprising that females are at increased risk of patellofemoral complaints and patellar instability. Additional malalignment factors include external tibial torsion, forefoot pronation (flat feet), and increased femoral anteversion. This has been

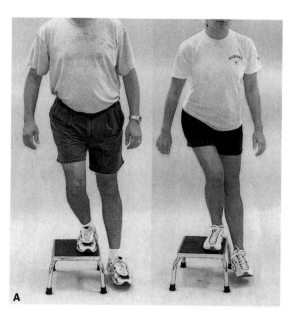
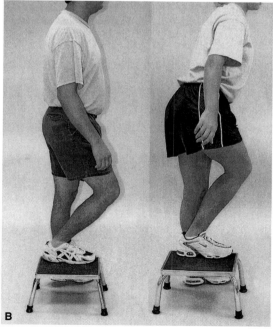

Figure 36-4. A, When instructed to do a mini-squat the male (left) demonstrates hip over knee over ankle alignment; the female (right) demonstrates femoral adduction and internal rotation and subsequent external rotation, valgus of the knee, and forefoot pronation. **B,** Seen from the side view, the female (right) is seen to have an anteriorly rotated pelvis, forward head, and forward trunk position compared with the male (left), who has a straight upright posture with normal lumbar lordosis. The anterior pelvis position creates lower extremity rotational compensation patterns. (Copyright 2001, ML Ireland.)

labeled "miserable malalignment syndrome" and is more frequently seen in females (Fig. 36-5).

Horton and Hall measured Q-angle in 50 males and 50 females.[39] Controlling for the effects of hip width and femur length, the relationship of Q-angle and gender was significant, with females having a larger Q-angle. The mean Q-angle for women was 15.8°±4.5° and for men was 11.2°±3.0°. How this relates to injury is not known. Females are reported to have greater width of the pelvis.[58,88] In this study, by clinical measurements, males were found to have greater hip width by 3 cm and longer femoral length by 5 cm. Ratios of hip width to femoral length were about equal—0.73 in males and 0.77 in females.

Alignment variations between men and women may have a direct effect on the biomechanical stresses felt by the ligaments about the knee. The tension force perceived by the medial collateral ligament (MCL) is a function of the alignment angle, the weight of the athlete, and the distance from the center of gravity. Since the valgus angle and the distance from the center of gravity is greater in the female knee, the MCL (and ACL for that matter) is subject to greater load than that in a male of similar weight.

Perhaps more important is the relative effect of increased valgus alignment and femoral offset of the female knee on the production of rotational forces (torque) on the ligaments about the knee. Most females have a lower center of gravity, a wider pelvis, shorter legs, and greater genu valgum compared to males[6,45] (Fig. 36-6). Since women have relatively wider hips, they have a relatively longer moment arm from the center of gravity to the lateral aspect of the proximal femur. Torque is related to the intensity of the force and the distance of that force from the center of rotation squared. This implies that even small variations in distance from the center of rotation can have a significant effect on stresses felt by the ligaments. More simply stated, a longer crank handle can put greater forces on a screw. In this case, the increased femoral offset and valgus alignment (longer crank handle) are important factors in creating elevated rotational stresses seen at the ACL (the screw).

In contact sports, the probability of injury increases with the weight of participants.[28] The likelihood of serious injury when the same gender and size compete is somewhat diminished; however, in contact sports with mismatched size, the smaller or less-skilled participant is more likely injured.[28] Since women are, in general, smaller at maturity,[11,14] the smaller female athlete is at increased risk when participating in contact sports with larger males.

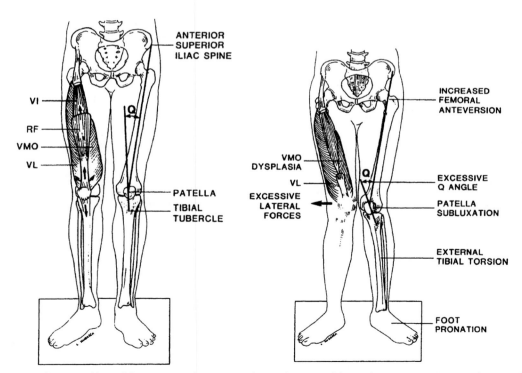

Figure 36-5. The miserable malalignment syndrome is made up of increased femoral anteversion, increased genu valgum, internal tibial torsion, and foot pronation (flat feet). This leads to excessive lateral forces, patellar subluxation, and pain. (From Fu FH, Stone DA (eds) Sports Injuries: Mechanism, Prevention, and Treatment, 2nd edition. Baltimore, Williams & Wilkins, 1994, p 159, with permission.)

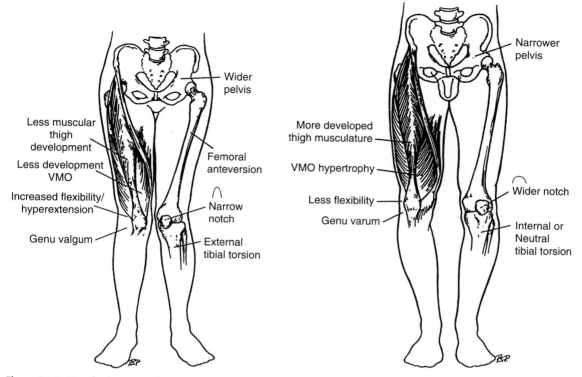

Figure 36-6. Females have a wider pelvis, a lower center of gravity, shorter legs, less-muscular thighs, increased flexibility, less-developed VMO, and genu valgum compared to males. (From Fu FH, Stone DA (eds) Sports Injuries: Mechanism, Prevention, and Treatment, 2nd edition. Baltimore, Williams & Wilkins, 1994, p 159, with permission.)

Since females in general are smaller, their ligaments are smaller and their bony anatomy is smaller. Nonetheless, these smaller ligaments are subject to similar stresses in twisting and cutting sports regardless of gender. However, a smaller ligament may not be a weaker ligament. Overall body size is also related to the size of important anatomic structures; that is, a tall athlete would be expected to have a long femur and a short athlete a shorter femur.

Within the knee, gender differences in the intercondylar notch shape and width as well as ACL size may place the female athlete at increased risk of injury.[65,102,103] Groups to compare should include race. Caucasians have greater anterior bowing of the femur and less depth of the intercondylar notch compared to blacks.[18] No gender studies comparing these factors have been done. Studies have revealed that a smaller absolute width or smaller notch width ratio is directly associated with an increased incidence of ACL injuries.[49,59,94] This is a small notch factor, not gender. If the forces across the knee for a given motion such as landing, twisting, and cutting are similar between males and females, it should not come as much of a surprise to observe an increased incidence of ACL injuries in the athletes with smaller liga-

ments. In addition, within the knee, notch shape may also be related to stresses seen by the ACL. Notch shape differences, "U" versus "C" versus "A," have not been shown to be a risk factor in ACL tears.[49] Notch width and notch width ratios and shapes are shown. The smaller A-shaped notch houses an ACL more likely to tear (see Fig. 36-6). The ratio of 0.136 and width of 9.8 mm is classified stenotic (Fig. 36-7A). The larger notch width measures 20.8, has a ratio of 0.3, and is U-shaped (Fig. 36-7B).

Variations in physiology and cyclic hormones may also have a significant effect on the different injury patterns seen between the male and female knee. Females appear to have increased ligamentous laxity and flexibility compared to males. There is controversy about whether this normal laxity predisposes the athlete to pathologic instability. Athletes with collagen disorders such as Ehlers–Danlos syndrome, Marfan syndrome, or generalized ligamentous laxity have a higher risk of joint dislocations throughout the body. The mild increase in baseline laxity in women compared to men may, therefore, contribute to the increased incidence of patellar subluxation and ligament sprains reported about the knee of female athletes.[27,86] This association between ligamentous laxity and

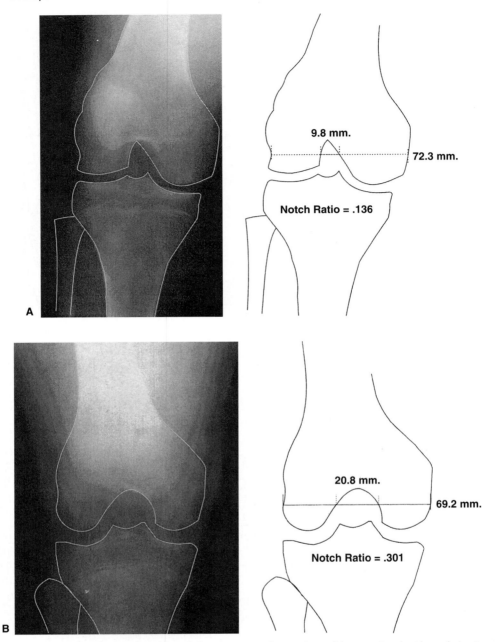

Figure 36-7. (**A** & **B**) Intercondylar notch width and shape may vary by gender and be associated with a relative increased risk of ACL injury. The notch width index (NWI) is measured at the level of the popliteal groove by dividing the notch width by the width of the condyles. An NWI less than 0.21 signifies stenosis and a relatively increased risk of ACL injury. (Copyright 2000, ML Ireland.)

injury is, however, controversial.[55,78] Some studies have shown no relationship between knee laxity and injury.[22,55] Indeed, other studies have shown that athletic women have less laxity than their sedentary counterparts. Nonetheless, the potential effect of increased laxity on pathologic instability must be considered.

Hormones such as estrogen may play an important role in ligamentous laxity and the associated risk of pathologic instability in female

athletes; however, the jury is still out. Women have the ability to attain a significant increase in ligamentous laxity during pregnancy because of the hormonal influences of such hormones as relaxin, estrogen, and progestins. The effect of relaxin during pregnancy demonstrates the hormonal effect of relaxation of all collagen tissue-symphysis, joints, and ligaments. Hormonal receptors, specifically estrogen receptors, have been identified on the ligaments, in particular the ACL.[64] It does not seem to be a unreasonable step to assume that cyclic hormones could play a similar role with laxity and therefore injury risk in the nonpregnant athlete. The definitive proof of this hypothesis has been rather elusive. Wojtys and colleagues from the University of Michigan claimed to have shown an increased risk of ACL injuries in female athletes from day 10 to day 14 of their cycle.[101] This corresponds to peaks in cyclic hormones. The statistical conclusions of this study, however, have been criticized recently. Studies on sheep fail to show effect of estrogen at a local tissue level.[96] Numerous studies are ongoing and the impact of cyclic hormones on the increased incidence of gender-related knee injuries remains to be proven. Indeed the impact of the findings would also be controversial. There is no evidence to support modification of practice or games during the athlete's monthly cycle.[31]

FUNCTIONAL ANATOMY AND PHYSICAL EXAMINATION

Although there is no significant difference in the anatomy between the genders, a brief review of anatomy will set the stage for understanding the classification of instability patterns as it relates to function. From a bird's eye view are seen the intra-articular structures of the anterior and posterior cruciate ligaments, medial—more attached and C-shaped, and the lateral meniscus, more mobile and covering a larger surface area of the tibial plateau (Fig. 36-8). The medial collateral ligament is divided into superficial (spanning from adductor tubercle to proximal tibial metaphysis under the pes anserinus) and deep (meniscofemoral and meniscotibial) ligament. The ACL is divided into 3 bundles—anteromedial, intermediate, and posterolateral—based on the attachments on the tibia. The anteromedial bundle is tight in flexion and extension and the posterolateral bundle is tight only in extension.[79,99] (Fig. 36-9) The anterior and posterior cruciate ligaments are intracapsular but extrasynovial.

The posterior cruciate ligament (PCL) has 2 bundles based on the femoral attachment posteromedially and anterolaterally. In full flexion, all fibers are taut and in extension only the posteromedial fibers are taut (Fig. 36-10).[82,99]

Patellofemoral Articulation

Anteriorly, the quadriceps tendon is formed from vastus medialis, vastus intermedius, vastus lateralis, and rectus femoris (Fig. 36-11).[99] Patellar tracking is influenced by static anatomic factors such as the trochlear groove depth and the relationship of the patellar tendon, patellar height, medial patellofemoral ligament, and lateral patellar retinaculum. Dynamic factors that influence patellar tracking are alignment, posi-

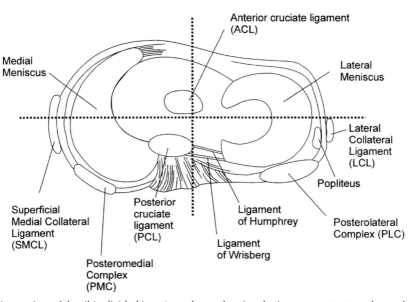

Figure 36-8. Bird's eye view of the tibia divided into 4 quadrants showing the important structures located in each quadrant: anteromedial (medial meniscus), anterolateral (lateral meniscus), posterolateral (lateral collateral ligament [LCL], popliteus, posterolateral complex [PLC], ligament of Humphrey, a ligament of Wrisberg), and posteromedial (posterior cruciate ligament [PCL], posteromedial complex [PMC], and superficial medial collateral ligament [SMCL]). (Adapted from Mueller W: The Knee: Form, Function, and Ligament Reconstruction. New York, Springer-Verlag, 1983, with permission.)

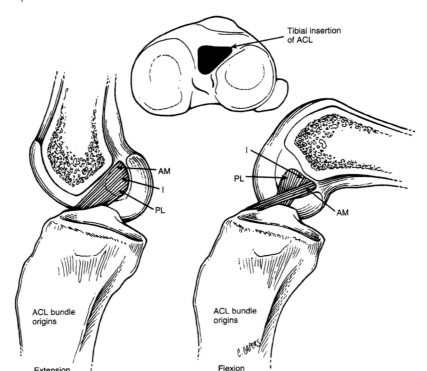

Figure 36-9. The ACL is divided into 3 bundles based on the tibial attachment: the anteromedial (AM), the intermediate (I), and the posterolateral (PL) bundles. With knee flexion, the posterior fibers loosen and the anteromedial fibers coil around the posterolateral ones. (From Baker CL, Jr: The Hughston Clinic Sports Medicine Book. Baltimore, Williams & Wilkins, 1995, with permission.)

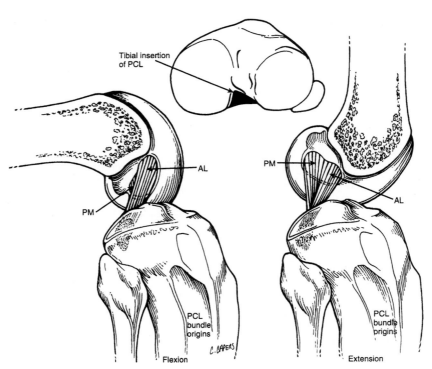

Figure 36-10. Attachment sites of the posteromedial (PM) and anterolateral (AL) bundles of the PCL. During knee flexion, the anterolateral fibers are progressively tensed. (From Baker CL, Jr: The Hughston Clinic Sports Medicine Book. Baltimore, Williams & Wilkins, 1995, with permission.)

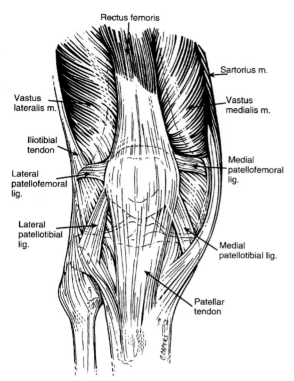

Figure 36-11. Muscular anatomy of the anterior aspect of the knee. (From Baker CL, Jr: The Hughston Clinic Sports Medicine Book. Baltimore, Williams & Wilkins, 1995, with permission.)

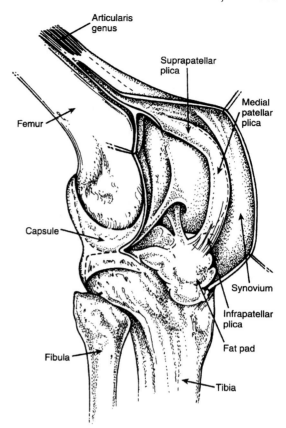

Figure 36-12. The plica is thought to act as a synovial-type tendon aponeurosis for the articularis genus muscle. (From Baker CL, Jr: The Hughston Clinic Sports Medicine Book. Baltimore, Williams & Wilkins, 1995, with permission.)

tion of the foot, strength, proximal hip position, core strength, and extrinsic forces. The synovial fold of suprapatellar plica is shown in Figure 36-12.[99] The plica can become symptomatic, most typically medial patellar plica into superior patellar plica. Inferiorly, the infrapatellar plica or ligamentum mucosum rests just behind the patellar tendon in the infrapatellar fat pad.

CLASSIFICATION OF KNEE INSTABILITIES

The significance of knee ligament instabilities can be better appreciated if one has an understanding of tibial movement on the femur and its relationship to the involved anatomic structure and findings on physical examination. The comprehensive classification of knee ligament injuries was described by Hughston and Andrews in 1976.[40,41] The American Medical Association (AMA) further defined sprains based on millimeters of opening and side-to-side differences are noted. A *sprain* is defined as an injury of ligamentous tissue. The AMA and medical aspect of sport 1968 handbook defines sprain and degrees of instability.[1] The amount of opening is estimated in millimeters as follows: mild[1+], less

than 5 mm; moderate[2+], 5 to 9 mm; severe[3+], greater than 10 mm; and gross, greater than 15 mm. Accordingly, diagnoses are listed as grades or severity of ligament injury (partial versus complete, functional versus nonfunctional): mild minimal tearing, less than 5 mm opening; moderate disruption or interstitial partial tearing, 5 to 10 mm; and severe, complete, greater than 10 mm with no end point.

Knee Motions

There are 6 degrees of freedom in knee motions. As described, these motions are rotations in the anterior posterior (sagittal) plane, medial lateral (coronal) plane, and compression distraction (axial) plane[9,105] (Fig. 36-13).

HISTORY AND PHYSICAL EXAMINATION

The patient can give the information necessary to make the correct diagnosis. The patient

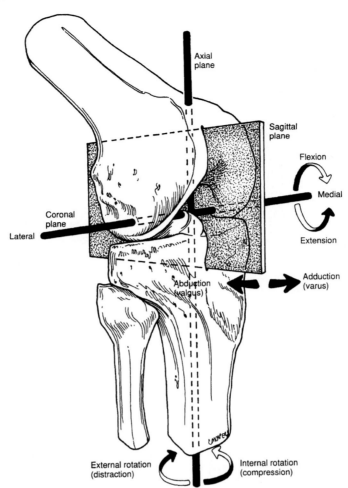

Figure 36-13. A 6-degrees-of-freedom model illustrates all possible rotations and translations about the knee. (From Baker CL, Jr: The Hughston Clinic Sports Medicine Book. Baltimore, Williams & Wilkins, 1995, with permission.)

should be asked to explain the mechanism of injury and describe her exact symptoms: pain, swelling, locking, or catching or getting stuck in one position. The patellofemoral disorder patient will grab the patella with her open hand and ACL patient may describe shifting and put her fists together, rotating them much like a pivot shift test is performed. Patients with plica syndrome often will point directly to the medial shelf plica. Meniscal tears in the adolescent female are very rare and the more likely diagnosis is symptomatic medial plica and/or patellofemoral stress syndrome. The specific primary diagnosis must be made to make the appropriate referral for rehabilitation. The history of ACL tear usually includes an awkward landing and feeling a "pop" or a shifting sensation. Often the athlete will try to return to the game, feel a second shifting sensation, and give up. This sensation is the functional pivot shift or anterior rotation of the lateral tibial plateau as the knee dislocates in extension, then with flex-

ion, reduces. There is usually swelling within a couple of hours. Patellar dislocation history is similar, with swelling, but the swelling occurs more quickly. If the patella is truly dislocated, reduction and another pop occurs with knee extension, which is opposite from what occurs in an ACL injury.

The order of the physical examination tests depends on the nature of the patient's injury. Routinely, the examination is started with the patient standing, walking, supine, then prone, if necessary. The most potentially painful tests should be done last.

Patellar Mobility and Tracking

The patella should move passively in the trochlear groove equally in medial and lateral directions. Estimation of quadrants of mobility or any asymmetry side to side or medially to laterally should be documented. Palpation should be done for pain over the patellar facet (patellofemoral stress syndrome or articular cartilage involvement) and tightness over the lateral retinaculum. Pain on palpation over the quadriceps tendon, patellar tendon, or tibial tubercle leads the examiner to the diagnosis of inflammation or injury at that level.

Patellar tracking is demonstrated by asking the patient to actively extend against the examiner's hand (Fig. 36-14). Observations of the patella staying in the trochlear groove and centrally tracking are made. A "J" sign occurs when the patella jumps laterally at about 30° of flexion into extension. The test is begun with the less painful or normal knee, and then proceeds to the injured knee. Range of motion should be checked passively and actively. The patient's heel is lifted (Fig. 36-15) to see if there is a symmet-

rical extension range, hamstring spasticity, or flexion contracture. This is done by putting the hand under the heel and gently bouncing the knee home (Fig. 36-15). Hamstring tightness is assessed and documented passively, flexing the hip to 90° and recording the knee flexion angle, in the case shown in Figure 36-16, 20°.

Q-angle measurement can be done with the patient standing or supine, or with the knee flexed over the table. The static Q-angle measurement does not give as much information as having the patient do a mini-squat and observing if the Q angle increases significantly or asymmetrically (see Fig. 36-5). The Q angle should be less than 12° to 15°. Measuring the Q angle clinically is done with the patient standing, seated, and supine. Measurements are erratic and examiner dependent. Alignment to determine torsion of the tibia and femur and leg-length discrepancy should be done routinely. Observation of foot alignment, pes cavus planus, forefoot pronation, and hindfoot varus/valgus is very important in the assessment of patellofemoral disorders.

Meniscal Examination

With the patient standing, instructions to flex as far as possible are given. The patient should be supported initially when she does this maneuver. Pain as the patient flexes medially with the feet externally rotated and laterally in the internally rotated position raises suspicion of meniscus tears of the respective compartments. Supine

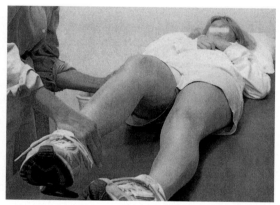

Figure 36-14. Instructing the patient to straighten the knee against the examiner's hand is helpful to assess patellar tracking. (Copyright 2002, ML Ireland.)

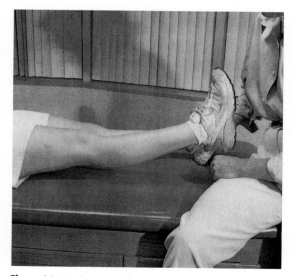

Figure 36-15. Bouncing the heel and driving the knee into extension is helpful to determine if there is an intra-articular process and subsequent hamstring spasticity. (Copyright 2002, ML Ireland.)

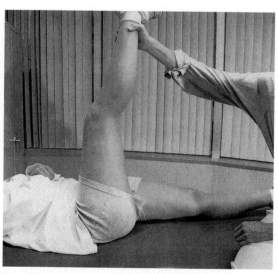

Figure 36-16. Assessment of hamstring flexibility is done by flexing the hip to 90°, then documenting an angle between the calf and thigh, extending the knee. This individual's hamstring angle is 20°. (Copyright 2002, ML Ireland.)

examination includes McMurray's test, which is positive with pain, and a "pop" over the joint line when the knee is flexed and extended with twisting and varus and valgus stresses applied. Hyperflexion of the knee in external rotation, reproducing pain posteriorly medially, may also indicate medial meniscus tear. A cystic lateral meniscus tear can often be palpated in the mid-third of the lateral joint line. Palpation of the posterior aspect of the joint to determine if there is a Baker's cyst is also suggested. The Apley grind and compression tests are done with the patient prone and are particularly helpful in distinguishing a MCL sprain (distraction by pulling up on the foot) from medial meniscus tear (compression by pushing down and rotating the foot).

Ligamentous Examination

Instabilities can be classified as rotatory, straight, or combined[50,71] (Table 36-2). By understanding the involved structures and their relationship to functional instability, appropriate treatment can be instituted. For example, ACL injury is anterolateral rotatory instability. The lateral tibia subluxes anteriorly relative to the femur. This phenomena creates the classic pivot shift when the subluxation is reduced with knee flexion.

The knee should be supported with a pillow or the examiner's leg, or placed over the side of the table. The most painful part of the examination should be done last. Valgus stress testing at 30° for MCL strain is done (Fig. 36-17). Varus testing at 30° for the lateral structures is also performed (Fig. 36-18). Anterior palpation of the medial tibial plateaus step off to determine any asymmetry or PCL injury is performed (Fig. 36-19). To reveal ACL injury, 3 tests are performed. To perform the anterior drawer test for ACL injury (Fig. 36-20), the examiner sits on the patient's foot and palpates the hamstrings, instructing the patient to relax her hamstrings. The tibia is then pulled forward, much like a drawer being pulled out of a chest of drawers. The Lachman test (Fig. 36-21) is the easiest test to determine ACL injury, and should be done first. The pivot shift can be performed in a reduction of the subluxation maneuver. The easiest method is to cradle the tibia with one arm and do a subluxation test where the tibia is being internally rotated by one arm while the lateral plateau is pushed anteriorly by the hand. If the

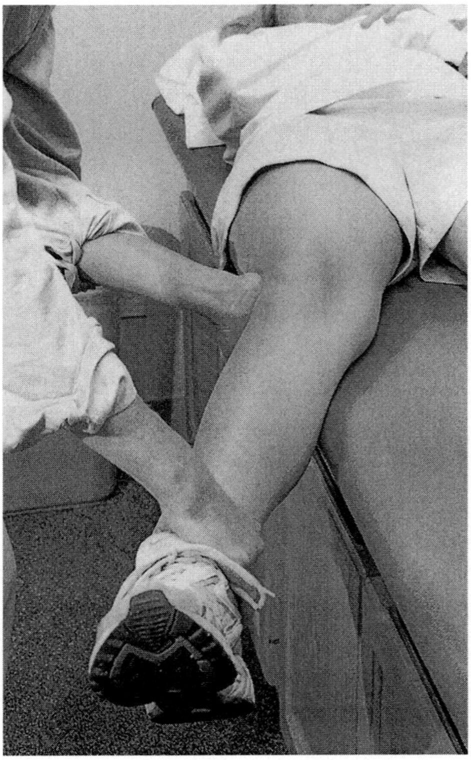

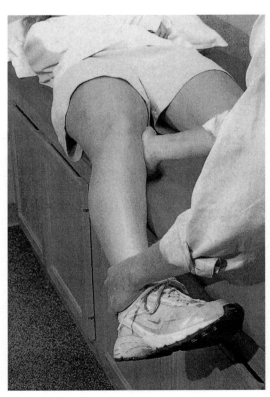

Figure 36-17. Testing of the medial collateral ligament is done with the leg over the side of the table at 0°, and as shown in this picture, 30°, applying valgus stress. (Copyright 2002, ML Ireland.)

Figure 36-18. Varus stress testing at 30°. For lateral instability at 0° and 30°, applying varus stress with the opposite hand stabilizing the knee is shown. (Copyright 2002, ML Ireland.)

Table 36-2. Classification of Knee Instabilities: Rotatory, Straight, or Combined

DIAGNOSIS	DIAGRAM	INVOLVED ANATOMIC STRUCTURE	PHYSICAL FINDINGS	MECHANISM AND FORCES
		Section 1. Anteromedial Rotatory Instabilities (AMRI)		
1+		PMC	1 + AD in ER	Contact: Lateral Force: Valgus
2+		PMC SMCL	1+ AD in ER 1+–2 + valgus 30°	Contact: Lateral Anterior Forces: Valgus Extension Tibia ER
		Section 2. Combined AMRI and ALRI		
3+		PMC SMCL ACL	3+ AD in ER 2+ AD in N 2+ valgus 30°	Contact: Lateral Forces: Valgus Extension Tibia ER
4+		PMC ACL PLC	3+ AD in ER 2+ AD in NR 2+ valgus at 30° 1+ recurvatum 1+ PS	Contact: Lateral Forces: Valgus Rotation Extension
		Section 3. Anterolateral Rotatory Instabilities (ALRI)		
1+		ACL Lateral capsule	+ AD in N and tibial IR PS	Noncontact Forces: Rotation Foot Planted
2+		ACL LCL PLC	+ AD + IR + Lachman + PS 1 + varus 30°	Noncontact or Contact: Medial Forces: Varus Extension Tibia IR
		Section 4. Straight Posterior		
Posterior		PCL ± Humphrey ± Wrisberg	PD 90° Neutral	Contact: Proximal Anterior Tibia Force: Posterior on Tibia Flexed or Hyperextension
		Section 5. Posterolateral Rotatory Instabilities (PLRI)		
1+		LCL PLC	ERR 2–3+ ADD at 30° PD Most 30° PLD 1+ RPS ER at 30° and 90°	Contact: Medial Forces Varus Extension

Table continued on following page

Table 36-2. Classification of Knee Instabilities: Rotatory, Straight, or Combined (*continued*)

DIAGNOSIS	DIAGRAM	INVOLVED ANATOMIC STRUCTURE	PHYSICAL FINDINGS	MECHANISM AND FORCES
Section 5. Posterolateral rotatory instabilities (PLRI)				
2+		PCL PLC	PD increased 30° more than 90° Moderate ER at 30° and 90°	Contact: Medial Forces: Varus Extension
3+		LCL PLC PCL PMC	ERR 2–3+ VAR 0° PD in Neutral Severe Hyperextension Rotation at 30° and 90°	Contact: Medial Anterior Forces: Hyperextension Varus
Section 6. Combined ALRI and PLRI				
		ACL PLC PCL Lateral Capsule	PS RPS Lachman ERR PLD PD Neutral ER at 20° Fx	Contact: Anterior Forces: Valgus Extension Hyperextension
Section 7. Straight Instabilities				
1+ Lateral (rare)		Isolated LCL	1+ ADD 30°	Contact: Medial Force: Varus
3+ Lateral		LCL PLC PCL ±ACL	2–3+ ADD 0° ERR PD in N AD in IR Hyperextension Injury with ACL	Contact: Medial Anteromedial Tibia Forces: Extension Varus
1+ Medial		SMCL	Abduction at 30°	Contact: Lateral Forces: Valgus
Posteromedial instability (PMI) (rare)		SMCL PMC PCL	Abduction 0° PD IR+ neutral AD in ER 2+ valgus at 30° and 0°	Contact: Anterior Forces: Valgus Extension

ACL is injured, subluxation occurs at 30° of flexion moving into extension. Reduction of the lateral tibial plateau occurs with increasing flexion past 30° (Fig. 36-22).

Radiographic Examination

Routine standing anteroposterior, lateral, notch, and bilateral patella views are obtained. A view routinely obtained is the merchant view (Fig. 36-23). The notch view is performed with the patient on the table in an all-fours position (Fig. 36-24). To have more reproducible angles with a notch view, use of a goniometer is suggested. The notch view gives measurements of the width and shape of the notch and can show osteochondritis dissecans. The lateral view is done with the knee in flexion (Fig. 36-25).

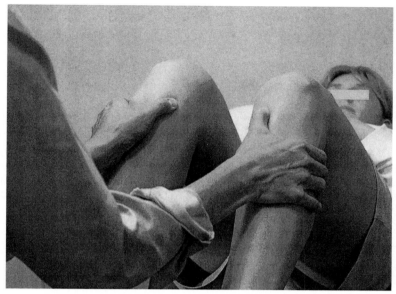

Figure 36-19. Palpation of both medial tibial metaphyses is performed with normal 5 to 10 mm anterior position of the plateau. If there is posterior position of the tibial plateau, this indicates PCL injury. (Copyright 2002, ML Ireland.)

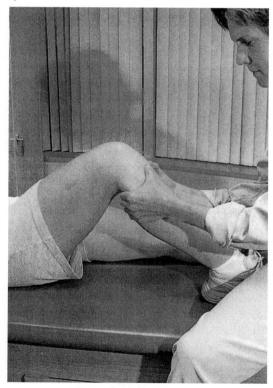

Figure 36-20. Anterior drawer test for an ACL tear is performed with the examiner seated on the patient's foot and the tibia pulled forward, much like taking a drawer out of a chest of drawers. (Copyright 2002, ML Ireland.)

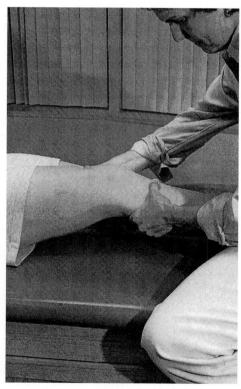

Figure 36-21. The Lachman test, performed at 30° of flexion, is the most sensitive for acute ACL injury. Determining if it is normal and symmetrical, with a firm end point or no end point, should be documented. A support can be placed behind the patient's knee. (Copyright 2002, ML Ireland.)

Standing 30° flexed posteroanterior views are also routinely obtained. To reproduce standard views, it is important to use a goniometer to document the knee flexion angle[90] (Fig. 36-26).

Magnetic resonance imaging (MRI) provides additional information if the diagnosis is not

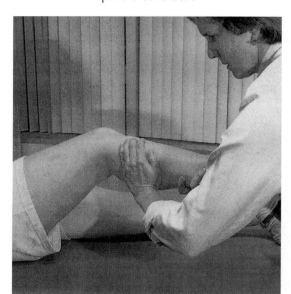

Figure 36-22. Pivot shift test is performed in a reduction or subluxation manner. In the subluxation test, the knee is brought from flexion to extension and tibia is internally rotated while axial load is applied. A "clunk" can be felt as the lateral tibial plateau subluxes anteriorly and a reduction can be felt as the tibia is externally rotated and flexed. (Copyright 2002, ML Ireland.)

clear. Referral to an orthopaedic surgeon prior to obtaining an MRI scan is most appropriate. A computed tomography (CT) scan for planning patellofemoral surgeries can be helpful. A technetium bone scan will give information about arthrosis, tumors, and overall homeostasis of the knee. Dye likens the homeostasis of the knee to an envelope.[20] The arthritic knee has a small envelope. One's physical activity must remain in this envelope or symptoms such as swelling, locking, and pain will occur.

SPECIFIC KNEE INJURIES

After a thorough history and complete examination are performed, the diagnosis usually becomes very clear. Care must be taken during the examination to identify associated proximal problems that might radiate to the knee, including hip, back, and knee pain, which may also occur in association with sciatic nerve, congenital, or post-traumatic alignment deformity such as tibial torsion or femoral anteversion or foot and ankle malalignment. Physical examination of the female knee should be no different than that of a male knee. The examination must be complete. Ligament and meniscal evaluation is best done with the athlete supine. What is her generalized ligamentous laxity and level of conditioning? Is she loose-jointed? Has she been training appropriately? A thorough patellofemoral examination includes assessment of tracking, tilt and instability, palpation of the medial patellar plica and patella articular facets, as well as an evaluation of the quadriceps mechanism (especially the vastus medialis obliquus muscle). Since pathology in these areas is seen more often in the female athlete, the following discussions will be limited to knee conditions that appear to be related to gender.

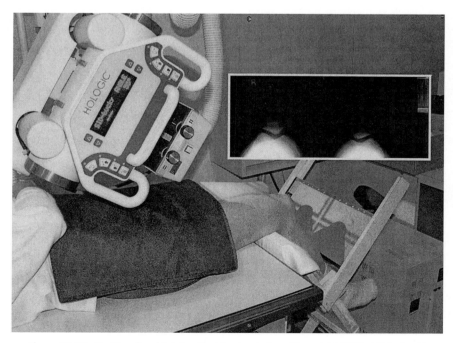

Figure 36-23. Position for obtaining the Merchant view. (Copyright 2002, ML Ireland.)

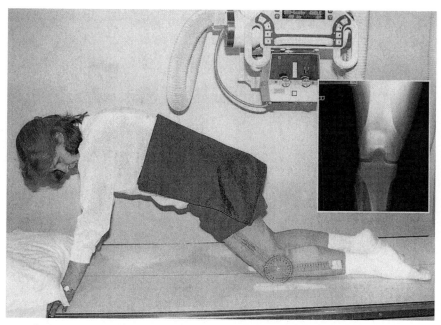

Figure 36-24. Position for obtaining the notch view. (Copyright 2002, ML Ireland.)

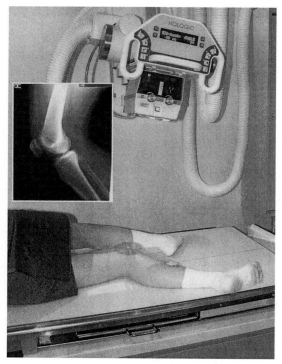

Figure 36-25. Position for obtaining the lateral view. (Copyright 2002, ML Ireland.)

Patellofemoral Disorders

The anterior knee is possibly the most common source of complaints or site of injury for the female athlete.[5,21,23,30,100] The causes of anterior knee pain are numerous but can usually be categorized as inflammatory or mechanical (Table 36-3). Rare causes of anterior knee pain such as tumors do not appear to have a gender predilection. A specific diagnosis should be made whenever possible so the treatment can be appropriately focused. An algorithmic approach to treatment is suggested and has been published.[56]

The less surgery performed on the patellofemoral joint, the better. The athlete may be unable to return to her prior level of competition following realignment and releases. In the adolescent, the nonoperative approach should be the rule. Patellofemoral stress syndrome is a clinical diagnosis and can include such pathologic processes as chondromalacia patella, symptomatic plica, lateral subluxation of the patella, and degenerative joint disease. Attempt to make the primary and specific diagnosis.

Patellar Instability

Patellofemoral instability occurs more frequently in females than in males. Females have a greater valgus alignment than males, which magnifies lateral directing forces. Females have a higher incidence of VMO hypoplasia and a lower baseline level of conditioning of all muscle groups, increasing their risk of instability. In patients with patellar subluxation, VMO activity is decreased.[89,104] The VMO is also the first component of the quadriceps to demonstrate atrophy in an injured knee and the last to return during rehabilitation.[5,91] Female athletes, in particular, tend to be especially susceptible to

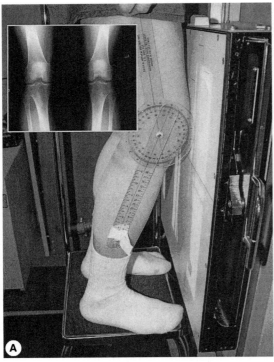 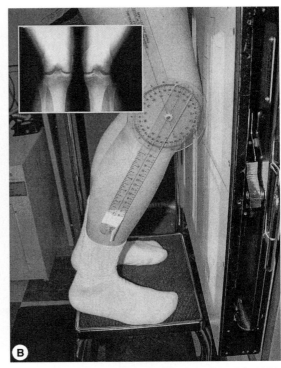

Figure 36-26. Position for obtaining Rosenberg views with goniometry. (**A**) 30° of flexion. (**B**) 45° of flexion. (Copyright 2002, ML Ireland.)

dysfunction after injury or surgery. Therefore, for female athletes it is necessary to focus on VMO strengthening for both prevention and treatment of patellar instability. Athletes may present with a complete dislocation of the patella. The presentation is usually obvious but can be missed without a careful history and physical examination. Reduction is frequently completed by the coach or trainer simply by extending the leg. If not, lifting the patella with medially directed pressure is usually all that is necessary. Complete roentgenograms, including anteroposterior, lateral, notch, and patellar sunrise or Merchant views, are important to rule out associated osteochondral fractures.[46]

Treatment is based on the presence of osteochondral loose bodies and risk of recurrence. Risk factors increasing the chance of recurrence include excessive genu valgum, increased Q angle, patella alta, generalized ligamentous laxity, a relatively low lateral femoral condylar height, a defect in the VMO insertion, VMO dysplasia, and abnormal patellar configuration (ie, a flat patella).[13,35,60] Symptomatic loose bodies should always be removed. For first-time dislocators with no risk factors or loose bodies, treatment is conservative, with knee immobilization in extension for 3 weeks. A lateral pad or taping is required to maintain the reduction while the medial structures heal. After immobil-

ization time, the program includes motion, quadriceps, and hip strengthening and taping or a knee sleeve with a lateral pad. Patients can generally return to competition in 8 to 12 weeks. Substantial risk factors for redislocation are present, and if redislocation occurs, open repair, proximal reefing, and/or distal tubercle transfer may be required. Acutely, repair is considered if the level of injury is favorable to repair by MRI and risk factors warrant acute surgery.

Lateral releases are only required if the lateral retinaculum is tight or the patella is tilted. If the patella glides 30% to 50% medially, no release is necessary. Lateral release is an operation for lateral retinacular tightness, not instability.[24] In a first-time dislocator, a distal bony patellar realignment procedure and proximal repair is rarely indicated. In skeletally immature patients, bone procedures are delayed until the physes are nearing or completely closed.

More commonly, female athletes present with complaints of chronic anterior knee pain and may note a sensation of "giving way." Care should be made to confirm that other important ligament stabilizers are intact. Giving way may be secondary to quadriceps weakness or true ligamentous laxity. In 1983 Mueller argued that sustaining both a patellar dislocation and ACL rupture simultaneously was not mechanically possible.[71] Subsequently, the two

Table 36-3. Differential Diagnosis: Anterior Knee Pain

MECHANICAL	INFLAMMATORY	OTHER
Repetitive Microtraumatic	*Bursitis*	*Referred Pain*
• Patella	• Prepatellar	• Lumbar disc herniation
Stability	• Retropatellar	• Others
Subluxation	Semimembranosus	
Dislocation	Pes anserinus	Reflex Sympathetic Dystrophy
Tilt		(Regional Pain Syndrome)
Rotation	Tendinitis	
Malalignment	• Quadriceps patella	Tumors
Fracture	• Pes anserinus	• Benign
Stress	• Semimembranosus	• Malignant
Bipartite	• Patella tendinitis	
Fibrous union		Pigmented Villonodular
Acute fracture	Neuromata/retinacular pain	synovitis
• Pathologic medial plica		
• Patellofemoral stress syndrome	Arthritis	
• Osteochondral fracture	• Osteo	
Trochlear groove	• Rheumatoid	
Patella	• Psoriatic	
• Loose bodies	• Others	
Cartilaginous		
Osteochondral	Syndromes	
• Osteochondritis dissecans	• Reiter	
Patella		
Trochlear groove		
• Skeletally immature		
Osgood-Schlatter's disease		
Sinding-Larsen-Johansson syndrome		

Acute Macrotraumatic Injury

• Extensor mechanism disruption
  Quadriceps rupture
  Patellar tendon rupture
    Inferior avulsion fracture
    Interstitial
  Skeletally immature
  Tibial tubercle fracture
• Patellar fracture
  Transverse
    Displaced/nondisplaced
  Comminuted
  Status Post ACL reconstruction
    with central third patellar
    tendon bone

Copyright 2001, ML Ireland.

injuries have been reported and discussed but, nonetheless, rarely occur together.

A positive apprehension sign is elicited by reproducing the subluxation event by pushing the patella laterally. Palpation of the medial plica is also done. Try to decide on the primary diagnosis—is it instability, plica, or articular cartilage? Occasionally the patella will be tilted laterally with the medial border raised. If the tilt can not be corrected past a neutral or flat position, the lateral retinaculum is tight, which can exacerbate lateral tracking. When placing the knee through a passive range of motion, the patella can occasionally be seen jumping back into the femoral groove with increasing flexion from an extended position, the so-called J-sign (Fig. 36-27). Alternatively, this can be observed as the athlete actively extends the knee from a flexed position while sitting or supine on commands to straighten the knee.

Standing, the athlete's patellae may point inward and toward each other. Although the athlete is not in valgus, she may demonstrate patellae that point toward each other, indicating femoral anteversion (Fig. 36-28A). When asked to flex the lower extremity, alignment of hip internal rotation varus and tibial external rotation further comprises normal patellar tracking (Fig. 36-28B). This is evidence of femoral anteversion. Flat feet or tibial torsion can further

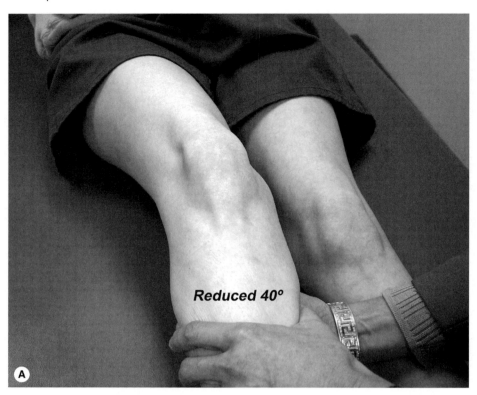

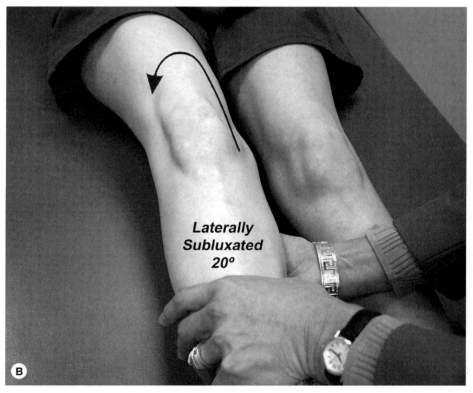

Figure 36-27. (**A** & **B**) A positive "J" sign is demonstrated as the patient's patella is at 40° of flexion and subluxes laterally at 20° of flexion. Asking the patient to straighten the leg against examiner's resistance can demonstrate this sign of lateral patellar instability. (Copyright 2002, ML Ireland.)

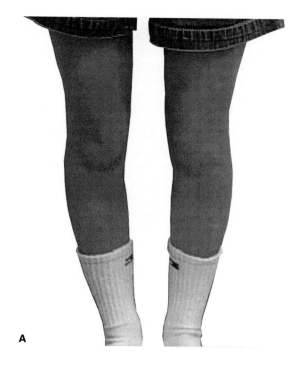

A

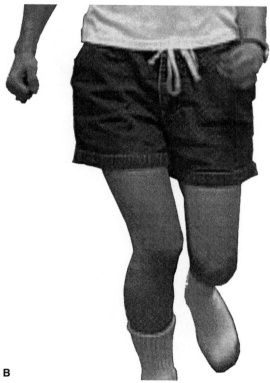

B

Figure 36-28. Individuals seen for anterior knee pain. **(A)** Although the alignment appears rather straight—no excessive genu valgum or valgus—there is significant internal rotation of the femora, indicating femoral anteversion. The patellae are pointing toward one another. **(B)** This is accentuated when the individual gets in a flexed position: the femur goes into further adduction and internal rotation. (Copyright 2002, ML Ireland.)

exacerbate the stresses on the patella. Documentation of the instability is not always simple. Variations in Q-angle clinical measurement are many. Slight hip rotation can alter the measurement. If the patella is subluxed, the measurement may also be in error. CT or MRI may more accurately document the patella-to-femur relationship. Overall valgus alignment is one important factor contributing to patellar instability. A shallow femoral groove, a flat patella, a hypotrophic lateral condyle, and patella alta are associated with patellofemoral instability.

Treatment of chronic patellar instability should always begin with a conservative course of rehabilitation focused on the VMO. McConnell has shown that patellar taping and mobilization associated with rehabilitation can provide symptomatic relief in a high percentage of patients.[66] Resistant cases may require surgical realignment. If patellar tilt exists alone with no evidence of lateral translation, an isolated lateral release using either arthroscopic or open techniques may provide long-term relief. Once again however, a lateral release is not a procedure for instability. If lateral translation is present, surgical realignment is required. Insall has reported excellent results with soft-tissue realignment where a lateral retinacular release is performed and the entire medial portion of the extensor mechanism including the VMO is reefed one half to three quarters over the patella.[47] If congenital bone deficiency or fixed alignment problems such as increased Q angle, flat patella, shallow patellar groove, hypoplastic lateral femoral condyle, and generalized ligamentous laxity are present, a distal realignment can be performed. Special caution should be used when considering surgical realignment in the skeletally immature. If forced in a child, treatment includes performing a soft-tissue procedure alone and waiting for skeletal maturity. In adults, the tibial tubercle can be osteotomized and shifted medially and/or anteriorly.[24] The damaged articular cartilage must be unloaded. Unfortunately, few studies exist showing the results of patellofemoral surgery on high-level athletes. Results can be disappointing. Patellofemoral pain may persist despite anatomic alignment improvements. Care should be taken in selecting patients for surgery.

Degenerative Joint Disease and Chondromalacia

Another possible component of patellofemoral syndrome is early degenerative changes of the articular cartilage of the patella. The female athlete commonly presents with complaints of dull aching pain beneath her kneecap. The pain is commonly worse when sitting in a chair with the knees flexed for an extended period of time, when rising from a chair, or when ascending stairs or a steep hill. Occasionally, she will note grinding sensations beneath her patella. The problem is most frequently seen in young adolescent females and there may be a component of malalignment or decreased conditioning.

During the physical examination, palpable grinding or audible popping may be appreciated through a range of motion. These signs do not correlate with location and severity of articular cartilage involvement. Hamstring tightness is often associated with effusion and arthritis. A symptomatic plica does not necessarily exclude the presence of chondromalacia but has been associated with various inflammatory processes about the knee. Routine roentgenographic studies, including patellar sunrise views, rarely show joint-space narrowing unless significant degeneration has occurred. MRI has been used successfully to document irregularities of the articular surface of the patella. Ultimately, the diagnosis of chondromalacia of the patella must be made by direct visualization using open or arthroscopic techniques. Outerbridge classified chondromalacia by grades of size and location of the lesion and the extent or depth of cartilage involvement.[52,84] These factors are important in gauging the prognosis and guiding the choices of treatment. For a majority of females who present with chondromalacia as young adolescents, only a relatively mild extent of cartilage softening or fibrillation is present (grade 1 to 2 chondromalacia). Eighty percent of patients will respond to a conservative course of decreased activity, anti-inflammatory medications, hamstring stretching, quadriceps strengthening, and core stabilization. Some athletes may receive benefit from a neoprene or elastic knee sleeve. However, the patient should decide if an open or closed knee sleeve is more comfortable. Deep squats and open chain extension exercises such as the leg extension machine significantly increase posterior directed stresses on the patellar. In turn, this will exacerbate knee pain and inflammation.

In resistant cases that fail 6 to 12 months of rehabilitation or that have significant degenerative changes (grade 3 and 4 chondromalacia), surgical intervention may be necessary. Diagnostic arthroscopy can define extent the lesion and can provide long-term relief if a simple cartilaginous flap is present that can be débrided. If no mechanical lesion is present and the chondromalacia is severe, the prognosis for complete relief of pain is poor. Cartilage abrasion, scraping, and drilling is not always successful and any cartilage that is removed does not regenerate. In the ideal case normal hyaline cartilage is replaced by less structurally sound fibrocartilage. If there is associated chondromalacia on the femoral side of the patellofemoral articulation, the prognosis is particularly guarded. Chondral and chondrocyte transplantation procedures have been less successful in the patellofemoral joint than in the medial and lateral sides of the knees. For resistant cases that have failed rehabilitation and arthroscopy, surgical elevation of the tibial tubercle to reduce the pressures on damaged cartilage on the undersurface of the patella may improve symptoms.

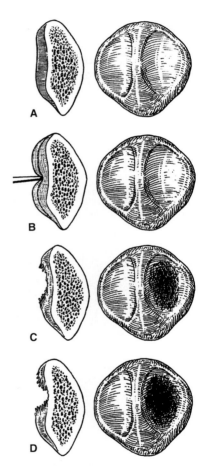

Figure 36-29. The Outerbridge classification of chondromalacic change is shown diagrammatically: **A**, normal articular cartilage of the patella; **B**, grade I: softening only, without fragmentation or fissuring; **C**, grades II and III: fissuring and fragmentation, with grade II being less than 1 inch and grade III being more than 1 inch. There is no exposed subchondral bone. **D**, grade IV: down to subchondral bone. Documentation of the grade and size of the arthritic change is helpful, particularly in the patellofemoral articulation, in predicting success and outlining a rehabilitation program. (From Outerbridge RE: The etiology of chondromalacia patellae. J Bone Joint Surg 43B:752-7, 1961.)

Patellectomy should only be a salvage procedure and should be considered only in rare cases. There is no guarantee of pain relief after patellectomy. Return to any athletic participation after patellectomy is all but impossible. Function of the knee will be permanently impaired.

Patellar Tendinitis, Osgood–Schlatter's Disease and Sinding—Larsen–Johansson Disease, and Jumper's Knee

An imbalance of flexor and extensor muscle strength and flexibility about the knee can lead to overuse and inflammation in the tendons and at the origins and insertions of the tendons to bone. The amount of overuse depends on a particular athlete's demands and the nature of her sport. Actively growing children develop a relative loss of flexibility because the muscle-tendon units take more time to stretch out and catch up to the length of the growing bone. Reduced flexibility has been associated with the prevalence of overuse injuries in this population: patellar tendinitis, Osgood–Schlatter's disease, and jumper's knee. These conditions continue to be significantly more common in males than females. Osgood–Schlatter's disease is a tibial tubercle apophysitis secondary to the traction forces of the extensor mechanism. Jumper's knee is an inflammation of the patellar tendon at its insertion onto the distal pole of the patella, while Sinding—Larsen–Johansson disease is an apophysitis of the distal pole of the patella.

Patellar tendinitis is a generalized inflammation that occasionally involves structural change (tendinosis) of the patellar tendon. Female athletes are at less risk of suffering from all of these extensor mechanism overuse injuries than their male counterparts. When these injuries are present, female athletes tend to suffer them earlier and to a milder degree. The reduced incidence is probably related to specific sports, intensity of participation, growth phases, and the relatively earlier maturation and physeal closure in females. As intensity and year-round demands increase for female athletes, one would expect the incidence to increase. The reduced severity is likely explained by the female athlete's smaller size and reduced torque production at the knee.[15] Most athletes respond to a conservative course of treatment, including ice, anti-inflammatory medications, hamstring stretching, and quadriceps and core strengthening. Topical nonsteroidal drugs and prolotherapy have also been advocated. Reduction in the intensity of activity may also be required. This may be accomplished by recommending that the athlete alternate seasons of athletic activity so that a competitive season is followed by a season of relative rest. Surgical débridement of the patella may provide relief in resistant cases after skeletal maturity. MRI is recommended to document the area of tendinosis prior to proceeding with débridement. Careful supervision of postoperative rehabilitation following a specific protocol is recommended to avoid recurrence.

Plicae

A plica is an intra-articular synovial fold,[44,85] In the knee, there are 4 possible sites for plicae: superior, medial, lateral, and anterior. Symptomatic plicae are most often seen in adolescent females competing in cheerleading, cross-country, and swimming. The medial plica is a band of synovium which crosses near the medial femoral condyle running between the patella and medial gutter. With deep flexion, the band can impinge on the medial femoral condyle and can occasionally be pinched between the medial facet of the patella and femoral condyle. With repetitive irritation and pinching, the synovial band becomes thickened and inflamed. With repetitive squatting, the athlete may complain of snapping, instability, or pain. The pain is usually quite focal along the medial border of the patella. A palpable plica that reproduces the pain and is asymmetrically thicker than the opposite knee's plica is indicative of the diagnosis. A complete knee examination should always be undertaken because intra-articular pathology can cause synovial and plical inflammation and mimic an isolated symptomatic plica. Most athletes with an isolated symptomatic plica will respond to a conservative course of ice, anti-inflammatory drugs, and quadriceps rehabilitation. Patellar taping or a knee sleeve with a lateral pad may also provide relief. Occasionally, an intra-articular steroid injection can provide long-term relief. In resistant cases, arthroscopic surgical resection of the plica is highly successful, assuming the diagnosis has been correctly made.

Iliotibial Band Tendinitis

Iliotibial band tendinitis is an inflammatory irritation of the structure at the level of the pelvic brim, the greater trochanter, the lateral femoral condyle, or Gerdy's tubercle as it inserts onto the tibia. Most commonly, pain is over the femoral epicondyle and occurs in sports involving repetitive running or landing. More frequently in women, contributing factors are a wider pelvis and more prominent trochanter.[43] Irritation occurs as the tight fascial band repetitively passes over the bony prominence. Athletes who are descending from a height with a relatively heavy load appear to irritate the band as it passes over the lateral femoral condyle. Localized pain on palpation over the lateral femoral condyle with flexion and extension of the knee confirms the diagnosis. Local anesthetic injection can assist in confirming the diagnosis.

Treatment is focused on relieving inflammation and stretching out the iliotibial band. Ice, anti-inflammatory medications, ultrasound, or electrical stimulation may be beneficial in relieving inflammation. The key to preventing recurrence is a program of stretching and strengthening the iliotibial band. Stretching can be done by having the patient put her body weight on her affected leg, which is positioned behind the unaffected leg, and leaning into the affected leg.[85] Leg abduction exercises and lateral step-ups are effective in strengthening the iliotibial band. In resistant cases, steroid injections can be made into the inflamed bursa. Care to avoid injection directly into ligaments or tendons is important. Relief of pain is diagnostic and, hopefully, will allow the athlete to more comfortably participate in her own rehabilitation. The majority of athletes improve with this treatment. In athletes who fail injections and conservative treatment, surgical releases can be performed, dividing the iliotibial band as it crosses the epicondyle.

Anterior Cruciate Ligament Tears

Perhaps the greatest concern regarding the female athlete's knee is the high rate of ACL injuries in noncontact sports. Reasons for the increased risk, as previously discussed, are multifactorial. Variables can be thought of as changeable (extrinsic), not changeable (intrinsic) or potentially changeable (Table 36-4).

The mechanism of ACL tear is captured on video in Figure 36-30. The position is typical: upright, weight forward, knee in extreme valgus, hip internally rotated, and femur adducted and tibial externally rotated.

Figure 36-31 presents postoperative views of a female basketball athlete who tore her ACL. With her knee in hyperextension, posterior bowing of her tibia is seen as she is supine passively (Fig. 36-31A) and standing (Fig. 36-31B). The extreme hyperextended position makes the knee more vulnerable to ACL tears because the hamstrings are at a mechanically less advantageous position and there is a tendency for more upright landings. On MRI the typical bone bruise pattern is seen at the mid-third lateral femoral condyle and posterior lateral tibial plateau (Fig. 36-31C,D).

Treatment choices and indications may be slightly different for the ACL-deficient female athlete. With less muscular power, relative hyperextension, increased ligamentous laxity, and greater valgus alignment, female athletes may be more likely to fail a conservative course of rehabilitation and bracing. Females may not be as good as males at "coping" with the ACL deficiency. If a female athlete suffers an ACL injury, her anatomic structure and ligament-dominated stability increase her likelihood of recurrent giving way, which reduces her likelihood of returning to sport at her previous level. One should base a decision to reconstruct on factors known to influence recurrence, including patient age, associated injuries, level of play, desire to return to competitive twisting and cutting sports, number of recurrent episodes, failure of conservative treatment, and willingness to undertake extensive rehabilitation. This decision is individual, not based on gender.

For the female athlete with an ACL injury, one should take extra steps to educate her to prevent injuring the contralateral knee. Positive reinforcement during rehabilitation is particularly effective for the female athlete. Graft selection for ACL reconstruction in female athletes has been debated. Autogenous hamstrings may minimize surgical scars and reduce the risk of postsurgical anterior knee pain. Proponents of autogenous bone—tendon—bone grafts note similar risks of anterior knee pain regardless of graft material, better initial graft fixation with bone—tendon—bone, and avoidance of injuring

Table 36-4. Factors Contributing to ACL Injuries

INTRINSIC	EXTRINSIC	COMBINED (POTENTIALLY CHANGEABLE)
Alignment	Strength	Proprioception
Hyperextension	Conditioning	Position sense/balance
Physiologic rotatory laxity	Shoes	Neuromuscular patterns
ACL size	Motivation	Order of firing
Notch size/shape		Acquired skills
Hormonal influences		
Inherited skills/coordination		

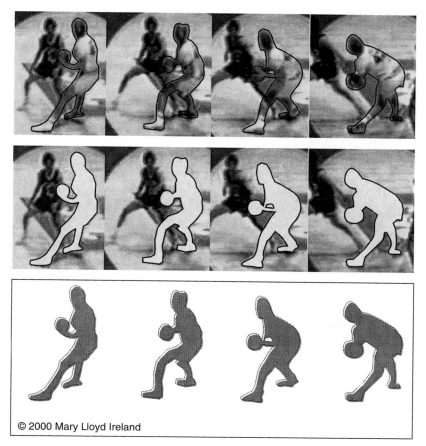

Figure 36-30. The mechanism of an ACL tear is captured on video. Injury to the left knee as observed from the back and left side of the athlete. She has just rebounded and stops to change direction to avoid the defending player. She lands in an upright position with less knee and hip flexion and a forward-flexed lumbar spine. After the ACL fails, she falls forward and knee valgus rotation and flexion increase. She is unable to upright herself and regain pelvis control to avoid ACL injury. (Copyright 2000, ML Ireland.)

the ACL-protective hamstrings. Other graft choices include a patellar tendon or hamstring graft harvested from the contralateral side, quadriceps tendon, or allograft. The preferred graft should be decided upon by the patient's informed understanding and the surgeon's own

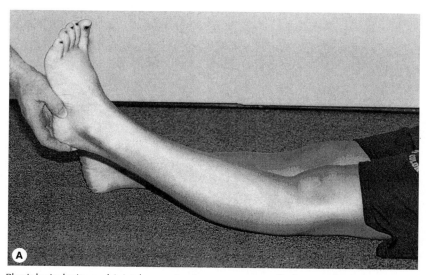

Figure 36-31. Physiologic laxity and joint hyperextension are common findings in the female athlete. (**A**) In the supine position, passive extension documents the hyperextension of the knee and posterior bowing of the tibia.

Illustration continued on following page

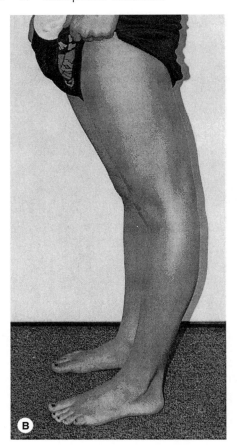

Figure 36-31 *(Continued).* **(B)** In the standing position, the hyperextension of the left knee is noted. A year after ACL reconstruction of the right knee, the patient has not regained all of her hyperextension and lacks approximately 20° of the hyperextension on her normal side.

experience. No studies comparing gender results from contralateral limbs have been published.[93] Clearly, there is no consensus at this time.

Gender Comparison Following ACL Reconstruction

Another study comparing male and female outcomes used the Cincinnati Knee Rating Scale, the Tegner Scale, and the ACL Quality of Life Scale to assess outcomes.[70,81,83,98] One hundred fifty-one athletes, 77 females and 74 males, were analyzed. No significant difference between acute and chronic female reconstructions was seen. Females tore their ACL at age 21.7 years, males at 26.5 years. Overall, no significant differences were seen between males and females using the Tegner and ACL Quality of Life scales. A significant difference was seen with the Cincinnati Knee Rating Scale, on which females scored lower on the involved side than males. In subgroups of athletes injured playing basketball or soccer, no differences were seen in any of the 3 scales.

In a prospective review of ACL reconstructions comparing patellar tendon autograft and hamstring autograft, gender differences were noted in KT-1000 testing.[16] Increased laxity in the hamstring tendon group was associated with the patient's sex. The mean difference side to side of 2.5 mm in females in the hamstring group was significantly greater than in females

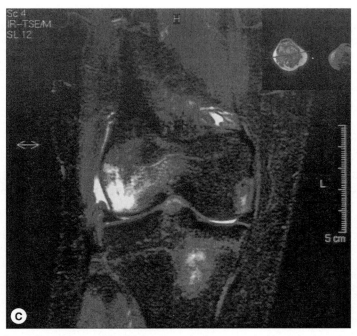

Figure 36-31 *(Continued).* **(C)** The MRI scan of her left knee acutely shows a typical bone bruise pattern with edema on the T_2-weighted images on the anteroposterior side of the femur and mid-portion and posterior aspect of the tibia seen on lateral view.

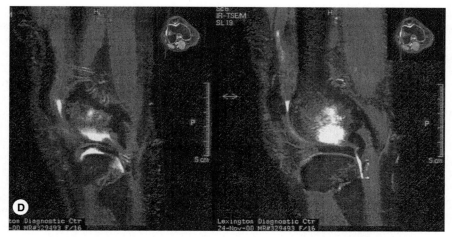

Figure 36-31 *(Continued).* **(D)** A subluxation event occurs as the ACL tears and the bone bruise pattern is consistent with a standing pivot shift. (Copyright 2002, ML Ireland.)

in the patellar tendon group ($P = 0.001$) and male patients in the patellar tendon ($P = 0.0003$) or hamstring group ($P < 0.0001$).

In a study comparing male and female outcomes after ACL reconstruction with ipsilateral central third patellar tendon bone, there were no significant differences.[4] Ninety-four patients, 47 of each sex, were rated by the Cincinnati Knee Rating Scale at 26 months postoperatively. Complications and outcomes were similar. Women required 6 more rehabilitation visits. The patellofemoral crepitus conversion rate was 7% in women and 15% in men. The failure rate was 6% for women and 4% for men. More outcome studies comparing gender in reconstructed knees are needed. A decision on rating scales must be made. There are established validated scales.[18,37,53,63,70,92,98] Decisions about which scale to use must be made for study design.

Other Ligament Injuries

Most ligament injuries are sport specific and not gender specific. Contact sports, including football and rugby, have the greatest incidence of medial collateral ligament (MCL) sprains. Because of their increased valgus alignment of the knee, it has been suggested that females should also be at increased risk of MCL injuries. Thus far, this has not been documented.[100] In swimmers performing the breaststroke, males tended to have increased complaints related to the MCL, while females tended to have complaints related to their patellofemoral joint.[97] No current literature documents a relationship between posterior cruciate ligament or lateral collateral ligament and gender.

Female athletes commonly sustain noncontact injuries, while males are more likely to sustain contact-related injuries to the knee. This is largely due to sport-specific factors rather than gender-specific factors. Gender influences can best be established by comparing males and females in similar sports or activities. For example, stress fractures and overuse injuries are related to poor conditioning seen in some female cadets, in comparison to male military cadets.[17,88] Female athletes are at risk of the same variety of knee injuries and complaints as male athletes, including fractures, knee dislocations, patellar instability, meniscal injuries, ligament injuries, muscle strains, overuse injuries, contusions, lacerations, abrasions, bursitis, and inflammation.

CONDITIONING AND EDUCATION

Level of fitness and conditioning, and knowledge of fundamental injury-prevention skills of movement and sport are important factors related to knee injuries. Admittedly this is a controversial subject and one must be careful NOT to stereotype female athletes as being less well conditioned or poorly skilled. Clearly this is not the case. Elite female athletes have, for the most part, trained hard, tuned their bodies, and optimized their skills to levels equivalent to those of their elite male counterparts. Nonetheless, young women historically have had reduced access to quality education and coaching. This is especially true for those just beginning their athletic activities.[14,17,25,34,100,102]

Studies from the military academies show a direct relationship between gender, conditioning level, and the incidence of stress-related and overuse injuries. In a random review of 74 female and 74 male young athletic cadets, an increased incidence of stress fractures and overuse injuries was found in females.[65] Interestingly, with preconditioning prior to boot camp or when the women became acclimated to the rigors of training, similar numbers of injuries were reported when comparing genders.[58,87] These studies did not specifically separate knee injuries; however, patellofemoral problems and acute knee ligament injuries have been related to poor conditioning. Indeed, preseason programs designed to address strength and balance have been instituted, with success in reducing the risk of knee injuries in some female collegiate athletes. Multicenter studies with higher numbers of participants are needed.

In addition to a relatively lower baseline level of conditioning found in female athletes, improper technical performance can increase an athlete's risk of injury.[34] Female athletes may not have enjoyed the benefits of their male counterparts of proper training under the supervision of a knowledgeable coach.[43] Only relatively recently have girls been welcomed into the beginner ranks of little league or soccer on equal footing with boys, entitling them to the same access to qualified coaches at a very young age. Improper technique and poor skills place the athlete at risk of injury because she may not perform the skill properly and safely, or use the recommended muscle firing pattern. The concept of safe landing position and position of no return should be understood (Fig. 36-32). The "ready position" is a bent hip and knee position seen in a number of sports, including basketball, volleyball, and tennis. In this knee-flexed position, the athlete can move quickly and safely. Not surprisingly, if one carefully observes collegiate men's and women's basketball and volleyball teams, one will quickly notice that the men are much more likely to assume the "ready position" than the women. The relative epidemic of ACL injuries in female athletes may be partially related to this type of variation in technique. It is now well accepted that proper training and conditioning programs are a necessity for any athlete, male or female.[57]

The effect of neuromotor training or retraining has proven to be effective in a number of studies. Caraffa and colleagues instituted prevention programs of conditioning and skills in soccer players and had a reduced incidence of major knee ligament injuries.[10] Johnson and coworkers from the University of Vermont were able to mimic these results in skiers by training skiers to avoid at-risk positions.[54] Noyes and

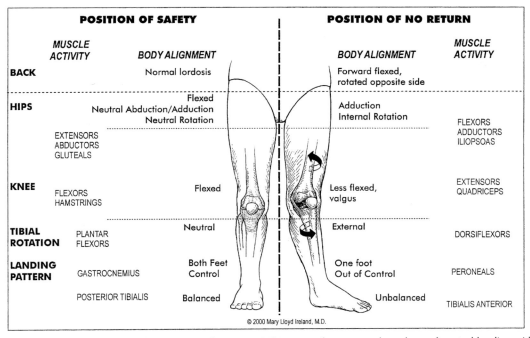

Figure 36-32. This diagram shows the "position of no return." This term refers to an awkward out-of-control landing with the leg pronated in valgus angulation, the body more upright and the leg in pronation and rotation, and the knee in valgus angulation, which places the ACL at risk of tearing. The safety position is more flexed, with the body over legs, and more balanced. (Copyright 2000, ML Ireland.)

colleagues definitively showed that an intense training program focused not only on muscular strength but also on landing skills and avoiding at-risk positions could significantly reduce the risk of ACL injuries in female athletes.[80] About the knee, poor conditioning can be associated with stress fractures, patellofemoral syndrome, iliotibial band syndrome, ligament injury, and so forth. Poor technique can lead to ligament injury, muscle strains, meniscal injuries, contusions, and other injuries.[6,45] It should not come as a surprise, therefore, that these are more commonly seen in female athletes. The good news is that conditioning and neuromotor skills training may hold the best potential to reduce the incidence of knee injuries in female athletes.

CONCLUDING REMARKS

In conclusion, gender does appear to play a significant role in the incidence of injuries as well as in the location and type of injuries sustained by the female athlete. A variety of factors, such as conditioning, flexibility, technical skills, and motor and neuromotor training, have the potential to be targets of preventive interventions. These could reduce the incidence of a number of knee-related complaints suffered more frequently by women. Nonetheless, structural anatomic variations between males and females such as valgus alignment, femoral offset, notch width, and ligamentous laxity may make it impossible for injury rates about the knee of male and female athletes to be identical. Intervention programs must be implemented. Sport-specific body awareness, strengthening, and landing strategies should be started at a young age and continued. Young female athletes should understand the risk of competing and be given the opportunity to reduce this risk by participating in specific programs.

References

1. American Medical Association: Standard Nomenclature of Athletic Injuries. Chicago, American Medical Association, 1966.
2. Arendt EA, Agel J, Dick R: Anterior cruciate ligament injury patterns among collegiate men and women. J Athletic Train 34(2):86–92, 1999.
3. Arendt E, Dick R: Knee injury patterns among men and women in collegiate basketball and soccer: NCAA data and review of literature. Am J Sports Med 23(6):694–701, 1995.
4. Barber-Westin SD, Noyes FR, Andrews M: A rigorous comparison between the sexes of results and complications after anterior cruciate ligament reconstruction. Am J Sports Med 25(4):514–26, 1997.
5. Beck X, Wildermuth BP: The female athlete's knee. Clin Sports Med 4(2)345–66, 1985.
6. Benas D: Special considerations in women's rehabilitation programs. In: Hunter LY, Funk FL (eds): Rehabilitation of the Injured Knee. St Louis, CV Mosby, 1985.
7. Bjordal JM, Arnly F, Hannestad B, Strand T: Epidemiology of anterior cruciate ligament injuries in soccer. Am J Sports Med 25(3):341–5, 1997.
8. Boden BP, Garrett WE, Jr: Mechanisms of injuries to the anterior cruciate ligament [abstr]. Med Sci Sports Exerc Suppl 28(5):S26, 1996.
9. Butler DL, Noyes FR, Grood ES: Ligamentous restraints to anterior-posterior drawer in the human knee: A biomechanical study. J Bone Joint Surg 62A:259, 1980.
10. Caraffa A, Cerulli G, Projetti M, et al: Prevention of anterior cruciate ligament injuries in soccer. A prospective controlled study of proprioceptive training. Knee Surg Sports Traumtol Arthrosc 4(1):19–21, 1996.
11. Carter JEL, et al: Anthropometry of Montreal Olympic athletes. In: Carter JEL (ed): Medicine and Sport, Vol. 16. Basel, S Karger, 1992.
12. Clarke KS, Buckley WE: Women's injuries in collegiate sports. Am J Sports Med 8(3):187–91, 1980.
13. Cofield RH, Bryan RS: Acute dislocation of the patella: results of conservative treatment. J Trauma 17(7):526–31, 1977.
14. Collins RK: Injury patterns in women's flag football, Am J Sports Med 15(3):238–42, 1987.
15. Colosimo AJ, Ireland ML: Isokinetic peak torque and knee joint laxity in elite female basketball and volleyball college athletes. Med Sci Sports Exerc 23 (suppl 4):135, 1991.
16. Corry IS, Webb JM, Clingeleffer AJ, Pinczewski LA: Arthroscopic reconstruction of the anterior cruciate ligament: A comparison of patellar tendon autograft and four-strand hamstring tendon autograft. Am J Sports Med 27(3):444–54, 1999.
17. Cox JS, Lenz HW: Women midshipmen in sports. Am J Sports Med 12:241–3, 1984.
18. Craig EA: Intercondylar shelf angle: A new method to determine race from the distal femur. J Forensic Sci Sept:777–82, 1995.
19. DeLee JC, Farney WC: Incidence of injury in Texas high school football. Am J Sports Med 2;20(5):575–80, 1996.
20. Dye SF: The knee as a biologic transmission with an envelope of function. Clin Orthop Rel Res 323:10–8, 1996.
21. Eisenberg I, Allen WC: Injuries in a women's varsity athletic program. Physician Sportsmed 5:112–20, 1978.
22. Franklin BA, Lussier L, Buskirk ER: Injury rates in women joggers. Physician Sportsmed 7:104–12, 1979.
23. Fulkerson JP: Disorders of the patellofemoral joint. Baltimore, Williams & Wilkins, 1997.
24. Fulkerson JP, Becker GJ, Meaney JA, et al: Anteromedial tibial tubercle transfer without bone graft. Am J Sports Med 18:490–7, 1990.
25. Garrick JG, Requa RK: Girl's sports injuries in high school athletics. JAMA 239:2245–8, 1978.
26. Gillette J: When and where women are injured in sports. Physician Sportsmed 2:61–3, 1975.
27. Glick JM: The female knee in athletics. Physician Sportsmed 1:35–7, 1973.
28. Goldberg B, Rosenthall PP, Nicholas JA: Injuries in youth football, Physician Sportsmed 12(8):112–20, 1978.
29. Gomez E, DeLee JC, Farney WC: Incidence of injury in Texas girls high school basketball. Am J Sports Med 24(5):684–7, 1996.

30. Gray J, et al: A survey of injuries to the anterior cruciate ligament of the knee in female basketball players. Int J Sports Med 6:314–6, 1985.
31. Griffin LY, Agel J, Albohm MJ, et al: Noncontact anterior cruciate ligament injuries: Risk factors and prevention strategies. J Am Acad Orthop Surg 8(3):141–50, 2000.
32. Gwinn DE, Wilckens JH, McDevitt ER, Ross G, Kao T: The relative incidence of anterior cruciate ligament injury in men and women at the United States Naval Academy. Am J Sports Med 28(1):98–102, 2000.
33. Hale RW: Caring for Exercising Women. New York, Elsevier, 1991.
34. Harmon KG, Dick R: The relationship of skill level to anterior cruciate ligament injury. Clin J Sport Med 8(4):260–5, 1998.
35. Hawkins RJ, Bell RH, Anisette G: Acute patellar dislocations: the natural history. Am J Sports Med 14(2)117–20, 1986.
36. Haycock CE, Gillette JV: Susceptibility of women athletes to injury, myths vs. reality, JAMA 236:163–5, 1976.
37. Hefti F, Muller W: Current state of evaluation of knee ligament lesions. The new IKDC knee evaluation form. Orthopade 22:351–62, 1993.
38. Hopper DM, Hopper JL, Elliott BC: Do selected kinanthropometric and performance variables predict injuries in female netball players? J Sports Sci 13(3):213–22, 1995.
39. Horton MG, Hall TL: Quadriceps femoris muscle angle: Normal values and relationships with gender and selected skeletal measures. Phys Ther 69(11):897–901, 1989.
40. Hughston JC, Andrews JR, Cross MJ, Moschi A: Classification of knee ligament instabilities. Part I. The medial compartment and cruciate ligaments. J Bone Joint Surg 58A:159, 1976.
41. Hughston JC, Andrews JR, Cross MJ, Moschi A: Classification of knee ligament instabilities. Part II. The lateral compartment. J Bone Joint Surg 58A:173, 1976.
42. Hungerford DS, Barry M: Biomechanics of the patellofemoral joint. Clin Orthop RelRes 144:9–15, 1979.
43. Hunter LY: Aspects of injuries to the lower extremity unique to the female athlete. In: Nicholas JA, Hershman EB (eds): The Lower Extremity and Spine in Sports Medicine. St Louis, CV Mosby, 1995, pp 90–111.
44. Hughston J, Andrews J: The suprapatellar plica and internal derangement. J Bone Joint Surg 55A:1318, 1973.
45. Hunter LY, et al: Common orthopaedic problems of female athletes, In: Frankel VH (ed): AAOS Instructional Course Lectures XXXI. St Louis, CV Mosby, 1992.
46. Hutchinson MR, Ireland ML: Patella dislocation, recognizing the injury and its complications. Physician Sportsmed 23(10):53–60, 1995.
47. Insall JN: Surgery of the Knee. New York, Churchill Livingstone, 1983, pp 191–261.
48. Ireland ML: Anterior cruciate ligament injury in female athletes: Epidemiology. J Athletic Training 34(2): 150–4, 1999.
49. Ireland ML, Ballantyne BT, Little K, McClay IS: A radiographic analysis of the relationship between the size and shape of the intercondylar notch and anterior cruciate ligament injury. Knee Surg Sports Traumatol Arthroscopy 9:200–5, 2001.
50. Ireland ML, Hutchinson MR, Williams RI, Gaudette M: The knee. In: The Injured Athlete, 3rd edition. Philadelphia, Lippincott-Raven, 1999, pp 353–419.
51. Ireland ML, Wall C: Epidemiology and comparison of knee Injuries in elite male and female United States basketball athletes (abstr). Med Sci Sports Exerc 14, 1990.
52. Ireland ML, Williams RI: Degenerative arthritis of the knee. In: Andrews JR, Timmerman LA (eds): Diagnostic and Operative Arthroscopy. Philadelphia, WB Saunders, 1997, pp 325–45.
53. Irrgang JJ, Snyder-Mackler L, Wainner RS, et al: Development of a patient-reported measure of function of the knee. J Bone Joint Surg 80A(8):1132–45, 1998.
54. Johnson R, et al: Vermont Safety Research. PO Box 85. Underhill Center, VT 00540.
55. Jones RE: Common athletic injuries in women. Chmpr Therapy. 6:47–9, 1980.
56. Kelly MA: Algorithm for anterior knee pain. AAOS Instructional Course Lectures 47:339–43, 1998.
57. Klafs CE, Lyon MJ: The Female Athlete. St Louis, CV Mosby, 1982.
58. Kowal DM: Nature and causes of injuries in women resulting from an endurance training program. Am J Sports Med 8(4):275–9, 1980.
59. LaPrade RF, Burnett QM: Femoral intercondylar notch stenosis and correlation to anterior cruciate ligament injuries: a prospective study. Am J Sports Med 22(2):198–203, 1994.
60. Larsen E. Lauridsen F: Conservative treatment of patellar dislocations: influence of evident factors on the tendency to redislocation and therapeutic result. Clin Orthop 171:131–6,1982.
61. Levy AS, Wetzler MJ, Lewars M, Laughlin W: Knee injuries in women collegiate rugby players. Am J Sports Med 22(3):360–2, 1994.
62. Lindenfeld TN, Schmitt DJ, Hendy MP, et al: Incidence of injury in indoor soccer. Am J Sports Med 22(3):364–71, 1994.
63. Lysholm J, Gillquist J: Evaluation of knee ligament surgery results with special emphasis on use of a scoring scale. Am J Sports Med 10(3):150–4, 1982.
64. Liu SH, Al-Shaikh RA, Panossian V, et al: Estrogen affects the cellular metabolism of the ACL. Am J Sports Med 25(5):704–9, 1997.
65. McBride JT, Meade WC, Ryan JB: Incidence and pattern of injury in female cadets at West Point Military Academy. In: Pearl AJ: The Athletic Female. Champaign, Ill, Human Kinetics Publishers, 1993, pp 219–34.
66. McConnell J: The management of chondromalacia patellae: a long term Solution. Aust J Phys Ther 32(4):215–23, 1986.
67. McKay GD, Payne WR, Goldie PA, et al: A comparison of the injuries sustained by female basketball and netball players. Aust J Sci Med Sport 28(1):12–7, 1996.
68. Messina DF, Farney WC, DeLee JC: The incidence of injury in Texas high school basketball: A prospective study among male and female athletes. Am J Sports Med 27(3):294–9, 1999.
69. Micheli L: Female runners. In: D'Ambrosia R, Drez D (eds): Prevention and Treatment of Running Injuries. Thorofare, NJ, Slack, 1982.
70. Mohtadi N: Development and validation of the quality of life outcome measure (questionnaire) for chronic anterior cruciate ligament deficiency. Am J Sports Med 26(3):350–9, 1998.
71. Mueller W: The knee: Form, function, and ligament reconstruction. New York, Springer-Verlag, 1983, pp 80–4.
72. Myklebust G, Engebretsen L: Registration of ACL-injuries in the 3 upper divisions in Norwegian team handball: A prospective study (abstr). Med Sci Sports Exer Suppl 25(5):S50, 1993.

73. Myklebust G, Maehlum S, Engebretsen L, et al: Registration of cruciate ligament injuries in Norwegian top level team handball. A prospective study covering two seasons. Scans J Med Sci Sports 7(5):289–92, 1997.

74. Myklebust G, Maehlum S, Holm I, Bahr R: A prospective cohort study of anterior cruciate ligament injuries in elite Norwegian team handball. Scand J Med Sci Sports 8:149–53, 1998.

75. National Collegiate Athletic Association: NCAA Injury Surveillance System. Overland Park, Kan, NCAA, 1997–1998.

76. National Collegiate Athletic Association: NCAA Injury Surveillance System. Indianapolis, Ind, NCAA, 1999–2000.

77. Natri A, Jarvinen M, Kannus P, et al: Changing injury pattern of acute anterior cruciate ligament tears treated at Tampere University Hospital in the 1980s. Scand J Med Sci Sports 5(2):100–4, 1995.

78. Nicholas JA: Injuries to knee ligaments. JAMA 212(13):2236–39, 1970.

79. Norwood LA, Cross MJ: Anterior cruciate ligament: Functional anatomy of its bundles in rotatory instabilities. Am J Sports Med 7:23, 1979.

80. Noyes, et al: The effect of neuromuscular training on the incidence of knee injury in female athletes. A prospective study. Am J Sports Med 27(6):699–706, 1999.

81. Noyes FR: The Noyes Knee Rating System: An Assessment of Subjective, Objective, Ligamentous, and Functional Parameters. Cincinnati Sportsmedicine Research and Education Foundation, Cincinnati, Ohio, 1990.

82. O'Brien WR, Friederich NF, Muller W, Henning CE. Functional anatomy of the cruciate ligaments. American Academy of Orthopaedic Surgeons Instructional Videotape. Park Ridge, Ill, AAOS, 1991.

83. Ott SM, Ireland ML, Ballantyne B, McClay I: Comparison of outcomes between males and females After ACL reconstruction. Med Sci Sports Med Exerc 32(5):S207, 2000.

84. Outerbridge RE: The etiology of chondromalacia patellae. J Bone Joint Surg 43B:752–7, 1961.

85. Patel D: Plica as a cause of anterior knee pain. Orthop Clin North Am 17(2):273, 1986.

86. Powers JA: Characteristic features of injuries in the knee of women. Clin Orthop and Rel Res 143:120–4, 1979.

87. Protzman RR, Bodnari LM: Women athletes. Am J Sports Med 8:53–5, 1980.

88. Protzman RR, Griffis C: Stress fractures in men and women undergoing military training. J Bone Joint Surg 59A:325, 1977.

89. Reynolds L, et al: EMG analysis of the vastus medialis obliquus and the vastus lateralis in their role in patellar alignment. Am J Phys Med 62(2):61–71, 1983.

90. Rosenberg TD, Paulos LE, Parker RD, et al: The forty-five degree posteroanterior flexion weight-bearing radio-graph of the knee. J Bone Joint Surg 70A(10):1479–83, 1988.

91. Santavirta S: Integrated electromyography of the vastus medialis muscle after meniscectomy. Am J Sports Med 7:40–2, 1979.

92. Shapiro ET, Richmond JC, Rockett SE, et al: The use of a generic, patient-based health assessment (SF–36) for evaluation of patients with anterior cruciate ligament injuries. Am J Sports Med 24(2):196–200, 1996.

93. Shelbourne KD, Urch SE: Primary anterior cruciate ligament reconstruction using the contralateral autogenous patellar tendon. Am J Sports Med 28(5):651–8, 2000.

94. Souryal TO, Moore HA, Evans JP: Bilaterality in anterior cruciate ligament injuries. Associated intercondylar notch stenosis. Am J Sports Med 22(2):198–203, 1994.

95. Stevenson H, Webster J, Johnson R, Beynnon B: Gender differences in knee injury epidemiology among competitive alpine ski racers. Iowa Orthop J 18:64–6, 1998.

96. Strickland S, Belknap TW, Levine RE, et al: Hormonal influences on mechanical properties of sheep knee ligaments (abstr). American Orthopaedic Society for Sports Medicine Final Program and General Session Abstracts and Outlines, Sun Valley, Idaho, June 18–21, 2000, p 205.

97. Stuhlberg SD: Breaststroker's knee: pathology, etiology, and treatment. Am J Sports Med 8(3):164–71, 1980.

98. Tegner Y, Lysholm J: Rating systems in the evaluation of knee ligament injuries. Clin Orthop 198:43–9, 1985.

99. Vaupel G, Dye S: Functional knee anatomy. In: Baker CL (ed): The Hughston Clinic Sports Medicine Book. Baltimore: Williams & Wilkins, 1995, pp 403–15.

100. Whiteside PA: Men's and women's injuries in comparable sports. Physician Sportsmed 8(3):130–40, 1980.

101. Wojtys EM, et al: Association between the menstrual cycle and anterior cruciate ligament injuries in female athletes. Am J Sports Med 26(5):614–8,1998.

102. Zelisko JA, Noble HB, Porter M: A comparison of men's and women's professional basketball injuries. Am J Sports Med 10:297–9, 1982.

103. Zillmer DA, Powell JW, Albright JP: Gender specific injury patterns in high school varsity basketball. J Women's Health 1(1):69–76, 1992.

104. Mariani P, Caruso I: An electromyographic investigation of subluxation of the patella. J Bone Joint Surg 61B(2):169–71, 1979.

105. Flandry F: A classification of knee ligament instability. In: Baker CL (ed): The Hughston Clinic Sports Medicine Book. Baltimore: Williams & Wilkins, 1995, pp 481–93.

Chapter 37

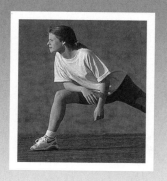

Foot and Ankle Injuries

Sandra A. Eisele, M.D.

This is an exciting time for women athletes, with new opportunities to reach ever-greater levels of performance. Women are training younger, harder, more intensively, and longer than ever before. The normal anatomy characteristic of women can predispose the athlete to injuries, and these anatomic characteristics must be better understood. However, most foot and ankle injuries in men and women are similar. This chapter will review special considerations involving the common injuries and treatment of the foot and ankle in female athletes.

FOOT AND ANKLE ANATOMY

The important aspects of the ankle and foot ligaments are summarized in Figure 37-1.

Ligaments

The ligaments span joints, supporting the bony anatomy and maintaining normal alignment of the underlying bony structure. The lateral ankle ligament complex, the syndesmotic ligament complex, the deltoid ligament, the calcaneonavicular or "spring" ligament, the bifurcate ligament, the interosseous talocalcaneal ligament, and the tarsal-metatarsal and intermetatarsal ligaments are the important structures. With the ankle in plantar flexion the anterior talofibular ligament is stretched parallel to the alignment of the leg. The most common plantar flexion inversion injury first tears this ligament and, secondarily, the calcaneofibular ligament. The syndesmotic ligament complex is most often injured in external rotation-type injuries, when the anterior inferior tibiofibular ligament is torn first, then the syndesmotic ligament and, with severe trauma, the posterior inferior tibiofibular ligament. The deltoid ligament, though rarely injured, is torn or sprained in external rotation-type injuries, so is often associated with syn-

desmotic injuries and proximal fibular fractures. The calcaneonavicular ligament helps the deep fibers of the deltoid ligament to support the head of the talus at the talonavicular joint. This ligament in itself can be torn or can stretch out, especially when associated with posterior tibial tendon insufficiency. This results in pain, swelling, and an acquired flat-foot deformity. The bifurcate ligament can be injured in the typical plantar flexion inversion injury, and an avulsion of the anterior process of the calcaneus can occur. This fracture is often missed, can cause persistent pain, and can develop into a nonunion that may require screw fixation or excision of the bony fragment. The talocalcaneal ligament can be torn in inversion injuries and contributes to persistent subtalar pain, synovitis, and subtalar instability. The tarsal-metatarsal ligaments maintain the important Lisfranc joints, and are injured with a forefoot abduction force or internal rotation of the leg with the foot planted. These ligaments also can be damaged with a fall onto the toes with the foot in plantar flexion. Since the joints can spring open and then return to near anatomic position, one must look for subtle widening of the intertarsal joints and metatarsals and small avulsion fractures at the bases of the metatarsals on plain radiographs. There is no ligament between the bases of the first and second metatarsals, so these bones often separate during this injury. Sprains, subluxations, and dislocations of the tarsal-metatarsal joints need immediate diagnosis and treatment.

Tendons

The extrinsic tendons of the foot and ankle are more easily injured than the intrinsics, and imbalance between these groups causes foot deformities such as hammertoes. The most common tendons injured are the Achilles, posterior tibial, and peroneal tendons.

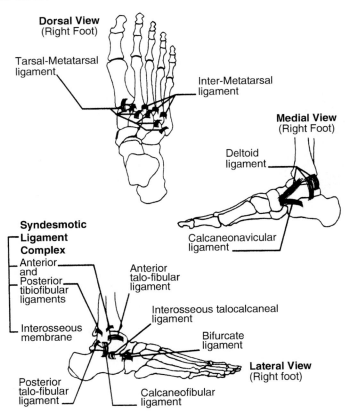

Figure 37-1. Ligaments of the ankle and foot.

The Achilles tendon is formed by the gastrocnemius and soleus muscles, and inserts on the posterior calcaneus after passing the posterior superior calcaneus. Overuse syndromes and tendinitis occur at the retrocalcaneal bursal area between the posterior superior calcaneus and the Achilles tendon (retrocalcaneal bursitis), as well as at the insertion of the Achilles tendon onto the calcaneus (insertional Achilles tendinitis). The Achilles tendon also can develop peritendinitis and tendinosis in the area 2 to 4 inches above the calcaneus.[26]

The posterior tibial muscle is part of the deep posterior compartment of the leg, and the tendon runs posterior to the medial malleolus to a broad insertion centered on the navicular. The posterior tibial tendon primarily inverts and plantar flexes the foot, and is the main dynamic stabilizer of the longitudinal arch. It can become inflamed from irritation as it passes posterior and below the medial malleolus. There is an area of relative hypovascularity posterior and distal to the medial malleolus, which is the most common location of tendinitis and tendon degeneration.[7]

The peroneal muscles form the lateral compartment of the leg, and the tendons course posterior to the lateral malleolus, with the peroneal brevis inserting at the base of the fifth metatarsal and the peroneal longus inserting on the plantar aspect of the first metatarsal head and medial cuneiform bone. Tendinitis and longitudinal tears occur in both these tendons, usually in the area near the tip of the lateral malleolus or distal to this location, on the lateral side of the calcaneus.[25] The groove the tendons travel through may be shallow, flat, or convex, predisposing the tendons to subluxation or dislocation.[6,16]

Some athletic activities may predispose to tendon injuries, for example, toe dancing predisposes to flexor hallucis longus tendinitis in ballet dancers. The flexor tendon sheath becomes stenotic, chronic inflammation of the tendon causes degeneration and thickening, and a "trigger toe" condition develops.

Joints

The ankle joint is a very tightly fitting joint, and range of motion is limited to dorsiflexion and plantarflexion. This joint is more stable in dorsiflexion than in plantar flexion because of the wider anterior width of the talus. The subtalar joint has limited inversion and eversion motion, has 3 facets, and allows for angular shifting necessary for the foot to accommodate to uneven ground. The configuration of the wedge-shaped bones of the midfoot maintains the transverse arch, and the longitudinal arch is maintained by bony configuration, ligamentous support, and dynamic support from the posterior tibial tendon.

The distal tibial and fibular growth plates are frequently injured in the child and adolescent. Ligaments are stronger than the cartilaginous growth plate (physis) and surrounding bone, and therefore the physis can break before a ligament tears or bone fractures.[29]

GENDER-SPECIFIC CONSIDERATIONS

There are no specific differences in foot and ankle anatomy related to gender, but other gender differences affect its structure and function. Some are hormonal, some structural, and some inherited.[29] There are also cultural factors that affect choice of shoe wear.

The female pelvis is wider and women tend to have more femoral anteversion at the hip, both of which contribute to an increased "Q angle."[4] This can result in peripatellar pain and patellar instability. Lower-extremity malalignment can result in genu valgum and a tendency to pronate the foot. The excessively pronated foot can be painful. The use of longitudinal arch supports or custom shoe inserts can correct the pronation, and often will alleviate knee pain as well as foot pain.

The use of high-fashion footwear is common among women. Many athletes wear athletic shoes much of the time, but fit and foot and shoe type must be evaluated. If there is a hereditary predisposition to foot deformity such as hallux valgus, more damage can occur. Parents and coaches must pay attention to what is worn off the court or playing field and encourage the use of properly fitting footwear.[8,12,27] Conditions such as metatarsus primus varus, hallux valgus, and juvenile bunion deformity affect women more than men, and may be symptomatic in many athletes.

ANKLE SPRAINS

The most common athletic injury in sports is the ankle sprain from a plantar flexion inversion positioning.[32] This injury was particularly common in gymnastics, basketball, volleyball, and soccer according to the National Collegiate Athletic Association Injury Surveillance System during the 1997–1998 season. The rate of ankle

sprains in adolescent girls has been reported to be slightly higher than that in adolescent boys, but treatment is similar.[28,33]

GRADING OF SPRAINS

Ankle sprains generally are classified in severity as grade 1, 2, or 3. On initial evaluation the physical examination will reveal the amount of swelling and ecchymosis, from which one can estimate how much tissue damage has occurred. One should also look for evidence of nerve damage, tendon injury, and injury to adjacent joints. If possible, anterior drawer and varus stress examinations should be done to detect instability. Radiographs will add information concerning bony injury as well as past injury to the joint. Based on the examination and radiographs, a treatment plan is then determined.[31]

A grade 1 ankle sprain is a partial rupture of the anterior talofibular ligament, with mild swelling, little functional impairment, and no instability on stress testing. A grade 2 sprain is a complete rupture of the anterior talofibular ligament and perhaps stretching of the calcaneofibular ligament, with more swelling and ecchymosis, an inability to be fully weight bearing, and mild instability with a positive anterior drawer test but negative talar tilt. A grade 3 injury is a complete rupture of the anterior talofibular and calcaneofibular ligaments, with severe swelling and pain, inability to bear weight, and positive anterior drawer and talar tilt tests. In a grade 3 injury the patient often can not tolerate stress testing, so stress testing may need to be done at a later time. In addition, the grade 3 sprain will cause swelling and tenderness medially, indicating the injury was rotational, causing stretching of the deltoid ligament.

TREATMENT

Nonsurgical treatment is recommended for essentially all ankle sprains initially, regardless of severity. The only controversy is in grade 3 sprains in elite athletes, in whom some would recommend early surgical repair. Grade 1 sprains can be treated with rest, ice, compression, and elevation and the athlete should be started on early physical therapy. The goal is to reduce the soft-tissue reaction to injury, begin the rehabilitative phase as soon as possible, and prevent reinjury. Grade 2 sprains need all the treatment described for grade 1 injuries, but may need an initial period of protection from weight bearing or brace immobilization. This will allow the healing process to begin and the pain to decrease before rehabilitation is begun. The treatment of severe grade 3 sprains is controversial. All the treatments for grades 1 and 2 sprains are needed, but the first phase often is immobilization. This can be in the form of a short-leg walking cast for 2 to 4 weeks or a functional brace that supports the ankle but allows earlier weight bearing and onset of the rehabilitative phase. Most studies show that functional bracing leads to the quickest return to full range of motion, improved strength, and return to work and recreational activity. Approximately 10% to 20% of all acute ankle sprains will develop chronic instability, on the basis of partial tearing and lengthening of the lateral ankle ligaments and abnormal proprioception in the ankle.[17]

COMPLICATIONS OF ANKLE SPRAINS

Other injuries can accompany the "simple" ankle sprain. Chondral or osteochondral fractures occur in approximately 6.5% of acute ankle sprains.[18] They often will heal with 6 weeks of immobilization and no weight bearing. The chronic osteochondral fractures, as well as those acute ones that are displaced, require surgical fixation or débridement.

The initial radiograph may show a fracture, sometimes very small, of the anterior process of the calcaneus, which is an avulsion of the bifurcate ligament. This injury will require about 6 weeks of cast immobilization, and then often will take several months to completely heal.

The initial radiographs should also be evaluated for a fracture of the lateral process of the talus. This is best seen on the mortise view. A small undisplaced fracture can be treated with cast immobilization for 6 weeks, but larger fractures require internal fixation, and comminuted fractures need to be excised.[9]

Persistent pain and swelling that may occur after ankle sprain may not respond to physical therapy, bracing, and anti-inflammatory medications. A magnetic resonance imaging (MRI) scan often is normal. These symptoms can be caused by anterolateral impingement or thickened synovium and scar tissue. This scar tissue develops from repetitive trauma to the anterior talofibular ligament or the inferior fibers of the anterior inferior tibiofibular ligament.[3,11] Arthroscopic débridement of this tissue usually provides relief. Anterior impingement is caused by bony spurs that are thought to develop from traction on the anterior joint capsule as it inserts into the distal tibia, and on the dorsal neck of the talus. These spurs limit joint motion and cause persistent pain in dorsiflexion; surgical removal of these spurs may be indicated.

Persistent lateral ankle pain and swelling can be caused by tears of the peroneal longus or brevis tendons. These conditions often occur at the time of an ankle sprain when the tendons sublux over the posterolateral edge of the fibula, causing a partial tear of the tendon that continues to degenerate. The superior peroneal retinaculum is torn, allowing the tendons to sublux, and then they resume their anatomic position. The tendon tears do not heal, requiring surgical débridement and repair, addressing associated conditions such as ligament instability and peroneal subluxation.[6,16]

ANKLE FRACTURES

The sudden onset of an acute fracture of the ankle is not specific to sport. Knowledge of the most common types of fractures in adults and children is essential in evaluating the athlete with an injured ankle.[30] Stress fractures also occur in the ankle. Injuries in the skeletally immature must be accurately assessed and anatomically reduced.[14]

Adult Fractures

There are many classifications of ankle fractures, and they are useful in determining the mechanism of injury, diagnosing associated injuries, and recommending the appropriate treatment and prognosis of the injury. Initial treatment should include splinting, rest, ice, compression, and elevation, and transportation to an emergency department for appropriate evaluation and radiographs.

Classification

The most widely used classification for ankle fractures is the Weber/AO classification, which is based on the level of the fibular fracture, as seen in Figure 37-2.[20]

The type A injury is a fibular fracture below the joint line and a vertical fracture of the medial malleolus. The type B injury is an oblique fracture of the fibula starting at the level of the tibiotalar joint and extending proximally, a tear of the deltoid ligament, or a medial malleolar fracture; it can also involve a posterior malleolar fracture. Type C injuries involve a fibular fracture above the tibiotalar joint, a transverse med-

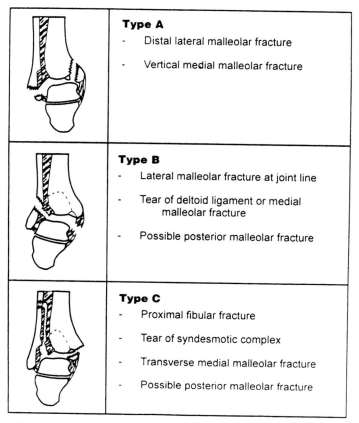

Type A
- Distal lateral malleolar fracture
- Vertical medial malleolar fracture

Type B
- Lateral malleolar fracture at joint line
- Tear of deltoid ligament or medial malleolar fracture
- Possible posterior malleolar fracture

Type C
- Proximal fibular fracture
- Tear of syndesmotic complex
- Transverse medial malleolar fracture
- Possible posterior malleolar fracture

Figure 37-2. The Weber/AO classification of ankle fractures. (From Poss R (ed): Orthopaedic Knowledge Update 3, Park Ridge, IL, American Academy of Orthopaedic Surgeons, 1990, pp 613–624. Adapted from Müller ME, et al. Manual of Internal Fixation. Heidelberg, Sprieger-Verlag, 1991.)

ial malleolar fracture, a posterior malleolar fracture, and rupture of the syndesmotic ligament. Not all the components described are present in each case, but these are associated injury patterns and are used as a guide to better evaluate each patient.

Treatment of ankle fractures depends primarily on the amount of displacement at the fracture sites and at the joint surface. Since a shift of the joint surface of only 1 mm has been shown to reduce tibiotalar surface contact area by 42%, joint subluxation can not be tolerated.[23] Isolated lateral malleolar fractures without lateral talar shift have recently been shown to be stable injuries that do not change the tibiotalar relationship, and can be treated nonoperatively.[13] Stable fractures also can be treated nonoperatively with cast or brace immobilization, but generally fractures displaced more than 2 or 3 mm or any fracture with a shift in the relationship of the articular surfaces of the joint should be surgically corrected.

Stress fractures of the ankle typically occur in the lateral or medial malleolus. The lateral malleolar fractures are transverse, just above the flare of the lateral malleolus, and are common in running and jumping sports. The medial malleolar fractures are rare, occur at the junction of the medial malleolus and tibial plafond, and occur in high-impact sports such as basketball and gymnastics. Stress fractures of the lateral malleolus usually heal with conservative treatment by eliminating the activity responsible for this injury for 4 to 6 weeks. Stress fractures of the medial malleolus heal much slower, often requiring many months of reduced activity for symptoms to disappear.

Age-Related Fractures and Conditions in Children and Adolescents

Tarsal Coalition

Tarsal coalition is an abnormal union between 2 or more tarsal bones, most commonly occurring between the calcaneus and the navicular, and in the area of the middle facet of the talocalcaneal joint.[5] The union can be bony, fibrous, or cartilaginous. The calcaneonavicular coalition becomes symptomatic between ages 8 and 12, and the talocalcaneal coalition becomes symptomatic about ages 12 to 16. These ages correspond to the age of bar ossification. On examination these adolescents are noted to have stiffness and pes planus, and some will have a classic spastic flat foot with excessive peroneal muscle spasm. Pain is usually located in the area of the midfoot, hindfoot, or subtalar joint. Treatment is initially conservative, with shoe modification and the use of custom-molded shoe inserts to limit motion in abnormal joints. If this does not result in pain relief then resection of the bar or subtalar or triple arthrodesis is necessary. If severe deformity is present, arthrodesis is the best choice.

Sever's Disease

Sever's disease occurs at the insertion of the Achilles tendon on the calcaneus. The posterior calcaneal apophysis is adjacent to this insertion, and with repetitive stress, such as running, this apophysis can become painful. In 1 series, the male:female ratio was 3:1 and the mean age of presentation 11 years and 10 months in boys and 11 years in girls.[19] This condition is self-limited in that as the growth plate closes the pain is relieved. In the symptomatic patient, treatment consists of heel lifts, dorsiflexion strengthening exercises, stretching exercises, nonsteroidal anti-inflammatory medications, and activity modification.[22]

FOOT INJURIES

Foot injuries are most common in sports such as running and basketball. In these high-impact activities 275% of body weight is transmitted across the metatarsal phalangeal joint, and the shear force is increased 50%.[21] These conditions can be due to overuse inflammation or be secondary to acute traumatic injuries.

Overuse Injuries

In the forefoot the most common overuse injuries are sesamoiditis and hallux rigidus. There may be a history of a specific injury episode, but usually there will be a gradual onset of pain in or under the first metatarsal head. There may be slight swelling of the metatarsal phalangeal (MTP) joint, and pain is particularly severe with the great toe in dorsiflexion. In this position the sesamoid bones are pulled onto the plantar aspect of the metatarsal head with tightening of the flexor hallucis brevis tendons.

With continued loading, osteochondral fracture of the sesamoids, most commonly the tibial sesamoid, can occur. Conservative treatment should include the use of metatarsal pads or custom-molded shoe inserts to relieve pressure on the sesamoid bones and limit MTP joint motion, nonsteroidal anti-inflammatory drugs for inflammation, and brace immobilization for the persistently painful sesamoid. If fracture occurs, bone grafting or sesamoid excision will provide pain relief.[10]

Hallux rigidus in the athlete usually results from many relatively minor sprains that cause a progressive stiffness of the joint and the development of spurs and, eventually, articular cartilage defects. Treatment consists of shoe modification with a rigid shank to limit MTP joint motion and use of a wide shoe toe box. If symptoms persist and joint changes have occurred, cheilectomy to remove spurs and a dorsal wedge of the first metatarsal head and base of the proximal phalange will relieve impingement pain and improve motion slightly.[21] Severe hallux rigidus with end-stage arthritis of the first MTP joint is best treated with arthrodesis.

Heel pain is common and encompasses a broad spectrum of conditions that cause pain on the plantar aspect of the heel. The most common is plantar fasciitis, or inflammation of the plantar fascia as it attaches onto the medial calcaneal tuberosity. This is common in the general population as well as in runners. With chronic inflammation in the plantar fascia, there often can be entrapment of the nerve to the abductor digiti quinti muscle, which contributes to the heel pain. Plantar calcaneal spurs can develop as a result of chronic inflammation and tightness, but are also common in the asymptomatic general population. Other conditions that cause plantar heel pain are fat-pad atrophy and stress fractures of the calcaneal spur. Treatment starts with simple measures, including wearing flat shoes with cushioned soles, use of shock-absorbing heel pads, heel-cord stretching exercises, nonsteroidal anti-inflammatory medications, and some alteration in athletic activity, at least until there is some improvement in the symptoms. Education about this condition is important, since it will often take 3 to 6 months for this condition to heal. Patients are relieved to hear that 95% of people with this condition will heal without surgery.[10] When surgery is indicated because of long-standing (longer than 12 months) symptoms unresponsive to multiple conservative treatments, plantar fascia release along with release of the fascia around the nerve to the abductor digiti quinti, and possible plantar calcaneal spur excision, is necessary to relieve symptoms.[15]

Talus Fractures

The importance of looking at radiographs in a suspected ankle sprain cannot be overstressed. The golfer whose ankle is depicted in Figure 37-3 sustained an inversion injury but plain radiographs did not demonstrate her initial talus fracture. Anteroposterior and lateral radiographs taken 1 month after injury, however, revealed a central displaced talus fracture. Healing occurred without operative treatment.

There can be difficulty in differentiating osteochondritis dissecans from an acute fracture of the talus. The 16-year-old football player whose ankle is depicted in Figure 37-4 sustained an ankle inversion injury, although the original radiographs were negative (Fig. 37-4A). A mortise view showed a small area of radiolucency, which was thought to be overlap from the tibia. Follow-up radiographs revealed a talus fracture of the lateral aspect, for which he was casted. He did not heal, and after 8 months radiographs showed a persistent radiolucency consistent with nonunion (Fig. 37-4B). MRI confirmed a fluid level around the minimally displaced fracture (Fig. 37-4C,D). Arthroscopic assessment showed the fragment, which was irregular but intact (Fig. 37-4E). The talus was drilled. At 4 months post-op, the patient was pain free and radiographs showed consolidation (Fig. 37-4F).

Acute Injuries

Acute injuries of the foot are classified according to location (forefoot, midfoot, and hindfoot) and diagnosis (sprains and fractures).

Sprains

Sprains of the first MTP joint, or "turf toe," have been prevalent in football players playing on artificial turf. This joint is also injured in soccer players, and occurs when the toe is acutely hyperextended. There is damage to the plantar plate and capsule, and in severe injuries sesamoid fractures or joint dislocation can occur. With careful initial evaluation to eliminate those with fractures, conservative care is recommended, with rest, ice, compression, and elevation, the use of a stiff shoe, taping to limit dorsiflexion, and therapy to reduce swelling and restore normal range of motion. Severe injuries can result in long-term symptoms from hallux rigidus or hallux valgus.[21]

Sprains of the midfoot occur primarily at the tarsal-metatarsal joints, also known as Lisfranc's joint. This injury occurs when the forefoot is suddenly abducted on the hindfoot, or when the athlete falls onto the foot when weight is localized on the ball of the foot with the foot and ankle in equinus. If the dorsal tarsal-metatarsal ligaments fail, dislocation of the joints can occur. Often the dislocation will reduce spontaneously, causing the radiographs to appear nearly normal. One must be suspicious of a very swollen, tender foot after injury and obtain a computed tomography (CT) scan to detect the subtle abnormalities in bony architecture. With any shift in the tarsal-metatarsal relationship, open reduction and internal fixation is required for optimal results.

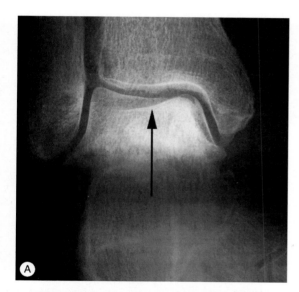

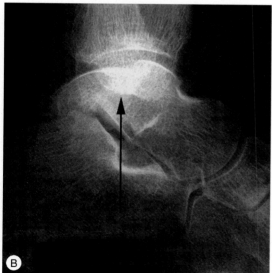

Figure 37-3. Anteroposterior **(A)** and lateral **(B)** views reveal a central displaced talus fracture in this golfer. These films were taken 1 month following the injury although initial films did not demonstrate the fracture. The patient was treated nonoperatively.

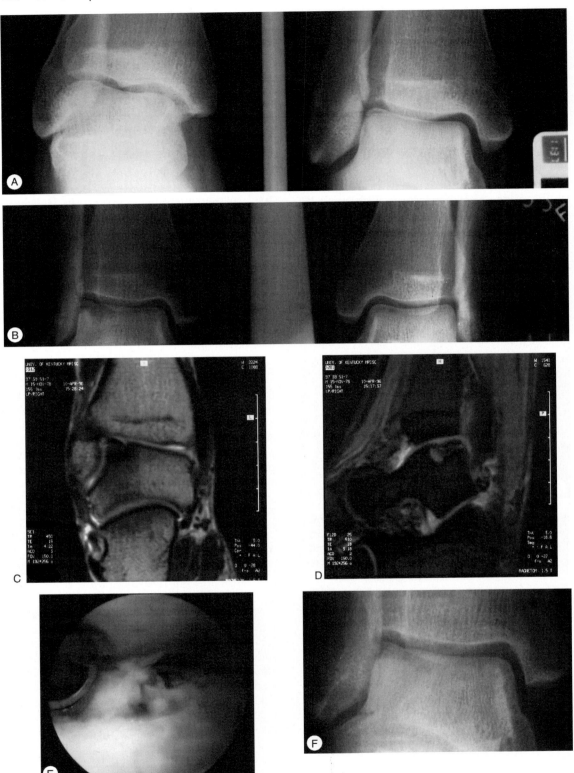

Figure 37-4. A 16-year-old football player with an ankle inversion injury. **(A)** Mortise view at the time of the injury shows a radiolucency on the lateral talus. Follow-up films taken 8 months later reveal an increase in the radiolucency with incomplete healing **(B)**. MRI scan shows a fluid level beneath the fragment, indicating a nonunion of the talus on the anteroposterior **(C)** and lateral **(D)** views. **(E)** Arthroscopy revealed an intact but depressed lateral osteochondral fracture. Débridement and drilling were performed. **(F)** Radiographs taken 4 months after surgery reveal good position of the fragment and healing.

Fractures

Fractures in the foot are evaluated for location (ie, intra-articular, shaft), alignment, and natural history. Generally, most extra-articular fractures in good alignment will heal with protected weight bearing for 4 to 6 weeks and gradual return to sporting activities. The notable exceptions to this are the fracture of the fifth metatarsal and the stress fracture of the navicular.

A fracture of the fifth metatarsal in the proximal shaft is known as a Jones fracture.[10] The healing potential in this area is poor, probably owing to a relatively poor blood supply. Often this fracture develops as a stress fracture, and symptoms start with a gradual onset of pain along the lateral side of the foot. An acute injury may cause a sudden increase in symptoms, and radiographs or a bone scan will be diagnostic. This acute fracture must be immobilized in a non-weight-bearing cast for approximately 8 weeks, or until radiographs show progressive healing. Alternatively, internal fixation with an intramedullary screw is effective in the athlete who does not tolerate non-weight bearing well and who needs to return to athletic activity as soon as possible. When nonunions develop in this fracture, treatment is intramedullary screw fixation, usually with bone grafting.

The fracture of the navicular in athletes is usually a stress fracture that may start out with nagging pain in the foot of varying location and mild associated swelling. Persistent pain should be investigated with plain radiographs and technetium bone scan (see Chapter 30). The fracture is not well visualized on radiographs. CT with coronal sections is the best way to diagnose this fracture, and a bone scan will also be abnormal. These nondisplaced fractures can be partial or complete, as well as an acute or chronic fracture that has not healed. The acute fracture can be treated nonoperatively with a non-weight-bearing cast for 6 to 8 weeks. The delayed union or nonunion will require internal fixation with or without bone grafting.[2]

TENDON INJURIES

Overuse injuries in the foot and ankle also include tendinitis, most commonly of the Achilles tendon, the posterior tibial tendon, and the peroneal tendons, and, least likely, of the flexor hallucis longus tendon. In all these tendons the injury severity can range from an inflammation of the paratenon, as seen around the Achilles tendon, to direct inflammation of the tendon fibers, to partial disruption of the tendon and fraying, to complete tear or incompetence of the tendon.

Achilles Tendinitis

Classic tendinitis occurs about 2 to 4 inches above the tendon attachment to the calcaneus. In this area the blood supply to the tendon is sparse, which may contribute to its weakness to injury and prolonged healing time. There are 3 levels of severity. First, *peritendinitis*, localized inflammation of the sheath around the tendon; second, *peritendinitis with tendinosis*, which includes some tendon degeneration, and third, *tendinosis*, referring to intratendinous degeneration and scar tissue formation. Factors that contribute to this condition include excessive heel varus or valgus deformity, increasing age, and muscle imbalance with tight gastrocnemius and soleus muscles. Treatment consists of heel-cord stretching, eccentric calf muscle training, custom-molded shoe inserts with a heel lift, ice treatments, anti-inflammatory medications, and alteration of training methods.[1] Persistent inflammation can lead to partial or complete rupture of the tendon, and then surgical repair will most likely be necessary.[26]

Posterior Tibial Tendon Dysfunction

Posterior tibial tendon dysfunction (PTTD) is often seen in middle-aged women, usually between 40 and 60 years of age. PTTD may occur in younger individuals who are flat footed and participate in a sport in which shoes are not worn. It is most often of insidious onset, without a specific injury episode. Symptoms start with pain and swelling on the medial side of the ankle and foot, into the longitudinal arch area. It is worse after activity, and may improve with reduced activity, but usually does not heal completely spontaneously. The persistent pain and swelling, and the inability to participate in any athletic or fitness activity, causes the patient to seek evaluation. Physical examination reveals pain over the posterior tibial tendon and loss of heel eversion on weight-bearing plantar flexion. Viewing the standing patient from behind, there will be more toes seen laterally if the tendon is ruptured. MRI is indicated if posterior tibial tendon rupture is suspected.

PTTD and attritional tear can occur. The typical tear is a longitudinal splitting in the tendon that starts in the area of the medial malleolus and extends distally to the insertion on the navicular. Once tendinosis has developed, the tendon is unable to support the longitudinal arch and an acquired flat foot deformity occurs. Without medial arch support, subluxation of the subtalar joint causes excessive heel valgus, and the midfoot gradually shifts into an abducted position. The end-stage result of severe PTTD is a rigid flat-foot deformity with the foot shifted laterally and weight bearing under a prominent head of the talus or navicular, or even on the medial malleolus.

PTTD is divided into 3 stages. Stage I involves pain and swelling and mild weakness of the tendon, without deformity. Stage II includes the symptoms of stage I, with a flexible flat-foot deformity. Stage III is when a rigid flat foot deformity has developed. Treatment depends on the stage of dysfunction, the age and activity requirements of the person, and the appearance of the tendon on the MRI study, which is the best diagnostic test to determine the extent of damage to the posterior tibial tendon.

Stage I PTTD is treated with nonsteroidal anti-inflammatory medications, a reduction of weight-bearing activity, and immobilization. A short-leg walking boot with adjustable ankle hinges works well for immobilization initially, with progressive increase in ankle motion as the inflammation subsides. Stage II PTTD can be treated as stage I, with less improvement in symptoms expected. Often surgical débridement and repair of the tendon with flexor digitorum longus tendon transfer may be necessary. This procedure will not correct the flat-foot deformity. If more correction is desired, a combination of posterior tibial tendon repair with tendon transfer and calcaneal osteotomy or lateral column lengthening is currently the procedure of choice. Surgical treatment in this stage is very controversial. At this time there is no clear evidence for choosing 1 over another. In stage III PTTD a bony fusion is necessary to correct deformity. Often a subtalar fusion with about 5° to 7° of heel valgus is the best treatment. When more extensive arthritis or subluxation is present, a double or triple arthrodesis may be necessary. The goal in treatment of PTTD is to make the diagnosis early, try to preserve posterior tibial function as much as possible, and prevent foot deformity from occurring.[7]

Peroneal Tendon Injuries

Peroneal longus and brevis tendinitis and tears often start with an injury such as an inversion-type ankle sprain. After the ligaments have healed, lateral pain and swelling continue. Tendinitis is treated conservatively, with emphasis on peroneal strengthening. Attritional-type tears due to tendon subluxation usually occur near the tip of the lateral malleolus, and cause persistent symptoms of pain and swelling along the course of these tendons, with weak foot eversion.[16] Chronic ankle instability may be present, with episodes of giving out. Stress radiographs will be helpful in making this diagnosis, and an MRI scan will show intratendinous degeneration and tearing. With tendon degeneration and fraying, surgical débridement and repair are necessary. It is important to detect all aspects of the injury, such as ankle instability or subtalar arthritis, and correct all conditions at the time of surgery, otherwise surgical results will be compromised.[6,16,24,25]

FOREFOOT CONDITIONS

Certain foot deformities are seen much more commonly in women than men, and are associated with foot pain and difficulty wearing shoes. Hallux valgus, hammertoes, metatarsalgia, and Morton's neuroma are all associated with the use of fashion footwear that has a high heel and a narrow toe box, and is generally too small for the foot. There seems to be a hereditary predisposition to developing bunion deformity and hammertoes, but high-fashion shoes only increase the problem. Juvenile bunion deformity results more from heredity than inappropriate shoes, but the use of the correct size and style of shoes can help alleviate symptoms.[8,12,27]

PREVENTIVE MEASURES

In reality, most foot and ankle problems are relatively mild, and if treated promptly will heal. Certain preventive measures can be taken to avoid causing or aggravating these problems. In a preparticipation physical examination preexisting conditions such as heel-cord tightness, hallux valgus, pes planus, pes cavus, and hammertoes should be noted and preventive measures taken to avoid injury and time lost during the season.

Simple measures such as placing emphasis on flexibility and strengthening exercises for the foot and ankle can be included in the routine warm-up program. Footwear on and off the playing surface should be the correct size and accommodate the individual needs of her foot and sport. Shoe inserts are often helpful, and can be simple cushioned heel pads, over-the-counter full sole inserts for impact absorption, full sole arch supports, or custom-molded shoe inserts for the foot for certain conditions.

A certified pedorthist is helpful in providing the appropriate shoe inserts. An individual who can make the orthotic comfortable and functional is key to success. The use of ankle taping and bracing for prophylactic purposes has been shown to prevent injuries, and is particularly important in the final rehabilitation phase after injury. Finally, all of these measures must be part of a carefully planned training program that allows the athlete to practice and compete at a rate that will not predispose her to the development of stress fractures, overuse injuries, and permanent limitations due to foot and ankle injuries.

References

1. Alfredson H, Pietila T, Jonsson P, Lorentzon R: Heavy-load eccentric calf muscle training for the treatment of chronic achilles tendinosis. Am J Sports Med 26:360–6, 1998.
2. Anderson RB: Injuries to the midfoot and forefoot. In Lutter LD, Mizel MS, Pfeffer GB (eds): Orthopaedic Knowledge Update Foot and Ankle. Rosemont, Ill, American Academy of Orthopaedic Surgeons, 1994, pp 255–68.
3. Bassett FH, Speer KP: Longitudinal rupture of the peroneal tendons. Am J Sports Med 21:354–7, 1993.
4. Beim G, Stone DA: Issues in the female athlete. Orthop Clin North Am 26:443–51, 1995.
5. Bowe JA: The pediatric foot. In Sullivan JA, Grana WA (eds): The Pediatric Athlete. Rosemont, Ill, American Academy of Orthopaedic Surgeons, 1990, pp 89–100.
6. Clarke HD, Kitaoka HB, Ehman RL: Peroneal tendon injuries. Foot Ankle 19:280–8, 1998.
7. Conti SF: Posterior tibial problems in athletes. Orthop Clin North Am 25:109–21, 1994.
8. Coughlin MJ, Thompson FM: The high price of high-fashion footwear. Instr Course Lect 44:371–7, 1995.
9. Davis Aw, Alexander IJ: Problematic fractures and dislocations in the foot and ankle of athletes. Clin Sports Med 9:163–81, 1990.
10. Dreeben S: Heel pain. In Lutter LD, Mizel MS, Pfeffer GB (eds): Orthopaedic Knowledge Update: Foot and Ankle. Rosemont, Ill, American Academy of Orthopaedic Surgeons, 1994, pp 179–91.
11. Ferkel RD, Jasulo GJ: Arthroscopic treatment of ankle injuries. Orthop Clin North Am 25:17–32, 1994.
12. Frey CC: Trends in women's shoewear. Instr Course Lect 44:385–7.
13. Harper MC: The short oblique fracture of the distal fibula without medial injury: an assessment of displacement. Foot Ankle 16:181–6, 1995.
14. Hunter-Griffin LY: Injuries to the leg, ankle, and foot. In Sullivan JA, Grana WA (eds): The Pediatric Athlete.

Rosemont, Ill, American Academy of Orthopaedic Surgeons, 1990, pp 187–98.
15. Karr SD: Subcalcaneal heel pain. Orthop Clin North Am 25:161–75, 1994.
16. Krause JO, Brodsky JW: Peroneus brevis tendon tears: pathophysiology, surgical reconstruction, and clinical results. Foot Ankle 19:271–9, 1998.
17. Lofvenberg R, Karrholm J, Sundelin G, Ahlgren O: Prolonged reaction time in patients with chronic lateral instability of the ankle. Am J Sports Med 23:414–7, 1995.
18. Mankey M: Fractures of the talus. In Lutter LD, Pfeffer GB (eds): Orthopaedic Knowledge Update: Foot and Ankle. Rosemont, Ill, American Academy of Orthopaedic Surgeons, 1994, pp 205–26.
19. Micheli LJ, Ireland ML: Prevention and management of calcaneal apophysitis in children: an overuse syndrome. J Pediatr Orthop 7(1):34–8, 1987.
20. Michelson J: Fractures of the ankle. In Lutter LD, Pfeffer GB (eds): Orthopaedic Knowledge Update: Foot and Ankle. Rosemont, Ill, American Academy of Orthopaedic Surgeons, 1994, pp 193–203.
21. Pedowitz WJ: Deformities of the first ray. In Lutter LD, Pfeffer GB (eds): Orthopaedic Knowledge Update: Foot and Ankle. Rosemont, Ill, American Academy of Orthopaedic Surgeons, 1994, pp 141–62.
22. Pizzutillo PD: Osteochondroses. In Sullivan JA, Grana WA (eds): The Pediatric Athlete. Rosemont, Ill, American Academy of Orthopaedic Surgeons, 1990, pp 211–33.
23. Ramsey PL, Hamilton W: Changes in tibiotalar area of contact caused by lateral talar shift. J Bone Joint Surg 58A:356–7, 1976.
24. Saltzman C, Bonar S: Tendon problems of the foot and ankle. In Lutter LD, Pfeffer GB (eds): Orthopaedic Knowledge Update: Foot and Ankle. Rosemont, Ill, American Academy of Orthopaedic Surgeons, 1994, pp 269–82.
25. Sammarco GJ: Peroneal tendon injuries. Orthop Clin North Am 25:135–45, 1994.
26. Scioli MW: Achilles tendinitis. Orthop Clin North Am 25:177–82, 1994.
27. Seale KS: Women and their shoes: unrealistic expectations? Instr Course Lect 44:379–84, 1995.
28. Sickles RT, Lombardo JA: The adolescent basketball player. Clin Sports Med 12:207–19, 1993.
29. Stanish WD: Lower leg, foot and ankle injuries in young athletes. Clin Sports Med 14:651–68, 1995.
30. Thordarson DB: Detecting and treating common foot and ankle fractures. Physician Sportsmed 24(9):29–38, Sept. 1996 and 24(10):58–64, Oct. 1996.
31. Trevino SG, Davis P, Hecht PJ: Management of acute and chronic lateral ligament injuries of the ankle. Orthop Clin North Am 25:1–16, 1994.
32. Yeung MS, Chan KM, So CH, Yuan WY: An epidemiological survey on ankle sprain. Br J Sports Med 28:112–6, 1994.
33. Zelisko JA, Noble HB, Porter MA: A comparison of men's and women's professional basketball injuries. Am J Sports Med 10:297–9, 1982.

Chapter 38

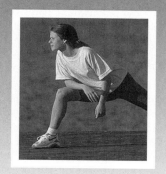

Head and Neck Injuries

William H. Brooks, M.D.

The degree of head-forward position that an athlete assumes is associated directly with the risk and occurrence of craniospinal injury. Further accentuation may be observed in those sports that are associated with speed in which the athlete does not wear protective headgear, such as soccer and field hockey, or is exposed to heightened risks of extremes of flexion, extension, or axial loading of the cervical spine, such as gymnastics, cheerleading, and diving. Although occurrences of craniospinal injuries are remote in noncontact sports, the frequency is sufficiently high that team physicians and others involved in the care of all athletes should be aware of the potential for cerebral and cervical spinal cord injury. The purpose of this chapter is to present a classification of brain and cervical spinal injuries based on the biomechanical mechanisms that are associated with specific pathophysiologic alterations. Additionally, guidelines for safe return to participation following these injuries will be presented. The specific aim is not to present a litany of injuries, but rather to familiarize the reader with a classification based on the neuropathologic entity and those biomechanical factors that give rise to it.

CEREBRAL INJURY

Biomechanical Mechanisms of Head Injury

Many factors are involved in determining what cerebral injuries may result from a specific mechanical input or force to the head and how those injuries occur. In addition to the characteristics of the mechanical force (load), the complex interaction of this input with the unique features of cerebral tissues are pivotal in determining whether the resultant injury will be associated with loss of consciousness and/or neurologic dysfunction.[16,20] Thus, the nature, direction, and severity of the mechanical force as well as the site of impact and subsequent movement of the head and neck all interact to produce a particular type of cerebral injury that may or may not be temporary.

Static Loading

Gradually applied mechanical input to the head (static loading) is seen infrequently in sporting events. Static loading may be compared to a progressive squeezing effect of the head. Such a mechanism may be observed when a horseback rider becomes trapped under the horse. This type of mechanical load rarely is associated with alterations in the level of consciousness, however, as the force is increased, comminuted fractures of the skull, cerebrospinal fluid leaks through the cribriform plate (nose) or temporal bone (ear), and focal cerebral injury may result.[29] These loading mechanisms may produce significant injury to the scalp and/or skull but, because of the relatively slow application, rarely result in cerebral injury and alterations in consciousness. Static loading is not seen in isolation, but potentially could be an uncommon contributing factor in producing head injury in the athlete.

Dynamic Loading

The most common mechanical forces associated with brain injury in sporting events are those that arise very rapidly (ie, in less than 200 msec) rather than slowly (within 200 to 500 msec) as observed with static loading. Impacts to the head that occur during athletic contests are dynamic events that may include contact phenomena and impulsive loading of the head and its contents.[32] Thus, dynamic loading consists of both impact to the head and movement (impulse) of the unrestrained head. Although contact phenomena only occur following impact, impulsive loading can arise by indirect impacts in which the head is set into motion without being struck. This may occur if an athlete is struck in the thorax or lumbar area when the head is freely movable or during sudden deceleration while restrained, thus resulting in severe flexion–extension movements of the head. Although impulsive loading infrequently occurs in the absence of impact in athletics the effects of inertial forces on the generation of brain injury are well documented.[6,7] Direct impact to the head is associated with 2 phenomena that alone or in combination can produce cerebral injury. The type of brain injury varies according to the contribution that is evoked from each of these phenomena. The first, *contact loading,* produces a complex of mechanical phenomena that may be observed both at and remote to the site of injury. The pathologic consequences of these specific phenomena (eg, skull fracture, cavitation, generation of shock waves) are dependent on the size of the impacting object and magnitude of the force.

Alterations of consciousness and neurologic deficits are observed uncommonly. The location, extent, and severity of skull fracture is dependent on the unique features of the contact load as well as characteristics of the impacted skull (Fig. 38-1). A significant impact to an area of thin bone will produce local bending of the skull, failure of the tensile strength of the bone, and, subsequently, linear fracture. Areas of thin bone adjacent to thicker portions of the skull receiving a direct impact also may break, hence a fracture may not always be found directly beneath the site of impact.

Propagation of a skull fracture from its origin tends to follow the line of less resistance toward the vertex or along the skull base. Concurrent with mechanical failure of tensile strength of the skull, contact loading also produces shock waves

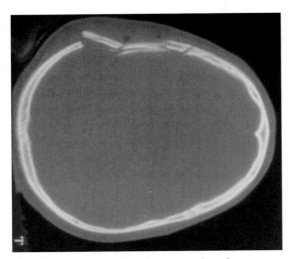

Figure 38-1. Temporal bone fracture resulting from contact load in a teenage athlete struck by a golf ball. No loss of consciousness occurred.

that transverse cerebral tissues and result in local and widespread pressure changes that may affect neuronal or axonal function (cavitation). Whereas the mechanical features of contact loading in producing skull fracture are accepted widely, the electrochemical effects of shock waves generated by this mechanism remain controversial.[13]

In addition to contact loading, direct impact to the head also is associated with *inertial loading.* Inertial loading, whether induced by direct impact to the head or impulsion induced by remote impact, involves 2 types of acute acceleration or deceleration motions of the head. Although the pathophysiologic consequences of acceleration are unrelated to the mechanisms of generation of inertial forces, these 2 types of acceleration differ in their ability to impart injury to brain tissue.

Acceleration of the head in a strict horizontal plane (translational acceleration or loading) differs markedly in injury-producing potential when compared to rotation of the head and neck (angular acceleration).[24,34] Experimental and clinical evidence has demonstrated that translational acceleration frequently is associated with the occurrence of focal structural damage (eg, cerebral contusions), yet rarely results in loss of consciousness. Rotational or angular acceleration forces are much more likely to result in cerebral concussion, unconsciousness, petechiae, subarachnoid hemorrhage, bilateral subdural hematoma, and diffuse cellular injury.[22,23] Moreover, the kinematics of rotational effects indicate that cerebral injury and subsequent alteration in neurologic function is related to the direction of angular motion. As the direction of angular force approaches the coronal plane, the degree of injury increases when compared to those injuries resulting from rotational forces applied in a sagittal plane. Thus, lateral rotational forces tend to produce brain injuries worse than those resulting from forces delivered in an anterior-posterior direction.[5,21]

Pure translational or angular acceleration is rarely, if ever, seen outside of the experimental laboratory. More commonly, a continuum or blend of acceleration–deceleration forces with contact phenomena are observed in sporting events. Indeed, both contribute to cerebral injury (Fig. 38-2). Therefore, any specific brain injury may be determined by the direct contribution of contact phenomena, the summary of interactive contribution of rotational and translational forces, the magnitude of impact loading, and the rate at which these mechanical forces are applied to the head.

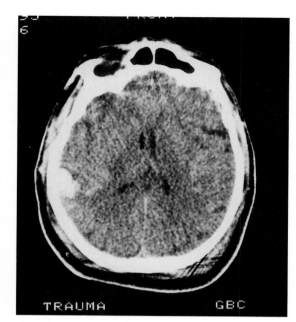

Figure 38-2. Rotational input with translational effects is the more common mechanism associated with athletic injuries to the head. This girl fell from a horse, sustaining a persistent neurologic deficit from focal and diffuse cerebral injury. She was wearing a helmet and sustained no skull fracture.

importantly, insight into how these forces may be prevented or at least lessened, thereby avoiding catastrophic and permanently disabling injuries.

Focal Versus Diffuse Axonal Injury

The consequences of mechanical loading of the head and brain may be considered to be focal or diffuse. The mechanisms associated with production of these injuries include both impact and impulsive loading, as discussed previously. Focal injuries of the brain usually are detectable easily by inspection of the standard diagnostic radiographic techniques of skull roentgenography, computed tomography (CT), and magnetic resonance imaging (MRI). These injuries include cerebral contusions and intracranial or intraparenchymatous hematoma, which make their presence known through local brain dysfunction specific to the area involved or through increased intracranial pressure, shifts of the brain, and secondary brain-stem compression (Fig. 38-3). Although these injuries may be produced solely through contact phenomena linked to impact, they rarely occur in isolation because impacts frequently are associated with inertial loading. Those types of injuries that arise from impact unassociated with inertial loading frequently do not present with immediate

Protective headgear is effective in reducing the occurrence of brain injuries to the degree by which it is capable of energy absorption and load distribution through the thickness of the helmet structure and its component materials. These features of all helmets lessen the risk of skull fracture by absorption and dispersion of contact-loading phenomena, yet offer little significant protection against angular acceleration forces.

The ongoing search for new materials that can be adapted to protective headgear should lead to more effective helmets. The principal challenge is to design a reasonably lightweight and nonbulky helmet that provides optimum protection yet allows the athlete to compete.

Classification of Brain Injury

The following classification is based on the mechanism of occurrence rather than anatomic location. The pathology of head and brain injuries also has been avoided in order to emphasize the biomechanical features of the production of cerebral injury. Underscoring the mechanistic forces involved in the traumatic production of cerebral dysfunction should provide not only a thorough understanding of how sport-related brain injuries arise, but, more

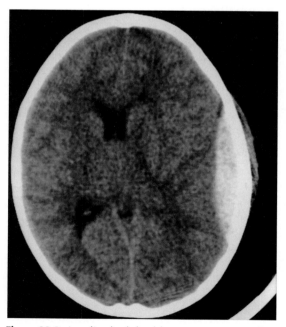

Figure 38-3. Localized subdural hematomas may produce increased intracranial pressure, shifting of the intracranial structures, and neurologic findings. In this manner, focal areas of injury (impact) may lead to diffuse cerebral dysfunction.

alterations in consciousness, although loss of consciousness may be observed if delayed brain-stem compression occurs secondary to an expanding intracranial hematoma or brain swelling.

Diffuse brain injuries represent a continuum of cerebral dysfunction associated with increasing inertial loading of the brain. More specifically, the rotational component of inertial or impulsive forces is the main factor in generating these types of brain injuries. Impacts obviously play an etiologic role in the generation of sport-related diffuse brain injuries, however, it is the subsequent generation of impulsion (inertial forces) imparted by these impacts that is pivotal in creating neurologic dysfunction (see Fig. 38-2). Diffuse brain injuries are widespread and associated with global disruption of cerebral function. They rarely are macroscopic although they may become so as the force increases. The earliest disruptions of cerebral dysfunction are physiologic disconnections of those electro-chemical processes that give rise to consciousness (ie, concussion). As acceleration forces increase and combine, anatomic disruption may occur, giving rise to persistent disconnection syndromes, neurologic deficits, and visual evidence of brain injury such as petechial and sub-arachnoid hemorrhages and bilateral subdural hematoma.

Consciousness

Although there are many definitions for consciousness, a particularly useful one in clinical practice describes a person who is conscious as being capable of interpreting and/or reacting to the environment. The physiologic basis for consciousness is linked to the molecular and biochemical characteristics of individual and interconnecting networks of neurons located in the cerebral hemispheres, hypothalamus-diencephalon, and brain stem. Thus, disruption of these interconnecting pathways or within the neuronal pool located in these areas of the brain would be anticipated to result in alterations in alertness and consciousness.

Focal head injuries induced by static or impact loads result in alterations in consciousness only through the production of mass lesions in the vicinity of the cerebral hemispheres that secondarily compress those areas of the brain stem associated with alertness, such as the reticular activating system. Diffuse cerebral injuries imparted by dynamic loading of the head result in widespread disruptions throughout the brain, hence they are associated with easily induced and early loss of consciousness.[4]

Whereas these interruptions may be transient with smaller loads, larger forces may produce anatomic lesions within these areas of the brain responsible for alertness and consequently lead to irreversible persistive coma.

Transient Alterations in Consciousness

The mildest, yet most common group of cerebral injuries encountered in sports medicine are those that present with alterations in thought and/or memory processing, known as transient alterations in consciousness (TAC). Often these syndromes are unrecognized or are not brought to the attention of the team physician or trainer because their chief manifestation is so transient. Following an injury, the athlete may have momentary confusion and disorientation that is unaccompanied by loss of consciousness. Lasting only a few moments, symptoms completely clear without sequelae and activity is resumed. A player may later state that her "bell got rung." Generally, this type of injury does not require medical evaluation or attention unless it occurs frequently. This would suggest improper technique or inappropriate participation in a particular sport.

More severe mechanical loading of the head may result in confusion, disorientation, and amnesia. Shortly after an impact and dynamic loading a player may experience a period of amnesia (post-traumatic amnesia). During this time she may continue to display coordinated although confused behavior. This period of amnesia resolves within minutes. Although those events leading up to the injury subsequently may be easily recalled, those immediately following the impact usually are lost to memory.

A third stage of TAC accompanies a more significant increase in mechanical loading and is manifest not only by confusion and disorientation, but by the presence of retrograde as well as post-traumatic amnesia. These players have no recall of events leading up to the period of injury, nor are they capable of recalling events after the impact. The length of confusion and alteration in consciousness may resolve quickly and the periods of amnesia shrink. However, some degree of retrograde as well as post-traumatic amnesia will persist. This particular stage of cerebral injury is heralded by the presence of retrograde amnesia and represents a continuum of alteration in cerebral function leading to a more severe diffuse injury and loss of consciousness.

The predominant characteristic of TAC is that although consciousness may not be lost, normal cerebral function and processing has been suspended temporarily as the result of mechanical loading of the head and brain. The persistent deficit that may result from this form of brain injury is confined solely to memory, thereby indicating a transient electrochemical disruption within the temporal lobe of the cerebral hemisphere. Such a physiologic or functional "injury" is most consistent with diffuse neuronal alterations inducible by inertial loads that accompany impact.

Cerebral Concussion

Although it should be differentiated from milder TAC, concussion represents a continuum in the cerebral response to mechanical loading. Concussion always is associated with retrograde and post-traumatic amnesia that persists longer than that observed in individuals sustaining lesser injury to the head. In general, the length of post-traumatic amnesia provides a good index as to the severity of the concussion syndrome.

Although experimental investigations have shown the anatomic presence of mild neuronal damage, concussion is associated with loss of consciousness that resolves within approximately 6 hours; hence, concussion primarily is a physiologic syndrome resulting from transient suspension of electrochemical processes necessary for consciousness and memory imprinting. It is of interest that those pathologic findings occasionally seen in experimental models of concussion are quite similar to those observed following inertial (rotation) loading of the head. Persons remaining unconscious from head injury longer than 6 hours should be considered to have sustained diffuse axonal injuries.

Immediate unconsciousness is the hallmark of concussion as compared to the milder TAC. Concurrent findings of nonreactive or asymmetrical pupils, decerebrate or decorticate posturing, and cardiovascular instability are short lived, thus providing a rapid differentiation from more serious cerebral injury. As the person regains consciousness she may be confused or disoriented, resembling those with more severe forms of TAC.

Post-traumatic and retrograde amnesia are present. The period of amnesia for events following the impact always is longer in duration than loss of memory for events immediately preceding the accident. Although the length of post-traumatic amnesia may be a reflection of the severity of the clinical syndrome of concussion, the presence and duration of retrograde amnesia is a better index of the pathophysiologic insult to the brain. Gradual clearing of consciousness is accompanied by resolution of amnesia, although with more severe concussion some loss of memory of the events surrounding the injury may persist.

In most incidences a player will have no long-lasting sequelae following concussion except a brief period of no recall of the injury. However, some may complain of persistent headache, photophobia, tinnitus, and difficulties with integration of thought processes.[9,11] These symptoms may last for several weeks before clearing; indeed, may resolve only partially. Additionally, some players may complain of subtle changes in their personality and deficits in short-term memory and learning capabilities. This constellation of symptoms may be found most frequently in players who have sustained more than 1 concussion. Recurrent concussion is associated with diminished intellectual function and impaired learning capabilities as measured by psychological and educational testing.[8,14] These observations support the hypothesis that even mild impact and inertial forces may produce subtle anatomic defects that interfere with integrated learning and other cerebral networks responsible for higher intellectual functioning. Concussions should be considered as important sequelae of head injury and call for appropriate medical evaluation prior to resuming competition. All symptoms should resolve before a player is allowed to participate in her sporting activity. To allow a player to compete without resolution of symptoms or while in an amnestic state invites further injury, which may lead to persistent neural dysfunction.

Diffuse Axonal Injuries

Diffuse axonal injuries (DAI) represent a transition between those electrochemical disconnection syndromes resulting from lesser mechanical loads as discussed and actual anatomic injuries induced following an impact to the head.

Thus, DAI form a continuum of responses in the cellular architecture of the brain to varying, yet significant forms of dynamic mechanical loads to the head. The classification of DAI is reflected in the degree of anatomic disruption of the neuron–axon complex and neuronal networks. As forces increase and combine the extent of destruction and neurologic consequences likewise increase. It should be emphasized that a diffuse axonal injury is primarily a clinical diagnosis that reflects a predicted anatomic defect based on experimental models of head injury.

In addition to axonal injuries, inertial and contact loading of the head may produce other undetermined structural alterations in the brain that may be associated with loss of consciousness, amnesia, and deficits in intellectual function. The clinical manifestations of DAI include increasingly prolonged loss of consciousness beyond 6 hours, peritraumatic amnesia of varying lengths of time, and, on occasion, persistive neurologic dysfunction and coma. Generally, DAI are classified as mild, moderate, or severe, reflecting both the length of unconsciousness and the loading force to the head.

Mild DAI are associated with loss of consciousness for periods of time extending from 6 to 24 hours. Initially, individuals with an axonal injury may demonstrate decerebrate or decorticate posturing indicative of brain-stem dysfunction, yet begin to improve within 24 hours. Full recovery may require days and usually is not attended with neurologic dysfunction with the notable exception of rather prolonged periods of amnesia.

A moderate diffuse axonal injury is the most frequent type of cerebral injury observed in athletes sustaining catastrophic head injuries. Fortunately, they are uncommon.

Moderate DAI are heralded by coma lasting longer than 24 hours and occasionally persisting for several days. Evidence of brain-stem dysfunction is evident immediately and may persist for several days. All too often these injuries are associated with permanent deficits in memory, cognitive and other higher intellectual functions, alterations in personality, and prolonged amnesia. Rarely do these individuals make an uneventful recovery. Whereas they may resume their education and assume a place in society, they generally are not capable of resuming their athletic careers.

Severe DAI rarely are seen in athletics. These injuries are associated with extremes of mechanical loads that are not achievable in most sporting activities other than motor sports. The most devastating form of nonfocal brain injury, severe DAI are characterized by immediate and profound coma that may persist for days to weeks, brain-stem signs of posturing and automatic nervous system dysfunction, and incomplete recovery of neurologic function. This form of diffuse axonal injury is associated with microscopically identifiable loss of axons and neurons.

DAI are seen infrequently in sporting events, yet should be considered as a continuation of the deleterious effects of mechanical loading to the head. The more common loading forces observable in athletes include varying combinations of impact and inertial loading that induce only physiologic deficits that are not permanent and resolve through the plasticity of neuronal networks and interconnections of dendrite–axonal systems. However, as mechanical loads increase and become more violent, anatomic lesions may be produced that are not repairable and thereby result in permanent neurologic deficits.

Postconcussive Syndrome

Approximately 25% to 30% of individuals have vague neurologic complaints that persist for several days after the usual symptoms associated with head injury seemingly have resolved. The athlete may complain of dizziness and unsteadiness, generalized weakness and clumsiness, photophobia and blurred vision, and difficulty with memory and cognition. These symptoms warrant consideration and should not be dismissed merely as a psychological response to injury. Similar symptoms are not observed in athletes who have sustained injuries to other parts of the body, therefore, represent yet another facet of mechanical loading to the brain. Those athletes who have suffered repeated TAC, concussion, or DAI may have persistence of these vague symptoms, thereby confirming the concept that the postconcussive syndrome is a reflection of biochemical and/or anatomic alterations in neural networks capable of influencing behavior and intellectual function.[18] Therefore, it is not uncommon for athletes to exhibit difficulties in the classroom following even the mildest of head injuries.

Individuals sustaining 3 or more concussions have been demonstrated to experience permanent difficulties in learning, recent memory, and general intellectual function. With more severe injuries psychiatric and social functional disorders may be evident and persistent for several weeks. Thus, it is important to identify those athletes who have sustained frequent and/or recurrent concussion in order to prevent intellectual deficits that may impede their continued education.

Second-Impact Syndrome

The existence of the "second-impact syndrome" remains controversial.[19] Nevertheless, there is sufficient evidence that a second impact to the head prior to full restoration of neurologic function and resolution of the biochemical alterations related to a concussion increases the likelihood of life-threatening cerebral edema and possibly death. It has been suggested that the second impact initiates the development of cerebrovascular instability and increased intracranial pressure that may result in brain-stem herniation and death. This syndrome is most prevalent in young males; less than 33%

occur in women. It is characterized by progressive neurologic deterioration following what seems to be a minor head injury. The symptoms of concussion rapidly give way to alterations in consciousness, coma, and death.

Fortunately, this syndrome rarely occurs. More importantly, it can be prevented entirely by a careful and conservative approach to allowing individuals to return to competition following a concussion, clearing them only after all symptoms related to a postconcussion syndrome fully resolve.

Criteria for Return to Competition

The negative effect on quality of student life following a head injury is reflected in neuropsychological difficulties, intellectual impairments, and social dysfunction. Obviously, most athletes who sustain a dynamic injury to the brain will recover without sequelae. There are a few, however, who, either as the result of a severe impact and inertial loading to the brain or recurrent injury, manifest permanent loss of cerebral function. By strict adherence to guidelines regarding when an athlete may safely return to competition subsequent to a head injury these long-term and devastating neurologic impairments should be avoided.[10]

At present no universally accepted rules that dictate when an athlete should or should not be permitted to continue to compete following a head injury exist. Most team physicians remain conservative in their recommendations based on observations that immediately after TAC or concussion thought processing is curtailed, thereby exposing the individual to greater risk of both repeated head injury as well as injury to other parts of the body. Moreover, repeated concussions are associated with impaired mental functioning. Indeed, the risk of occurrence of a second and/or third concussion is much greater after having sustained the initial insult than had the athlete never received the first. These observations clearly warrant a conservative estimation as to when the injured athlete may safely return to competition. All symptoms related to the head injury must resolve before the possibility of allowing a student-athlete to resume activity can be considered. Recommended guidelines for returning to competition are presented in Table 38-1.

INJURY TO THE CERVICAL SPINE

Those sporting activities that are typically described as noncontact are not commonly associated with catastrophic cervical spine and/or spinal cord injury. Nevertheless, the occurrence of injuries involving the cervical spine without spinal cord involvement is sufficiently frequent to warrant a thorough understanding of the mechanisms involved in the production of these accidents. The purpose of this section is to review those mechanisms by which cervical spine injuries occur, present a classification of resulting neurologic syndromes, and suggest guidelines regarding when an athlete may resume activity subsequent to sustaining a cervical injury.

In general, although measurements to determine the presence of and degree of spinal segmental instability are readily available, undue reliance should not be placed on determination of these parameters. For example, overdistraction of the spine may result in a profound neurologic deficit yet be attended with a roentgenogram that is normal with regard to measurements designating instability. Asymmetry is more important than measurements. All individuals who appear to have sustained a neck injury, as manifest by pain, limitation of motion, and muscular spasm, or who complain of symptoms suggesting nerve root or spinal cord injury should be suspected of having a cervical fracture until conclusively proven otherwise.

Biomechanical Mechanisms of Cervical Spine Injury

The spine responds to mechanical loading as determined by the interrelationships of the articular surfaces in conjunction with the mechanical (tensile) properties of connecting structures.[28,36] The anatomic configuration of the facets of the cervical spine permits considerable ranges of sagittal motion, however, pure rotation or lateral bending (flexion) is not possible because of the medial slope of the articulating surfaces. Additionally, flexion and extension are restricted significantly during rotation or lateral bending. Axial rotation likewise is limited by the anatomic configuration of the interarticular facets. The interplay of these planes of movement has been demonstrated to be complex; each movement actually consists of a compromise of at least 2 types of movements, called "coupling." Thus, when analyzed in accordance with the phenomenon of "coupling" movement of the cervical spine may be considered as translational or rotational about 3 interconnected perpendicular planes (anterior-posterior, lateral, and rotational). The specific coupling phenomena and the limits of movement in each of these planes is determined by

Table 38-1. Suggested Criteria for Return to Competition Following Cerebral Injury

TRANSIENT ALTERATION OF CONSCIOUSNESS		
Mild–moderate	Momentary (<30 sec) confusion, disorientation, automatic behavior, and rapidly resolving post-traumatic amnesia.	May return to play if absolutely asymptomatic, including no headache, no deficits in recall, orientation, or concentration after rest period of 2–5 minutes and exertion.
Severe	Prolonged (>1 min) confusion, disorientation, post-traumatic amnesia that may persist for minutes (typically <15 min).	May return to play after asymptomatic for 1 week or cleared by neurologic evaluation.
CONCUSSION		
Mild	Although loss of consciousness may not be experienced, a prolonged post-traumatic amnesia lasting less than 30 minutes is observed. Concurrent headache, disorientation, dizziness, tinnitus, and dilated, but reactive pupils usually are present.	Return to play is dependent on neurologic evaluation and resolution of all symptoms, and generally requires 1 week of rest.
Moderate	Loss of consciousness that clears within 5 minutes, post-traumatic amnesia lasting in excess of 1 hour, and the presence of retrograde amnesia. Symptoms of increased intracranial pressure (eg, flux in pupillary size and reactivity, decerebrate or decorticate posturing, and cardiovascular instability) may be observed temporarily. Concurrent complicants of headache, disorientation, vertigo, tinnitus, and nausea or vomiting are seen frequently.	Return to play after 1 month if asymptomatic and cleared by neurological evaluation.
Severe	Loss of consciousness persists longer than 5 minutes and is associated with both retrograde and post-traumatic amnesia that may persist more than 1 hour. Amnesia of the events surrounding the incident may be permanent. Ancillary symptoms (headache, dizziness, etc) also are present.	Return to play is dependent on neurologic examination and rarely should be permitted within 1 month.
DIFFUSE AXONAL INJURY		
Mild	Loss of consciousness extends between 6 and 24 hours. Associative symptoms of brain stem and/or cerebral hemispheric dysfunction are present but improve within 24 hours. Full recovery may take several days and is associated with prolonged periods of amnesia.	Return to play is questionable and is dependent on neurologic evaluation. Competition should not be permitted for the remainder of the season.
Moderate	Loss of consciousness persists greater than 24 hours and frequently is associated with prolonged neurologic deficits. Intellectual and cognitive function may be impaired.	All sporting activities with a potential for head injury should be terminated regardless of the degree of recovery.

the anatomic configuration of the particular cervical level.[3,15]

In addition to the unique anatomic constructs of the cervical vertebrae and vertebral coupled segments, movement of the neck is influenced by the ligamentous and muscular supporting structures and intervertebral discs. Unlike the remainder of the spinal column, the interspinal, intertransverse, and joint capsular ligaments, ligamentum flava, and supraspinal (ligamentum nuchae) are relatively weak. Although these structures may play a role in "checking" the extremes of normal, volitional movement, their collective tensile strength is insufficient to afford significant protective value in preventing spinal injury. Because the posterior longitudinal ligament possesses less tensile strength than the anterior longitudinal ligament, there is less resistance to flexion than extension. In extreme cases, flexion is limited by contact between the chin and sternum. Extension beyond the anatomic limits of the vertebral segments and ligamentous tensile strength may be prevented by the relatively strong anterior cervical muscles and annular connections of the intervertebral disc with the vertebral endplate. Indeed, it is the abilities of the cervical paraspinal muscular and intervertebral discs to absorb loads applied to the cervical spine that primarily limit neck injuries. The interconnecting complexities of the coupled vertebral segment, supporting muscular and ligamentous components, and the intervertebral disc become more significant as loading that exceeds the rotational and/or translational tolerance of the particular segment occurs. Thus, the failure of the anatomic construct will be determined not only by the magnitude of the load (force) but also by the direction by which it is applied.

During athletic competitions the cervical spine frequently is exposed to a variety of external forces that may result in anatomic injury if the load is sufficient. These injuries may be induced by compressive (axial) loading, inertial loading, or impulsive loading. Most frequently, energy applied to the neck is absorbed by the cervical muscles, intervertebral discs, and, to a lesser extent, the ligaments.

Movement of the neck in response to translational or rotational forces also helps in dissipating potentially harmful loads. It is when the force applied is in excess of the toleration (elastic capabilities) of the involved structures that injury to the cervical spine and neural structures will occur.

Compressive (Axial) Loading

Although not the most common mechanism for all neck injuries, compressive loading of the vertex with the cervical spine slightly flexed (axial loading) carries the greatest potential for cervical dislocation and neurologic injury.[25] When the neck is slightly flexed the cervical spine is straightened. Compressive forces applied along the axis of the straightened spine results in loading of the coupled segments in a vertical plane. When the energy-absorbing abilities of the supportive structures are exceeded, vertebral fracture, ligamentous disruption, and injury to annular components of the intervertebral disc may occur. Continued compression of the coupled segment leads to dislocation or subluxation, thereby increasing the potential for producing spinal cord or nerve root injury. This is the common mechanism by which cervical fracture and/or spinal cord injury arises in contact sports such as football, rugby, and diving. Whether this mechanism is relevant in the production of cervical spine injuries in other sporting activities remains to be proven. Nevertheless, regardless of the athletic endeavor, striking the vertex with the neck slightly flexed poses great risk for cervical spine and/or spinal cord injury. All those involved in sporting events that are associated with a potential for bodily contact should be adequately forewarned of the potential danger of this mechanism of cervical injury.

Inertial Loading

Compressive forces associated with extremes of flexion frequently result in posterior ligamentous disruption, compression fracture of the anterosuperior vertebral margin, and possible retrolisthesis of the posterior portion of the vertebral body. Although the articular facets may sublux with sudden extremes of flexion, the laminar arch typically remains intact. Vertical compression with the neck held in normal, lordotic position most frequently is unassociated with fracture of the vertebral body because of the energy-absorbing properties of supportive muscular structures and the ability of the laterally bending spine to deflect the load from the coupled segment. However, with forced cervical flexion in conjunction with contact loading subtle alterations such as slight anterior displacement of the vertebral body, widening of the space between the spinous processes, and opening of the apophyseal joints may occur.[35] Therefore, it is apparent that cervical fracture with or without subluxation is produced through the combined loads of contact and impulsion (inertial loading). Hyperextension injury to the neck associated with and produced by contact loading occurs by force applied to the face or forehead. These injuries may result in disruption of the anterior longitudinal ligament, strain of the muscles in the anterior cervical triangle, and infolding of the ligamentum flavum. Concurrently, fractures of the spine may occur through the pedicle of the vertebral segment and, in conjunction with ligament injuries, result in severe neurologic deficits or death. More frequently, the only evidence of cervical spine injury in those sustaining a neck injury is radiographic evidence of a widening of the disc space.[2] Recognition of this subtle finding on a lateral neck roentgenogram should raise the suspicion of instability and indicates immediate immobilization. Compression of the vertex concurrent with extension of the neck may result in fractures of the posterior elements of the vertebrae, including the lamina, articular facets, and lateral mass (pedicle). Typically, the vertebral body is not involved. It would be anticipated that this particular mechanism may not result in spinal cord injury yet may result in nerve root compression related to disruption and compression of the facets, uncinate process, and transverse process.

Concomitant with fracture of the vertebrae and musculoligamentous injuries, this mechanism of neck injury may result in intimal tears of the vertebral artery resulting in subsequent thrombosis and cerebral vascular ischemic infarction and/or death (Fig. 38-4). Although symptoms of brain-stem dysfunction may develop promptly, it is not rare for ischemic symptoms to occur many hours after such an injury. It is presumed that the delay in symptoms results from propagation of thrombus from the vertebral artery into the basilar artery.[31]

In addition to rare vascular complications associated with hyperextension injuries of the neck, this mechanism commonly is observed to result in spinal cord injury in those individuals with a congenitally narrowed spinal canal. Although it has been suggested that the presence of a shallow or congenitally narrowed spinal canal does not predispose one to neuro-

logic injury with axial loading (compressive loading),[25] hyperextension injuries frequently result in a variety of spinal cord injury syndromes in those harboring this anomaly. Typically, these individuals are found to have neurologic abnormalities that seem to exceed those anticipated by the magnitude of the injury (eg, the presence of a spinal cord syndrome arising in an athlete struck in the face or forehead by what observers judged to be a "minor" impact) (Fig. 38-5). Most commonly, this congenital defect remains undisclosed until an individual sustains a spinal cord injury following inertial loading. The presence of a shallow spinal canal may be diagnosed with lateral cervical spine roentgenography as determined by the ratio of the vertebral body to the anterior-posterior distance of the spinal canal (Fig. 38-6) or by measuring the sagittal distance from the posterior margin of the vertebral body to the junction of the lamina and spinous process (normal sagittal distance greater than 13 mm) or by CT of the cervical spine. The most reliable seems to be determination of the vertebral/spinal canal

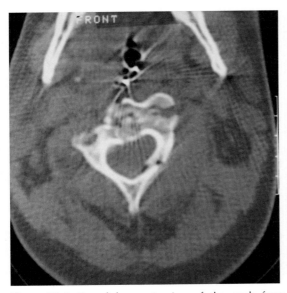

Figure 38-4. Forced hyperextension of the neck from striking the forehead occurred after a fall from the high bar. Neurologic signs of brain-stem ischemia were observed 12 hours after the event although no deficit was initially present.

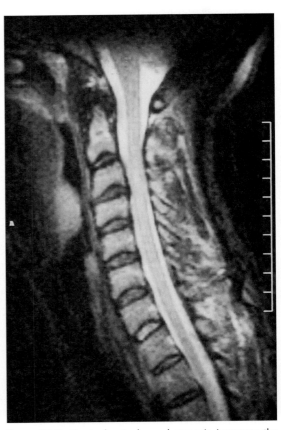

Figure 38-5. Cervical spinal canal stenosis increases the risk for spinal cord injury in individuals sustaining impulsive loading of the neck. This competitor fell as her horse slipped. She landed on her shoulder and hip (lateral impulsion), but did not hit her head. Quadriplegia resulted.

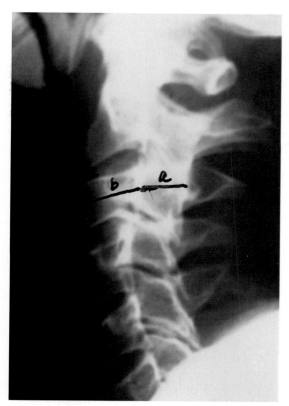

Figure 38-6. Spinal canal stenosis is present if the ratio of the distance from the midpoint of the posterior margin of the vertebra to the nearest point of the anterior margin of the spinous process (a) is less than the width of the corresponding vertebral body (b). The ratio of a:b should be greater than 0.9.

ratio.[27] It remains problematic as to whether these individuals, once identified through preseasonal x-ray examination, should be allowed to participate in sporting activities associated with risk for neck injury. Lateral bending or "side" bending rarely results in spinal injury yet frequently is associated with stretch of the brachial plexus.[12] Symptoms associated with these injuries include a reduction in the cervical range of motion, paresthesia, weakness, and sensory loss in the distribution of the brachial plexus. Most frequently the upper trunk or lateral cord of the plexus is involved, as manifest in proximal arm and shoulder weakness. Fortunately, these injuries are usually short lived. Permanent neurologic defects are rare.

Impulsive Loading

Flexion/extension injuries to the cervical spine can occur without direct application of force. Similar to inertial loading associated with cerebral injury, rapid acceleration–deceleration loads to the cervical spine can result in significant injury without contact loading.[17,26,30] This mechanism typically is observed when an athlete is struck in the thorax and sudden hyperextension or flexion results. Indeed, any sudden movement of the neck induced as a consequence of impulsive or inertial loading regardless of the magnitude of energy is prone to result in this particular injury. For example, a fall striking the shoulder or buttock can result in impulsive linked injuries of the cervical spine. These hyperextension injuries may produce tears of the longus colli and sternocleidomastoid muscles, injury to the intervertebral disc and longitudinal ligament, and in severe injuries, hemorrhage in the esophagus and retropharyngeal space. Spinal cord injury, while rare, can arise as the vertebral arteries are compressed at the occipital-axis junction.

Symptoms associated with these injuries include neck pain and stiffness; paresthesias and numbness in the arms and/or hands; headache; interscapular pain; and vertigo, tinnitus, and blurred vision. It should be emphasized that these mechanisms also may produce cerebral injuries, hence it is not uncommon to observe both cervical and cerebral complaints in athletes sustaining impulsive injuries.

Examination will reveal the presence of marked restriction in the normal range of motion secondary to paracervical muscular spasm. Roentgenographic findings include reversal of the normal lordic curvature, straightening of the spine, and an increase in the prevertebral space.

Spinal Cord Injury Syndromes

Like the brain, the spinal cord displays considerable elasticity.[1] The cervical spinal cord lengthens and shortens without tension under normal circumstances because there is a slight excess of spinal cord length when compared to the overall length of the vertebral central canal when measured in the neutral position. During normal ranges of motion (ie, flexion and extension), the initial change in spinal cord length results from a reduction in the slack normally present. Increases in the inertial or impulsive load that exceed the elastic properties of the cord will result in internal disruption and subsequent neurologic injury. Neurologic involvement also may occur when the cord rapidly decelerates by striking a fractured or dislocated vertebra (contact loading). In general, the calculated elastic modulus is low, thereby underscoring the hazardous nature of large deformations that may occur from relatively small loads. The classical examples of these mechanisms of cervical spinal cord

Table 38-2. Clinical Syndromes of Cervical Spinal Cord Injury

Nerve root syndrome	The clinical findings correlate with dysfunction (motor, sensory, and/or reflex) of 1 or multiple nerve roots (brachial plexus).
Central spinal cord syndrome	Neurologic functions mediated by the more central portion of the cervical spinal cord are altered. Involvement of the upper extremities (arm and/or hand) is greater than loss of function of the legs. Bladder and bowel function usually is altered.
Acute anterior spinal cord syndrome	Injury to the anterior portions of the spinal cord results in immediate complete paralysis associated with hypesthesia and hypalgesia distal to the level of injury, yet touch, proprioception, and vibratory perception are preserved.
Complete transection	Complete loss of motor and sensory function distal to the area of spinal injury may be anatomic or physiologic.

injury arise with axial loads (contact loading), impulsive loads (flexion-hyperextension), and inertial loads resulting in fracture dislocation of the cervical vertebra.

Classification of spinal cord injury based on the presumed force and direction of its application is primarily descriptive and connotes little in the way of prognosis or mechanism of injury. Four neurologic syndromes of cervical injury have been suggested (Table 38-2). Although classification of spinal cord injuries into syndromes has provided clinical-anatomic correlations, the usefulness of such a classification in treatment has not been appreciated. Thus, determination as to whether an individual has sustained a central spinal cord injury or an anterior spinal cord syndrome is of little practical importance. The most useful method of classification remains whether the injury is a complete cord injury with loss of sensory and motor function or an incomplete cord injury in which there is some preservation of sensation and/or motor power caudal to the level of injury. Only 15% of patients with symptoms and signs of complete loss of spinal cord function during the initial assessment regain any function, whereas those with incomplete loss may regain as much as 70% to 80% of lost neurologic function.

The initial assessment, immobilization techniques, and subsequent methods of determining the necessity for specific treatment modalities are beyond the scope of this chapter. This information is available in standard textbooks of neurosurgery.

Criteria for Return to Competition

The criteria for permitting an athlete who has sustained a neck injury to return to competition must be conservative. It is better to err on the side of restraint than expose one to further and perhaps more serious injury. In general, all athletes who have sustained a cervical injury should be evaluated thoroughly by the team physician before returning to play. All individuals rendered unconscious should be considered to have sustained a cervical injury, indicating appropriate immobilization and transport to a medical facility. Only after complete resolution of symptoms and/or medical evaluation, including cervical roentgenography, should an athlete be permitted to play.

A team physician may be called on to render a decision as to whether an athlete who has sustained a cervical fracture may return to competition after adequate healing has occurred. A completely healed fracture that has been shown to result in no abnormal subluxation as determined by lateral flexion/extension roentgenography and no limitation in active range of motion of the neck, and that was unattended with any neurologic syndrome should pose no particular contraindication to competition in noncontact sports. However, each case should be individualized.

Repeated neck injuries should raise the question as to whether an individual should continue in a particular discipline. These persons should be evaluated thoroughly before permission can be given to continue. Particular attention should be directed to teaching proper techniques of participation, achieving a suitable physique, and obtaining radiographic evidence of occult anomalies that would preclude activity.[33]

CONCLUDING REMARKS

The characteristics of sport-related injuries that involve the central nervous system may be predicted to a large extent by knowledge of the forces and loads applied to the brain and spinal cord. In addition to contact, impulsion is an important factor in inducing injury to these structures. The neuropathologic alterations produced by these forces are specific to the particular load, the direction of its application, and the tensile features of the brain and cervical spinal cord. Return to competition will be dependent on the nature of the injury and should be individualized, with a strong argument for conservatism.

References

1. Breig A (ed): Biomechanics of the Central Nervous System. Chicago, Yearbook Medical Publishers, 1960, pp 62–95.
2. Cintron E, Gilula LA, Murphy WA: The widened disc space: a sign of cervical hyperextension injury. Radiology 141:639–44, 1981.
3. Fielding JW: Normal and selected abnormal motions of the cervical spine from the second to the seventh cervical vertebra. J Bone Joint Surg 46A:1779–91, 1964.
4. Gennarelli TA, Segana H, Wald U: Physiological response to angular acceleration of the head. In Grossman RG, Gildenberg PL (eds): Head Injury: Basic and Clinical Aspects. New York, Raven Press, 1982, pp 129–40.
5. Gennarelli TA, Thibault LE, Adams JH: Diffuse axonal injury and traumatic coma. Ann Neurol 12:564–74, 1982.
6. Goldsmith W: Biomechanics of head injury. In Perrone N, Anliker M (eds): Biomechanics, Its Foundations and Objectives. New York, Prentice-Hall, 1970.
7. Goldsmith W: Some aspects of head and neck injury and protection. In Nuri A (eds): Progress in Biomechanisms, Leiden, The Netherlands, Sijthoff and Noordhoff, 1979, pp 33–377.
8. Gronwall D, Wrightson P: Delayed recovery of intellectual function after minor head injury. Lancet 2:605–9, 1974.
9. Gronwall D, Wrightson P: Memory and information processing capacity after closed head injury. J Neurol Neurosurg Psychiatry 44:889–95, 1982.
10. Guskiewicz KM, Riemann BL, Perrin DH: Alternative approaches to the assessment of mild head injury in athletes. Med Sci Sports Exerc 19(suppl 7):3213–21, 1997.
11. Guthkelch AN: Posttraumatic amnesia, postconcussional symptoms and neurosis. Eur Neurol 19:91–102, 1980.
12. Hershman EB: Injuries to the brachial plexus. In Torg JS (ed): Athletic Injuries to the Head, Neck, and Face. Philadelphia, Mosby-Year Book, 1991, pp 338–67.
13. Holbourn AHS: Mechanics of head injury. Lancet 2:438–41, 1943.
14. Jennett B: Late effects of head injury. In Critchley M, O'Leary JL, Jennett B (eds): Scientific Foundations of Neurology. Philadelphia, FA Davis, 1971, pp 441–51.
15. Jones MD: Cineradiographic studies of the normal cervical spine. Cal Med 93:293–6, 1960.
16. King AI, Ruan JS, Zhdu C: Recent advances in biomechanics of brain injury research. J Neurotrauma 12:651–58, 1995.
17. LaRocca H: Acceleration injuries of the neck. In Keener EB (ed): Clinical Neurosurgery: Proceedings of the Congress of Neurological Surgeons. Baltimore, Williams & Wilkins, 1978, pp 209–17.
18. Levin HS: Neurobehavioral Consequences of Closed Head Injury. Oxford, UK, Oxford University Press, 1988.
19. McCrory PR, Berkovic SF: Second impact syndrome. Neurology 50:677–83, 1998.
20. Meaney DF, Smith DH, Schreiber DI: Biomechanical analysis of experimental diffuse axonal injury. J Neurotrauma 12:689–94, 1995.
21. Ommaya AK: Biomechanics of head injury: experimental aspects. In Nahum AM, Melvin J (eds): The Biomechanics of Trauma. New York, Appleton & Lange, 1985, pp 245–69.
22. Ommaya AK, Faas F, Yarnell PR: Whiplash injury and brain damage: an experimental study. JAMA 204:285–9, 1968.
23. Ommaya AK, Genarelli T: Cerebral concussion and traumatic unconsciousness. Brain 97:633–54, 1974.
24. Ommaya AK, Hirsch AE: Tolerances of cerebral concussion from head impact and whiplash in primates. J Biomech 4:13–22, 1971.
25. Otis JC, Burstein AH, Torg JS: Mechanisms and pathomechanisms of athletic injuries of the cervical spine. In Torg JS (ed): Athletic Injuries to the Head, Neck, and Face. Philadelphia, Mosby-Year Book, 1991, pp 438–68.
26. Patrick LM: Studies of hyperextension and hyperflexion injury in volunteers and human cadavers. In Gurdjian ES, Thomas LM (eds): Proceedings of the Workshop of the American Association of Neurologic Surgeons and the National Institutes of Health. Springfield, Ill, Charles C Thomas, 1970, pp 92–107.
27. Pavlov H: Radiographic evaluation of the cervical spine and related structures. In Torg JS (ed): Athletic Injuries to the Head, Neck, and Face. Philadelphia, Mosby-Year Book, 1991, pp 384–411.
28. Roaf R: A study of the mechanics of spinal injuries. J Bone Joint Surg 42B:810–23, 1960.
29. Russell WR, Schiller F: Crushing injuries of the skull; clinical and experimental observations. J Neurol Neurosurg Psychiatry 12:52–60, 1949.
30. Shea M, Wittenberg RH, Edwards WT: In vitro hyperextension injuries in the human cadaveric cervical spine. J Orthop Res 10:911–20, 1992.
31. Simeone FA, Goldberg HI: Thrombosis of the vertebral artery from hyperextension injury to the neck. J Neurosurg 29:540–4, 1967.
32. Thibault LE, Gennarelli TA: Biomechanics and craniocerebral trauma. In Povlishock J, Becker D (eds): Central Nervous System Trauma Status Report. NINCDS, 1985, pp 370–90, 1985.
33. Torg JS, Ramsey-Emphein JA: Suggested management guidelines for participation in collision activities with congenital developmental, or post injury lesions involving the cervical spine. Med Sci Sports Exerc 29(suppl l7):5256–72, 1997.
34. Unterharnschiedt F, Higgins LS: Neuropathologic effects of translational and rotational acceleration of the head in animal experiments. In Walker AE, Caveness WF, Critchley MaCD (eds): The Late Effects of Head Injury. Springfield, Ill, Charles C Thomas, 1969, pp 158–67.
35. Webb JK, Broughton BK, McSweeney T, Park WM: Hidden flexion injury of the cervical spine. J Bone Joint Surg 58B:322–7, 1976.
36. White AA, Panjabi MM: Clinical Biomechanics of the Spine, 2nd edition. Philadelphia, JB Lippincott, 1990.

Chapter 39

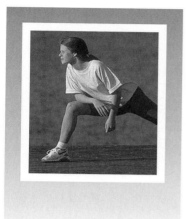

Shoulder Injuries

Mary Lloyd Ireland, M.D.
Kenneth B. Tepper, M.D.
John A. LeBlanc, B.S., D.O.

FUNCTIONAL ANATOMY AND BIOMECHANICS

The shoulder is a complex arrangement of joints and articulations with a greater range of motion than any other joint in the body. Synchronous motion among the various joints and articulations is required, otherwise instability or breakdown of the shoulder complex will occur. A basic understanding of functional anatomy of the shoulder is necessary for the accurate diagnosis of the various disorders that may occur.

The shoulder complex includes the glenohumeral, acromioclavicular, and sternoclavicular joints, as well as the scapulothoracic and sub-acromial articulations. The bony architecture of the clavicle, acromioclavicular joint, and scapula is easily palpable and serves as landmarks for identification of soft-tissue structures. The ligaments that stabilize the clavicle are named for their bony attachments. These are the coracoclavicular ligament composed of the medial coronoid and lateral trapezoid ligaments, the coracoacromial ligament, and the acromioclavicular ligament (Fig. 39-1).[1] The coracoacromial arch consists of these stabilizing ligaments and their connections to the acromion and clavicle.

The rotator cuff is composed of 4 muscles: the supraspinatus, infraspinatus, teres minor, and subscapularis (Fig. 39-2).[4] The only internal rotator,

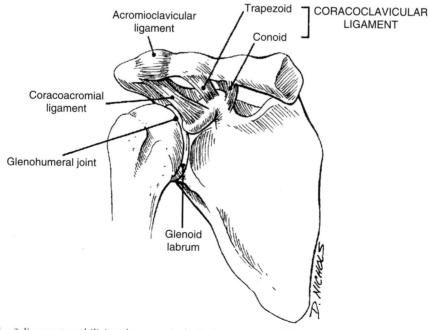

Figure 39-1. The 3 ligaments stabilizing the acromioclavicular and coracoid bones are named for their attachments. The coracoclavicular ligament has lateral trapezoid and medial conoid portions. (From Andrews JR, Zarins B, Wilk KE: Injuries in Baseball. Philadelphia, Lippincott-Raven, 1998, p 41, with permission.)

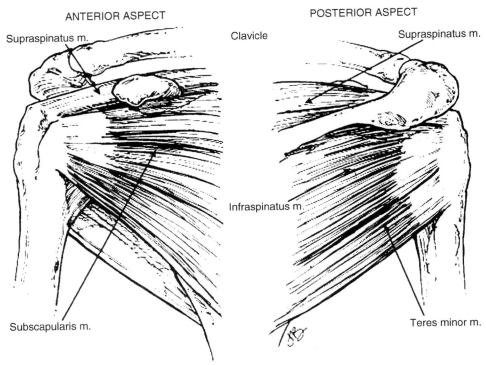

ANTERIOR ASPECT

Supraspinatus m.

Subscapularis m.

POSTERIOR ASPECT

Clavicle

Supraspinatus m.

Infraspinatus m.

Teres minor m.

Figure 39-2. Anteriorly, the subscapularis is the only internal rotator of the rotator cuff, concerting onto the lesser tuberosity. The other 3 portions of the rotator cuff are external rotators (from superior to inferior): supraspinatus, infraspinatus, and teres minor, with insertions onto the greater tuberosity. (From Baker CL: The Hughston Clinic Sports: Medicine Book. Baltimore, 1995, Williams & Wilkins, p 230, with permission.)

the subscapularis, originates from the subscapular fossa on the anterior aspect of the scapula and inserts on the lesser tuberosity. The other 3 rotator cuff muscles are the external rotators, depressors, and stabilizers of the humeral head. They can be thought of as a "soft-tissue sandwich" passing underneath the compressive roof of the acromial arch and functioning to move and rotate the humeral head below (Fig. 39-3).[22]

The supraspinatus originates superior to the scapular spine in the supraspinatus fossa and passes under the acromion on its way to insertion on the greater tuberosity. The supraspinatus counteracts the superior pull of the deltoid. The supraspinatus cannot initiate abduction. The posterior 2 rotator cuff muscles—infraspinatus and teres minor—are external rotators of the humeral head (Fig. 39-4).[42] The infraspinatus originates inferior to the scapular spine in the infraspinatus fossa of the scapula and inserts on the greater tuberosity. The teres minor originates from the lateral border of the scapula and inserts on the lower facet of the greater tuberosity. The labrum surrounds the glenoid and provides static stability by deepening the socket, acting as a buttress, and serving as an attachment for the glenohumeral ligaments (Fig. 39-5).[1] The most important structure in anterior dislo-

cation is the anterior inferior glenohumeral ligament. The rotator interval involves the capsule between the superior glenohumeral ligament and the subscapularis. The normal interval prevents inferior subluxation of the humeral head. The middle glenohumeral ligament crosses the subscapularis tendon anteriorly.

The face of the glenoid can be thought of as a clock face. The side view of the right shoulder in Figure 39-6 shows the orientation during arthroscopy. The lesions of the labrum are named according to their relationship to the clock face (Fig. 39-6). A SLAP (superior labrum, anterior posterior tear) lesion is located in the 10:00 to 3:00 position. Instability can be associated with SLAP lesions. An anterior inferior glenohumeral dislocation results in an anterior inferior labrum detachment referred to as a *Bankart lesion.* Weight lifters are more susceptible to lesions in the posterior superior labrum. Posterior inferior labral lesions are rare.

Shoulder function results from a sequence of linking movements throughout the kinetic chain. Scapulothoracic musculature provides the stability of the scapula to the chest, with the thoracolumbar spine allowing the shoulder to be supported in space. The movements of the scapula are protraction, retraction, rotation

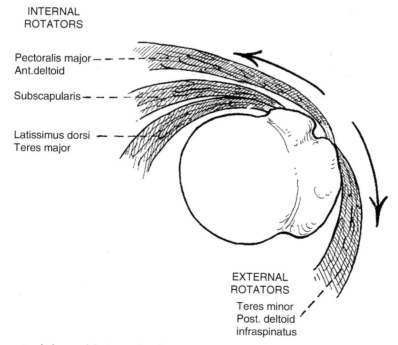

Coracoacromial
arch

Rotaor
interval

Greater
tuberosity

Supraspinatus
Infraspinatus
Teres minor

Subacromial
bursa

Subscapularis
(lesses tuberosity)

Biceps (long head)

Subacromial bursa between overlying coracoacromial arch and underlying cuff tendons attached to
greater and lesser tuberosities.

Figure 39-3. This side view of the coracoacromial arch and rotator cuff insertions shows the posterior position of the external rotators, supraspinatus, infraspinatus, and teres minor. The rotator interval is between the subscapularis and superior glenohumeral ligament. The bursa lies in the subacromial space and can be likened to a soft-tissue "sandwich" composed by the fixed coracoacromial arch, coracoacromial ligament superiorly and humeral head inferiorly. (From DeLee JC, Drez D: Orthopaedic Sports Medicine. Philadelphia, WB Saunders, 1994, p 624, with permission.)

(upward and downward), depression, and elevation. The largest and most easily seen muscle is the trapezius, which has its origin at the spinous processes of the thoracic vertebra and its insertion on the distal clavicle. The upper fibers elevate the scapula.[44,59,64] Elevation of the scapula is assisted by the levator scapulae, and the rhomboideus minor and major (Fig. 39-7).[41] Opposing muscles that depress the scapula are the subclavius, which crosses the sternoclavicular joint, pectoralis minor, lower fibers of the pectoralis major, serratus anterior, latissimus

INTERNAL
ROTATORS

Pectoralis major
Ant.deltoid

Subscapularis

Latissimus dorsi
Teres major

EXTERNAL
ROTATORS

Teres minor
Post. deltoid
infraspinatus

Figure 39-4. The important balance of the internal and external rotators is shown diagrammatically. The 4 muscles for the rotator cuff are external rotators of supraspinatus, infraspinatus, teres minor, and internal rotator of subscapularis. Other internal rotators of the shoulder are pectoralis major, anterior deltoid, subscapularis, latissimus dorsi, and teres major. (From Hollinshead WH, Jenkins DB: Functional Anatomy of the Limbs and Back. Philadelphia, WB Saunders, 1981, p 106 with permission.)

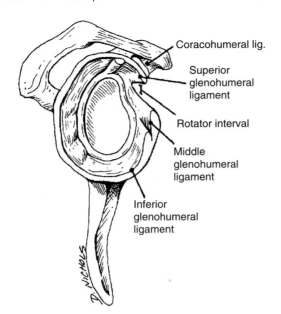

Orientation of glenohumeral ligament

Figure 39-5. With the humeral head removed, the glenoid concavity is deepened by the labrum and ligaments attach anteriorly onto the labrum in a superior, medial, and inferior fashion. (From Andrews JR, Zarins B, Wilk KE: Injuries in Baseball. Philadelphia, Lippincott-Raven, 1998, p 44, with permission.)

dorsi, and trapezius (Fig. 39-8).[41] The upper part of the trapezius, lower part of the trapezius, and serratus anterior act as upward rotators (Fig. 39-9).[41] The serratus anterior originates

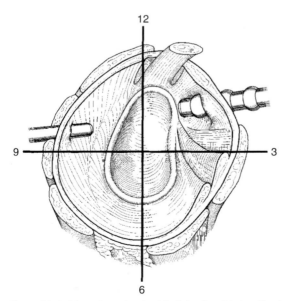

Figure 39-6. The orientation in this right glenoid visualized arthroscopically shows a clock schematic for classification of labral tears. Lesions in throwers typically are in the 12 to 3 o'clock position, and SLAP lesions in the 3 to 6 o'clock position anterior inferior. (Copyright 1998, ML Ireland, MD.)

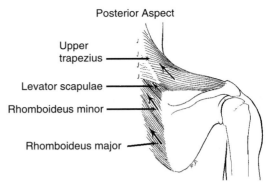

Figure 39-7. Scapular elevators and the direction of their forces. (From Hollinshead WH: Anatomy for Surgeons, Vol 3. New York, Harper & Row, 1969, p 327 with permission.)

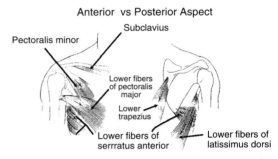

Figure 39-8. Scapular depressors and the direction of their forces. (From Hollinshead WH: Anatomy for Surgeons, Vol 3. New York, Harper & Row, 1969, p 328, with permission.)

from the ribs anteriorly and inserts on the inferior scapular angle. The serratus acts to protract and upwardly rotate the scapula.[67] Injury to the long thoracic nerve (C5–C7) causes winging of the scapula and significant disability. The downward rotators include the rhomboideus minor and major, levator scapulae, pectoralis minor, and lower pectoralis major (Fig. 39-10).[41] The protractors of the shoulder are the pectoralis minor and major and serratus anterior muscles (Fig. 39-11).[41] The opposing retractors of the scapula are the rhomboideus minor, middle

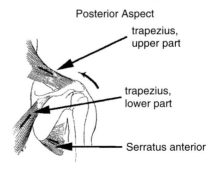

Figure 39-9. Upward rotators and the direction of their forces. (From Hollinshead WH: Anatomy for Surgeons, Vol 3. New York, Harper & Row, 1969, p 329 with permission.)

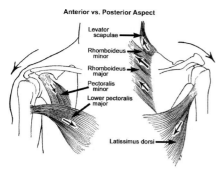

Figure 39-10. Downward rotators and the direction of their forces. (From Hollinshead WH: Anatomy for Surgeons, Vol 3. New York, Harper & Row, 1969, p 329, with permission.)

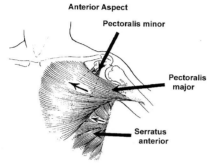

Figure 39-11. Scapular protractors. (From Hollinshead WH: Anatomy for Surgeons, Vol 3. New York, Harper & Row, 1969, p 330, with permission.)

trapezius, rhomboideus major, and upper latissimus dorsi (Fig. 39-12).[41]

The forces for shoulder function are generated mainly in the legs, hips, and trunk. The scapula helps to control the forces and motion at the shoulder joint and serves as a pivot point. Altered scapular motion and scapular dyskinesias may be seen in 67% to 100% of shoulder injuries. Efficient rotator cuff function requires a stable scapular base. Disorganized muscle activation patterns are observed early in shoulder injuries.

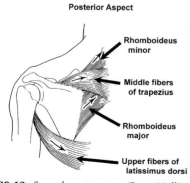

Figure 39-12. Scapular retractors. (From Hollinshead WH: Anatomy for Surgeons, Vol 3. New York, Harper & Row, 1969, p 331, with permission.)

Table 39-1 presents a summary of shoulder examination testing based on enervation, myotomes, and technique for testing.[70]

PHYSIOLOGIC VARIATIONS AND GENDER DIFFERENCES

The female athlete, as a rule, has looser joints than the male athlete. There are familial and gender influences. In a study of 100 patients with generalized joint laxity who presented with musculoskeletal complaints, it was concluded that hypermobility syndrome occurs as an isolated condition and is genetically distinct from other connective tissue disorders.[28] An association of dominant inheritance in familial generalized articular hypermobility has been reported.[9] There are reports of recurrent dislocation of the patella and shoulder associated with familial laxity.[16] Increased generalized ligamentous laxity has been reported in patients with idiopathic scoliosis.[81] In a study of normal shoulders and shoulders with instability and impingement, patterns of flexibility, laxity, and strength were evaluated.[82] The study concluded that isokinetic testing may be helpful to screen for instability and impingement.

In a study comparing shoulder laxity and pain in competitive swimmers, 40 senior national elite swimmers completed a questionnaire and underwent clinical stability tests. The clinical score of glenohumeral laxity and presence of shoulder pain that interfered with practice or competition was statistically significant.[56] Therefore, shoulder laxity may be a common denominator in the cause of significant shoulder pain interfering with practice in the swimming athlete. The question remains, does underlying laxity predispose to the symptomatic instability?[3] Thirty-six competitive swimmers with shoulder pain, the majority of whom were women, were evaluated for impingement and increased glenohumeral translation. The Hawkins test for impingement was more sensitive than other tests.[39,61,62] The direction of shoulder laxity in swimmers in this series was predominantly anterior inferior and associated conditions existed (eg, shoulder pain from coracoacromial impingement with associated increased glenohumeral translation and apprehension). The goal is to determine the underlying or primary process. In the young athlete glenohumeral instability is usually the primary problem. A study of 150 asymptomatic shoulders in 75 school children revealed "instability in 57% of the shoulders in boys and in 48% of shoulders in girls." The mean age of the boys was 14.4 years and girls 16.6 years. A posterior drawer sign was found in 63 of the 300

Table 39-1. Shoulder Muscle Testing Chart

MUSCLE	INNERVATION	MYOTOMES	TECHNIQUE FOR TESTING
Trapezius	Spinal accessory	C2–C4	Patient shrugs shoulders against resistance.
Sternomastoid	Spinal accessory	C2–C4	Patient turns head to one side with resistance over opposite temporal area.
Serratus anterior	Long thoracic	C5–C7	Patient pushes against wall with outstretched arm. Scapular winging is observed.
Latissimus dorsi	Thoracodorsal	C7–C8	Downward backward pressure of arm against resistance. Muscle palpable at Inf. angle of scapula during cough.
Rhomboids	Dorsal	(C4) C5[a]	Hands on hips pushing elbows backward against resistance.
Levator scapulae	Scapular		
Subclavius	Nerve to subclavius	C5–C6	None
Teres major	Subscapular (lower)	C5–C6	Similar to lat. dorsi; muscle palpable at lower border of scapula.
Deltoid	Axillary	C5–C6 (C7)	With arm abducted 90°, downward pressure is applied. Anterior and posterior fibers may be tested in slight flexion and extension.
Subscapularis	Subscapular (upper)	C5	Arm at side with elbow flexed to 90°. Examiner resists internal rotation.
Supraspinatus	Suprascapular	C5 (C6)	Arm abducted against resistance (not isolated). With arm pronated and elevated 90° in plane of scapula, downward pressure is applied.
Infraspinatus	Suprascapular	C5 (C6)	Arm at side with elbow flexed 90°. Examiner resists external rotation.
Teres minor	Axillary	C5–C6 (C7)	Same as for infraspinatus
Pectoralis major	Medial and lateral pectoral	C5–T1	With arm flexed 30° in front of body, patient, adducts against resistance.
Pectoralis minor	Medial pectoral	C8, T1	None
Coracobrachialis	Musculocutaneous	(C4) C5–C6 (C7)	None
Biceps brachii	Musculocutaneous	(C4) C5–C6 (C7)	Flexion of the supinated forearm against resistance.
Triceps	Radial	(C5) C6–C8	Resistance to extension of elbow from varying position of flexion.

[a]Numbers in parentheses indicate a variable but not rare contribution.
From Rockwood CA, Matsen FA III (eds): The Shoulder, Vol I. Philadelphia, WB Saunders, 1990, with permission.

shoulders. Generalized joint laxity was not a feature of subjects whose shoulder had positive instability signs.[24]

Females test weaker in upper body strength than males. Lower extremity gender differences are much less than those of the upper extremity and equalize more quickly with a strengthening program.

PHYSICAL EXAMINATION

In general, the physical examination is used to confirm the diagnosis suggested by the history.[4,12,22,29,32,37] With a combination of careful history and physical examination, a diagnosis can be obtained. There are many excellent review articles about the physical examination of the shoulder. These articles all emphasize the importance of making the diagnosis. Oftentimes there are many abnormal physical examination tests, and from these results the examiner must decide the initial abnormality that started the shoulder complex. Unfortunately, many of the physical examination tests do not isolate the primary or initial diagnosis. A detailed history and repeat examinations are required.

Access to the entire upper body, including both shoulders, is essential. Examination requires a table that will support both supine and prone testing. Systematic examination of the entire shoulder complex should be performed routinely. Examination comprises inspection, palpation, assessment of range of motion, strength testing, and finally, special provocative testing. Measurements should be taken the same way at each examination, recorded, and compared to the uninvolved side.

Inspection

Inspection requires complete access to the upper body. Female athletes are best evaluated in a gown or halter top that exposes both shoulders and scapulae. Systematic inspection may reveal asymmetry, atrophy, hypertrophy, prominences, depressions, or swelling, which should be noted. Scars suggest prior injury or surgery. Hypertrophy may be normal in the throwing and overhead athlete, however, atrophy in the supraspinatus and infraspinatus fossa may suggest rotator cuff pathology or suprascapular nerve entrapment. Deformity suggests an acute or chronic injury such as glenohumeral or acromioclavicular joint dislocation. Rupture of the long head of the biceps tendon would be demonstrated by asymmetrical distal biceps enlargement.

The lower extremity is often overlooked, and also requires careful observation. Trunk and core imbalances will result in abnormal shoulder biomechanics. The entire kinetic chain requires evaluation. Posture should be evaluated for trunk kyphosis or lordosis. Hip weakness may manifest as a Trendelenburg gait. The scapula may have a drooping or abnormally protracted attitude. All areas found to be abnormal on the physical examination must be addressed in the rehabilitation program.

Palpation

All joints and articulations require palpation, assessing for instability and pain with motion. The examination proceeds systematically from proximal to distal, starting with the sternoclavicular joint, progressing to the clavicle and acromioclavicular joint, and ending with the acromion and coracoid. Tenderness with deformity over a joint suggests dislocation or subluxation, while pain without deformity suggests arthritis. Posterior sternoclavicular dislocations require urgent medical attention as neurovascular compromise may occur. Tenderness surrounding the coracoid is nonspecific and can occur with anterior subluxation, acromioclavicular separations, and joint coracoid impingement. Joint line tenderness may suggest a labrum tear. The rotator cuff is assessed just lateral to the acromion. Discomfort suggests rotator cuff tendonitis or tear.

Range of Motion

Active and passive range of motion is assessed. Forward flexion, abduction, and internal and external rotation with the arm in 90° of abduction are recorded bilaterally. The scapula should be stabilized to assess true glenohumeral motion. Greater external rotation on the dominant side of an overhead or throwing athlete is common and is usually normal, however, if a significant internal rotation deficit exists, the posterior capsule may be contracted. Asymmetry and limitations are documented.

Palpation throughout range of motion may reveal crepitus emanating from the glenohumeral, acromioclavicular, or scapulothoracic joint or from the subacromial space. The quality of the scapulothoracic motion is assessed dynamically. The athlete is then asked to perform repetitive circular motions; dyskinesia suggests shoulder pathology or nerve injury. Flexibility of the hip and core should also be assessed.

Strength

Muscle strength is determined and recorded for the deltoid, supraspinatus, and involved external and internal rotators. The muscles work in patterns, and do not function in an isolated manner. Various grading systems have been described.[70,71] The sides should be compared and determinations recorded.

The distant kinetic chain also should be evaluated. Hip strength is quickly assessed by having the patient perform a one-legged squat to 45° of knee flexion followed by extension. The proper position is one of hip over knee over ankle. Hip and leg rotation indicate weak hip abductors.

Order and Principles of Physical Examination

The most painful part of the examination should be done last. The goal of the examination is to determine the primary diagnosis. Is the involved joint glenohumeral, acromioclavicular, or sternoclavicular? Is the structure involved labrum or capsuloligamentous? Is the rotator cuff pathology articular or bursal? Is it inflammation or a tear, partial or complete? After a thorough history is taken, the patient is asked to actively move the shoulder while the examiner checks for ranges of motion of abduction, forward flexion, and internal and external rotation. Any asymmetry should be noted. Scapulothoracic motion is then assessed with several maneuvers. The patient should wear a halter or swim suit top to better assess scapulothoracic motion (Fig. 39-13). The patient is instructed to stand and to push backward against the examiner's hand. Scapular asymmetry and motion away from the spine is observed. While the patient performs a push-up against a wall, flexes forward, pushes her palms together, puts her hands on her waist, and pushes backward against the examiner's hand, the examiner assesses scapular movement and observes for symmetric protraction, retraction, upward and downward elevation, and rotation. The distance from the spinous processes to the scapula is measured. Scapular winging is observed. Trigger points are palpated. Next, the

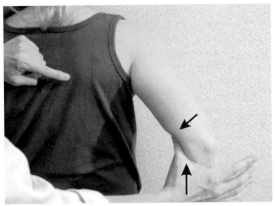

Figure 39-13. Observation for scapular motion is done as the patient is instructed to push against the examiner's hand. (Copyright 2002, ML Ireland, MD.)

patient is examined seated, supine, and prone while she goes through a series of range of motion and strength testing.

Correlation of the deficient anatomic structure as it relates to the physical examination allows the examiner to determine the diagnosis and better design the rehabilitation program and/or surgery. This helps to reveal what positions to avoid based on the apprehension positions obtained during the examination (Table 39-2).[33]

The labrum is a fibrocartilaginous structure that attaches to the glenoid, improving stability by deepening the concavity of the glenoid. Variations of labral attachments at the biceps anchor and anterior superior and middle glenohumeral ligaments are frequently seen. SLAP tears are better understood as arthroscopic techniques have become more common and instrumentation and techniques have advanced.

Tears of the labrum are associated with instability in 50% of cases. Snyder classified labral tears into 4 types (Fig. 39-14)[1,76]: type I, labral frame with no detachment; type II, detachment of superior labrum and biceps anchor; type III, Bucket handle tear, intact biceps anchor; type IV, bucket handle tear extending into the biceps tendon.

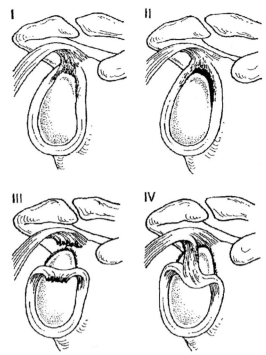

Figure 39-14. Synder classification of labral tears. (From Snyder SJ, Karzel RP, Del Pizzo W, et al: SLAP lesions of the shoulder. Arthroscopy 6:274–9, 1990, with permission.)

PROVOCATIVE TESTS

Instability and Labral Injury

Numerous tests exist to help identify and quantify instability and labral pathology. The patient is sometimes able to voluntarily demonstrate posterior or multidirectional instability. Generalized ligamentous laxity may be present with instability and should be assessed. Elbow hyperextension greater than 10°, abduction of the thumb to touch the forearm, metacarpophalangeal joint hyperextension, and knee hyperextension greater than 10° are clues that generalized ligamentous laxity exists.

Table 39-2. Anatomic Considerations in Shoulder Stabilization

POSITION OF ABNORMAL TRANSLATION	DEFICIENT ANATOMIC STRUCTURE
Inferior subluxation (in adduction)	Rotator interval
Translation at 45°	Middle glenohumeral ligament
Translation at 90°	Anterior, inferior glenohumeral ligament
Inferior subluxation (in abduction)	Axillary recess
Posterior translation at 90°	Posterior, inferior glenohumeral ligament
Posterior translation at 45°	Mid-posterior capsule

From Guandre CA: Arthroscopic shoulder stabilization. Operative Tech Sports Med 10(1): 18–24, 2002, with permission.

Stability Testing

Glenohumeral translation is evaluated. The patient is seated and a Lachman or drawer test of the shoulder is performed. The scapula is stabilized and anterior, posterior, and inferior forces are applied to the humeral head. Excursion is noted and compared to the uninvolved side (Fig. 39-15). A grading system from 0 to III has been described. Grade 0 is normal. Grade I demonstrates up to 50% translation and is a normal excursion in anterior translation. In grade II the humeral head rides over the glenoid and spontaneously reduces; posteriorly, grade II is generally normal. In grade III, the humeral head dislocates and remains dislocated upon the release of force.[27] Grading the difference and direction from the involved side to the uninvolved side is done and documented.

The sulcus sign is tested with the athlete's arm at the side. A longitudinal force is applied and the displacement between the humeral head and the lateral acromion is noted. Greater than 1 cm of excursion is pathologic and suggests inferior and multidirectional instability. Similar testing with the arm in 30° of external rotation will assess the rotator interval.[36]

Anterior Apprehension Test. The patient is supine or sitting and the arm is in 90° of abduction and 90° of elbow flexion. The scapula is stabilized and while the shoulder is maximally externally rotated an anterior force is applied to the proximal humerus (Fig. 39-16). With anterior instability, the athlete becomes apprehensive

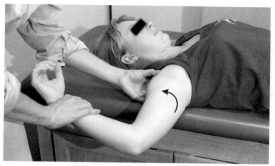

Figure 39-16. In a supine position, the arm is abducted and externally rotated and the humeral head is translated anterior to reproduce anterior instability or anterior labral symptoms. (Copyright 2002, ML Ireland, MD.)

and exhibits anxiety as it feels as if the shoulder will subluxate or dislocate. Speer and coworkers demonstrated that in patients who underwent anterior capsular reconstruction who had sustained a prior dislocation, true apprehension without pain was present in 96% of patients preoperatively. However, if pain is present, rotator cuff pathology needs to be considered as this shoulder position places stress on the rotator cuff and the anterior capsule. In subjects requiring anterior capsular reconstruction who have not had a complete dislocation, true apprehension without pain will be felt in only 42%, while pain will be present in 84%.[77]

Posterior Apprehension Test. The athlete is supine or seated and the shoulder is placed in 90° of forward flexion and then internally rotated. A posterior force is applied at the elbow; the athlete may feel as if the shoulder is going to subluxate or dislocate. In some cases the patient can demonstrate posterior instability voluntarily moving her shoulder into horizontal adduction and internal rotation.

Palpating the humeral head and applying posterior force, the humeral head is pushed posteriorly and a "pop" is felt, indicating posterior instability and a posterior labral tear. If one is thinking about instability, attempts at distraction and reproducing the direction of instability posteriorly are made, going into horizontal adduction and internal rotation with posterior palpation. The anterior direction is external rotation, abduction, and anterior palpation for any humeral head luxation or labral "pop". With the patient in the prone position, posterior instability is checked. The posterior glenohumeral joint is palpated as force is directed posteriorly (Fig. 39-17).

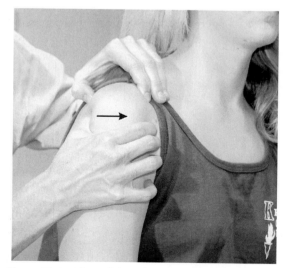

Figure 39-15. The stability of the shoulder is tested in the seated position by performing anterior humeral head translation with the right hand while stabilizing the acromion. (Copyright 2002, ML Ireland, MD.)

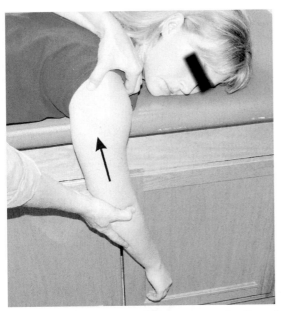

Figure 39-17. In the supine position posteriorly directed forces are placed on the forearm while the glenohumeral joint is palpated with the left thumb. Reproduction of symptoms of humeral head luxation confirms posterior instability or labrum tear. (Copyright 2002, ML Ireland, MD.)

Labral Testing

To test for labral injuries, axial loading is performed and the arm is maximally horizontally abducted, internally rotated, and externally rotated. If there is pain in maximal internal rotation, this is more indicative of labral tear than in external rotation. Conditions of the rotator cuff may also cause pain with rotation maneuvers. No one test is specific for rotator cuff, labrum, or capsule. Many tests named after the examining physician have been reported. The principles of the test must be understood and the steps taken to reproduce symptoms described.

Oftentimes there are injuries to the labrum and articular side of the rotator cuff. The vicious cycle of injury in a younger person will usually start with instability, leading to rotator cuff weakness, then compression impingement, pain, and muscular imbalance. The labral injury can occur at the time of the initial instability episode.

The labral tests may be thought of as comparable to meniscal tests of the knee. Compression and rotation of the humeral head on the torn labrum produces pain, popping, and reproducible symptoms. Supine and prone tests are done similar to stabilization tests but axial loading and compression forces are applied instead of distraction.

With the patient supine, testing for stability is done again. While the examiner stabilizes the scapula with his or her hand, the arm is externally rotated and abducted. Pain and apprehension or a labral "pop" indicate anterior instability.

Relocation Test. The relocation test is performed similar to the apprehension test. When symptoms begin to occur, a posterior force is applied to the proximal humerus and the symptoms of apprehension or pain diminish or resolve.[46] If apprehension complaints resolve, the likelihood of anterior labral pathology is high.[77]

O'Brien's Test. The arm is placed in 90° of forward flexion, internally rotated with the thumb pointing downward, and then adducted 15° to 20° across the chest. The examiner applies a downward force at the hand. The thumbs-down position loads the biceps–glenoid–labrum complex, and places compressive loads on the acromioclavicular joint. Deep pain relieved with external rotation is suggestive of a SLAP lesion. Acromioclavicular joint pathology will cause more superficial pain. Pain must be relieved in the thumb-up position for the test to be positive.[65,66]

SLAP Test. The arm is in 90° of abduction with the hand fully supinated. The examiner's hand is placed on the shoulder with the thumb in the axilla. The examiner applies a downward force to the supinated hand, while applying an upward force with the thumb. Pain is suggestive of a type II or IV SLAP lesion.

Anterior Glide Test. The seated athlete places her hand on the ipsilateral hip with her fingers anterior and her thumb posterior. While stabilizing the scapula, an upward and forward force is applied at the elbow by the examiner. The athlete may have pain or a "click" with anterior superior lesions, SLAP tears, and middle glenohumeral ligament avulsions. With a positive test, there is a high probability of a labral lesion. The reported specificity is 91% and sensitivity 79%.[47]

Crank Test. An upright examination test has been reported by Liu.[52] Sensitivity and specificity is very high in this test, which is performed with the patient in an upright position. The examiner performs the crank test by elevating the patient's arm 260° in the scapular plane and loading against the axis of the humerus with one hand, while externally and internally rotating the patient's other hand.

Load and Shift Test. This test allows the examination of any part of the labrum. The arm and elbow are abducted to 90°. The examiner places a thumb in the axilla and directs a force toward the area to be tested.

Rotator Cuff Injury

Supraspinatus Injury

Supraspinatus testing is done with the patient in the empty can position. (Fig. 39-18). With the palm parallel to the floor, the deltoid is tested. In the "empty can" position, there is lessening of the subacromial space and rotator cuff weakness is detectable. Neer, Welsh, and Hawkins popularized names for impingement signs in which the arm is placed into a hyperabducted forward elevated position, causing the supraspinatus to be "impinged" by the fixed bony acromion and coracoacromial ligament.[37,89] In the standing position, the arm is horizontally adducted and internally rotated (Fig. 39-19). If this reproduces pain, this indicates subacromial bursal and rotator cuff involvement. Pain can often radiate into the upper arm.[38] In the supine position, the rotator cuff and subacromial space can be palpated for crepitus, popping, and reproducible pain in internal and external rotation (Fig. 39-20). Differences in location in glenohumeral labral popping and subacromial location can be felt by an experienced examiner. The examiner should pick several of the impingement tests and become proficient at these, describing what test is being done, rather than just giving the name of the tests.

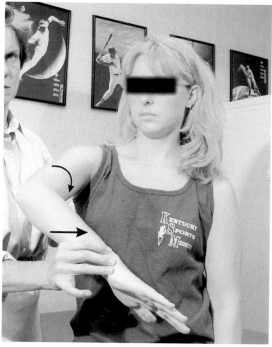

Figure 39-19. Impingement is tested for by horizontally adducting the shoulder and internally rotating the humerus. Reproduction of pain in the upper arm indicates subacromial rotator cuff involvement. (Copyright 2002, ML Ireland, MD.)

Subscapularis Injury

Tests for subscapularis function include internal rotation testing with arms behind the back or the lift-off test. The subscapularis can be palpated anteriorly and there can be pain over the subscapularis tendon when there is inflammation or a tear. There is usually no palpable deformity. The lift-off test is performed by asking the patient to put the back of her hand behind the low back and lift her hand away from the spine while the examiner pushes on the palm.[30] The patient will have pain and be unable to push her arm back. Burkhart described the Napoleon sign, in which the patient is asked to put her hand on her abdomen and push toward the abdomen. The arm should stay in a straight line. If it does not, this indicates subscapularis involvement.

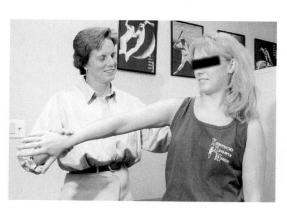

Figure 39-18. The rotator cuff is tested with the arm in slight horizontal adduction and a thumb-down position. Weakness and pain are consistent with rotator cuff dysfunction. (Copyright 2002, ML Ireland, MD.)

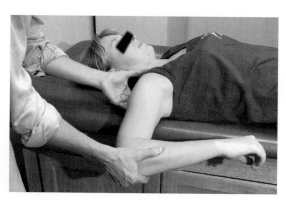

Figure 39-20. Palpating the subacromial space by internally rotating the humerus is done to distinguish primary rotator cuff involvement. Crepitus is often palpated in the subacromial space. (Copyright 2002, ML Ireland, MD.)

Biceps Tendon Injury

In the past, biceps tendinitis and instability were more often diagnosed. In overhead throwers, the biceps tendon is rarely involved by itself and is often associated with either an articular-sided supraspinatus disorder or a SLAP tear. In repetitive activities that involve elbow flexion, pronation, or supination, primary biceps problems can occur. Localized tenderness on palpation over the bicipital groove is seen. Feeling a "pop" and ecchymosis in an individual with an associated rotator cuff tear indicates a proximal biceps rupture.

In the Speed test, the patient resists forward elevation of the arm with the hand held in supination and the elbow extended.[31] In the Yergason test, the patient flexes the elbow to 90° and is instructed to supinate the forearm against resistance.[87] Yergason and Speed tests are positive if pain is felt over the biceps tendon proximally in the bicipital groove.

IMAGING

Roentgenography

Plain roentgenography provides important information in assessment of the injured shoulder. Referral to a standard atlas helps the x-ray technician to position the patient for the view desired.[57] Views must be obtained in the antroposterior and lateral directions. Failure to obtain adequate views in at least 2 planes may result in missed fractures or dislocations, partic-

ularly posterior lesions. Routine anteroposterior views are obtained in the plane of the thorax in internal rotation (Fig. 39-21).

The Stryker view (Fig. 39-22) was described by Hall and coworkers.[35] The axillary lateral view shows a notch in the posterolateral humeral head, known as a Hill–Sachs lesion (Figs. 39-23 and 39-24).

Standing outlet views also can be obtained (Fig. 39-25). The West Point view was described by Rokous and coworkers with the beam directed to view to anterior glenoid rim (Fig. 39–26 A,B).[69,70] A modified axillary lateral view with the arm in external rotation will distinguish a Hill–Sachs lesion, a posterolateral humeral head fracture, from anterior instability (Fig. 39-27). The patient depicted in Figure 39-28 with anterior instability had a normal axillary view, but the modified axillary view in external rotation revealed flattening of the humeral head, consistent with a Hill–Sachs lesion. The axillary lateral view on the left shows no Bankart lesion and a normal humeral head; in the externally rotated position, however, a Hill–Sachs lesion is revealed. A West Point view can also be obtained to show humeral head lesions.

Magnetic Resonance Imaging

Magnetic resonance imaging (MRI) gives the clinician another test to determine the correct diagnosis. Referral to an orthopaedic surgeon who treats many athletes with shoulder problems should be done prior to ordering an MRI scan. MRI performed at a facility where the

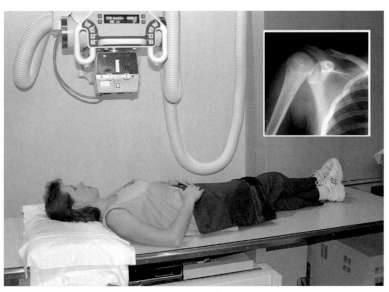

Figure 39-21. The position of the patient and normal roentgenographic findings are shown in the internal rotation anteroposterior view. (Copyright 2002, ML Ireland, MD.)

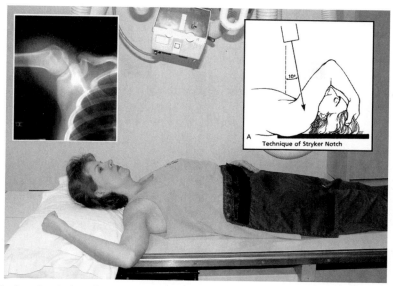

Figure 39-22. The Stryker view is described as 45° of abduction, as shown in the diagram. The modified Stryker view allows better roentgenographic imaging of the acromioclavicular joint and posterior glenoid. (Copyright 2002, ML Ireland, MD.)

quality is inferior and the reading radiologist cannot be contacted by the ordering physician is not of benefit. If the ordering physician cannot read the MRI scan, referral to a physician treating shoulder problems is appropriate. Intra-articular gadolinium-enhanced MRI gives more meaningful information if a labral tear is suspected.

A study comparing MRI and clinical examination found that physical examination is more accurate in predicting glenoid labrum tears than MRI.[53] The other conclusion was that in this era of cost containment, the diagnostic workup, without expensive ancillary services, allows the patient's care to proceed in the most timely and economical fashion. However, a letter to the editor regarding questions on the Liu study reported that reanalysis of MRI interpretation revealed discrepancies. The MRI studies were not blinded in scoring and the study was retrospective.[74] Vigorous review of any published article must be done by all interested readers.

Several studies have been performed comparing intra-articular injection, arthrography, and MRI to non-intra-articular MRI. A study from the Hospital for Special Surgery concluded that with appropriate pulse sequences, unenhanced (non-intra-articular injected) MRI of

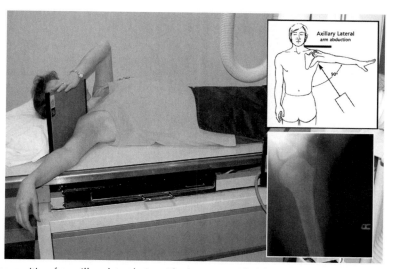

Figure 39-23. Supine position for axillary lateral view. The beam is angled from inferior to posterior and the arm is palm down, relatively internally rotated. (Copyright 2002, ML Ireland, MD.)

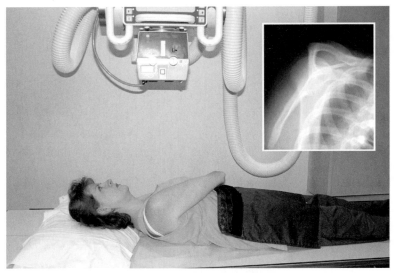

Figure 39-24. Supine outlet view position. The subacromial space and morphology of the acromion is well visualized. (Copyright 2002, ML Ireland.)

the shoulder is an accurate technique for detection and localization of labral injuries.[34]

In another study from the Hospital of Special Surgery of non-contrast-enhanced superior labral lesions, MRI, and arthroscopy, the conclusion was that high-resolution non-contrast-enhanced MRI can accurately diagnose superior labral lesions and aid in surgical management. MRI had a specificity of 89.5% and an accuracy of 95.7% in this study of 102 patients.[19]

In another study of 57 subjects, routine MRI provided the best results in rotator cuff tears as opposed to labral injuries. Three injury groups were compared: labral tears, rotator cuff disease, and other pathologic conditions. In a study conducted at the University of Calgary MR Center, MRI did not appear to be an accurate, effective tool for assessing shoulder pathologic conditions in which the clinical picture is not clear.[79] Comparing MRI and arthroscopic evaluation in the 11 labral tears identified by MRI, accuracy

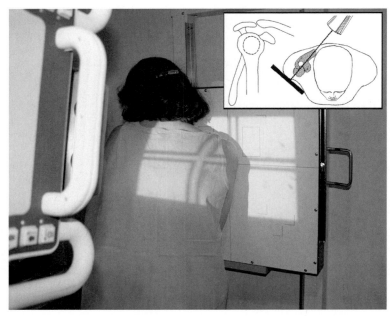

Figure 39-25. Standing outlet views can also be performed as shown by position and diagrammatically. (Copyright 2002, ML Ireland, MD.)

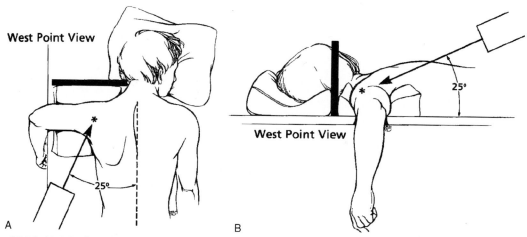

Figure 39-26. (A & B) The West Point view is obtained in the prone position, tangential, with the beam directed tangentially to the anterior inferior rim of the glenoid. Calcifications and Bankart lesions can best be seen in this view. (From Rokous FR, Feagin JA, Abbott HD: Modified axillary roentgenogram. Clin Orthop 82:84–6, 1972, with permission.)

was 62%, sensitivity 73%, and specificity 58%. In rotator cuff tears identified by MRI, accuracy was 68%, sensitivity 96%, and specificity 49%.

In another study correlating 88 patients, MRI, and arthroscopic surgery, MRI accurately predicted anterior labrum tears with a sensitivity of 96%, specificity of 86%, and accuracy of 92%. MRI was less predictive of tears of the superior labrum and was unreliable in the prediction of posterior or inferior labral tears.[51]

It is the authors' opinion that intra-articular gadolinium enhancement improves the accuracy and sensitivity of labral tears. In a study of 159 patients, 52 underwent arthroscopy after MRI arthrography. Arthrography was found to be a useful and accurate technique in the diagnosis of SLAP lesions, giving information regarding the exact location of the tear and the greater involvement of the biceps tendon.[11]

Computed Tomography

Computed tomography (CT) is still used by some to assess glenoid version and the labrum. However, the information obtained from MRI, which includes the rotator cuff, biceps, subscapularis, and capsule, makes the MRI superior to CT.

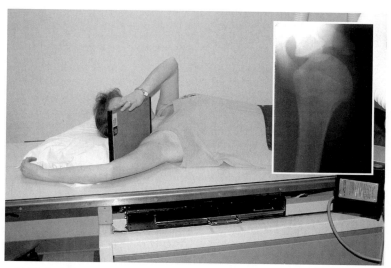

Figure 39-27. To reveal Hill–Sachs lesions, a modified axillary view is obtained with the arm in external rotation. Flattening of the posterior humeral head indicates anterior instability. (Copyright 2002, ML Ireland, MD.)

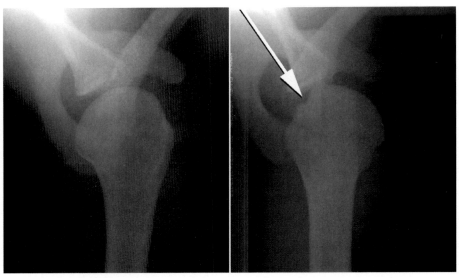

Figure 39-28. This football athlete with anterior instability had a normal axillary appearance on the left, but the external rotation view revealed humeral head flattening (arrow), consistent with a Hill–Sachs lesion. (Copyright 2002, ML Ireland, MD.)

EPIDEMIOLOGY

Injury rates are extremely difficult to calculate because of the many diagnoses recorded. For information that will assist in prevention, one must strive to make the primary diagnosis. The National Collegiate Athletic Association (NCAA) rates comparing genders for shoulder injury in 1999 to 2000 are shown in Table 39-3.[60] The categories are shoulder, clavicle, scapula, acromioclavicular joint separation, and other.

In sports that are comparable in competition, basketball and soccer, the rates for injuries to the clavicle, scapula, and acromioclavicular joint are extremely low but are greater in women than men. Classification of injuries is by body part: shoulder, clavicle, scapula, and acromioclavicular joint separation. The highest rate of shoulder injury is in men's football, 5.85, followed by wrestling, 5.51. However, in basketball, the injury rates are greater in the shoulder for women and men in practice and games. In soccer, the men and women's injury rates are the same in practice but greater in men and in games. Lacrosse has a greater injury rate of the shoulder in men compared to women.

Several series comparing gender and shoulder injury rates have been reported. In an epidemiologic survey of shoulder complaints in upper arm sports events, 372 athletes responded. In this survey, 35% (130) were female and 65% (242) were male.[54] Forty-four percent[163] in this survey had shoulder problems. The sport with the highest percentage of injury was volleyball, followed by swimming.

In a survey of recreational cyclists, the shoulder was more often injured in females compared to males. Neck injuries were also greater in females compared to males and occurred at the highest rate.[85]

In a study of alpine skiing, gender comparisons were made. Males were injured more often than females. In falls, the top 3 diagnoses were rotator cuff contusion, 24%, anterior glenohumeral dislocation, 22%, and acromioclavicular joint separation, 20%. Of the anterior glenohumeral dislocations, 61 of 85 (72%) were primary dislocations. Males were affected in 83.5% of injuries and females in 16.5%. Similar percentages were seen in acromioclavicular joint separations.[49]

DIFFERENTIAL DIAGNOSIS

The primary diagnosis in shoulder problems must be made. In the face of shoulder laxity in the female athlete, the incorrect diagnosis of subacromial impingement or rotator cuff dysfunction as the primary problem is often made. In the young athlete, repetitive movements that may cause humeral head subluxation and physiologic laxity predispose to a vicious cycle that results in rotator cuff dysfunction. Understanding the cascade of events that occur in swimming, gymnastics, cheerleading, and tennis is necessary in treating the athlete with shoulder problems (Fig. 39-29).

In a patient performing repetitive training activities, physiologic laxity can lead to micro-

Table 39-3. NCAA Injury Rates for Shoulders, 1999–2000

	SHOULDER		CLAVICLE		SCAPULA		AC SEPARATION		OTHER[a]	
	PRACTICES	GAMES	PRACTICES	GAMES	PRACTICES	GAMES	PRACTICES	GAMES	PRACTICES	GAMES
Gymnastics Women	0.30	0.48	0.00	0.00	0.00	0.00	0.00	0.00	0.05	0.00
Men	1.82	0.85	0.10	0.00	0.00	0.00	0.20	0.00	0.00	0.00
Basketball Women	0.14	0.41	0.00	0.03	0.00	0.00	0.00	0.07	0.08	0.07
Men	0.09	0.33	0.01	0.00	0.01	0.00	0.00	0.03	0.06	0.09
Soccer Women	0.09	0.40	0.01	0.11	0.00	0.00	0.00	0.07	0.15	0.26
Men	0.09	0.66	0.04	0.12	0.00	0.00	0.01	0.20	0.09	0.00
Lacrosse Women	0.16	0.47	0.00	0.00	0.00	0.00	0.03	0.00	0.03	0.00
Men	0.23	2.22	0.01	0.08	0.00	0.00	0.08	0.82	0.05	0.00
Field Hockey—Women	0.02	0.00	0.00	0.09	0.00	0.00	0.00	0.00	0.07	0.00
Volleyball—Women	0.55	0.51	0.00	0.00	0.00	0.00	0.01	0.00	0.06	0.00
Softball—Women	0.29	0.44	0.01	0.03	0.02	0.00	0.00	0.01	0.02	0.00
Spring Football—Men	1.13	0.00	0.16	0.00	0.04	0.00	0.15	0.00	0.08	0.00
Wrestling—Men	0.85	5.51	0.01	0.51	0.02	0.10	0.07	0.82	0.20	0.41
Football—Men	0.50	5.85	0.04	0.56	0.00	0.04	0.09	1.42	0.18	0.30
Ice Hockey—Men	0.22	2.28	0.05	0.75	0.00	0.14	0.04	1.40	0.06	0.14
Baseball—Men	0.39	0.81	0.00	0.02	0.00	0.01	0.01	0.00	0.01	0.01

All data are shown as rate per 1000 athletic exposures for 1999–2000.
[a]Other: Principal body part injured
From NCAA Injury Surveillance System, 1999–2000. Copyright 2002, ML Ireland, MD.

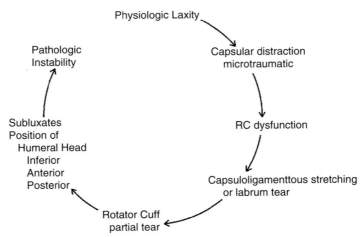

Figure 39-29. The vicious cycle in which physiologic laxity can lead to pathologic instability is shown schematically.

traumatic capsular distraction, as well as rotator cuff dysfunction and stretching of the capsule or labral tear. Because of these distraction forces and repetitive tensile forces on the rotator cuff, a partial articular-sided rotator cuff tear occurs. The humeral head can then become unstable in an anterior, posterior, or inferior direction, or in all 3 directions. As the activity continues, pathologic instability develops. The physician must decide the direction and degree of instability, and whether this instability is acute or chronic, and make a specific diagnosis. The TUBS pattern (*t*raumatic, *u*nidirectional, *B*ankart, *s*urgery) is the easiest instability pattern to treat, in that it is a one-event, one-direction problem that is treated with surgical repair of the injured structures. The AMBRI pattern (*a*traumatic, *m*ultidirectional, *b*ilateral *r*ehabilitation, *i*nferior capsule shift), seen commonly in the female athlete,[37] is a result of repetitive movements in a multidirectionally lax shoulder. Decisions for treatment and specific movements to avoid in rehabilitation are based on the severity and direction of the instability. To ensure all factors are included in the history and physical examination, the acronym MADAME (mechanism, acuteness, degree/directional, age, multiplicity, effort) should be kept in mind.

In the younger athlete, a capsuloligamentous or labral lesion is the most likely the primary diagnosis. Subsequently, rotator cuff involvement can occur. In middle-aged and older athletes, a rotator cuff injury is usually the primary problem. This injury can result from subacromial space compression from above with associated subacromial bursitis and impingement of the bony acromion, clavicle, and coracoacromial ligament. Impingement signs and a diagnostic injection into the sub-acromial space will help confirm the diagnosis of subacromial impingement. In the past, subacromial decompressions have been done very frequently. Now, with better understanding of the shoulder and the higher incidence of glenohumeral instability and labral pathology, there are fewer diagnoses of subacromial impingement and subsequently subacromial decompression is less common. Impingement syndrome should not be used as a diagnosis much like anterior knee pain should not be used. A specific diagnosis should be made. If there is rotator cuff strain or tendinitis tendinopathy, this should be listed as the diagnosis, not impingement syndrome.

In overhead throwing athletes, internal impingement has been reported.[45] Internal impingement is articular-sided rotator cuff involvement in an associated posterior superior glenoid labrum tear and is distinct from sub-acromial impingement[23] (Fig. 39-30). The cause of this lesion is thought to be excessive external rotation, but underlying instability has also been discussed.

INSTABILITY

The anatomic problem should be considered when performing a shoulder examination for instability (Table 39-4). If the humeral head translates at 90°, classic anterior inferior instability with involvement of the anterior inferior glenohumeral ligament is diagnosed. If there is inferior subluxation in adduction, the rotator cuff interval is the deficient structure. Translation at 45° involves the middle glenohumeral ligament. Posterior translation at 90° involves the posterior inferior glenohumeral lig-

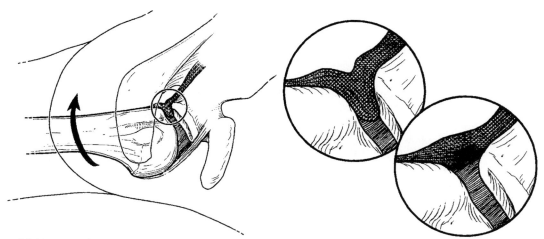

Figure 39-30. Internal impingement is defined as articular-sided infraspinatus and posterior superior labrum tear. The greater tuberosity impinges on the posterior superior aspect of the glenoid rim and labrum with the arm in abduction, external rotation, and extension. (From Edwards TB, Walch G: Posterosuperior glenoid impingement: Is microinstability really the problem? Operative Tech Sports Med 10(1):40–6, 2002, with permission.)

ament. Posterior translation at 45° involves the mid-posterior capsule.

LAXITY AND INSTABILITY

Laxity is the quality or condition of being lax or loose. *Instability* is defined as a lack of stability; it reflects the quality of unstableness, as in lack of firmness or steadiness.[84]

Operative management should be considered only when nonoperative measures have been exhausted. Numerous procedures, both open and arthroscopic, have been described for treatment of instability. Open techniques have been considered the "gold standard" and include capsulolabral reconstruction, subscapularis transfer, and coracoid transfer. Although successful in treating the instability, open procedures have a variable success rate in terms of return to

Table 39-4. Abnormal Shoulder Exam: Differential Diagnosis — Make the Primary Diagnosis

INVOLVED JOINT	DIAGNOSIS	PATHOMECHANICS	MOST COMMON SPORTS

Glenohumeral	Instability
	  Direction
	    Unidirectional
	    Multidirectional
		Contact
		Noncontact
			Collision—Football,
			Gymnastics, cheerleading,
			swimming

	Labral tear Articular side Rotator cuff tear	Distraction/compression Distraction	Throwing, weight lifting Throwing, baseball
Subacromial	Bursal-sided rotator Cuff involvement from bony impingement	Microtraumatic Compression	Tennis, golf
	Subacromial arch AC Joint Arthrosis/osteolysis	Compression	Weight lifting Older age
Acromioclavicular	Arthrosis	Macro and micro contact Loading	Weight lifting
	Instability, sprain	Macro contact	Rugby, ice hockey, equestrian
Scapulothoracic	Neurologic Long thoracic nerve involvement	Serratus anterior weakness	Baseball, archery
	Physiologic dysfunction	Underlying lack of strength	Swimming, tennis

previous level of sport participation in the throwing and overhead athlete. Many of the quoted studies on open procedures were performed decades ago and do not hold up to current peer review. Outcome shoulder measurement instruments continue to evolve. By today's standards, a surgical procedure is not considered successful if less than a perfectly functioning shoulder results. Arthroscopic procedures successfully repair the labrum and capsule. Advances in arthroscopy over the past 2 decades have allowed not only a better understanding of shoulder pathology, but also new and exciting treatment options. Appropriate patient selection (ie, making the correct diagnosis) and proper arthroscopic technique are crucial to achieve results equal or superior to those reported for open procedures.

The contraindications to arthroscopic reconstruction have decreased over the years as our understanding of anatomy and pathoanatomy has improved, through careful analysis of arthroscopically reconstructed failures. Structures that can be easily addressed arthroscopically include the anterior, posterior, and superior labrum, the capsule, the rotator interval, and the rotator cuff. Arthroscopic procedures allow for an anatomic reconstruction and have a lower morbidity, improved cosmesis, and increased postoperative range of motion. Current techniques can lead to success rates greater than 90°. The disadvantage is that arthroscopic reconstruction is technically demanding.

Open procedures are best able to address glenoid and humeral bone loss, version abnormalities, and the inability to achieve stability arthroscopically. Glenoid loss of greater than 20% to 25% has been described as having an inverted pear configuration by Burkhart.[13] With this degree of glenoid bone deficiency, recurrence rates of 67% have been seen, with an 87% recurrence rate in contact athletes. Significant glenoid bone loss requires an open procedure such as a coracoid (Latarjet) transfer to the anterior inferior glenoid to restore the glenohumeral arc of motion. Burkhart has also shown that when an engaging Hill–Sachs lesion is present, higher failure rates will occur.[13] The orientation of the Hill–Sachs lesion is viewed arthroscopically in 90° of abduction and external rotation. Lesions that are parallel to the anterior glenoid rim are defined as engaging. These lesions may be treated with a capsular shift procedure to restrict the humeral arc or by lengthening the glenoid arc by the Latarjet coracoid transfer. Typically more than 90% of open procedures are successful.

The goals of both open and arthroscopic procedure are uniform. Muscular injury is to be avoided during dissection and arthroscopic portal placement. The glenoid needs to be prepared down to a bleeding surface for labral repair. The labrum needs to be completely mobilized to allow for ligament tensioning. The labrum should be fixed to the rim of the glenoid. Capsular redundancy is eliminated. The rotator interval may require closing. Associated pathology is addressed. Appropriate rehabilitation is mandatory. An arthroscopic procedure is less painful and typically the patient feels ready to do more than the biology of healing will allow. The choice of an arthroscopic versus an open procedure is dependent on the skill of the surgeon and whether all pathology can be appropriately addressed.

BANKART LESIONS

Bankart lesions occur following an anterior shoulder dislocation.[7] The labrum and anterior inferior glenohumeral ligaments are avulsed, sometimes with a piece of glenoid. Bankart lesions are shown diagrammatically in Figure 39-31. The classic Bankart lesion is a labrum tear with periosteal rupture. A bony Bankart lesion is a piece of anterior inferior glenoid with labrum still attached. A Perthes lesion is stripping of the soft tissue of the anterior inferior glenohumeral ligament with labrum stripped away from the glenoid.[68] The anterior inferior glenohumeral ligament, inferior capsule, and posterior inferior glenohumeral ligament all sustain injury with an anterior glenohumeral dislocation. This complex can be likened to a hammock that should tighten up in external rotation. If there is an avulsion of the labrum and anterior inferior glenohumeral ligament or glenoid bone, as well as stretching of the capsule, recurrent dislocations and increasing instability will occur. The inherent instability and mismatch of the humeral head in the glenoid eventually makes the shoulder the most unstable joint in the body.

Cadaveric ligament sectioning studies have shown that an injury to the posterior inferior ligaments must also occur to allow dislocation. Anterior dislocation in teenagers and young adults has a high recurrence rate. More than 80% of athletes younger than 20 and 30% of nonathletes younger than 20 had a recurrent dislocation.[75] Baker and colleagues demonstrated that intra-articular pathology is common following shoulder dislocation, with labral

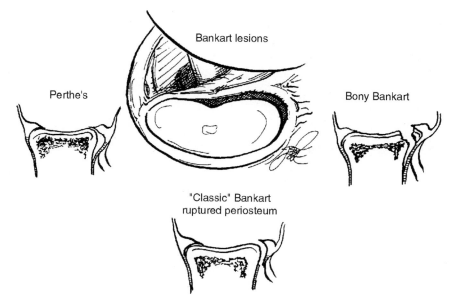

Figure 39-31. Glenoid lesions associated with anterior instability are shown and include Bankart lesion of ruptured periosteum, bony Bankart lesion, and Perthes lesion or soft-tissue stripping. (Courtesy of Stephen J. Snyder, MD.)

tears present in 39 of 45 first-time anterior dislocations.[6] Traditional treatment following a first-time dislocation was conservative with strengthening and protective bracing.[15] Because of the time lost from athletics and the high propensity of redislocation, a more aggressive approach has been observed.[2,21,48,50]

Arthroscopic treatment allows for identification of all intra-articular pathologies. If no significant glenoid bone deficiency exists and an engaging Hill–Sachs lesion is not encountered, arthroscopic stabilization is performed. The labrum and capsule need to be mobilized until the subscapularis is visualized. The capsuloligamentous structures are then advanced to the anatomic position on the glenoid rim. These structures should not be attached in a medial position on the glenoid neck. Associated capsular laxity may be suture plicated or a thermal capsulorrhaphy may be performed. Evaluation of the rotator interval should also be performed. Chondral injuries may be mechanically débrided to prevent mechanical symptoms.

ANTERIOR INSTABILITY

Traumatic unidirectional anterior instability is often a result of injury from contact/collision sports. The individual depicted in Figure 39-32 has a history of 50 dislocations with her arm in a position of external rotation and abduction. She can easily reduce the dislocations. Her examination is consistent with anterior instability with significant apprehension when her humerus is abducted, externally rotated, and backwardly flexed. The Stryker view (Fig. 39-32A) demonstrates radiolucency of the humeral head consistent with a Hill–Sachs lesion (posterolateral impaction fracture). The Axillary lateral view (Fig. 34-32B) shows a Bankart lesion with rounding off of the anterior glenoid. Arthroscopic findings confirm the roentgenographic findings. The Hill–Sachs lesion (Fig. 39-32C) indicates a compression fracture of the posterior lateral humeral head. The Bankart lesion of the anterior inferior glenoid labrum and the anterior inferior glenohumeral ligaments that were stripped off of the glenoid rim are shown in Figure 39-32D. Arthroscopic stabilization was performed using suture anchors to approximate the unstable soft tissues (Fig. 39-32E–G).

Open Bankart repair and capsular shift may be performed as well.[7] Postoperative rehabilitation is essential. Return to activity is allowed after approximately 4 months.

SLAP (SUPERIOR LABRUM ANTERIOR POSTERIOR) LESIONS

SLAP lesions occur commonly in the throwing athlete and were first classified by Snyder and coworkers.[76] The SLAP lesions have been classified as types I to IV. Fifty percent of the time SLAP lesions are associated with instability.

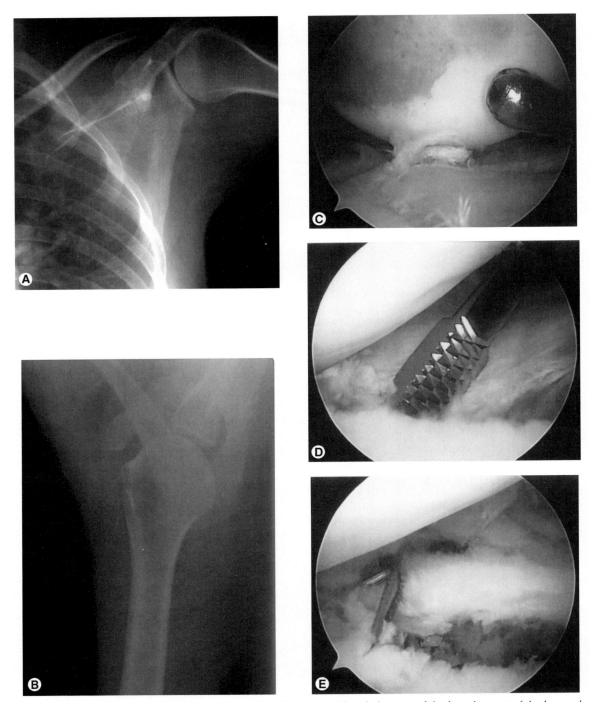

Figure 39-32. (A–G) The Stryker view suggests a Hill-Sachs lesion, with radiolucency of the lateral aspect of the humeral head. **(A)** Rounding-off of the glenoid anteriorly is consistent with recurrent anterior dislocation episodes and severe anterior instability. **(B)** Arthroscopic findings confirm the Hill–Sachs lesion **(C)** and Bankart lesion **(D)**. **(E)** next page.

Illustration continued on following page

Classic labral tear signs exist. Early intervention for SLAP lesions may prevent progression to more serious types. These lesions are most common in overhead throwers.[54] Softball pitchers do not develop SLAP lesions because this position involves underhand throwing. In the overhead/throwing athlete, SLAP lesions generally occur posteriorly (Snyder type II). The type II lesion has 3 subtypes: anterior, posterior, and anteroposterior.[58] Operative management needs to address the "peel-back" mechanism, which is caused by a torsional force transmitted through

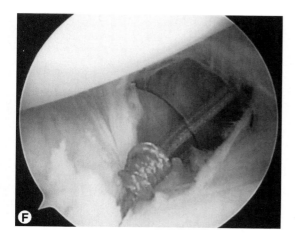

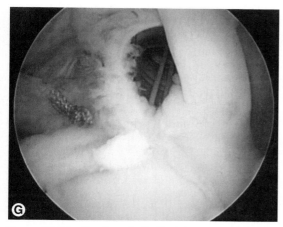

Figure 39-32. *(Continued).* **(E–G)** Arthroscopically aided stabilization was performed with suture anchors into the glenoid and passing them through the labrum. (Copyright 2002, ML Ireland, MD.)

the biceps tendon. This occurs as a result of an acquired tight posterior capsule increasing posterior superior forces of the humeral head on the glenoid labrum. The "peel-back" mechanism is dynamic and is visualized arthroscopically by abducting and externally rotating the arm. The labrum will be seen rotating medially over the glenoid. The criteria used in assessment of a posterior superior and combined SLAP lesion include (1) a positive "peel-back" sign; (2) a displaceable biceps root; (3) a positive "drive-through" sign; and (4) a superior sublabral sulcus greater than 5 mm. In an isolated anterior or superior lesion, the only positive finding may be the "drive-through" sign.[14]

Different implants have been developed to manage labral lesions, including suture anchors and translabral tacks. The objective is reattachment of the labrum to the glenoid. Suture anchors, while more technically demanding, have a higher reported success rate than translabral tacks. After preparing the superior glenoid down to bleeding bone with a motorized shaver, an anchor is placed directly inferior to the biceps root with a simple translabral suture loop placed directly posterior to the biceps root. Other suture anchors and suture loops are used as needed to repair the labrum and neutralize the "peel-back" mechanism and eliminate the "drive-through" sign.

Rehabilitation begins immediately with passive external rotation followed by progression to overhead motion and strengthening. Light throwing is begun 3 months post operatively and return to throwing at full speed from the mound is allowed at approximately 7 to 8 months.

POSTERIOR LABRAL TEARS

Posterior labral tears most often occur in football, hockey, and lacrosse athletes. Injury occurs with a posteriorly directed force to a shoulder prepared for collision and contact. The humeral head shears off the posterior central labrum and a posterior glenoid chondral lesion may occur. The lesion may also occur as a result of wear and tear of the posterior joint. Pain develops when the labrum detaches and is typically present with bench pressing, throwing, or posterior loading in sport participation. Conservative treatment can be successful and includes avoiding provocative activities. Physical therapy is usually not helpful. Surgery is considered with continued pain and difficulty with participation in the sport. The goals are the same as with other labral injuries. Repair of the torn posterior labrum to the glenoid can be addressed with either an open or an arthroscopic procedure. The advantages of arthroscopic repair are that a much bigger surgical dissection is avoided and the labrum is much better visualized arthroscopically. A postoperative rehabilitation program is initiated and return to contact athletics is possible at 4 months.

ACUTE POSTERIOR DISLOCATION

The high school junior depicted in Figure 39-33 dislocated her dominant shoulder throwing the discus. She released the discus as her arm went into adduction and internal rotation. Roentgenograms taken in the emergency department showed a posterior dislocation (Fig. 39-33A). The glenoid is shown by the arrows. Closed reduction was done. The patient was evaluated in the office and was found to

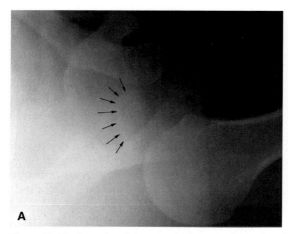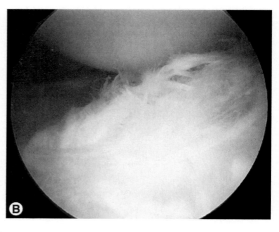

Figure 39-33. Posterior dislocation is shown radiographically. The arrows outline the glenoid and the humeral head is posteriorly dislocated. **(A)** Arthroscopic view of posterior labrum tear. **(B)** Patient underwent open anterior reconstruction.

have a greater posterior instability than the multidirectional laxity exhibited on the opposite side. Arthroscopy showed a posterior superior glenoid labrum tear, which was débrided (Fig. 39-33B). An open posterior capsular reconstruction was performed. She did not return to discus throwing but has had no subsequent posterior dislocations. Her main complaints now are of tightness and mild pain.

HABITUAL POSTERIOR INSTABILITY

The cheerleader and dance athlete depicted in Figure 39-34 is able to posteriorly dislocate her shoulder on command. When she puts her arm

in a horizontally adducted position and internally rotates, the humerus slips out posteriorly (Fig. 39-34A). Axillary lateral roentgenograms show a reverse (arrow) Hill–Sachs lesion with radiolucency of the anterior aspect of the humerus consistent with posterior instability (Fig. 39-34B). The patient was symptomatic on her right side and underwent arthroscopy and open posterior capsulorrhaphy. She has done well but has not had surgery on her opposite side.

The patient in Figure 39-35 dislocated her shoulder while playing volleyball at school. She underwent right open anterior reconstruction and was seen for problems of recurrent dislocation. Her examination was bilaterally symmetrical and revealed a multidirectional

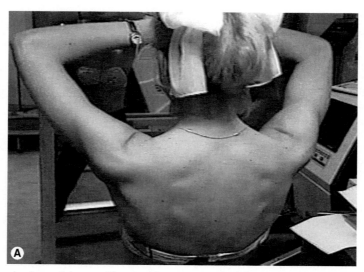

Figure 39-34. This cheerleader and dance athlete is able to posteriorly dislocate her shoulder on command. She puts her arm in a horizontally adducted position and internally rotates, and the humerus slips out posteriorly. Axillary lateral roentgenograms **(A)**

Illustration continued on following page

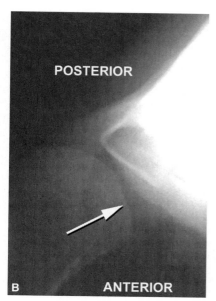

Figure 39-34 *(Continued).* show a reverse (arrow) with flattening and radiolucency of the humeral head **(B)**.

component to her instability. The position she rested her shoulders in caused the humeral head to be in an anterior inferior luxated position (Fig. 39-35A). Instructing her to sit up straight and essentially move the scapula underneath the humeral head resulted in improved glenohumeral coaptation (Fig. 39-35B). Significant widening of her surgical scar consistent with capsular looseness and elastin insufficiency may be noted. A strengthening program and counseling on her posture was begun. She was placed in a figure-of-8-splint. No surgery was suggested.

MULTIDIRECTIONAL INSTABILITY

The pathoanatomy of multidirectional instability is believed to be increased capsular volume as a result of redundancy of the inferior glenohumeral ligament complex.[8] Nonoperative treatment includes patient education, physical therapy for rotator cuff exercises, and more than 6 months of treatment prior to consideration of surgery. Nonoperative treatment has been shown to have an 80% satisfactory outcome. Surgery specifically addresses the tightening of loose ligaments through labral repair (if needed) and ligament plication. The rotator interval may require closing. If the surgeon chooses to address these patients with an open procedure, diagnostic arthroscopy is recommended to identify all pathology. Arthroscopic treatment of capsular redundancy and rotator interval defects

by laser shrinkage is as effective as open procedures.[88] The internal may require plication.

Multidirectional instability can also be addressed by an open inferior capsular shift. The rotator interval is closed and the capsule is then split in a T fashion from the glenoid or humeral side. The capsule is released both inferiorly and posteriorly and is then advanced and closed.

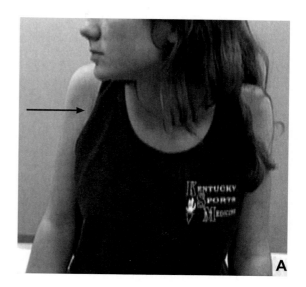

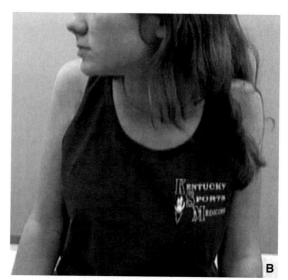

Figure 39-35. This patient dislocated her shoulder while playing volleyball at school. She underwent right open anterior reconstruction and was seen for problems of recurrent dislocation. Her examination was bilaterally symmetrical, showing a multidirectional component to her instability. The position she rested her shoulders in caused the humeral head to be in an anterior inferior luxated position. **(A)** The instructions to sit up straight and essentially move the scapula underneath the humeral head resulted in improved glenohumeral coaptation. **(B)** Note the significant widening of her surgical scar, which is consistent with capsular looseness and elastin insufficiency.

This procedure has been reported as 86% successful at 2 years.[20, 63]

THERMAL CAPSULORRHAPHY

The use of heat to treat shoulder instabilities is an old concept. Hippocrates treated recurrent shoulder dislocations with a hot probe in the axilla.[72] Heating of the capsular tissue of the shoulder has been performed with laser and radiofrequency probes. Radiofrequency probes are more commonly used today because of their lower cost, greater safety, and ability to provide temperature feedback. The pattern used in shrinkage is a grid, leaving a normal strip of tissue and a thermally modified strip of tissue.[55] Thermal energy applied to the shoulder capsule causes the highly ordered structure of collagen to break down and shrink, denaturing its type I collagen. Differences in the composition of collagen elastin fibers have been found in studies comparing stable and unstable shoulders.[73] In unidirectional and multidirectional instability, larger collagen fibril diameters and a greater proportion of cystine and elastin form a more stable collagen cross-link.

Histologic evaluation of the capsule after laser treatment shows collagen without its distinctive fiber structure and fusion of its bundles. There is cell death of the synoviocytes, fibroblasts, smooth muscles cells, and endothelial cells. Repair of these tissues becomes evident at 3 months.[40]

Initial improved stability from thermal capsulorrhaphy is thought to be due to capsular thickening, scar formation, and reduction in afferent sensory stimulation to reduce painful stimuli. These factors contribute to improved stability, strength, and function.[25,26,78,80]

There have been reports of adhesive capsulitis and arthrofibrosis and restricted range of motion following thermal modification. Other complications are injury to the axillary nerve by the transmission of heat.[80] Fortunately, this is usually temporary. Capsular necrosis may also occur. With the tissue necrosis that occurs after thermal modification prior to its remodeling, the timing of movement and return to sport is critical. Immobilization typically is done for 3 weeks, followed by a range of motion program to regain external rotation, with eventual return to full activities, at the earliest, after 4 months. An accelerated and basic rehabilitation program in overhead athletes has been reported by Wilk.[86] There is concern that return to sport too rapidly will result in initial cellular death and weakening of the capsule.

Use of thermal modification in the female athlete is of concern. The principles of stabilizing deficient structures anteriorly with arthroscopic or open repair are much more sound than those of thermal modification. In the authors' practice, use of thermal modification of the shoulder is rarely done. Many collegiate softball and volleyball athletes have had thermal modification. There are no long-term studies of the performance of these individuals. The significant potential complications of capsular necrosis, axillary nerve injury, and continued instability are of enough concern to cause reconsideration of thermal's use.

ROTATOR CUFF TEARS: CLASSIFICATION AND MANAGEMENT

The rotator cuff acts as a fine tuner of the shoulder to keep the humeral head seated in the glenoid throughout its multiple positions. The rotator cuff can be inflamed, partially torn, or completely torn. In the unstable shoulder, the rotator cuff is weak, but this is secondary to the instability. The rotator cuff can be involved on the subacromial side or the articular side. The diagnosis should describe the pathologic change in the involved structure. This allows better communication among the patient, therapist, and physician. The symptoms of the complete rotator cuff tear include night pain and weakness in external rotation and abduction. Oftentimes, there is a palpable defect in the rotator cuff or associated proximal biceps tendon rupture. The typical location of the tear is in the supraspinatus. The subscapularis—the only internal rotator of the rotator cuff—should be examined, whether involved with an isolated tear or biceps tendon instability.

Plain roentgenograms often show osteopenia and proximal migration of the humeral head. In chronic rotator cuff tears, there often is arthropathy with significant spurring and an abnormal shape to the humeral head. Further diagnostic imaging to document rotator cuff tear is indicated if the patient desires surgery. Arthrography is inexpensive and remains a good test to document a complete rotator cuff tear. MRI can be helpful to document the injury as partial versus complete, as well as to determine the size of the rotator cuff tear and the degree of its retraction. In some centers, ultrasonography is utilized to diagnose rotator cuff tear.

The primary indication for surgical intervention remains night pain, but with advances in arthroscopic techniques, more rotator cuff surgeries are being performed. In rotator cuff tear patients who do not desire surgery, range of motion exercises should be performed in a functional arc of less than 90° to maintain scapulothoracic control and improve rotator cuff strength. Injection with steroid and anesthetic can help control night pain. Injection is done posteriorly into the subacromial space, but in a complete rotator cuff tear, this would also involve the glenohumeral articulation.

Open repair of the rotator cuff was reported by Codman in 1911.[17,18] Neer's results reported in 1972 showed improvement of results with the addition of anterior acromioplasty.[61] Advances in arthroscopic techniques have allowed rotator cuff repairs to be done entirely through the scope or in a mini-open fashion. These procedures do not require an approach that detaches the deltoid origin. This has greatly improved the functional outcome of this procedure, but not the timing of return to activity.

Studies comparing open versus arthroscopically aided rotator cuff repair have reported equal results.[5,83] The return to full activities following rotator cuff surgery is not influenced by the choice of technique. The injured cuff must heal back to the greater tuberosity in order to provide adequate function. Postoperatively, the time to return to a sport like golf is 6 months and to throwing sports 9 months, maybe never.

Classification of rotator cuff tears is by the pattern of the tear: transverse, crescent, L-shaped, linear in line with the fibers, and triangular (Fig. 39-36). The tear pattern is assessed and sutures are placed through the tendon. More than likely, anchors are placed in the greater tuberosity to bring the rotator cuff back down to its insertions. In explaining the rotator cuff tear to patients, one can describe the analogy of a window shade that should be all the way down to the sill but has now retracted, because the origin of the supraspinatus is still in place. This can be helpful in the process of discussing treatment options also. A massive rotator cuff tear (Fig. 39-37) with significant retraction of the supraspinatus, involvement of the biceps tendon with partial or complete rupture, and involvement of the subscapularis can be encountered. Primary repair may not be possible in these chronic situations. Tenderness over the acromioclavicular joint results from sprain, osteolysis, or arthrosis. In the chronically painful acromioclavicular joint, injection is diagnostic and therapeutic. Osteolysis (weightlifter's shoulder) is more common in males.

ADHESIVE CAPSULITIS

Adhesive capsulitis is seen more often in females than males. This diagnosis is most common in the perimenopausal female and can be associated with systemic conditions such as diabetes. The mainstay of treatment is aggressive physical therapy, emphasizing passive rotation and abduction. An early intra-articular injection with

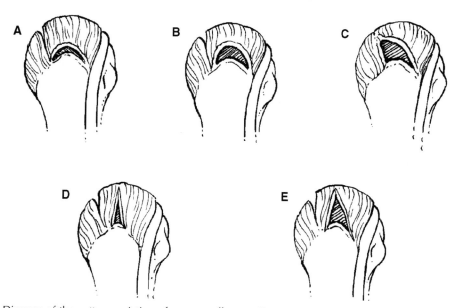

Figure 39-36. Diagram of the pattern variation of rotator cuff tears. **(A)** Transverse-shaped tear. **(B)** Crescent-shaped tear. **(C)** L-shaped tear. **(D)** Linear tear in line with the tendon fibers. **(E)** Triangular tear. (From Jobe FW: Operative Techniques in Upper Extremity Sports Injuries. St Louis, CV Mosby, 1996, p 225, with permission.)

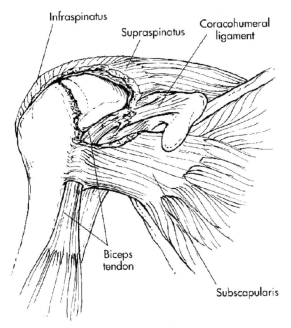

Figure 39-37. A massive rotator cuff tear involving the subscapularis, supraspinatus, and infraspinatus muscle tendons. There is retraction of the supraspinatus tendon, subluxation of the biceps tendon, and contraction of the coracohumeral ligament. (From Jobe FW: Operative Techniques in Upper Extremity Sports Injuries. St Louis, CV Mosby, 1996, p 228, with permission.)

anesthetic and steroids is diagnostic and therapeutic.

The adhesive capsulitis process may take a year to run its course. Typically patients respond to a therapy regimen and surgery is infrequently indicated.

FRACTURES

Gender comparisons are not usually made in fracture series. Regardless of gender, fracture management is similar.

The cheerleader depicted in Figure 39-38 was doing gymnastics in a parking lot and landed awkwardly on her left upper extremity. She was unable to move her shoulder. Roentgenograms revealed a displaced Salter II fracture of the proximal humerus (Fig. 39-38A). Closed reduction and percutaneous pinning was performed (Fig. 39-38B). The patient did well and pins were removed 6 weeks postoperatively. She was able to return to gymnastics and cheerleading. Remodeling of the proximal humeral epiphysis allows acceptance of a large amount of deformity. Because of the significant displacement and acute deformity in this situation, closed reduction was performed.

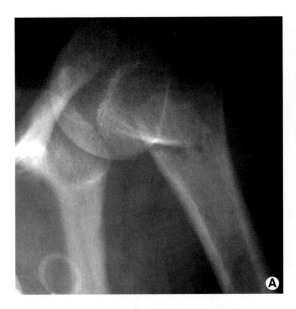

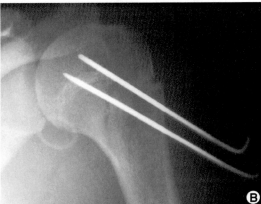

Figure 39-38. (A) Roentgenography revealed a displaced Salter II fracture of the proximal humerus. (B) Closed reduction and percutaneous pinning was performed. (Copyright 2002, ML Ireland, MD.)

The diver depicted in Figure 39-39 sustained a clavicle fracture when she was involved in a motor vehicle accident and struck the dashboard. This high-energy trauma resulted in a displaced mid-third clavicle fracture (Fig. 39-39A). After initial figure-of-8 splinting and use of a sling, there was no evidence of healing at 6 months following her injury (Fig. 39-39B). Her physical examination at the time of open reduction and internal fixation and iliac crest bone grafting showed gross movement at the fracture site (Fig. 39-39C). A plate was used and autogenous iliac crest bone grafting was performed (Fig. 39-39D). The plate was removed 18 months postoperatively. Follow-up roentgenograms revealed clavicular union and filling in of the screw holes (Fig. 39-39E).

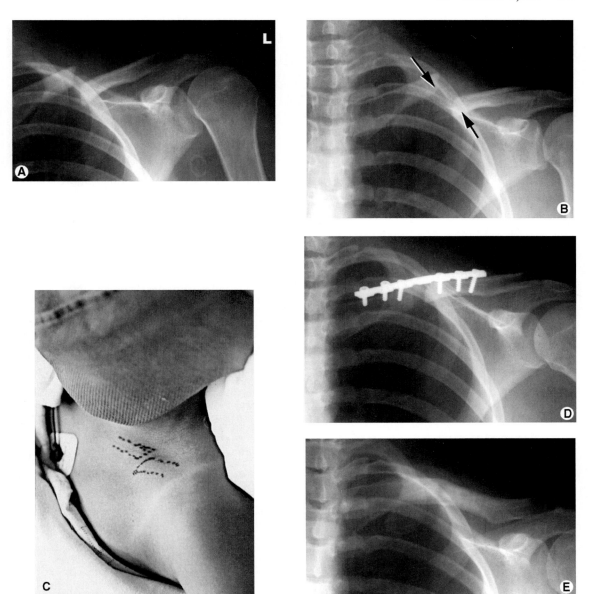

Figure 39-39. This diver sustained a clavicle fracture when she was involved in a motor vehicle accident and struck the dashboard. **(A)** This high-energy trauma resulted in a displaced mid-third clavicle fracture. **(B)** After initial figure-of-8 splinting and use of a sling, there was no evidence of healing (arrows) at 6 months following her injury. **(C)** At the time of surgery, physical exam showed gross motion at the nonunion site. **(D)** Plate was used and autogenous iliac crest bone grafting performed. **(E)** Plate was removed after 18 months and follow-up roentgenograms revealed clavicular union and filling in of the screw holes. (Copyright 2002, ML Ireland, MD.)

CONCLUDING REMARKS

Understanding the functional anatomy and biomechanics of the sport will allow the practitioner to make the correct primary diagnosis. (Is the diagnosis a primary instability or a labrum or rotator cuff tear?) Making every effort to determine the primary diagnosis will allow for implementation of the correct treatment and rehabilitation program with possible surgery. The advances in arthroscopy for diagnosis and

treatment of shoulder disorders are quite exciting. Earlier surgical intervention is occurring more frequently today. The arthroscopic treatment of anterior stabilization or rotator cuff repair does not allow for an earlier return to sports as compared to the open techniques. The principles of repairing injured structures based on arthroscopic findings has allowed improved function of the shoulder postoperatively. In treating athletes with shoulder problems, one must be aware of the advances that have been made in rehabilitation after arthroscopic techniques. We should also be wary of newer and often unfounded basic science techniques such as thermal capsular modification. The health care provider must be aware of the advances that allow for predictable return to activity with a consideration of the demands placed on the patient's shoulder while performing sports.

References

1. Andrews JR, Zarins B, Wilk KE: Injuries in Baseball. Philadelphia, Lippincott-Raven, 1998.
2. Arciero R, Wheeler J, Ryan J, McBride J: Arthroscopic Bankart repair vs. nonoperative treatment for acute, initial anterior dislocation of the shoulder. Am J Sports Med 22:589–94, 1994.
3. Bak K, Fauno P: Clinical findings in competitive swimmers with shoulder pain. Am J Sports Med 25(2):254–60, 1997.
4. Baker CL: The Hughston Clinic: Sports Medicine Book. Baltimore, Williams & Wilkins, 1995.
5. Baker CL, Liu SH: Comparison of open and arthroscopically assisted rotator cuff repairs. Am J Sports Med 23:99–104, 1995.
6. Baker CL, Uribe JW, Whitman C: Arthroscopic evaluation of acute initial anterior shoulder dislocation. Am J Sports Med 18:25–8, 1990.
7. Bankart A: The pathology and treatment of recurrent dislocation of the shoulder joint. Br J Surg 26:23–9, 1938.
8. Beasley L, Faryniarz DA, Hannafin JA: Multidirectional instability of the shoulder in the female athlete. Clin Sports Med 19(2):331–49, 2000.
9. Beighton PH, Horan FT: Dominant inheritance in familial generalized articular hypermobility. J Bone Joint Surg 52B:145, 1970.
10. Beltran J, Rosenberg ZS, Chandnani VP, et al: Glenohumeral instability: Evaluation with MR arthrography. Radiographics 17(3):657–73, 1997.
11. Bencardino JT, Beltran J, Rosenberg ZS, et al: Superior labrum anterior-posterior lesions: diagnosis with MR arthrography of the shoulder. Radiology 214(1):267–71, 2000.
12. Boublik M, Hawkins RJ. Clinical examination of the shoulder complex. J Orthop Sports Phys Ther 18(1)379–85, 1993.
13. Burkhart SS, DeBeer JF: Traumatic glenohumeral bone defects and their relationship to failure of arthroscopic Bankart repairs: Significance of the inverted-pear glenoid and the humeral engaging Hill–Sachs lesions. Arthroscopy 16(7):677–94, 2000.
14. Burkhart SS, Morgan CD: The peel-back mechanism: its role in producing and extending posterior type II SLAP lesions and its effect on SLAP repair rehabilitation. Arthroscopy 14:637–40, 1998.
15. Burkhead WJ, Rockwood CH: Treatment of instability of the shoulder with an exercise program. J Bone Joint Surg 74A:890–6, 1992.
16. Carter C, Sweetnam R: Recurrent dislocation of the patella and of the shoulder: Their association with familial joint laxity. J Bone Joint Surg 42B:721, 1960.
17. Codman EA: The Shoulder: Rupture of the Supraspinatus Tendon and Other Lesions In or About the Subacromial Bursa. Boston, Thomas Todd, 1934.
18. Codman EA: Complete rupture of the supraspinatus tendon. Operative treatment with report of two successful cases. Boston Med Surg J 164:708–10, 1911.
19. Connell DA, Potter HG, Wickiewicz TL, et al. Noncontrast magnetic resonance imaging of superior labral lesions. Am J Sports Med 27(2):208–13, 1999.
20. Cooper RA, Brems JJ: The inferior capsular shift procedure for multidirectional instability of the shoulder. J Bone Joint Surg 74A(suppl):1516–21, 1992.
21. DeBerardino TM, Arciero RA, Taylor DC, Uhorchak JM: Prospective evaluation of arthroscopic stabilization of acute, initial anterior shoulder dislocations in young athletes: Two- to five-year followup. Am J Sports Med 29(5):586–92, 2001.
22. DeLee JC, Drez D: Orthopaedic Sports Medicine, Vol. 1. Philadelphia, WB Saunders, 1994.
23. Edwards TB, Walch G: Posterosuperior glenoid impingement: Is microinstability really the problem? Operative Tech Sports Med 10(1):40–6, 2002.
24. Emery RJH, Mullah AB: Glenohumeral joint instability in normal adolescents: Incidence and significance. J Bone Joint Surg 73B(3):406–8, 1991.
25. Fanton GS: Arthroscopic electrothermal surgery of the shoulder. Operative Tech Sports Med 6:139–46, 1998.
26. Fanton GS, Wall MS, Markel MD: Electrothermally assisted capsule shift (ETAC) procedure for shoulder instability. In: The Science and Applications of Electro thermal Arthroscopy. Menlo Park, Calif, Oratec Interventions, 1998.
27. Field LD, Warren RF, O'Brien SJ, et al: Isolated closure of rotator interval defects for shoulder instability. Am J Sports Med 23(5):557–63, 1995.
28. Finsterbush A, Pogrund H: The hypermobility syndrome: Musculoskeletal complaints in 100 consecutive cases of generalized joint hypermobility. Clin Orthop Rel Res 168:124–7, 1982.
29. Fu FH, Stone DA: Sports Injuries: Mechanisms, Prevention, Treatment. Philadelphia, Lippincott Williams & Wilkins, 2001.
30. Gerber C, Krushell RJ: Isolated rupture of the tendon of the subscapularis muscle. Clinical features in 16 cases. J Bone Joint Surg 73B:389–94, 1991.
31. Gilcreest E, Albi P: Unusual lesions of muscles and tendons of the shoulder girdle and upper arm. Surg Gynecol Obstet 68:903–17, 1939.
32. Gillogly SD, Andrews JR: History and physical examination of the throwing shoulder. In: Andrews JR, Zarin B: Injuries in Baseball. Philadelphia, Lippincott-Raven, 1998, pp 57–74.
33. Guanche CA: Arthroscopic shoulder stabilization. Operative Tech Sports Med 10(1):18–24, 2002.
34. Gusmer PB, Potter HG, Schatz JA, et al: Labral injuries: Accuracy of detection with unenhanced MR imaging of the shoulder. Radiology 200(2):519–24, 1996.
35. Hall RH, Isaac F, Booth CR: Dislocations of the shoulder with special reference to accompanying small fractures. J Bone Joint Surg 41A(3):489–94, 1959.
36. Harryman DT, Sidler JA, Harris SL, Matsen FA: The role of rotator interval capsule in passive motion and stability of the shoulder. J Bone Joint Surg 74A(1):53–66, 1992.
37. Hawkins RJ, Bokor DJ: Clinical evaluation of shoulder problems. In: Rockwood CA, Matsen FA (eds): The Shoulder, Vol. 1. Philadelphia, WB Saunders, 1990, pp 149–77.
38. Hawkins RJ, Hobeika P: Physical examination of the shoulder. Orthopaedics 6(10):1270–8, 1983.
39. Hawkins RJ, Kennedy JC: Impingement syndrome in athletes. Am J Sports Med 8:151–8, 1980.
40. Hayashi K, Massa D, Thabit G III, et al: Histologic evaluation of the glenohumeral joint capsule after the

laser-assisted capsular shift procedure for glenohumeral instability. Am J Sports Med 27:162–7, 1999.

41. Hollinshead WH: Anatomy for Surgeons, Vol. 3. New York, Harper & Row, 1969.

42. Hollinshead WH, Jenkins DB: Functional Anatomy of the Limbs and Back. Philadelphia, WB Saunders, 1981.

43. Ireland ML, Ahuja GS: Physical examination of the painful shoulder. J Musculoskel Med 181–99, 1999.

44. Jobe CM: Gross anatomy of the shoulder. In: Rockwood CA, Matsen FA (eds): The Shoulder. Philadelphia, WB Saunders, 1990, 34–97.

45. Jobe CM, Sidles J: Evidence for a superior glenoid impingement upon the rotator cuff. J Shoulder Elbow Surg 2:S19, 1993.

46. Jobe FW, Bradley JP: Rotator cuff injuries in baseball. Prevention and rehabilitation. Sports Med 6:378–87, 1988.

47. Kibler WB: Specificity and sensitivity of the anterior glide test in throwing athletes with superior glenoid labral tears. Arthroscopy 11:296–300, 1995.

48. Kirkley A, Griffin S, Richards C, et al: Prospective randomized clinical trial comparing the effectiveness of immediate arthroscopic stabilization versus immobilization and rehabilitation in first traumatic anterior dislocations of the shoulder. Arthroscopy 15(5):507–14, 1999.

49. Kocher MS, Feagin JAJ: Shoulder injuries during alpine skiing. Am J Sports Med 24(5):665–9, 1996.

50. Larrain MV, Botto GJ, Montenegro HJ, Mauas DM: Arthroscopic repair of acute traumatic anterior shoulder dislocation in young athletes. Arthroscopy 17(4):373–7, 2001.

51. Legan JM, Burkhard TK, Goff WB, et al: Tears of the glenoid labrum: MR imaging of 88 arthroscopically confirmed cases. Radiology 179:241–6, 1991.

52. Liu SH, Henry MH, Nuccion SL: A prospective evaluation of a new physical examination in predicting glenoid labral tears. Am J Sports Med 24(6):721–5, 1996.

53. Liu SH, Henry MH, Nuccion S, Shapiro MS: Diagnosis of glenoid labral tears: A comparison between magnetic resonance imaging and clinical examinations. Am J Sports Med 24(2):149–54, 1996.

54. Lo YPC, Hsu YCS, Chan KM: Epidemiology of shoulder impingement in upper arm sports events. Br J Sports Med 24(3):173–7, 1990.

55. Lu Y, Hayashi K, Edward RB, et al: The effect of monopolar radiofrequency treatment pattern on joint capsular healing: In vitro and in vivo studies using an ovine model. Am J Sports Med 28:711–9, 2000.

56. McMaster WC, Roberts A, Stoddard T: A correlation between shoulder laxity and interfering pain in competitive swimmers. Am J Sports Med 26(1):83–6, 1998.

57. Merrill V: Roentgenographic Positions and Standard Radiologic Procedures. St Louis, CV Mosby, 1975.

58. Morgan CD, Burkhart SS, Palmeri M, Gillespie M: Type II SLAP Lesions: Three subtypes and their relationship to superior instability and rotator cuff tears. Arthroscopy 14:553–65, 1998.

59. Mortensen OA, Wiedenbauer M: An electromyographic study of the trapezius muscle. Anat Rec 112:366–7, 1952.

60. National Collegiate Athletic Association: NCAA Injury Surveillance System. NCAA, Indianapolis, Ind, 1999–2000.

61. Neer CS II: Anterior acromioplasty for the chronic impingement syndrome in the shoulder: a preliminary report. J Bone Joint Surg 54A:41–50, 1972.

62. Neer CS II: Impingement lesions. Clin Orthop 173:70–7, 1983.

63. Neer CS II, Foster CR: Inferior capsular shift for involuntary inferior and multidirectional instability of the shoulder: A preliminary report. J Bone Joint Surg 62A:897–908, 1980.

64. Nuber GW, Jobe FW, Perry J, et al: Fine wire electromyographic study of the trapezius muscle (abstr) Anat Rec 112:366–7, 1952.

65. O'Brien SJ, et al: A new effective test for diagnosing labral tears and acromioclavicular joint pathology. Paper presented at the annual American Shoulder and Elbow Surgeons Meeting. Atlanta, Ga, 1996.

66. O'Brien SJ, Pagnani MJ, Fealy S, et al: The active compression test: A new and effective test for diagnosing labral tears and acromioclavicular joint abnormality. Am J Sports Med 26(5):610–3, 1998.

67. Perry J: Biomechanics of the shoulder. In: Rowe C (ed): The Shoulder. New York, Churchill Livingstone, 1998.

68. Perthes G: Uber Operationen bei Habitueller Schulterlxation. Deutsch Ztschr Chir 85:199–227, 1906.

69. Rokous FR, Feagin JA, Abbott HD: Modified axillary roentgenogram. Clin Orthop 82:84–6, 1972.

70. Rockwood CA, Matsen FA III (eds): The Shoulder, Vol 1. Philadelphia, WB Saunders, 1990.

71. Rockwood CA, Matsen FA III (eds): The shoulder, Vol 2. Philadelphia, WB Saunders, 1990.

72. Rockwood CA Jr, Wirth MA: Subluxations and dislocations about the glenohumeral joint. In: Rockwood CA, Green DP, Bucholtz RW, Heckman JD (eds): Rockwood and Green's Fractures in Adults, 4th edition, Philadelphia, Lippincott-Raven, 1996, p. 194.

73. Rodeo S, Suzuki K, Yamauchi M, et al: Analysis of collagen and elastic fibers in shoulder capsule in patients with shoulder instability. Am J Sports Med 26:634–43, 1998.

74. Seeger LL, Yao L, Gold RH: Letters to the editor. Am J Sports Med 25(1):141–4, 1997.

75. Simonet WT, Cofield RH: Prognosis in anterior shoulder dislocation. Am J Sports Med 12(1):1984.

76. Snyder SJ, Karzel RP, Delpizzo W, et al: SLAP lesions of the shoulder. Arthroscopy 6:274–9, 1990.

77. Speer KP, Hannafin JA, Altcheck DW, et al: An evaluation of the shoulder relocation test. Am J Sports Med 22:177–83, 1994.

78. Thabit G: The arthroscopically assisted holmium: YAG laser surgery in the shoulder. Operative Tech Sports Med 6:131–8, 1998.

79. Torstensen ET, Hollinshead RM: Comparison of magnetic resonance imaging and arthroscopy in the evaluation of shoulder pathology. J Shoulder Elbow Surg 8(1):42–5, 1999.

80. Vangsness CT Jr, Ennis M, Taylor JG, Atkinson R: Neural anatomy of the glenohumeral ligaments, labrum and subacromial bursa. Arthroscopy 11:180–4, 1995.

81. Veliskakis KP: Increased generalized ligamentous laxity in idiopathic scoliosis. J Bone Joint Surg 55A:435, 1973.

82. Warner JJP, Micheli LJ, Arslanian LE, et al: Patterns of flexibility, laxity, and strength in normal shoulders and shoulder with instability, and impingement. Am J Sports Med 18(4):366–75, 1990.

83. Weber SC, Schaefer R: "Mini-open" versus traditional open repair in the management of small and moderate size tears of the rotator cuff. Arthroscopy 9:365–6, 1993.

84. Webster's New World Dictionary, Third College Edition. Cleveland, Simon & Schuster, 1988.

85. Wilber CA, Holland GJ, Madison RE, Loy SF: An epidemiological analysis of overuse injuries among recreational cyclists. Int J Sports Med 16:201–6, 1995.

86. Wilk KE: Rehabilitation after shoulder stabilization surgery. In Warren RF, Craig EV, Altchek DW (eds): The Unstable Shoulder. Philadelphia, Lippincott-Raven, pp. 367–402, 1999.

87. Yergason RM: Rupture of biceps. J Bone Joint Surg 13:160, 1931.

88. Lyons TR, Griffith PL, Savoie FH III, Field LD: Laser-assisted capsulorrhaphy for multidirectional instability of the shoulder. Arthroscopy 17(1):25–30, 2001.

89. Neer CS II, Welsh RP: The shoulder in sports. Orthop Clin North Am 8:583–91, 1977.

Chapter 40

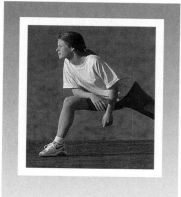

Elbow Injuries

James R. Andrews, M.D.
James A. Whiteside, M.D.

The elbow of the female athlete has not received the attention given the shoulder and knee, but without the elbow's controlled kinetic chain action to complement and augment upper extremity performance, athletic activities that require elbow flexion and extension would be significantly restricted. A thorough understanding of the sports-related biomechanical, strength, and structural variations of the elbow of the female athlete is essential to the diagnosis and treatment of elbow injuries.

ANATOMY

The elbow joint allows movement in one plane only: flexion and extension. In athletic motions valgus deviation occurs. Figure 40-1 shows anterior and medial views of the elbow.

The elbow is composed of the humeroradial, humeroulnar, and proximal radioulnar joints.

The capitellum of the humerus lies laterally and the trochlea lies centrally and medially.[10] The proximal ulna articulates with the trochlea by

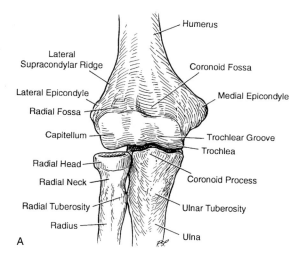

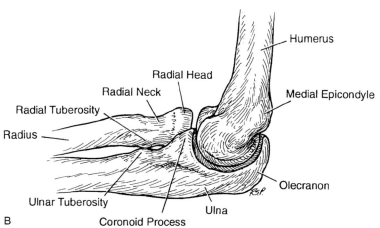

Figure 40-1. Bony configuration of the elbow is shown anterior to the articulations. Radial–ulnar, radial–humeral, and proximal radial–ulnar joints are shown anteriorly **(A)** and medially from the side **(B)**. The coronoid fossa and olecranon fossa allow for bony contact in flexion and extension. The smooth articulation of the distal humerus, capitellum, and spool-like trochlea, radial head, and proximal ulna are necessary for normal function and range of motion of the elbow. The distal humerus is shown anteriorly with the capitellum laterally and the trochlea medially. (Illustrated by Rich Pennell, CMI. From Andrews JR, Zarins B, Wilk KE (eds): Injuries in Baseball. Philadelphia, Lippincott-Raven, 1998, pp 199–209, with permission.)

way of the coronoid process anteriorly and the olecranon process posteriorly. The proximal radioulnar joint (Fig. 40-2) allows for rotary movement of the radial head in the annular ligament upon the radial notch of the ulna. Osseous stability is maintained by the trochlea–coronoid and capitellum–radius articulations. Varus–valgus stability is enhanced by locking the olecranon into the olecranon fossa.

Soft-tissue structural stability is minimal and is provided by the thin anterior joint capsule and the overlying brachialis and the equally thin posterior capsule and overlying triceps. Ligamentous support is provided principally by the ulnar collateral ligament (UCL) medially. The UCL extends from the medial epicondyle of the humerus to the medial side of the coronoid process and olecranon of the ulna. The anterior portion of the UCL is taut in both flexion and extension. The posterior component is taut only in flexion. The transverse portion of the UCL appears to be noncontributory to either flexion or extension. Medial stability is enhanced by the flexor–pronator mass, which arises from the medial epicondyle. Lateral soft-tissue stability is provided by the radial collateral ligament (RCL), which originates from the lateral epicondyle and inserts into the annular ligament over the radial head.[33] A few RCL fibers course distally to insert on the radial border of the ulna along with the anconeus. Together, the RCL, wrist extensors, and anconeus function as relatively weak, but significant, stabilizers against varus stress.

Musculotendinous support of the elbow is less in the female than in the male.[42] The muscles are the biceps, brachialis, and brachio-

radialis anteriorly. The flexor–pronator group, originating from the medial epicondyle, serves as a dynamic stabilizer to resist valgus forces.

Proprioceptive neuromuscular control of joint stability is provided by afferent sensory mechanoreceptors in ligaments, tendons, muscles, joints, and skin. The mechanoreceptors, especially those in ligaments, yield neurologic feedback mediating and implementing muscular stabilization of a joint. With ligamentous injury, proprioceptive deficits reduce neuromuscular control of a joint, causing functional instability.[1,19,29,49]

EXAMINATION

When evaluating the female athlete with an elbow injury, the history should elicit the usual data: age, handedness, sport, and level of proficiency. Questioning must determine *what* area of the elbow is primarily involved, *how* the injury happened (not just the sport), *when* the injury occurred, and *where* the injury took place. Next it is ascertained if the injury is new, old, or recurring, and if any treatment—injection or oral medication—has been utilized. After this information is obtained, and before the physical examination begins, inquiries are made concerning each compartment of the elbow.

The shoulder and arms are visualized, inspected, tested, and compared. The carrying angle, range of motion, and forearm girth are measured bilaterally. Pronation, supination, and intrinsic hand muscle function are noted. Neck and shoulder function are evaluated and palpation is performed to determine the area of maximum elbow pain or tenderness.[20] Temperature and sensory variations are noted. Strength and stability are assessed. Obvious deformities are treated expeditiously.

Plain x-ray films, bilateral if called for, including anteroposterior, right and left oblique, lateral, and olecranon (axial) views are obtained. Comparison views of both right and left valgus stress roentgenograms that reveal a unilaterally increased medial opening are evidence of a UCL sprain. Computed tomography (CT) scans are useful for detecting fractures, osteophytes, and osteoid osteomas. Single-photon emission computed tomography (SPECT) bone scans are sensitive in locating stress fractures. Saline–gadolinium-enhanced magnetic resonance imaging (MRI) will reveal bone and soft-tissue abnormalities and, in a high percentage of cases, will indicate the presence of undersurface, partial, or complete tears of the UCL.

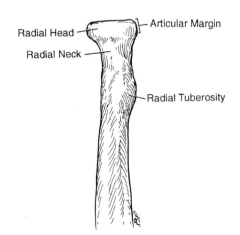

Figure 40-2. The proximal radius is shown with radial head, neck, articular margin, and radial tuberosity. (Illustrated by Rich Pennell, CMI. From Andrews JR, Zarins B, Wilk KE (eds): Injuries in Baseball. Philadelphia, Lippincott-Raven, 1998, pp 199–209, with permission.)

CHARACTERISTICS

The elbow exhibits laxity to varus–valgus stress and may functionally extend 5° to 10° beyond 180° of extension. A valgus carrying angle of 10° to 20° in the female athlete is evident in both elbows. The female baseball pitcher may develop exaggerated valgus deviation in her throwing arm. Loss of elbow extension in the female thrower is uncommon. Incomplete extension in the feamle athlete usually indicates a congenital anomaly, post-traumatic injury, fracture, or ligamentous damage as a sequel to dislocation. Incomplete extension with swelling often is associated with reactive synovitis of uncertain cause or collagen disease (eg, rheumatoid arthritis). In both sexes there is a 6° valgus deviation of the distal humerus and 6° to 9° of valgus extension and obliquity of the distal medial trochlea.[5] In the female, an increased carrying angle could represent an increase in osseous obliquity or simply increased laxity. The distal humeral growth centers fuse at approximately 13 years of age in the female; the medial epicondyle fuses at 14 years.[22] Isometric muscle testing has shown the summit of the strength curve for the female to be at 90°. There are no sex differences in the number of muscle fibers and strength per cross-sectional area.

Another difference relates to muscle mass and muscular definition. The gender difference in the female may reflect less upper body muscle and a greater body surface area: mass ratio. The female has a lower proportion of lean tissue in her upper body.

Hyperextension

The single most identifiable characteristic of the postadolescent female athlete is the persistence of joint hyperextension or increased range of motion.[9] Although capsular laxity is an asset in endeavors that require repetitive motion as in playing a musical instrument, it is a liability when joints must yield support, as in the martial arts.[28] (Fig. 40-3). Elbow hypermobility is hyperextension beyond 180°, that is, the angle between humerus and ulna is greater than expected. In the sitting position, elbow hyperextension is exaggerated when the arm is externally rotated at the side, the hand hypersupinated, the wrist dorsiflexed, and the upper body weight transferred to the palm. In this situation, with elbow laxity, the antecubital area becomes prominant anteriorly (Fig. 40-4). If valgus laxity is added, elbow strength and stability are dramatically reduced. The female gymnast who performs handstands

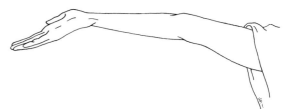

Figure 40-3. The abducted and externally rotated right upper extremity of the female illustrates about 15° of elbow hyperextension with the hand supinated almost 90°.

on the upper bar of uneven parallel bars contracts the biceps, brachialis, and brachioradialis muscles.[26] Hyperextension of the elbow is suspected when hyperextension of the knees (back knee) is present. When hypermobility is present in both parents, the incidence of pulled elbow (nursemaid's elbow) in children is significantly increased. In this entity, extension and traction on the hand with the forearm pronated allows the radial head to be pulled out distally from the annular ligament.[3] Hypermobility allows for relief by supination and when pressure is applied over the head of the radius.

SPORTS ACTIVITY

The female athlete is no longer confined to non-contact sports. Inevitably, musculoskeletal trauma is produced in the form of sprains, strains, contusions, lacerations, fractures, avulsions, and inflammatory reactions[8] (Table 40-1).

Typically, the repetitive, forceful stress of overuse produces an inflammatory soft-tissue response, especially in tendons, at the muscle–

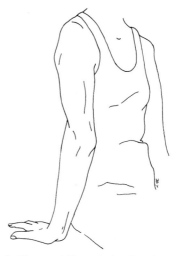

Figure 40-4. Hypermobility of the female right upper extremity is revealed as the humerus is externally rotated, the elbow hyperextended, and the forearm externally rotated on the dorsiflexed hand.

Table 40-1. Pathologic Conditions Occurring More Commonly in the Female Elbow

CONDITION	COMMENT
Thoracic outlet syndrome	Pain from the neck and shoulder involving arm extension at the elbow
Lateral epicondylitis	Work or sport requiring repetitive wrist extension
Fibromyalgia	Musculoskeletal stiffness with an elbow trigger point
Lupus erythematosus	Skin lesions about the elbow and forearm
Benign rheumatoid nodules	Nodules about the elbows, feet, and forearms
Rheumatoid arthritis[2]	Involving joints other than those seen in osteoarthritis
Mesenchymal syndrome of Nirschl[35]	Multiple sites of tendinosis, including the elbow
Stress fractures[41,43]	Eating disorders; increased mechanical loading, as in gymnastics
Neisseria gonorrhoeae infection[50]	Occasional nonarticular septic involvement of the elbow
Regional pain syndrome (reflex sympathetic dystrophy)	Limitation or immobility of the elbow joint
Joint stiffness[51]	After reduction and immobilization

tendon junction, at the tendon–osseous interface, or in the tendon itself. A peritenovitis may develop with only a subclinical, intratendinous inflammatory reaction that is insufficient to mimic the full-blown immunologic cascade. The result of incomplete healing is degenerative rather than inflammatory. The cystic, relatively acellular area, now correctly identified as tendinosis, becomes susceptible to ballistic forces, which may lead to rupture. Disruption of the distal biceps tendon, as occurs in weightlifting, and UCL injury in throwing sports are rare in the female athlete.

The structures in and about the elbow that are conventionally involved when the female athlete is injured are best addressed under the headings of the four anatomic compartments of the elbow.

Anterior Compartment

The anterior compartment of the elbow of the female athlete is particularly vulnerable to capsular and distal bicipital injury because of joint hypermobility and relatively inadequate biceps and brachialis strength. The capsule of the anterior compartment, which is covered by the brachialis, is relatively thin and easily stretched (inflamed) by forced hyperextension when attempting multiple pull-ups. In addition, acute stetching anteriorly may damage blood vessels and cause injury to the biceps tendon at its insertion in the tuberosity of the radius. When performing curls in weightlifting, a flexor–pronator muscle mass strain typically occurs at the muscle–tendon junction. Violent anterior stretching may result in injury to the anterior bundle of the UCL when a valgus stress is added to the back handspring. In the drive phase of sculling, bicipital tendinitis may develop after repetitive forceful, concentric flexion of the elbow by the biceps. Actual rupture of the distal

biceps tendon from its insertion on the radius is rare in the female rower. Such an avulsion rarity may, however, be present in the user of anabolic steroids and suspected in the female weightlifter or competitive bodybuilder who presents with anterior elbow tenderness, weakness, and swelling. Demonstration of bicipital tendon involvement may require MRI[17,47] or special roentgenographic views.[18]

The overworked fast-pitch softball pitcher with a windmill delivery may develop upper extremity muscular weakness. This leads to faulty mechanics that, with repetition, may produce a stress fracture of the proximal ulna. An indication is the clinical finding of persistent anterior elbow pain and tenderness on pronation or supination.

In platform diving, the arms are extended and the hands "punch" the water. The high forces at water entry drive the elbow into hyperextension. The biceps and brachialis must be strengthened in training to prevent this hyperextension.[4]

In throwing the javelin, the arm is abducted, posteriorly flexed, and externally rotated and the wrist supinated to facilitate the palm-up grasp of the spear. Repeated throwing from this position in the lax shoulder of the female may produce recurrent anterior subluxation of the radiohumeral head that impinges on the musculo- cutaneous nerve. Such an intermittent, but cumulative injury can compromise distal biceps and brachialis function, causing stretching of the anterior capsule and hyperextension.

The competitive female gymnast possesses hypermobility of the elbows. When performing maneuvers that require sustaining body weight, like handstands on the beam or vaulting, strength and proper technique are required to control hyperextension of the elbows that ordinarily would stretch the anterior capsule and strain the flexor–pronator muscle mass. However, should the hyperextension be uncontrolled and explosive or traumatic, as in a fall from the bars or a missed pass in floor exercise, the tip of the olecranon may drive the trochlea up and over the coronoid process. Such a mechanism may produce an anterior and superior displaced coronoid tip fracture, as well as anterior bulging, characteristic of a posterior dislocation of the elbow.

Lateral Compartment

On the radial aspect of the elbow, which assumes 60% of the vertical load, compression of the convex capitellum into the concave radial head often occurs in concert with medial valgus laxity in throwing sports and in weight-bearing maneuvers on the extended arm. In basketball, repeated passing or attempting long shots, which require forceful extension of the forearm, at times produces radiocapitellar articular cartilage wear and tear. This damage is reflected as localized lateral pain, tenderness, and often reduced range of motion. In the immature female, radial head overgrowth and premature physeal closure may be seen.[16] The young basketball player who, chasing a loose ball, falls on the extended arm with pronation of the forearm, may sustain a radial head fracture. Posterolateral instability may result from excessive abduction force and contraction of the extensor muscles with the arm extended, causing injury to the lateral collateral ligament, radiohumeral joint, subluxation, or fracture of the lateral humeral condylar physis.[36]

For the young female gymnast, by far the most severe and often career-ending lateral compartment disorder is osteochondritis dissecans (OCD).[11,16,37] Repetitive compression and large shear forces on the radiocapitellar joint in weight-bearing maneuvers are believed to be partially responsible. These forces are believed to compromise the epiphyseal–transchondral blood supply.[23] Symptoms may be minimal or they may be acute with painful synovitis, swelling, and limitation in range of motion. Often surgical intervention is needed for the placement of pins or débridement to remove a large fragment.[12] Young girls may be diagnosed as having Panner's osteochondritis, but if activity is curtailed the need for surgical intervention can be avoided.

In performing a screening examination for cheerleading candidates, a 12-year-old girl was noted to have exaggerated carrying angles and incomplete supination and extension. Here congenital lateral joint hypoplasia must be considered along with dislocation of the radial head, which is the most common congenital anomaly about the elbow.[1] Other skeletal abnormalities

to be looked for are the generalized hypermobility and ophthalmologic involvement of Ehlers–Danlos syndrome and the cracked nails seen in the nail–patella syndrome.

Inflammation of the lateral epicondyle occurs in tennis players ("tennis elbow"); whereas, medial epicondyle inflammation is associated with throwing sports. Previously related to repeated supination in learning to hit a one-handed backhand, the incidence of tennis-induced epicondylitis (or lateral tendinosis) has decreased because young tennis players are now taught to use a 2-handed backhand grip. However, lateral epicondylitis has increased and is seen in professional billiard players and in workplace maneuvers (computers) and in those who lug heavy bags or briefcases. Persistent lateral pain and inability to return to sports, even following rehabilitation, may require lateral release, débridement, and reattachment of the common extensor tendon to the lateral condyle. Rarely does lateral release, when carefully performed, lead to posterior lateral rotatory instability. For the lateral epicondylitis that is refractory to treatment, consideration is given to the racquetball or squash player who not only extends the wrist concentrically to hit but also bumps into the side wall, contusing the area of the anconeus muscle. If that proves not to be the case and if pressure applied over the proximal extensor muscles in the forearm produces pain and extensor or supinator weakness is noted, then entrapment of the deep motor branch of the radial nerve (posterior interosseous nerve, PIN) may be the cause. In bodybuilders entrapment occurs from extensive forearm muscle hypertrophy. The PIN may be compressed and irritated in serving in volleyball by thickened fibrous bands that develop at the supinator and at the interval between the brachialis and the biceps tendon with repetitive wrist flexion and extension.[7] A rarer cause of failed treatment of lateral epicondylitis results from persistence of a lateral synovial fold, or plica, that becomes thickened and inflamed as a result of flexion and extension with the forearm in pronation.[15] Repetitive resistance training using French curls and extensions for biceps strengthening may be the cause.

Posterior Compartment

Except for triceps tendinitis, posterior compartment injuries, in contradistinction to the other 3 elbow areas, are primarily osseous. Female baseball players develop posterior medial osteophyte formation. More likely than the baseball thrower, the female with joint laxity who serves and spikes in volleyball or swims the backstroke is apt to drive the medial border of the olecranon into the medial wall of the olecranon fossa and produce osteophytes and loose bodies. This entity, identified as valgus extension overload (VEO), has little gender preference.[48] The female, because of her natural increased carrying angle and relative valgus instability, along with her earlier musculoskeletal development, may be prone to develop VEO at an early age.

The early-adolescent girl who is learning to serve and hit overheads in tennis or to throw a softball may incur posterior elbow symptoms similar to those of the VEO syndrome. Another, similar, clinical picture permits differentiation. Bilateral comparison roentgenograms and MRI scans confirm the diagnosis of olecranon apophysitis in the female tennis player 15 years old or younger or the gymnast who vaults and performs tumbling floor exercises. Repetitive traction on the unfused olecranon by the triceps in forceful explosive extension can proceed to avulsion (Salter type I stress fracture) through the less strong physis.[14,44] Should the olecranon physis be closed, repetitive forceful triceps traction can cause a stress reaction in the body of the olecranon. More often, an actual fracture of the olecranon occurs in the older female athlete from a fall when striking the tip of the olecranon on a hard surface like ice, as seen in figure skaters, the wooden floor of the basketball court, or the hard ground, seen in motocross racers.

Triceps tendinitis occurs typically at the muscle–tendon attachment near the insertion of the triceps into the olecranon. Triceps tendinitis, if not the result of local trauma, is related to overuse and abuse, especially that experienced when repeatedly performing passive resistance-type forearm extension and curls on a bench or doing multiple push-ups, chin-ups, and dips. Weight training for female collegiate sports is now a requirement, particularly for the stick sports of lacrosse and field hockey and the racquet sports of tennis and squash.[27] The development of chronic soreness, aching, and extension weakness in the posterior compartment often indicates a protracted form of triceps tendinitis (more accurately defined as tendinosis).

It is becoming commonplace for the lowest person (foundation) in the pyramid cheerleading squad to develop triceps tendinitis because of forceful raising and then balancing the up-persons overhead in a prolonged, extended-forearm position. The female bodybuilder or shotputter who has received repeated local corticosteroid injections for triceps tendinitis and who may have used anabolic steroids may sustain a partial or complete tear in the distal triceps muscle–tendon–osseous unit.

The female martial arts student may strike the point of her elbow on the padded mat hard enough to develop sufficient compression and shear forces to cause an effusion and present with the clinical picture of olecranon bursitis.

The most common elbow dislocation is posterior. Classically, the athlete falls with the forearm in extension and in varus while pronated. The anterior capsule and collateral ligaments are disrupted and the brachialis is stretched or torn. Fracture of the medial epicondyle, radial head, or coranoid is a more severe outcome. Female mountain climbers, road bikers, racing cyclists, and cross-country joggers are prone to falls that cause an elbow dislocation. In the young pre-teen female, a fall on the outstretched extremity, even in roughhousing play, may result in a supracondylar fracture of the distal humerus. An elbow dislocation presents significant roentgenographic findings. Frequently, that is not the case in supracondylar fractures, where clinical suspicion often precedes identification of the subtle findings.[45]

Case History

This 14-year-old cheerleader was doing tumbling runs when she landed awkwardly on her dominant right upper extremity. Her father and coach attempted to straighten the elbow in the gymnasium. When she was evaluated in the emergency department, her radial pulse was absent and a small area of purple skin discoloration was noted in the antecubital fossa (Fig. 40-5A). Roentgenograms revealed a postero-lateral elbow dislocation (Fig. 40-5B). Documentation of the vascular injury was done by physical examination. A closed reduction in the emergency department under intravenous sedation was performed. Angiography showed lack of filling of the brachial artery (Fig. 40-5C). Owing to loss of the radial pulse and her young age and dominant extremity, the vascular surgeon recommended an anterior exploration. A thrombectomy and brachial vein patch and anterior capsule repair were done. Her postoperative range of motion was limited to 45° to 90° (Fig. 40-5D and E). Despite recommendations to not return to cheerleading, she did return. Her postoperative roentgenograms show ectopic ossification about the elbow (Fig. 40-5F). Her radial pulse was restored and the hand remained vascular, but she has permanent limitations in her range of motion. She is without pain.

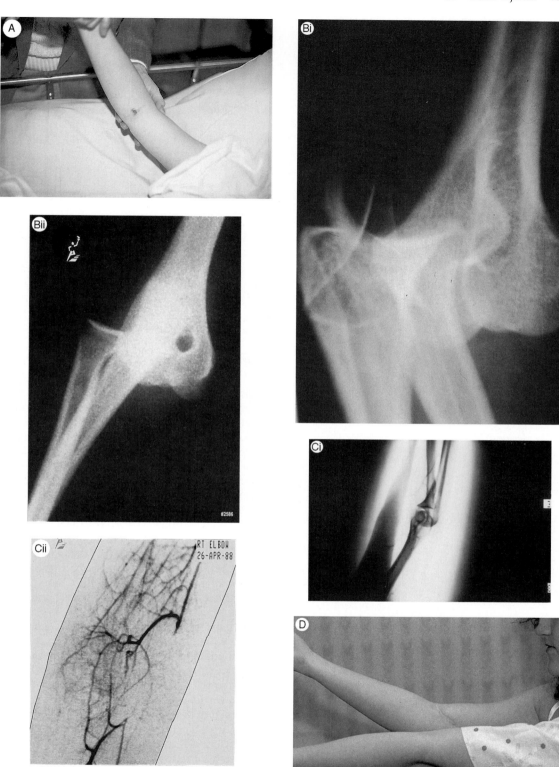

Figure 40-5. A 14-year-old cheerleader who sustained a fall during a tumble run. **(A)** Area of discoloration in the antecubital fossa. **(Bi,Bii)** Roentgenogram showing posterolateral elbow dislocation. **(Ci,Cii)** Angiogram showing lack of filling of the brachial artery. **(D & E)** Following anterior exploration, postoperative range of motion is limited to 45° to 90°.

Illustration continued on following page

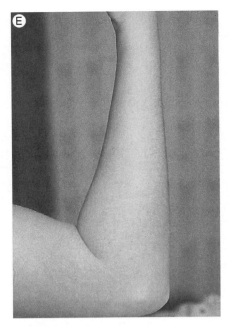

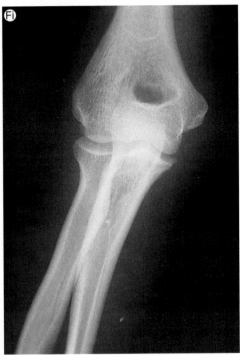

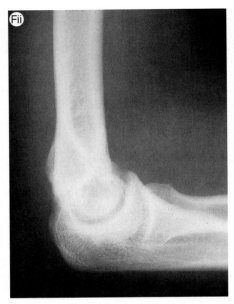

Figure 40-5 *(Continued)*. **(Fi,Fii)** Postoperative roentgenogram showing ectopic ossification about the elbow.

Medial Compartment

The medial elbow compartment is subject to valgus traction and, by skeletal design, compresses the lateral compartment. The anterior bundle of the UCL, because of its superior strength and stiffness, functions as the primary soft tissue stabilizer of the elbow.[39] A UCL injury in the female, although rare, occurs as the result of repetitive overuse, as in serving in tennis, in javelin throwing, and in bench-pressing. As more and more girls and young women play baseball, UCL injuries from overuse and abuse may become more prevalent and need surgical correction. Skeletal maturity determines the extent and kind of UCL pathology. If the elbow is immature with open physes, valgus stress, both cumulative and acute, will avulse the medial apophysis but maintain an intact UCL. The result, however, is an unstable elbow. A proportionate force in the early adolescent may avulse only the superior portion of the apophysis, along with the flexor–pronator muscle mass, and leave the UCL intact. In this instance, the elbow remains stable. In the female 15 years old and older, a similarly applied valgus force can produce partial undersurface or complete tearing of the UCL, resulting in functional instability. The production of undersurface UCL tears in the female is facilitated by the repetitive rigor of training in swimming the backstroke. A complete UCL tear may result from arm wrestling or a forceful throw in water polo or after sustaining many minor episodes of UCL intrasubstance sprains.

Unfortunately, this female athlete did not receive proper emergent treatment and reduction was attempted in the gymnasium. It is not known when the vascular injury occurred, whether at the time of dislocation or during the many attempts at relocation. Proper supervision of the education and practices of coaches in providing emergent care should be a goal of health professionals.

Medial traction apophysitis ("little leaguer's elbow"), which is characterized by fragmentation, irregularity, and painful separation of the apophyseal plate, is seen in young female baseball pitchers. In the older female adolescent, medial elbow symptoms from repetitive traction may spare the UCL and produce an inflammatory response or strain of the flexor–pronator mass known as medial epicondylitis (tendinosis). Poor mechanics on the downswing may cause lateral epicondylitis in the left elbow of a right-handed golfer, and opening up of the hips too early or repeatedly hitting divots may result in medial epicondylitis of the right elbow. Medial flexor–pronator muscle strain is seen in the tennis player who persistently hits forehands late down the line in an inside-out fashion with the elbow in front of the racquet head and in the right-handed baseball batter who swings late. The advanced female gymnast, or even the older, retired, occasional gymnast who presents with physiologically increased elbow valgus, recurvatum, or laxity, is notorious for the development of medial overload symptoms. In addition, those whose routines require powerful weight-bearing moves, as seen in vaulting, balance beam workouts, and tumbling, are prone to medial elbow injury.

Ulnar nerve dysfunction occurs congenitally as a result of subluxation or dislocation of the ulnar nerve from the epicondylar groove of the distal medial humerus. Ulnar nerve symptoms may develop in active athletics when combined with valgus instability, direct trauma, and localized soft-tissue scar formation. Fibrous compression and irritation of and tension on the ulnar nerve in the groove produces forearm paraesthesias and pain commonly referred to as the *cubital tunnel syndrome*. Ulnar nerve dysfunction, which may also result from involvement of zone I above or zone III below the cubital tunnel in females who play "ultimate frisbee" or who box should not be considered the cause or result of a single pathologic entity. Rather, ulnar nerve neuritis often is merely the most obvious component in a multifactorial complex of physical and exertional insults. Clearly, other causes, such as stress fracture, UCL sprain, full passive movement strain, or any combination of these, could be the reason that surgical transfer of the ulnar nerve alone is not always successful in alleviating medial compartment symptoms.

Compression of the median nerve at the level of the flexor–pronator forearm muscles produces vague postexertional pain in the volar aspect of the medial forearm and distant paresthesias. Such symptoms characterize the rare pronator teres syndrome. These musculoskeletal changes may be related to increased female participation in competitive race car driving and excessive weight training, which require repetitive forearm pronation and forceful gripping.

PREVENTION AND CARE

Prevention of elbow injuries includes general health measures, including nutrition and weight control, plus the proper and systematic development of the individual's strength, range of motion, and neuromuscular control.[3] The latter are enhanced by repetitive maneuvers and informed coaching. With the exception of significant augmentation of muscle mass about the elbow, the elbow of the female athlete responds to strength, endurance, and flexibility training, and incorporates motor work into biomechanical skills.[34]

The elbow of the female athlete is subject to force, overuse, concentric and eccentric stretch, and thermal injuries. Strains, sprains, contusions, lacerations, fractures, and infections are seen in athletes of both sexes. The female athlete is, however, not likely to incur the myositis ossificans that results from a karate-chop contusion of the brachioradialis.

The female athlete will react appropriately to routine therapeutic modalities, closed chain exercises, and passive resistance exercises as employed by the trainers and physical therapists who care for and treat musculoskeletal injuries. Guidelines for the use of wrapping, taping, bracing, and padding about the elbow are comparable for all athletes.

Rehabilitation protocols for treatment of specific elbow injuries are tailored to conform to the individual's needs. Response to treatment is also individually determined.

References

1. Agnew DK, Davis RJ: Congenital unilateral dislocation of the radial head. J Pediatr Orthop 13:526–8, 1993.
2. Alarcon-Segovia D: Rheumatoid arthritis, epidemiology, etiology, rheumatic factors, pathology, pathogenesis. In: Schumacher HR (ed): Primer on the Rheumatic Diseases. Atlanta; Orthopaedic Foundation, 1988, pp 83–99.
3. Amir D, Frankl U, Pogrund H: Pulled elbow and hypermobility of joints. Clin Orthop 257:94-9, 1990.
4. Anderson SJ, Rubin BD: Evaluation and treatment of injuries in competitive divers. In: Bruschbacher RM, Branddom RL (eds): Sports Medicine and Rehabilitation: A Sport-Specific Approach. Philadelphia, Hanley & Belfus, 1994, pp 111–22.
5. Anderson TE: Anatomy and physical exam of the elbow. In: Nicholas JA, Hershman EB (eds): The Upper Extremity in Sports Medicine, 2nd edition. St Louis, Mosby-Year Book, 1995, pp 261–74.

6. Andrews JR, Satterwhite YE: Elbow forearm trauma. In: Current Review of Sports Medicine. Chapter 3, November 1993, pp 1–12.

7. Andrews JR, Schemmel SP, Whiteside JA, Timmerman LA: Evaluation, treatment, and presentation of elbow injuries in throwing athletes. In: Nicholas JA, Hershman EB (eds): The Upper Extremity in Sports Medicine. Chapter 35. St Louis: CV Mosby, 1995, pp 749–88.

8. Andrews JR, Whiteside JA: Common elbow problems in the athlete. J Orthop Sports Phys Ther 17:289–95, 1993.

9. Andrish JT: Upper extremity injuries in the skeletally immature athlete. In: Nicholas JA, Hershman EB (eds): The Upper Extremity in Sports Medicine. St Louis, CV Mosby, 1990, pp 673–88.

10. Articulation of the upper limb (Chapter 5) and Muscles and fascia of the forearm (Chapter 6). In: Gray's Anatomy, 29th edition. Philadelphia, Lea & Febiger, 1991, pp 317–40 and 460–72.

11. Bauer M, Jonsson K, Josefsson PO, Linden B: Osteochondritis dissecans of the elbow: a long-term follow-up study. Clin Orthop 284:156–60, 1992.

12. Baumgarten TE, Andrews JR, Satterwhite YE: The Arthroscopic classification and treatment of osteochondritis dissecans of the capritellum. Am J Sports Med 26(4):520–3, 1998.

13. Brodgon BG, Crow NF: Little leaguer's elbow. Am J Roentgenol 8:671–3, 1960.

14. Chan D, Aldridge MJ, Maffulli N, Davis AM: Chronic stress injuries of the elbow in young gymnasts. Br J Radiol 64:1113–8, 1991.

15. Clarke RP: Symptomatic lateral synovial fringe (plica) of the elbow joint. Arthroscopy 42:112–6, 1988.

16. DeSilva MF, Williams JS, Fadale PD, et al. Pediatric throwing injuries about the elbow. Am J Anthopol 27(2):90–6, 1998.

17. Falchook FS. Zlatkin MB, Erbacher GE, et al: Rupture of the distal biceps tendon: evaluation with MR imaging. Radiology 190:659–63, 1994.

18. Fritz RC: MR imaging of sports injuries of the elbow. Magnetic Reson Imaging Clin N Am 7(1):51–72 viii, 1999.

19. Gregg P: Peripheral neural mechanisms in proprioception. J Sports Rehabil 3:2–17, 1994.

20. Hoppenfeld SL: Physical Examination of the Spine and Extremities. Norwalk, Conn, Appleton-Century-Crafts, 1976, p 36.

21. Hutchinson M, Ireland ML: Knee injuries in female athletes. Sports Med 14(4):288-302, 1995.

22. Ireland ML, Hutchinson MR, Andrews JR, et al: Elbow Injuries: Injuries in Baseball. Chapter 26. Philadelphia, Lippincott-Raven, 1998, 283–305.

23. Jackson DW, Silvino N, Reiman P: Osteochondritis of the female gymnast's elbow. Arthroscopy 5:129–36, 1989.

24. Kessler KJ, Uribe JW, Vargas L: Tendon rupture: new mechanism of injury. Contemp Orthop 29:134–6, 1994.

25. Klemme WR, Peterson SA: Avulsion of the triceps brachii with selective radial neuropathy: case report. Orthopedics 18:285–7, 1995.

26. Koh TJ, Grabiner MD, Weiker GG: Technique and ground reaction forces in the back handspring. Am J Sports Med 20:61–6, 1992.

27. Kramer UMJ, Ratamese N, AC Fry, et al: Influence of resistance training volume and periodization and performance adaptations in collegiate women tennis players. Am J Sports Med 28(5):626–33, 2000.

28. Larsson LG, Baum J, Mudholkar GS, Kollia GD: Benefits and disadvantages of joint hypermobility among musicians. N Engl J Med 329:1079–82, 1993.

29. Lepart SM, Pincivaro DM, Giraldo GL, Fu FH: The role of proprioception in the management and rehabilitation of athletic injuries. Am J Sports Med 25(1):130–7, 1997.

30. Lui SH, Henry M, Bower R: Complications of type I coronoid fractures in competitive athletes. Report of two cases and review of the literature. J Shoulder Elbow Surg 5(3):223–7, 1996.

31. Mackie SJ, Tauton EE: Injuries in female gymnasts: trends suggest prevention tactics. Physician Sportsmed 22:40–5, 1994.

32. Miller AE, MacDougall JD, Tarnopolsky MA: Gender difference in strength and muscle fibre characteristics. Eur J Appl Physiol Occup 66:254–62, 1993.

33. Netter FH: The CIBA Collection of Medical Illustrations, Vol 8. Musculoskeletal System, Part 1, Anatomy, Physiology, and Metabolic Disorders. Upper Limb and Elbow Joint. Summitt, NJ, CIBA Geigy Corp., 1987, pp 42–3.

34. Nindl BC, Mahas MT, Harmon EA, Patton JF: Lower and upper body anaerobic performance in male and female adolescent athletes. Med Sci Sports Exerc 24:235–41, 1995.

35. Nirschl RP: Patterns of failed healing in tendon injury. In: Leadbetter WB, Buckwalter JS, Gordon SL (eds): Sports Induced Inflammation. Park Ridge, Ill, American Academy of Orthopaedic Surgeons, 1990, pp 577–85.

36. O'Driscoll SW, Bell DF, Morrey BF: Posterolateral rotatory instability of the elbow. J Bone Joint Surg 73A: 440–6, 1991.

37. Peterson RK, Savoil FH 3rd, Field LO: Osteochondritis dissecans of the elbow. Instr Course Lect 48:393–8, 1999.

38. Quick facts 2000: Olympic Games Sydney Organizing Committee for the Olympic Games Sydney, Australia. Internet Sports Med 9/18/2000,11:15AM.

39. Regan WD, Korinek SL, Morrey BF, An KN: Biomechanical study of ligaments around the elbow joint. Clin Orthop 291:170–9, 1991.

40. Rosenberg ZS, Beltran J, Cheung YY, et al: The elbow: MR features of nerve disorders. Radiology 188(1):235–40, 1993.

41. Sallis RE, Jones K: Stress fractures in athletes. Postgrad Med 89:185–8, 191–2, 1991.

42. Shangold MM, Mirkin G (eds): Women and Exercise: Physiology and Sports Medicine. Philadelphia, FA Davis, 1994.

43. Sinha AK, Kaeding CC, Wadley GM: Upper extremity stress fractures in athletes: clinical features of 44 cases.

44. Stevens MA, El-Khoury GY, Kathol MH, et al: Imaging features of avulsion injuries. Radiographics 19(3): 655–72, 1999.

45. Swischuk LE: Elbow injury. Pediatr Emerg Care 9:113–5, 1993.

46. Tsunoda N, O'Hagan F, Sale DG, MacDougall JD: Elbow flexion strength curves on untrained men and women and male bodybuilders. Eur J Appl Physiol 66:235–9, 1993.

47. Van der Wall H, Frater CJ, Magee MA, et al: A novel view for the scintigraphic assessment of the elbow. Nucl Med Commun 20(11):1059–65, 1999.

48. Wilson FD, Andrews JR, Blackburn TA, McCluskey G: Valgus extension overload in the pitching elbow. Am J Sports Med 11(2):83–8, 1983.

49. Women's greatest challenges: finding places to play soccer. USA Today Aug 1:1c, 2c, 1994.

50. Wyngaarden JB, Smith LH, Bennett JC: Cecil Textbook of Medicine, 19 edition. Philadelphia, Saunders, 1992, pp 1755–59.

51. DeLee JC, Green DP, Wilks KE: Fractures and dislocations of the elbow. In: Rockwood CA Jr, Green DP (eds): Fractures in Adults, 2nd ed. Philadelphia, Lippincott, 1984, Chapter 9, p 616, Vol. 1.

Chapter 41

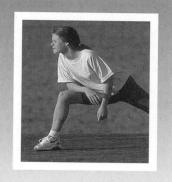

Hand and Wrist Injuries

Frank C. McCue, III, M.D.
Robert R. Bell, M.D.
Duc Tien Nguyen, M.D.

Injuries to the hand and wrist are among the most common an athlete will encounter. The hand is characteristically in front of the athlete in most sports and frequently absorbs the initial contact. There is a tendency to minimize the severity and importance of these injuries since the injury does not totally disable the athlete. The key to proper treatment is careful evaluation and accurate diagnosis; only then can precise and proper treatment be implemented. The goal is restoration of maximal function, both on and off the field. Conservative treatment is preferable for the majority of injuries; however, in a small percentage of patients, surgical treatment may be needed in the acute or chronic reconstructive setting. In this chapter, we will review the more commonly seen injury patterns to the hand and wrist of athletes' bony anatomy and ligamentous structure.

FRACTURES OF THE WRIST

Scaphoid Fractures

The scaphoid is the most commonly fractured carpal bone. Often, the trauma causing the injury is minor and many times the injury is written off as a sprain, resulting in delayed diagnosis. The mechanism of injury is forced hyperextension with the wrist in ulnar deviation.[58] The predominant blood supply of the scaphoid enters through its distal aspect.[23,24,54] The proximal pole receives no direct vascular supply, but derives its supply from interosseous vessels, which pass in a retrograde fashion. This vascular configuration provides the anatomic basis for the high rate of nonunion and avascular necrosis characteristic of the proximal pole. Patients usually present with pain localized in the snuffbox region. Anteroposterior, lateral, and ulnar deviation views, to assess the scaphoid, are needed to make a diagnosis of scaphoid fracture.

A clenched-fist view can also be useful in diagnosing scaphoid fractures associated with scapholunate dissociation. Bone scans are also useful in the diagnosis of scaphoid fractures. They are especially useful after 72 hours in those patients suspected of having a scaphoid fracture, but not having the fracture readily visible on plain roentgenography. Uncomplicated scaphoid fractures have a union rate of 95% with early diagnosis and immobilization. Several factors are associated with higher rates of nonunion. Fractures involving the proximal pole have a higher incidence of delayed union, nonunion,[15] and avascular necrosis.[18] Displacement of more than 1 mm and a diagnosis delay of greater than 4 weeks also adversely affect healing potential.[21] Treatment options depend upon location of fracture, alignment, and displacement. Potentially unstable (ie, vertical oblique) fractures or fractures older than 3 weeks should probably be treated initially with long arm thumb spica casts and be followed closely for potential displacement.[25] Acute, displaced, or angulated fractures involving the middle third of the scaphoid should undergo open reduction and internal fixation.[51] Kirschner wires and Herbert screws[30] are effective fixation. Acute fractures involving the proximal third should also be treated with long arm thumb spica immobilization for approximately 6 weeks followed by short arm thumb spica cast immobilization. Fractures involving the distal third acutely can be treated with short arm thumb spica casts. Displaced fractures of the proximal third can be treated with retrograde fixation.[30] Displaced intra-articular fractures of the distal third can undergo open reduction and internal fixation for best results as well. Fractures of the distal third will show clinical signs of union at 6 weeks, whereas fractures involving the proximal third can take as long as 4 months to achieve union. If there is no evidence of union after 6 months, bone grafting and internal fixation as needed should be considered.

Following removal of immobilization, the athlete is placed on a supervised program of strengthening and range of motion exercises. The wrist should be protected with a splint for athletic activities until strength of the injured wrist reaches that of the opposite uninjured wrist. Protection should continue for a minimum of 3 months following cast removal.

Lunate Fractures

Kienböck in 1910 described a malady involving the lunate carpal bone that today bears his name.[34] Kienböck attributed the progressive collapse to avascular necrosis. Today, there are still many possible mechanisms to account for this disorder. Zapico suggested that a lunate with a more apical proximal articular surface is most susceptible to avascular necrosis.[3] Hulten noted that there is an increased incidence of avascular necrosis of lunate in wrists that show ulnar minus variant.[34] Most investigators agree that some form of repetitive compressive traumatic forces lead to microfractures of the lunate, with eventual collapse.[2,8,22,56] It is continued stress that prevents healing of the lunate. The patients usually present complaining of vague pain or stiffness in the wrist. Plain radiographs may reveal no changes in the lunate, but often ulnar minus variant is noted. Magnetic resonance imaging (MRI) can be useful, as well as bone scanning in the acute setting.[7] With time, progressive x-ray changes will include sclerosis followed by cyst formation with fragmentation and collapse of the lunate. Kienböck's disease can be divided into 4 stages as described by Stahl.[62] In stage I, linear compression fractures are noted, but there is otherwise normal density of the lunate. In stage II, there is increased density and sclerosis of the lunate, but no collapse is noted. Stage III is heralded by collapse of the lunate and in stage IV there are extensive osteoarthritic changes involving the articulations about the lunate. Treatment can be correlated to stage of disease. For stages I to III joint leveling procedures are quite useful. These entail either radial shortening or ulnar lengthening.[4] Trumble found that bone leveling procedures were as effective as scaphoid-trapezium-trapezoid (STT) fusions in relieving lunate loading.[65] Their study showed that only 2 mm of shortening was required to maximize lunate decompression. In some cases of stage III with extreme collapse, excision of the lunate can be utilized with interposition arthroplasty utilizing auto- or allograft tendon. Intercarpal fusion may be utilized with or without lunate excision, either STT or scaphocapitate fusion.[69] Almquist

has described shortening of the capitate in the treatment of Kienböck's disease.[2] In stage IV when advanced perilunate osteoarthritic changes are present, proximal row carpectomy can be useful to maintain wrist motion. An alternative method of treatment is complete wrist fusion in patients with stage IV Kienböck's. Return to sports participation will require healing from the procedure performed and physical therapy to allow the patient to reach strength in the operated wrist equivalent to that in the opposite wrist.

Hamate Fractures

There are 2 primary types of hamate fractures, those that involve the body and those localized to the hook of the hamate.[58] On physical examination, these 2 fractures are quite similar, with pain localized to the ulnar half of the wrist. Fractures of the body of the hamate can be quite difficult to diagnose. Often fractures of the base of the ulnar metacarpals may accompany fractures of the body of the hamate.[44] For isolated fractures of the body, immobilization for 4 to 6 weeks is often sufficient. For fractures displaced greater than 2 mm, open reduction and internal fixation is often required. Following fixation, immobilization for 6 weeks in a short arm cast is necessary. Fractures of the hook of the hamate may easily be missed when they are not clinically suspected.[10] These fractures are often seen in golfers, but may also be noted in tennis, baseball, softball, and squash players. Ulnar nerve involvement as well has been reported and is attributed to hemorrhage within Guyon's canal. Flexor tendon ruptures have been noted owing to attrition against rough fracture surfaces.[1] Radiographically, carpal tunnel projections are useful in the diagnosis. Typically, fractures of the hook of the hamate will progress to nonunions if left untreated. This is in large part due to poor blood supply of the hook. The recommended treatment acutely is for cast immobilization to allow the hook to heal. Most cases are seen in the late setting with persistent pain following nonunion. The recommended treatment is for excision of the hook of the hamate fragment in these cases.[55]

Capitate Fractures

Fractures of the capitate are similar in many ways to fractures of the scaphoid. The most common mechanism of fracture is forced dorsiflexion or palmar flexion of the wrist. On physical examination, point tenderness is usually elicited over the bases of the third and fourth metacarpal rays in the vicinity of the capitate.

Plain roentgenograms are useful in the diagnosis, but on occasion bone scans can be useful in the diagnosis of occult fracture. The blood supply of the proximal pole of the capitate is retrograde from vessels entering at the wrist.[49] This explains the increased incidence of avascular necrosis of the proximal pole of the capitate following fracture. Fractures of the capitate similar to fractures of the scaphoid can be involved in perilunate dislocation injuries. Avascular necrosis of the capitate has been reported in collegiate gymnastics.[19] Murakami and Nakajima reported 2 cases.[19] Each case presented with initial wrist pain chronic in nature. Neither patient had specific trauma that they could recall. Physical examination usually shows limitation of motion of the wrist and tenderness of the capitate. Radiographic evaluation reveals resorption of the proximal pole of the capitate. Resection and interpositional tendinous grafts have been utilized in combination with capitohamate fusion, with good relief of pain. Treatment of nondisplaced fractures of the capitate involves immobilization for approximately 6 weeks. Displaced fractures of more than 2 mm require open reduction and internal fixation with Kirschner wires or Herbert screws. Attention should be given to the possibility of avascular necrosis of the proximal pole. Criteria for return to sports participation similarly involves the attainment of strength equal to that of the opposite wrist and splint protection for approximately 3 months following removal of the surgical immobilization device.

Pisiform Fractures

Fractures of the pisiform are uncommon. They account for approximately 1% of carpal fractures.[20] The most common mechanism of injury is that of a direct blow. Pisiform fractures are often missed because of the difficulty in radiographic evaluation. Thirty-degree supinated oblique views can be quite useful in observing the pisotriquetral articulation. For acute fractures cast immobilization has been recommended, however, many fractures result in nonunion or post-traumatic pisotriquetral arthritis. If these late sequelae are symptomatic, then excision of the pisiform is usually successful in reducing pain and improving function of the wrist.[29] It appears to have little effect on the overall palmar flexion strength of the wrist.

Triquetrum Fractures

Fractures of the triquetrum usually result from hyperextension leading to impingement of the triquetrum upon the distal ulna. This usually will lead to an avulsion fracture from the dorsal cortex of the triquetrum. These fractures routinely respond to 3 weeks of short arm cast immobilization. Nonunion of these dorsal avulsion fractures has rarely been implicated as a cause for persistent symptoms.[5] The criteria for return to sport participation involve the athlete utilizing a cast or splint for protection during athletic participation. The athlete can resume activity when discomfort has decreased to the extent that it does not interfere with sport-specific activity.

CARPAL INSTABILITIES AND DISLOCATIONS

Scapholunate Instability

Scapholunate instability is the most common form of carpal instability. The diagnosis is often missed in the acute setting because of the patient's own delays in presenting for evaluation. Many athletes will write this injury off as a wrist sprain. Evaluation of these patients will usually find pain, swelling, and tenderness over the region of the scapholunate articulation. There is usually a history of a fall or a direct blow to the hand causing a hyperextension-type injury of the wrist. Watson has described a test in which the examiner stabilizes the scaphoid with his or her thumb over the volar pole of the scaphoid while the wrist is held in ulnar deviation.[68] The hand is then brought into radial deviation, with pain being produced as force is transmitted to the torn scapholunate ligament. Radiographic findings can be quite subtle. An anteroposterior view may show gapping between the scaphoid and lunate interval. A gap of 3 mm or more is abnormal. This is known as the "Terry Thomas sign" after the famous British comedian's dental diastema. The scaphoid will appear shortened owing to its subluxation into a more vertical position. A ring sign may be present representing the cortical projection of the distal pole. The crescent ring to proximal pole distance is normally greater than 7 mm or is within 4 mm of the opposite wrist. On the lateral view, a scapholunate angle of more than 70° (normal 30° to 60°) is also quite suggestive of scapholunate dissociation.[42] On occasion, plain radiographs will not show changes consistent with a scapholunate dissociation; however, the patient will complain of a "clunk" with motion of the wrist and may have a positive Watson maneuver. In these instances special radiographic studies may be necessary.

Bone scanning and arthrography can aid in localizing the area of injury.[31,50] Treatment of scapholunate instability depends in part upon the time from injury. Acute injuries, or those diagnosed within 4 weeks, may be treated by cast immobilization, closed reduction with percutaneous pinning,[51] or open reduction with repair of the involved ligaments and percutaneous pinning. In the acute setting, our preferred method is for open reduction. Return to sports usually requires 1 or 2 months of rehabilitation. We usually will utilize an orthosis for 6 months until the patient demonstrates maximum strength and range of motion. For chronic injuries we determine whether degenerative changes have occurred. In those patients with a chronic injury without degenerative changes, there are several treatment options. Blatt described a dorsal capsulodesis technique in which the dorsal capsule acts as a check-rein to prevent volar rotation of the distal pole of the scaphoid.[6,9] A variety of intercarpal arthrodeses have been performed to correct late scapholunate instability.[66,68] These limited wrist arthrodeses attempt to control the rotary subluxation of the scaphoid. Scapholunate joint arthrodesis would seem to be the most appropriate procedure as this is where the pathology lies.[66] Rosenwassen and coworkers noted good success with Herbert screw fixation of the scaphoid and lunate.[61] Peterson and Lipscomb described the STT arthrodesis.[57] Watson and Hempson have published extensively on his success with this procedure.[68] Many surgeons utilize a partial styloidectomy at the time of the initial STT arthrodesis to help prevent radioscaphoid wear. Return to sports participation is similar to that for patients with acute injures treated with open reduction and pinning. For patients with scapholunate dissociation and established arthrosis, the patients probably have already experienced significant limitation of sports activity. The proximal row carpectomy appears to have good results.[28] However, it does result in decreased grip strength. The procedure should be done before degenerative changes involve the capitate or the lunate fossa of the radius. These salvage-type procedures are probably not consistent with maintaining athletic activities at a higher level.[17] In patients with generalized arthrosis of the midcarpal and radiocarpal joints and particularly in individuals desiring to return to heavy activity, wrist arthrodesis should be the procedure of choice. For patients with scapholunate advanced collapse (SLAC) deformity, the 4-corner fusion with removal of the scaphoid has been described.[67]

Triquetrolunate Instability

Triquetrolunate injuries are being diagnosed with increasing frequency. The more severe forms of triquetrolunate dissociation may progress to a volar intercalated segmental instability (VISI) deformity.[28,52] Partial or complete disruption of the lunotriquetral interosseous ligament alone will not lead to the VISI deformity pattern. With complete disruption of the lunotriquetral interosseous ligament and the palmar lunotriquetral ligament there can be evidence of volar intercalated segmental instability seen on the roentgenogram. Reagan has described a ballottement test for determination of injuries to the lunotriquetral articulation.[59] The lunate is firmly stabilized with the thumb and index fingers of one hand while the triquetrum and pisiform are forced dorsally and palmarly with the other hand. A positive test will elicit pain with crepitus and a feeling of laxity at the lunotriquetral articulation. Radiographic evaluation includes anteroposterior and lateral films. On the lateral film, the scapholunate angle may be decreased to less than 30°. The lunate in a static VISI deformity will be in a palmar flexed position and somewhat dorsally subluxed. A bone scan can be particularly useful as a screening tool in patients with ulnar-sided wrist pain. Arthrography may show a tear of the lunotriquetral interosseous ligament. Arthrography should be combined with a physical examination, as there is a high false-positive rate on arthrograms in asymptomatic wrists. Treatment requires arthrodesis of the triquetrum and lunate, arthroscopic débridement and pinning, or open ligament repair. A trial of conservative therapy including immobilization and anti-inflammatory medication can be attempted. For patients with fixed VISI deformity Taleisnik has recommended fusion of the radiolunate articulation.[64] In patients with positive ulnar variance, a bone scan can help aid in the diagnosis of ulnar impaction associated with triquetrolunate instability. In these patients, ulnar shortening should be included as much of the symptomatology can result from ulnar impaction. Following removal of the patient's cast, normally 1 to 2 months are necessary to show significant improvement in strength and range of motion. Participation in sports activities will require an orthosis for approximately 6 months until demonstration of maximal strength and functional range of motion.

Triquetrohamate Instability

Patients with triquetrohamate dissociation have a characteristic "clunk" that can be both audible and palpable. This clunk can be reproduced with active radial and ulnar deviation of the wrist. Lichtman and coworkers stated that the ulnar arm of the arcuate ligament extending from the capitate to the triquetrum is torn, causing this instability pattern.[40] With this ligament divided, the triquetrum no longer moves smoothly through its helicoid articulation with the hamate, but instead jumps "from the low to the high position with sudden abrupt movement." Cineradiographs can be useful in visualizing this abnormal kinematic pattern of the carpus. Treatment initially can be symptomatic, with immobilization and steroid injection of the midcarpal joint if the patient is not significantly symptomatic to warrant surgical treatment. For those patients who have sufficient disability to require surgical intervention, intercarpal arthrodesis of the triquetrohamate joint is carried out. Usually, the capitate and lunate are added to the fusion to help increase the chances for successful union. Further studies of the kinematics of the midcarpal joint are underway, and many centers are studying possible soft-tissue corrections.

Carpal Dislocations

Dislocations involving the carpal bones can either be pure ligamentous injuries or combined fracture-dislocations. Johnson has described the pure ligamentous injuries as lesser arc injuries and those that involve fractures as greater arc injuries.[32] The fractures may occur through the radial styloid, the scaphoid, the capitate, the hamate, or the triquetrum, and can be associated with perilunate or volar lunate dislocation. The initial emergency department radiographs may not detect the full nature of the carpal dislocation or instability pattern as dorsal dislocations may partially reduce. Methods of treatment range from simple closed reduction, to closed reduction with percutaneous fixation, all the way to open reduction including both dorsal and volar incision. Most investigators now agree with Linscheid and Dobyns that open reduction with repair of the ligaments and internal fixation is the treatment of choice with the most predictable rate of healing.[42]

STRESS SYNDROMES OF THE WRIST

Madelung's Deformity

An acquired form of Madelung's deformity described in gymnast is thought to be due to repetitive overload of the ulnar aspect of the distal radius.[70] It is much more common in females and is often bilateral. As described in *The Young Gymnast*, alterations include early fusion of the ulnar half of the distal physis with ulnar and volar angulation of the distal radial articular surface. There may be a decrease in rotation of the forearm, especially pronation. Prominence of the ulnar styloid can be noted on physical examination. Discomfort is usually slow to develop unless there is added repetitive trauma. Mild deformity is not usually accompanied by discomfort. Thus treatment is often not sought unless some traumatic episode precipitates symptoms. There is little indication to treat patients with mild deformity. Surgical intervention would be indicated in the child age 10 or less with significant deformity who is likely to have further deformity and in the teenage or adult patient with significant deformity and loss of function. There are several procedures described for the treatment of Madelung's deformity. The use of physiolysis followed by placement of interpositional material to inhibit recurrent tethering of the physis would seem appropriate. Also, the use of external fixator distractor techniques, which can correct multiplanar deformity, would also seem to be a reasonable choice. Corrective osteotomy of the distal radius with either closed or opening wedge techniques is useful in skeletally mature patients. This is often used in conjunction with excision of the distal ulna, ulnar osteotomy, or the Suave-Kapandji procedure. Return to sports activity following surgical intervention for such a deformity in the young patient is controversial. There are splints available that limit wrist dorsiflexion, but counseling would be needed for the patient wanting to return to a sport that requires excessive repetitive overload of the wrist. Koh and coworkers[37] revealed that stresses across the wrist exceed 2.4 times body weight in some floor exercises.

Scaphoid Impaction Syndrome

Repetitive hyperextension of the wrist can result in the impaction of the dorsal rim of the scaphoid against the dorsal lip of the radius.[14] Such stresses result in pain and point tenderness over the dorsal scaphoid rim reproduced by hyperextension. Radiographs often will demonstrate hypertrophic changes at the dorsal scaphoid rim best seen on the lateral view with the wrist in flexion. Patients may develop irritation of the dorsal capsule known as "dorsiflexion jam syndrome." This occurs often in gymnasts who require repetitive dorsal wrist positioning such as that associated with the use of the vault.

Irritation of the posterior interosseous nerve should be included in the differential diagnosis. Treatment initially involves taping or dorsal block splinting as well as anti-inflammatory medication and rest. Surgical exploration is occasionally required. Cheilectomy should be performed in those patients with hypertrophic changes on the dorsal scaphoid rim.[14,19] Excision of the posterior interosseous nerve innervation to the dorsal wrist capsule can aid in the relief of symptoms. Gradual return to sports participation may commence after rehabilitation of the wrist to return strength and motion. Splinting to prevent recurrent hyperdorsiflexion should be utilized.

Distal Radial Physeal Stress Syndrome

Repeated microtrauma to the wrist can functionally disrupt small vessels to the physis. This can result in a radiographically demonstrable widened and irregular physis. This widening of the physis of the distal radius has been described in athletes participating in sports requiring repetitive compressive stresses as well as those who participate in activities that lead to repetitive distraction loads across the wrist.[71] Patients complain of wrist pain, primarily dorsal, that usually occurs hours into a workout and gradually progresses. Tenderness may be elicited with forced dorsiflexion as well as palpation of the dorsal wrist in the region of the physis. Radiographic findings consist of widening of the distal radial physis, especially on the radial and ulnar margins. Irregularity of the metaphysis and haziness of the physis may be noted. Treatment consists of reduction of activity level. In more recalcitrant cases casting or splinting to support the wrist may be utilized, along with anti-inflammatory medication. In 1985 Roy and coworkers, reviewed 21 gymnasts who had wrist pain thought to be related to stress changes of the distal radial physis.[60] Despite the chronicity of the problem, none of these patients demonstrated permanent growth alteration of the affected limb. Return to full activity may commence after the patient has been pain free for approximately 2 to 4 weeks. Many patients, however, will have symptoms lasting longer than 6 months.

Ulnar Impaction Syndromes

Transmission of load through the triangular fibrocartilage complex and the ulna depends on the position of the wrist and forearm. Glisson found that in the neutral position, the ulna bears 15% of loads applied through the wrist. With ulnar deviation of 25° or pronation of 75°, this load increases to 24% and 37%, respectively.[21,28] Certain athletic events involve use of the hand and wrist in ulnar deviated or pronated positions. This results in an increased load transmission through the ulnar aspect of the wrist, which can lead to tears of the triangular fibrocartilage, ulnotriquetral ligament attrition, and the impaction changes of chondromalacia, subchondral sclerosis, and subchondral cyst formation of the opposing articular surfaces of the lunate, triquetrum, or ulna.[19] On physical examination, patients often have symptoms elicited over the ulnar aspect of the wrist with tenderness of the proximal lunate and triquetral region. Pain is exacerbated by forced ulnar deviation of the wrist. Radiographic examination frequently reveals an ulna-plus configuration and can show signs of sclerosis of the ulnar head,[19] the proximal lunate, or the triquetrum. Arthrography is useful in the evaluation of the triangular fibrocartilage complex.[52] MRI has been utilized for evaluation purposes as well. Treatment begins with conservative modalities, including rest, anti-inflammatory medications, and splinting. Patients that fail conservative management and have continued symptoms severe enough to limit or abolish physical activities related to the patient's sport can be considered for surgical intervention. Arthroscopic débridement of partial tears of the triangular fibrocartilage complex can be beneficial. Repair of peripheral tears of the triangular fibrocartilage complex is appropriate.[19] For patients with ulnar impaction, distal ulnar shortening should be considered for ulna-plus configuration. Return to sports participation will require healing of osteotomies in the case of ulnar shortening, followed by rehabilitation to achieve maximal strength and range of motion. Splints and taping to help prevent increased ulnar deviation and dorsiflexion can help in preventing recurrence of the ulnar impaction syndrome.

TENDINITIS AND TENDON INJURIES OF THE WRIST

Tendinitis is the most frequently reported problem requiring medical attention. Symptoms are usually attributed to overuse. The athletes typically complain of pain localized to one area that is made worse by activity. On physical examination there can be swelling noted in conjunction with tendinitis. In severe cases, a "wet leather" feeling as the tendon moves through its swollen sheath is noted. Roentgenograms typically are negative except in chronic cases, in which calcifications may be present in the soft tissue.

de Quervain's Disease

Stenosing tenosynovitis of the dorsal compartment of the wrist is a common cause of wrist pain and disability in the athlete. The pathology involves the fist extensor compartment, which contains the abductor pollicis longus, which often is divided into multiple slips, and the extensor pollicis brevis.[12] Twenty to 30 percent of the population have a fist compartment that is subdivided by a longitudinal ridge and septum into 2 tunnels.[28] Patients present with local swelling and tenderness at the radial styloid. A positive Finkelstein test, in which ulnar deviation of the wrist with the thumb adducted into the palm causes pain in the area around the radial styloid, is considered indicative of de Quervain's tenosynovitis. First-compartment tenosynovitis must also be differentiated from intersection syndrome, in which pain and swelling are found 4 cm proximal to the wrist involving the second extensor compartment. In the older athlete, degenerative changes of the carpometacarpal joint of the thumb must also be considered. Treatment consists of splinting, anti-inflammatory medications, avoidance of activity, and local steroid injection into the first dorsal compartment. Patients who fail a 6-week trial of conservative therapy may then be considered for surgical intervention. Surgery involves adequate decompression of the first dorsal extensor compartment. Frequently there are multiple slips of the abductor pollicis longus and the extensor pollicis brevis may be in a separate tunnel. Care should be taken that all slips of both tendons are released.[42] Attention to the superficial sensory branches of the radial nerve is quite important. Taping or splinting can be utilized as needed for comfort following return to sports. We generally allow return to sports participation as soon as the athlete feels comfortable.

Intersection Syndrome

The intersection syndrome involves pain in the area where the abductor pollicis longus and extensor pollicis brevis of the first compartment cross over the underlying wrist extensors. This syndrome had been described in gymnasts and weight lifters as well as in oarsmen secondary to the repetitive wrist activity required for these sports. Swelling and tenderness are noted over the dorsal radial aspect of the forearm typically 4 to 6 cm proximal to Lister's tubercle.[19] Crepitus or the "wet leather" feeling distinguishes this syndrome and actually may result in an audible "squeak." Cooney described a syndrome of inflammation of Wood's bursa, which he termed "squeaker's syndrome" because of the occasionally audible tendon rub that sounds like a squeak.[14] Treatment initially includes splinting in neutral or slight dorsiflexion, anti-inflammatory medications, local heat, and restriction of activity. If symptoms persist, local corticosteroid injections can be useful. If conservative therapy fails, surgical exploration for lysis of adhesions can be considered, but this is rarely necessary in our experience.

Subluxation of the Extensor Carpi Ulnaris

Subluxation of the extensor carpi ulnaris has been noted in several athletic activities.[11] It is heralded by a painful snap over the dorsal ulnar aspect of the wrist. It typically occurs with supination and ulnar deviation. The injury results from rupture of the ulnar portion of the septum of the sixth dorsal compartment, which then allows the extensor carpi ulnaris to subluxate in supination. The subluxation can be reduced with pronation of the wrist and forearm. On clinical examination, supination and pronation will cause the subluxation and reduction, respectively. In the acute setting, patients can be treated with immobilization in a long arm cast with the wrist in pronation to reduce the tendon.[71] This immobilization can continue for 6 weeks, at which time therapy and splinting can be utilized. Chronic cases may respond to taping of the wrist and hand to prevent the exaggerated position leading to the subluxation. If the patient continues to have subluxation, then the fibro-osseous tunnel can be reconstructed utilizing a flap of the extensor retinaculum, as described by Spinner and Kaplan.[62] For the athlete to return to a particular sport, we require that range of motion and strength reach 80% of the level of the opposite extremity.

Flexor Carpi Ulnaris and Flexor Carpi Radialis Tendinitis

Tendinitis involving the wrist flexors has been noted with increasing frequency because of the repetitive nature of many athletic events and the increased importance put upon athletic endeavors, with more and more practice sessions. On physical examination, patients will have localized swelling and tenderness in the region of the wrist flexor. There will be increased pain with resisted wrist flexion and resisted radial or ulnar deviation depending upon which tendon is primarily involved. This form of tendinitis frequently can co-exist with other conditions of the wrist, such as arthritis at the scaphotrapezial articulation, scaphoid fractures, and carpal tunnel syndrome. As a diagnostic maneuver, injection of local anesthetic into the painful area or corticosteroid into the painful area frequently can help to resolve symptoms, along with a splinting program and anti-inflammatory medication. The wrist is splinted in a neutral position to limit the inciting activities. Further diagnostic studies can include plain roentgenography, which may show evidence of calcification at the insertion of the flexor carpi ulnaris or flexor carpi radialis tendon or may show evidence of scaphotrapezial arthritis, scaphoid fracture, or arthritis at the pisotriquetral joint. For cases that do not respond to conservative care, surgery may be necessary to excise calcific deposits and release the flexor sheath. For severe cases involving the flexor carpi ulnaris, excision of the pisiform may be necessary.[53] The patient may return to sports participation as soon as full range of motion and strength return, usually within 4 to 6 weeks following surgery.

GANGLION

The ganglion is the most common soft tissue mass involving the hand and wrist. Patients will often present with a tender palpable soft-tissue mass on the dorsum and occasionally on the volar aspect of the wrist. The majority of ganglia arise from periscaphoid articulations. Treatment can involve aspiration with installation of corticosteroid. The recurrence rate following this procedure is 50%, however.[28] In athletes who will be continuing with repetitive stress on the wrist, the failure rate is even higher. Surgical treatment involves excision of the ganglion, including its stalk and capsular base. With this technique a success rate of over 90% should be expected. Volar ganglia often are intermingled with the branches of the radial artery, and very careful dissection to avoid injury to the radial artery as well as the palmar cutaneous branch of the median nerve should be used. Excision of dorsal ganglia can be associated with irritation of the sensory branch of the radial nerve. For athletes we recommend rehabilitation for another 2 to 4 weeks to regain strength and motion, at which time they may return to their particular sport with taping to prevent excessive forces on the wrist.

CARPAL VASCULAR THROMBOSIS

Blunt trauma to the palm can lead to the development of thrombosis in the ulnar artery at Guyon's canal or irritate the persistent median artery in the carpal tunnel.[16,39] This will incite an acute neuropathy that frequently requires early surgical intervention. The sensory branches of the ulnar nerve are typically affected. Occasionally, the median nerve may be affected. Patients may present with a tender mass in the hypothenar region. Patients may also have ischemic symptoms with pallor and numbness resulting from compression of the adjacent nerves. Arterial thrombosis occurs secondary to blunt trauma sustained during athletic activity. Occasionally, thrombosis can occur secondary to fractures of the hook of the hamate.[13] On physical examination, some patients will have positive Tinel's sign in the region of the ulnar nerve. Allen's test will show abnormal filling through the ulnar artery as compared with brisk refilling through the radial artery. Ultrasonography and angiography can also help in establishing the diagnosis. Surgical intervention involves removal of the thrombosed portion. Some investigators have recommended reanastomosis or grafting to re-establish blood flow.[26] Numerous studies have demonstrated that simple resection, however, is curative.[27] Typically, patients are restricted from athletic participation for 6 weeks after surgery. The region of the palm is then protected with taping or splinting for approximately 3 months after surgery.

FRACTURES OF THE HAND

Fractures involving the phalanges and metacarpals are quite common injuries in the athlete. There are no differences in the types of fractures seen in the athlete as compared to the nonathletic population. The difference is that with the athlete the treatment may be altered somewhat in order to allow earlier return to competition. It is important, however, to keep in mind that the treatment should not jeopardize the eventual outcome following fracture healing. Rotation as well as angulation must be assessed carefully. When the fingers are flexed, they should point toward the region of the scaphoid tubercle just inside the thenar crease. Most fractures of the phalanges and metacarpals can be treated with simple immobilization. It is important to realize anatomic relationships when immobilizing the hand. The unique shape of the metacarpal head allows for a cam effect by which the collateral ligaments tighten with flexion at the metacarpophalangeal (MCP) joint. Thus, injuries that require immobilization across the MCP joint should be immobilized with the MCP joint in at least 50° to 70° of flexion. Similarly the intrinsic-plus position should dictate that the digits at the interphalangeal joints be placed in slight flexion. Fractures involving the index and middle finger metacarpals have much less forgiveness than those involving the ring and little fingers because of the relatively immobile carpometacarpal joints of the former 2 digits. Careful clinical evaluation should be performed on all athletes presenting with swelling, pain and deformity in the hand. Injury to the soft tissue, including neurologic and vascular structures as well as tendinous structures, should not be overlooked when a fracture is being assessed. To prevent infection, open wounds should not be probed on the sidelines. These patients should be taken to a proper area for cleansing of the wound, careful evaluation clinically, and then finally evaluation of the open wound. Radiographic evaluation should include at least posteroanterior, lateral, and oblique views of the hand. A lateral view of the hand in 10° of supination is useful for identifying injuries to the more ulnar digits, whereas a lateral view in 10° pronation can be useful for the more radial digits. There are many options avalable for the treatment of phalangeal and metacarpal fractures. No single method of treatment should be applied to all fractures involving the phalanges and metacarpals. The various modes of treatment fall into 3 broad categories. These are closed reduction, closed reduction and fixation, and open reduction and fixation. Most fractures can be treated by closed reduction and simple immobilization. The fracture must be stable after reduction in order for this method to be succesful. In general, transverse fractures fall into this category. Spiral or oblique fractures are somewhat more unstable and it may not be possible to hold them with simple splinting or casting. For those fractures that can be reduced closed, but are unstable, closed reduction and percutaneous pin fixation is quite useful and causes less soft-tissue damage than open reduction and internal fixation. For those fractures in which closed reduction is unsuccessful, open reduction and internal fixation should be utilized. This is especially the case in fractures involving the articular surfaces. The use of the AO system is technically quite difficult and there is a very narrow margin for error. In this section, we will attempt to address the more commonly seen fracture patterns and their treatment.

Fractures of the Distal Phalanx

Fractures of the distal phalanx are typically seen following crush-type injuries. Many of these injuries involve lacerations of the nail bed and thus would be classified as open fractures that require special treatment. If the nail plate is intact and a subungual hematoma is noted, this should be evacuated. This can be done either with a paper clip that has been heated or a small battery-operated disposable cautery. The nail bed will heal nicely in closed injuries. For open injuries with nail bed damage, the nail bed should be carefully repaired using 6–0 absorbable sutures with loupe magnification. The wound should be irrigated and with the open nature of the fracture, antibiotics should be given to the patient at the time of nail bed repair and for 48 hours post-nail bed repair. For those patients that suffer avulsion of the nail plate at its base, it should be carefully removed, scrubbed, and sutured back into place. This will help serve as a protective splint. It usually takes about 3 to 4 months for a new nail to grow. The common tuff fracture needs merely simple protection for comfort. Shaft fractures of the distal phalanx are usually stable and can be treated with a simple dorsal or volar splint. Mallet finger injuries will be discussed later with tendon injuries.

Middle and Proximal Phalanx Fractures

Fractures involving the phalanges can involve the shaft or be intra-articular, involving either the base or the condyles. Truly undisplaced intra-articular fractures may be treated by careful splinting. Frequent clinical and radiographic evaluations are important to ensure that fracture displacement does not occur. For displaced intra-articular fractures, anatomic reduction of the joint surface is necessary. This often requires open reduction and internal fixation. Fractures involving the condyles of the proximal or middle phalanges are typically unstable and require fixation. Large fragments may be fixed with AO mini-fragment screws. Otherwise, Kirschner wires provide quite adequate fixation. Fractures of the base of the phalanx usually represent avulsion of the collateral ligament. Small or nondisplaced fragments can be managed with buddy taping. Fragments involving more than 25% of the articular surface or displaced more than 2 mm away from the base of the proximal phalanx are best treated with open reduction and internal fixation. Severely comminuted intra-articular fractures are a difficult problem for the hand surgeon. They are usually the result of a so-called jamming injury. Open reduction and internal fixation should only be attempted when the treating surgeon believes that this is efficacious. For those fractures that are too severely comminuted for individual fixation, traction or external fixation with traction in an effort to restore the joint congruity is probably the best method. Transverse fractures are, in general, stable. These may be treated with splints that immobilize a joint above and a joint below. Spiral or long oblique fractures are sometimes unstable. If successful closed reduction is not possible, we prefer percutaneous pin fixation with smooth Kirschner wires. If a satisfactory closed reduction cannot be achieved, then we use open reduction and internal fixation, preferably with AO mini-fragment lag-screw fixation, however, Kirschner wire fixation is adequate. Transverse fractures of the neck of the proximal or middle phalanx are often easily reduced, but difficult to hold. If a reduction can be obtained and maintained, we will follow these closely. If any evidence of loss of reduction is noted, then they would best be treated with percutaneous pin fixation or open reduction and internal fixation. Intra-articular fractures of the metacarpal are less common than phalangeal intra-articular fractures. For head fractures that are displaced, open reduction and internal fixation is the best treatment. For minimally displaced fractures, closed treatment with early motion is possible. For severely comminuted metacarpal head fractures, traction may yield the best results. The most commonly seen metacarpal fracture is probably that of the metacarpal neck, the so-called boxer's fracture. Because of the amount of motion granted at the carpometacarpal joint of the little and ring fingers, more angulation is acceptable. Most investigators agree that 30° of apex dorsal angulation is acceptable in the ring finger and up to 40° is acceptable in the small finger.[28] No more than 10° to 15° is acceptable for the index or middle fingers. Transverse metacarpal shaft fractures can be difficult to hold. In general, 20° of angulation is acceptable for the small finger, 10° for the ring finger, and only slight angulation for the middle and index fingers. For border digits percutaneous Kirschner wires fixing the metacarpal to the adjacent intact metacarpal may be all that is necessary. Spiral fractures of the metacarpal shaft usually do not tend to angulate. Up to 5 mm of shortening is believed to be acceptable to most investigators.[28] Careful attention to rotation should be paid. Fractures involving the thumb metacarpal shaft may allow for up to 30° of angulation because of the great range of motion afforded to the thumb. One of the most commonly talked about fractures is Bennett's fracture.[28] This is an intra-articular fracture. The shaft is subluxed dorsally by the pull of the abductor pollicis longus on this fracture. It is typically difficult to hold anatomic reduction with any sort of cast. The treatment options thus include closed reduction and percutaneous pin fixation or open reduction and internal fixation. If adequate reduction cannot be obtained by closed reduction then open reduction and internal fixation would be our choice. This may either be performed with Kirschner wires or AO screws. Patients suffering multiple fractures within the same hand often need stable internal fixation, as there is often associated soft tissue injury. These fractures represent a greater risk to the hand for stiffness than isolated fractures. Rigid internal fixation will allow early range of motion exercises of the finger to prevent stiffness. Protective splinting should be utilized for an adequate period when return to sports participation following rehabilitation will apply great stresses to the hand.

DISLOCATIONS AND LIGAMENTOUS INJURIES IN THE HAND

Dislocations and ligamentous injuries in the hand are probably the most common athletic injuries of the entire upper extremity. They range in complexity from the simple "jam injury" to the complex irreducible MCP joint dislocation. Evaluation of the patient with a swollen, painful proximal interphalangeal (PIP) or MCP joint begins with testing for the point of maximal tenderness to determine the site of injury. Following this determination, the joint should be tested for stability of the collateral ligaments and the volar plate. Radiographs of the digit are quite useful in determining the extent of injury. Small chip fractures can leave clues as to injuries of the collateral ligaments, volar plate, or tendons. Stress radiographs can be used to differentiate partial from complete collateral ligament tears. It has been concluded that laxity greater than 20° is diagnostic of complete ligament rupture.[35] Athletes are particularly prone to injuries of the collateral ligaments of the distal joints. The most common mechanism is longitudinal force created by a ball striking the end of the finger or "jamming" the digits into an opposing player. These injuries are quite common in basketball, softball, and soccer. Initially, the collateral ligament is stressed, leading to partial or complete rupture. Further force may lead to dislocation of the joint. Pain, swelling, and loss of motion are typically noted following the "jamming" injury. For partial tears, most agree that buddy taping for 3 to 6 weeks is quite adequate. The patient may be allowed to participate when soreness allows. Active motion is encouraged from the outset. The treatment of complete tears of the collateral ligaments is somewhat more controversial. It has been shown that continuous buddy taping for 6 weeks leads to acceptable outcome in the majority of complete collateral ligament ruptures involving the PIP joint.[28] The surgical repair of collateral ligaments is delicate to say the least. Some investigators recommend surgical repair for complete rupture of the radial collateral ligament of the index finger, where the stability is of the utmost importance. Isolated injury of the collateral ligament of the MCP joint is relatively uncommon. Most of these injuries appear to involve the radial collateral ligament. The mechanism of injury is usually an ulnarly directed force on the MCP joint of the athlete. On physical examination, tenderness may be noted in the web space between 2 metacarpal heads. Pain with stressing of the MCP joint will be noted in the vicinity of the collateral ligament. Radiographs may demonstrate a small fragment that has been avulsed from the metacarpal head. Treatment for those injuries not involving significant avulsion fractures involves splinting of the joint in 60° of flexion for 3 weeks. If there is a large fragment that shows displacement greater than 2 mm, or if the fragment involves more than 25% of the articular surface, it should be reduced and fixated through operative methods. Many of these injuries are missed in the acute setting and thus present in the chronic setting. At this point, there are several treatment options. Initially, a period of immobilization with steroid injection may relieve symptoms. If the pain persists, the surgical intervention may be necessary. There are 2 main choices: ligament reconstruction and ligament resection.

Dorsal Dislocation of the Proximal Interphalangeal Joint

Dorsal dislocation is by far the most common type of dislocation of the PIP joint. Physicians often do not see the finger in the dislocated position because of the fact that trainers and coaches frequently will "fight" over the opportunity to reduce the player's dislocated finger. It is imperative for the treating physician to determine the initial displacement of the finger as dorsal or volar. The treatment options are vastly different for the 2 different entities. The mechanism of injury is typically that of axial loading causing hyperextension of the joint. In order for the dorsal dislocation to occur, the volar plate must be torn either directly from the bone or by avulsion along with a small chip of bone.

Occasionally excessive scarring will occur at the site of the volar plate injury, producing a flexion contracture, which McCue has referred to as a pseudoboutonniere deformity.[47] Treatment of the uncomplicated dorsal dislocation is directed toward healing of the volar plate while preventing recurrent dislocation. A volar splint in 25° of flexion will allow return to participation in most sports. Splinting can be continued for up to 2 weeks followed by buddy taping until painless motion is possible. Some investigators recommend only buddy taping for 3 to 6 weeks for stable uncomplicated dislocations.[28] For those patients suffering damage to the proximal membranous portion of the volar plate producing a pseudoboutonniere deformity, dynamic splinting to correct the PIP joint flexion contracture is necessary. A reverse knuckle-bender splint or a safety-pin-type splint is useful in these cases. For deformities resistant to stretching that maintain beyond 40° of flexion contracture, surgical treatment as described by McCue and coworkers may be necessary.[47]

Volar Dislocation of the Proximal Interphalangeal Joint

Pure volar dislocation of the PIP joint is a relatively uncommon injury. For this type of dislocation to occur, the central slip must be disrupted, creating the potential for a boutonniere deformity. Most investigators now choose to treat this form of dislocation with closed methods following reduction.[28] The presence of a small dorsal chip fracture at the base of the middle phalanx is not an indication for open reduction and internal fixation, unless it is significantly displaced and is not reduced with PIP joint extension. For the uncomplicated volar dislocation, we immobilize the PIP joint in full extension for 6 weeks in combination with active and passive flexion exercises of the distal interphalangeal (DIP) joint, similar to the treatment of a boutonniere lesion. Significantly displaced dorsal avulsion fractures should be openly reduced and fixated as this represents a disruption of the central slip. For the athlete to return to sports participation, splinting must be maintained for 6 weeks. This is difficult in many types of ball-handling sports. It is important for the patient to follow the exercise for the DIP joint to help prevent volar displacement of the lateral bands.

Rotary Subluxation of the Proximal Interphalangeal Joint

Rotary subluxation of the PIP joint is quite uncommon.[28] The mechanism of injury is typically a twisting-type force applied to the digit. This results in buttonholing of one condyle of the head of the proximal phalanx through a tear in the extensor hood between the central slip and the lateral band. These latter structures usually are intact. Radiographically, the lateral view is of utmost importance. A true lateral film of both the proximal phalanx and middle phalanx will not be possible as one will be rotated owing to the rotary subluxation. These dislocations are sometimes irreducible by closed methods. To reduce these dislocations the MCP and PIP joints should be flexed to 90°.[20] This helps to relax the volarly displaced lateral band and allows the condyle to disengage. Successful reduction should be confirmed by postreduction radiographs. Full active and passive motion of the PIP joint is then allowed. We treat injuries with buddy taping and early motion. The buddy taping should be continued for 3 to 6 weeks. If the subluxation cannot be reduced with closed methods, then open reduction will be required through a curved dorsal incision. It is typically easy to reduce the condyle under direct vision by retracting the lateral band from its position about the condyle. Careful inspection of the collateral ligaments should be performed at the time of open reduction. Postoperatively a splint is worn on the involved digit for 2 weeks and then early range of motion is begun with buddy taping for 2 to 4 weeks.

Dorsal Fracture/Dislocations of the Proximal Interphalangeal Joint

Dorsal fracture/dislocations of the PIP joint typically result from longitudinal compression-type injuries. When the volar articular surface of the base of the middle phalanx is fractured, the remaining portion of the middle phalanx subluxes dorsal to the head of the proximal phalanx. If the fracture fragment involves less than 40% of the articular surface then these are typically stable following closed reduction, as the collateral ligaments will still be attached to the majority of the middle phalanx.[28] Clinically, the PIP joint is swollen and there is severe pain with attempted motion. Radiographs are of the utmost importance to diagnose the accompanying fracture with the dislocation. For fractures that are reducible with closed techniques and remain stable, dorsal extension block splinting as described by McElfresh and colleagues is quite useful and yields good results. Postreduction films in the splint should show congruent reduction. The "V" sign described by Light is present when an inadequate reduction has occurred.[41] If the radiographs reveal a satisfactory reduction a short arm cast may be applied incorporating a 1-inch-wide padded aluminum splint extending over the dorsum of the involved digit. The PIP joint is splinted in the degree of flexion required to maintain a congruent reduction. This typically is about 50° to 60° initially. The proximal phalanx must be held firmly with tape, thus allowing PIP joint flexion, but not extension beyond the selected degree. The patient should be followed at weekly intervals to ensure that congruent reduction is maintained. The flexion can be reduced by approximately 10° to 15° each week so that at the end of the 4 to 6 weeks of treatment, full extension has been achieved. At the time of splint removal, buddy taping is then instituted for an additional 2 to 3 weeks. For patients in whom a satisfactory closed reduction cannot be achieved or maintained, open reduction or volar plate arthroplasty as described by Eaton should be undertaken.[20] Recently, we have utilized a dynamic PIP external fixator (Biomet, Warsaw, Ind.) with excellent results.

Dorsal Dislocation of the Metacarpophalangeal Joint

Dorsal dislocations of the MCP joint can be either simple or complex. It is extremely important to determine whether the dislocation is a simple subluxation that can be reduced by closed manipulation or a complex irreducible dislocation. If one attempts longitudinal traction and further hyperextension to reduce a simple dislocation it can very easily be turned into a complex irreducible dislocation. Most investigators agree that the most important factor in irreducibility is the interposition of the volar plate between the proximal phalanx and the head of the metacarpal.[33] If further hyperextension or longitudinal traction is applied, the volar plate can be "sucked" into the joint space, leading to an irreducible dislocation pattern. Closed reduction of the MCP subluxation is undertaken with the wrist and interphalangeal joints in flexion to relax the flexor tendons. The base of the proximal phalanx is then pushed volarly across the articular surface of the metacarpal head, keeping the phalanx in contact with the head of the metacarpal throughout the entire maneuver to prevent re-entrapment of the volar plate. Following reduction, radiographs should be taken to confirm the reduction and rule out associated fractures. Postreduction, a short period of immobilization with the MCP joint in 50° to 70° of flexion is acceptable. Many investigators advocate immediate active motion utilizing buddy taping to prevent hyperextension.[28]

Irreducible MCP dislocations are thought to be secondary to interposition of the volar plate between the base of the proximal phalanx and the head of the metacarpal, as described by Kaplan.[33] The metacarpal head is thought also to be caught in a buttonhole position between the constriction of the flexor tendon and lumbrical volarly. On clinical examination, the exaggerated hyperextension position seen in simple subluxations will not be noted. For complete dislocation, the joint is only slightly hyperextended, with the proximal phalanx lying on the dorsum of the metacarpal head. A typical finding for complex dislocations also is that of puckering of the volar skin. Radiographic evaluation will often show a sesamoid trapped within a widened joint space. The sesamoid is situated within the volar plate and thus is a sign of entrapment of the volar plate within the joint.[28] Treatment initially consists of an attempt at closed reduction, even if puckering is noted. If closed reduction fails, then an open reduction should be undertaken. The dorsal approach is thought to be a safer approach because it avoids the neurovascular bundle situated on the volar aspect just beneath the puckered skin.[28] If there is a concomitant fracture of the metacarpal head, the dorsal approach tends to provide better access as well. Other investigators have advocated the volar approach because it is a more direct approach to the pathology, since the volar plate is entrapped within the joint.[33] Postoperatively, a bulky hand dressing is applied, which allows early motion of the hand. Buddy taping is continued for 3 to 4 weeks to prevent hyperextension.

Volar Dislocation of the Metacarpophalangeal Joint

Volar dislocations of the MCP joint are quite rare.[71] Closed reduction may be attempted by hyperflexing the MCP joint and pushing the proximal phalanx back into place. Failure to achieve a congruent reduction is an indication for open reduction. Some investigators have noted that both volar and dorsal exposures are necessary, however, most would attempt a volar incision first and then perform dorsal exposure if necessary.[28,71]

Ulnar Collateral Ligament Rupture

Rupture of the ulnar collateral ligament, known as gamekeeper's thumb or skier's thumb, is one of the most common injuries to the thumb. The mechanism of the injury is usually a fall on the outstretched hand. This can commonly occur in skiing, softball, soccer, or any activity in which the hand is put at risk. In field hockey and lacrosse, ulnar collateral injuries can occur when players fall on their sticks. Most ruptures occur at the distal portion of the ligament. They can also occur with avulsion of a small fragment of the bony insertion from the base of the proximal phalanx. The ulnar collateral ligament and the accessory collateral ligament form a box with their connection to the volar plate. The volar plate contributes to stability in extension. Stener found that a torn ulnar collateral ligament reflected proximally in 25 of 39 patients in whom he explored the ligament following disruption.[63] He further found that the ligament protruded from beneath the proximal edge of the adductor aponeurosis, blocking realignment of the disrupted ulnar collateral ligament, which precluded closed treatment. Clinically, patients will present complaining of an extension abduction-type injury. They will have pain localized to the region of the ulnar collateral ligament. Further physical examination may find a palpable swelling at the proximal edge of the adductor aponeurosis consistent with a Stener lesion.[63] The stability of the MCP joint should be tested in flexion to isolate the ulnar collateral ligament and in extension to assess the accessory ligament as well as the volar plate. Palmer and Louis showed that the MCP joint opens at least 35° following sectioning of the ulnar collateral ligament and adductor aponeurosis. Comparison should be made with the uninjured thumb. Anteroposterior and lateral roentgenograms are also necessary as the ligament can be avulsed through bone. Injuries with less than 35° of instability may be treated with thumb spica cast. The thumb should be immobilized for 3 weeks and then placed in a protective spica splint for an additional 2 weeks to allow rehabilitative exercises outside the splint. Injuries that result in greater MCP joint instability should be treated surgically because of the high incidence of Stener lesions.[63] Fractures displaced more than 2 mm or rotated and fractures involving greater than 25 percent of the articular surface also should be repaired. Those fractures displaced more than 5 mm can present with a Stener-type lesion owing to the proximal displacement.[48] Chronic reconstruction has not been as successful as early surgery and this is another reason for earlier surgical intervention. Protective taping can be utilized once the patient has finished this period of spica cast immobilization and spica splinting as for uncomplicated sprain injuries. Taping should continue as long as the patient has soreness with abduction and extension of the thumb.

Radial Collateral Ligament Rupture

Radial collateral ligament injuries are much less common than those of the ulnar collateral ligament. There does not appear to be a situation analogous to the Stener lesion on the radial side of the thumb. Theoretically, nonoperative treatment for complete ruptures of the radial collateral ligament would be more likely to be successful. Some investigators, however, still advocate primary repair for complete ruptures.[72] Following either conservative or surgical intervention, immobilization in a thumb spica cast for 3 to 4 weeks is required followed by a splinting and taping program similar to that outlined for ulnar collateral ligament injury.

Carpometacarpal Joint Injuries

The articular surfaces of the carpometacarpal (CMC) joint of the thumb appear as 2 opposed saddles. The concave nature of these articular surfaces affords a degree of inherent stability to the joint. Roentgenographs are useful to rule out the more common Bennett's fracture/dislocation. Posteroanterior radiographs of both thumbs with the distal phalanges pressed firmly together to stress the CMC joint are useful in defining partial tears of the volar ligament. Treatments of the partial injuries involve immobilization in a thumb spica cast. For complete dislocation, closed reduction should be performed; a spica cast also can be utilized. The patient should be followed regularly to ensure that congruous reduction is maintained. If the metacarpal is not well seated, then Kirschner wires can be used to ensure reduction. If with closed reduction and pinning there is still a tendency for the metacarpal to sit in a dorsal or lateral position then open reduction and reconstruction of the volar ligament should be undertaken. Most investigators utilize the flexor carpi radialis tendon split longitudinally to reconstruct the volar ligament, as described by Eaton.[20] Following either conservative or surgical treatment, protective splinting should continue until full strength and motion has been achieved. Taping can be utilized as long as there is soreness with abduction or extension of the first metacarpal.

TENDON INJURIES IN THE HAND

Mallet Finger

The mechanism of injury for mallet finger is thought to be forceful flexion of the DIP joint.

The injury usually occurs when the extensor tendon is taut, as in catching a ball or striking an object unexpectedly with the finger extended. The forcible flexion leads to disruption of the extensor tendon as it inserts into the dorsal base of the distal phalanx. The tendon fibers may be stretched ruptured or may avulse a small fragment of the distal phalanx. Radiographs are needed to assess for volar subluxation when a large bony fragment has been avulsed. Clinical examination will reveal tenderness over the DIP joint and a droop of the distal phalanx. Typically, there is a 10° to 20° loss of extension in partial injuries and a 40° to 60° loss of extension for complete ruptures. Most investigators now agree that only the DIP joint needs to be immobilized.[28] Several methods of splinting are available, including a dorsal padded splint, a volar padded splint, and a Stack plastic splint. We prefer a custom-molded splint to hold the DIP joint in extension. In special cases, percutaneous Kirschner-wire fixation across the DIP joint can be utilized. The DIP joint must be held in extension continuously for 6 to 10 weeks. At no point in the process should the DIP joint be allowed to drop into flexion. At the end of the splinting process, 4 weeks of additional nighttime extension splinting of the DIP joint are necessary. Patients should be cautioned against exerting strong pressure on the DIP joint to achieve flexion following removal of the splint. A gradual increase in flexion typically occurs with time. Most patients will have some cold weather intolerance postsplinting. For mallet finger associated with avulsion of a small fragment of bone, we recommend similar conservative therapy with splinting. Even large fragments tend to remodel quite nicely. The only indication for open reduction at this time is the mallet finger associated with a volar subluxation of the distal phalanx that does not reduce with splinting. Patients with fractures treated nonoperatively have been found to have better motion than those treated surgically.[47] Athletes typically are able to perform with the splint in place. For contact sports, sometimes padding of the splint is necessary. For patients presenting with a late mallet finger, even at 2 to 3 months, splinting for 6 to 10 weeks has still been effective. Surgical options include dermodesis, reefing of the scarred tendon, or arthrodesis, which is more commonly employed for patients with post-traumatic arthritis.[28]

Flexor Digitorum Profundus Avulsion

Avulsion of the flexor digitorum profundus (FDP) tendon is a common injury in athletes.

The classic mechanism is grabbing the jersey of an opponent, hence the common name, "jersey finger." The ring finger is the most frequently injured finger. Leddy and Packer identified 3 different types of FDP avulsion.[38] Type I injuries retract into the palm. This severs the blood supply to the tendon and leads to extensive scarring within the tendon sheath. With time, the distal end of the retracted tendon softens and deteriorates. Repair within 7 to 10 days is required. Type II injuries are typically entrapped at the chiasma of the flexor digitorum superficialis. Sometimes a small fleck of avulsed bone can be seen on the lateral radiograph. The blood supply from the vincula is intact with this type of injury, thus deterioration of the tendon is less likely. Treatment for type II injuries can be done as late as 3 months after injury. Type III injuries involve a large bony fragment avulsed from the base of the distal phalanx. This usually is lodged at the level of the A4 pulley. Similar to type II injury, the blood supply is intact with these as well. Patients present with tenderness, usually greatest over the stump of the FDP tendon. Testing of the isolated FDP will show absence of function. Radiographs should be taken in order to determine if an avulsed fragment or larger fracture from the distal phalanx is present. Operative treatment is required in order to achieve a good result. As stated previously, the blood supply to the tendon may be tenuous, therefore surgical intervention should be undertaken within 7 days. Postoperatively, the patient will have to refrain from competition until complete healing has occurred because of the forces placed upon the repair. It usually requires 8 weeks of protection prior to return to competition. Protection of the repair should be continued for at least 3 months. There are several protocols that can be utilized in the initial postoperative setting. Some surgeons prefer 3 weeks of immobilization, after which a mobilization program is set into motion. Others utilize early motion, within a few days of surgery, with splinting as described by Kleinert.[36] Many of these injuries are not seen until months after the initial incident. In the late setting, there are several options available, including doing nothing, arthrodesis of the DIP joint, tendon grafting, and a staged grafting procedure utilizing silicone rod implants.[28] Reconstruction of the FDP through or around an intact superficialis should be undertaken with some trepidation, as there is significant risk to PIP joint motion.

Boutonniere Injuries

Boutonniere injuries are caused by disruption of the central slip combined with a disruption of the triangular ligament on the dorsum of the middle phalanx. With time, the lateral bands shift to a position volar to the axis of the PIP joint and thus become flexors of the PIP joint. The deformity leads to flexion of the PIP joint with complete loss of extension. The displaced lateral bands tenodeses the DIP joint in extension limiting flexion, which becomes the most disabling portion of deformity. The patient presents with a swollen painful PIP joint and does not show the classic boutonniere deformity until later. Early diagnosis hinges on noting that the primary point of tenderness is on the dorsum of the PIP joint near the insertion of the central slip. Radiographs of the involved finger in some instances will show a small avulsion fracture arising from the dorsum of the base of the middle phalanx. Treatment in the acute stage involves splinting of the PIP joint in full extension for at least 6 weeks. Active and assisted flexion of the DIP joint is key to allow mobilization of the lateral bands and prevent their volar migration. Night splinting should continue for at least 4 weeks following the initial 6 weeks of full-time splinting. There are a number of splints available. Injuries that present with a displaced avulsion fracture of significant size and displacement require open reduction and internal fixation. It is important to repair the triangular ligament at the same time to prevent volar subluxation of the lateral bands. Postoperative splinting of the PIP joint in extension is undertaken. For chronic boutonniere injuries presenting with a fixed flexion contracture, treatment begins with dynamic splinting to achieve PIP joint extension prior to any surgical intervention that may later be needed. Mild deformities respond to conservative dynamic splinting alone. Techniques for surgical reconstruction include extensor tenotomy as described by Eaton and Littler when DIP joint flexion is of primary concern.[43] Release and dorsal shift of the lateral band as described by Littler has also been effective. For patients with marked extensor lag at the PIP joint who have severely deficient central slip, tendon grafts as described by Littler have also been useful.[28,43] Patients with adequate tendons may undergo reefing and reconstruction or shortening of the extensor tendon. Procedures involving tendon repair require 4 to 6 weeks of immobilization postoperatively. Procedures that utilize tenotomy or lysis require early active and passive range of motion exercises.

PROTECTIVE SPLINTING

The wrist and hand are exposed in almost all sporting activities, and as outlined there are many forms of injury that can occur. The goal of protective splinting is to return the athlete to participation as quickly, but safely, as possible. The splints are a calculated alteration in the traditional treatment and should only be used to allow the patient to return to the particular sport if there is no appreciable risk of compromising the healing of the particular injury. A decision must be made whether the athlete's injury can be safely protected. The simplest form of splinting is prophylactic taping. The wrist should be placed into the desired position. An underwrap is optional. The methods of taping vary, but typically a figure-of-8 technique is utilized. Taping can help to restrict motion and give support to the wrist for comfort and some protection from further injury. The wrist is positioned to relax the involved tendons. For example, radial deviation is utilized for de Quervain's disease to relax the affected tendons of the first extensor compartment. Protective splints can be molded from semirigid material such as silicone or synthetic fiberglass.[45] Trainers and physicians should be familiar with the regulations that pertain to protective splinting. Padded aluminum splints are readily available and versatile. Buddy taping of the digits can be performed easily with cloth tape.[45] It is important to place cotton or other material between the digits to avoid maceration. Premade Velcro buddy taping devices are available.

CONCLUDING REMARKS

The athlete is susceptible to a wide variety of injuries to the hand and wrist. Because of its position in front of the body, the hand is at risk in both contact and noncontact sports. Those responsible for evaluation of injuries to the athlete's hand or wrist should be familiar with the multitude of possible injuries. At times, slight departures from traditional treatment methods may be utilized to return an athlete to competition. However, these departures should never increase the risk of compromised healing or functional loss with regard to the particular injury. The tendency for injuries of the hand to be viewed as trivial is probably the primary factor leading to suboptimal results. The key to

proper care is early accurate diagnosis that allows the implementation of proper treatment.

References

1. Alho A, Kanhaanjaa U: Management of fractured scaphoid bones: A prospective study of 100 fractures. Acta Orthop Scand 46:737–43, 1975.
2. Almquist EE, Burns JF: Radial shortening for the treatment of Keinbock's Disease—a 5 to 10 year follow up. J Hand Surg 7:348–52, 1982.
3. Antuna Zapico JM: Malacia del semi lunar. Thesis, Universidad de Valladolid. Valladolid (Spain), Industrias y Editorial Sever Cuesta, 1966.
4. Armstead R B, Linscheid RL, Dobyns JH, et al: Ulnar lengthening in the treatment of Kienbock's disease. J Bone Joint Surg 64A:170–8, 1982.
5. Bartone NF, Grieco RV: Fracture of the triquetrum. J Bone Joint Surg 38A:353–6, 1956.
6. Bell R, Rhoades C: Treatment of scapholunate disassociation by dorsal capsulodesis. Presented at the American Society of Surgery of the Hand, Kansas City, 1993.
7. Bellinghausen HW, Weeks PM, Young LV, et al: Roentgen rounds No. 62. Orthop Rev 11:73, 1982.
8. Blaine ES: Lunate osteomalacia. JAMA 96:492, 1931.
9. Blatt G: Capsulodesis in reconstructive hand surgery: Dorsal capsulodesis for the unstable scaphoid and volar capsulodesis following excision of the distal ulna. Hand Clin 3:81–102, 1987.
10. Bowen TL: Injuries of the hamate bone. Hand 5:235–8, 1973.
11. Burkhart SS, Wood MB, Linscheid RL: Posttraumatic recurrent subluxation of the extensor carpi ulnaris tendon. J Hand Surg 7:1, 1982.
12. Bruman M: Stenosing tendovaginitis of the dorsal and volar compartments of the wrist. Arch Surg 65:752, 1952.
13. Bruman JL, Janes JM: Injuries of the superficial palmar arch. J Trauma 3:505–16, 1963.
14. Cooney W: Sports injuries to the upper extremity. Sports Injuries 76(4):45–50, 1984.
15. Cooney WP, Dobyns JH, Linscheid RL: Nonunion of the scaphoid. Analysis of the results from bone grafting. J Hand Surg 8:343–54, 1980.
16. Costigan DG, Riley JM Jr, Coy FE Jr: Thrombofibrosis of the ulnar artery in the palm. J Bone Joint Surg 41A:702–4, 1959.
17. Crabbe WA: Excision of the proximal row of the carpus. J Bone Surg 46B:708–11, 1964.
18. Dickinson JC, Shannon JG: Fractures of the carpal scaphoid in the Canadian Army. Surg Gynecol Obstet 79:225–39, 1944.
19. Dobyns J, Gabel G: Gymnast's Wrist. Hand Clin 6:3:493–505, 1990.
20. Eaton R: Joint Injuries of the Hand. Springfield, Ill, Charles C Thomas, 1971.
21. Eddeland A, Eiken O, Hellgren E, et al: Fractures of the scaphoid. Scand J Plast Reconstr Surg 9:234–9, 1975.
22. Gelberman RH, Bauman TD, Menon J: The vascularity of the lunate bone and Kienböck's disease. J Hand Surg 5:272–8, 1980.
23. Gelberman RH, Menon J: The vascularity of the scaphoid bone. J Bone Joint Surg 5:508–13, 1980.
24. Gelverman RH, Gross MS: The vascularity of the wrist. Clin Orthop 202:43, 1986.
25. Gellman H, Caputo RJ, Carter V, et al: Comparison of short and long thumb-spica casts for nondisplaced frac-

tures of the carpal scaphoid. J Bone Surg 71A:354–7, 1989.

26. Given KS, Puckett CL, Kleinert HE: Ulnar artery thrombosis. Plast Reconstr Surg 61:405–11, 1978.

27. Goren MD: Palmer intramural thrombosis in the ulnar artery. Calif Med 89:424–5, 1958.

28. Green DP (ed): Operative Hand Surgery, 2nd edition. New York, Churchill Livingstone, 1988.

29. Grundy M: Fractures of the carpal scaphoid in children. Br J Surg 56:523–4, 1969.

30. Herbert TJ, Fisher WE: Management of the fractured scaphoid using a new bone screw. J Bone Joint Surg 66B:114–23, 1984.

31. Hudson RM, Caragol WJ, Faye JJ: Isolated rotary subluxation of the carpal navicular. Am J Roentgenol 126:601, 1976.

32. Johnson RP: The acutely injured wrist and its residuals. Clin Orthop 149:33–44, 1980.

33. Kaplan E: Dorsal dislocation of the metacarpophalangeal joint of the index finger. J Bone Joint Surg 39:1081–6, 1957.

34. Keinböck R: Uber Traumatische Malazie Des Monbeins, Und Ihre Folfezustaude: Eufartungsformen Und Kompressions Frakturen. Fortschr Roengenstr 16:77, 1910.

35. Kiefhaber T, et al: Lateral stability of the proximal interphalangeal joint. J Hand Surg. 11:661–9, 1986.

36. Kleinert H, Verdan C: Report of the committee on tendon injuries. J Hand Surg 8:794–8, 1983.

37. Koh TJ, Grabiner MD, Weiken GG: Technique and ground reaction forces in the back handspring. Am J Sports Med 20; 61–6, 1992.

38. Leddy J, Packer J: Avulsion of the profundus tendon insertion in athletes. J Hand Surg 2:66–9, 1977.

39. Levy M, Pauker M: Carpal tunnel syndrome due to thrombosed persisting median artery. A case report. Hand 10:65–8, 1978.

40. Lichtman DM, Schneider JR, Mack GR, Swafford AR: Ulnar midcarpal instability. J Hand Surg 6:515–23 1981

41. Light T: Buttress pinning techniques. Orthop Rev 10:49–55, 1981.

42. Linscheid RL: Scapholunate ligamentous instabilities (dissociations, subdislocations, dislocations). Ann Chir Main 3:323–30, 1984.

43. Littler J, Eaton R: Redistribution of forces in the correction of the boutonniere deformity. J Bone Joint Surg 49:1267–74, 1967.

44. Marck KL: Variations of stenosing tenosynovitis at the radial styloid process. J Bone Joint Surg 33A:340, 1951.

45. Mayer V, Gieck JH: Rehabilitation of hand injuries in athletes. Clin Sports Med 5(4):783–93, 1986.

46. Mayfield JR: Mechanism of carpal injuries. Clin Orthop 149:45–54, 1980.

47. McCue FC, Meister K: Common sports hand injuries. Sports Med 15:281–9, 1993.

48. McCue F, Hakala M, Andrews J, Gieck J: Ulnar collateral ligament injuries of the thumb in athletes. J Sports Med 2:70–80, 1974.

49. Murakami S, Nakajima H: Aseptic necrosis of the capitate bone. Am J Sports Med 12 (2):170–3, 1984.

50. Nielsen PT, Hedeboe J: Posttraumatic scapholunate dissociation detected by wrist cineradiography. J Hand Surg 9A:135–8, 1984.

51. O'Brien ET: Acute fractures and dislocations of the carpus. Orthop Clin North Am 15:237–58, 1984.

52. Palmer AK, Levinsohn EM, Kuzma GR: Arthrography of the wrist. J Hand Surg 8:15–23, 1983.

53. Palmieri TJ: Pisiform area pain treatment by pisiform excision. J Hand Surg 7:477, 1982.

54. Panagis JS, Gelberman RH, Taleisnik J, Baumgartner M: The arterial anatomy of the human carpus, Part II: the interosseous vascularity. J Hand Surg 8:35, 1983.

55. Parker RD, Berkowitz MS, Brahms MA, Bohl WR: Hook of the hamate fractures in athletes. Am J Sports Med 14:517–23, 1986.

56. Perrson M: Casual treatment of lunatomalacia. Acta Chir Scand 100:531–44, 1950.

57. Peterson HA, Lipscomb PR: Intercarpal arthrodesis. Arch Surg 95:127, 1967.

58. Polivy KD, Millender LH, Newgberg A, et al: Fractures of the hook of the hamate: a failure of clinical diagnosis. J Hand Surg 10A:101–4, 1985.

59. Reagan DS, Lincheid RL, Dobyns JH: Lunotriquetral sprains. J Hand Surg 9A:502–14, 1984.

60. Roy S, Caine D, Sikger K: Stress Changes of the sital radial epiphysis in young gymnasts. Am J Sports Med 13(5):301–8, 1985.

61. Rosenwasser MP, Miyasaka KC, Strauch RJ: The Rasl procedure: reduction and association of the scaphoid and lunate using the Herbert screw. Tech Hand Upper Ext Surg No. 4, pp 263–7, December 1997.

62. Stahl F: On lunomalacia (Kienbock's disease), a clinical and roentgenological study, especially on its pathogenesis and the late results of immobilization treatment. Acta Chir Scand (Suppl) 126:1–133, 1947.

63. Stener B: Displacement of the ruptured ulnar collateral ligament of the metacarpophalangeal joint of the thumb. J Bone Joint Surg 44:869–79, 1962.

64. Taleisnik J: Management of common hand and wrist disorders. St Luke's Hospital Symposium. Houston, Tex, April 1997.

65. Trumble T, et al: A biomechanical comparison of the methods for treating Kienbock's disease. J Hand Surg 11A:88–93, 1986.

66. Watsom HK: Limited wrist arthrodesis. Clin Orthop 149:126–36, 1980.

67. Watson HK, Ballet FL: The SLAC wrist: scapholunate advanced collapse pattern of degenerative arthritis. J Hand Surg 9A:358–65, 1984.

68. Watson HK, Hempton RR: Limited wrist arthrodesis. I: The triscaphoid joint. J Hand Surg 5:320–72, 1980.

69. Watson HK, Rye J, DiBella A: An approach to Kienböck's disease: Triscaphe arthrodesis. J Hand Surg 10A:179–87, 1985.

70. Weiker G: Hand and wrist problems in the gymnast. Clin Sports Med 11(1):189–202, 1992.

71. Wood MD, Dobyns JH: Sports-related extra-articular wrist syndromes. Clin Orthop 202:93–102, 1986.

72. Woods D, et al: Radial collateral ligament injuries of the thumb metacarpophalangeal joint. AAOS Meeting, San Francisco, 1987.

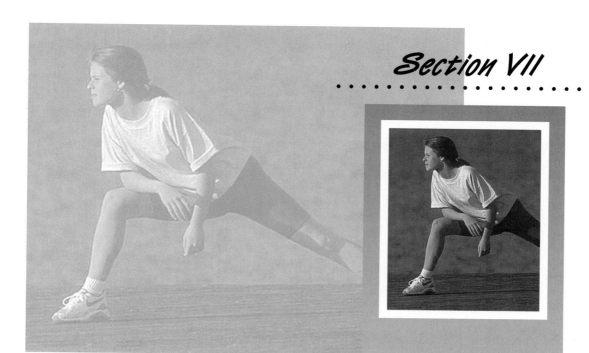

Rehabilitation and Strength Issues

Chapter 42

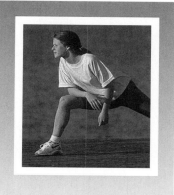

Sport-Specific Rehabilitation Programs

Susan K. Hillman, M.S., M.A.

Fortunately, injury is not common to all sports participants. However, if and when an injury does happen, the athlete encounters a number of obstacles to overcome. This chapter will address the general principles to be considered in developing a rehabilitation or "retraining" program following injury. Program design, open and closed kinetic chain exercises, sport specificity, and functional activities will be discussed.

PROGRAM DESIGN

Following injury or surgery, the involved tissues need time for repair. The tissues involved, the extent of the trauma, and the general health of the individual may affect tissue healing. The chief objective in designing a rehabilitation program is *safety*. Throughout the program, care must be taken to provide a gradual and systematic progression from the initial stage of healing to the final return to competition. The athlete, guided by the physician and sports therapist, must consider the stage of the tissue-healing process and select exercises and activities to enhance and not jeopardize the continued repair. High loads and unexpected occurrences will often be encountered by the participating athlete, yet the aim of the rehabilitation process is to sufficiently and progressively load the tissues in preparation for the unexpected nature of sport participation prior to her full return to competition.

Principles of Program Design

Each sports medicine professional will have his or her own technique of rehabilitation program design. Factors that influence the program will include skills of the therapist, time needed versus time available for one-on-one therapy, and motivation level of the patient. An attempt will be made to explain general principles and phases of typical rehabilitation programs. Keep in mind, each athlete will be different; your task is to suit the program to the needs of the athlete.

Principle One: Focus on the Therapeutic Objectives

Always select exercises that are consistent with the objectives of the particular stage of the reconditioning process. The athlete is usually a very busy person; often her class schedule, work schedule, and personal time conflict with the rehabilitation time. If possible, provide exercises that relate directly to one or more of the therapeutic objectives for that time period. If you are unfamiliar with the exact objectives during a period of time in the reconditioning process, consult the orthopedic surgeon for his or her objectives for the athlete.

Principle Two: Vary the Exercises and Challenges

Considering the fact that most athletes are highly competitive, active individuals, an injury that sidelines them from participation can be devastating. One common problem found in many reconditioning programs is a lack of variety. In the early stages of the recovery process, competitive challenges certainly would not be wise, yet each activity and exercise employed should contribute to a goal, and those activities should be varied. If the program fails to challenge the athlete or if it becomes boring and repetitious the athlete often fails to follow through with the program, and less than satisfactory return to sport results. To avoid losing motivation of the athlete through the rehabilitation program, the exercises should be varied on a daily basis. No two programs should be allowed to be exactly alike; each visit should be a new adventure while the goals of the program remain the focus.

Principle Three: Properly Utilize the Kinetic Chain

All exercises and skills can be analyzed according to the *kinetic chain*. Kinetic energy is energy produced by movement; a series of body segments connected by joints can be envisioned as a chain. The kinetic chain thus may be described as the movement of body segments. Movement produced by the foot while the athlete is seated, as in knee extension (Fig. 42-1), represents the *open kinetic chain*; movement of the athlete's body over the stationary foot, as in a squat exercise (Fig. 42-2), represents the *closed kinetic chain.*

The importance of the kinetic chain in developing an exercise program can be clearly understood as one evaluates the function of the body during the sport skills to be performed. Additionally, one must realize that muscles work differently when the chain is open as opposed to when the chain is closed. In general, during closed kinetic chain exercise, more muscle activity occurs, more coordination and balance (proprioception) is required, and the exercise often resembles a motor pattern found in the particular sport for which the athlete is training. These principles are of particular concern in working

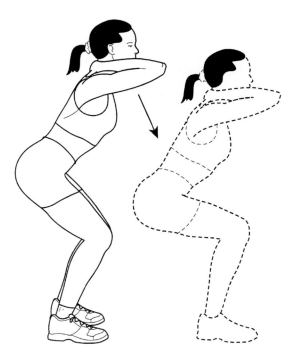

Figure 42-2. The squat exercise.

with the lower extremity, leading one to realize the importance of closed kinetic chain exercises during the rehabilitation process. On the other hand, the upper-extremity skill patterns used in most sports involve a large range of motion with tremendous speed of motion. Less balance and little weight bearing is needed of the upper extremities in the racket and throwing sports. Thus, exercises involving the open kinetic chain will prove to be most functional and sport specific, yet to enhance the stability of the joint one might employ closed kinetic chain exercises.

Principle Four: Follow the KISS Principle

Throughout the reconditioning process, the major focus should always be to return to competitive form in a specific sport. Many exercises can be found that fail to have any direct application to any sport skill. Some such exercises are essential for building a strong base (see discussion of resistance training, below), however, the majority of exercises should be functional and sport specific—thus the KISS principle: "keep it sport specific."

Principle Five: Always Provide a Progression

Throughout the process of reconditioning the athlete, a progression must be provided. An

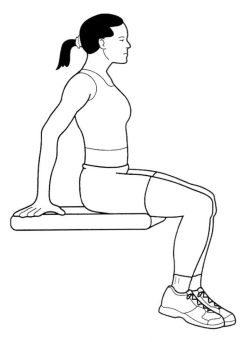

Figure 42-1. Knee extension exercise.

exercise that has no subsequent exercise or skill has no place in a well-planned reconditioning program. Progressions are increases. Increases may be of weight lifted, repetitions performed, minutes sustained, distance thrown, and height jumped, among others. Each step in the progression must be clearly understood and measured if possible. In moving from a low level up the progression ladder, single increases should be made. It would not be wise to increase both the weight being lifted and the number of repetitions being performed. It would be equally unwise to increase both the speed of a throw and the distance being thrown. Single increases not only reduce the pain and soreness associated with increases in activity, but also allow a better understanding of the cause of difficulty if problems arise.

An excellent example of a progression for a throwing athlete can be seen in all levels of baseball. The athlete begins at a shortened distance, throwing a set number of repetitions at a predetermined speed (half speed, for example) with a specified rest period between sets of throws. The progression increases the number of sets thrown but keeps all other parameters the same. After the athlete satisfactorily performs the number of sets at that initial distance, the distance is increased but the number of sets is reduced to the original starting point. The progression is repeated at that distance and the entire process continues until the athlete is able to throw from her game position with ease and accuracy. Using the baseball throwing program as a model, a possible progression for the overhead in tennis is expressed in Table 42-1.

This sample program illustrates the concept of progressing the athlete while keeping as many variables as consistent as possible. The tennis overhead is dependent on a well-placed ball to hit. During stages 1 and 3, a ball machine is used to project the ball to the athlete. The ball projection speed should be set to "lob" the ball to the athlete. During the stage 2 and stage 4 practices, an assistant is used to project the balls to the athlete. This assistant should be highly skilled in the sport to provide as much control as possible and should attempt to project the ball with the same speed and line of projection as practiced in the previous stage using the ball machine.

Similar progressions may be developed for any specific sport skill, keeping in mind the variables that can be controlled and varying only 1 element in each phase.

STAGES OF THE REHABILITATION PROGRAM

Each rehabilitation program may be divided into 3 major stages: the early stage (tissue healing), the middle stage (range of motion and motor control), and the final late stage (resistance training and functional activities). These stages are followed by the return to sport participation. In the following sections, objectives of each stage of the process are identified and suggestions for exercises introduced.

Early Stage: The Healing Phase

The principal objective of this stage of the reconditioning process is to provide an environment for healing. During this period the athlete rests and the injured part is often immobilized by a cast, brace, wrap, or other means.

Following any trauma, including surgery, the involved tissues do need rest. Rest need not be total inactivity, but can be mild exercise of the noninvolved body parts. Care must be taken to follow the physician's orders regarding immobilization and weight-bearing status if applicable. Following surgery or severe trauma, rest for 4 to 6 weeks is not uncommon, although the athlete may be permitted to exercise the noninvolved extremities or the cardiovascular system if that exercise does not jeopardize the healing of the injured tissues. During this early stage the athlete may be introduced to simple, low- or no-impact proprioceptive skills to begin to develop balance and coordination in normal daily activities. Proprioception activities may take on many forms depending on the extremity involved and the range of joint motion permitted. Body position and joint position sense may be re-established without risking further injury.

Middle Stage: Range of Motion, Motor Control, and Cardiopulmonary Function

The objectives of this stage include (1) return of full range of motion of the involved area, (2) regain proper motor control of the injured area and adjacent musculature, and (3) increase cardiopulmonary (heart and lung) function to allow continual total-body exercise for sport-specific time periods.

Range of Motion

When the physician gives permission to begin light activities, the general rule is to begin

Table 42-1. Overhead Stroke in Tennis: A Progression

Stage One: From a position approximately 5 feet behind the net. Ball machine projecting balls within racket reach of overhead. Practice days are numbered:

Day 1.   Hit 20 balls, attempt to keep ball within the singles court.
Rest 5 minutes.
Hit 20 balls within the singles court.

Day 2.   Hit 20 balls, within singles court.
Hit 20 balls, toward right side of singles court.
Rest 5 minutes.
Hit 20 balls, toward left side of singles court.

Day 3.   Repeat day 2 program until reaching 90% accuracy.

Day 4.   Repeat day 2 program with 30, 40, and 50 balls.

Stage Two: From same court location. Assistant projecting balls to require movement to position for return:

Day 1.   Hit 25 balls into singles court.
Rest 5 minutes.
Hit 25 balls into singles court.
Rest 2 minutes.
Hit 25 balls into singles court.

Day 2.   Hit 25 balls into singles court.
Rest 2 minutes.
Hit 25 balls into right side of singles court.
Rest 2 minutes.
Hit 25 balls into left side of singles court.

Day 3.   Repeat day 2 activities until reaching 90% accuracy in each task.

Day 4.   Repeat day 2 activities using 30, 40, and 50 balls.

Stage Three: From a position within 2 feet of the baseline. Using ball machine to project balls within racket reach of overhead. Practice days are numbered:

Day 1.   Hit 20 balls, attempt to keep ball within the singles court.
Rest 5 minutes.
Hit 20 balls within the singles court.

Day 2.   Hit 20 balls, within singles court.
Hit 20 balls, toward right side of singles court.
Rest 5 minutes.
Hit 20 balls, toward left side of singles court.

Day 3.   Repeat day 2 program until reaching 90% accuracy.

Day 4.   Repeat day 2 program using 30, 40, and 50 balls.

Stage Four: From same court location. Assistant projecting balls to require movement to position for return:

Day 1.   Hit 25 balls into singles court.
Rest 5 minutes.
Hit 25 balls into singles court.
Rest 2 minutes.
Hit 25 balls into singles court.

Day 2.   Hit 25 balls into singles court.
Rest 2 minutes.
Hit 25 balls into right side of singles court.
Rest 2 minutes.
Hit 25 balls into left side of singles court.

Day 3.   Repeat day 2 activities until reaching 90% accuracy in each task.

Day 4.   Repeat day 2 activities using 30, 40, and 50 balls.

---

regaining range of motion in the affected area. Full movement may be difficult because of surgery, immobilization, or a simple loss of motor control. Range of motion of the area should progress to full joint motion without pain unless there are limitations following surgery. When range of motion is limited, passive range of motion exercise may be prescribed. In passive range of motion exercises someone other than the injured individual moves the joint through the range of motion. As scar tissue becomes more elastic and motor control returns, the athlete will be able to progress from passive to active motions (where the athlete moves her own joint through the range of motion) and finally to resistive motions. Proprioceptive neuromuscular facilitation (PNF) is a technique in which manual resistance is applied to an extremity while the athlete moves through a specific range of motion. PNF as well as other forms of manual resistance will allow the sports therapist to guide the development of range of joint movement while beginning the process of strengthening.

Motor Control

During the progression to active exercises, the sports therapist observes the quality of motion to ensure the return of excellent motor control. Motor control is often "lost" following trauma or surgery. All too often, chronic injury is attributed to poor motor control prior to the actual structural damage. Usually, skilled athletes will be able to recognize faulty motor patterns once the proper pattern of movement is understood. Strengthening a muscle group that is poorly functioning is unwise and a waste of valuable time. An example of poor motor patterning is an abnormal walking pattern (limp) or a more subtle substitution of shoulder protraction to avoid full elbow extension in a forward reach. All motor patterns should be watched carefully for abnormalities and substitutions. Gradual challenges of the control can be provided, acting as both the start of resistance training as well as in the development of the motor control system.

Observation of movement patterns should begin in the early stages of the reconditioning process, but also continue into sport-specific retraining of exact skill patterns. Videotape analysis of high-speed movement patterns may assist the sports therapist and/or coach to understand some of the more subtle flaws in the skill performance. The athlete seeing a video of her performance may become more aware of the proprioceptive information being received from her body during performance. Sports therapists unfamiliar with the highly specialized sport skills should seek assistance from coaches, athletes, and athletic trainers more familiar with the sport.

Cardiopulmonary Development

Following any period of immobility the cardiopulmonary system declines. During this middle stage of the reconditioning process, the athlete may begin work to recondition this vital component of total fitness. If the injury involved the lower extremity or the trunk, adaptations must be made to allow progressive work for the heart and lungs without compromising the postinjury exercise progression. A variety of exercises can be used to build cardiovascular condition. Some of those exercises include jogging, swimming, bicycling, stairclimbing, use of cross-country ski machines and rowing machines, and running in the swimming pool

(with or without a buoyancy vest). The goal is to provide an exercise the athlete can perform for 20 minutes or longer without stress to the injured area.

Late Stage: Resistance Training and the Functional Exercise Pyramid

The therapeutic objective of this stage of the program is to provide a gradual return to sport-specific situations. This stage encompasses a large gamut of exercises, from the general exercises needed as a base from which to build, to the final goal of full functional return to the particular sport.

As the tissues heal it is important to provide mild stress to assist in the realignment of fibers within the tissues. This stage must be carefully monitored to be certain an unsafe overload situation does not occur. This last phase of the reconditioning process will consume the majority of the rehabilitation time and may extend from about week 6 to, in extreme cases, week 24 or longer.

During the initial time in this phase, exercises must be performed to continue to regain control of the injured part. A gradual increase in muscle activity will begin, using the large muscle groups in straight-line movement patterns. This is the first step in building strength for specific sports: building a solid strength base or *foundation*. This foundation is typically built over time, gradually increasing the weight being lifted or the number of repetitions or sets being performed. The athlete should follow the physician's advice and consult the athletic trainer and/or sports therapist for exercises to be included. As the athlete progresses through the building of a strong foundation, additional sport-specific, *functional* exercises will be included on a daily basis, while the foundation exercises will be continued on a less frequent weekly or biweekly basis. The exact combination of foundation and functional exercises will be determined by the injury, the status of the healing, and the physical abilities of the athlete.

Functional Exercises and the Functional Exercise Pyramid

A *functional exercise* is a motor skill with direct relevance to a specific task or skill. Functional exercises usually resemble, fully or in part, a specific sport skill or technique. This does not mean that exercises that resemble exercises in the weight room are not functional exercises. Strength-training techniques as well as sport-skill techniques fall into the functional exercise category.

During this phase of the rehabilitation process, strength development continues and as the tissues can tolerate changes in movement patterns, functional skills are incorporated into the program. The functional activities may be subdivided into 3 levels of activities. This division allows the athlete some sense of achievement while progressing toward the ultimate goal of return to competition.

Poorly planned exercise programs can subject the body to stresses before the athlete has conditioned sufficiently to accept those demands, sometimes resulting in reinjury or, more often, associated stress injuries. Athletes who always seem to be hurt are often found not to rest following an injury, but return to sport participation without progressing through a retraining program first, which results in another injury or chronic irritation such as tendinitis. The better procedure would follow rest with specific exercises designed to progress the athlete back to playing status.

Figure 42-3 illustrates the pyramid approach to program design.

Level I: Functional Exercises. Within level I functional exercises, the athlete will begin using patterns of movement under very low load conditions. In working with the lower extremity, the pool is a very useful tool to allow replication of motor patterns without the weighted condition found on land.

Level I exercises should be performed slowly, with emphasis on the execution of the pattern of movement. Increases in speed, distance, time, and load will be accomplished in levels II and III.

Level II: Functional Exercises. As one progresses through level I without difficulty (pain, swelling, excessive fatigue), the exercises may be progressed to the next level. Many of the functional exercises will be continued from level I, with adjustments made in the progressions identified earlier. As changes in the program are made, records of those changes must be made. In increasing the speed of a movement, one may use 1/4 speed, 1/2 speed, 3/4 speed, and full speed as the delineators. This identification system, however, varies from individual to individual and must be an intrinsic measure. Other changes, distance, time, and load, can be measured very objectively and records of those changes well understood.

In progressing from the slow-speed, low-load, low-repetition exercises one should initially increase only 1 of the parameters at a time. If one increases the speed of movement through the pattern, the weight being lifted through the pattern (tension or other load), and the number of times the pattern was performed, soreness would usually result. This soreness may be so severe that the program must be cut back or canceled until the athlete feels better again. This yo-yo training is not only difficult to keep track of, but also very harmful and unsafe for the athlete.

Level III: Functional Exercises. This final level of functional exercises will bring the athlete to the intensity of exercise that prepares her for the return to the sport. Continued challenges should be given to the athlete at this level while keeping the environment as safe as possible. With a gradual building of the stresses, the athlete's body should now be able to withstand the demands of nearly the level of competition.

Because of the wide variety of sport skills and techniques, the sports therapist must work closely with the athlete and gain assistance from the sport coach to provide suitable drills and exercises to prepare for the athlete's full return to participation. Situations often occur where the athlete expresses a concern with a particular motion or skill technique. When the athlete fears a particular position, motion, or skill, the sports therapist must analyze the problem and find some way to replicate the physical loads to gradually prepare the athlete to overcome this anxiety and safely perform the skill.

Often, the exact mechanism causing the injury is well remembered by the athlete. An avoidance of this sport skill or situation during the recovery process can be a sign of trouble. Special attention must be paid to the psychological status of the athlete as well as extreme care taken to provide a safe environment to develop the physical abilities needed to perform that skill without risk of injury. Seeking the assistance of

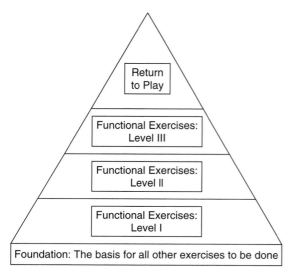

Figure 42-3. Skill development pyramid.

the sport psychologist is often extremely beneficial.

The Final Stage of Reconditioning: Return to Sport Participation

As the athlete progresses through the phases of the rehabilitation process, sufficient sport-specific challenges should have been met. These sport-specific drills prepare the athlete for her return to the competitive environment of sport, but not without yet another progression.

In some rather rare cases, the athlete may be able to fully return to sport practice, yet in most cases a selective return to participation is warranted. The athlete, coach, and athletic trainer should consult on the number of drills, type of drills, and length of time the athlete is allowed to participate. As the partial return is well tolerated, more drills may be allowed until the final goal of full participation is reached.

An interested, yet unvalidated observation of athletes returning to sport participation following orthopaedic surgery is that most athletes' sport skills continue to develop for 2 to 4 games. These game skills fail to fully develop during regular practice sessions and very few individuals return to play at their full functional ability in the first competition. This observation warrants further study and consideration for allowing the athlete to engage in off-season competitive games should the sport have such leagues or events.

CONCLUDING REMARKS

Throughout an athlete's career, training is a natural part of the participation process. Retraining following an injury or surgery follows many of the same principles as training, with special consideration given to the healing of damaged tissues.

With consideration given to providing the tissues an optimal environment for healing, followed by closely supervised stretching, re-education, and re-training programs, the athlete will have the best potential for full return to her chosen sport.

A wide variety of exercises exist, sometimes with the result of confusing the rehabilitating athlete. Exercises can be analyzed to determine whether biomechanical benefits warrant including them in the rehabilitation program. Each stage of the rehabilitation program should have clearly defined objectives. Progress into subsequent stages will be guided by the performance on objectives at the previous level. Through the late stages of the retraining program, exercises should become very specific to the sport and skills needed. Exercises should be functional in nature, they should be challenging yet safe, and very importantly, they should be enjoyable. The athlete should find rehabilitation an interesting divergence during this period of relative loss, not a further punishment for being injured.

Selected Readings

Baechle TR (ed): Essentials of Strength Training and Conditioning. Champaign, Ill, Human Kinetics, 1994.

Burk D: Year-round program design for Canyon High School football players. Strength and Conditioning 17:7–15, 1995.

Chu D: Jumping Into Plyometrics. Champaign, Ill, Human Kinetics, 1992.

Jobe FW, Bradley JP: Rotator cuff injuries in baseball: Prevention and rehabilitation. *Sports Med* 6: 378–87, 1988.

Lephart SM: Proprioceptive considerations for sport. J Sport Rehabil 3:1, 1994.

Pappas AM, Zawacki RM, McCarthy CF: Rehabilitation of the pitching shoulder. Am J Sports Med 13:223–34, 1985.

Perry J: Anatomy and biomechanics of the shoulder in throwing, swimming, gymnastics, and tennis. Clin Sports Med 2:247–70, 1983.

Shelbourne KD, Nitz P: Accelerated rehabilitation after anterior cruciate ligament reconstruction. Am J Sports Med 18:292–9, 1990.

Shelbourne KD, Klootwyk TE, De Carlo MS: Update on accelerated rehabilitation after anterior cruciate ligament reconstruction. J Orthop Sports Phys Ther 15: 303–8, 1992.

Shelbourne KD, Klootwyk TE, De Carlo MS: Clinical development of preoperative and postoperative ACL rehabilitation. In Feagin JA (ed): The Crucial Ligaments. New York, Churchill Livingstone, 1994, pp 737–50.

Tullos HS, King JW: Throwing mechanisms in sports. Orthop Clin North Am 4: 709–21, 1973.

Chapter 43

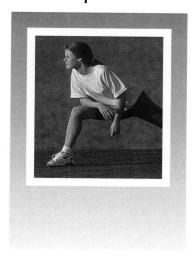

Rehabilitation Concerns
LOWER EXTREMITY

Mark R. Hutchinson, M.D.
Mary Lloyd Ireland, M.D.
Scott Crook, P.T., C.S.C.S.

Female athletes have concerns regarding their participation in sports, their risk of specific types of athletic injuries, and their optimal rehabilitation from injury. Females have wider hips and increased knee valgus, and smaller bones and bony structures (eg, the femoral notch), increased ligamentous laxity, and decreased muscle mass in the lower extremity (Fig. 43-1) compared with men. Each anatomic variance implies differences in injury risk and injury patterns. Increased ligamentous laxity can lead to instability, especially of the patellofemoral joint,

in females, who already have increased valgus angulation at the knee and increased forces causing lateral subluxation. These variations in alignment are further magnified if muscle imbalances are present.

Proximal pelvic alignment and control of pelvic flexion and rotation dictate lower extremity position. In the male, the hip is well centered over the ankle (Fig. 43-2, left). In the female (Fig. 43-2, right), the femur is in varus and is internally rotated, creating valgus knee alignment, and the tibia is in external rotation

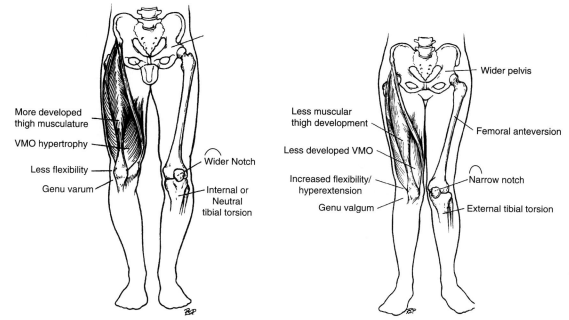

Figure 43-1. The male alignment, shown on the left, is overall straighter, the pelvis narrower, and the thigh musculature more developed. The male has less flexibility, genu varum, and internal or neutral tibial torsion. The female alignment, shown on the right, has a relatively wider pelvis and the thigh musculature is less developed. The female has increased flexibility, hyperextension of the knees, genu valgum, and external tibial torsion. (From Fu FH, Stone D (eds): Sports Injuries: Mechanisms, Prevention, Treatment. Baltimore, Williams & Wilkins, 1994, with permission.)

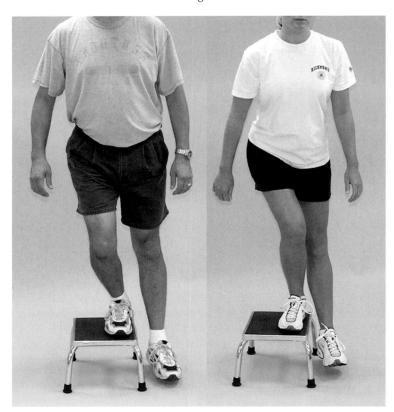

Figure 43-2. These individuals were instructed to perform a step-down maneuver. Anatomically, the alignment of the male, on the left, shows a straight-as-an-arrow hip over knee over ankle. The female, on the right, demonstrates hip adduction and internal rotation with anteriorly rotated pelvis, excessive genu valgum, and external tibial rotation and subsequent pronation of the foot.

subsequent to forefoot pronation. In Figure 43-3, depicting the step-down maneuver, the female, on the right, has an anteriorly rotated pelvis and greater lumbar lordosis, and her trunk is forward. Diagrammatically (Fig. 43-4), the position that is safe is the neutral spinal alignment, shown on the left. In the high-risk position the pelvis is anteriorly rotated with the head forward and the spine in hyperlordosis, shown on the right.

Rehabilitation programs are based on groups of muscles functioning in synchrony. No muscle functions in isolation. Use of proper trunk, pelvis, and lower extremity position is critical in prevention of lower extremity injuries in rehabilitation programs. The proper position of the lumbar spine and pelvis in the lunge is shown in Figure 43-5, which depicts a model holding the Swiss ball upward and directly forward. Another lunge position, again utilizing upper and lower body coordination, is shown in Figure 43-6, which demonstrates the proper bending technique with the back straight and the knee bent. In a proper squat, the hip is over knee, which is over the ankle. Commands emphasizing straight alignment without rotation should be used.

More sophisticated physioball activities incorporate the back and upper and lower extremities.

Doing hip extensions while balancing on the ball will enforce lumbosacral control. The instructions are to flex the knees and hips, then extend, while maintaining balance (Fig. 43-7). The weakness of hip abductors and external rotators seen in the female athlete may increase the risk of injury. Bridging activates hip abductors (Fig. 43-8) The instructions are to keep the left greater trochanter off of the ground, maintaining balance with support from the right arm with the right hand flat on the floor. As the athlete improves in strength, doing this exercise without the support of the upper extremity will become possible. Incorporation of balance by using the ball for "perturbation activities" is shown in Figure 43-9. The subject is instructed to balance while maintaining trunk position as well as foot position on the bigger and smaller balls.

Anatomic gender variations are not the only factors that influence the risk of injury and rehabilitation of the female athlete. Physiologic issues (such as amenorrhea) have been associated with increased rates in overuse injuries (such as stress fractures) in women. Sociological and psychological obstacles unique to the female athlete may also need to be addressed during rehabilitation. In general, the fundamentals of

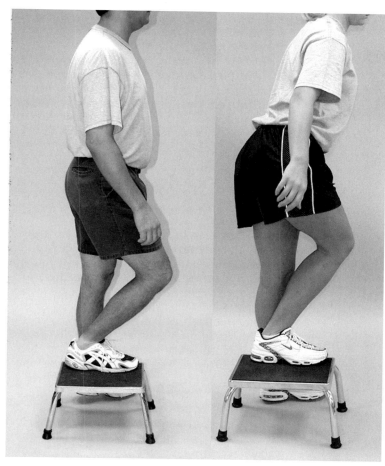

Figure 43-3. From the side, the anterior pelvis rotation can be seen in the female, on the right. The male, on the left, has a straighter alignment with the lumbar spine and pelvis in neutral position. On the right, the female shows an anteriorly rotated pelvis and excessive lumbar lordosis, which sets up the more distal limb alignment.

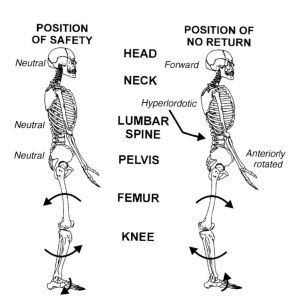

Figure 43-4. In the "position of no return" (ie, the high-risk position), the head is forward, the lumbar spine hyperlordotic, and the pelvis anteriorly rotated. Internal rotation of the relatively straight knee and subsequent tibial external rotation and foot pronation are also seen. The safe position shown on the left is more neutral and more flexed.

rehabilitation, including motion, strengthening, and modalities (electrical stimulation, massage, cryotherapy, and ultrasound), are as applicable to females as they are to males. Nonetheless, addressing certain gender concerns and differences can optimize the rehabilitation of the female athlete. While some overlap with other chapters in this book on topics such as anatomy, specific injuries, and specific sports is unavoidable, we have made every effort to stay focused on the rehabilitation concerns of the female athlete.

PREVENTION AND THE IMPORTANCE OF CONDITIONING AND EDUCATION ON FEMALE INJURY PATTERNS

Prevention is very important in all aspects of medicine. By identifying risk factors and addressing them with directed and proper training techniques and conditioning, injuries can be obviated and the need for later treatment or time loss from sport can be avoided entirely. For most

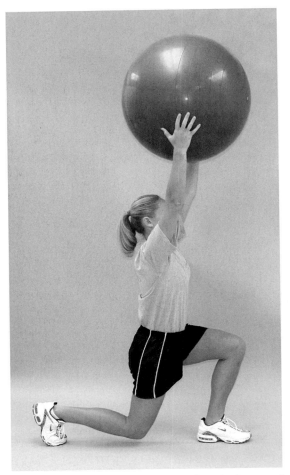

Figure 43-5. The subject shows excellent body control position in this forward lunge, balancing the ball directly overhead.

women, the baseline level of conditioning is significantly less than that of their male counterparts.[11,14,21,76,78] More specifically, this reduced level of conditioning has been related to knee injuries[6,35] as well as overuse injuries and stress fractures.[44,62,64] Adequate conditioning improves performance and reduces the risk of injury.[26] Fortunately, females in comparison to males have demonstrated a greater potential to make significant improvements in their status of conditioning with focused training.[7]

Excellent comparative studies have been done in the military setting that confirm the benefit of conditioning for women.[3,14,21,24,64] At the United States Naval Academy, stress-related injuries were seen more frequently in women. However, as the women became more acclimated to the rigors of training, the rates of serious injuries were similar between the sexes.[44,64] One of the major factors noted in that study was that the development of these injuries was directly related to the rapid onset of training without allowance for a progressive exposure to stress, rest, and the development of tolerance.[44]

In the university setting, we noted an increased incidence of stress fractures and overuse complaints in collegiate division 1 basketball and volleyball players about 3 to 4 weeks into their preseason workouts. Education of the coaches about the injury patterns in their own players and available medical reports provided the impetus for them to modify their practice plan. Every third or fourth day was designated a day off or a reduced-stress day where the athletes focused on lower-stress conditioning exercises. The intensity of the third or fourth week of practice was also reduced.[5] These interventions and a continued focus on conditioning have been effective in reducing the incidence of overuse injuries in these athletes.

Other factors that must be addressed to prevent or reduce the incidence of injury in the female athlete include education in proper sport-specific skills and rehabilitation techniques, nutrition, amenorrhea, and pregnancy. While these topics are addressed elsewhere in this text, it is important for the therapist, trainer, or physician to obtain a thorough history to assess whether these factors may not only contribute to the injury, but also play a part in the rehabilitation. Often, the personal aspect of the player–trainer or player–physician relationship provides the best opportunity to address sensitive issues involving menstrual irregularities, nutrition, eating disorders, and sexuality.

The female athlete may be at increased risk of injury because of errors in their performance of sport-specific and rehabilitative skills.[5] In comparison to male athletes, the average female athlete has less experience in sports, may have begun training and sports-specific skills at a later age, and may have less access to good coaching, athletic trainers, and facilities.[5,16,20,23,39,42,53] Female athletes may not have access or previous experience in the weight room. It is therefore especially important for female athletes to review proper sport-specific skills and techniques to operate specific weight training and rehabilitation equipment. Ensuring proper technique can reduce the incidence of injury in sports and in the weight room.

Pregnancy introduces an entire new set of factors into injury risk and prevention. Physically fit women with normal pregnancies who exercise regularly have larger babies, shorter labors, and decreased incidence of complications compared to those without planned exercise programs.[17,18,38,40,77] Various investigators

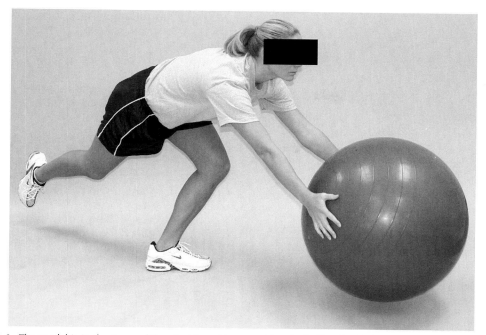

Figure 43-6. The model is in the "around the clock" position, touching the ball to the floor and extending the right leg.

have outlined some special considerations with regard to exercise during pregnancy.[25,31,41,50,56,66]

The musculoskeletal conditions associated with pregnancy have been summarized by Ireland and Ott.[37] Caution should be used when recommending high-intensity exercise, as it may decrease blood flow to the fetus or elevate core body temperature, with possible detri-

mental effects.[25,60,65] Mild to moderate exercise, however, in the low-risk pregnant female is not deleterious to the fetus and may be beneficial in maintaining fitness and easing labor. If the pregnant athlete can carry on a conversation during her workout then she has not exceeded her maximal physical effort.[25] The American College of Obstetricians and Gynecologists have created a set of guidelines for exercise during

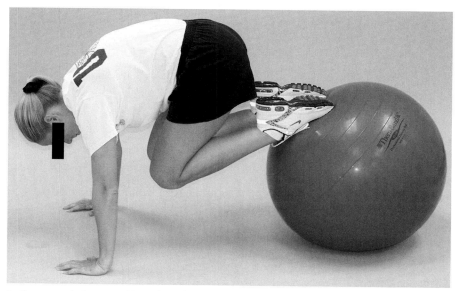

Figure 43-7. In the prone balance position, the subject maintains control, going from hip flexion and knee flexion into extension combines for core stabilization, balance, and neuromuscular control.

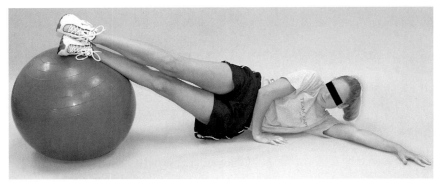

Figure 43-8. In bridging, the left greater trochanter is lifted off the floor while maintaining balance on the ball; support is given by the upper extremity. As advanced control occurs, less hand support is required.

pregnancy and postpartum.[2,75] Contraindications to exercise during pregnancy are pregnancy-induced hypertension, preterm rupture of membranes, preterm labor during the prior or current pregnancy or both, incompetent cervix/cerclage, persistent second- or third-trimester bleeding, and intrauterine growth retardation (see Chapter 20).

OVERCOMING SOCIOLOGICAL AND PSYCHOLOGICAL OBSTACLES

In general, the fundamentals of rehabilitation of the lower extremity, including motion, strengthening, and modalities, are no different

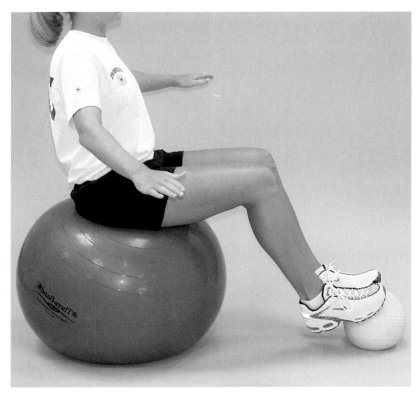

Figure 43-9. Incorporating balance while seated on an unstable base is shown. Such advanced Swiss ball maneuvers incorporate position awareness and strength. Modifications of these exercises can be made to maintain the interest of the patient.

for male and female athletes. However, associated factors such as anatomy, physiology, conditioning, and education are different. In addition, sociological and psychological obstacles may further complicate the rehabilitation of female athletes. The physician, therapist, or trainer should be aware of these obstacles to be able to overcome them and optimally rehabilitate the female athlete.

Historically, the athletic female has been plagued by a variety of psychosocial barriers that have reduced her effectiveness in athletic training, performance, and rehabilitation. In the past, competitive or aggressive females were thought to be unladylike. Females who participated in sports were more likely to have their womanhood questioned.[8] Social pressures often forced young girls into less aggressive roles. Some females feared being called a "tomboy" or becoming muscle bound if they exercised. In recent decades, participation of females in organized athletics has received better acceptance and has been encouraged. Participation and success in athletics can be used as a springboard to deal with stress, competition, and the challenges of professional life.[58] Young female participants in athletics have been shown to improve their self-confidence as well as overall performance.[13,44,70] Enlightening a female athlete to these benefits and providing continued acceptance and encouragement can further maximize motivation for rehabilitation and performance.

Interestingly, the way that the reinforcement and encouragement is provided may also be critical when rehabilitating a female athlete. Positive reinforcement is key. Negative reinforcement or critique tends to erode the female's self-confidence more quickly than her male counterpart's.[13] Three factors may make female athletes more susceptible to situational vulnerability and a reduction of self-confidence. First, females tend to do poorly on gender-type tasks considered to be masculine or gender-role inappropriate. Second, they tend to be more sensitive to social evaluation than males. Third, females do better in achievement situations when they receive objective, immediate, and accurate feedback concerning their performance.[13] To overcome these obstacles, rehabilitation should be designed as a series of progressive, realistic, and attainable goals so that the athlete can visualize her improvement. More frequent rehabilitative sessions with more frequent objective evaluation and positive reinforcement are beneficial. Objective tests, including biofeedback, appropriate functional testing, and isokinetic studies may also be of particular benefit in providing accurate and immediate feedback.

GENDER-SPECIFIC INJURIES AND REHABILITATION

Most injuries seen in female athletes are strains, sprains, and contusions, which are the same types of injuries seen in predominantly male sports. The specific incidence and types of injuries are primarily related to the sport and not the gender of the participant. Nonetheless, subtle and sometimes less than subtle differences can be seen when comparing the two sexes. This section will discuss those variations by anatomic location and provide suggestions regarding rehabilitation of the female athlete.

The Hip and Thigh

The hip is not commonly the source of lower extremity complaints by athletes of either gender. The knee, ankle, calf, and foot are much more commonly involved. Low back pathology with associated radiculopathy should be ruled out in anyone who complains of hip pain. Most causes of hip pain are not specifically gender related. They include such diagnoses as contusions, myositis ossificans, iliopectineal bursitis, osteitis pubis, muscle strains or tears, groin strains, sacroiliac joint sprains, traumatic or avulsion fractures, dislocations, or Legg-Calvé-Perthes disease. At least 4 pathologies about the hip, however, appear to be related in some way to gender. They include stress fractures, snapping hip syndrome, and trochanteric bursitis, as well as slipped capital femoral epiphyses.

Since women in general are at greater risk for stress fractures, it is important to rule out a stress fracture when one is suspected. Female athletes with a history of amenorrhea or oligomenorrhea should be placed in a high-risk category and be evaluated by dual photon absorptiometry.[9] Stress fractures can occur in the femur or pelvis.[9,12,45,47,48] Pavlov and colleagues[61] postulated that the higher incidence of pelvic stress fractures in females might be explained by differences in gait between men and women runners. Physiologic factors such as bone density and hormonal balance may also play significant roles. Stress fractures should always be considered in the differential diagnosis of a female athlete with hip pain. The treatment is generally conservative, and most athletes respond to 3 to 5 months of reduced-impact activity. Stress fractures of the femur most commonly occur in runners. A stress fracture of the tension side of the femoral neck (the lateral side) is considered ominous and at high risk of progression to a complete fracture. These may require surgical pinning.

Regarding rehabilitation and training, the athlete must understand that rapid increase of mileage or intensity probably precipitated the injury and must not be repeated in the future.[9] When the injury has healed, a progressive program of gradual increase in distance and intensity is recommended. A gradual transition from soft to harder running surfaces may also be of benefit.

Females, by design, have a wider pelvis and greater varus angulation at the hip. This, in turn, leads to a relatively greater trochanteric prominence.[30] These factors have been associated with an increased number of overuse syndromes about the hip and knee.[32] The relative trochanteric prominence may place female athletes, especially female runners, at increased risk of trochanteric bursitis compared to their male counterparts.[29,36] Typically, the pain of the snapping hip occurs at the level of the greater trochanter secondary to friction as the iliotibial band rides over the bony prominence of the trochanter. Weakness of the hip abductors allows for a relative lowering of the contralateral side of the pelvis during the stance phase, which further accentuates the trochanteric prominence and tightens the iliotibial band over the trochanter. Occasionally, an audible snap can be heard, hence the name "snapping hip syndrome."

The Ober test is a diagnostic test that can assist in the diagnosis of iliotibial band irritation. The patient lies on the asymptomatic side with the downside leg being flexed at the hip and knee. The extremity being tested is brought into extension and full abduction at the hip and flexion at the knee. With the knee still in flexion, the leg is allowed to adduct maximally. To be diagnostic, the pain or pop created as the iliotibial band passes over the greater trochanter should mimic the patient's complaints. Treatment is focused on abductor strengthening and stretching of the tight iliotibial band. Lateral step-ups, with emphasis on holding the pelvis level on a step approximately 8 to 12 inches high, are an effective means of strengthening the muscle. Stepping in side-to-side box and diamond patterns with elastic tubing tied around the thighs to provide resistance can add more functional strengthening activities. Crossover stretching, placing the affected leg behind the good leg, helps stretch the iliotibial band. Dynamic balance training can include standing on the involved side and kicking with the contralateral leg in 4 different directions or using Swiss ball exercises. Swiss ball exercises allow for strengthening of hip and core musculature to increase functional body control of both muscle groups. Ice, massage, anti-inflammatory medications, modalities, or local steroid injections may also be of benefit. Rarely surgical releases may be necessary. Hip strengthening and iliotibial band stretching in the conditioning should be included in the preparticipation regimens of female athletes who are at risk of hip problems or have a history of hip problems.

Slipped capital femoral epiphysis, the most common hip disorder seen in adolescents, may be related to hormonal, genetic, and mechanical factors. As the name implies, the proximal femoral physis is compromised and the epiphysis of the proximal femur slips medially and posteriorly. If missed or severe, this can lead to significant life-long morbidity. Males are affected twice as frequently as females, and black males have an unusually high incidence. Surgical pinning is general recommended to prevent further slippage and deformity.[51]

THE KNEE

Perhaps the most common site of injury in the lower extremity as well as the site of greatest gender variation in injury patterns is the knee. Female athletes are at increased risk of anterior cruciate ligament (ACL) injury and patellofemoral disorders. Females may also be at increased risk of overuse injuries when reduced conditioning is a factor. Any athlete, male or female, with little previous experience in the weight room or with rehabilitative techniques should receive proper instruction. Initial therapy should be monitored closely to ensure proper technique as the athlete acclimates to the equipment and protocols. Some weight-training techniques or machines are of particular concern.

Certain exercises may exacerbate and not rehabilitate problems in the knee. With increasing knee flexion, as is seen with deep squats or leg presses, the patellofemoral contact areas increase.[1] When the athlete flexes her knee to 90° or more, the increased surface area of contact and elevated posteriorly directed forces exacerbate pain from patellofemoral syndrome and decrease the effectiveness of the exercise. Greater posteriorly directed pressures are seen in open-chain exercises such as the maneuvers performed on the knee extension machine. Such open-chain exercises have been incriminated as a common cause of anterior knee pain in female athletes who use weight equipment.[19,28,46,65] The motor imbalance of open-chain exercises on the knee with unbalanced quadriceps activity appears to be the main factor that magnifies the direct and shear forces perceived by the patellofemoral articulation. In the ACL-deficient athlete, open-chain knee extensions may actually sublux the knee anteriorly owing to the lack of an opposing reduction hamstring pull.

A more focused approach to quadriceps rehabilitation for the female athlete at risk of or with the symptoms of patellofemoral syndrome includes standing terminal extension exercises, straight-leg raises with or without ankle weights, and mini-squats or mini-leg presses, which avoid deep flexion. Squats and leg presses beyond 90° of flexion should be avoided to minimize stresses at the patellofemoral articulation. Avoidance of high-resistance open-chain exercises (eg, extension machines) in an arc of motion between 90° and full extension in patients who have patellofemoral disease is also suggested.[33] Open-chain exercises near full extension are probably also safe and effective. Swimming or stationary bicycling with moderate resistance and a high seat also are usually well tolerated.

Modifications in rehabilitation can also be undertaken for the female athlete with abnormal patellar tracking. Patellar instability may present with nonspecific anterior knee pain and be confused with patellofemoral syndrome or chondromalacia. The athlete may also complain of instability or "giving way." Physical examination generally reveals apprehension to lateral glide of the patella and perhaps an abnormal alignment or Q-angle. Many patellar-tracking abnormalities can be addressed conservatively although some require surgical intervention. The only active muscle that resists lateral subluxation is the vastus medialis obliquus (VMO). Conservative treatment is generally dedicated to strengthening the VMO and stretching tight lateral tissue.

A focused approach to rehabilitation of the female athlete with patellar maltracking should address the VMO. Simple straight-leg raising and terminal extension exercises are not optimal ways to rehabilitate the VMO.[52] Instead, the femur should be externally rotated to decrease the lateral pull of the tensor fascia lata and stretch the VMO. The external rotation of the femur with knee extension forces the hip adductors to fire when performing the leg raise. Since the VMO may have dual innervation with knee extenders and hip adductors, this may further accentuate its rehabilitation. Stretching of the tight lateral structures by forcing the patella medially is also important. Adjunctive techniques, including oral anti-inflammatory medications, modalities, patella taping, knee sleeves

with lateral J-pads, electric stimulation, and biofeedback, may also be of benefit in allowing the athlete to eliminate pain to optimally strengthen the VMO.

The trunk and hip musculature should not be forgotten when addressing the knee. Control of the femur in all planes of movement is affected by strength of the trunk or core musculature and the hip musculature. Lack of control at the hip results in the femur becoming a long lever arm and, thus, increases forces occurring at the knee. These forces often take the knee into positions that increase the probability of both traumatic and overuse injuries. Strengthening of the hip and core musculature should be done in a way that integrates the entire kinetic chain in all planes of movement. These are best done with closed kinetic chain and functional sports-specific exercises.

Finally, the lowest end of the kinetic chain should be evaluated. Foot alignment can affect tibial rotation and, in turn, knee stresses. Excessive pronation is commonly the culprit. The examiner should be aware of the "miserable malalignment syndrome." This combination of pes planus, tibial torsion, and femoral anteversion can lead to anterior knee pain. Strengthening of the hip and core musculature should be done in a way that integrates control of the entire kinetic chain in all planes of movement. These are best done with closed-chain exercises and Swiss ball exercises as mentioned previously.

The position of the foot must also be considered. Excessive pronation may result in increased moment of adduction and internal rotation at the knee. The use of orthotics may be beneficial to accommodate for malalignment at the foot, thus reducing forces up the kinetic chain.

THE ANKLE AND FOOT

Ankle and foot injuries in female athletes are related more to specific sports demands than to gender differences between males and females. Marked stunting of lower leg growth in young female gymnasts has been reported but is probably secondary to repetitive trauma to the distal tibial physis rather than any gender specific etiology.[72] Metatarsal and hindfoot stress fractures are more common in unconditioned females but appear to occur at similar rates once conditioning has occurred.[44] Early reports of increased ligamentous laxity in women suggested a predisposition to ankle sprains in women.[35] This has not been substantiated by epidemiologic studies.[10,76] Both sexes have an increased incidence of ankle sprains in running sports. Conditioning may again be a factor.[36] Since female athletes tend to begin training at a lower level of conditioning, ankle strengthening and proprioceptive skills training should be a required component of the female athlete's preseason and in-season conditioning plans. This may help to reduce the incidence of ankle injuries. Large rubber bands are inexpensive and effective in strengthening ankle invertors, evertors, plantar flexors, and dorsiflexors. Proprioceptive training also can be performed inexpensively with ankle alphabets (drawing the alphabet with the great toe), mini-tram activities, or homemade balance boards. Additional proprioceptive activities include tandem balancing with progression to toe raising and eventually single-leg balancing. A partner can provide additional challenges by performing light pushes in alternating directions for rhythmic stabilization. Playing catch while maintaining balance increases difficulty by requiring the ability to focus on another object.

Ankle impingement syndromes are seen in sports in which extreme ankle motion is desired.[34] Pointing the toes appears to be an especially valuable characteristic in female aesthetic sports such as dance, diving, artistic gymnastics, and rhythmic gymnastics. The position of forced plantar flexion may result in irritation of the posterior capsule or fracture of a posterior talar ossicle (the os trigonum).[22] Treatment is generally conservative and symptomatic, with abstention from those activities that exacerbate the pain. Physical therapy modalities and non-steroidal anti-inflammatory medications may reduce the inflammation. Once symptoms have subsided, a course of stretching of both the anterior and posterior capsule as well as strengthening of the anterior dorsiflexors can prevent recurrence. If symptoms continue, the os trigonum can be removed surgically.

Anterior capsular impingement may occur when a gymnast "lands short" during dismounts or tumbling routines, causing the foot to be hyperdorsiflexed.[69] Treatment is similar to that for posterior impingement, with strengthening of the plantar flexors in contrast to dorsiflexors of the ankle. Pads taped to the anterior aspect of the ankle can decrease symptoms and reduce hyperdorsiflexion at landing. Pads taped to the anterior aspect of the ankle can decrease symptoms and reduce the excessive dorsiflexion at landing. Proper education in landing techniques can further reduce recurrence.

Forefoot problems, including bunions, bunionettes, corns, and calluses, are more common in female than male athletes and are related at least in part to improper or inappropriate shoe wear.[63] Ballet dancers, partially because of the fit of their toe shoes and their relative lack of support, have a high incidence of foot disorders.[67] Athletes with a tendency toward these disorders should be cautioned during preseason examinations to be careful about their athletic and street shoe selection.[27] The shoes should allow for appropriate width of the forefoot so that no rubbing of the first metatarsophalangeal joint occurs and all toes can lie comfortably in the toe box with no overlap. Arch support in the case of overpronated feet can also reduce symptoms in the forefoot. Lower heels or flats reduce the forces on the forefoot and thus the incidence of forefoot problems. Once symptoms from bunions, bunionettes, or hammertoes develop, they should be treated promptly with shoe modifications, padding, ice, or taping. Surgical procedures may alter the mechanics of the forefoot and should be used with extreme caution in athletes with high foot demands.[27,34,67]

REHABILITATION OF SPORTS-SPECIFIC INJURIES

The classic sequence of rehabilitation and restoration of an injured athlete to her previous level of sport for most injuries begins by obtaining an accurate diagnosis through history, evaluation of the mechanism of injury, and physical examination. Initially, the athlete reduces her level of activity to avoid re-exacerbating the injury. Treatment is focused on reducing the inflammatory response with ice, compression, and elevation. Once the early period is past, rehabilitation focuses on increasing range of motion and flexibility, increasing strength, and finally increasing power and proprioception. The speed at which one proceeds through this sequence depends on the severity and type of injury and the athlete's response. Finally, when the athlete has achieved near-normal function, she is ready to be challenged with progressive sport-specific skills to enable her to return to competitive sport. Premature return may compromise the athlete's safety and risk exacerbation of the injury. Functional testing is recommended to compare the injured to the uninjured side, to ensure that the athlete is ready to return to her sport.

Knowledge of the skills unique to a particular sport (ie, does the sport demand flexibility, power speed, agility, running, landing?) can assist in determining the focus and demands of the rehabilitation. The physical demands of sports whose participants are primarily female (ie, artistic gymnastics, dance and ballet, cheerleading, rhythmic gymnastics and synchronized swimming) differ from those undertaken primarily by men, and their rehabilitation plans must be tailored to women; however, sports-specific rehabilitation for any given sport in which both genders participate is similar.

Ballet and Dance

Dance and ballet demand a high degree of flexibility and fine motor control. Certain required positions such as plié and en pointe place stresses on the lower extremity unlike any other sport or activity. Obtaining external rotation of the hips, or "turnout," is a primary goal of the ballet dancer,[54] and dancers with poor "turnout" attempt to make up for it by flexing the knees and hips and "screwing" the knees.[68] This, in turn, can lead to patellar instability, meniscus tears, and ligament strains. Strains on the hip can cause tendinitis, muscle strains, or bursitis.

Appropriate rehabilitation is focused on the specific complaints. Regaining the initial flexibility of the entire lower extremity is important and can reduce the recurrence of complaints and avoid associated injuries. Rehabilitation is performed in the athlete's "adjusted" axis of rotation, that is, strengthening is performed in a turned-out position for ballet dancers. Educating the athlete as to the performance of safe and proper techniques is also important. Judicious use of modalities and oral anti-inflammatory medications can speed the recovery, reduce the pain, and allow improved rehabilitation.

For classical ballet, young girls should not be allowed to go to pointe dancing before they have developed proper balance, coordination, mental maturity, physical strength, and mastery of the basic dance steps.[4] Indeed, advancing a dancer beyond his or her ability and training can lead to both acute and chronic injuries.[59] Those injuries include stress fractures, tendinitis, myositis, arthritis, synovitis, corns and calluses, and toenail pathologies. To reduce the incidence of such injuries, care must be taken to enforce the criteria for allowing en-pointe activities. In addition, flexibility and strength of the leg, foot, and ankle should be maintained. Proper warm-up should be instituted and meticulous care of the foot, nails, and skin should be practiced. Shoes should be carefully sized and adjusted. Proper technique should be emphasized. When injuries related to en-pointe activities occur, reduction of time spent in the exacerbating position is necessary, but stopping participation completely is not usually required. When the athlete is ready to return, she should be able to demonstrate the proper position without pain and the time allowed in that position should be increased progressively.

Cheerleading

Cheerleading as a sport has significant components of gymnastics and dance. Skills involving the lower extremity include flexibility, proprioception and balance, running, twisting, jumping, and landing. In addition, unlike most seasonal sports, cheerleading is a year-round activity, making cheerleaders prone to overuse injuries. The lower extremity is involved in a majority of those injuries, with sprains and strains about the ankle and knee predominant.[55] A 2-year retrospective chart review at the Kentucky Sports Medicine Clinic revealed over 70 injuries to cheerleaders, a majority of which involved the knee. Ligament sprains made up 34%, inflammation or plica irritation made up 31%, and patella subluxation and instability made up 26%.

When rehabilitating the injured cheerleader, great emphasis must be placed on flexibility and full return of proprioception and balance. Without complete motor control and balance, the athlete is at increased risk of reinjury or potentially a new injury from missed landings or falls from mounts, tosses, or towers. Return to at-risk activities should be slow, progressive, spotted, and supervised. Because of the increased incidence of overuse injuries, time should be set aside throughout the year for conditioning. In addition, because of the increased incidence of medial plica problems and patellar instability, conditioning should include quadriceps rehabilitation focused on the VMO muscle.

Field Hockey

Lower extremity skills required for field hockey include running, cutting, and stopping. In addition, the athlete is at risk of contusions secondary to stick use and collisions. In field hockey, ankle injuries are common and knee injuries occur at rates similar to those in male soccer (32% and 27% of all injuries, respectively).[10,76] However, female soccer athletes have twice the risk of ACL injuries compared to their male counterparts. The epidemic of ACL injuries in women involved in twisting and cutting sports has been discussed elsewhere in this book. Neuromuscular retraining may reduce the risk of ACL injuries in these athletes.

The injured field hockey athlete should be able to sprint at full speed prior to return to competition. More importantly, she should pass a series of agility tests that include box drills, alternating leg cross-overs, and running backward. Because of the increased incidence of ankle sprains in women involved in running and cutting sports, the female field hockey athlete should also include ankle conditioning and proprioceptive training in the preseason and in-season conditioning regimen.

Gymnastics: Artistic and Rhythmic

Although men and women participate in artistic gymnastics, the events are gender specific. Women participate in the balance beam, uneven parallel bars, vault, and floor exercises. The lower extremity demands of the sport include strength, flexibility, twisting, landing, proprioception, and balance. Rhythmic gymnastics, while eliminating the risk of falls from apparatus, adds the need for the fine motor skills of catching equipment (even with the lower extremities) as well as flexibility and aesthetic requirements of ballet and dance.

A majority of injuries that occur in artistic gymnastics involve the lower extremity, particularly the knee.[10] Most are secondary to overuse with associated intrinsic factors, including patellar malposition, limb deformity, muscular imbalance, malalignment, symptomatic plica, and muscle tightness.[74] Many, however, are quite significant. In one year of the National Collegiate Athletic Association Injury Surveillance Study, female gymnasts had the highest incidence of ACL ruptures of all sports studied.[57]

When returning an injured gymnast to sport, especially apparatus, it is important to confirm that she has regained her complete proprioceptive and balance skills. Focused attention in rehabilitation prior to apparatus includes balance board training, mini-trampoline workouts, and balance-beam workouts with the beam on the floor rather than on its normal mount. Once appropriate skills are demonstrated, the athlete can progressively return to apparatus with spotters. Preventing future injuries includes general conditioning and working on eliminating muscle imbalances and areas of limited flexibility. The predominance of injuries about the knee, especially related to the patellofemoral joint, would suggest emphasis on quadriceps conditioning focused on the VMO. Neuromuscular retraining to prevent ACL injuries would be ideal. In addition, rhythmic gymnasts should emphasize proper techniques in attaining ballet positions.

Softball

The incidence of injuries to the lower extremity in females increases in direct relationship to the need for cutting activities in that sport. Softball has a lower incidence of serious knee injuries in comparison to women's soccer or women's basketball.[57] For female softball athletes, 82% of all injuries that required time-loss from sport involved the upper extremity.[15,49]

For the lower extremity, softball demands running and agility, but minimal twisting and cutting. Sport-specific skills that should be included in the final phase of rehabilitation include running bases, sliding, and side-to-side agility that mimics moving to the ball in the infield or outfield. Ankle conditioning and proprioceptive training may be valuable in reducing the incidence of ankle injuries.

Swimming

Very little information is available on the injury patterns in synchronized swimming. Certainly, the sport demands no specific impact, landing, running, or twisting and cutting, which should significantly reduce the occurrence of major ligamentous injury of the knee or lower extremity. Knee injuries in swimming are closely related to the biomechanics of the stroke and kick. Breaststroker's knee may be secondary to a collateral ligament sprain or to patellofemoral syndrome.[43,73] In fact, it would appear that patellar instability and pain along the medial patella facet are more common in females, while medial collateral ligament sprains are more common in men.[71] This would imply that rehabilitation and conditioning of the quadriceps and VMO might reduce the incidence of knee complaints in selected female swimmers.

Synchronized swimming is yet another "aesthetic sport" that, like diving and gymnastics, encourages the participant to hold the foot in a pointed, plantar-flexed position. Attempts at prevention or reduction of the associated posterior ankle impingement should include plantar flexion and dorsiflexion flexibility and strengthening.

CONCLUDING REMARKS

In summary, while the fundamentals of rehabilitation should not vary between male and female athletes, the female gender introduces a number of factors that should be accounted for to optimize rehabilitation success and return to sport. Being astute to specific anatomic, physiologic, and conditioning factors helps the treating medical professional to understand baseline gender variations in risk of injuries. Awareness of injury patterns, sport-specific risks, and injury rates can help the trainer, therapist, or clinician to focus on certain aspects of the rehabilitation to optimize care and avoid reinjury. Knowledge of psychological and sociological factors can increase the clinician's understanding of the athlete and help her to be an active participant in her rehabilitation.

References

1. Aglietti P: A new patellar prosthesis. Clin Orthop Rel Res 179:175–87, 1975.
2. American College of Obstetricians and Gynecologists: Exercise during pregnancy. ACOG Technical Bulletin No 189. Washington, DC: ACOG, 1994.
3. Baechle TR: Women in resistance training. Clin Sports Med 3:791–880, 1984.
4. Beaumont CW, Idzikowski S: A Manual of Theory and Practice of Classical Theatrical Dancing. New York, Dover Publications, 1970.
5. Beck JL, Wildermuth BP: The female athlete knee. Clin Sports Med 4(2):345–66, 1985.
6. Benas D: Special considerations in women's rehabilitation programs. In Hunter LY, Fu FJ (eds): Rehabilitation of the Injured Knee. St Louis, CV Mosby, 1985, pp 393–405.
7. Berg K: Aerobic function in female athletes. Clin Sports Med 3(4):779–89, 1984.
8. Berlin P: The woman athlete. In Gerber EW, et al (eds): The American Woman in Sport. Reading, Mass, Addison-Wesley, 1974.
9. Brunet ME, Hontas RB: The thigh. In Delee JC, Drez D(eds): Orthopaedic Sports Medicine. Philadelphia, WB Saunders, 1994, pp 1086–111.
10. Clarke KS, Buckley WE: Women's injuries in collegiate sports. Am J Sports Med 8:187, 1980.
11. Collins RK: Injury patterns in women's flag football. Am J Sports Med 15(3):238–42, 1987.
12. Cook SD, Harding AF, Thomas KA, et al: Trabecular bone density in menstrual function in women runners. Am J Sports Med 15:503–7, 1987.
13. Corbin CB: Self confidence of females in sport and physical activity. Clin Sports Med 3(4):895–908, 1984.
14. Cox JS, Lenz HW: Women midshipmen in sports. Am J Sports Med 12:241–3, 1984.
15. DeGroot H, Mass DP: Hand injuries in softball players using a 16 inch ball. Am J Sports Med 16(3):218–24, 1988.
16. Eisenberg I, Allen WC: Injuries in a women's varsity athletic program. Physician Sportsmed 5:112–20, 1978.
17. Erdelyi GJ: Gynecological survey of female athletes. J Sports Med Phys Fitness 2:174, 1962.
18. Erkkola R: The influence of physical training during pregnancy on physical work capacity and circulatory parameters. Scand J Clin Lab Invest 36–47, 1976.
19. Ficat RP, Hungerford DS: Disorders of the Patellofemoral Joint. Baltimore, Williams & Wilkins, 1977.
20. Franklin BA, Lussier L, Buskirk ER: Injury rates in women joggers. Physician Sportsmed 104–12, 1979.
21. Garrick JC, Requa RK: Girl's sports injuries in high school athletics. JAMA 239:2245–8, 1978.
22. Gelabert R: Preventing dancing injuries. Physician Sportsmed 8:69–76, 1980.
23. Gillette J: When and where women are injured in sports. Physician Sportsmed 2:61–3, 1975.
24. Good JE, Klein KM: Women in the military academies: US Navy (part I of 3). Physician Sportsmed 17:99–106, 1989.
25. Goodlin RC, Buckley KK: Maternal exercise. Clin Sports Med 3(4):881–93, 1984.
26. Griffin LY: The female as a sports participant. J Med Assoc Ga 81(6):285–7, 1992.
27. Griffin LY: The female athlete. In Delee JC, Drez D (eds): Orthopaedic Sports Medicine. Philadelphia, WB Saunders, 1994, pp 1086–111.
28. Grood ES: biomechanics of knee extension exercise. J Bone Joint Surg 66:725–34, 1984.
29. Gross ML, Nasser S, Finerman GA: Hip and pelvis. In Delee JC, Drez D (eds): Orthopaedic Sports Medicine. Philadelphia, WB Saunders, 1994, pp 1063–5.
30. Hale R: Factors important to women engaged in vigorous exercise. In Strauss R (ed): Sports Medicine. Philadelphia, WB Saunders, 1984, pp 250–69.
31. Hall DC, Kaufman DA: Effects of aerobic and strength conditioning of the pregnancy outcomes. Am J Obstet Gynecol 157(5):1199–203, 1987.
32. Haycock C, Gillete, G: Susceptibility of women athletes to injury: myth versus reality. JAMA 236:163–5, 1976.
33. Hungerford DS, Lennox DW: Rehabilitation of the knee and disorders of the patellofemoral joint. Orthop Clin North Am 14:397–402, 1983.
34. Hunter L, Andrews J, Clancy W. Funk F: Common orthopaedic problems in the female athlete. Instr Course Lect 31: 126-151, 1982.
35. Hunter L: Women's athletics: the orthopaedic surgeons point of view. Clin Sports Med 3(4):809–27, 1984.
36. Hunter LY: Aspects of injuries to the lower extremity unique to the female athlete. In Nicholas JA, Hershman EB (ed): Lower Extremity and Spine in Sports Medicine. St Louis, CV Mosby, 1986, pp 90–111.
37. Ireland ML, Ott SM: The effects of pregnancy on the musculoskeletal system. Clin Orthop Rel Res 372:169–79, 2000.
38. Ireland ML: Special concerns of the female athlete. In Fu FH, Stone DA (ed): Sports Injuries: Mechanism, Prevention, and Treatment, 2nd edition. Baltimore, Williams & Wilkins, 1994, pp 153–87.
39. Jackson DS, Furman WK, Berson BL: Patterns of injuries in collegiate athletes: a retrospective study of injuries sustained in intercollegiate athletics in two colleges over a two year period. Mt Sinai J Med 47:423–6, 1980.
40. Jarrett R, Spellacy W: Jogging during pregnancy. Obstet Gynecol 61:705, 1983.
41. Jarski RW, Trippett DL: The risks and benefits of exercise during pregnancy. J Fam Prac 30(2):185–9, 1990.
42. Jones RE: Common athletic injuries in women. Compr Ther 6:47–9, 1980.
43. Kennedy JC, Hawkins P, Krissoff WB: Orthopaedic manifestations of swimming. Am J Sports Med 6(6): 309–22, 1978.
44. Kowal DM: Nature and causes of injuries in women resulting from an endurance training program. Am J Sports Med 8(4):265–9, 1980.
45. Latshaw RF, Kantner TF, Kalenak A, et al: A pelvic stress fracture in a female jogger. Am J Sports Med 9:54, 1981.
46. Lieb FJ, Perry J: Quadriceps function: anatomical and mechanical study using amputated limbs. J Bone Joint Surg 50A:1535–48, 1968.
47. Linnell S, Stager J, Blue P, et al: Bone mineral content and menstrual irregularity in female runners. Med Sci Sports Exercise 16:343–8, 1984.
48. Lombardo SJ, Benson DW: Stress fractures of the femur in runners. Am J Sports Med 10:219, 1982.
49. Loosli AR: Injuries to pitchers in women's collegiate softball. Am J Sports Med 20:35–7, 1992.

50. Lotgering FK, Gilbert RD, Longo LD: The interactions of exercise and pregnancy: a review. Am J Obstet Gynecol 149:560, 1984.
51. Macewen GD, Bunnell WP, Ramsey PL. The hip. In Lovell WW, Winter RB (eds): Pediatric Orthopaedics. Philadelphia, JB Lippincott, 1986.
52. McConnell J: The management of chondromalacia patellae: a long term solution. Austral J Phys Ther 32(4)215–23, 1986.
53. Micheli L: Female runners. In D'Ambrosia R, Drez D (eds): Prevention and Treatment of Running Injuries. Thorofare, NJ, Slack, 1982.
54. Micheli LJ, Gillespie WJ, Walaszek A: Physiologic profiles of female professional ballerinas. Clin Sports Med 3(1):199–209, 1984.
55. Mueller FO: Cheerleading Injury Research. Chapel Hill, NC, National Center for Catastrophic Sports Injury Research, University of North Carolina, 1992.
56. Mullinax KM, Dale E: Some considerations of exercise during pregnancy. Clin Sports Med 5(3):559–70, 1986.
57. National Collegiate Athletic Association: NCAA Injury Surveillance System. Overland Park, Kan, NCAA, 1993.
58. Nilsson S, Roass AA: Soccer injuries in adolescents. Am J Sports Med 6(6):358–61, 1978.
59. Nixon JE: Injuries to the neck and upper extremity in dancers. Clin Sports Med 2:459, 1983.
60. Orseli RC: Possible teratogenic hyperthermia and marathon running (letter). JAMA 243:332, 1980.
61. Pavlov H, Nelson TL, Warren RF, et al: Stress fractures of the pubic ramus. J Bone Joint Surg 64A: 1020, 1982.
62. Pearl A: The Athletic Female. Champaign, Ill, Human Kinetics, 1992.
63. Potera C: Women in sports: the price of participation. Physician Sportsmed 14:149–53, 1986.
64. Protzman RR, Griffis C: Stress fractures in men and women undergoing military training. J Bone Joint Surg 59A:825, 1977.
65. Reilly DJ, Martens M: Experimental analysis of quadriceps muscle force and patellofemoral joint reaction force for various activities, Acta Orthop Scand 43:126–37, 1972.
66. Sady SP, Carpenter NW: Aerobic exercise during pregnancy: special considerations. Sports Med 7(6):357–75, 1989.
67. Sammarco G: Diagnosis and treatment in dancers. Clin Orthop Rel Res 187:176–87, 1987.
68. Sammarco GJ: Dance injuries. In Nicholas JA, Hershman EB (eds): The Lower Extremity and Spine in Sports Medicine. St Louis, CV Mosby, 1986, pp 1406–20.
69. Snook G: Injuries in women's gymnastics. Am J Sports Med 7(4):242–4, 1979.
70. Stark JA, Toulesse A: The young female athlete: physiological considerations. Clin Sports Med 3(4):909–20, 1984.
71. Stuhlberg SD: Breaststroker's knee: pathology, etiology, and treatment. Am J Sports Med 8(3):164–71, 1980.
72. Theintz GE, Howard H, Weiss U: Evidence for reduction of growth potential in adolescent gymnasts. J Pediatr 122:306–13, 1993.
73. Vlzsolyi P: Breaststroker's knee: an analysis of epidemiology and biomechanical factors. Am J Sports Med 15(l): 63–71, 1987.
74. Walsh WM, Human WW, Shelton GL: Overuse injuries of the knee and spine in girl's gymnastics. Clin Sports Med 3(4)829–50, 1984.
75. White J: Exercising for two: what's safe for the active pregnant woman. Physician Sportsmed 20(5):179–86, 1992.
76. Whiteside PA: Men's and women's injuries in comparable sports. Physician Sportsmed 8(3):130, 1980.
77. Woodward SL: How does strenuous maternal exercise affect the fetus: a review. Birth 18:17, 1981.
78. Zelisko JA, Noble HB, Porter M: A comparison of men's and women's professional basketball injuries. Am J Sports Med 10:297–9, 1982.

Chapter 44

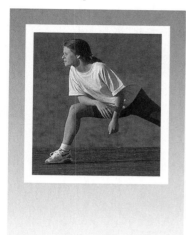

Rehabilitation Concerns
UPPER EXTREMITY

Kevin E. Wilk, P.T.
Mandy Kimball, M.S., P.T., A.T.C.

Female participation in sports continues to grow. Overhead sports such as softball, swimming, diving, gymnastics, tennis, and volleyball continue to be popular sports among female athletes. According to National Collegiate Athletic Association (NCAA) data, the academic years 1998 to 1999 saw 145,832 females participating in intercollegiate sports.[44] In contrast, during the 1988 to 1989 season, only 90,180 females participated in sports. This represents a 62% increase in collegiate female athletes. In the 1998 to 1999 season, there were 3216 college teams consisting of 48,131 athletes who participated in gymnastics, swimming/diving, softball, tennis, and volleyball. Nearly 15,000 females participated in collegiate softball, and 13,154 in volleyball.

According to the NCAA Injury Surveillance Data for 1998 to 1999, the number of shoulder complex injuries in females was 138, while for males it was 574 for all sports. The injury ratio of males to females varies significantly for each sport; shoulder injuries in soccer indicated a male:female ratio of 1.4:1, basketball 1:1.6, gymnastics 1:1, and baseball/softball 1.5:1.[45]

Participation in overhead sports frequently leads to shoulder and elbow injuries. The repetitive microtraumatic forces often result in overuse injuries to the upper extremity. Additionally, sports such as diving and gymnastics can generate large macrotraumatic forces, which may lead to gross tissue injuries such as dislocations, fractures, and ligamentous ruptures.

Anatomic variations of the upper extremity between women and men may increase the female athlete's risk of sustaining specific injuries. At the shoulder joint these anatomic differences include less-developed muscular mass, greater glenohumeral mobility, smaller bony structures, increased ligamentous laxity, and increased scapular mobility. At the elbow joint these anatomic differences include increased valgus alignment, increased elbow flexion, greater elbow hyperextension, less-developed muscular mass of the arm and forearm, and less-developed ligamentous structures. Thus, it appears that the female athlete exhibits greater joint mobility, which may compromise static joint stability, placing greater demands on the dynamic stabilizers.

Although there appear to be numerous anatomic factors that may predispose the female athlete to specific injuries, there also appear to be other possible predisposing factors. These factors are physiologic, sociological, and psychological in nature. Physiologic factors include muscle performance, neuromuscular control, proprioception, technique and skill level. Sociological factors include peer pressure, family concerns, and financial and educational gains. Lastly, psychological factors include body image, dietary practices, femininity concerns, and self-image concerns.

The purpose of this chapter is to discuss the specific rehabilitation concerns for the upper extremity in the female athlete. Additionally, discussion of specific injuries in various sports, such as gymnastics, softball, swimming, tennis, golf, and volleyball, will be included. The goal of this chapter is to stimulate interest and establish a foundation for future research in the area of upper extremity injuries in the female athlete.

UNIQUE FEATURES AND CLINICAL MANIFESTATIONS OF UPPER EXTREMITY INJURIES IN THE FEMALE ATHLETE

Clinically, the most striking differences between male and female subjective pain relate to the nature, location, and description of the pain. The male overhead athlete complains most frequently of posterosuperior shoulder pain (ie, internal impingement),[24,39,60] whereas the female overhead athlete notes diffuse shoulder pain. Occasionally, the female athlete will note diffuse shoulder weakness, with episodes of "dead arm syndrome." Furthermore, female overhead athletes frequently complain of clicking in the front of the shoulder, over the biceps brachii tendon. These subjective complaints are unique to the female athlete and uncommon to the male athlete. The subjective complaints of diffuse shoulder soreness, pain, and a "dead arm feel" are characteristic of glenohumeral joint hypermobility. Due to the hypermobility of the glenohumeral joint, there is an increased demand placed on the dynamic stabilizers of the shoulder joint complex.

Second, based on clinical examinations, it has been noted that the female overhead athlete exhibits greater joint laxity than the male overhead athlete. On arthroscopic examination, Crockett and coworkers[9] have noted that the female exhibits a less-developed anterior inferior glenohumeral joint ligament (AIGHL) complex,[48] particularly the anterior and posterior bands. Thus, the hammock effect of these 2 structures in supporting the humeral head is less efficient than it is in someone who exhibits a significant AIGHL complex (Fig. 44-1). Furthermore, Crockett and coworkers[9] have noted a larger rotator cuff interval. Harryman and coworkers[21] have reported that the larger the rotator cuff interval, the greater the humeral head displacement inferiorly and posteriorly. It has been our clinical experience that the female overhead athlete exhibits greater mobility in all directions and thus generalized shoulder laxity. However, this does not mean that the female exhibits more instability episodes. Brown and coworkers noted that females exhibited an increase in generalized laxity relative to males, but the increased laxity was not synonymous with instability.[7] However, we agree with the basic concept of Brown and coworkers that an increase in joint laxity places greater demands on the other stabilizing structures, such as the rotator cuff and biceps, and thus may lead to associated lesions. We refer to this as the sequelae of hypermobility of the glenohumeral joint.

Third, a frequent clinical complaint of the female overhead athlete is bicipital tendon pain, or "groove pain." Often, the female athlete will exhibit hypermobility of the proximal biceps tendon; the complaints are clicking, popping, tenderness and pain, which is worse with excessive external rotation. Treatment options for this lesion will be discussed later in the chapter.

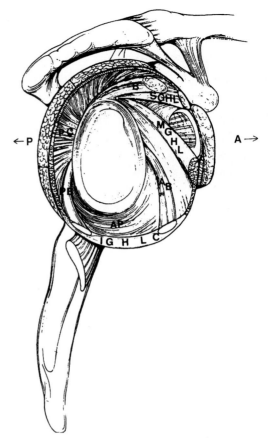

Figure 44-1. The glenohumeral joint capsule. Anatomy of the inferior glenohumeral ligament. Three distinct bands are seen: anterior band (AB), posterior band (PB), and axillary pouch (AP). (From O'Brien SJ, Neves MC, Arnoczky SP, et al: The anatomy and histology of the inferior glenohumeral ligament complex of the shoulder. Am J Sports Med 18:449–556, 1990, with permission.)

Another lesion of the biceps brachii is bicipital tendinitis. This lesion is again often seen in female athletes, specifically volleyball, softball, and swimming athletes. It is our belief that often the bicipital tendinitis is secondary to some other injury, such as a superior labrum tear anterior-posterior (SLAP) lesion or rotator cuff injury, or may be due to subtle instability. Knatt and coworkers[29] have noted a glenohumeral biceps reflex in the female. They noted that when the anterior capsule was stimulated, the biceps contracted the fastest of all the muscles around the shoulder joint. Guanche and coworkers[20] reported the biceps brachii contracted in 2.5 msec compared to 3.0 to 3.2 msec for the surrounding rotator cuff muscles. Therefore, we believe the biceps contracts first and stays contracted longer, thus possibly causing overuse tendinitis. We frequently see this in the hypermobile female athlete.

The female overhead athlete also exhibits a slightly different wear pattern than the male overhead athlete. Crockett and coworkers [9] have noted less rotator cuff pathology, less-defined internal impingement lesions, and slightly less glenoid labrum fraying. These may all signify greater glenohumeral joint laxity and less opportunity for significant wear patterns.

Fifth, the female athlete frequently exhibits hypermobility of the scapula. This may be due to the increase in generalized laxity and less-developed upper extremity musculature. The increase in scapular mobility may affect glenohumeral joint stability. Excessive scapular mobility may affect the orientation of the glenohumeral joint, and thus the ability of the shoulder muscles to stabilize the glenohumeral joint capsule effectively.

SPORT-SPECIFIC INJURIES SEEN IN THE FEMALE ATHLETE

Swimming Injuries

At the recreational level, swimming is an extremely popular activity, with more than 120 million Americans reporting that they swim regularly. More than 165,000 regularly compete in swimming. In 1998 and 1999, 10,012 female athletes participated in collegiate swimming.[44] McFarland and Wosik[37] have reported that the injury rate in collegiate swimmers was relatively low and that swimming is relatively safe compared to other collegiate sports. Although the rate of injury is relatively low, injuries are common. It is also estimated that up to 40% to 60% of competitive swimmers experience shoulder pain to the extent that their training is interrupted.[11,38,43] The most common shoulder injuries seen in the female swimmer are mechanical impingement, overuse tendinitis, glenohumeral instability, and muscular asymmetries. Mechanical subacromial impingement may result from a variety of causes. Several investigators believe the most important cause to be improper or deteriorated stroke mechanics.[6,16,52,53] Other causes relate to muscular weakness and fatigue. Overuse tendinitis may occur in any of the shoulder girdle musculature. Most commonly, it affects the biceps brachii, rotator cuff, and periscapular muscles. Overuse tendinitis may be due to improper stroke mechanics, muscular weakness/imbalances, instability, or repetitive microtraumatic forces. Anterior glenohumeral laxity is frequently seen in all swimming strokes, but it seems to be much more prevalent in back-strokers.[12,27] The swimmer may experience a spectrum of symptoms, from anterior shoulder pain and tendinitis, to palpable and sometimes voluntary subluxations. Lastly, postural faults and muscular asymmetry are common in swimmers.[28] The swimmer often exhibits well-developed upper back musculature such as the latissimus dorsi, increased thoracic kyphosis, forward shoulder posturing with associated pectoris minor tightness, frequent thoracic outlet symptoms, and gross scapular hypermobility. Beach and coworkers reported a correlation between muscles fatigue and the onset of shoulder pain.[2] The muscles that fatigued were the external rotators and abductors.

Successful clinical treatment of these lesions is dependent on the identification of the predisposing factors and accurate diagnosis. There are several key rehabilitation concepts to consider when treating the female swimmer. First, there must be assurance that proper swimming mechanics are being performed. In particular, a sufficient body roll and rotation is performed during the recovery phase; this minimizes the amount of horizontal abduction necessary for initiating the recovery. A body roll of 40° to 60° is recommended.[2,26] In addition, proper hand placement and position is critical, as is proper kick, head position, and breathing technique. Most swimmers exhibit excessive glenohumeral joint mobility, therefore, a program that emphasizes stabilization is critical. Specific exercises for the rotator cuff, especially the external rotators, the scapular retractors, depressors, and protractors, are also indicated. Flexibility exercises for the pectoralis minor muscles, scalene muscles, and sternocleidomastoid muscles are useful in correcting postural faults. Training exercise drills that emphasize muscular endurance is vital for distance swimmers. Lastly, and perhaps most importantly, is a proper training program of swimming, weight training, and stretching. Frequently, the swimmer overtrains, resulting in overuse conditions and diminished performance. The swimmer should consider cross-training activities or land workouts to improve shoulder strength and swimming techniques.

Softball Injuries

Most upper extremity injuries in softball players appear to occur to the glenohumeral joint. Loosli and coworkers performed an injury survey of 8 college teams during the 1989 NCAA Tournament.[32] The shoulder was the most commonly injured joint, with the diagnoses of shoulder tendinitis and strain being most common. It appears that pitchers are more susceptible than catchers. Barrentine and coworkers[1] have reported significant forces and stresses at the shoulder joint during the windmill softball pitch.

Barrantine and colleagues[1] have described 4 phases of the windmill pitch: windup, stride, delivery, and follow through (Fig. 44-2). During the delivery phase, the shear forces at the shoulder and elbow joint are quite high. During the delivery phase, shoulder flexion angular velocity is $5260° ± 2390°$/sec. In addition, glenohumeral joint superior compressive force is 98% of body weight, which may predispose the pitcher to subacromial impingement, biceps tendinitis, and SLAP lesions. Shoulder internal rotation torque is $4.4 ± 1.5$ times body weight and shoulder adduction/horizontal adduction torque is 3.3 times body weight. Thus, tremendous forces are generated at the anterior aspect of the glenohumeral joint. At the elbow joint approximately 70% of body weight is compressing the ulna into the humerus, and elbow flexion torque is 4.6 times body weight. This elbow flexion torque may explain the high incidence of biceps tendinitis seen in the windmill pitcher.

Maffet and colleagues[34] have described the electromyographic activity of the shoulder musculature during the windmill softball pitch. Interestingly, the posterior deltoid exhibited the highest level of electromyographic activity ($102 ± 42\%$ MMT [manual muscle test]) of all muscles studied. This occurred during the 3 to 12 o'clock position (see Fig.44-2). The supraspinatus and infraspinatus were most active (78% and 93%, respectively) during the 6 to 3 o'clock position. During the delivery phase (12 o'clock position to ball release) the subscapularis (81% MMT), pectoralis major (76% MMT), and serratus anterior muscles (61% MMT) were most active.

As noted by Loosli and coworkers,[32] the most common injuries occurring to the softball pitcher are shoulder tendinitis, bicipital tendinitis, and shoulder strains. It appears the female windmill pitcher is susceptible to overuse injuries and injuries related to hypermobility of the glenohumeral joint. The injuries we see most often are rotator cuff tendinitis, subacromial impingement, bicipital tendinitis, and rotator cuff strain.

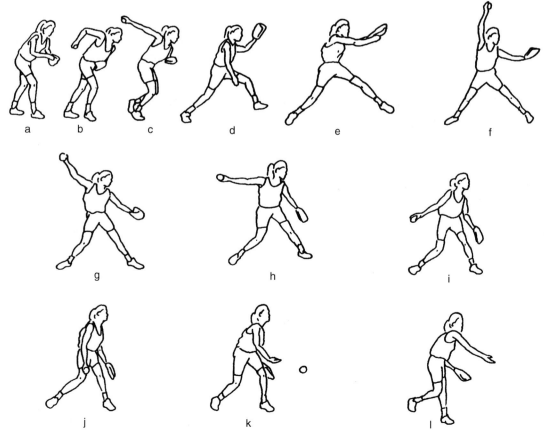

Figure 44-2. Four phases of the windmill pitch: Wind-up **(A–C)**, stride **(D–F)**, delivery **(G–J)**, follow through **(K–L)**. (From Barrantine SW, Fleisig GS, Whiteside VA, et al: Biomechanics of windmill softball pitching with injury mechanisms at the shoulder and elbow. J Orthop Sports Phys Ther 28:405–14, 1998, with permission of the Orthopaedic and Sports Sections of the American Physical Therapy Association.)

Occasionally, we see a windmill pitcher who exhibits posterior elbow pain due to excessive compression with forceful extension.

Specific rehabilitation guidelines for the windmill pitcher are numerous. A thorough clinical examination with careful subjective history is critical in establishing a successful rehabilitation program. Often, the first treatment suggestion is abstaining from pitching or throwing for a brief period of time (2 to 8 weeks) to allow the inflamed tissues to calm down. The use of anti-inflammatory medications can be helpful. Our treatment for the female softball player has been improving dynamic stabilization of the glenohumeral joint, enhancing posterior rotator cuff strength, improving scapular muscle strength, and enhancing shoulder proprioception. Once a foundation of muscular strength has been established, the athlete can be progressed to an isotonic strengthening program. The program we utilize is called the "Throwers' Ten" exercise program. This core exercise program has been established on the basis of several electromyographic studies.[4,22,42,57] Once the athlete can perform isotonic exercises without pain, she may be progressed to plyometrics and then to an interval throwing program. Brief examples of exercise drills for each of these concepts will be discussed later in this chapter.

Gymnastics Injuries

Shoulder injuries in gymnasts result more frequently from overuse than from any specific traumatic episode. This reflects the training intensity inherent in this particular sport. The incidence of shoulder pathology is slightly higher in male gymnasts; this due to the stress imposed on the shoulder during events such as the rings and high bar. Also, the types of shoulder injuries vary significantly between males and females, with males experiencing an increased incidence of macrotraumatic injuries, such as dislocations and subluxations.

During the 1998 to 1999 intercollegiate season, 90 colleges participated in female gymnastics, with 1490 athletes. Conversely, during the same season, only 26 colleges fielded a male gymnastics team, consisting of 375 athletes.[44] Pettrone and Ricciardelli[49] and Lowry and coworkers[33] have reported that the incidence and severity of injury increase with the gymnast's skill and experience. The difficulty demands of advanced skill execution in terms of strength, flexibility, complexity, and coordination also place gymnasts at frequent risk for more severe injuries. Pettrone and Ricciardelli[49]

reported a positive correlation between duration and frequency of practice and injury rate. Gymnasts who train more than 20 hours/week are also at greater risk of both acute and chronic injuries. Competitive gymnasts invest at least 20 hours/week in their sport and often train 50 weeks/year with no off season.

Several investigators have reported that the shoulder joint is susceptible to chronic injuries, such as overuse tendinitis, strains, and other microtraumatic lesions. Wadly and Albright reported the shoulder joint the fourth most commonly injured joint in female intercollegiate gymnasts over a 4-year period, with low back, ankle, great toe, shoulder, and knee injuries occurring in lesser numbers.[59] Lindner and Cain analyzed injury patterns of female competitive club gymnasts and noted that the most common injuries were fractures of the wrist, fingers, and toes, followed by sprains of the ankle and knee.[31] Shoulder injuries were not common.

Elbow injuries can be seen in female gymnasts. One common elbow injury is osteochondritis dissecans of the humeral capitellum. Jackson and coworkers[23] reported on 10 cases (ages 10 to 17 years of age) in high-performance gymnasts. Priest[50] reported on 32 elbow injuries in 30 female gymnasts. Thirty of the 32 injuries were fractures or dislocations. The author had several recommendations for preventing these injuries, including use of experienced spotters, thicker pads, and teaching proper falling techniques.

In the female gymnast, glenohumeral joint laxity is not uncommon; hypermobility is, in fact, the general rule. Because of the finely tuned quality and high degree of dynamic stabilization inherent in these athletes, symptomatic hypermobility is rarely a problem. Rather, female gymnasts usually complain of isolated or diffuse shoulder pain, tendinitis pain, and occasionally labrum lesion symptoms such as popping or catching. Rehabilitation of the shoulder joint in gymnasts includes reduction of pain and inflammation, enhancing dynamic stabilization, and improving scapular strength. Emphasis should be placed on closed kinetic chain exercises.[65] Exercise drills such as hand weight-bearing shifts, dips, push-ups, handstands, and pommel horse push-offs should be integrated into the functional progression. In the authors' experience, the lower the skill level of the gymnast, the more the athlete requires strength and stabilization training. Conversely, higher-level (elite) gymnasts often require rest, technique modification, and fine-tuning of surrounding musculature.

Golf Injuries

Golf is one of the most practiced recreational sports today because of its appeal to people of all ages, genders, and levels of fitness. Women's competitive golf has increased steadily over the past few years. Data from the NCAA during the 1998 to 1999 intercollegiate season reported 716 men's golf teams, with 7695 players and 364 women's golf teams with 2933 players.

The average golf professional plays almost every day between 6 and 10 hours a day to improve the quality of his or her game. Because of the repetitious nature of the golf swing and also the significant amount of time required to improve and maintain skill, it is no surprise that most injuries to the golfer are caused by overuse. Reports of the prevalence of injury vary, from 62% of both males and females[36] to 23% of male and 29% of female golfers.[56] Both professional and amateur female golfers have reported increased injuries to the upper extremity and fewer injuries of the spine when compared to male golfers. This may be due to the higher swing velocity and greater use of trunk rotation during the downswing phase of male golfers. Jobe and coworkers found that men and women have similar firing patterns at the shoulder during the golf swing.[25]

Because golf is not as taxing on the shoulder as traditional overhead sports, these athletes can often participate in golf for a longer duration. This added dimension of longevity may perpetuate the wear and tear on the active shoulder. The older golfer tends to have more degenerative changes to the acromioclavicular joint, the labrum, and the articular surfaces of the glenohumeral joint. However, the younger golfer typically has greater laxity of the capsule and thus more frequently suffers from tendinitis of the rotator cuff and posterior capsulitis.

Most golf injuries to the shoulder occur during the backswing. Both shoulders are predisposed to impingement-type problems as a result of the awkward position of forward flexion and internal rotation at extreme ranges of horizontal adduction. Typically, it is the lead arm that suffers greatest injury. Tightness of the posterior cuff and the large decelerative forces placed on the lead arm often cause posterior cuff tendinitis or internal impingement. Internal impingement, where the posterior cuff is impinged on the posterior superior labrum, may result in an undersurface rotator cuff lesion.

The elbow is another common site of pathology. Medial epicondylitis, also known as "golfers elbow," occurs after the excessive muscle contraction or suddenly applied forceful resistance during the swing. Lateral epicondylitis is also prevalent, with equal frequency of medial epicondylitis in both males and females. Of all golf injuries, wrist injuries are the most common among professional golfers (37.4%).[56] During the repeated golf swings, the range of motion of the wrists often exceed their functional capabilities, leading to overuse and traumatic injuries.

Glazebrook and colleagues found differences in muscle activity patterns of subjects with and without medial epicondylitis.[19] The symptomatic subjects had greater electromyographic activity of the wrist flexors during the address and swing phases. This increase in muscle activity may be the predisposing factor that leads to medial epicondylitis.

Successful treatment of golf tendinitis and impingement pathologies involves modifying the activity of the golfer. This may consist of shutting the athlete down from golf for a brief period or altering the pathologic mechanics of the swing. Often instructing the golfer to shorten the backswing motion allows for a decrease in symptoms. In addition, greater trunk flexion will allow for a more upright shoulder turn initiated from trunk rotation. Thus, strengthening the core of the body will allow more force production from the larger musculature as opposed to the distal arm muscles.

Use of ice and heat along with anti-inflammatory medications will help during the recovery period. Flexibility issues must be addressed, focusing on the posterior cuff and capsule. Strengthening of the entire shoulder complex with an emphasis on the scapular stabilizers and the posterior cuff is necessary. The posterior cuff should be trained eccentrically in order to prepare these muscles for the large decelerative forces of the arm and club during the swing. As the golfer progresses with the rehabilitative process, a gradual return to activity may be initiated to ensure symptom-free return to play.

Tennis Injuries

Tennis is an extremely popular sport among both males and females of all ages. During the 1998 to 1999 intercollegiate season, 877 colleges produced women's tennis teams, with 8492 athletes; this compared to 769 men's tennis teams, composed of 7729 players.[44] A survey conducted by Priest and Nagel of 84 world-class tennis players reported that 74% of men and 60% of women had shoulder or elbow pain in the dominant arm that affected tennis play.[51] Injuries to both the shoulder and elbow of the dominant arm were reported at 21% and 23% of the world-class male and female players, respectively.

Because of the great forces required of the upper extremity, most injuries incurred by tennis players involve the shoulder and elbow. The injuries to the shoulder typically involve the rotator cuff and/or the biceps tendon. The overhead nature of the serve causes these structures to be placed in a compromised position between the humeral head and the coracoacromial arch. The progression that has been reported in the literature begins with tendinitis, causing impingement, developing into partial and full-thickness tearing of the rotator cuff.[10]

The primary mechanisms for these overuse tendinitis injuries of the tennis athlete is the intrinsic tendon loading from the high-intensity decelerative function of the posterior cuff as well as anterior shoulder instability. The increased stress placed on the dynamic stabilizers of the glenohumeral joint may lead to microtraumatic tendon injury and further compromise joint stability and overhead function. For the skilled tennis player, there is a relatively consistent pattern of muscular activity during the tennis serve and ground strokes.[69] However, for the untrained and less-skilled tennis player, the muscular activity is more varied and often greater in certain muscle groups.[40] This represents how less-than-optimal timing and a lack of whole-body contributions to force generation and deceleration subject an individual's shoulder to overuse injury.

Another common overuse injury in tennis involves the elbow. Lateral epicondylitis, also known as "tennis elbow," primarily involves the extensor carpi radialis brevis. It is often thought that inappropriate mechanics on the backhand groundstroke, specifically the leading elbow backhand, is the major cause of tennis elbow. Nirschl and Sobel showed that the incidence is dependent on skill level, with recreational and novice players suffering greater occurrence. Conversely, the highly skilled players had a higher rate of medial epicondylitis owing to the powerful and repetitive nature of the serve.[47]

Slowing the degenerative process and facilitating the repair process of the body are the primary goals in the treatment of these overuse injuries. Often shutting the player down is necessary to calm the inflamed tissue. It may be possible to allow the player to continue with groundstrokes and limit the amount of overhead serves. The focus of the rehabilitation program should be placed on the dynamic stabilizers of the shoulder. Specific exercises will be discussed later in this chapter. In addition, the posterior cuff strength of the athlete must be addressed. As the posterior cuff works in deceleration of the arm in the swinging motion, this type of exercise should be incorporated into

the program. Evaluating the equipment is necessary for the injured player. A stiffer racquet is less forgiving and may contribute to an overuse condition. A more flexible racquet will soften the initial impact of the ball and thus decrease the shock imparted on the arm. In addition, it is also recommended that the tension on the strings of the racquet be reduced following return to play after an upper extremity overuse injury. Upon return to competition, an interval tennis program should be utilized to properly prepare the athlete for full symptom-free participation.

Volleyball Injuries

In 1975, volleyball became the first professional team sport to have men and women competing on the same team. In 1981, the NCAA held its first volleyball championship for women. Since then, the sport has seen tremendous growth. During the 1998 to 1999 intercollegiate season, there were 960 women's volleyball teams, fielding 13,194 athletes; this compares to 79 men's teams, comprising 1124 athletes.[44] According to the National Federation of State High School Associations (NFSHA), volleyball is the third most popular sport among high school girls.[46] During the 1998 to 1999 volleyball season, there were 53 shoulder injuries and only 3 elbow injuries reported by the NCAA surveillance system. The most common injuries are tendinitis and strains. This may be due to the fact that most volleyball injuries to the shoulder are overuse in nature. Typically, tendinitis of the rotator cuff or the biceps tendon is seen. This may be caused by the frequent cycles of abduction and external rotation followed by forceful extension and internal rotation as the ball is contacted during spiking and overhead serving.

Several researchers have collected data on the incidence of suprascapular neuropathy.[13,41,54,61,68] All of the studies showed that this pathology was found mostly in elite competitive volleyball players. Suprascapular neuropathy occurs when the suprascapular nerve is compressed at the spinoglenoid notch. Although this is often a painless condition, isolated weakness of the infraspinatus is present. Because of this weakness of the external rotators, a muscular imbalance may develop, thus requiring treatment to prevent any secondary pathology. Treatment involves addressing this abnormal muscle ratio with strengthening exercises that focus on the external rotators of the shoulder.

Hand injuries occur frequently in volleyball; however, they usually do not prevent the athlete's playing or practicing. Bhairo found that sprains and strains were the most common type of injuries, followed by fractures and then contusions.[3] Taping of wrists and fingers may help prevent and manage these injuries.

The rehabilitation program for the female volleyball player is similar to that for other female overhead athletes. It is important to focus on scapular strengthening along with strengthening of the posterior cuff musculature. The rehabilitation program for these females must also include power drills to prepare the player for spikes and serves.

SPECIFIC REHABILITATION PRINCIPLES FOR THE FEMALE ATHLETE

We have identified 8 unique anatomic and physiologic factors present in the female overhead athlete. Based on these 8 factors we have developed 8 rehabilitation concepts to address their unique factors (Table 44-1). First, the treatment program should emphasize dynamic stabilization to control and minimize glenohumeral laxity. To improve dynamic stabilization of the shoulder several progressive steps must be accomplished successfully. Initially, muscular balance of the surrounding musculature must be accomplished, particularly the muscular strength ratio of the external and internal rotators.[66] Based on isokinetic testing, we have determined the ratio for overhead athletes should be 65% to 75% when tested at 180° or 300°/sec.[64] Thus, if the ratio is below this value, the athlete must be established on a progressive strengthening program to accomplish this balance. Once muscular balance is achieved, then coactivation drills may be initiated. We perform static rhythmic stabilization (RS) drills initially, then progress to proprioceptive neuromuscular facilitation (PNF) drills with RS

throughout the arc of motion (Fig. 44-3). These drills should be progressive from midrange positions and then advanced to end-range stabilization in order to maximally challenge the dynamic stabilizers. In addition, closed kinetic chain drills are effective in enhancing dynamic stabilization as well. We prefer the use of an unstable platform or ball to challenge the neuromuscular system. Drills such as push-ups on a ball, push-ups on a balance system, and arm stabilizations onto a ball into the wall (Fig. 44-4) are examples.

Next, some female athletes exhibit hypermobility of the proximal biceps tendon. Because of the repetitive subluxations of the tendon, the tendon can become painful and inflamed. During the acute inflammatory process we believe it is important for the rehabilitation specialist to attempt to control recurrent biceps tendon subluxations. Specific techniques include limiting external rotation to neutral when performing strengthening exercises (Fig. 44-5). In addition, shoulder-strengthening exercises should be performed in neutral position in the scapular plane at 30° to 45° abduction to place the biceps tendon on slack. Consideration should be given to performing joint approximation or closed kinetic chain exercises initially until the tendon inflammation diminishes. The athlete is then progressed to isotonic strengthening. Murphy has suggested the use of an upper arm strap (similar to a tennis elbow strap) to assist in stabilization of the biceps tendon in the intertubercular groove (Fig. 44-6).[43] Clinically, he has noted improvement in his patients while using the strap.

Third, frequently we see female athletes who exhibit hypermobility of their scapula with poorly developed scapular musculature. Thus, the rehabilitation goal is to improve scapular muscle strength and enhance scapular stability. Scapular stability is critical to the function of the shoulder joint and arm, especially in the over-

Table 44-1. Rehabilitation Concepts That Address the Unique Anatomic and Physiologic Factors of Female Athletes

UNIQUE ANATOMIC AND PHYSIOLOGIC FACTORS	REHABILITATION CONCEPTS
Increased shoulder laxity	Emphasize dynamic stabilization
Biceps tendon hypermobility	Limit external rotation
Scapular hypermobility with poorly developed scapular musculature	Improve stability
Less developed shoulder girdle musculature	Enhanced proprioception, neuromuscular control and dynamic stability
Less developed glenohumeral capsule	Emphasize rotator cuff strength and performance
Stable foundation	Emphasize scapular stability and "core" stability
Frequent diagnoses "overuse tendinitis"	Proper training and techniques
	Preparticipation conditioning
Increased laxity with muscular fatigue	Improve shoulder muscular endurance

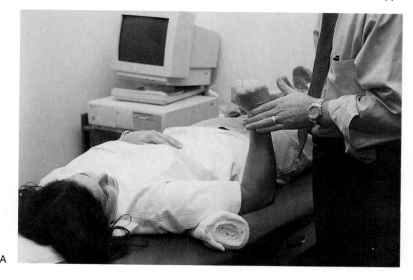

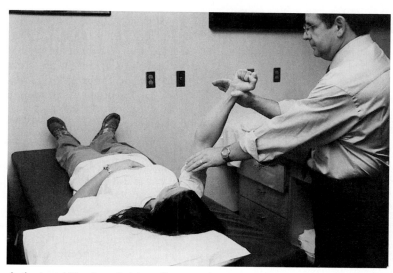

Figure 44-3. A, Static rhythmic stabilizations. **B,** Manually resisted PNF D$_2$ drills with rhythmic stabilizations.

head athlete. Initially, it is vital to re-establish a proper force-couple relationship of the scapular muscles.

The scapular muscles act within a typical force-couple pattern, whereas the balance of forces produce a rotary movement. Hence, it is vital to have achieved balance of these components of the force couple prior to initiating aggressive movements or activities. The critical muscle groups to assess and most often treat are the scapular depressors, the retractors, and lastly the protractors. The exercises that utilize these movements are prone horizontal abduction with full external rotation, press-ups, prone horizontal abduction with neutral rotation, seated rowing, and for the scapular protractors, supine punches, push ups, and a dynamic hug.

Once we believe we have re-established a stable base of support for upper extremity function, the more challenging exercise drills are initiated for the scapular muscles. We perform neuromuscular control drills for the scapular muscles (Fig. 44-7). This maximally challenges the scapular muscles, but perhaps more importantly, challenges the athlete's proprioceptive system.

Fourth, most female athletes exhibit less-developed shoulder girdle musculature than their male counterparts. Therefore, when training or rehabilitating a female athlete it is imperative to enhance proprioception and neuromuscular control. Blasier and colleagues[5] have shown that individuals with increased generalized laxity exhibit proprioception inferior to that of individuals who do not exhibit excessive laxity. This has

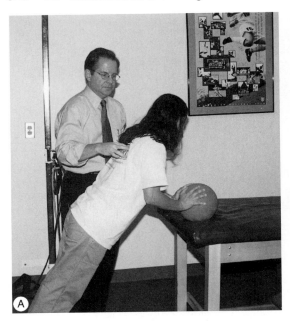

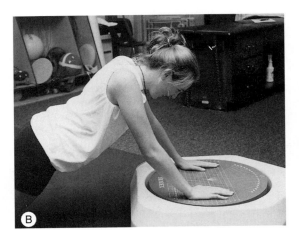

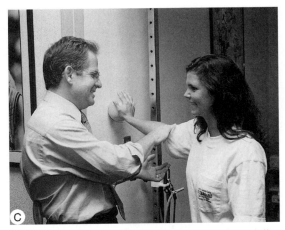

Figure 44-4. **A**, Push-up drills on a ball. **B**, Push-up drills on a balance system. **C**, Rhythmic stabilizations with a ball on a wall.

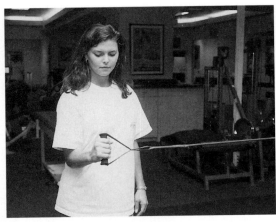

Figure 44-5. Tubing external rotator to neutral position.

significant relevance to the female athlete with excessive laxity. Specific drills we initially prefer are passive–active joint repositioning assessments and drills (Fig. 44-8). Lephart and colleagues[30] have utilized a mechanical motorized proprioception testing and training device. This exercise can also be performed on an isokinetic device (Fig. 44-9). From static dynamic joint repositioning, we progress to PNF patterns and closed kinetic chain exercises (unstable surfaces), as discussed earlier. Next, we would integrate perturbation training. These drills challenge the athlete's neuromuscular system at end ranges of motion, where most athletes experience difficulty. For the overhead athlete a drill we utilize is external rotation with exercise tubing with RS/perturbation at the end range (Fig. 44-10). This can also be accomplished using a lightweight plyoball against a wall (Fig. 44-11). Another exercise drill that produces significant improvements in the neuromuscular system is the use of plyometrics. The progression we use with plyometrics is 2-hand drills first, then one-hand standing drills, then lastly entire-body

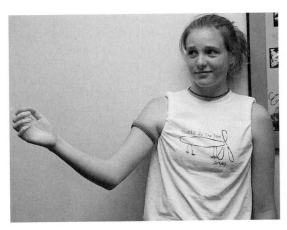

Figure 44-6. Upper arm strap.

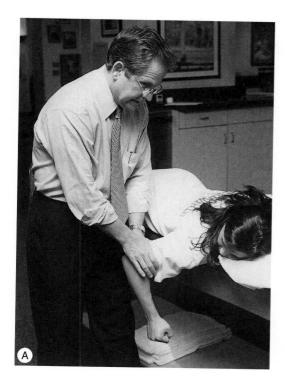

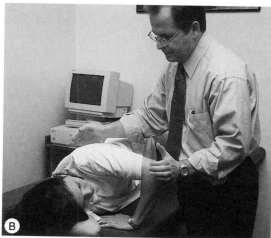

Figure 44-7. A, Manual resistance prone rows. **B**, Neuromuscular control drill of the scapula.

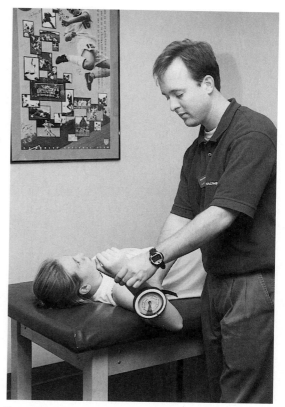

Figure 44-8. Passive–active joint repositioning.

overhead athletes exhibit weakness of the external rotators and scapular muscles. This appears especially true for female overhead athletes. Thus, the rehabilitation specialist must emphasize external rotation strengthening. Fleisig and coworkers[14] reported the most effective exercises for the external rotators based on electromyographic analysis. They determined sidelying external rotation, prone rowing into external

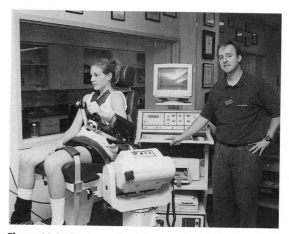

Figure 44-9. Passive–active joint repositioning on an isokinetic machine.

one-hand drills. The use of plyometric training has been shown to improve kinesthesia[15,55] as well as enhance throwing distance and internal rotation strength.[15] For a complete description of specific plyometric drills, the reader is encouraged to examine the articles by Chu,[8] Gambett,[17] and Wile and coworkers.[67]

Fifth, as previously mentioned, the female athlete generally exhibits a lesser developed muscular of the shoulder girdle, specifically, the posterior shoulder and scapular region. It has been the experience of the authors that most

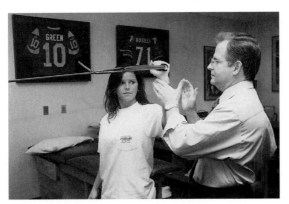

Figure 44-10. Tubing external rotation with end-range rhythmic stabilization.

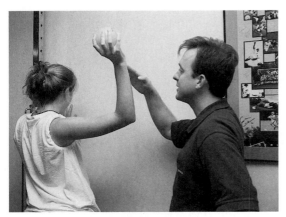

Figure 44-11. Plyoball wall dribble with end-range rhythmic stabilization.

Table 44-2. Typical Periodization Model for a Professional Baseball Player

EMPHASIZE DYNAMIC STABILIZATION
Muscular balance
Coactivation drills
Rhythmic stabilization drills
Closed kinetic chain exercises

BICEPS TENDON HYPERMOBILITY
Limit external rotation
Exercise in neutral rotation
Joint approximation drills

SCAPULAR HYPERMOBILITY—IMPROVE STABILITY
Normalize force couples "balance"
Neuromuscular control drills
Restore stable base

ENHANCE PROPRIOCEPTION AND NEURO- MUSCULAR CONTROL
Joint reposition drills
Perturbation training
Plyometric training

EMPHASIZE ROTATOR CUFF STRENGTH AND PERFORMANCE
External rotator strengthening
Internal rotator strengthening
Coconcentration drills

EMPHASIZE CORE STABILITY
Trunk strength
Control pelvis
Legs to create rotational movements

PROPER TRAINING AND TECHNIQUE (PREPARTICIPATION CONDITIONING)
Year round program (periodization)
Conditioning drills
Technique, skill training drills

IMPROVE SHOULDER MUSCULATURE ENDURANCE
Endurance drills
Upper body ergometry
Increased repetitions

rotation, and prone horizontal abduction to 100° with full external rotation to be the most effective. Additionally, standing external rotation with exercise tubing resistance and a towel roll placed between the humerus and body enhanced electromyographic activity by 18% to 23% compared to no use of a towel roll. Enhancement of internal rotator strength should also be performed, but caution must be exercised not to offset the desired unilateral muscle ratio of the external and internal rotators.

Sixth, all overhead athletes require a stable base of support for the upper extremity to act from. That base of support is not only the scapula but also the core of the body, which includes the trunk and pelvis.[63] We have referred to this as "core stability." Pelvis stability may be even more critical for the female athlete. Exercises such as abdominal sit-ups, low back extensions, and gluteal muscle training are all vital aspects of establishing core stability.

Furthermore, we prefer utilizing a balance beam to enhance gluteal and pelvic control. Specific drills on the balance beam include the dip walk, lateral step-ups, and stabilization in the "balanced position." Once baseline core stability is achieved advanced exercises, such as the 2-hand overhead soccer throw with step-up onto a box or plyo sit-ups, may be initiated.

The seventh concept is the importance of a well-structured year-round conditioning pro-

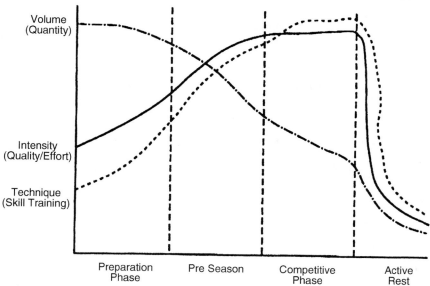

Figure 44-12. The periodization model. (From Matveyev L: Fundamentals of Sports Training. Moscow, Russia, Progress Publishers, 1977, with permission.)

gram. The program must utilize the principles of periodization. The periodization model specifies various phases during the year; most often the program will use 4 specific training sessions during the calendar year. Table 44-2 presents a typical periodization model for the professional baseball player. This model can be modified to fit any athlete. These 4 phases are the competitive (in-season) phase, the postcompetition (recovery) phase, preparation, and the transitional phase.[35] The periodization model is based on controlling and adjusting 3 variables: volume of work, intensity of effort, and skill technique training. As illustrated in Figure 44-12, volume and technique are inversely related, whereas intensity and technique are directly related. In some year-round sports, such as professional tennis, golf, and gymnastics, the periodization concept is difficult to implement. In these sports, athletes are expected to perform at a high level for 10 to 11 months of the year. This expectation is unrealistic and cannot be accomplished for a long period or over a career. Usually the athlete will exhibit peaks and valleys in performance during the year. Also as a result of high-intensity training over a long period of time, injury may occur. The conditioning program and specific exercises should change based on the time of year. The objectives of using the periodization model are to (1) control peaking of athletic skills, (2) prevent under- or over-training, (3) minimize boredom of training, and (4) enhance cross-training effects.

Lastly, a critical rehabilitation concept is enhancing muscular endurance. It has been shown that once the surrounding shoulder musculature is fatigued, proprioception is significantly diminished[58] and laxity increases significantly.[18,62] It appears that both laxity and proprioception are critical elements to the female overhead athlete. Thus, when training or rehabilitating, the female athlete should include endurance muscle training. We utilize several forms of exercises to enhance endurance. They include upper body ergometry, use of a VersaClimber machine, high-repetition sets, and specific plyometric-type drills. These drills include plyoball wall dribbling, plyoball wall throws, and 2-hand side-to-side throws (Fig. 44-13).

The Prevention and Conditioning Program

The primary objectives of the conditioning program for any athlete is injury prevention and performance enhancement. These 2 concepts are closely related. A thorough conditioning program will help prevent injuries; in turn, a healthy athlete who trains properly should improve athletic performance and experience a long productive career. The SAID principle, *s*pecific *a*daptation for *i*mposed *d*emands, refers to the concept that to be proficient at a skill or task, the training of that specific activity must exceed the normal limits in order for improvement to occur.

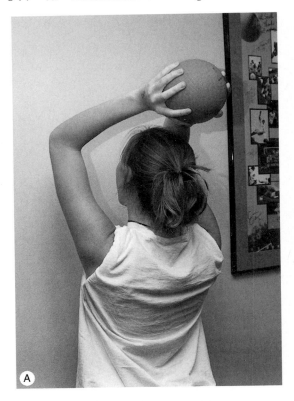

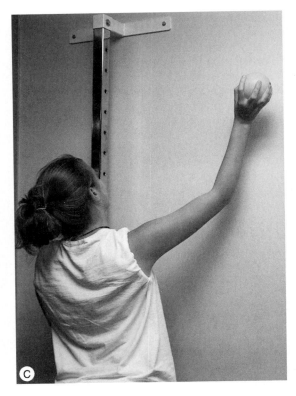

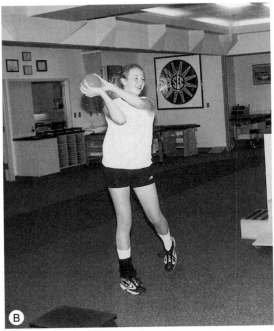

Figure 44-13. A, Plyometric wall drill: wall dribbling. **B,** Plyometric wall drill: 2-hand soccer throw. **C,** Plyometric 2-hand side-to-side throw.

Therefore, the conditioning program for individual sports along with positions within each sport will vary greatly; however, there are gener-al principles for all athletes. A conditioning program for any athlete must include the following components: strength, endurance, power, speed, flexibility, neuromuscular training, and skill/coordination training. The athlete's program should represent a balance between these concepts. Overemphasis in one area may lead to injury or suboptimal performance. Also, the conditioning program should vary throughout the year. This concept of periodization has previously been discussed.

Because the shoulder and elbow represent the final link of the kinetic chain, the entire body must be incorporated into the conditioning program. As mentioned earlier in the chapter, core strength provides a stable base of support from which the rest of the body may function. Strength from the legs and trunk of the body will help dissipate stress to the upper extremities and allow for improved power and function during sport-specific activities.

CONCLUDING REMARKS

The upper extremity of the female has unique characteristics that make the rehabilitation of these athletes a challenge. The key to designing an effective program for either rehabilitation or the prevention of injury is understanding these unique characteristics and considering their effects on the function of the upper extremity in the involved sport. By obtaining a thorough evaluation and application of the 7 basic principles of rehabilitation, the female will be given the optimal opportunity to return to full participation in athletic activity.

References

1. Barrantine SW, Fleisig GS, Whiteside VA, et al: Biomechanics of windmill softball pitching with injury mechanisms at the shoulder and elbow. J Orthop Sports Phys Ther 28:405–14, 1998.
2. Beach ML, Whitney SL, Dickoff-Hoffman SA: Relationship of shoulder flexibility, strength, and endurance to shoulder pain in competitive swimmers. J Orthop Sports Phys Ther 16:262–9, 1992.
3. Bhairo NH, Nijsten MWN, van Dalen KC, et al: Hand injuries in volleyball. Int J Sports Med 13:351–4, 1992.
4. Blackburn TA, McLeod WIB, White B: EMG analysis of posterior rotator cuff exercises. J Athletic Train 25:40–5, 1990.
5. Blasier RB, Carpenter JE, Huston LJ: Shoulder proprioception: effects of joint laxity, joint position, direction of motion. Orthop Rev 23:45–50, 1994.
6. Blatz D: Swimmer's shoulder. Swimming World 25:41, 1985.
7. Brown GA, Tan JL, Kirkley A: The lax shoulder in females. Clin Orthop 372:110–22, 2000.
8. Chu D: Plyometric exercise. Nat Strength Cond J 6:56–9, 1984.
9. Crockett HJ, Andrews JR, Wilk KE: Arthroscopic findings of the glenohumeral joint in male vs. female overhead athletes. Presented at the American Sports Medicine Institute Fellow Research Day, July 30, 1999.
10. Ellenbecker TS: Shoulder injuries in tennis. In Andrews JR, Wilk KE (eds): The Athlete's Shoulder. Churchill Livingstone, New York, 1994, p 399.
11. Falkel JE: Swimming injuries. In Sanders B (ed): Sports Physical Therapy. Norwalk, CT, Appleton & Lange, 1009, p 477.
12. Falkel JE, Murphy TC: Swimming injuries. In Malone T (ed): Sports Injury Management Series. Baltimore, Williams & Wilkins, 1988.
13. Ferretti A, DeCarli A, Fontana M: Injury of the suprascapular nerve at the spinoglenoid notch. The natural history of infraspinatus atrophy in volleyball players. Am J Sports Med 26(6):759–63, 1998.
14. Fleisig GS, Zheng N, Barrantine SW, et al: Kinematic and kinetic comparison of full effort and partial effort baseball pitching, 20th annual American Society of Biomechanics, Atlanta, October 18, 1996.
15. Fortun CM, Davis GJ, Kernozck TW: the effects of plyometric training on the shoulder internal rotators. Phys Ther (Abstr) 78(51):587, 1998.
16. Fowler P: Swimmer problems. Am J Sports Med 7:141, 1979.
17. Gambetta V: Conditioning of the shoulder complex. In Andrews JR, Wilk KE (eds): The Athlete's Shoulder. Churchill Livingstone, New York, 1994, p 643.
18. Gladstone J, Andrews JR, Wilk KE: The effects of muscular fatigue on glenohumeral kinematics in the overhead professional baseball pitcher. A radiographic study. Presented at the ASMI Fellow Research Day, July 12, 1996.
19. Glazebrook MA, Curwin S, Islam MN, et al: Medial epicondylitis: An electromyographic analysis and an investigation of intervening strategies. Am J Sports Med 22(5):674–9, 1994.
20. Guanche C, Knatt T, Solomonow M, et al: The synergistic action of the capsule and the shoulder muscles. Am J Sports Med 23(3):301–6, 1995.
21. Harryman DT, Sidles JA, Harris SL, et al: Role of the rotator cuff interval capsule in passive motion and stability of the shoulder. J Bone Joint Surg 74A:53–66, 1992.
22. Hintermeister RA, Lange GW, Schultheis JM, et al: EMG activity and applied load during shoulder exercises using elastic resistance. Am J Sports Med 26(2):210–20, 1998.
23. Jackson DW, Silvino N, Reiman P: Osteochondritis in the female gymnast elbow. Arthroscopy 5(2):129–36, 1989.
24. Jobe CM: Superior glenoid impingement. Clin Orthop 330:98–107, 1996.
25. Jobe FW, Perry J, Pink M: Electromyographic shoulder activity in men and women professional golfers. Am J Sports Med 17(6):782–7, 1989.
26. Johnson JE, Sim FH, Scott SG: Musculoskeletal injuries in competitive swimmers. Mayo Clin Proc 62:289, 1987.
27. Kibler WB: The role of the scapula in athlete's shoulder function. Am J Sports Med 26:325–37, 1998.
28. Kennedy JC, Craig AB, Schneider RD: Swimming. In Schneider RC, Kennedy JC, Plant ML (eds): Sports Injuries: Mechanisms, Prevention and Treatment. Baltimore, Williams & Wilkins, 1985.
29. Knatt T, Guanche C, Solomonow M: The glenohumeral biceps reflex in the feline. Clin Orthop 314:247–52, 1995.
30. Lephart SM, Warner JJP, Borsa PA, et al: Proprioception of the shoulder in healthy, unstable and surgically repaired shoulders. J Shoulder Elbow Surg 3:371–81, 1996.
31. Lindner KJ, Cain DJ: Injury patterns of female competitive club gymnastics. Can J Sport Sci 15(4):254–61, 1990.
32. Loosli AR, Regua RK, Garrick JG, et al: Injuries to pitchers in women's collegiate fast pitch softball. Am J Sports Med 20:35–7, 1992.
33. Lowry CB, LeVeau BF: A retrospective study in gymnastic injury to competitors and non-competitors in private clubs. Am J Sports Med 110:237, 1982.
34. Maffett MW, Jobe FW, Pink MM, et al: Shoulder muscle firing patterns during the windmill softball pitch. Am J Sports Med 25:369–74, 1997.
35. Matveyev L: Fundamentals of Sports Training. Moscow, Russia, Progress Publishers, 1977.
36. McCarroll JR, Rettig AC, Shelbourne KD: Injuries in the amateur golfer. Phys Sports 18(3):121–6, 1990.
37. McFarland EG, Wosik M: Injuries in female collegiate swimmers due to swimming and cross training. Clin J Sport Med 6(3):178–82, 1996.
38. McMaster WC: Painful shoulder in swimmers: a diagnostic challenge. Physician Sportsmed 14:108, 1986.
39. Meister K: Current concepts: Injuries to the shoulder in the throwing athlete. Part one. Am J Sports Med 28(2):265–75, 2000.
40. Miyashita M, Tsunoda T, Sakurai S, et al: Muscular activities in the tennis serve and overhand throwing. Scand J Sports Sci 2(52), 1980.
41. Montagna P, Colonna S: Suprascapular neuropathy restricted to the infraspinatus muscle in volleyball players. Acta Neurol Scand 87(3):248–50, 1993.

42. Moseley JB, Jobe FW, Pink M, et al: EMG analysis of the scapular muscles during a shoulder rehabilitation program. Am J Sports Med 20:182–4, 1992.

43. Murphy TC: Shoulder injuries in swimming. In Andrews JR, Wilk KE (eds): The Athlete's Shoulder. New York, Churchill Livingstone, 1993, pp 411–24.

44. National Collegiate Athletic Association's Championship Sports Participation Data, 1982–1999.

45. National Collegiate Athletic Association's Injury Surveillance Data, 1998–1999.

46. National Federation of State High School Associations. Indianapolis, Ind, 1999.

47. Nirschl RP: Prevent and treatment of elbow and shoulder injuries in the tennis player. Clin Sports Med 7:289–308, 1998.

48. O'Brien SJ, Neves MC, Arnoczky SP, et al: The anatomy and histology of the inferior glenohumeral ligament complex of the shoulder. Am J Sports Med 18:449–556, 1990.

49. Pettrone FA, Ricciardelli E: Gymnast injuries: The Virginia experience. Am J Sports Med 15:59, 1987.

50. Priest JD: Elbow injuries in gymnastics. Clin Sports Med 4(1):73–83, 1985.

51. Priest JD, Nagel DA: Tennis shoulder. Am J Sports Med 4:28–42, 1976.

52. Richardson AB: The biomechanics of swimming: the shoulder and knee. In Cuillo JV (ed): Swimming. Clin Sports Med 5:103, 1986.

53. Richardson AB, Jobe FW, Collins HR: The shoulder in competitive swimming. Am J Sports Med 8:158, 1980.

54. Sandow MJ, Illic J: Suprascapular nerve rotator cuff compression syndrome in volleyball players. J Shoulder Elbow Surg 7(5):516–21, 1998.

55. Swanik KA, Lephart SM, Swanik CB, et al: The effects of shoulder plyometric training on proprioception and muscle performance characteristics. J Athletic Train 34:59, 1999.

56. Theriault G, Lacoste E, Gaboury M, et al: Golf injury characteristics: A survey from 528 golfers. Med Sci Sports Exerc 28(5):565–9, 1996.

57. Townsend H, Jobe FW, Pink M, et al: EMG analysis of the glenohumeral muscles during a rehabilitation program. Am J Sports Med 19:264–9, 1991.

58. Voight ML, Hardin JA, Blackburn TA, et al: The effects of muscle fatigue on and the relationship of arm dominance to shoulder proprioception. J Orthop Sports Phys Ther 23:348–52, 1996.

59. Wadley GH, Albright JP: Women's intercollegiate gymnastics. Injury patterns and "permanent" medical disability. Am J Sports Med 21(2):314–20, 1993.

60. Walch G, Boileau P, Noel P, et al: Impingement of the deep surface of the supraspinatus tendon on the posterosuperior glenoid rim: an arthroscopic study. J Shoulder Elbow Surg 1:238–45, 1992.

61. Wang DH, Koehler SM: Isolated infraspinatus atrophy in a collegiate volleyball player. Clin J Sport Med 6(4):255–8,1996.

62. Wickiewicz TH, Chen SK, Otis JC, et al: Glenohumeral kinematics in a muscle fatigue model: A radiographic study. Presented at the 1994 Specialty Day Meeting. AOSSM, New Orleans, February 1994.

63. Wilk KE: Physiology of baseball. In Garret WE, Kirkendall DT (eds): Exercise and Sports Science. Philadelphia, Lippincott, Williams & Wilkins, 2000, pp 708–31.

64. Wilk KE, Andrews JR, Arrigo CA, et al: The strength characteristics of internal and external rotator muscles in professional baseball players. Am J Sports Med 21(1):61–6, 1993.

65. Wilk KE, Arrigo CA, Andrews JR: Closed and open kinetic chain exercises for the upper extremity. J Sports Rehabil 5:88–102, 1996.

66. Wilk KE, Arrigo CA, Andrews JR: Current concepts: The stabilizing structures of the glenohumeral joint. J Orthop Sports Phys Ther 25:364–79, 1997.

67. Wilk KE, Voight ML, Keirns MA, et al: Stretch-shortening drills for the upper extremity: theory and clinical application. J Orthop Sports Phys Ther 17:225–39, 1993.

68. Witvrouw E, Cools A, Lysens R, et al: Suprascapular neuropathy in volleyball players. Br J Sports Med 34(3):174–80, June 2000.

69. Yoshizawa M, Itani T, Jonsson B: Muscular load in shoulder and forearm muscles in tennis players with different levels of skill. In Jonsson B (ed): Biomechanics X-B. Champaign, Ill, Human Kinetics, 1987.

Chapter 45

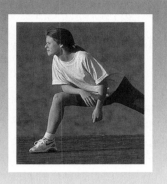

Evaluation of Strength

George J. Davies, M.Ed., P.T., S.C.S., A.T.C., C.S.C.S.
Terry R. Malone, Ed.D., P.T., A.T.C.

Evaluation of strength is but one part of the comprehensive examination or serial reassessment of the female athlete. This chapter begins with the traditional concepts and then introduces an integrated algorithm of functional testing and rehabilitation.

OVERVIEW OF CONSIDERATIONS OF STRENGTH TESTING

Strength can be defined in various ways; however, for the purposes of this chapter we are going to focus primarily on strength as it relates to the female athlete. Therefore, evaluation of strength is going to focus on isometric, isotonic, and isokinetic testing of selected muscle groups. Furthermore, various modes of muscle actions can be assessed, including isometric, concentric, and eccentric actions, acceleration, deceleration, and plyometrics. The assessment of muscle performance for a particular activity should be contraction specific. However, most muscles actually function in sporting activities in multiple contraction modes. Therefore, multiple assessment techniques are probably most appropriate.

EVALUATION OF STRENGTH

There are various methods of evaluating strength, including manual muscle testing, hand-held dynamometry, hand-grip dynamometry, and cable tensiometry, 1- or 10-repetition-maximum progressive resistive exercise isotonic testing, computerized isokinetic dynamometry, and functional performance testing of activities of daily living, ergonomics, tests of agility, and sport-specific testing.

Manual Muscle Testing

Manual muscle testing (MMT) is a commonly used method of assessing muscle strength in a clinical setting; however, for testing female athletes, it may be relatively unreliable because of the large forces produced. Various MMT systems have been developed over the years, with each having advantages and disadvantages.[5] MMT is useful when screening many athletes within a limited time frame, or with limited equipment or facilities, as is often the case when performing preseason screening of female sports teams. MMT can also be used as part of the initial assessment of an injury and for serial reassessment during a rehabilitation program.[5]

Hand-Held Dynamometry

Hand-held dynamometry (HHD) is used to objectively quantify MMT, and its use has increased in popularity over the last several years. HHD has many of the advantages and disadvantages of MMT. It allows relatively quick and reliable isometric assessment of many muscle groups.

Cable Tensiometry

Cable tensiometers are rarely used today because they only measure isometric strength and are not as reliable as computerized testing. They are somewhat difficult to position and to use reliably.

1- or 10-Repetition-Maximum Progressive Resistive Isotonic Exercise Testing

Traditional 1- or 10-repetition-maximum progressive resistive exercise isotonic testing has for many years been considered the standard for strength testing.[2, 22] If only weights are available, then such testing can be used for strength assessment. However, isotonic testing only maximally tests a muscle at its weakest point in its range of motion (ROM) and does not control "ease" or speed of movement related to movement assessment. It is also difficult to assess true maximal efforts, particularly eccentric (lowering) capabilities. Therefore, isotonic testing is of limited value in strength testing.[6,22]

Open Kinetic Chain Computerized Isokinetic Dynamometry

Computerized isokinetic dynamometer testing has been used regularly for over 20 years. Open kinetic chain (OKC) isokinetics has been demonstrated to be valid and reliable in many studies during this time frame.[21,23,35,36,43,44,49,54,57,60] There are specific limitations with OKC isokinetics,[6,11] however, there are also many reasons to include OKC isokinetic testing in a testing process.[6,15,63] These reasons include the following:

1. The need to perform isolated testing of specific muscle groups (isolation of pathology/involvement).
2. The need to identify muscle groups away from the specific site of injury to determine *other* associated weaknesses.
3. Closed kinetic chain (CKC) or total extremity testing may not demonstrate the true weakness that exists because of compensation by proximal and distal muscles for weak/involved/inhibited structures.
4. Performing OKC exercises allows the clinician to have significant clinical control.
5. There is a correlation between OKC testing and CKC functional performance.[15]

OKC isokinetic testing can be performed either concentrically (shortening contractions) or eccentrically (lengthening actions). Eccentric isokinetic testing is a more recent modality, thus there is less information available; in addition, there have been some controversial findings regarding its application. A detailed description of eccentric testing is beyond the scope of this article, so the reader is referred to the review by Davies and Ellenbecker for more details.[7]

Conversely, concentric isokinetic testing has been well researched, documented, and described. Several studies have demonstrated the correlation between OKC concentric isokinetic testing and functional performance.[51,56,58]

Furthermore, a recent study by Wilson and coworkers[63] demonstrated the correlation of concentric testing to quantifying the rate of force development. Wilson and coworkers[63] performed research to quantify the rate of force development (RFD) and maximum force in isometric, concentric, and stretch–shortening (eccentric) cycle contraction modes and to determine their relationships to dynamic performance (sprinting). Of the 20 force-time variables calculated, only the concentric tests were significantly correlated to performance and able to discriminate effectively between good and poor performers. Therefore, their results were strongly supportive of the use of concentric RFD testing for assessing dynamic performance.

Closed Kinetic Chain Computerized Isokinetic Dynamometry

Closed kinetic chain (CKC) computerized isokinetic dynamometer testing is a relatively recent development that has obviously been created as a means to assess CKC function. As the popularity of CKC rehabilitation has grown during the last several years, so has the need for objective CKC testing.

Davies and Heiderscheit[16] recently performed reliability testing on a Lido Linea CKC Computerized Isokinetic dynamometer, which is dedicated to performing CKC testing. The reliability using a repeated-measures paradigm and velocity spectrum testing for CKC ranged from 0.85 to 0.94.

Comparison Between Open and Closed Kinetic Chain Computerized Isokinetic Dynamometer Testing

Recently, the first research[11,12] comparing OKC and CKC computerized isokinetic dynamometer testing has been presented and published. Interestingly, there are significant differences between OKC (isolated joint testing) and CKC (multiple joint testing) (Table 45-1). The data in this table demonstrate the need for performing both OKC and CKC strength testing. An integrated approach is required to be reflective of "strength" in relation to activity.

Functional Testing Algorithm

Davies[10,11,13,14] has developed a progressive functional testing algorithm (FTA) that can be used as one method of integrating the evaluation of strength in the female athlete. An overview of the FTA will be presented and then emphasis will be placed on the integration of strength testing components. The FTA is predicated on a systematic progressive testing sequence going from controlled testing to more functional testing. The FTA for the lower extremity is described in Figure 45-1. It must be recognized that this is an evolving sequence and is presented to demonstrate the need for integration of testing into rehabilitation regimens.

Table 45-1. Comparison of Lido Linea Closed Kinetic Chain (CKC) Computerized Isokinetic Testing and Cybex Open Kinetic Chain (OKC) Computerized Isokinetic Testing[a]

CYBEX (OKC)	DEFICIT	LINEA (CKC)	DEFICIT
PT 60°/sec quads U: 142 ft-lbs I: 101 ft-lbs	29%	PF 10 in/sec U: 462 lbs I: 420 lbs	9%
PT BW 60°/sec quads U: 95% I: 66%	31%	PF %BW 10 in/sec U: 298 lbs I: 266 lbs	11%
PT 180°/sec U: 99 ft-lbs I: 78 ft-lbs	21%	PF 20 in/sec U: 374 lbs I: 331 lbs	11%
PT BW 180°/sec U: 64% I: 48%	25%	PF %BW 20 in/sec U: 239 lbs I: 253 lbs	11%
PT 300°/sec U: 80 ft-lbs I: 64 ft-lbs	20%	PF 30 in/sec U: 302 lbs I: 253 lbs	16%
PT BW 300°/sec U: 51% I: 41%	20%	PF %BW 30 in/sec U: 193 lbs I: 171 lbs	11%

[a]Based on 300 patients having undergone surgery for heterogenous knee pathologies.
PT Peak torque; PF Peak force; U Uninvolved leg; I Involved leg; BW Body weight

The FTA testing strategies are based on the principles of progression and control. Each test in the testing sequence must be performed at a minimum level before progression to the next higher level in the FTA can occur. The criteria for the patient to progress from one level of the FTA to the next level is presently predicated on empirically based clinical experience, limited published research, and correlational research presently in progress. Table 45-2 describes these criteria.

The overview of the FTA presented below is brief because the evaluation of strength of the female athlete has to be performed within the context of various evaluation strategies and tools. The evaluation of strength is only one of the many parameters that needs to be assessed, whether it be for preseason screening, preoperative evaluation, serial reassessments during rehabilitation, or evaluating parameters for discharge and return to activity.

The primary components of the FTA are basic measurements, strength testing, and functional testing.

Basic Measurements

Basic measurements are the traditional measurements commonly used to evaluate patients, such as goniometric measurements and anthropometric measurements. Oftentimes, anthropometric measurements are used to assess muscle symmetry. Furthermore, occasionally anthropometric measurements or girth measurements are used to reflect "strength." However, because of the composition of girth measurements (adipose tissue, muscle, skin, etc), the measurements are neither very reliable nor totally reflective of muscular status.

Typically, if the patient has a 10% or greater deficit in these measurements, then physical therapy/rehabilitation is continued. When a deficit of less than 10% is present, the patient is progressed to the next level of the testing algorithm.

KT1000 Tests

If the patient has an anterior cruciate ligament (ACL) injury, KT1000 tests are performed to evaluate the laxity of the knee and/or the

Table 45-2. Functional Testing Algorithm Progression Criteria

TESTS	EMPIRIC GUIDELINES
Sport-specific testing	
Lower extremity functional test	M < 1:30 min; F < 2:00 min
Functional hop test	< 15% bilateral comparison +norms
Functional jump test	< 20% normative (height) data
Standing CKC	< 25% bilateral comparison
OKC test	< 25% bilateral comparison
Supine CKC test	< 30% bilateral comparison
Digital balance evaluator	< .6
KT1000 test	< 3 mm bilateral comparison
Basic measurements	< 10% bilateral comparison
Subjective (analog pain scale)	Pain < 3 (0–10)

integrity of an ACL-reconstruction graft. If the patient's manual maximum KT1000 value presents a difference of 3 mm or less early in the rehabilitation, then the rehabilitation program is progressed according to the clinic's protocol.

Kinesthetic/Proprioception/Balance Testing

Different methods are used to assess proprioception. If the patient has significant deficits, the patient is not progressed in rehabilitation until the deficits are within the normal limits of the test parameter.

There is some controversy regarding the method of testing lower extremity function because of the various studies that have researched the effects of CKC exercises in rehabilitation.[4,8,17,18,26,30,40,41,48,50,52,65] Therefore, the FTA acknowledges the advantages and disadvantages of testing of both OKC and CKC and consequently incorporates both modes of testing.

Closed Kinetic Chain—Supine Isokinetic Testing

Strength/power testing of CKC is initiated with the subject in the supine position using isokinetics.[10–14] We begin with this position because it is a relatively safe starting position as most

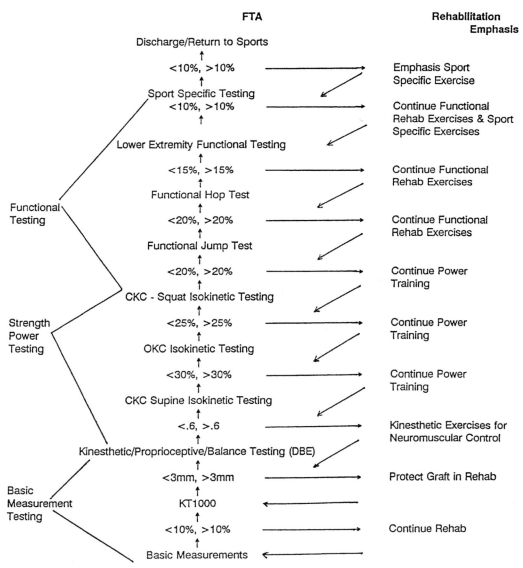

Figure 45-1. Functional testing algorithm.

variables (weight-bearing status, ROM, speeds, varus/valgus and rotational stresses, translatory joint forces, etc) are controlled. The CKC position allows for axial loading through the joint and consequently minimizes rotations and theoretically enables increased joint compressive forces to assist with joint stabilization.[33,42,53] In the CKC position there is some level of coactivation of the muscles around the knee, thereby creating a dynamic stabilization phenomenon as well.[20,55] When the patient has a deficit greater than 30%, various rehabilitation intervention strategies are performed, with emphasis on bilateral CKC exercises. Once the deficit improves to less than 30% bilaterally, the patient is progressed to the next stage of the FTA strength testing for OKC.

Descriptive data for CKC computerized isokinetic testing of the lower extremities of female athletes is given in Table 45-3.[12–14]

Open Kinetic Chain Isokinetic Testing

OKC isokinetic testing is performed because it allows for individual isolation of a muscle and therefore the ability to selectively isolate and evaluate portions of the kinetic chain. As with CKC isokinetic testing, we believe this is a safe test because each of the following variables is controlled: weight-bearing status, ROM, speeds, varus/valgus and rotational stresses, and translatory joint forces. If a proximally placed pad is used,[32,37,61] higher speeds[61,64] and limited ROM[29,37] then OKC isokinetic testing is also safe following ACL reconstruction.[6,15]

Admittedly, muscles do not work in isolation functionally; but the only way one can determine if a deficit exists within the kinetic chain is to perform isolated muscle group power assessments. Although some research indicates there is limited correlation between OKC testing and functional performance,[1,27] there are several studies that demonstrate that a correlation does exist. In other words, if one tests well with OKC isokinetics, he or she will perform well in a variety of functional tests.[3,31,58,59,62] Research by

Davies and coworkers[10–14] demonstrates that doing CKC isokinetic testing of several muscle groups in a functional lower extremity pattern alone does not identify existing weaknesses in major muscle groups. Therefore, isolated muscle group testing must be performed.

Standardized isokinetic testing to determine total leg strength as described by Nicholas and coworkers,[45] Gleim and coworkers,[25] and Davies[11, 12] can be used for testing various lower extremity muscles.

To allow progression through the FTA, the patient must have a deficit of less than 25%. If a deficit exists, then specific OKC exercises or specific exercises targeted to isolate and strengthen the weak muscles are included in the rehabilitation program. Once the deficits are minimized, the patient is progressed to the weight-bearing test position.

Descriptive data for OKC computerized isokinetic testing of quadriceps and hamstrings of the female athlete are included in Table 45-4.[6]

Closed Kinetic Chain—Squat Isokinetic Testing

The next progression is to test the patient in the CKC weight-bearing position and perform squat isokinetic testing.[46,47] This position still provides control of most variables but it places the patient into the functional weight-bearing position. The variables of ROM, speeds, varus/valgus, and rotational forces are still well controlled and can be limited.

The fully weight-bearing CKC position allows for a "controlled functional assessment." The patient should have less than a 25% deficit before progressing to the next stage of the FTA, which includes functional testing.

Functional Jump Test

The functional jump test (using both legs), the next phase of testing, leads to the progressive series of functional tests.[6,34]

Once functional testing begins, there is no longer control of most stresses to the extremity. Shock-type weight-bearing occurs, ballistic con-

Table 45-3. Descriptive Data for Closed Kinetic Chain Computerized Isokinetic Testing of the Lower Extremities in Female Athletes[a]

SPEEDS	FORCES/BW
Slow (10 in/sec)	≈2 1/2 BW
Medium (20 in/sec)	≈2 BW
Fast (30 in/sec)	≈1 1/2 BW

[a]Lido Linea CKC Isokinetic dynamometer.

Table 45-4. Descriptive Data for Open Kinetic Chain Computerized Isokinetic Testing of the Quadriceps in Female Athletes

SPEEDS	TORQUE/BW
Slow (60°/sec)	≈ 90% BW
Medium (180°/sec)	≈ 60% BW
Fast (300°/sec)	≈ 45% BW

Table 45-5. Descriptive Normative Data for the Functional Jump Test for Female Athletes

DISTANCE JUMPED NORMALIZED TO PERCENT OF BODY HEIGHT
Jump Test (2 legs) 90% of height

centric and eccentric muscle actions occur, ROM varies, there is no control over speed, and there are significant varus/valgus and rotational stresses imposed on the extremity. Therefore, we progress from the "controlled stress-test" environment to an "uncontrolled stress-test" situation.

In the functional jump test the female patient should jump at least 80% of the descriptive normative value, which is based on the patient's height (Table 45-5).[16]

If the patient still has a deficit of greater than 20%, then various exercises emphasizing power activities and plyometrics are incorporated into the rehabilitation program.

Once the patient can jump to within 20% of the descriptive value given in Table 45-5, she progresses to the next stage of the functional jump test, which is to isolate demand to the involved extremity.

Functional Hop Test

The functional hop test is performed with all of the same considerations as the functional jump test except that it is performed unilaterally.[6,19,28,34]

The patient is expected to hop within 15% of her ability with the uninvolved leg and to within 10% to 15% of the descriptive value in Table 45-6.

If the patient cannot meet the aforementioned criteria, rehabilitation is continued with emphasis on single-leg power exercises and plyometrics. Once the patient performs with less than a 15%

Table 45-6 Descriptive Normative Data for the Functional Hop Test for Female Athletes

Distance Hopped Normalized to Percent of Body Height	
Hop Test (1 leg) (U)	70–80% / height
Hop Test (1 leg) (I)	70–80% / height
Athlete should also be within 10–15% in a bilateral comparison	

U-Uninvolved leg
I-Involved leg

Table 45-7. Components of the Lower Extremity Functional Test

Sprint front	
Sprint retro-run	
Side shuffles	both ways
Cariocas	both ways
Figure 8s	both ways
45° < cuts	both ways
90° < cuts	both ways
Cross-over steps	both ways
Sprint front	
Sprint retro-run	

deficit, she is progressed to the next stage of the FTA, the lower extremity functional test.

Lower Extremity Functional Test

In order to incorporate the various functional activities[24,38,39] that are inherent in many sports, a lower extremity functional test (LEFT) is performed.[6,13] This is an agility-type test as well as an anaerobic assessment.

The test involves a series of different movements to functionally stress the lower extremity to replicate various sports performance movements. Table 45-7 lists the components of the LEFT test. Table 45-8 lists the descriptive normative data for the LEFT test.[6,13,66]

Sport-Specific Testing

When the athlete has passed the hierarchy of tests designed to progressively stress her from controlled to noncontrolled environments, then sport-specific testing is performed in order to determine the athlete's readiness to return to her specific sports activity. Although this chapter focuses on lower extremity testing, a similar approach to testing is applied to the upper extremity.[9]

Acknowledgments

Thanks to Kris Lawson, MA, PT, and the Gundersen Sports Medicine Center, La Crosse,

Table 45-8 Descriptive Data for Lower Extremity Functional Testing in Female Athletes — Time to Complete the Test

Female athletes < 25 years old	Female athletes > 25 years old
100 seconds—good	120 seconds—good
120 seconds—average	150 seconds—average
140 seconds—below average	180 seconds—below average

WI, and Debbie Anderson, Lexington, KY, for their assistance in the preparation of this manuscript.

References

1. Anderson MA, Gieck JH, Perrin D, et al: The relationship among isometric, isotonic and isokinetic concentric and eccentric quadriceps and hamstring force and three components of athletic performance. J Orthop Sports Phys Ther 14:114–20, 1991.
2. Baechle TR: Essentials of Strength Training and Conditioning. Champaign, Ill, Human Kinetics, 1994.
3. Barber SD, Noyes FR, Mangine RE, et al: Quantitative assessment of functional limitations in normal and anterior cruciate ligament deficient knees. Clin Orthop Rel Res 225:204–14, 1990.
4. Bynum EB, Barrack RL, Alexander AH: Open versus closed chain kinetic exercises after anterior cruciate ligament reconstruction. Am J Sports Med 23(4):401–6, 1995.
5. Daniels L, Worthingham C: Muscle Testing; Techniques of Manual Examination, third edition. Philadelphia, WB Saunders, 1986, pp 1–3.
6. Davies GJ: A Compendium of Isokinetics in Clinical Usage and Rehabilitation Techniques, fourth edition. Onalaska, Wisc, S & S Publishers, 1992.
7. Davies GJ, Ellenbecker TS: Eccentric isokinetics. Orthop Phys Ther Clin North Am 1:297–336, 1992.
8. Davies GJ, Romeyn RL: Prospective, randomized single blind study comparing closed kinetic chain versus open and closed kinetic chain integrated rehabilitation programs of patients with ACL autograft infrapatellar tendon reconstructions. (unpublished research)
9. Davies GJ, Hoffman SD: Neuromuscular testing and rehabilitation of the shoulder complex. J Orthop Sports Phys Ther 18:449–58, 1993.
10. Davies GJ, Malone T: Proprioception, open and closed kinetic chain exercises and application to assessment and rehabilitation (Instructional Course). Proceedings of the AOSSM, July 1994.
11. Davies GJ: The need for critical thinking in rehabilitation. J Sports Rehab 4:1–22, 1995.
12. Davies GJ: Descriptive study comparing open kinetic chain and closed kinetic chain isokinetic testing of the lower extremity in 200 patients with selected knee pathologies [Abstract]. Proceedings of the 12th International Congress of the World Confederation for Physical Therapy, APTA, Washington, DC, p 906, June, 1995.
13. Davies GJ: Functional testing algorithm for patients with knee injuries. [Abstract]. Proceedings of the 12th International Congress of the World Confederation for Physical Therapy, APTA, Washington, DC, p 912, June, 1995.
14. Davies GJ, Malone, T: Proprioception, open and closed kinetic chain exercises and application to assessment and rehabilitation (Instructional Course) Proceedings, AOSSM, July 1995.
15. Davies GJ, Heiderscheit B, Clark MA: Open kinetic chain assessment and rehabilitation. Athletic Training: Sports Health Care Perspectives. 1(4):347–70, 1995.
16. Davies GJ, Heiderscheit, BC. Reliability of the Lido Linea closed kinetic chain isokinetic dynamometer. J Orthop Sports Phys Ther 25(2):133–136, 1997.
17. DeCarlo M, Porter DA, Gehlsen G, Bahamonde R: Electromyographic and cinematographic analysis of the lower extremity during closed and open kinetic chain exercise. Isokin Exerc Sci 2:24–9, 1992.
18. DeCarlo M, Shelbourne KD, McCarroll JR, Rettig AC: Traditional versus accelerated rehabilitation following ACL reconstruction: A one-year follow-up. J Orthop Sports Phys Ther 15:309–16, 1992.
19. DeCarlo M, Sell KE: Range of motion and single-leg hop values for normals and patients following anterior cruciate ligament reconstruction [Abstract]. J Orthop Sports Phys Ther 19:73, 1994.
20. Draganich LF, Jaeger RJ, Kralj AR: Coactivation of the hamstrings and quadriceps during extension of the knee. J Bone Joint Surg 71A:1075–1081, 1989
21. Farrell M, Richards JG: Analysis of the reliability and validity of the kinetic communicator exercise device. Med Sci Sports Ex 18:44, 1986.
22. Fleck SJ, Kraemer WJ: Designing Resistance Training Programs. Champaign, Ill, Human Kinetics, 1987.
23. Francis K, Hoobler T: Comparison of peak torque values of the knee flexor and extensor muscle groups using the Cybex II and Lido 2.0 isokinetic dynamometers. J Orthop Sports Phys Ther 8:480, 1987.
24. Gauffin H, Peterson Y, Tegner Y, Tropp H: Function testing in patients with old rupture of the anterior cruciate ligament. Int J Sports Med 11:73–7, 1990.
25. Gleim GW, Nicholas JA, Webb JN: Isokinetic evaluation following leg injuries. Physician Sportsmed 6:74–82, 1978
26. Graham VL, Gehlsen GM, Edwards JA: Electromyographic evaluation of closed and open kinetic chain knee rehabilitation exercises. J Athletic Training 28:23–30, 1993.
27. Greenberger HB, Paterno MV: Comparison of an isokinetic strength test and functional performance test in the assessment of lower extremity function [Abstract]. J Orthop Sports Phys Ther 19:61, 1994.
28. Greenberger HB, Paterno MV: The test-retest reliability of a one-legged hop for distance in healthy young adults. J Orthop Sports Phys Ther 19:62, 1994.
29. Grood ES, Suntay WJ, Noyes FR, Butler DL: Biomechanics of the knee-extension exercise. J Bone Joint Surg 66A:725–34, 1984.
30. Gryzlo SM, Patek RM, Pink M, Perry J: Electromyographic analysis of knee rehabilitation exercises. J Orthop Sports Phys Ther 20:36–43, 1994.
31. Harter RA, Osternig LR, Singer KM, et al: Long-term evaluation of knee stability and function following surgical reconstruction for anterior cruciate ligament insufficiency. Am J Sports Med 16:434–43, 1988.
32. Howell SM: Anterior tibial translation during a maximum quadriceps contraction: Is it clinically significant? Am J Sports Med 18:573–8, 1990.
33. Hsieh H, Walker PS: Stabilizing mechanisms of the loaded and unloaded knee joint. J Bone Joint Surg 58A:87–93, 1976.
34. Hu HS, Whitney SL, Irrgang J, Janosky J: Test-retest reliability of the one-legged vertical jump test and the one-legged standing hop test [Abstract] J Orthop Sports Phys Ther 15:51, 1992.
35. Jackson AL, Highgenboten C, Meske N, et al: Univariate and multivariate analysis of the reliability of the kinetic communicator. Med Sci Sports Exerc (Suppl) 19:23, 1987.
36. Johnson J, Siegel D: Reliability of an isokinetic movement of the knee extensors. Res Q 49:88, 1978.
37. Jurist KA, Otis JC: Anteroposterior tibiofemoral displacements during isometric extension efforts. Am J Sports Med 13:254–8, 1985.
38. Lephart SM, et al: Functional assessment of the anterior cruciate insufficient knee [Abstract]. Med Sci Sports Exer 20:2, 1988.

39. Lephart SM, Perrin DH, Fu FH, Minger K: Functional performance tests for the anterior cruciate ligament insufficient athlete. J Athletic Training 26:44–50, 1991.

40. Lutz GE, Palmitier RA, An KN, Chao EYS: Closed kinetic chain exercises for athletes after reconstruction of the anterior cruciate ligament [Abstract]. Med Sci Sports Exerc 23:413, 1991.

41. Lutz GE, Palmitier RA, An KN, Chao EYS: Comparison of tibiofemoral joint forces during open kinetic chain and closed kinetic chain exercises. J Bone Joint Surg Am 75A:732–9, 1993.

42. Markolf KL, Bargar WL, Shoemaker SC, Amstutz HC: Role of joint load in knee stability. J Bone Joint Surg 63A:579–85, 1981.

43. Mawdsley RH, Knapik JJ: Comparison of isokinetic measurements with test repetitions. Phys Ther 62:169, 1982.

44. Molnar GE, Alexander J, Gudfeld N: Reliability of quantitative strength measurements in children. Arch Phys Med Rehabil 60:218, 1979.

45. Nicholas JA, Strizak AM, Veras G: A study of thigh muscle weakness in different pathological states of the lower extremity. Am J Sports Med 4:241–8, 1976.

46. Ohkoshi Y, Yasada K: Biomechanical analysis of shear force exerted to anterior cruciate ligament during half squat exercise. Orthop Trans 13:310, 1989.

47. Ohkoshi Y, Yasuda K, Kaneda K, et al: Biomechanical analysis of rehabilitation in the standing position. Am J Sports Med 19:605–10, 1991.

48. Palmitier RA, An K-N, Scott SG, Chao EYS: Kinetic chain exercise in knee rehabilitation. Sports Med 11:402–13, 1991.

49. Perrin DH: Reliability of isokinetic measures. Athletic Training 23:319, 1986.

50. Renstrom P, Arms SW, Stanwyck TS, et al: Strain within the anterior cruciate ligament during hamstring and quadriceps activity. Am J Sports Med 14:83–7, 1986.

51. Sachs RA, Daniel DM, Stone ML, Garfein RF: Patellofemoral problems after anterior cruciate ligament reconstruction. Am J Sports Med 17:760–4, 1989.

52. Shelbourne KD, Nitz P: Accelerated rehabilitation after anterior cruciate ligament rehabilitation. Am J Sports Med 18:292–9, 1990.

53. Shoemaker SC, Markolf KL: Effects of joint load on the stiffness and laxity of ligament-deficient knees. J Bone Joint Surg Am 67A:136–46, 1985.

54. Snow DJ, Johnson K: Reliability of two velocity-controlled tests for the measurement of peak torque of the knee flexors during resisted muscle shortening and resisted muscle lengthening. Phys Ther 68:781, 1988.

55. Solomonow M, Baratta R, Zhov BH, et al: The synergistic action of the anterior cruciate ligament and thigh muscles in maintaining joint stability. Am J Sports Med 15:207–13, 1987.

56. Tegner Y, Lysholm J, Lysholm M, Gillquist J: A performance test to monitor rehabilitation and evaluate anterior cruciate ligament injuries. Am J Sports Med 14:156–9, 1986.

57. Timm K: Reliability of Cybex 340 and MERAC isokinetic measures of peak torque, total work, and average power at five test speeds. Phys Ther 69:782, 1988.

58. Timm KE: Post-surgical knee rehabilitation: A five year study of four methods and 5,381 patients. Am J Sports Med 16:463–8, 1988.

59. Wiklander J, Lysholm J: Simple tests for surveying muscle strength and muscle stiffness in sportsmen. Int J Sports Med 8:50–4, 1987.

60. Wilk KE, Johnson RE: The reliability of the Biodex B–200 (Abstact). Phys Ther 68:792, 1988.

61. Wilk KE, Andrews JR: The effects of pad placement and angular velocity on tibial displacement during isokinetic exercise. J Orthop Sports Phys Ther 17:23–30, 1993.

62. Wilk KE, et al: The relationship between subjective knee scores, isokinetic (OKC) testing and functional testing in the ACL-reconstructed knee J Orthop Sports Phys Ther 20(2):60–73, 1994.

63. Wilson GJ, Tyttle AD, Ostrowski KJ, Murphy AJ: Assessing dynamic performance: A comparison of Rate of force development tests. J Strength Cond Res 9(3):176–81, 1995.

64. Wyatt MP, Edwards AM: Comparison of quadriceps and hamstring torque values during isokinetic exercise. J Orthop Sports Phys Ther 3:48–56, 1981.

65. Yack HJ, Collins CE, Whieldon TJ: Comparison of closed and open kinetic chain exercise in the anterior cruciate ligament-deficient knee. Am J Sports Med 21:49–54, 1993.

66. Tabor MA, Davies GJ, Kernozek, Negrete RJ, Hudson V. A multicenter study of the test-retest reliability of the lower extremity functional test. Accepted for publication in the J Sport Rehabil August, 2002.

Chapter 46

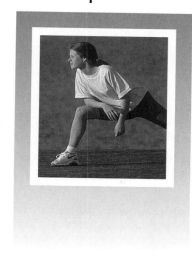

Upper and Lower Extremity Proprioception Testing and Practical Use

Scott M. Lephart, Ph.D., A.T.C

Susan L. Rozzi, Ph.D., A.T.C

NEUROLOGIC BACKGROUND INFORMATION

Terminology

The role of proprioception is currently attracting a considerable amount of attention in both research and clinical sports medicine and orthopaedic communities as it relates to joint injury and management.[1–8,11,14–15,19–21,28–29,35–42, 48–51,54–56,58–60] Proprioception is considered a specialized variation of the sensory modality of touch, which encompasses both joint position sense and joint motion sense, also known as *kinesthesia*. Proprioception has also been defined as a compound sense, relying on simultaneous activity in a number of types of afferent neurons resulting in a complex efferent neurosensory– efferent neuromotor loop that is responsible for precise movements and dynamic joint stabilization.[23]

Anatomy and Histology

Afferent neurons, originating in the skin, muscle, and articular tissues, provide information on both joint movement and joint position.[30] The contribution to proprioception by cutaneous afferents is considered relatively minor, while the muscle spindle receptors play a far more important role. Muscle spindle afferents respond as a function of muscle length, while their signal of joint movement is said to be unconfounded and unidirectional. Stimulation of the afferent neurons from a stretched muscle results in a sensation of joint movement, kinesthesia.[23] The sensitivity of the muscle spindle afferent neurons increases with the active tensing of the muscle. Moreover, this increase in

sensitivity was shown to dramatically increase joint proprioceptive acuity attributed solely to changes in muscle spindle afferent neurons.[18] The afferent neurons, located in muscle tissue, also play a major role in providing information of joint position sense. The work of Clark and colleagues[13] demonstrated no decrease in joint position sense following the blocking of cutaneous and capsular afferents in the knee, emphasizing the role of the muscle receptors. However, isolated stimulation of the muscle spindle afferents, independent of cutaneous, subcutaneous, and joint tissue afferents, results in poor proprioceptive acuity, suggesting that muscle afferents rely on the simultaneous stimulation of neighboring afferent neurons.[45]

The mechanoreceptors originating in the joint capsule, bone, and ligaments also provide afferent contributions to joint proprioception. The 2 classes of sensory, afferent neurons originating in joint tissue are group 2 afferents and group 3 and 4 afferents. Group 2 includes those neurons having large-diameter, rapidly conducting axons, while group 3 and 4 afferents are composed of neurons of small-diameter, thin or unmyelinated axons. Ruffini afferents and paciniform afferents compose group 2. Ruffini afferents are found in the "flexion" side of the joint and respond proportionally to the stress of the tissue. As a function of location, Ruffini afferents serve a role in proprioception only at the extreme ranges of joint extension and may be considered range limit detectors. Widely distributed about the joint, paciniform afferents sense joint compression through end-range joint movement or local compression stimuli. The properties of group 3 and 4 afferents are less proprioceptive and more pain sensing.

Rather than signaling direction of movement, these afferents signal the presence of noxious intense stimuli, potentially providing for extreme-range joint protection.[23]

Mechanoreceptor nerve endings are also located in the ligamentous tissue of joints and in tendons. The presence and the role of mechanoreceptors in the anterior cruciate ligament (ACL) of the knee joint has been well established.[52,53] Rapidly adapting pacinian corpuscles, which respond to joint acceleration and deceleration, have been found in both the joint capsule and ligamentous insertions.[2] However, noxiceptors have been documented to be sparse and even absent in knee ligaments, especially the ACL.[10] Fortunately, pain receptors play only a minimal role in providing joint proprioception and resulting joint protection.

Physiology

In normal, healthy joints, the afferent pathway receives information from stimulated sensory receptors located in the skin, joint, and ligamentous tissue and transports the information to the central nervous system. At the central nervous system the afferent pathway synapses with the efferent pathway. Efferent stimulation travels to the muscles surrounding the stimulated joint and the reflex loop is completed. Information received by the central nervous system is also transported up the spinal cord for cortical programming.

Following injury to ligamentous tissue there is partial deafferentation of the mechanoreceptors, resulting in proprioceptive deficits. These proprioceptive deficits affect both the afferent and efferent pathways. Because the afferent pathway has been compromised, the traumatized joint may demonstrate decreased kinesthesia and joint position sensibility. Disruption of the efferent pathway potentially results in decreased neuromuscular control that is demonstrated by diminished protective joint reflexes. Decreased neuromuscular control, in concert with the mechanical joint instability attributed to trauma, results in functional instability. Functional instability is the precursor to repetitive ligamentous injury and to exacerbation of joint instability (Fig. 46-1).

PROPRIOCEPTION TESTING OF THE UPPER AND LOWER EXTREMITY

Proprioception is a complex neurosensory and neuromuscular mechanism that is most effec-

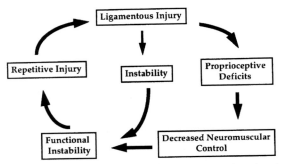

Figure 46-1. The effects of joint injury on functional instability.

tively studied through the combined assessment of both the afferent and efferent pathways. The afferent and efferent pathways are evaluated through the assessment of joint position sense and kinesthesia, muscle activity, and balance and postural sway. Assessment of the afferent pathway provides information of joint proprioceptive acuity both consciously and unconsciously. The efferent pathway is studied by measuring muscle activity and response following joint stress. Evaluation of balance includes assessment of performance criteria that reflects the function of both the afferent and efferent pathways.

Assessment of the Afferent Pathway

Assessment of the afferent pathway is achieved through examination of kinesthesia and joint position sense. Kinesthesia is determined by establishing the threshold to detection of passive motion (TTDPM).[3–5,36–38,40–42,54–56] TTDPM assesses the ability to perceive passive joint motion through stimulation of joint receptors while providing little stimulation of muscle receptors.

Joint position sense is examined by measuring either reproduction of passive positioning (RPP) or reproduction of active positioning (RAP).[6,56] RPP assesses the ability to accurately reproduce a set position angle in the arc of available motion. Performed actively, reproduction of joint position provides for stimulation of joint receptors, in addition to muscle receptors. Compared to passive repositioning, active joint position assessment may be more representative of joint function. Although both TTDPM and RPP testing assess the afferent pathway, the results are test specific. Barrack,[2] in a study of ballet dancers, described no correlation between TTDPM and RPP test scores for either a test group or a control group.

The Proprioception Testing Device (PTD) is an instrument that was designed specifically to assess kinesthesia and joint position sense in the

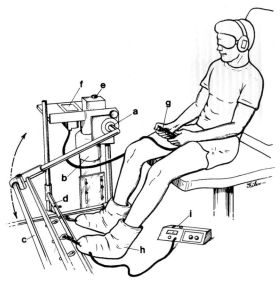

Figure 46-2. Knee joint proprioception testing using the University of Pittsburgh's Proprioception Testing Device (PTD). (From Lephart SM, et al: Proprioception following anterior cruciate ligament reconstruction. J Sport Rehabil 1:188–96, 1992, with permission.)

research setting (Fig. 46-2). Test–retest reliability of the PTD has been established with a correlation coefficient of 0.92.[41] TTDPM is defined by the degrees of joint movement occurring between the time movement is initiated by the device and when the subject disengages the drive shaft upon the sensation of passive joint motion. Assessment of TTDPM in the shoulder joint typically involves movement into internal and external rotation from a set reference angle.[42] When testing the knee joint, movement into flexion and into extension at the

2 test angles of 15° of knee flexion (near terminal range of motion) and 45° of knee flexion (midrange of motion) are most commonly utilized.[36–38,41] Lephart and coworkers[41] demonstrated increased kinesthetic awareness in the ACL-reconstructed knee of individuals when tested from the starting position of 15° of knee flexion compared to tests at 45°. These results are consistent with histologic studies that suggest active tensioning of the muscle, as seen near terminal range of motion, increases the sensitivity of muscle spindle afferents. At these terminal ranges of motion Ruffini afferents will also respond to tissue stress.

In addition to assessing kinesthesia, the PTD permits assessment of joint position sense by measuring reproduction of passive positioning (RPP). RPP is assessed in the knee joint from the starting positions of 45° and 15° of knee flexion moving into both flexion and extension. From the starting angle the subject's limb is either flexed or extended into a test angle and then immediately returned to the start angle. The subject then permits the device to move the limb in the test direction until the previously presented test angle is sensed. At this point the subject disengages the device, motion ceases, and the angle is recorded. The difference between the presented test angle and that achieved by the subject is recorded as degrees of error.[11]

Kinesthesia and joint position sense can also be measured clinically using the Biodex System 2 Isokinetic Testing Device (Biodex, Shirley, NY) (Fig. 46-3). TTDPM, RPP, and RAP testing capabilities for a number of joints have been integrated into this isokinetic testing device and accompanying computer software package.

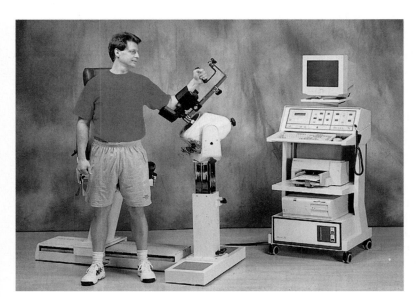

Figure 46-3. Upper extremity proprioception testing and training using the Biodex System 2 Isokinetic Dynamometer. (Courtesy of Biodex Medical Systems, Inc, Shirley, NY.)

Assessment of the Efferent Pathway

As mentioned earlier, the efferent pathway is measured by assessing muscle activity, which provides a direct assessment of the efferent response to afferent stimulation.[7,29] Muscle activity is traditionally assessed utilizing electromyography (EMG), which is the study of the motor unit action potential. Surface electrode placement or fine-wire indwellings record muscle activity during a given task. EMG permits the clinician to investigate preactivated muscle tension, reflex muscular contractions, and the firing sequences of muscle groups. Using the mean absolute value (MAV), comparisons can be made between ipsilateral and contralateral limb muscles.[58]

In addition to EMG, reactive neuromuscular activity can be assessed by measuring static and dynamic balance. Balance has been defined to include 3 equally important components: the ability to maintain a position, the ability to voluntarily move, and the ability to react to a perturbation.[9] Balance is mediated by the same peripheral afferent mechanism that mediates joint proprioception while relying on input from multiple sensory sites, both internally and externally. Motivation, concentration, muscle strength, and visual acuity are a few variables required for maintaining balance.[28] Balance and postural sway can be measured with the use of commercially available devices or with subjective means, such as the single leg (stork) stand or the Rhomberg test. Assessment of the efferent pathway through balance testing may provide information more representative of lower extremity function compared to results obtained in the open kinetic chain test position.

Testing of balance and postural sway can be performed statically and dynamically by employing commercially available balance testing devices or may be assessed subjectively with clinical balance tests. Objective balance and postural sway measurements can be obtained through the use of any of the following commercially available devices: The Biodex Stability System (Biodex, Shirley, NY), The Chattecx Dynamic Balance System (Chattecx Corporation, Hixson, TN), and the Kinesthetic Ability Training (KAT) balance platform (BREG Inc. Carlsbad, CA).

The Biodex Stability System (Biodex, Shirley, NY) consists of a moveable balance platform that provides up to 20° of surface tilt in a 360° range to stimulate joint receptors and promotes reflex muscular contractions necessary for joint stability (Fig. 46-4). The platform is interfaced with computer software, which enables the

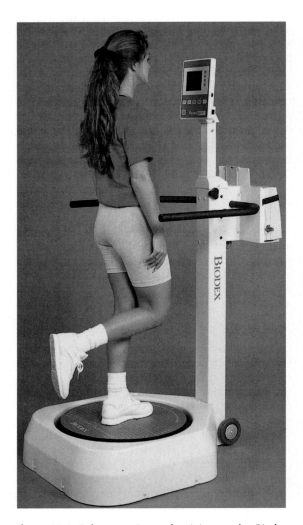

Figure 46-4. Balance testing and training on the Biodex Stability System (Biodex Medical Systems, Inc, Shirley, NY). (From Lephart SM, Henry TJ: Functional rehabilitation for the upper and lower extremity. Orthop Clin North Am 6(30):579–92, 1995, with permission.)

device to perform as both a training tool and an objective quantifier of balance ability. Reliability of the Stability System has been established with an intraclass correlation coefficient ranging from 0.6 to 0.95.[47] The Chattecx Dynamic Balance System measures postural sway during both static (stable platform) and dynamic (movable platform) tests.[34] This system uses 4 independent force-measuring transducers to record postural stability with displacement from the center point of balance determining postural sway. The reported reliability of the Chattecx Dynamic Balance System ranges from poor to excellent ($r = 0.06$ to 0.90), with the wide range appearing to be primarily a function of test condition.[44] The BREG Kinesthetic Ability Trainer (KAT) balance platform uses an inflatable air bladder located under a balance platform to allow for variations in platform stability. Bladder pressure, displayed in pounds per square inch (psi), may be used for control of platform position and stability, in addition to being a means of subject feedback. The KAT has a software program designed for balance testing and training in both the static and dynamic modes. The software assesses balance ability by calculating a balance index. The balance index is calculated as the sum of the absolute tilt values, obtained by measuring the distance from the center of the circular platform to the tilt position for each tilt during the test trial, divided by the duration of the test.[43]

Numerous studies incorporate subjective measures of balance in determining lower extremity proprioceptive abilities.[1,35] The ease of administration of these tests has made them appealing in the clinical setting in addition to the research venue. The accuracy of static, subjective balance measurements has been questioned and recently investigated. Using the Chattecx Balance System, Lebsack and Perrin[34] reported a moderate correlation when the objective postural sway measures were compared to subjective balance scores obtained under multiple test conditions.

CLINICAL PROPRIOCEPTION RESEARCH

Knee Joint

Evaluating the afferent neuromuscular pathway by assessing proprioception has provided important information for researchers and clinicians. Barrack and colleagues[3] and Lephart and coworkers[41] have both demonstrated that proprioception of the knee joint does not appear to be related to limb dominance. However, proprioception appears to be related to gender, as the authors' research has demonstrated inferior joint kinesthesia in female soccer and basketball athletes compared to their male counterparts.[49] While enhanced kinesthesia and joint position sense have been described in gymnasts and dancers, the question remains as to whether these discrepancies are the result of a genetic predisposition or are a function of training.[4] Although contrary to the work of Skinner and coworkers,[54] the authors' current research suggests that knee joint proprioception of healthy athletes is abated by muscular fatigue.[48] In addition to muscular fatigue, knee joint proprioception appears to be altered by joint trauma, as research has established kinesthesia and joint position sense deficits in the ACL-deficient knee.[3,15,41,60] However, surgical reconstruction of the assaulted ligamentous tissue appears to restore some degree of kinesthesia and joint position sense in the affected joint.[41]

Examination of the efferent pathway via muscle activity assessment provides information of muscle recruitment in normal and pathologic joints. Muscle activity in normal healthy male and female soccer and basketball athletes appears to differ.[49] Utilizing EMG, the authors assessed the muscle activity of 6 knee joint stabilizing muscles during the performance of a functional landing task. Compared to their male counterparts, the female athletes in this study produced significantly greater EMG peak amplitude and area of the lateral hamstring subsequent to landing, suggesting they have developed an alternative means of achieving knee joint functional stability.[49] In the fatigued state, these athletes demonstrated an increased time to contraction of the medial hamstring and lateral gastrocnemius muscles, 2 muscles that function to control anterior tibial translation during functional activities. These findings are in agreement with other workers[46,61] who have demonstrated delayed firing of the hamstring musculature subsequent to an imposed joint load.

Tibone and colleagues[58] utilized EMG analysis to investigate muscle activity in the ACL-deficient limb during both straight-ahead running and during "cutting" activities. Relative to the lateral hamstring, the medial hamstring demonstrated prolonged firing during the stance phase of the running gait cycle. During the functional activity of "cutting," no changes in EMG activity between the injured and the contralateral limb of ACL-deficient subjects was evident.[58] However, this lack of altered muscular activity in the ACL-deficient subjects is inconsistent with the findings of other researchers.[12,46] Branch and colleagues[12] analyzed quadriceps, hamstring, and gastrocnemius activity in ACL-deficient and normal subjects who performed side-step cutting both with and without a functional knee brace. The ACL-deficient subjects demonstrated decreased quadriceps and gastrocnemius activity with increased medial hamstring activity. Additionally, the application of a functional brace while cutting did not appear to enhance muscle stimulation or serve to promote joint stability in the ACL-deficient joints.[12]

For the ACL-insufficient individual, the most consequential neurosensory–neuromuscular capability may be the ability of the hamstring to fire reflexively.[59] A shorter duration between joint displacement and reflexive muscular contraction results in less joint trauma and an increased sense of joint stability. Beard and colleagues designed a device to test this important time frame.[8] The VICON Interfaced Knee Displacement Equipment (VIKDE) is a stationary frame that includes an EMG unit to measure activity of the medial and lateral hamstring muscles while subjects single-leg stand in the apparatus. The VIKDE randomly discharged a posteroanterior shear force of approximately 100 N to the posterior tibia. Reflex hamstring contraction latency (RHCL), defined as the time interval between the first recorded displacement of the tibia to the first discernible reflex reaction of the hamstrings (EMG) signal, is recorded. Of the patients with ACLD, 94% had increased RHCL on the involved side compared to the uninvolved side. The RHCL of the uninvolved limb of the ACL-deficient individuals did not differ significantly from those of the normal subjects.[8]

Ankle Joint

As seen in the knee joint, trauma to the static stabilizers of the ankle joint affects both the afferent and efferent neurologic pathways. Assessing the afferent pathway, Garns and Newton[19] noted decreased kinesthetic awareness, while Glenncross and Thorton[21] noted decreased reproduction of passive position, in the involved ankle of subjects with unilateral ankle sprains. Following ankle joint ligamentous trauma the application of ice is effective in allowing for pain-free activity. However, ice application prior to sport participation has been suggested to affect proprioceptive acuity adversely and thereby predispose participants to injury. LaRiviere and Osternig[33] tested ankle joint reproduction of active position after the pretest conditions of a 5-minute ice immersion, a 20-minute ice immersion, and following no ice treatment. Their results revealed no significant difference between test conditions, suggesting either resilience of the joint receptors or compensation for affected receptors by unaffected afferent receptors.[33]

In the ankle joint, the efferent neuromuscular pathway is commonly assessed through the quantification of balance ability. In addition to deficits in joint proprioception, aberrations and deficiencies in neuromuscular control have been documented subsequent to ankle joint ligament injury.[1,14,16,24,31,50] We investigated single-leg balance ability of individuals with a self-reported functionally unstable ankle and noted inferior balance ability of the involved limb when compared to the contralateral lower extremity and when compared to a randomly selected limb of a healthy individual.[50] The functional instability documented in our subjects is consistent with the results of other similar investigations and what is reported clinically by the practitioner. Therefore, rehabilitation programs addressing proprioceptive and neuromuscular deficits are commonly recommended in an effort to restore functional joint stability. Researchers have investigated the effect of balance training as a rehabilitation tool in healthy individuals and in those with ankle instability. Hoffman and Payne[24] investigated the effects of a progressive training program on the balance ability of subjects absent of ankle pathology. Assessed with the Kistler force platform, the balance ability of the trained group demonstrated significant improvements in both the medial–lateral and anterior–posterior parameters of postural sway compared to the untrained group, demonstrating that healthy noninjured individuals can improve proprioceptive acuity through training.[24] These findings are consistent with those of Balogun and coworkers, whose normal healthy subjects demonstrated improvements in both balance performance (assessed using the noncriterion one-legged stance timed balance test) and strength of the lower extremity muscles following 6 weeks of wobble board training.[1] In our investigation of the effects of balance training, we selected a 4-week-long balance training program rather than a commonly reported 6-week-long program. Interestingly, the authors' research suggests that the 4-week-long balance training program they utilized effectively improved both unstable and healthy ankle joint neuromuscular control, as assessed through single-leg balance ability.[50] Cox and colleagues[16] also investigated the effects of balance training but their results were inconsistent with previous reported studies. For this study of healthy subjects, training consisted of single-limb static balance on either a hard surface or a foam surface. Objective balance assessment by the Chattecx Dynamic Balance System demonstrated no significant pre- to post-test mean score improvement within either training group. The assessment of balance training seems to be a function of the mode of training. When balance training is generally static, dynamic assessment may not be specific enough to detect changes in performance. When normal subjects trained with dynamic balance exercises using visual feedback of their center of gravity, there was no change in static stability when measured pre- and post-therapy, although dynamic stability measures improved significantly.[24]

Shoulder Joint

Although fewer in number, studies of shoulder joint proprioception demonstrate trends seen at the knee and ankle joints. Lephart and coworkers[42] studied shoulder joint kinesthesia and joint position sense in normal, unstable, and reconstructed individuals and concluded that in overhead throwing athletes and normal subjects, upper extremity dominance does not appear to influence shoulder joint kinesthesia. Assessed from a starting position of 30° of external rotation, kinesthesia and joint position sense were significantly diminished in the unstable shoulder when compared to the healthy contralateral limb. Additionally, the authors' work has revealed that following reconstructive surgery of the unstable shoulder, kinesthesia and joint position sense appear to return to normal values. This later finding suggests that retensioning of the capsule and ligaments facilitates afferent receptor response by allowing for mechanoreceptor deformation.[42]

Ligamentous laxity and resulting joint instability of the shoulder affects the efferent response to afferent stimulation. Distraction-induced capsuloligamentous laxity commonly seen in the throwing athlete can result in altered muscle firing patterns. Glousman and colleagues[22] examined the EMG of shoulder musculature during throwing in athletes with unilateral shoulder joint instability. Compensating for the lax dynamic stabilizers, these athletes demonstrated excessive supraspinatus activity, especially in the late cocking phase, in addition to decreased internal rotator activity throughout the entire throwing motion. These altered firing patterns appear to contribute to the existing ligamentous laxity to create an increasingly unstable shoulder joint.

Supported by the previously reviewed research, it can be concluded that injury to ligamentous tissue of the knee, ankle, and shoulder joints results in proprioceptive deficits that affect both the afferent and efferent pathways. When coupled with mechanical joint instability, these proprioceptive impairments result in a functionally unstable joint. Restoring the strength of the muscles around the unstable joint is insufficient in restoring joint stability. Proprioceptive training addressing both the altered afferent and efferent pathways is the key to attaining a functionally stable joint.

PROPRIOCEPTIVE TRAINING

Goals of Training

Assessment of proprioception provides valuable information for rehabilitative and preventative conditioning programs. Altered afferent pathways, revealed with kinesthesia and joint position testing, and affected efferent pathways may be retrained through proprioceptive rehabilitation. The primary goals of proprioceptive rehabilitation need to address both the afferent and efferent neurologic pathways and should be aimed at stimulating visual, vestibular, and peripheral afferent mechanoreceptors (Fig. 46-5). The rehabilitation program should begin with activities that permit simultaneous stimulation of the mechanoreceptors and progress to those activities that restrict sensory input, such as performing balancing activities with the eyes closed. The 3 levels of motor control—cognitive programming, brain stem involvement, and spinal reflexes—can be addressed through the use of various rehabilitative activities. Proprioception training exercises also

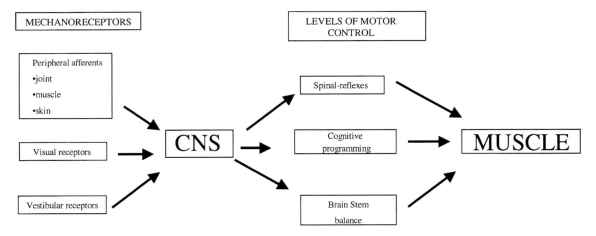

Figure 46-5. Neuromuscular control pathways. (From Lephart S, Henry TJ: The role of proprioception in the management and rehabilitation of athletic injuries. Am J Sports Med 25(1):131, 1997, with permission.)

need to stimulate both the conscious and unconscious pathways.

Proprioceptive training should begin early in the rehabilitation program, continue throughout, and become increasingly more difficult in the program's later stages. Early-stage proprioception training includes simple tasks such as balance training and joint repositioning, which stimulate mechanoreceptors and address all 3 levels of motor control. The later stage of training, the functional or sport-specific stage, aims at refining joint position awareness to initiate muscle reflex stabilization and prevent reinjury.

Lower Extremity

Proprioceptive rehabilitation of the lower extremity is most appropriately performed in the functional, closed kinetic chain position. Closed kinetic chain activities are reflective of the stresses placed upon the joint during normal lower extremity function. The orientation of the lower extremity joints during closed kinetic chain activities also permits muscle firing patterns necessary for joint stabilization.[39]

Beginning with the early phases, lower extremity proprioception rehabilitation should emphasize static and dynamic balance training. Progression of static balance activities should be from bilateral to unilateral activities, from eyes-open activities to eyes-closed activities, and from activities performed on a stable surface to those on an unstable surface.[28] Since the skills of walking, running, cutting, and pivoting may be considered a series of losses and gains in balance, lower extremity rehabilitation must include dynamic balance training. Dynamic balance control activities should follow a progression from slow-speed to fast-speed activities, from low-force to high-force activities, and from controlled to uncontrolled activities.[28]

Upper Extremity

Unlike the lower extremity, proprioceptive training of the upper extremity is beneficial when performed in both open and closed kinetic chain positions. Both modes of training are felt to be valuable for maximally stimulating glenohumeral mechanoreceptors. Development of joint position sense can be attained with passive and active joint repositioning, most appropriately performed in the functional position and near the end ranges of motion. Performed in either an open or closed kinetic chain, activities that necessitate reflex muscular stabilization should be encouraged. These reflex stabilization activities stimulate the afferent pathways and retrain the efferent pathways required for dynamic joint stability. Shoulder plyometrics have recently been suggested as a means to restore the reactive neuromuscular mechanism responsible for joint stabilization.[11]

References

1. Balogun JA, Adesinasi CO, Marzouk DK: The effects of a wobble board exercise training program on static balance performance and strength of lower extremity muscles. *Physiother Can* 44(4):23–30, 1992.
2. Barrack RL, Lund PJ, Skinner HB: Knee joint proprioception revisited. *J Sports Rehab* 3(1):18–42, 1994.
3. Barrack RL, Skinner HB, Brunet ME, et al: Proprioception in the anterior cruciate ligament deficient knee. *Am J Sports Med* 17:1–6, 1989.
4. Barrack RL, Skinner HB, Brunet ME, Cook SD: Joint kinesthesia in the highly trained knee. *J Sports Med Phys Fitness* 24:18–20, 1983.
5. Barrack RL, Skinner HB, Cook SD: Proprioception of the knee joint: paradoxical effect of training. *Am J Phys Med* 63(4):175–81, 1984.
6. Barrett DS: Proprioception and function after anterior cruciate reconstruction. *J Bone Joint Surg* 73B:833–7, 1991.
7. Beard DJ, Kyberd PJ, Fergusson CM, Dodd CA: Proprioception after rupture of the anterior cruciate ligament: an objective indication of the need for surgery? *J Bone Joint Surg* 75B:311–5, 1993.
8. Beard DJ, Kyberd PJ, O'Connor JJ, et al: Reflex hamstring contraction latency in anterior cruciate ligament deficiency. *J Bone Joint Surg* 12:219–28, 1994.
9. Berg K: Balance and its measure in the elderly: A review. *Physiother Can* 41:240–6, 1989.
10. Biedart RM, Stauffer E, Friederich NF: Occurrence of free nerve endings in the soft tissue of the knee joint. *Am J Sports Med* 20(4):430–3, 1992.
11. Borsa PA, Lephart SM, Kocher MS, Lephart SP: Functional assessment and rehabilitation of shoulder proprioception for glenohumeral instability. *J Sports Rehabil* 3(1):84–104, 1994.
12. Branch TP, Hunter R, Donath M: Dynamic analysis of ACL deficient legs with and without bracing during cutting. *Am J Sports Med* 17:35, 1989.
13. Clark FJ, Horch KW, Bach SM, Larson GF: Contribution of cutaneous and joint receptors to static knee-position sense in man. *J Neurophysiol* 42:877–88, 1979.
14. Cornwall MW, Murrell P: Postural sway following inversion sprain of the ankle. *J Am Podiatric Med Assoc* 81:243–7, 1991.
15. Corrigan JP, Cashman WF, Brady MP: Proprioception in the cruciate deficient knee. *J Bone Joint Surg* 74B:247–50, 1992.
16. Cox ED, Lephart SM, Irrgang JJ: Unilateral balance training of noninjured individuals and the effects on postural sway. *J Sport Rehabil* 2:87–96, 1993.
17. Dick R: Gender specific knee injury patterns in collegiate basketball and soccer athletes [abstr]. *Med Sci Sports Exerc* 25:S, 1993.
18. Gadevia SC, McCloskey DI: Joint sense, muscle sense, and their combination as positions sense, measured at the distal interphalangeal joint of the middle finger. *J Physiol (Lond)* 260:387–407, 1976.
19. Garns SN, Newton RA: Kinesthetic awareness in subjects with multiple ankle sprains. *Phys Ther* 68:1667–71, 1988.

20. Giannantonio FP, Swanik CB, Lephart SM, et al: Long term resistance training and its effects on neuromuscular characteristics in females. *J Athletic Training* 33(2):S72, 1998.

21. Glenncross D, Thorton E: Position sense following joint injury. *J Sports Med Phys Fitness* 21:23–7, 1982.

22. Glousman R, Jobe F, Tibone J, et al: Dynamic electromyographic analysis of the throwing shoulder with glenohumeral instability. *J Bone Joint Surg* 70A:220–6, 1988.

23. Grigg P: Peripheral neural mechanisms in proprioception. *J Sports Rehabil* 3(1)2–17, 1995.

24. Hoffman M, Payne VG: The effects of proprioceptive ankle disk training on healthy subjects. *J Orthop Sports Phys Ther* 21(2):90–3, 1995.

25. Ireland ML: Special concerns of the female athlete. In: Fu FH, Stone DA (eds): Sports Injuries: Mechanism, Prevention, and Treatment, 2nd edition. Baltimore: Williams & Wilkins, 1994, pp 153–87.

26. Ireland ML, Wall C: Epidemiology and comparison of knee injuries in elite male and female United States basketball athletes. [abstr]. *Med Sci Sports Exer* 22:S82, 1990.

27. Ireland ML, Williams P: Epidemiology of injury and illness at the United States olympic sports festival 1990 [abstr]. *Med Sci Sports Exer* 25:S158, 1993.

28. Irrgang JJ, Whitney SL, Cox ED: Balance and proprioceptive training for rehabilitation of the lower extremity. *J Sports Rehab* 3(1):68–83, 1994.

29. Jennings AG, Seedhom BB: Proprioception in the knee and reflex hamstring contraction latency. *J Bone Joint Surg* 76B:491–4, 1994.

30. Kennedy JC, Alexander IJ, Hayes KC: Nerve supply of the human knee and its functional importance. *Am J Sports Med* 10:329–35, 1982.

31. Konradsen L, Ravn JB: Ankle instability caused by prolonged peroneal reaction time. *Acta Orthop Scand* 61:388–90, 1990.

32. Lanese RR, Strauss RH, Leizman DJ, Rotondi AM: Injury and disability in matched men's and women's intercollegiate sports. *Am J Public Health* 80:1459–62, 1990.

33. LaRiviere J, Osternig LR: The effect of ice immersion on joint position sense. *J Sports Rehabil* 3(1):58–67, 1994.

34. Lebsack D, Perrin DH: Comparison of subjective and objective assessment of balance. *J Athletic Training* 29:170, 1994.

35. Lentell GL, Katzman LL, Walters MR: The relationship between muscle function and ankle stability. *J Orthop Sports Phys Ther* 11(12): 605–11, 1990.

36. Lephart SM, Fu FH, Irrgand JJ, Borsa PA: Proprioception characteristics of trained and untrained college females [abstr]. *Med Sci Sports Exerc* 23(4):S113, 1991.

37. Lephart SM, Fu FH: The role of proprioception in the treatment of sports injuries. *Sports Exerc Injury* 1:96–102, 1995.

38. Lephart SM, Fu FH, Borsa PA: Proprioception in sports medicine. In *Advances in Operative Orthopaedics.* Vol 2. St Louis, Mosby-Year Book, 1994, pp 77–94.

39. Lephart SM, Henry TJ: Functional rehabilitation for the upper and lower extremity. *Orthop Clin North Am* 26(3):579–92, 1995.

40. Lephart SM, Kocher MS: The role of exercise in the prevention of shoulder disorders. In: Matsen FA, Fu FH, Hawkins RJ (eds): *The Shoulder: A Balance of Mobility and Stability.* Rosemont, Ill, American Academy of Orthopaedic Surgeons, 1992, pp 597–619.

41. Lephart SM, Kocher MS, Fu FH, et al. Proprioception following anterior cruciate ligament reconstruction. *J Sports Rehabil* 1:188–96, 1992.

42. Lephart SM, Warner JJ, Borsa PA, Fu FH: Proprioception of the shoulder joint in healthy, unstable, and surgically repaired shoulders. *J Shoulder Elbow Surg* 3(6):371–80, 1994.

43. Loose GM, et al: Correlation of lower extremity injury to balance indices: An investigation utilizing an instrumental unstable platform. American Orthopaedic Society for Sports Medicine, New Orleans, 1994.

44. Mattacola CG, Lebsack DA, Perrin DH: Intertester reliability of assessing postural sway using the Chattecx balance system. *J Athletic Training* 29(2):170, 1994.

45. Moberg E: The role of cutaneous afferents in position sense, kinesthesia, and motor function of the hand. *Brain* 106:1–19, 1983.

46. Nyland JA, Shapiro R, Stine RL, et al: Relationship of fatigued run and rapid stop to ground reaction forces, lower extremity kinematics, and muscle activation. *J Orthop Sports Phys Ther* 20(3):132–7, 1994.

47. Pincivero D, Lephart SM, Henry T: Learning effects and reliability of the Biodex Stability System. *J Athletic Training* 30:S35, 1995.

48. Rozzi SL, Lephart SM, Fu FH: Effects of muscular fatigue on knee joint laxity and neuromuscular characteristics of male and female athletes. *J Athletic Training* 34(2):106–14, 1999.

49. Rozzi SL, Lephart SM, Gear WS, Fu FH: Knee joint laxity and neuromuscular characteristics of male and female soccer and basketball players. *Am J Sports Med* 27(3):312–9, 1999.

50. Rozzi SL, Lephart SM, Sterner R, Kuligowski L: Balance training for persons with functionally unstable ankles. *J Orthop Sports Phys Ther* 29(8),478–86, 1999.

51. Safran MR, Caldwell GL, Fu FH: Proprioception considerations in surgery. *J Sports Rehabil* 3(1):105–15, 1994.

52. Schultz RA, Miller DC, Kerr CS, Micheli L: Mechanoreceptors in human cruciate ligaments. A histological study. *J Bone Joint Surg* 66A:1072–6, 1984.

53. Schutte MJ, Dabezies EJ, Zimny ML, Happwl LT: Neural anatomy of the human anterior cruciate ligament. *J Bone Joint Surg* 69A:243–7, 1987.

54. Skinner HB, Barrack RL, Cook SD: Age-related decline in proprioception. *Clin Orthop* 184:208–11, 1984.

55. Skinner HB, Barrack RL, Cook SD, RJ Haddad Jr: Joint position sense in total knee arthroplasty. *J Orthop Res* 1:276–83, 1984.

56. Smith RL, Brunolli J: Shoulder kinesthesia after anterior glenohumeral dislocations. *Phys Ther* 69:106–12, 1989.

57. Tenvergent EM, Ten Duis HJ, Klasen HJ: Trends in sports injury, 1982–1988: An in-depth study in four types of sport. *J Sports Med Phys Fitness* 32:214–20, 1992.

58. Tibone JE, Antich TJ: Electromyographic analysis of the anterior cruciate ligament-deficient knee. *Clin Orthop Rel Res* 288:35–9, 1993.

59. Walla DJ, Albright JP, McAuley E, et al: Hamstring control and the unstable anterior cruciate ligament-deficient knee. *Am J Sports Med* 13:34–9, 1985.

60. Wojtys EM, Huston LJ: Neuromuscular performance in normal and anterior cruciate ligament-deficient lower extremities. *Am J Sports Med* 22:89–104, 1994.

61. Wojtys EM, Wylie BB, Huston LJ: The effects of muscular fatigue on neuromuscular function and anterior tibial translation in healthy knees. *Am J Sports Med* 24:615–21, 1996.

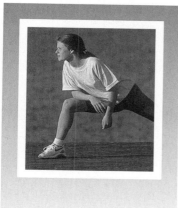

Chapter 47

Upper and Lower Extremity Strength Training

Scott Crook, P.T., C.S.C.S.

Female athletes are participating in greater numbers in strength and conditioning programs to help improve their athletic performance and prevent injury. Proper training methods are essential in helping them meet their goals. The purpose of this chapter is to discuss training methods to help female athletes maximize their athletic potential and minimize the potential for injury during their training program or sport.

GENDER DIFFERENCES

It is important to understand the physical differences between males and females when incorporating training programs to prepare females for their sport. The physical dimensions of males are approximately 7% to 10% larger than those of females at maturity.[2] The effects of testosterone enable men to be taller, with longer limbs. Males typically have a wider shoulder girdle and a narrower pelvis.[2] Females are influenced by estrogen, and have narrower shoulders, a wider pelvis (relative to their height), and greater carrying angles at the elbows.[2,8–10] These physical characteristics may contribute to structural malalignment, which may predispose the athlete to injury. Strength and conditioning programs can be beneficial in accommodating for malalignment, and thus may better prepare the athlete for her sport and lessen the potential for injury.

Testosterone and estrogen also affect muscular development, as males have the advantage of testosterone to help increase muscle mass.[2] Females can increase muscle fiber diameter and mass, but not to the same extent as males because of lower testosterone levels.[11,14] Therefore, females can participate in strength programs without the fear of losing their femininity by becoming overly muscular or bulky.

There are numerous studies regarding muscular strength differences between males and females. Females have the same biologic ability to gain strength as males.[13] They demonstrate equal strength per unit of cross-sectional area of muscle.[13] One study suggests that when statistically controlled, the lower extremity strength differences between males and females are not significant. However, the same study suggests that males are stronger in the upper extremities per unit of muscular weight.[7]

In summary, females can benefit from strength training to help improve their athletic performance, but their lower levels of testosterone keep them from achieving the levels of muscular hypertrophy that would be achieved by males. Many females find this socially beneficial, as they do not need to fear losing their feminine qualities.

CORE STRENGTHENING

The core of the athletic body is made up of the cervical spine, trunk, hips, and pelvic musculature. These structures are essential for control of gravity, posture, and balance. The body's center of gravity is located within the core, and control of the center of gravity is essential for performance in all sports. The core also plays a major role in transfer of forces from the lower extremities to the upper extremities, and vice versa.

Therefore, strengthening of the core should not be neglected, and is essential in providing a foundation for strengthening of the upper and lower extremities. Many of the core strengthening exercises incorporate the extremities into functional patterns, and thus work to gain strength simultaneously in the core and extremities.

Core strengthening should include all planes of motion, including the transverse plane, which is necessary for rotational movements. Rotational movements are a major component of many sport activities. Since most athletic activities are done in a standing position, the core should also be trained in that manner. However, sport activities also require having body control while in the air, so the core should also be trained to prepare for that aspect of sport. Use of machines, or single-plane exercises done in a sitting position may isolate muscles or motions by stabilizing the pelvis. This takes away the proprioceptive aspect of the training and reduces the effect on spatial awareness.[4]

Some excellent methods for training the core include medicine ball or Swiss ball exercises. Medicine ball exercises are performed in a standing position, which is functional to many sports. They can be done with a partner or done individually. Done individually, a dumbbell can be used for resistance if a medicine ball is not available.

Individual exercises include torso circles (Fig. 47-1), which are done standing with feet shoulder width apart. The arms are extended and the ball is rotated in a circular movement in front of the body. Other exercises from the same position include figure-of-8 patterns in front of the body, side-to-side twists, vertical chopping from overhead to between the knees, and diagonal chops from over one shoulder to outside the opposite knee. The variables of these exercises include the speed with which they are performed, the position of the arms, which create longer or shorter lever arms to affect the resistance, and the amplitude of the movement pattern. Those variables allow for a wide variety of resistances, even if the weight is constant. Initially, the weight should be very light (2 to 4 pounds), with a gradual progression up to as much as 10 pounds as long as the athlete demonstrates good technique.

Partner exercises are done with the medicine ball either handed off or passed to the partner. A medicine ball rebounder/trampoline works very well for medicine ball passes, if one is available. Partner hand-off exercises include the medicine ball half twist, and medicine ball full twist. The partners stand back to back, one arm's length apart. For the half twist, the individual twists to one side and hands off to the second partner, who rotates to the other side and returns the handoff. The ball moves around the outside of the 2 partners. The full twist is done with the individual rotating further to hand the ball off to the opposite side of the partner, who then turns the opposite way to perform the full twist and return the handoff. The ball moves in a figure-of-8 pattern between the 2 partners. Initially 2 to 4 pounds is adequate weight with progression up to as much as 10 pounds as technique allows.

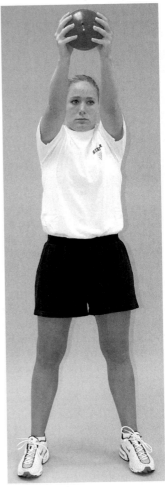

Figure 47-1. Torso circles require stabilization of the entire body against the forces generated by the circular movement of the weighted object.

Medicine ball passes allow for higher-intensity and higher-velocity strengthening. They are, in essence, plyometrics for the core and upper extremities. Because of their intense nature, it is important that adequate warm-up be performed before beginning these exercises. Some useful medicine ball passes include chest passes, overhead passes, diagonal passes, and side passes. The key to gaining the greatest effect is to be in position to have the ball returned to the position of release. The individual will absorb the energy from the ball as it moves to the starting position and provides a stretch to preload the muscles and create the plyometric effect. The position of the feet should be staggered to help maintain balance while absorbing the energy of the ball. Chest passes are performed as the individual starts from the chest and passes the ball chest-high to the partner. Overhead passes are performed with the individual starting with the ball behind the head. The ball is passed overhead, to just above the head of the partner. Diagonal passes and side passes can be combined with partners. The first partner starts with the ball above the shoulder on one side, and with the trunk rotated to the same side. She then rotates and throws the ball with 2 hands across the body to the partner with the goal being to throw to waist height on the opposite side. The second partner catches the ball waist high, and absorbs the energy with trunk rotation. The second partner will be performing a side pass as the ball is returned from waist high. Her goal is to return the ball to just above the shoulder of the first partner to preload the body for the next diagonal pass.

The initial weight will range from 2 to 4 pounds, with the maximum weight usually around 8 pounds. The ideal number of sets and repetitions will be in ranges of 2 to 4 sets and 10 to 20 repetitions. Three days per week is appropriate because of the plyometric effect. Medicine ball exercises can be customized to simulate sport-specific movement patterns and the number of exercises that can be performed is limited only by one's imagination.

Swiss ball exercises use a large rubber or plastic ball and allow for a variety of positions, including working from a sitting position, supine on the ball or floor, and prone over the ball, including a walkout position on the hands. The appropriate size of the ball can be determined by having the individual sit on the ball. The hips and knees should be flexed approximately 90° with the feet flat on the floor.

Swiss ball exercises have the ability to enhance proprioception in the extremities as well as improving spatial awareness in the core. Many of the exercises involve strengthening and stabilization of the upper and/or lower extremities in addition to the core strengthening. Medicine balls, dumbbells, resistance tubing, and other forms of resistance can be added to the exercises to increase the difficulty.

Exercises involving sitting on the ball require body control to compensate for the unstable base of support. Sitting or lying supine on the ball, one can perform reactive activities that challenge the abdominal musculature and core proprioceptive abilities (Fig. 47-2). If the individual walks out from the ball in the supine position, moving the center of gravity off the ball, she may perform bridging activities, and must demonstrate greater control in the extensors of the core to compensate for the unstable position (Fig. 47-3). Lying supine on the floor with the feet on the ball requires stabilization of the core

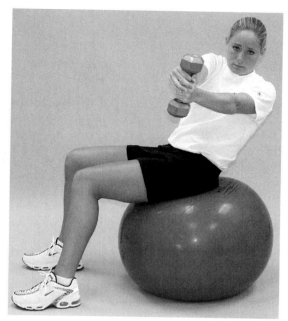

Figure 47-2. Sitting on the Swiss ball emphasizes control of the anterior and oblique abdominal musculature.

extensors and lower extremities. When exercising prone over the ball, one challenges the reactive abilities of the trunk extensors. Walking out from the ball in the prone position requires stabilization of the core flexors, as well as stabilization of the scapular stabilizers and proprioception in the upper extremities (Fig. 47-4). Weakness in the abdominal musculature is demonstrated by poor technique, as the trunk will tend to sag in the lumbar region. This will result in compression of the lumbar facets and the individual may complain of back pain while exercising. Reducing the distance of the walkout will modify the exercise to decrease the difficulty. Moving the center of gravity further away from the ball increases the degree of difficulty with all Swiss ball exercises. Again, as with the medicine ball exercises, the number of exercises is only limited by one's imagination. The above position descriptions are basic suggestions for a starting point with the exercises.

Core stability is essential before progressing into training of the extremities, and provides a vital link in performance of all athletic activities. Incorporation of the exercise activities for core strengthening will help provide a better foundation for performance of upper and lower extremity strength training. They will also transcend into better athletic performance, and better body control will make the athlete less likely to be injured.

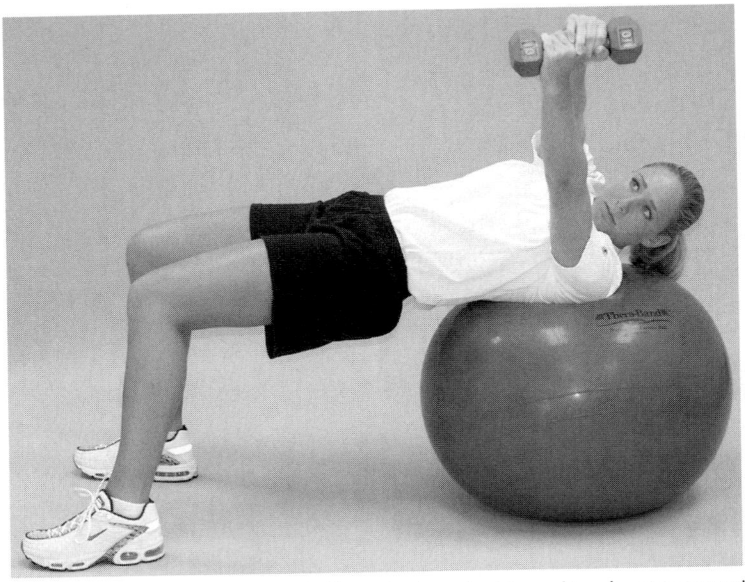

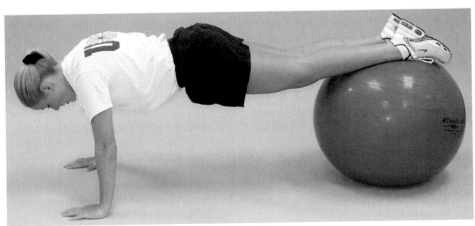

Figure 47-3. The supine-bridge position on the Swiss ball emphasizes the hip and trunk extensors, with additional control required in the lower extremities.

FUNCTIONAL STRENGTHENING FOR ATHLETICS

Females are participating in sports that are physically demanding, and are working hard to prepare for the demands of their sport. To prepare for a sport, one must understand the demands of the sport. These include the primary planes of movement, the aerobic and anaerobic demands, and the areas and mechanisms of potential injury. It is important to incorporate the concept of periodization to allow for peak performance at the most important times.

Understanding the demands of the sport requires examination of the movement patterns that are required to perform the sport. Examination of the dominant planes of movement will determine the areas of focus for the strength program. Velocity of movement is also relevant to help the athlete prepare for the high-velocity demands of the sport. The athlete must also be prepared for the aerobic and anaerobic demands. The athlete who is in better overall condition is less likely to be injured.

Females have higher injury rates for the lower extremities,[8-10] and thus would benefit from strength training designed to prevent injury as well as improve performance. A program emphasizing core stability and enhanced proprioception will benefit the athlete. It is important

Figure 47-4. The prone-bridge position on the Swiss ball emphasizes scapular stabilization, upper extremity proprioception, and the anterior core musculature. Proper technique requires maintaining the core and lower extremities in a straight plane.

to continue the program during the season to help maintain the benefits of the program.

FREE WEIGHTS VERSUS MACHINES

The most functional method of strength training involves the use of free weights.[3,6] The advantages provided by machines are the reasons why they are not very functional. Machines are excellent at isolating muscle groups in isolated arcs of motion. However, the body rarely works in an isolated fashion. Movement patterns in sports require integrated movement patterns, through many planes of movement. Furthermore, the motor cortex is set up to work in terms of movement patterns and synergistic movements instead of movement of individual muscles.[12] The use of free weights, including barbells, dumbbells, and medicine balls, allows for the greatest freedom of movement patterns, and requires the greatest neuromuscular control.[3,6] The control required to stabilize the weight enhances proprioception and works all of the stabilizers needed for body control in athletics. Exercise machines often provide support to all body parts except for the designated muscle. This does nothing to improve body control or proprioception, and may train the body to work in unnatural movement patterns. Therefore, use of free weights is more beneficial for sport-specific conditioning.

MULTIJOINT EXERCISES

Multijoint exercises can be defined as exercises using more than one joint in motion contributing to the movement of the object of resistance. These exercises include all upper body presses, squats, lunges, and upper and lower extremity combination exercises such as the snatch and the clean and jerk. These exercises should be done early in the exercise session as they use multiple muscle groups. Use of exercises that isolate muscle groups may fatigue the muscle group, which may be an important component of a multijoint exercise. That would limit the performance during the exercise and lessen the challenge to the other muscle groups. It also could create potential for injury with an important muscle group being unable to support the joint during the exercise.

A good rule with multijoint exercises to help achieve muscle balance in the upper extremities is to work in opposite directions for each exercise. Example: For every pushing exercise such as the military (overhead) press, one should perform a pulling exercise such as latissimus pulldowns. This concept works groups of muscle on both sides of the body for both power movements and stabilization.

Muscle balance in the lower extremities is achieved with closed chain exercises. Closed chain exercises utilize cocontractions of the lower extremity musculature with most exercises. Furthermore, they utilize muscle groups of all the lower extremity joints with most exercises. They are more sport specific, as most sporting activities require closed chain positions during play, including all running and jumping activities. Example: A single-leg squat (Fig. 47-5) utilizes all muscles about the hip, as well as both the quadriceps and hamstrings musculature. All the muscles of the lower leg and foot are working to provide balance and control at the ankle.

Single-leg activities for lower extremity strengthening are very sport specific owing to most ground-based sports generating most of the force one leg at a time.[15] Running and direction changes require single-leg force production, and when both feet are on the ground simultaneously, the weight is usually not evenly distributed.[15] Weight is constantly being shifted from one side to the other, and movement occurs through all planes of movement. Therefore, it is important to include and emphasize single-leg activities for lower extremity strengthening. Another benefit to single-leg conditioning is that the external resistance is

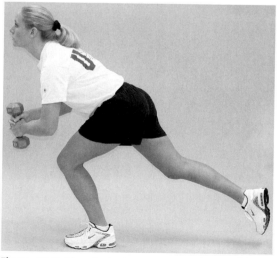

Figure 47-5. The single leg squat exercise emphasizes balance as well as strengthening of the entire lower extremity kinetic chain.

usually done adequately with dumbbells. This lessens the need for equipment (barbells), and also reduces the heavy loads on the body. Use of dumbbells also allows athletes to perform the exercises without needing a spotter. Forward and multidirectional lunges fall into this category as most of the weight is shifted to the lunging lower extremity. Single-leg standing with a reach around the clock is an excellent exercise to improve balance and proprioception in the standing leg (Fig. 47-6). The athlete actually works toward the inwardly rotated, valgus position of the knee often described as a mechanism of injury.[8–10] However, this exercise allows the athlete to learn how to use the muscles in that position, and develop their proprioceptive abilities.

Basic Multijoint Exercise Recommendations

Basic upper body strengthening can be done with 4 basic multijoint exercises. Two pushing exercises, (1) bench press, and (2) military, incline, or overhead press, are balanced by 2

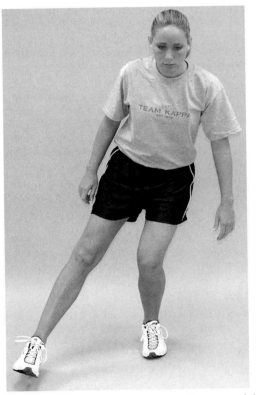

Figure 47-6. Single-leg standing with reaching around the clock emphasizes balance and proprioception while allowing the knee to move into positions that will be encountered while participating in sporting activities.

pulling exercises, (3) rowing, or forward-bent rowing, and (4) latissimus pull-downs.

Basic lower body strengthening can be done with 3 basic multijoint exercises: (1) squats, or single-leg squats, (2) forward or side lunges, and (3) leg presses. The leg press can emphasize different muscles by changing the angle of the press. The deeper leg press with the feet further in front of the body emphasizes the hip extensors (gluteals) and hamstrings. The more shallow leg press, with the feet lower on the press platform, will emphasize the quadriceps, and gastrocnemius-soleus muscle groups.

SINGLE-JOINT EXERCISES

Single-joint exercises are effective for isolating muscle groups. This is beneficial for working underdeveloped muscle groups to help with overall muscle balance. It is also beneficial for strengthening of musculature to provide specific support and prevent injuries. The rotator cuff is a good example of musculature providing support to the glenohumeral joint. It is also a frequent site of injury with overhead sports.

Single-joint exercises can also be done to emphasize certain muscle groups for bodybuilding or body-shaping purposes. As previously mentioned, these exercises are best done at the end of the exercise session to prevent the fatiguing of specific muscle groups that are important components of other exercises.

The most important single-joint exercises for injury prevention are directed at the rotator cuff. The rotator cuff blends into the glenohumeral joint capsule and functions to centralize the head of the humerus during upper extremity movements. The rotator cuff can be overpowered by the larger pectoralis major, latissimus dorsi, and deltoid musculature if it is not of adequate strength. Inability to maintain centralization of the humeral head may result in injury to the rotator cuff as the humeral head rides upward and impinges the rotator cuff on the acromion. Also, overstretching of the glenohumeral joint capsule may occur if the humeral head is allowed to move too far in an anterior or posterior direction. This is applicable to females, as they tend to have greater laxity in their joints than their male counterparts.

Rotator cuff exercises can be performed with resistive bands and can also be done effectively with light dumbbells. The starting weight may be as light as 1 to 3 pounds, and the resistance will usually not exceed 8 to 10 pounds, as these muscles are very small. Two effective exercises that can be done in a side-lying position are side-lying external rotation (Fig. 47-7) and side-lying abduction. The abduction exercise should be done with the arm straight in the 0° to 45° arc of motion, as gravity will have its greatest effect in that arc of motion. This arc of motion also is lower than the common arc of impingement (90° abduction). The abduction exercise can be done with the thumb pointing straight ahead. Another variation would be starting with the thumb turned downward toward the hip to begin the exercise, with rotation to thumb upward at the end of the exercise, which puts more emphasis on the external rotators.

The lower extremities are covered fairly well with multijoint exercises, but the gastrocnemius-soleus muscle group may be a good target for single-joint exercises. These muscles are involved to a lesser extent by the multijoint exercises. They function to help with push-off and drive during jumping and running activities. They also provide support for the knee from below with their absorption of ground forces. Calf raises and walking on the toes are 2 exercises to help isolate the gastrocnemius-soleus musculature. Standing with the foot flat and leaning forward with the knees, hips and trunk extended emphasizes gastrocnemius-soleus strengthening as the musculature must decelerate the forward movement of the body's center of gravity. This simulates function well as the gastrocnemius-soleus functions to decelerate forward movement of the tibia during the stance phase of gait when the foot is flat on the ground.

Isolated strengthening of the hamstring musculature may be beneficial with the use of hamstring curls. Swiss ball exercises emphasizing the hamstrings include supine bridging (single- or double-leg). These are done lying on the floor with the feet upon the ball. The subject lifts the hips and holds the position for 2 to 4 seconds. An exercise performed in a similar position on the Swiss ball is the hamstring curl, which is done by lifting the hips, then flexing the hips and knees and rolling the ball back toward the hips as the hips remain 4 to 6 inches above the floor. Returning to the extended position for the lower extremities completes the exercise.

Quadriceps isolated strengthening can be done with knee extensions. However, this exercise may not be recommended for those who have had anterior cruciate ligament injuries owing to the increased anterior shear forces on the tibia at the knee.[16] The patellofemoral compressive forces are also increased significantly during the knee extension exercise. The arc of motion that is most detrimental for the anterior cruciate ligament and the patellofemoral articulation in the open chain is from 45° flexion to full extension. Thus, if this exercise is used, it is best to avoid the final 45° of extension. Another argument against the use of knee extensions is the question: How much does the exercise simulate actual functional activities of the knee? The knee functions primarily with the foot on the ground, in the closed chain position. So, open chain knee extensions have very little functional value. An alternative method of quadriceps strengthening involves standing on one leg and reaching forward with the opposite leg approximately 1 inch above the floor. The standing leg flexes at the knee and the knee moves forward over the toes. Generally, the knee moving forward over the toes will place additional stress on the patellofemoral articulation. However, this

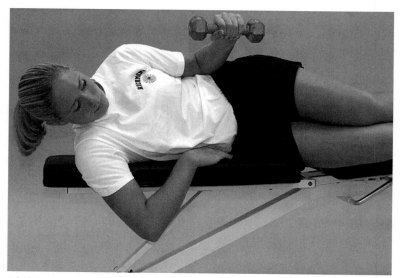

Figure 47-7. Side-lying external rotation with a dumbbell is an excellent exercise for rotator cuff strengthening.

functionally simulates the position of the knee when descending steps, and thus has value for preparing a person for activities of daily living. No external resistance is necessary as the subject increases the demand by reaching further forward.

Single-joint exercises can be used to enhance the exercise program, but care should be taken when choosing the exercises. They should always be done toward the end of the exercise session to avoid fatigue of musculature that is an important component of another multijoint exercise.

PLYOMETRICS

Plyometric training is a valuable method for improving explosive strength. It uses the elastic potential of the muscle and the nervous system to train the athlete to become more explosive. The object is to train the athlete to utilize the elastic energy of the muscle, and train the neurologic system to be more responsive. The key is to reduce the time for the muscle transition from the eccentric (landing/absorbing) phase to the concentric (push-off) phase.[5] It is important to have a solid strength base before beginning plyometrics, and they should be trained in conjunction with a strength program.

Before beginning a plyometric program the athlete should demonstrate balance and body control. Previous studies have suggested that the athlete be able to squat 2 to 2.5 times her body weight. These standards may be higher than necessary.[5] The ability to control a single-leg squat demonstrates body control and balance. The athlete should be able to perform 10 single-leg squats to 45° knee flexion, with good control and without losing their balance. The athlete should always demonstrate good technique and control of the exercise. The gradual progression of activities allows the athlete to master one phase of the plyometrics before progressing to more advanced techniques.

Plyometric Progression

Phase 1: Jumps up to a platform. The platform height is 6 to 12 inches. Emphasis is on sticking the landing and absorbing the landing (Fig. 47-8). The emphasis should be on landing softly and quietly. The impact forces are reduced with jumps up to a platform, as the body does not have as far to fall after the jump. This exercise can be useful for female athletes to help train body control and proper posture when landing from jumps.

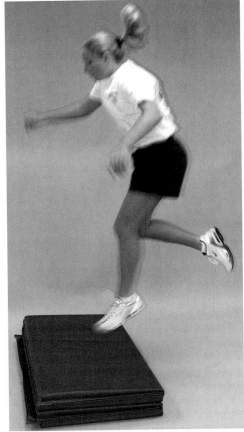

Figure 47-8. Jump up to a mat or platform allows the subject to emphasize control of the landings with reduced impact.

Phase 2: Low-intensity jumping. This involves low-amplitude jumping such as jumping rope or ricochet jumps. Ricochet jumps are low-amplitude jumps done very quickly over a line, using either alternate legs or both at the same time.

Phase 3: Jumps in place. Jumping and holding the landing is done for 2 to 4 seconds before jumping again. Eventually the athlete progresses to more rapid jumping, working toward less ground time and more time in the air. The focus should be on landing in the same area.

Phase 4: Bounding activities. Double-leg bounding activities are done first. Included in this phase are double-leg lateral hops over boxes or cones and power skipping. Power skipping is taking the activity of skipping and emphasizing additional vertical or horizontal displacement. The aim is to spend as much time in the air, with as little time on the ground, as possible.

Phase 5: Single-leg activities. The exercise begins with alternate-leg bounding (or long stride running with maximal length of stride and minimal ground time). Progression is to single-leg bounding with increasing distances to increase the intensity.

Phase 6: Depth jumps or shock jumps. These are not recommended in most cases. They have a high neurologic demand and a higher risk of injury. The athlete should demonstrate proficiency at the previous phases before attempting this level. These should be monitored individually to select the appropriate level of exercise. Depth jumps include jumping down from boxes with immediate rebound jumps. Choosing the proper height of the box is essential. First the athlete's vertical jump is measured. Next a height is set for the box to perform a depth jump (usually 12 inches to start). Measure the vertical jump height again, including the jump down from the box. If the vertical jump is the same or less than before, the athlete is not demonstrating adequate control and will not benefit from the exercise. That athlete will also be increasing her risk of injury. If the vertical jump is improved, the athlete demonstrates adequate control to perform the exercise. The box height is raised and the vertical jump retested until the athlete is no longer improving in vertical jump height. The height for the depth jump is chosen based on the maximal vertical jump height performed using the box.

The volume of plyometric exercises can be measured by the number of contacts in an exercise session. Initially the number of contacts should be limited to 70 to 90 in a session, with many of the contacts being the lower-intensity exercises. Eventually, the volume can progress to as much as 200 to 250 contacts in a session. However a variety of intensities should be done within a training session. Depth jumps should be limited to no more than 30 contacts in a session. The frequency can be up to 3 times per week, but 3 days rest should be allowed after depth jumps.[5] Plyometrics should be performed in cycles lasting 4 to 6 weeks, with at least 2 weeks off for recovery between cycles.

Use of plyometrics during a competitive season should be limited to 100 to 120 contacts per session. The frequency should be limited to 2 times per week. Owing to the extended recovery time needed, depth jumps should be avoided during in-season conditioning.

Upper extremity plyometrics are best done using a medicine ball and were previously discussed in this chapter in the section on core strengthening.

PERIODIZATION

Periodization is the use of a plan to incorporate training methods into a time frame to allow for peak performance at the most important time. Manipulation of training variables allows for improvement in performance, with the goals being peak performance during the competitive season. Variation of the program prevents boredom, and stimulates growth and physical improvement.

The annual training cycle can be broken down into 3 phases: (1) preparatory phase, (2) competitive phase, and (3) transition phase.[1] The preparatory phase is designed to improve general physical conditioning and work capacity. It also works to develop the motor abilities required by the sport. The preparatory phase can be separated into 2 subphases, the general and specific preparatory phases. The goal of the general preparatory subphase is to develop the highest level of physical conditioning and work capacity. It begins after the transition phase (4 to 6 weeks after the end of the competitive season). The specific preparatory subphase is working toward becoming more sport specific to prepare for the competitive season.[1] This subphase should cover the last 6 to 8 weeks prior to the beginning of practice time for the competitive season.

The competitive phase occurs during the preseason practice and competitive season. Owing to the demand of the sport, the intensity of training should be reduced by 25% to 30%. Even greater tapering may be done prior to the final competition to allow for full recovery and peak performance.

Some valuable in-season exercises for females may include single-leg squats, jumps up to a platform, and single-leg standing with reach around the clock. This exercise is performed as the athlete stands on one leg and reaches forward with the opposite leg. The object is to reach in the direction of the numbers on a clock face. The athlete is instructed to keep the reaching leg 1 inch above the floor throughout the exercise. The intensity is increased as the athlete reaches further. This exercise improves dynamic balance and proprioception in the lower extremities. These exercises are best done after practice to avoid excessive fatigue during the practice session. They should be limited to 2 to 3 times per week, and should not be done on the day before a competition.

The transition phase is the phase immediately after the end of the season. It will last from 3 to 5 weeks and the emphasis in this phase is recovery from the season and active rest. Focus on rehabilitation of any injuries sustained during the season and light workouts to minimize any effects of inactivity.[1]

Periodization is important to maximize the effects of strength training. Unfortunately, many athletes participate in their sport on a year-round basis. It is important that they prioritize the time of year for peak performance and work in a program to help them peak at the proper time.

CONCLUDING REMARKS

Females are able to reap the benefits of strength training to help improve athletic performance and better prepare them to prevent injury. The relatively wider pelvis, greater femoral anteversion, and valgus alignment in the female place the knee in a position more prone to injury,[8–10] which may make them more susceptible to injury. Therein lies the importance of the proprioceptive exercise activities. Their tendency toward increased joint laxity and flexibility may serve them well in some sports, but may create problems that can be worsened with improper strength training techniques. Females who tend to have increased joint laxity or flexibility should avoid the extremes of motion with heavier strength training. Although strength throughout the range of motion may be desirable, the risks may outweigh the benefits when placing large amounts of shear stress on joints that are already lax.

Finally the importance of core strength cannot be underestimated for providing a solid foundation for all strength training and athletic performances. Core strength and proprioception training should be a part of all strength training programs.

References

1. Bompa TO: Periodization training for peak performance. In: Foran B (ed): High Performance Sports Conditioning. Champaign, Ill, Human Kinetics Publishers, 2001, pp 267–82.
2. Carbon RJ: The female athlete. In: Bloomfield J, Fricker PA, Fitch KD (eds): Textbook of Science and Medicine in Sport. Champaign, Ill, Human Kinetics Publishers, 1992, pp 467–8.
3. Gambetta V: A leg to stand on. In: Gambetta V (ed): The Gambetta Method: Common Sense Training for Athletic Performance. Sarasota, Fla, Gambetta Sports Training Systems, Inc., 1998, pp 35–7.
4. Gambetta V: From the core. In: Gambetta V (ed): The Gambetta Method: Common Sense Training for Athletic Performance. Sarasota, Fla, Gambetta Sports Training Systems, Inc., 1998.
5. Gambetta V: Leaps and bounds. Gambetta V (ed): The Gambetta Method: Common Sense Training for Athletic Performance. Sarasota, Fla, Gambetta Sports Training Systems, Inc., 1998.
6. Harman E: The biomechanics of resistance exercise. In: Baechle TR (ed): Essentials of Strength Training and Conditioning/National Strength and Conditioning Association. Champaign, Ill, Human Kinetics Publishers, 1994, p. 34.
7. Hoffman T, Stanffer RW, Jackson AS: Sex difference in strength. Am J Sports Med 7:265–7, 1979.
8. Ireland ML: Anterior cruciate ligament injury in female athletes: epidemiology. J Athletic Training 34(2):150–4, 1999.
9. Ireland ML: Special concerns of the female athlete. In: Fu FH, Stone DA (eds): Sports Injuries. Baltimore, Williams & Wilkins, 1994, pp 153–87.
10. Ireland ML, Gaudette M, Crook S: ACL injuries in the female athlete. J Sport Rehabil 6:97–110, 1997.
11. Mayhew JL, Gross PM: Body composition changes in young women with high resistance weight training. Res Q 45:433–40, 1974.
12. Noth J: Cortical and peripheral control. In: Komi PV (ed): Strength and Power in Sport. Cambridge, Mass, Blackwell Scientific Publishers, 1991, p 11.
13. O'Shea JP, Wegner J: Power training and the female athlete. Physician Sports Med 9:109–20, 1981.
14. Oyster N: Effects of heavy resistance weight training program on college women athletes. J Sports Med 10:79–83, 1979.
15. Santana JC: Single-leg trianing for 2-legged sports: efficacy of strength development in athletic performance. Strength Condition J 23(3):35–7, 2001.
16. Wilk KE, Andrews JR: The effects of pad placement and angular velocity on tibial displacement during isokinetic exercise. J Orthop Sports Phys Ther 17(1):24–30, 1993.

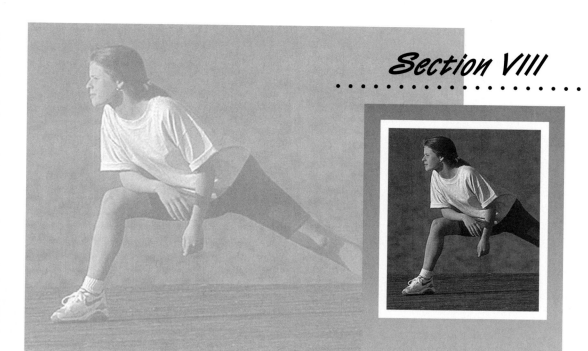

Sport-Specific Conditions

Chapter 48

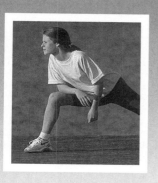

Basketball

Leigh Ann Curl, M.D.

Since the passage of Title IX legislation in 1972, women's sports have grown in both number and popularity. Basketball is perhaps the sport that has made the greatest gains both on a recreational and professional level.

At the high school level, the number one sports by teams and participants for girls is basketball. Based on participants, football is the numbers one sport for boys, with players numbering 1,002,734. In basketball, the numbers are 541,130 for boys and 451,600 for girls. The numbers of schools participating in basketball are 16,852 for boys and 16,526 for girls. This information is from the 1999–2000 Athletics Participation Summary of the National Federation of State High School Associations (National Federation of State High School Associations, P.O. Box 690, Indianapolis, Indiana 46206, *www.nfhs.org*, 2000).

At the collegiate level, according to the National Collegiate Athletic Association (NCAA), the number of basketball athletes is 14,445 for women and 15,874 for men.[46] The divisions for women's sports are: Division I: 317 teams, 4565 athletes; Division II: 284 teams, 3976 athletes; Division III: 410 teams, 5904 athletes; and overall, 1011 teams with 14,445 athletes. Those for men's sports are: Division I: 321 teams with 4815 athletes; Division II: 287 teams with 4391 athletes; Division III: 381 teams with 6668 athletes; and overall, 989 teams with 15,874 athletes.

With this growth and popularity has come the recognition of specific injury patterns, particularly as they relate to the female player. While female players sustain injuries in a pattern similar to male players when evaluated by anatomic area (Table 48-1),[46] women sustain a higher number of sprains and strains, and more significantly, a higher number of more serious knee injuries. In this chapter, common basketball injuries will be discussed, with specific attention to those injuries that have been found to be more common among female players.

INJURIES BY AGE OR LEVEL OF PARTICIPATION

When comparing studies looking at injury rates at different levels of competition, it is difficult to draw definite conclusions because of the fact that the definition of "injury" varies from study to study. Some consider "injury" any trauma resulting in evaluation by a trained medical professional. Others consider an event an "injury" only when it results in restriction from a game or practice. Furthermore, the reported "rate" may be the percentage of participants injured in a season, or the number of injuries per 1000 athlete exposures, or some other defined number.

In a study of youth players (ages 5 to 12), girls had a 13.5% rate of injury (any problem requiring evaluation), with 2.7% losing playing time because of their injury.[18] Female high school players were found to have a 25% injury rate (injury preventing participation), with 16% of injuries occurring during games compared to 9% during practice.[14] On a collegiate level, most statistics are from NCAA surveillance data. Data from the period of 1988 to 1993 showed a 20% injury rate (any problem causing loss of participation one or more days beyond day of injury) among 20 female collegiate teams, with 2.5 injuries per 1000 exposures.[9] At the professional level, one study[60] found 51.2 injuries (any event requiring evaluation) per 1000 exposures, while another[63] indicated an injury rate 60% higher than that for their professional male counterparts. At the professional level, almost twice as many injuries occurred during games as compared to practice.

Thus, while the data are variable, it is clear that there are injuries at all levels of participa-

Table 48-1. NCAA Injury Surveillance System Reports of Injuries in Males and Females, Practices and Games, With Female:Male Ratios, 1999–2000

| INJURY TYPES AND BODY PARTS | PRACTICES | | | GAMES | | |
	MALES	FEMALES	F:M RATIO	MALES	FEMALES	F:M RATIO
Laceration	0.12	0.02	0.17	0.55	0.38	0.69
Ligament sprain (incomplete tear)	1.58	1.54	0.97	3.26	3.10	0.95
Ligament sprain (complete tear)	0.08	0.18	2.25	0.18	0.62	3.44
Muscle–tendon strain (incomplete tear)	0.55	0.88	1.60	1.22	0.45	0.37
Muscle–tendon strain (complete tear)	0.01	0.02	2.00	0.03	0.07	2.33
Dislocation (partial)	0.12	0.14	1.17	0.03	0.24	8.00
Dislocation (complete)	0.07	0.05	0.71	0.33	0.14	0.42
Fracture	0.28	0.16	0.57	0.97	0.79	0.81
Stress fracture	0.11	0.21	1.91	0.18	0.07	0.39
Concussion	0.14	0.22	1.57	0.58	0.86	1.48
Lower back	0.24	0.23	0.96	0.37	0.21	0.57
Pelvis, groin, hip	0.16	0.18	1.13	0.46	0.28	0.61
Upper leg	0.21	0.43	2.05	0.55	0.21	0.38
Knee	0.46	0.68	1.48	1.13	1.97	1.74
Patella	0.08	0.11	1.38	0.15	0.17	1.13
Lower leg	0.17	0.25	1.47	0.21	0.14	0.67
Ankle	1.28	1.32	1.03	2.62	2.14	0.82
Heel/Achilles	0.06	0.12	2.00	0.00	0.14	
Foot	0.22	0.29	1.32	0.64	0.59	0.92
Neck	0.01	0.03	3.00	0.09	0.03	0.33
Shoulder	0.09	0.14	1.56	0.33	0.41	1.24
Clavicle	0.01	0.00	0.00	0.00	0.03	
Acromioclavicular joint separation	0.00	0.00		0.03	0.07	2.33
Elbow	0.04	0.03	0.75	0.21	0.10	0.48
Forearm	0.01	0.01	1.00	0.00	0.00	
Wrist	0.05	0.01	0.20	0.30	0.10	0.33
Hand	0.05	0.01	0.20	0.12	0.17	1.42
Finger(s)	0.11	0.06	0.55	0.24	0.24	1.00
Thumb(s)	0.05	0.11	2.20	0.15	0.24	1.60
Head	0.16	0.25	1.56	0.91	1.03	1.13
Eye	0.06	0.04	0.67	0.21	0.21	1.00

Data from 1999–2000 NCAA Injury Surveillance System.

tion. It also seems apparent that more injuries occur during game competition than in regular practice time.

INJURIES BY ANATOMIC REGION AND TYPE

The NCAA Injury Surveillance System reports from 18% of its member institutions, classifying injuries based on rate of members per 1000 athletic exposures and into types and body parts. Comparing practices and games, the statistics for females and males are shown in Table 48-1.[46] More injuries occur during games, and the rates of complete tear of the ligament, muscle tendon strain, and dislocation are significantly greater in females than males. During the 1999 to 2000 season, stress fractures and concussions were also greater in females than males during practice. Based on the anatomic region during practice, females were injured twice as often as

males in the upper leg, heel/Achilles tendon, neck, and thumb.

Facial Injuries

Basketball is a contact sport, and a number of eye and maxillofacial injuries occur during participation each year. Injury can occur as a result of contact with an opponent's elbow or fingers, the floor, surrounding chairs, walls, or tables, or the ball itself. Basketball is second only to baseball in the number of eye and mouth injuries that occur during organized sports in the United States, and up to 10% of all basketball injuries involve the face or scalp.[19] Despite this, the use of facial protective equipment is not mandatory during organized participation.

Eye

It is estimated that 7500 eye injuries occur each year while playing basketball.[19,31] In one report, nearly 30% of all eye injuries evaluated by a single ophthalmologist were sustained while playing basketball, with 6% requiring surgery and 3% resulting in permanent visual loss.[33] The International Federation of Sports Medicine places basketball players in the "high-risk" category for eye injury. Most injuries result either from a direct blow, such as an elbow to the head, or from being poked by a finger.

The most common eye injury sustained is a corneal abrasion. Frank tears, hyphema, lens injury, and posterior segment injury occur less frequently. Corneal abrasion presents with pain and photophobia, and is readily identified by fluorescein examination. Most abrasions respond to patching for 24 to 48 hours in conjunction with topical antibiotics. As with any eye injury, the orthopedist should not hesitate to refer the player for ophthalmologic evaluation.

More recently, corneal tear or rupture has occurred following a direct blow to the eye in players who have undergone previous laser keratotomy for the treatment of near-sightedness. This has occurred as late as 10 years after the procedure, and thus suggests persistent corneal weakness, and subsequently persistent risk of critical injury, following this procedure.[29]

Zagelbaum and coworkers in a prospective study of eye injuries in the National Basketball Association (NBA) found somewhat similar results.[62] Of the 1092 injuries sustained by the NBA players, 59 (5.4%) involved the eye. Eighteen (30%) occurred while the player was on offense. The most common diagnosis was abrasion or laceration to the eyelid (50.9%). Seventeen (28.8%) involved contusions to eyelid or periorbital regions and 7 (11.9%) were corneal abrasions. Fifty-seven players (96%) were not wearing protective eyewear at the time of injury.[62]

Most eye injuries can be prevented with the use of commercially available eye protectors with polycarbonate lenses. Protectors designed specifically for basketball are available. They protect the eye and distribute forces to the stronger surrounding nasal and orbital bones. Although they can initially be bothersome to the player, their use should be encouraged, particularly among "high-risk" players (eg, centers and forwards, those with previous or recurrent eye injury, those with a history of keratotomy).

Upper Face

Nasal and orbital fractures also occur during basketball. Nasal fractures are more common. Players will have a bloody nose with associated swelling, pain, crepitus, and occasionally an obvious deformity. Roentgenographic evalu-ation should be followed by reduction by a trained specialist if required. Players who cannot breathe through the nose after injury, even following 0.25% phenylephrine hydrochloride to shrink the mucosa, should be referred for urgent evaluation. An obstructed naris in this setting may be a sign of septal hematoma, which has a subsequent risk of septal necrosis. Following nasal fracture, participation can resume at the athlete's comfort level with a special protective mask or nasal bridge.

Orbital blowout fractures can be significant, resulting in ocular muscle entrapment with resulting enophthalmos and diplopia. Appropriate referral is required for the management of these injuries, and the athlete should not be allowed to continue participation in this situation unless appropriately cleared.

Lower Face

The mouth is the most frequently injured area of the body in athletes participating in team sports.[19] While the overall number of injuries has decreased with the required use of mouth protectors in sports such as hockey and lacrosse, no such regulations are in place for basketball, and therefore preventable injuries continue to occur. The anterior maxilla is the most common location of injury. Fracture of the alveolar bone can occur, with associated damage to the teeth.

Tooth avulsions and fractures are not uncommon. An avulsed tooth should be replaced into the socket as soon as possible to maximize the chance of salvage. As with eye injury, prompt referral to a specialist should be routine management. Fortunately, the majority of oral injuries can be prevented by the routine use of mouth guards and their voluntary use should be encouraged.

Spinal Injuries

Basketball players are not at specific or increased risk for cervical or thoracolumbar spine injuries. However, low back pain secondary to muscle sprain is the most common spine complaint seen in this group. While this may be related to the jumping and rotational components of activity, no specific risk factors relating to basketball itself have been identified.[21]

The management of low back pain or other spinal complaints should include a complete neurologic examination. The treating physician should be aware of the potential for spondylolysis or other bony abnormality. Generally, pain secondary to muscular sprain is responsive to nonsteroidal anti-inflammatory drugs, stretching, and abdominal strengthening. The athlete may continue participation as the degree of discomfort allows.

Upper Extremity Injuries

Basketball players require excellent hand–eye coordination and the full use of both upper extremities. Players require the ability to position both hands above the head for skills such as rebounding and shooting, but also must be able to work at positions lower than this for skills such as passing and dribbling. Because of this, injury to any part of the extremity, even the nondominant one, can be quite limiting.

Shoulder

There are no specific shoulder injuries unique to or commonplace among basketball players. Treating physicians or trainers should be comfortable evaluating and managing shoulder complaints that would be seen in general practice. Rotator cuff symptoms (secondary to inflammation and/or impingement) may occur as a result of overhead drills and shooting, particularly during the preseason. Treatment should include rest or avoidance of repetitive overhead activity in conjunction with a cuff strengthening and stretching protocol.[3]

Shoulder instability, either frank dislocation or subluxation, is an uncommon problem among basketball players. Management of these problems should be consistent with routine clinical practice. Similarly, acromioclavicular joint injury is rare but may occur following significant contact to the top of the shoulder and is usually managed conservatively.

Elbow

As with the shoulder, basketball players are not at increased risk of particular elbow injuries. The one exception may be the occurrence of medial epicondylitis ("little leaguers elbow") among youth and adolescent players before the age of skeletal maturity.[31] This may occur following shooting, which places stress upon the open physis. Medial elbow pain associated with elbow flexion contracture is the hallmark of this condition. Roentgenograms may show physeal irregularity or widening. Treatment is avoidance of activity until pain free.[7]

Wrist

Injuries to the hand and wrist are common upper extremity injuries in basketball players.

Aside from athletic tape, protective splints are not allowed during play at the professional and collegiate levels, and among most interscholastic conferences. Because of this, the prevention and treatment of these injuries, particularly treatment to allow continued participation, can be challenging. Appropriate treatment should aim to avoid chronic problems; the treating physician should avoid the temptation to sacrifice appropriate immobilization in order to return a player to competition earlier.

Wrist injury typically results from a fall onto the court with an outstretched arm. The wrist is forced into dorsiflexion. Injury can be either bony or ligamentous, with the most common result being either a scaphoid fracture or intercarpal scapholunate ligament tear. Even so, these injuries are relatively rare among basketball players.

A player with wrist pain after a fall should be examined, and the site of pain should be localized. The presence or absence of snuffbox tenderness should be determined, and specific roentgenograms should be obtained. Identified fractures should be treated per routine general practice, and because of the restrictions on the use of protective splints, participation is typically restricted until complete healing has occurred. If the diagnosis is uncertain or if the identified injury is one not commonly treated by the team physician, referral to a hand specialist should be made.

Thumb

Injuries to the thumb and digits are more common than injuries to the wrist. The thumb and digits are exposed and at risk to injury by being caught on another player's jersey or body or by being hit or jammed by the basketball. The most common thumb injury is bony or ligamentous damage at the thumb metacarpophalangeal (MCP) joint and trapeziometacarpal joint.[61] A player presenting with pain and swelling in this area following trauma requires examination to localize the site of pain, followed by roentgenography to evaluate for fracture or dislocation. If roentgenograms are normal, the possibility of ligamentous injury, particularly to the thumb MCP ulnar collateral, should be entertained ("gamekeeper's" or "skier's" thumb). A valgus or radial stress examination should be performed with the MCP joint in 15° to 20° of flexion. Examination may be facilitated by local radial and median nerve block at the wrist.

The treatment of partial tears of the ulnar collateral ligament is somewhat open to debate.

Some advocate 1 to 3 weeks of thumb-spica casting and others advocate functional splinting or taping to prevent recurrent MCP hyperabduction and extension. While splinting or taping may allow return to play if the level of player discomfort allows, there is a definite risk of converting a partial injury to a complete one.[48]

Complete tears (no ligamentous "end-point" to stress testing, more than 35° of valgus opening, or 15° of increased opening compared to the contralateral side) is generally treated by operative repair.[61] While taping with delayed reconstruction (to allow completion of the season) can be done, a delay in surgical repair of a complete tear will decrease the possibility of performing direct repair at surgery. Therefore, acute repair of all complete injuries is recommended.[30]

Digits

Proximal interphalangeal (PIP) joint injuries are the most common digital injuries, and include both bony and capsuloligamentous components. Evaluation should include determination of the direction of the injuring force and documenting the presence of any deformity (or the position of the joint if a previous court-side reduction was done). Examination should attempt to localize tenderness over the collaterals, the volar plate, and/or the dorsal extensor slip. Stability and range of motion should be assessed and may be facilitated by digital block anesthesia.

In the acute court-side setting, reduction of PIP dislocation (usually dorsal) can be done with longitudinal traction and flexion. Anesthetic is not typically required. Following successful reduction, if no deformity persists and the joint is not unstable, return to competition can be allowed with the digit functionally splinted (buddy taped) to an adjacent digit. Obviously, this decision should be made with the player's level of skill and competition in mind. Subsequent treatment should include roentgenography to ensure adequate reduction followed by active motion with or without an extension block splint to prevent recurrent dislocation.

Roentgenograms should be obtained for all PIP injuries with significant pain or swelling. Examination will not allow reliable determination of the presence or absence of underlying fracture.[38,61] Displaced fractures resulting in joint incongruity and instability need to be recognized early (before 7 to 10 days) because they require operative treatment, which is more difficult and less optimal after this time period.

The most common distal interphalangeal (DIP) joint injury is a closed avulsion of the extensor tendon from its distal phalanx insertion, which results in the loss of active DIP extension ("mallet finger"). This typically results from a direct blow to the finger from the basketball, which causes sudden flexion of the DIP joint. Roentgenograms should be obtained to rule out the presence of fracture. A displaced fracture fragment involving more than 25% to 30% of the joint surface or any fracture associated with joint subluxation or incongruity should undergo operative fixation. Otherwise, treatment involves continuous splinting (most recommend a dorsal based splint) of the DIP joint in full extension for 4 to 6 weeks, followed by nighttime splinting for an additional 2 to 4 weeks. Care must be taken to avoid excessive skin pressure in these splints. Continued game participation can be difficult because of restrictions on the use of even plastic or fully covered splints, but immobilization in extension with multiple layers of circumferential wide athletic tape may be possible. This, however, is not as reliable as formal splinting, and the risk of reinjury and the development of a chronic problem is higher. Therefore, the chosen treatment protocol should consider the player's age and level of competition.

A number of other hand injuries have occurred among basketball players, including carpometacarpal dislocation, extra-articular phalanx fracture, flexor digitorum profundus tendon avulsion, and DIP dislocation, but they are much less common than the injuries discussed above. The reader is referred elsewhere for discussion of these injuries.[61]

Lower Extremity Injuries

The most common and typically the most serious injuries sustained by basketball players are those involving the lower extremities, particularly the knee. A number of studies have documented the higher incidence of significant knee injuries among female basketball players when compared to males. In the paragraphs below, the common lower extremity injuries that occur in basketball will be discussed, with an emphasis on knee injuries.

Hip and Thigh

Injury to the hip adductor muscles ("groin pull") and to the hamstrings are commonplace in both female and male players. They occur most frequently during the preseason and therefore lack of proper conditioning or overexertion are thought to be contributing factors. Early management can usually avoid the development of chronic symptoms.

Both adductor muscle and hamstring injuries occur when repetitive forces or a single large force act to cause injury to the musculotendinous junction. With groin injury, this occurs with the flexed and abducted hip position (such as during defensive stance). For hamstring injury, sudden knee extension with the hamstrings attempting to decelerate or maintain knee flexion (as occurs during sprinting) can result in injury. Pain and tenderness will be localized to the involved muscle group, and active muscle contraction will provoke discomfort.[8]

Severity is graded into categories of mild (grade I or II, incomplete tear of the musculotendinous junction) and severe (grade III, complete tear). Management includes early rest and avoidance of provocative activities, combined with gentle stretching of involved muscle groups to deter contracture. Oral nonsteroidal anti-inflammatory drugs and local thermal therapy may be advantageous. With severe acute injury (within the first 7 to 10 days), heat should be avoided as this may provoke increased tissue swelling and pain. As motion, strength, and the degree of comfort permits, the athlete can gradually return to full participation. The use of local compressive wraps may offer symptomatic relief. A significant increase in pain after

participation should be a signal to slow down the player's return to full progression.

The degree of symptoms and expected time to recovery generally correlate directly to the severity of initial injury. With mild injury, the athlete may be able to continue play while undergoing treatment, while more severe injury may initially require complete restriction from activity, with full return not occurring until 4 to 8 weeks after initial injury. The key to successful treatment is to avoid too early a return to full activity. An early return may result in persistence of symptoms and recurrence of the injury, which then becomes a chronic performance-limiting problem.

Knee

While it is generally true that most musculoskeletal injury patterns are sport specific and not gender specific, it has recently been recognized that there is a gender-specific pattern of knee injuries concerning female basketball players, with women sustaining an increased number of knee and anterior cruciate ligament (ACL) injuries compared to men.[4,15,37,49,63]

The rates from NCAA of ACL tears in women and men from 1989 until 1999 are shown in Figure 48-1.[46] Significantly greater rates of ACL tears have been seen in basketball. Over this period, the average ratio of women to men was 3.5, with rates of 0.28 for women and 0.08

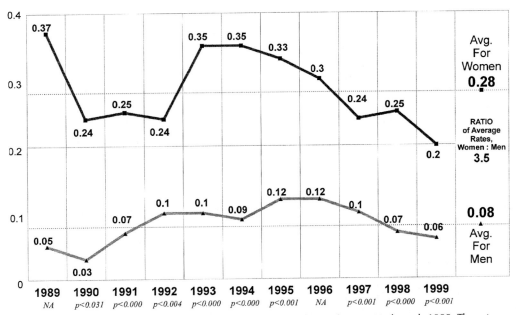

Figure 48-1. Rates of ACL injury according to the NCAA Injury Surveillance from 1989 through 1999. The rates are noted on the chart, and the p values are provided below the dates. For 2 years, 1989 and 1996, p values are not available, but for all other years, the differences are statistically significant.

for men. Unfortunately, this disparity in rates does not seem to be changing despite earlier playing and improved coaching and conditioning for females.[4,27,46] There were also 16% more collateral injuries, 85% more meniscal injuries, and 350% more ACL injuries. Expressed in other terms, there was one ACL injury for every 247 activity sessions (game or practice) for women compared to one in every 952 sessions for men. The majority (71%) of ACL injuries occurred with a noncontact mechanism (landing from a jump, pivoting, or decelerating), which was similar to the rate in men (61% noncontact injuries). Similar gender differences in knee and ACL injuries have been found among professional players[15] and among elite US players.[27] In the study of US elite players, a survey of US Olympic Trial participants, a history of knee injury was reported in 53% of female players compared to 13% of male players and 3.1% and 7.5%, respectively, had had previous knee surgery.[27]

A player sustaining ACL injury usually has a classic mechanism as described above, knee pain, and an acute hemarthrosis. The initial court-side examination is critical and often the most reliable as it can be done before significant swelling and increased muscle guarding develop. The diagnosis should be suspected with a positive Lachman test (increased anterior translation at 30° of knee flexion, soft endpoint). A pivot shift can be attempted but often is not possible in the acute setting because of guarding. Associated injury to the menisci or the collaterals is common. If the diagnosis is in doubt, repeat examination as symptoms improve may be helpful or magnetic resonance imaging can be performed. The player should be held from practice or competition unless the ACL is thought to be intact and assessment on the sideline indicates normal agility.

Unfortunately, an ACL tear means the end of an athlete's basketball season or career unless ACL reconstruction is done. Bracing does not allow players to return to full participation without recurrent subluxation, which risks acute reinjury or chronic joint deterioration.[20,55] Because of the significance of ACL injury, an explanation for the increased risk of female players to injury is being sought.

The reason for this increased incidence of knee injury in female basketball players is not yet fully understood, but many potential theories have been offered: poorer muscular strength and coordination, lower skill level, inexperience, differences in style of play or technique, valgus lower extremity limb alignment, increased joint laxity, hormonal effects, smaller ligaments, and narrow femoral notch dimensions.[1,4,24,44,47,49,51,53,57] The persistence of what has been sometimes termed an "epidemic" of knee injuries during the current era when women have often been participating since early childhood and have access to better coaching argues against the concept that inexperience and skill level are significant factors. Instead, much recent research has focused on defining the neuromuscular performance characteristics and intrinsic hormonal and structural factors that may predispose to ACL injury.

A number of researchers have studied the size of the femoral notch as a risk factor for ACL injury, with 2 main hypotheses in mind: (1) a small notch would indicate smaller and therefore weaker ACL more prone to injury, and (2) a small, stenotic notch would predispose a normal-sized ligament to impingement and subsequent injury with rotational or translational movements. While a small notch has not been shown to indicate a small ligament,[45] it has been shown that athletes with intercondylar notch stenosis have an increased risk of ACL injuries.[32] Notch stenosis is a relative risk for both men and women as, despite the fact that women may tend to have smaller notches than their male counterparts, the range of notch width indices in males and females overlap considerably.[54,58]

The potential role of hormonal fluctuations has gained interest with a recent report that ACL injuries tended to occur during the ovulatory phase of the menstrual cycle in women.[16] It has also been shown that the ACL has the most laxity during the premenstrual phase of the cycle.[59] The normal ACL has estrogen receptors that may help regulate the collagen composition of the ligament. Although not yet proven, the normal fluctuation of estrogen levels during the menstrual cycle may potentially render the ligament more susceptible to injury at certain phases of the cycle.[36]

Perhaps the most intriguing recent research has focused on neuromuscular performance characteristics as contributing risk factors for injury. It has been theorized that gender-related differences in muscle recruitment order, reaction time, and strength may be responsible for physiologic differences, resulting in men and women performing certain skills such as jumping or turning differently. These differences in turn may be responsible for the disproportionate number of ACL injuries in women.

Huston and Wojtys[26] demonstrated that, compared to male athletes, women tended to have more inherent anterior tibial laxity and less muscle endurance and strength. In addition, the female athletes demonstrated a tendency to rely more on their quadriceps muscles to stabilize their knees against anterior tibial translation as opposed to males, who generated earlier and higher levels of hamstring force during the same activity. This "quadriceps first" pattern of muscle recruitment to stabilize the knee may not only be less effective in preventing excessive anterior tibial translation but may actually assist the movement and subsequently increase the risk of ACL injury.

This study raises the question as to the potential to utilize specific training programs to alter these neuromuscular performance patterns and diminish the risk of knee injury in female athletes. In one of the initial studies addressing this issue, modification of techniques used during basketball play among women (such as a flexed-knee landing instead of a straight-knee landing, and a flexed-knee 3-step stop instead of a one-step stop) reduced the rate of ACL injury in division I female collegiate players by 89% over a 10-year period.[17] More recently, Hewett and coworkers found that a specific plyometric jump training program successfully reduced impact forces at the knee and was able to significantly reduce the risk of knee injury in female high school basketball and soccer players.[22,23]

Overall, despite the voluminous research on ACL injury, there is still little information to allow one to clearly identify potential "at-risk" female players, and subsequently little information upon which to develop specific predictable preventative measures. While gender-specific differences in structural and hormonal factors may be significant, the neuromuscular performance characteristics may be the most amenable to intervention via specific training programs aimed at muscle conditioning, balance, and recruitment patterns. Further research in this area clearly needs to be done if the medical community is to be successful in preventing this critical injury among female athletes.

While ACL injuries receive great attention because of their clinical significance, injuries to the meniscus, the collateral ligaments, and patellofemoral mechanism occur at least twice as often.[4] Posterior cruciate injuries are rare.[4,44] Meniscal injuries can be treated conservatively and the athlete may continue participating as long as pain permits and mechanical symptoms such as locking are absent or minimal. The decision to delay treatment should be made on an individual basis, recognizing the potential risk of tear progression or conversion of a repairable tear to an irreparable one. Collateral injury, most commonly injury to the medial collateral ligament from a valgus stress, is managed by

return to activity as knee motion, stability, and the degree of discomfort allow.[35] Protection with a hinged sport brace or taping is usually recommended with grade II and III injuries.

Most patellofemoral injuries in basketball are overuse injuries resulting from the repetitive stresses of jumping, pivoting, and cutting. Tendinitis in either the quadriceps or patellar tendon ("jumper's knee") is the most common problem among jumping athletes.[43] The injury occurs as a result of failure of the healing response to keep pace with the repetitive stress injury at the tendon–bone interface. Rarely is the pathology completely intratendinous. The development of this problem is associated with a sudden increase in activity, particularly in poorly conditioned or previously inactive players. Correspondingly, this condition is prevalent during the preseason. Proper conditioning, with attention to extensor mechanism flexibility and strengthening, is the key to prevention.[11] Recently, researchers have been evaluating more proximal musculature such as the hip, back, abdominals, and gluteals (ie, core musculature) with the thought that weakness or asymmetry in these muscles may predispose the athlete to injury. Evaluation of these muscle groups should not be overlooked.[5]

Once symptoms develop, rest, oral non-steroidal anti-inflammatory drugs, local modalities (heat, ultrasound), and gentle stretching and strengthening should be undertaken. Injection of corticosteroid should be avoided because of the risk of tendon rupture. Return to activity should progress as pain allows. Fortunately, most players respond to conservative measures and rarely require surgical débridement to effect resolution.[11]

Leg

The most common leg conditions are tibial stress fractures and "shin splints" (tibial periostitis, medial tibial stress syndrome). While stress fractures have been shown to occur at a higher rate in female compared to male runners or military recruits,[40] no specific predisposition has been demonstrated for female basketball players. Both stress fractures and shin splints represent overuse injuries and therefore are common in the preseason or in previously inactive players, but can also develop in otherwise highly trained athletes. Play on hard surfaces or with poorly cushioned footwear also play a role.

Both conditions present with anterior leg discomfort that is typically most significant at the start of an activity session and decreases with time. While it can be difficult to distinguish the two, it is important to do so as continued participation in the face of an underlying stress fracture risks progression to frank fracture. A significant component of rest pain should raise one's suspicion of an underlying stress fracture, as should increasing pain during a practice or game session. On clinical examination, periostitis pain usually localizes to the posteromedial tibial cortex, whereas stress fracture pain often involves this site as well as the anterior tibial cortex, with the symptoms being more point specific. Plain roentgenograms may be unremarkable or show periosteal reaction in both cases, but intramedullary changes or a frank linear cortical lysis are diagnostic of stress fracture. Most commonly, tibial stress fracture involves the junction of the distal and middle thirds of the tibia. If the diagnosis remains in doubt, radionuclide bone scanning should be done.[52]

Both conditions should be treated by limitation of exercise to nonimpact activities such as swimming or stationary cycling. With shin splints, stretching and local heat or ice massage may be helpful. Activity during this period should be pain free. Return to play should be gradual. Modifications to footwear and exercise surface should be made if possible if these are contributing factors.[2]

Foot and Ankle

Injury to the ankle represents the most common injury among basketball players, both male and female.[13,63] In a study of Swedish elite players, 59% of all female and 49% of all male injuries were to the ankle, compared to 17% and 19%, respectively, for knee injury.[10] The most common injury is lateral ligamentous injury (lateral ankle sprain), with fracture and other injuries occurring much less frequently.

Lateral ankle sprain results from an inversion stress that occurs from landing on the outside border of the foot, or on another player's foot. The ligaments involved are the anterior talofibular (ATFL) and the calcaneofibular (CFL) ligaments, and injury can be partial or complete. Less frequently, the deltoid or distal talofibular ligament will be involved. Initial evaluation should document areas of swelling and tenderness, and roentgenograms should be obtained to rule out underlying fracture (particularly of the talus, calcaneal process, distal fibula, and tuberosity of the fifth metatarsal).

While complete lateral ligamentous injury results in producible anterior or varus instability to examination, the treatment of both complete and incomplete injury follows the same general protocol: ice, elevation, and compression to reduce swelling, followed by the progression of weight bearing and activity as tolerated. While severe sprains may benefit comfort-wise from a short period (less than 7 to 10 days) of soft or rigid casting, no long-term benefit is realized over early mobilization.[50] The period of activity progression should include peroneal muscle strengthening and proprioceptive training to regain control of the ankle and prevent recurrence. The use of taping or functional bracing may offer improved comfort and protection from reinjury during early return to activity. There is some evidence that the use of prophylactic bracing or taping may reduce the incidence of ankle sprains in basketball players and football players, while high-top shoes alone may be insufficient.[6,25,56] In addition, specific training of the peroneal muscles, the functional evertors of the ankle, may reduce the rate of ankle injury.[41]

Aside from ankle sprains, 2 other common foot and ankle injuries that occur in basketball players represent stress or overuse injury: Achilles tendinitis and stress fracture of the fifth metatarsal. Achilles tendinitis can be insertional or intratendinous, involving the area 3 to 5 cm above the calcaneal insertion. Palpation will localize the involved site. Both conditions should be managed by rest, gentle stretching, nonsteroidal anti-inflammatory drugs, local ice massage, and heel lifts. As the pain improves, progressive strengthening exercises, including eccentrics, should be incorporated. Shoe modification to avoid pressure at the Achilles insertion may benefit those with insertional pain. The use of injectable steroids should be avoided in both cases because of the risk of catastrophic rupture. Return to activity should be gradual and pain free. Persistence of activity with pain risks progression to frank rupture. In refractory cases, surgical débridement may be indicated, with the highest rate of success occurring in those players with insertional tendinitis and an underlying Haglund's deformity.[39]

Stress fracture of the fifth metatarsal involves the proximal diaphysis, and it should be distinguished from an acute fracture of the proximal metaphyseal–diaphyseal junction (a true Jones' fracture). It is critical to understand the differences between these fractures and those of the proximal metatarsal tuberosity as their respective treatment considerations are quite different. Review of these fractures and their nomenclature is found elsewhere.[34] Proximal diaphyseal stress fractures can be categorized as complete or incomplete, acute or chronic (nonunion). While treatment variables can seem complex, there is increasing evidence that this fracture is best treated by early intramedullary screw fixation to prevent delayed union and to decrease the risk of refracture following return to activity.[12,42,60] With operative fixation, return to activity can occur as early as 7 weeks postoperatively.

CONCLUDING REMARKS

The sport of basketball has experienced a tremendous increase in popularity in recent years. Public support for the women's game has grown, and female players now have the opportunity to participate in organized competition from a young age.[28] The net result is continued improvement in the overall level of skill and competition. Despite this progress, it remains concerning that female players at all levels of competition sustain an alarming number of knee injuries.

Acklowledgment

Thanks to Mary Lloyd Ireland, MD, and Kittie H. George for assistance in this manuscript preparation.

References

1. Anderson A, Lipscomb A, Liudahl K et al: Analysis of the intercondylar notch by computed tomography. Am J Sports Med 15:547–52. 1987.
2. Andrish J: The leg. In: DeLee J, Drez D (eds): Orthopaedic Sports Medicine. Principles and Practice. Philadelphia, WB Saunders, 1994, pp 1603–31.
3. Arendt E: Orthopedic issues for the active and athletic women. Clin Sports Med 13(2):483–503, 1994.
4. Arendt L, Dick R: Knee injury patterns among men and women in collegiate basketball and soccer. NCAA data and review of literature. Am J Sports Med 23:694–701, 1995.
5. Ballantyne BT, Leetun DT, Ireland ML, McClay IS: Differences in core stability between male and female collegiate basketball athletes as measured by trunk and hip muscle performance. Med Sci Sports Exerc 33S(5):200, 2001.
6. Barrett J, Tanji J, Drake C: High- versus low-top shoes for the prevention of ankle sprains in basketball players: A prospective randomized study. Am J Sports Med 21(4):582–5, 1993.
7. Bennett J: Articular injuries in the athlete. In: Morrey B (ed): The Elbow and Its Disorders, 2nd edition. Philadelphia, WB Saunders, 1993, p 583.
8. Brunet M, Hontas R: The thigh. In DeLee J, Drez D (eds): Orthopaedic Sports Medicine. Principles and Practice. Philadelphia, WB Saunders, 1994, pp 1086–1112.
9. Clarke K, Buckley W: Women's injuries in collegiate sports. A preliminary comparative overview of three seasons. Am.J Sports Med 8(3):187–91, 1980.
10. Colliander E, Eriksson E, Herkel M, et al: Injuries in Swedish elite basketball. Orthopedics 9(2):225–7, 1986.
11. Colosimo A, Bassett F: Jumper's knee: Diagnosis and treatment. Orthop Rev 19(2):139–49, 1990.
12. DeLee J, Evans J, Julian I: Stress fractures of the fifth metatarsal. Am J Sports Med 11(5):349–53, 1983.
13. Garrick J: The frequency of injury, mechanism of injury, and epidemiology of ankle sprains. Am J Sports Med 5:241-2, 1977.
14. Garrick J, Requa R: Girls' sports injuries in high school athletics. JAMA 239:2245–8, 1978.
15. Gray J, Taunton J, McKenzie D, et al: A survey of injuries to the anterior cruciate ligament of the knee in female basketball players. Int J Sports Med 6:314–6, 1985.
16. Griffin L: ACL injuries in women: To prevent these injuries, we must understand their causes. Orthopedics Today 18(2):74–5, 1998.
17. Griffis N, Verquist S, Yearout K: Injury prevention of the ACL. American Orthopaedic Society for Sports Medicine Annual Meeting. Traverse City, Mich, 1989
18. Gutgesell M: Safety of a preadolescent basketball program. Am J Dis Child 145:1023–5, 1991.
19. Guyette R: Facial injuries in basketball players. Clin Sports Med 12(2):247–64, 1993.
20. Halling A, Howard M, Cawley P: Rehabilitation of anterior cruciate injuries. Clin Sports Med 12(2):329–48, 1993.
21. Herskowitz A, Selesnick H: Back injuries in basketball players. Clin Sports Med 12:293–306, 1993.
22. Hewett T, Riccobene J, Lindenfeld Y: A prospective study of the effect of neuromuscular training on the incidence of knee injury in female athletes. 24th Annual Meeting of the American Orthopaedic Society for Sports Medicine. Vancouver, British Columbia, 1998.
23. Hewett T, Stroupe A, Nance T, et al: Plyometric training in female athletes: Decreased impact forces and increased hamstring torques. Am J Sports Med 24(6):765–73, 1996.
24. Houseworth S, Mauro V, Mellon B: The intercondylar notch in acute tears of the anterior cruciate ligament: A computer graphics study. Am J Sports Med 15:2221–9, 1987.
25. Hunter D: Ankle taping versus ankle bracing: a prospective study on the prevention of injuries. 24th Annual Meeting of the American Orthopaedic Society for Sports Medicine. Vancouver, British Columbia, 1998.
26. Huston L, Wojtys E: Neuromuscular performance characteristics in elite female athletes. Am J Sports Med 24(4):427–36, 1996.
27. Ireland M, Wall C: Epidemiology and comparison of knee injuries in elite male and female basketball athletes. Med Sci Sports Exerc 22(2):S582, 1990.
28. Ireland ML: Basketball. In Garrett W (ed): Women's Health in Sports and Exercise. American Academy of Orthopaedic Surgeons, Rosemont, Ill, 2001, pp 229–43.
29. Jeffers J: Sports related eye injuries: presentation, management, and prevention. Seventh Annual Professional Sports Care Sports Medicine Symposium. Teaneck, NJ, 1994.
30. Kozin S, Bishop A: Gamekeeper's thumb: Early diagnosis and treatment. Orthop Rev 23(10):797–804, 1994.
31. Krivickas L: Basketball. In: Agostini R (ed): Medical and Orthopedic Issues of Active and Athletic Women. Philadelphia, Hanley & Belfus, 1994, pp 465–77.
32. LaPrade R, Burnett Q: Femoral intercondylar notch stenosis and correlation to anterior cruciate ligament injury: A prospective study. Am J Sports Med 22:198–203, 1994.
33. Larrison W, Hersh P, Kunzweiler T, et al: Sports-related ocular trauma. Ophthalmology 97:1265–9, 1990.

34. Lawrence S, Botte M: Jones' fractures and related fractures of the proximal fifth metatarsal. Foot Ankle 14(6):358–65, 1993.
35. Linton R, Indelicato P: Medial ligament injuries. In: DeLee J, Drez D (eds):Orthopaedic Sports Medicine. Philadelphia, WB Saunders, 1994, pp 1261–74.
36. Liu S, Al-Shaikh R, Panossian V, et al: Estrogen affects the cellular metabolism of the anterior cruciate ligament: A potential explanation for female athletic injury. Am J Sports Med 25(5):704–9, 1997.
37. Malone T, Hardaker W, Garrett W: Relationship of gender to ACL injuries in intercollegiate basketball players. J South Orthop Assoc 2(1):36–9, 1992.
38. McCue F, Andrews J, Hakala M, et al: The coach's finger. J Sports Med 2:270–5, 1974.
39. McDermott E: Basketball injuries of the foot and ankle. Clin Sports Med 12(2):373–93, 1993.
40. Meyer S, Saltzman C, Albright J: Stress fractures of the foot and leg. Clin Sports Med 12(2):395–413, 1993.
41. Milia M, Ashton-Miller J, Siskosky M, et al: On the muscular protection of ankles. 24th Annual Meeting of the American Orthopaedic Society for Sports Medicine. Vancouver, British Columbia, 1998.
42. Mindrebo N, Shelbourne K, VanMeter C, et al: Outpatient percutaneous screw fixation of the acute Jones' fracture. Am J Sports Med 21(5):720–3, 1993.
43. Molnar T, Fox J: Overuse injuries of the knee in basketball. Clin Sports Med 12(2):349–62, 1993.
44. Moyer R, Marchetto P: Injuries of the posterior cruciate ligament. Clin Sports Med 12(2):307–15, 1993.
45. Muneta T, Takakuda T, Yamamoto H: Intercondylar notch width and its relation to the configuration and cross-sectional area of the anterior cruciate ligament: A cadaveric knee study. Am J Sports Med 25(1):69–72, 1997.
46. National Collegiate Athletic Association: NCAA injury surveillance system. Indianapolis, Ind, NCAA, 2000.
47. Nicholas J. Injuries to knee ligaments: Relationship to looseness and tightness in football players. JAMA 212:2236–9, 1970.
48. Pichora D, McMurtry R, Bell M: Gamekeeper's thumb: A prospective study of functional bracing. J Hand Surg Am 14(3):567–73, 1989.
49. Reider B, D'Agata SD: Factors predisposing knee injury. In DeLee J, Drez D (eds): Orthopaedic Sports Medicine. Principles and Practice. Philadelphia, WB Saunders, 1994, pp 1134–45.
50. Renstrom P, Kannus P: Injuries of the foot and ankle. In: DeLee J, Drez D (eds): Orthopaedic Sports Medicine. Philadelphia, WB Saunders, 1994, pp 1705–67.
51. Rozzi S, Lephart S, Gear W, et al: Knee joint laxity and neuromuscular characteristics of male and female soccer and basketball players. The American Orthopaedic Society for Sports Medicine Specialty Day, Annual Meeting of the American Academy of Orthopaedic Surgeons. New Orleans, 1998.
52. Rupani H, Holder L, Espinola D, et al: Three-phase radionuclide bone imaging in sports medicine. Radiology 156:187–96, 1985.
53. Shambaugh J, Klein A, Herbert I: Structural measures as predictors of injury in basketball players. Med Sci Sports Exerc 23:522–7, 1991.
54. Shelbourne K, Facibene W, Hunt J: Radiographic and intraoperative intercondylar notch width measurements in men and women with unilateral and bilateral anterior cruciate ligament tears. Knee Surg Sports Traumatol Arthrosc 5(4):229–33, 1997.
55. Shelton W, Barrett G, Dukes A: Early season anterior cruciate ligament tears: A treatment dilemma. Am J Sports Med 25(5):656–8, 1997.
56. Sitler M, Ryan J, Wheeler B: The efficacy of a semirigid ankle stabilizer to reduce acute ankle injuries in basketball: a randomized clinical study at West Point. Am J Sports Med 22(4):454–61, 1994.
57. Souryal T, Freeman T: Intercondylar notch size and anterior cruciate ligament injuries in athletes: A prospective study. Am J Sports Med 21:535–9, 1993.
58. Teitz C, Lind B, Sacks B: Symmetry of the femoral notch width index. Am J Sports Med 25(5):687–90, 1993.
59. Thomas R, Cascio B, Faegin I: The influence of the menstrual cycle on ACL laxity. The American Orthopaedic Society for Sports Medicine Specialty Day, Annual Meeting of the American Academy of Orthopaedic Surgeons. New Orleans, 1998.
60. Torg J, Pavlov H, Torg E: Overuse injuries in sport: The foot, Clin Sports Med 6(2):291-320, 1987.
61. Wilson R, McGinty L: Common hand and wrist injuries in basketball players. Clin Sports Med 12:265–91, 1993.
62. Zagelbaum B, Starkey C, Hersh P, et al: The National Basketball Association eye injury study. Arch Ophthalmol 113(6):749–52, 1995.
63. Zelisko J, Noble H, Porter M: A comparison of men's and women's professional basketball injuries. Am J Sports Med 10:297–9, 1982.

Chapter 49

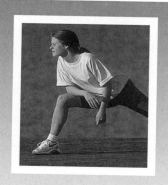

Cheerleading

Mark R. Hutchinson, M.D.

Cheerleading is an activity that began at the turn of the century in association with American football. Specifically, a University of Minnesota fan stood in his seat at a football game and encouraged the crowd to repeat a verse to show support for their team. From those humble beginnings, a competitive, athletic sport has blossomed that has nearly a million participants in the United States, including club, elementary, high school, college, and professional levels.[7]

Webster's New Collegiate Dictionary[30] defines a sport as a physical activity engaged in for pleasure or diversion. Certainly cheerleading qualifies as a sport by definition. It also qualifies as a sport because of its risk of injury secondary to participation. Cheerleaders have greater time lost from sport than most sport participants when an injury occurs. Their injury rates, however, appear to be slightly less than those of many more recognized sports. Recent studies show that an alarmingly high number of catastrophic injuries in female athletes are related to cheerleading.[3,21] In general, cheerleading injury patterns and injury types have not been well reported in the literature. This is partially due to the fact that most early epidemiologic studies focused on higher-profile sports. It is also due to the poor level of respect, in general, that the sports medicine community has shown cheerleaders as athletes. This chapter will review the unique aspects of cheerleading as a sport and the injury patterns seen in its participants.

CHEERLEADING: THE SPORT

Cheerleading has seen a dramatic rise in popularity over the last several years. The early days of fan chants and supportive phrases have given way to a sport filled with athleticism. The intermittent groups of exuberant fans competing with the opposite team to see who could scream louder has given way to organized regional and national competitions.

Important components of championship cheerleading teams include cheers and chants, gymnastic and tumbling runs, partner stunts, pyramid building, and pom-pom and dance routines. Each component introduces unique injury risks to the sport. Injury patterns in cheerleading parallel those of gymnastics (knee injuries from twisting and cutting, wrist and upper extremity injuries from using the arms as weight-bearing structures, and back injuries from repetitive hyperextension); dance (foot, ankle, and hip injuries from repetitive impact and overuse); and weight-lifting (upper extremity and low back injuries from serving as the base of partner stunts or pyramids). While men participate in cheerleading at the collegiate level, relatively few participate at the high school or club level. Indeed, the injury patterns in male cheerleaders are different from the injury patterns in females as they are more likely to have upper extremity injuries secondary to repetitive lifting. Since the proportion of females participating in cheerleading is significantly greater than males, injuries associated with the female gender are more common in the sport of cheerleading as a whole.

Cheerleading Compared to Other Sports

Little literature is available comparing the risk of cheerleading to other athletic activities. Much of the literature that is available is, instead, anecdotal and focused on isolated case reports.[9,16,22,26–28] A few studies have analyzed cheerleading as a sport but without comparison to other sports.[2,6,10,20,31] One exception to that trend is a study by Axe and colleagues,[1] who reported on 619 athletes from 23 sports, including cheerleading, and found that cheerleading had the highest average days lost (28.8 days) per injury (Table 49-1). One might argue that a single athlete with a particularly long time loss from sport could skew those data. At the

Table 49-1. Severity of Injuries: Average Days Lost from a Variety of Sports

SPORT	DAYS LOST
Cheerleading	*28.8*
Girls' basketball	12.8
Wrestling	12.3
Boys' cross country	12.0
Girls' tennis	10.5
Boys' basketball	9.2
Miscellaneous (boys)	8.8
Volleyball	8.4
Girls' lacrosse	8.3
Girls' cross country	8.2
Boys' track	7.2
Miscellaneous (girls)	6.7
Girls' swimming	5.9
Boys' soccer	5.7
Football	5.6
Boys' lacrosse	5.5
Baseball	5.4
Softball	3.8
Field hockey	3.5
Girls' track	3.2
Boys' swimming	2.8
Boys' tennis	1.4
Girls' soccer	0

From Axe MJ, Newcomb WA, Warner D: Sports injuries and adolescent athletes. Delaware Med J 63(6):359–63, 1991, with permission.

Kentucky Sports Medicine Clinic, the author reviewed the injury patterns of 74 high school cheerleaders and confirmed the elevated days lost from sport per injury found by Axe and coworkers (35 days compared to 28.8 days).[12,13]

When making injury risk comparisons across sports, it is important to use similar-size populations or define the injury risk in terms of the number of athletic exposures; if this is not done, the conclusions achieved may not be valid. Indeed, when comparing different studies it is also important to confirm that a similar definition of injury was used in each. In Axe's study of 870 injuries, 40% were caused by football and only 1% were caused by cheerleading.[1] Unfortunately the authors failed to report the total number of participants in each sport or the number of athletic exposures, which would allow us to compare the injury risk to other sports. Similarly, Rettig and colleagues[25] reported that of 213 hand injuries reported to their clinic, 37% were secondary to football, 22% were secondary to basketball, and less than 1% were associated with cheerleading. They also made no mention of the uninjured population or the number of athletic exposures. While of interest to a practicing physician as they give a picture of a sports medicine practice, the studies do not allow us to compare various sports.

In 1982, the National Collegiate Athletic Association (NCAA) created an injury surveillance system that defines injury risk in various sports in relation to the number of athletic exposures. Rates of injury of 16 sports are recorded and reported yearly.[23] Unfortunately, to date, the NCAA has not included cheerleading in their surveillance, therefore, no collegiate cheerleading injury rates are available.

Mueller[19] has reported the most extensive studies on cheerleading injury research and found in 58,738 cheerleaders who participated in the Universal Cheerleading Association's summer camps an injury rate of 0.31 per 100 participants. Assuming each camp session is approximately 1 week in length with morning and afternoon sessions qualifying as athletic exposures, each athlete would have 12 to 14 athletic exposures per week. The total risk translates to 0.24 injuries per 1000 athletic exposures at summer camp (range 0.22 to 0.26). In the course of a school year, Mueller found injury rates of 13.3 per 100 participants for collegiate cheerleaders and 3.3 per 100 participants for high school cheerleaders.[19] Including practices, games, and competitions, cheerleaders may have from 100 to 200 athletic exposures per year, translating to between 0.07 and 0.13 injuries per athletic exposure for collegiate cheerleaders and 0.01 and 0.03 injuries per 1000 athletic exposures for high school cheerleaders.

In the 16th Annual Report of the National Center for Catastrophic Sports Injury Research,[21] Mueller and Cantu noted that while football accounts for the largest number of catastrophic injuries, gymnasts and hockey players are at greater risk per 100,000 participants. Alarmingly for female athletes, cheerleading accounted for 46.2% of all direct catastrophic injuries in the high school population and 76.2% of catastrophic injuries to females at the college level. It was felt that a major factor in this increase was the change in emphasis in cheerleading on a greater amount of gymnastic stunts and the relatively poor availability of competent coaches to teach skills.

Cheerleaders: At Risk?

While similar in some ways to gymnastics and dance, cheerleading differs from many sports in its year-round demand. Cheerleaders are asked to perform throughout 3 seasons and then peak for national competitions in the spring. The summer season may be allotted for rest but is frequently filled with cheerleading camps focused on optimizing the next year's performance and techniques. The constant "in-season" state does not allow appropriate down time for recuperation or conditioning, which, in turn, can lead to overuse injuries. The number of cheerleading injuries that are seen in hospital emergency departments has grown from 5000 in 1980 to 16,000 in 1994.[2,11,21] At the Kentucky Sports Medicine Clinic, the author performed a retrospective survey of high school cheerleading athletes.[12,13] Overuse injuries predominated and 83.8% of athletes reported at least one injury that required time loss from sport in their career. The athletes reported practice times averaging 12 hours per week and had been involved in cheerleading for an average of 6 years. A few had begun at a club level at the age of 3!

At many schools and programs, cheerleading is not considered a sport but rather an extracurricular activity. This can place the cheerleading athlete at several disadvantages and increase her risk of injury. When defined as an activity, cheerleading may not fall under state athletic associations' guidance and regulations. Coaches or sponsors may not have appropriate background and training to educate these athletes in safe and proper techniques. This varies from state to state and from school to school but it does increase the injury risk to the athlete. In addition, the risk may be elevated because of poor access to equipment or physical plant. Most schools, even those that consider cheerleaders athletes, do not provide on-site athletic trainer coverage for cheerleading events.[5,11] This inherently increases the response time for any major injury.

Many school athletic programs' budgets are financially strapped and cannot afford to have practice mats available for a school "activity." Cheerleading athletes frequently find themselves practicing in whatever space is available when the prime sports take the gymnasium or practice facility. The space is frequently the hard concrete floor of a hallway, basement, or corner of the gym. The practice surface itself can lead to overuse injuries.

Historically, another source of injuries to cheerleaders was the use of the trampoline or mini-trampoline to perform stunts and tricks. Catastrophic injuries to the head and neck were occasionally reported.[4,11,16,17] This led to the development of safety guidelines as well as state and local rulings that virtually banned the use of the mini-trampoline in cheerleading performances and practices.

CHEERLEADING INJURIES

Existing research on sport-specific injuries in cheerleading has been obtained using 3 epi-demiologic techniques: retrospective case review, retrospective interview, and prospective surveillance. When assessing data from such studies it is important to understand the value and restrictions of each style. For example, retrospective case reviews analyze the number of injuries reporting to a single physician or group of physicians, emergency departments, or hospitals. While important in analyzing facility use or referral base, the results may be skewed to more severe injuries or to a specific geographic area. They may, therefore, not be generalizable to a larger population. Retrospective interviews or questionnaires, while giving a broad overview of the question, may introduce memory bias where specific numbers may not be accurate. Prospective surveillance provides the most valid information but requires a network of trainers, coaches, and physicians that carefully collect data under a rigid defined set of protocols and guidelines. Prospective studies tend to be expensive and more time-intensive.

Catastrophic Injuries and Fatalities

Head and neck injuries constitute a small portion (7%) of all cheerleading-related injuries, but can be very severe and have catastrophic and potentially fatal consequences. Cantu and Mueller have been collecting data from the National Center for Catastrophic Sports Injury Research since 1982.[2,20] The pyramid stunt was responsible for 50% of the head and neck injuries. Ten of 20 head and neck injuries occurred while doing pyramids, and 2 of these injuries were deaths. The direct fatalities (defined as being caused by performing the activities of the sport) and catastrophic injuries (those resulting in transient or permanent severe functional spinal cord disability) and the indirect fatalities (caused by systemic failure as the result of exertion while participating in sport) are shown in Table 49-2.[2] From 1982 through 1997, 60 direct fatalities and catastrophic injuries and 25 indirect fatalities occurred among high school and college female athletes, including cheerleaders. Cheerleading accounted for 34 (57%) direct fatalities and catastrophic injuries. These injuries occurred from gymnastics-type activities such as flips, mini-trampoline diving, and pyramid stunts. Recommendations that pyramid building and tossing of cheerleaders be banned have been made and many high school associations have adopted them. The American Association of Cheerleading Coaches and Advisors has implemented a safety certification program. The recommendations to reduce the numbers of injuries have been made and are

Table 49-2. Fatalities and Catastrophic and Serious Injuries in U.S. Female Student-Athletes, 1982–1997

DIRECT FATALITIES[a] AND CATASTROPHIC INJURIES[b]			INDIRECT FATALITIES[c]	
High School				
Cheerleading	18		Basketball	8
Gymnastics	9		Swimming	5
Track	3		Track	4
Swimming	2		Cheerleading	3
Basketball	2		Soccer	1
Softball	2		Cross country	1
Field hockey	2		Volleyball	1
Volleyball	1			
Total	39			23
College				
Cheerleading	16		Tennis	1
Gymnastics	2		Basketball	1
Field hockey	1			
Downhill skiing	1			
Lacrosse	1			
Total	21			2

[a]Caused by performing the activities of a sport.
[b]Resulting in transient or permanent severe functional spinal cord disability.
[c]Caused by systemic failure as a result of exertion while participating in a sport.
From Cantu RC, Mueller FO: Fatalities and catastrophic injuries in high school and college sports, 1982–1997: Lessons for improving safety. Physician Sportsmed 27(8):47, 1999, with permission.

quoted from Cantu and Mueller's work (Table 49-3).[2] The fact that cheerleading injuries are a leading cause of direct fatalities and catastrophic illnesses in high school and college is very alarming. Prevention of injuries should be the goal.

Mechanism of Injuries

A retrospective questionnaire performed at the Kentucky Sports Medicine Clinic showed that a majority of injuries (67%) were secondary to gymnastic maneuvers and tumbling.[12,13] Falls from mounts and partner stunts caused 16% of injuries, followed distantly by cheers and chants. Mueller's surveillance studies of high school and college cheerleaders and cheerleaders at summer camps showed, instead, a predominance of injuries secondary to partner stunts (Table 49-4).[19] Mueller also found partner stunts to be associated with the more serious injuries.

Other factors associated with injuries in cheerleading include overuse, experience, conditioning, supervision, surface, and equipment. Experience may be related to the number, type, and severity of injuries. More experienced cheerleaders are apt to attempt more dangerous stunts associated with partners. The least-experienced cheerleaders, however, appear to be injured more frequently.[19] This may be due to poor supervision or training techniques, attempting stunts that they are not qualified for, or poor conditioning. Various studies have shown that female athletes tend to begin at a lower state of condition, making them prone to injuries, especially overuse injuries.[18,24] The

Table 49-3. Safety Initiative Recommendations

- Coaches should supervise all practices and be safety certified.
- Cheerleaders should have a preparticipation exam, be trained in gymnastics, spotting, and conditioning, and participate only in stunts that they have mastered.
- Stunts should be limited (eg, pyramids should be limited to 2 levels and performed on mats).
- Emergency procedures should be written and available.
- Cheerleaders who have signs of head trauma should receive immediate medical attention and return to cheerleading only with permission from a physician.

From Cantu RC, Mueller FO: Fatalities and catastrophic injuries in high school and college sports, 1982–1997: Lessons for improving safety. Physician Sportsmed 27(8): 47, 1999, with permission.

Table 49-4. Mechanism of Various Cheerleading Injuries

	HIGH SCHOOL	COLLEGIATE
Cheers/chants	14.7%	8.5%
Spotting	14.7%	3.4%
Landing techniques	8.8%	1.7%
Tumbling	17.7%	20.5%
Partner stunts	29.4%	41.9%
Pyramids	8.8%	5.2%
Other	5.9%	18.8%

From Mueller FO: Cheerleading Injury Research. Universal Cheerleading Association Publications, Memphis, 1993, with permission.

Table 49-5. Percentage of All Cheerleading Injuries by Anatomic Location

ANATOMIC LOCATION	PERCENT OF INJURIES
Head and neck	7%
Elbow	5%
Wrist	8%
Hand	13%
Back	12%
Abdomen	2%
Hip	2%
Groin	2%
Leg	2%
Thigh	0%
Knee	15%
Ankle	22%
Foot	2%

From Hutchinson MR: Cheerleading injuries: Patterns, prevention, and case reports. Physician Sportsmed 25(9): 83–96, 1997, with permission.

same studies go on to show that with proper conditioning gender differences disappear.

Injury Patterns by Anatomic Location and Type

In comparison to central or upper extremity injuries, the lower extremity accounts for the greatest percentage of high school cheerleading injuries. Specifically, ankle injuries are most common, followed by knee injuries (Table 49-5).[14] At the collegiate level, an increase in upper extremity injuries is seen.[15,19] This increase is probably correlated with the increase in partner stunts and catches required at that level.

The most common types of cheerleading-related injuries are ligament sprains and muscular strains (Table 49-6). Fractures and dislocations are also surprisingly common. The specific percentages and relationships depend on the definition of injury used in each survey and the population evaluated. For example, fractures and more severe injuries were more likely to require evaluation in an emergency department or by a physician, suggesting increased percentages of those injuries in studies based on physi-

cian chart reviews or emergency department reports. Those results might not accurately present the actual incidence of those injuries in comparison to all injuries. Indeed, it is not surprising to find that if a time loss from sport is required as a definition of injury the percentage of abrasions, lacerations, and contusions decreases (Table 49-6).

Cheerleaders may also be at increased risk of nonmusculoskeletal injuries. High school and college-aged females are at increased risk of eating disorders or the female athlete triad, which includes disordered eating, amenorrhea, and osteoporosis. Female participants in aesthetic sports such as ballet, figure skating, gymnastics, and cheerleading are at increased risk of this problem. Athlete education, coaches' awareness, and maintained clinician identification and early treatment are essential to prevent the potential catastrophic end result of the female athlete triad.

Prevention

Safety guidelines for cheerleaders vary tremendously from state to state, school to school, and organization to organization.[11,17] After the death of a cheerleader performing a pyramid stunt, North Dakota and Minnesota legislatures banned the use of pyramids at the high school and college level.[2] The state of Illinois banned performing basket tosses at the high school level after a separate catastrophic incident. Unfortunately, safety guidelines instituted by athletic associations, school boards, cheerleading training organizations, and state legislatures have been infamous for banning stunts because they were arbitrarily determined to be unsafe.[29] The decisions to abolish certain moves or stunts have not always been based on sound scientific research.

The American Association of Cheerleading Coaches and Advisors (AACCA) have created a safety manual that addresses many issues surrounding optimizing the safe and healthy participation in cheerleading.[7] Important issues

Table 49-6. Cheerleading Injuries by Type

	INJURIES WITH TIME LOSS	INJURIES REGARDLESS TIME LOSS
Sprains and strains	52%	31%
Abrasions and lacerations	2%	22%
Fractures and dislocations	29%	6%
Contusions	7%	22%
Other	10%	19%

From Hutchinson MR: Cheerleading injuries: Patterns, prevention, and case reports. Physician Sportsmed 25(9):83–96, 1997, with permission.

include optimizing the environment and safety equipment, assuring supervision by qualified coaches, maximizing the level of conditioning to prevent overuse injuries, progressing gradually and safely to increasingly difficult skill levels, and educating athletes regarding health risks and safety precautions. Another valuable reference for cheerleaders and coaches is the United States Gymnastics Federation's Gymnastic Safety Manual.[8] A condensed version of the AACCA's recommendations[7] to prevent injuries includes the following:

1. Preseason history and physical examinations should be done on all athletes.
2. Emphasis on optimizing conditioning is important.
3. Coaches should be qualified to teach cheerleading and gymnastics and supervise all activity in a safe facility with the best equipment available.
4. Athletes should demonstrate mastery of stunts in a safe, progressive fashion . . . simplest to most difficult.
5. Mini-trampolines and flips or falls off pyramids and shoulders should be prohibited.
6. Pyramid and partner stunts over shoulder level should not be performed without mats or spotters.
7. Emergency procedures and plans should be carefully outlined prior to any practice or performances.

Perhaps one of the best ways to avoid certain injuries in any sport is to target the most common or most preventable injuries with proactive programs. In cheerleading, the most common type of injury is overuse. We recommend to all cheerleaders to participate in a general conditioning program prior to participation and during the course of their season (Table 49-7). This should include aerobic training for endurance, general conditioning and strengthening, and focused strength training targeting sport-specific muscle groups. For example, cheerleaders who lift and serve as bases for stunts should include upper body strengthening, low back and core strengthening, and lower extremity strengthening exercises. Cheerleaders who serve on top of a mount should optimize proprioceptive skills. Targeting specific high-demand regions is effective; however, balance between agonist and antagonist muscles is encouraged. Imbalance can lead to overuse injuries of the weak muscle or poor flexibility around a specific joint. Perhaps more important is the concept that cheerleaders must condition the entire kinetic chain of muscles that makes their skill elements possible. Lifting a partner overhead requires coordination and strength in the ankle, leg, knee, hip, back, and arms. A weak link in the chain will predispose to injury at that or adjacent levels.

Certain common injuries should also be addressed proactively to reduce their incidence and prevalence in this population. Low back strains and injuries are quite common in cheerleaders. Abdominal strengthening and core stabilization exercises should be part of a cheerleader's daily workout. Female athletes and cheerleaders in particular secondary to their repetitive squatting have an increased incidence of anterior knee complaints. Specific diagnoses such as plica syndrome, chondromalacia, and patellofemoral syndrome are common. Prevention includes quadriceps strengthening focused on the vastus medialis obliquus muscle as well as hamstring stretching for flexibility.

A major challenge when taking care of competitive cheerleading athletes is not only to convince them that preventative exercise is in their

Table 49-7. Exercise Plan Targeting a Reduction in Common Cheerleading Injuries

EXERCISE	FREQUENCY	GOAL
Aerobic training	3 times/week	Increase baseline condition
Biking or swimming	3 times/week	Increase condition and endurance while avoiding impact injuries
Stomach crunches	5 times/week	Increase core strength and reduce low back complaints
Low back extensions	5 times/week	Increase core strength and reduce low back complaints
Hip flexibility and strength	3 times/week	Increase core strength
Mini-squats, lunges, leg presses	3 times/week	Increase functional quadriceps strength to reduce patellofemoral complaints and improve power
Straight leg raises in external rotation and adductor squeezes	5 times/week	Increase quadriceps strength focused on vastus medialis obliquus to reduce patellofemoral complaints
Ankle strengthening and proprioceptive skills	3 times/week	Increase inversion and eversion strength and improve propioception to reduce ankle sprains
Rotator cuff program and scapular stabilizers strengthening	5 times/week	Reduce shoulder impingement and instability complaints (special emphasis for bases and tumblers)

From Hutchinson MR: Cheerleading injuries: Patterns, prevention, and case reports. Physician Sportsmed 25(9): 83–96, 1997, with permission.

best interest but also finding the appropriate time and sequence to accomplish the workout. Since cheerleaders perform throughout the school year and compete in the spring, they rarely have down time to recuperate much less work out. We recommend a lower-impact cardiovascular training program in the off-season and preseason. Very little impact or lifting or intense skill activity should be done during this time. This allows them a down season to let their bodies recuperate from the previous season. The cardiovascular conditioning can include swimming and biking, as well as rehabilitation focused on areas of identified weakness. When they return the next season, their general baseline condition will begin at a higher level. Ideally this preseason conditioning will reduce the incidence of overuse injuries.

When cheerleaders return to training in the fall, daily conditioning and strengthening is initiated as the first part of each practice. As the habit of including maintenance conditioning activities into their daily routine takes hold, the athlete's core strength improves and the balance of agonist and antagonist muscles is maintained. In addition, we recommend that when the athletes return to practice, the intensity of practice is balanced with days off for recuperation and readjustment to the daily grind of impact demands. Ideally, this means for the first 2 to 3 weeks, every third day is a "low-impact" day where conditioning and coaching can occur but impact is minimized. After 2 or 3 weeks, the interval can be changed to every fourth day. It is recommended that athletes have low-impact days or days off at least once a week throughout the season.

Perhaps the greatest concern of injuries in cheerleaders is the relative high risk of catastrophic injury. It is clear that while these athletes are injured less frequently, the injuries tend to be more severe. The fact that cheerleading accounts for not only the highest percentage but also the majority of catastrophic injuries for both high school and college female athletes should awaken supervisory bodies to the need for safety interventions, including safe practice areas and qualified coaches. The best way to accomplish this is to welcome cheerleading into the family of accepted sports and allow it to be supervised by state and national athletic associations, yet few states have taken these steps.

In conclusion, cheerleaders are athletes who carry certain injury risks secondary to their participation in sport. Awareness of the injury patterns, use of safe equipment in a supervised environment, progressive introduction of more difficult stunts, and increased focus on maintaining strength and conditioning can hopefully reduce the incidence of injury in this athletic population.

References

1. Axe MJ, Newcomb WA, Warner D: Sports injuries and adolescent athletes. Delaware Med J 63(6):359–63, 1991.
2. Cantu RC, Mueller FO: Cheerleading. Clin J Sports Med 4:75–6, 1994.
3. Cantu RC, Mueller FO: Fatalities and catastrophic injuries in high school and college sports, 1982–1997: Lessons in improving safety. Physician Sportsmed 27(8):35–49, 1999.
4. Consumer Products Safety Commission, Product Summary Report. Washington, DC, National Injury Information Clearinghouse, 1987.
5. Cox JS, Lenz HW: Women midshipmen in sports. Am J Sports Med 12:241–3, 1984.
6. DeBenedette V: Are cheerleaders athletes? Physician Sportsmed 15(9):214–7, 1987.
7. George GS (ed): American Association of Cheerleading Coaches' and Advisors' Cheerleading Safety Manual. Memphis, Universal Cheerleading Association Publications, 1990.
8. George G (ed): United States Gymnastics Federation Gymnastics Safety Manual. Indianapolis, United States Gymnastics Federation, 1985.
9. Hage P: Cheerleading: new problems in a changing sport. Physician Sportsmed 9(2):140–5, 1981.
10. Hage P: Cheerleaders suffer few serious injuries. Physician Sportsmed 11(1):25–6, 1983.
11. Hunt V: Cheerleading takes on athleticism, increases need for attention to safety. NATA News. Dallas, National Athletic Trainers Association, February 1999, pp 8–12.
12. Hutchinson MR: Injuries in cheerleading: diagnosis and prevention. Physician Sportsmed 9(25):83–96, 1997.
13. Hutchinson MR, Ireland ML, et al: Injuries in cheerleading (abstr). Med Sci Sport Exerc 26(5 suppl):S109, 1997.
14. Hutchinson MR, Ireland ML: Knee injuries in female athletes. Sports Med 19(4):288–302, 1995.
15. Ireland ML, Hutchinson MR: Upper extremity injuries in young athletes. Clin Sports Med 14(3):533–69, 1995.
16. Lockey MW: The sport of cheerleading. J Mississippi State Med Assoc 32(10):375, 1991.
17. Marcaccini M: Let's make cheerleading a sport. Women's Sports Fitness 1:78, 1987.
18. Meade KM: Something to cheer about: Preventing and treating cheerleading injuries. Adv Directors Rehabil 7(2):24–5, 1998.
19. Mueller FO: Cheerleading Injury Research. Memphis, Universal Cheerleading Association Publications, 1993.
20. Mueller FO, Cantu RC: National Center for Catastrophic Sports Injury Research: Tenth Annual Report. Chapel Hill: University of North Carolina, 1993.
21. Mueller FO, Cantu RC: National Center for Catastrophic Sports Injury Research—16th Annual Report. Chapel Hill, North Carolina, University of North Carolina (World Wide Web. UNC/DEPTS/NCCSI), 1999.
22. Nash HL: Cheerleading not as safe as it once was. Physician Sportsmed 13(11):39–40, 1985.
23. National Collegiate Athletic Association (NCAA): NCAA Injury Surveillance System. Overland Park, Kan, NCAA, 1993.

24. Protzman RR, Bodnari LM: Stress fractures in men and women undergoing military training. J Bone Joint Surg 59A:825, 1977.
25. Rettig AC, Ryan RO, Stone JA: Epidemiology of hand injuries in sport. In: Strickland JW, Rettig AC (eds): Hand Injuries in Athletes. Philadelphia, WB Saunders, 1992, pp 37–48.
26. Ross T: Cheerleading and club sports. Law and Sports Conference Proceedings. Winston-Salem: Sports and the Courts Inc, 1986, pp 100–6.
27. Shields RW, Jacobs IB: Median palmar digital neuropathy in a cheerleader. Arch Phys Med Rehabil 67:824–6, 1986.
28. Tehranzadeh J, Labosky DA, Gabriele OF: Ganglion cysts and tear of triangular fibro-cartilages of both wrists in a cheerleader. Am J Sports Med 11(5):357–9, 1983.
29. Webb J: Message from the AACCA president. In: George S (ed): AACCA Cheerleading Safety Manual. Memphis, UCA Publications, 1990.
30. Webster's New Collegiate Dictionary, 8th edition. Springfield, Mass, G & C Merriam, 1981.
31. Whiteside JA, Fleagle SB, Kalenak A: Fractures and refractures in intercollegiate athletes: an eleven year experience. Am J Sports Med 9(6):369–77, 1981.

Chapter 50

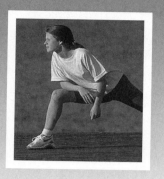

Cycling and In-Line Skating

Renata J. Frankovich, M.D.

Cycling and in-line skating are similar in many ways. Participation in these activities spans a wide age range and is predominantly for recreational purposes. Cyclists and in-line skaters often share the same roadways or pathways, although in-line skaters typically travel at speeds slightly less than cyclists. A smaller but growing number compete at various levels and in various forms of cycling and in-line skating. Both activities are environmentally conscious forms of transportation that are also very economical. For fitness training, cycling and in-line skating are excellent aerobic activities.

CYCLING

Equipment

Bicycle technology has evolved over the past 20 years to produce variations of the traditional bicycle design that meet specific demands of cyclists with different needs. There are 4 basic bicycle types: mountain, touring, hybrid, and racing. The mountain bike is a durable, stable all-terrain bicycle favored by those who seek a comfortable commuter bike and those who cycle rugged, uneven terrain. The touring bike was developed for longer rides and is a more responsive bike. It has thinner wheels than a mountain bike and drop handle bars. The hybrid bike is a cross between the mountain and touring bicycle with smoother fat tires that make road cycling easier but still allow dirt riding. This type of bike is suitable for long-distance touring, off-road use or for commuting. Racing bikes have steeper frame angles and narrow tires designed for quicker handling and speed but are less comfortable for the rider. Equipment design has evolved from the standard double-triangle steel bike design (Fig. 50-1) to new frame geometries with advanced materials and braking systems for all types of bicycles, especially the competitive high-priced racing bicycles.

Along with advancements in bicycle design, improvements have been made in pedal systems. Toe clips or toe baskets have been replaced by clipless pedal systems for the serious cyclist, allowing for improved power transmission from the foot to the pedal. Other advantages of clipless pedal systems include no interference by straps, improved clearance while cornering, lighter-weight shoes, and easy entry and exit out of the pedals.[3] The first generation of clipless pedal systems locked the cyclist's foot securely onto the pedal in one position through a fixed shoe cleat–pedal interface. The fixed, rigid positioning of the foot was found to contribute to overuse injuries, particularly in the knee.[14] Floating clipless pedals were developed in response to this problem. They allow for variable amounts of rotation at the shoe cleat–pedal interface, which can then be adapted to suit individual kinematics.

There are bicycles designed specifically for women, even though many women buy a traditional frame designed for a male cyclist. The bicycle designed for a female cyclist may include some or all of the following: a step-through frame design (top tube angled down), higher-rise stem, narrower handlebar, frame geometry proportioned to the female, shorter crank arm, wide gear range, and contoured and padded saddle. These features are marketed to provide a more comfortable and efficient ride for women. There are no studies in the scientific literature comparing performance, comfort, or injury patterns of a bicycle designed for women compared with a traditional bicycle design.

Proper Fit of the Bicycle

Bicycle fit is an important issue influencing the cyclist's comfort, predisposition to injury and performance. The cyclist's optimum position on the bicycle is determined by a biomechanical analysis of the individual's anatomic variants, equipment choices, and level of participation.

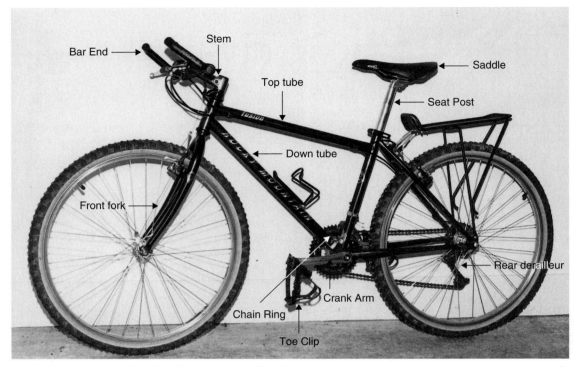

Figure 50-1. Anatomy of a bicycle. This is a mountain bicycle.

Static bicycle fitting is used predominantly because of convenience and is a reasonable first step to fit a bicycle. However, cycling is a dynamic process and occasionally observing the cyclist on the road is necessary to fine-tune fit, especially in the elite cyclist. Frame size, saddle height position, fore and aft positioning, saddle tilt, foot placement on the pedals, and upper body positioning all need to be considered for optimum bike fit.

Correct frame size depends on whether a road bike or mountain bike is being fitted. The bike should be straddled and the distance between the crotch and the top tube should be 3 to 6 inches for a mountain bike and 1 to 2 inches for a road bike (Fig. 50-2).[4] Riders of newer bikes with nontraditional top tube geometry may not be able to use this method and may have to rely on comfort and balance to select the right frame size. Test riding all bikes is recommended prior to purchase.

Saddle position is a critical factor in enabling a cyclist to maximize transmission of power to the pedals. However, the positions that enable the cyclist to produce the most power also put the most stress through the knee.[30] A convenient method of determining saddle height is to measure knee flexion at the bottom dead center (6 o'clock position) of the pedaling stroke. The degree of knee flexion can be measured using a goniometer. The landmarks used are the greater trochanter, the lateral condyle of the knee, and the lateral malleolus of the ankle (Fig. 50-3). The optimal position, taking into account both

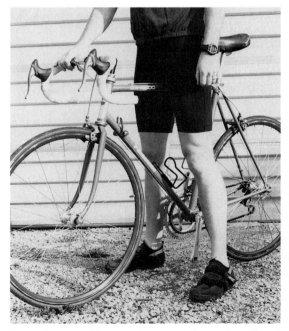

Figure 50-2. To determine the correct frame size, allow 1 to 2 inches between the crotch and the top of the frame for a road bicycle. For mountain bicycles, allow 3 to 6 inches.

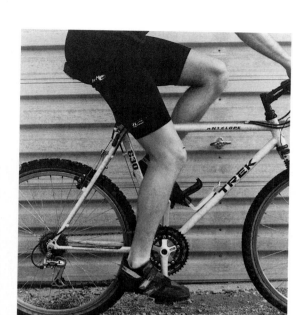

Figure 50-3. To determine the proper saddle height, put the pedal at the 6 o'clock position (bottom dead center). The extended leg should be flexed 25° to 30°. The angle is measured using the greater trochanter, the lateral femoral condyle, and the lateral malleolus as landmarks. Some mountain bikers prefer a lower saddle height, as shown in this photograph.

power and comfort, is 25° to 30° of flexion.[14] Adjustments are made by 1/4-inch increments until a comfortable position is found. An alternative method is to have the cyclist pedal backward with the heel on top of the pedal. The saddle height is set at the point where the knee is barely extended and the hips are not rocking side to side.[4] When the cyclist is actually riding, the ball of the foot will be on the pedals instead of the heel and the knee will be in approximately 25° to 30° of flexion. To improve off-road stability and increase maneuverability, some mountain bikers prefer a seat lower than the described method would recommend.[18] Saddles that are too high tend to cause posterior knee pain while saddles that are too low tend to produce anterior knee pain.

The fore–aft position of the saddle is determined by the length of the femur, crank arm, and foot when the ischial tuberosities are weight bearing and the ball of the foot is over the pedal axle. The ideal fore–aft position occurs when a line drawn anterior to the patella (of the front leg) down toward the pedal falls at the end of the crank arm when the crank arm is horizontal (3 and 9 o'clock positions) (Fig. 50-4).[4,14] Mountain bikers often move the saddle back 1/2 inch from this position to improve rear wheel traction while climbing.[18] To ensure that the saddle is level or slightly upward, a carpen-

ter's level can be used. This ensures that the weight is distributed over the widest part of the saddle. Occasionally women may want the front of the saddle tilted down for comfort.[18]

Foot placement depends on the type of pedal system being used. For platform pedals or pedals with toe clips or straps, the widest part of the foot should be centered over the pedal axle.[18] For clipless pedals, the cleat should be placed so that the foot is aligned over the pedal so that the metatarsal head of the great toe is over the axle of the pedal. Cleat position should be adjusted for any anatomic variants that were noted on physical examination and adjusted so that the foot placement on the pedals reflects the cyclists natural foot position while standing. Cyclists with marked pronation, excessive toeing out, or varus alignments may need spacers between the pedal and the crank arm.[14]

Upper body position is determined by less exact methods and is influenced by the cyclist's flexibility and comfort.[4] Top tube length, stem length, and saddle fore–aft position influence upper body position. The optimum upper body position should allow for a comfortable fit with arms relaxed and elbows slightly bent. Elbows should not interfere with knee movement. Torso angle measured against the top tube varies depending on the participation level of the cyclist and the style of cycling.[4] A more

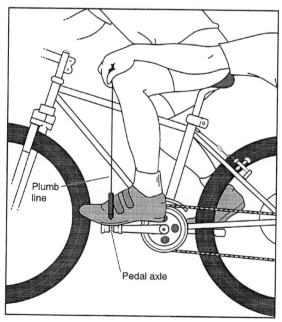

Figure 50-4. To determine the fore–aft position, the crank arms should be at the 3 and 9 o'clock positions. The saddle should be moved forward or backward until a plumb line from the anterior aspect of the patella falls directly over the pedal axle under the forward foot.

upright position preferred by beginner cyclists provides stability and comfort. Increasing upper body lean forward enables a more aerodynamic position for the competitive cyclist. To further reduce aerodynamic drag, aerodynamic or clip-on handlebars have become popular in triathlon and time-trial cycling. These new handlebars reduce the body's frontal area and allow the wind to be directed around the body without negatively impacting physiologic responses to exercise.[4] Handlebar height depends on the type of bicycle but generally a drop handle bar is positioned 1 to 2 inches below the top of the saddle.

Cycling Biomechanics

The cycling gait can be broken down into the propulsive phase and the recovery phase. The propulsive phase begins just after the top dead center (12 o'clock). It has a weight-bearing component when the power generated by the lower extremity is transmitted through the foot to the pedal. During increases in foot pressures there is compensatory pronation at the foot, internal rotation of the tibia, and adduction of the hip.[5] Pedaling force decreases after the cyclist reaches the bottom of the pedaling stroke (6 o'clock).[11] This bottom dead center position marks the transition into the recovery phase where the cyclist starts pulling up on the pedal to overcome gravity and inertia. Overuse injuries are more commonly related to the propulsive phase because of the higher torque and forces generated through the musculoskeletal system during this phase.[12]

Etiology of Injuries

Cyclists are at risk for both traumatic and overuse injuries. Trauma from falls and collisions results in a spectrum of injuries from minor abrasions to more serious life-threatening conditions. Although there are similarities between off-road cycling injuries and road-biking injuries, there are environmental and terrain factors that also play variable roles in these injuries. On the other hand, overuse injuries result from training errors, improper bike fit, and anatomic malalignments. The management of cycling injuries requires a basic knowledge of the sport of cycling, cycling equipment, and cycling biomechanics.

Traumatic Injuries

Traumatic injuries are not uncommon in cycling. In the United States over 500,000 people are treated in emergency departments each year for bicycle-related injuries.[40] Bicycle crashes account for approximately 1000 deaths annually.[40] Head injury is one of the most serious injuries that a cyclist can incur. Head injuries account for one third of all bicycle-related emergency department visits, two thirds of hospital admissions, and three quarters of deaths.[40] Peak incidence of cycling injuries occurs in youth,[42] with 80% being between 5 and 14 years of age.[38] Of bicycle-related deaths, approximately three quarters occur in children less than 19 years of age.[44] In the majority of the studies, there is an increased incidence in males injured compared to females, especially in the pediatric population.[22] The male death rate from bicycling injuries is also greater than the female death rate because males have a greater exposure rate and case fatality rate.[21] Lofthouse[22] summarized specific anatomic injury patterns from a number of studies and found upper extremity injuries to account for 36.0%, head and face injuries 31.8%, lower extremity injuries 25.8%, and thorax injuries 6.4%. Contusions represent 39.2% of these injuries, abrasions 36.1%, lacerations 23.2%, and fractures 16.1%.

In a survey of off-road cyclists, 85.7% reported injuries sustained during the preceding 12 months.[20] Significant traumatic injuries accounted for 20.4% of these injuries. Minor injuries such as abrasions, contusions, and lacerations accounted for 60% to 70% of injuries, while fractures (20% to 30%) and concussions (3% to 12%) were less common. The majority of fractures were to the upper extremity.[19,20] The shoulder is at risk for injury when a cyclist falls and lands on the shoulder, resulting in clavicle fractures, acromioclavicular separations, and shoulder dislocations.

Injuries are caused by a number of factors related to the cyclist, the equipment, and the terrain. A survey of recreational and competitive off-road cyclists identified loss of control, high-speed descent, and competition as contributing factors to injuries.[20] Downhill rides account for the majority of injuries in off-road cycling. Mechanical problems, including flat tires, are also more common during downhill races.[19] Accidents in which the rider is thrown forward over the handlebars result in more severe injuries than when the rider falls off the bike to the side.[19] One study found that female cross-country racers were more likely to be thrown forward off their bikes and injured than males.[19]

Prevention of traumatic injuries includes proper bicycle maintenance, developing good bicycle-handling skills, and using protective equipment, especially a helmet. In an extensive review of the literature, Thompson and Patterson[40,41] found substantial evidence supporting the use of bicycle helmets that meet national standards. Helmet use is protective in bicycle falls, collisions with objects, and collisions with motor vehicles. Head injury is reduced by 85%, brain injury by 88%, and severe brain injury by at least 75% with helmet use.[40] Helmets have also been shown to reduce injuries to the upper and mid facial regions by two thirds.[39] However, bicycle helmets do not provide protection for the lower part of the face.[39] Helmets that extend around the mandible and/or face shields may be more protective. The role of other types of protective gear like chest, shoulder, and extremity padding is unclear but likely decreases more superficial injuries.

Overuse Injuries

Overuse injuries in cycling are found in the lower extremity, the spine, the upper extremity, and the saddle region.[25,33,45] Overuse injuries have been reported by 85% of cyclists, 36% of whom required medical treatment.[46] Interactions between the cyclist, the bicycle, and the terrain on which she rides account for the overuse injuries found in cycling. Errors in bicycle fit and/or anatomic variants not accounted for can contribute to injuries to the knee (Table 50-1), hip and pelvis (Table 50-2), and lower leg (Table 50-3). Overuse upper extremity injuries and injuries affecting the spine are related to weight bearing on the handlebars and vibrations transmitted from rough terrain to the cyclist (Tables 50-4 and 50-5). Females were 1.5 times more likely to develop neck and 2.0 times more likely to develop shoulder overuse injuries.[46] Training errors such as increasing frequency, intensity, and duration too quickly, along with riding in too high a gear, also contribute to overuse injuries.

If bicycle fit cannot correct an alignment problem, cycling orthotics should be considered. Orthotics made for running are not appropriate for cycling because they are different in a number of ways.[14] Pedal contact with the foot occurs under the metatarsal heads and therefore forefoot posting, not rearfoot posting as is done in running, is needed to correct the alignment. The cycling orthotic is a full-length orthosis, making it longer than the running orthotic, which is often three-quarter length. Cycling orthotics must be made from more rigid materials like polypropylene to minimize any dampening effect of force generated by the lower extremity to the pedal.

The evaluation of a cycling overuse injury should begin with a detailed history of the cyclist's training pattern. The physical examination should look for anatomic variations with the cyclist standing and sitting with the hip and knee flexed at 90°, knees shoulder-width apart, and the ankle in neutral position. Bicycle fit should be evaluated.

Putting the rider in neutral position on the bicycle can often treat an overuse injury. If the rider is in neutral position and sustains an injury, then adjustments may need to be made for anatomic malalignments by adjusting the saddle and the pedals. Upper extremity problems like ulnar nerve compression and neck soreness often respond to measures that decrease the cyclist's reach, such as raising the handlebars so that the elbows are slightly bent.

Treatment of overuse injuries in cyclists must be comprehensive. Traditional modalities such as ice, anti-inflammatory medications, stretching, muscle strengthening and balance, and formal physical therapy may all be useful in treating the injury. Additional treatment options specific to cycling can be found in Tables 50-1 to 50-5. Training issues also need to be addressed, with an emphasis on preseason conditioning, gradual increase in mileage, hill climbing, and intensity. However, if the bicycle and the cyclist are left out of the evaluation and treatment plan, the overuse injury is likely to recur.

Protective Equipment

The bicycle helmet is the most important piece of safety equipment the cyclist should wear. Only helmets that meet the safety standards of the American National Standards Institute (ANSI) and the Snell Memorial Foundation should be worn. The helmet should touch the head at the crown, sides, forehead, and posterior aspect of the head. It should fit squarely on top of the head, covering part of the forehead (Fig. 50-5). The straps should fit snugly. The helmet should not move when pushed side to side. When a helmet sustains a crash, it should be returned to the manufacturer for inspection and/or replacement.[9] In addition to a helmet, protective eyewear should be worn to shield against sun radiation, objects like bugs and stones, and irritants like rain.[9] Standards for protective eyewear are set by the ANSI, the American Society of Testing and Materials (ASTM), and the Canadian Standards Association (CSA).

Cycling clothes should be bright to enhance the cyclist's visibility. Shorts are typically made of Lycra or similar stretch material and contain

Table 50-1. Cycling Overuse Injuries of the Knee: Etiology and Treatment[14,15,18,25,33,45]

INJURY	ETIOLOGY	TREATMENT
Anterior Knee		
Patellar tendinitis	Training errors	Low-resistance cycling
Patellofemoral pain	Lack of conditioning	Avoid hills
Quadriceps tendinitis	Improper bicycle fit	Correct bicycle fit
	Saddle too low	Adjust saddle position to 25° to 30° knee flexion
	Saddle too far forward	
	Anatomic malalignment	Strengthen quadriceps
	Internal tibial rotation	Maintain hip and calf strength
	Pronation	Adjust cleat position for anatomic variation
	Valgus alignment	Orthotics
Medial Knee		
Medial synovial plica	Training errors	Restrict cycling to pain-free easy spinning
Medial patellofemoral ligament	Lack of conditioning	
	Improper bicycle fit	Avoid hills
	Cleats externally rotated	Correct bicycle fit
	Anatomic malalignment	Orthotics to correct pronation
	Pronation	Arthroscopy—medial wall synovectomy and excision or
	Valgus knees	release of medial patellofemoral ligament
	Internal tibial rotation	
Pes anserine bursitis	Training errors	Correct bicycle fit
	Lack of conditioning	Orthotics to correct pronation
	Improper bicycle fit	Stretch medial hamstrings and pes anserine muscles
	Saddle too high	
	Trauma from bicycle frame	Friction massage
	Anatomic malalignment	Steroid injection
	External tibial rotation	
	Pronation	
	Leg-length discrepancy	
Lateral Knee		
Iliotibial band friction syndrome	Training errors	Low-resistance cycling
	Lack of conditioning	Avoid hills
	Improper bicycle fit	Correct bicycle fit
	Saddle too high	Adjust saddle height to 30° to 35° knee flexion
	Saddle too far back	
	Cleats too internally rotated	Adjust cleat position into neutral or slight external rotation
	Anatomic malalignment	
	Internal tibial rotation	
	Pronation	Switch to floating pedals
	Iliotibial band tightness	Add spacers between pedal and the crank arm to widen stance
		Deep-tissue massage
		Injection
Posterior Knee		
Biceps tendinitis	Training errors	Low-resistance cycling
	Lack of conditioning	Correct bicycle fit
	Improper bicycle fit	Adjust saddle height to 30° to 35° knee flexion on long leg
	Saddle too high	Adjust cleat position for anatomic variation
	Saddle too far back	
	Cleats too internally rotated	
	Anatomic malalignment	Switch to floating pedals
	Varus alignment	Spacers
	Short leg length	Orthotics for leg-length discrepancies

a crotch pad for cushioning. Gloves with padded palms are used to prevent shock transmission up the upper extremity to the shoulders and neck.

Concluding Remarks

Bicycling is a multipurpose activity, utilized as a form of recreation, competition, and transporta-

Table 50-2. Cycling Overuse Injuries of the Hip/Pelvis: Etiology and Treatment[14,15,18,25,33,45]

INJURY	ETIOLOGY	TREATMENT
Trochanteric bursitis	Tight iliotibial band Narrow stance	Spacer between pedal and crank arm to widen stance
Ischial tuberosity Irritation	Saddle position Saddle tilt, shape, or texture Prolonged sitting on saddle	Change saddle shape Adjust saddle position Rest from cycling
Gluteal muscle strain	Long rides	Increase upright position Limit length of rides

Table 50-3. Cycling Overuse Injuries of the Lower Leg: Etiology and Treatment[14,15,18,25,33,45]

INJURY	ETIOLOGY	TREATMENT
Posterior tibialis Tendinitis	Pes planus foot Floating pedals Toed-out cleats	Orthotics
Achilles tendinitis	Excessive ankling Flexible foot Pes planus Soft shoe Foot too far back on pedal Short leg Excessive toe-in	Orthotics Rigid supportive shoe Move foot forward on pedal Correct leg-length discrepancy

Table 50-4. Cycling Overuse Injuries of the Spine: Etiology and Treatment[14,15,18,25,33,45]

INJURY	ETIOLOGY	TREATMENT
Low back pain	Excessive vibration Cyclist too far forward Improper saddle position Inflexibility Leg-length discrepancy Pre-existing back pain	Wider tires Lower inflation Front suspension Decrease reach Correct saddle position Raise handlebars Upright handlebars Alternate hand position
Neck pain	Excessive vibration Excessive neck extension Improper bicycle fit Helmet too low on forehead	Wider tires Lower inflation Front suspension Padded gloves and/or grips Decrease reach Raise handlebars Upright handlebars Mirror on helmet Lighter helmet Alternate hand position

tion. Physicians often prescribe cycling as part of rehabilitation therapy as well. Given the high number of repetitive pedal revolutions in cycling and given the many variables involved in bicycle fit, it is not uncommon for an avid cyclist to sustain an overuse injury. The physician must understand the biomechanics of cycling in order to make appropriate adjustments to bicycle fit for the cyclist.

IN-LINE SKATING

History of the Sport

The original in-line skate dates back to 1823 when an English inventor Robert John Tyers placed 5 wheels in a row on the bottom of a shoe. The current version of in-line skates was created in 1980 by Scott and Brennan Olson of

Table 50-5. Cycling Related Neuropathy: Etiology and Treatment[14,15,18,25,33,45]

INJURY	ETIOLOGY	TREATMENT
Pudendal neuropathy	Improper saddle position	Change saddle tilt Wider saddle Padded saddle Padded cycling shorts
Ulnar or median neuropathy	Excessive vibration Handlebars too low Reach too long	Wider tires Lower inflation Front suspension Padded gloves and/or grips Decrease reach Raise handlebars Upright handlebars

Minneapolis, who started the Rollerblade brand of in-line skates. They added wheels to ice-hockey boots so that they could simulate ice skating on land.[32] Since that time, participation has grown steadily in the United States and Canada.[26] Although in-line skating is predominantly a recreational activity, other forms of participation are also popular. Some use it as a form of transportation, while others use it to cross-train aerobically. Twenty percent of in-line skaters play roller hockey[35] and there is even a professional roller hockey league. In-line skating has also

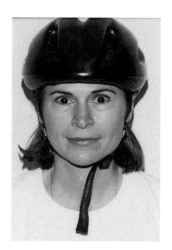

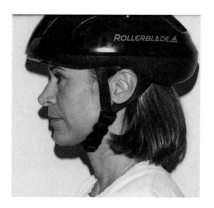

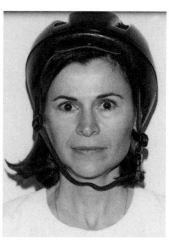

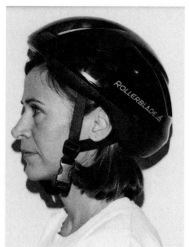

Figure 50-5. (Top) Proper helmet fit. (Bottom) Improper helmet fit. Note how the helmet covers the forehead and the straps fit snugly around the chin in the properly fitting helmet compared to the poorly fitting helmet.

become a popular extreme sport, which emphasizes tricks like jumps, spins, and other artistic forms. Recently amateur in-line skating races have been organized, often in conjunction with running road races.

Demographic Characteristics of In-Line Skaters

The number of in-line skaters has grown steadily in the United States from 6.2 million people in 1991 to 22.5 million people in 1995.[37] In 1993, 77% of in-line skaters were younger than 25 years of age, with 39% of these between 6 and 11 years of age.[35] Equal numbers of men and women participate in the sport. Over one third of skaters live in households with an annual income exceeding $50,000. In-line skating is an activity enjoyed by all ages.

Equipment

The in-line skate consists of a boot constructed similar to either an ice-skate boot (lace-up closure) or a downhill ski boot (buckle closure). The boot is made of polyurethane, leather, or plastic. There are typically 4 polyurethane wheels attached to the bottom of the boot in a linear fashion. Five wheels are used when greater speed is desired. This linear arrangement of the wheels differentiates in-line skates from roller skates, in which the wheels are aligned in parallel. The wheels can vary in diameter and density, with softer wheels used for recreational skating, offering a smoother ride, less speed, and better maneuverability. Variations in speed can also be achieved by using wheel bearings that vary in frictional resistance. For example, low-friction bearings are used to provide a faster spinning wheel to gain more speed.

Most skates have a braking system that is placed at the rear of the skate of the dominant leg, usually the right leg. The brakes are activated by dorsiflexing the ankle, in a repetitive pumping type of action, to bring the rear brake to the ground. The process of stopping is augmented by lowering the center of gravity of the body by flexing at the knee and the hip and leaning back with the arms forward for balance. Some skates have an adjustable feature that allows the skater to adjust the position of the brakes so that more or less dorsiflexion at the ankle is required to initiate the stopping process.

Protective equipment available for in-line skating includes a helmet, knee pads, elbow pads, and wrist guards (Fig. 50-6). There is no specific helmet designed for in-line skating and

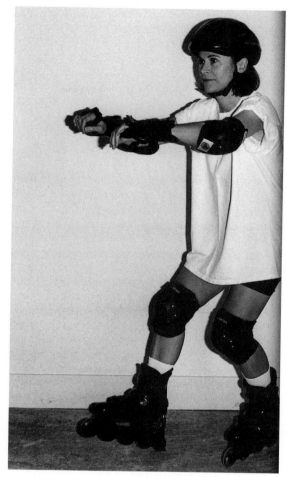

Figure 50-6. Technique of stopping using the rear brake pad. Complete protective gear is being worn: helmet, elbow pads, wrist guards, and knee pads.

those who do wear headgear while skating tend to use a bicycle helmet. Wrist guards have a hard plate over the volar aspect of the wrist that stabilizes the wrist in extension. The protective effect of wrist guards is thought to be prevention of extreme wrist extension, dissipation of forces by increasing the surface contact area and reducing the friction between the contact point and the ground, and reduction of abrasions and contusions sustained during a fall. Elbow and knee pads are designed as a hard protective cup-like shell that is secured over the elbow or knee via a sleeve or Velcro fastener.

Physiology

In-line skating is an aerobic activity suitable for improving cardiorespiratory fitness. It has been shown to be similar to treadmill running in terms of physiologic responses.[43] For equivalent training volume and intensity, running and in-line skating can achieve similar improvements in maximal oxygen consumption (VO_2max).[24] Some highly conditioned athletes, like competitive cross-country skiers, find it difficult to cross-train with the newer in-line skates because of the high speeds attained with minimal effort.

Injury Epidemiology

Studies of in-line skating injuries have predominantly taken place in the emergency department setting, focusing on traumatic and more severe injuries. There is no published literature on overuse injuries or injuries presenting to other ambulatory care facilities. A national probability sample for product-related injuries in emergency departments of US hospitals has been obtained from the National Electronic Injury Surveillance System (NEISS) database.[36] During a 12-month period beginning July 1, 1992, an estimated 31,000 skaters were injured severely enough that they presented to the emergency department.[36] In 1995 that number rose to 99,500,[37] an increase that reflects increased participation in the sport. The percentage of in-line skaters injured while skating has been reported to be 27%[48] in one survey and 38% in another survey study,[1] of which only 6% of the injured sought formal medical care. The ratio of males to females injured varies in the literature and depends on the mean age of the study population.[1,8,23,27,31,36,37] The trend is that the proportion of males injured in the pediatric population is greater and the proportion of females injured in the adult population is greater. This phenomenon may be related to increased risk-taking behaviors in younger males and lower fitness levels in older females.

Injury Distribution and Type

The anatomic distribution and the types of injuries sustained during in-line skating have been documented in a number of studies that have reported on injuries presenting to the emergency department.[1,6,8,23,31,36,37] The results of a representative study are shown in Table 50-6. Approximately two thirds of in-line skating injuries are to the upper extremity; one third of total injuries occur at the wrist. The proposed mechanism for upper extremity injuries is a fall on an outstretched hand, a natural response to bracing for a fall. Head injuries account for approximately 5% of the total injuries. Fractures and/or dislocations comprise 40% to 69% of injuries presenting to the emergency department. Soft-tissue injuries such as contusions, sprains, lacerations, and abrasions each account for approximately 10% to 20% of total injuries. Hospital admission was required for about 3.5% of skaters.[36]

Retrospective analysis of injury type in a general population of in-line skaters differs from the emergency department data. Fracture rates were found to be lower, 3%[1] and 13.4%,[48] in in-line skaters who were surveyed while skating in parks. Only about one third of those injured sought formal medical care, probably because abrasions and contusions were the most prevalent injuries cited.

Factors Contributing to Injury

There are numerous factors that may contribute to the risk of injury in in-line skating. High speeds can be all too easily achieved, especially going downhill. The average speed of an in-line skater is 10 to 17 miles/hr but speeds of up to 30 miles/hr can be reached.[34] Speed was cited

Table 50-6. Anatomic Distribution of Injuries Sustained During In-Line Skating Expressed as a Percentage of the Total Number of Injured In-Line Skaters

UPPER EXTREMITY	% OF TOTAL INJURIES	LOWER EXTREMITY	% OF TOTAL INJURIES
Wrist	37%	Ankle	7%
Elbow	9%	Knee	5%
Face	8%	Lower leg	5%
Head	5%	Upper leg	2%
Shoulder	5%	Foot	1%
Trunk	5%	Pubic area	<1%
Hand	4%	Not specified	<1%
Finger	4%		
Upper arm	<1%		
Mouth	<1%		
Neck	<1%		

From Schieber RA, Branche-Dorsey CM, Ryan GW: Comparison of in-line skating injuries with roller skating and skateboarding injuries. JAMA 271:1856–8, 1994, with permission.

as the cause of injury by 35% of injured in-line skaters.[29] The technique used for stopping or slowing down to control speed may be another factor. The techniques used for stopping include use of a rear brake pad 52.3%, spin stop 13.3%, t-stop 11.1%, going off into the grass 14.6%, and falling 3.5%.[48] Spin stops are achieved by changing momentum by skating in a tight circle, while a t-stop is performed by dragging a skate behind the body, with the dragging skate perpendicular to the lead skate. Both the spin stop and the t-stop are advanced maneuvers. Stopping using the rear brake pad system is difficult to master as well (see Fig. 50-6) and may not be achieved instantaneously, even if skilled. Ice skaters who in-line skate cannot rely on their ice-skating skills to stop since the techniques are different.

Skating is usually done on hard paved surfaces that have additional hazards that may be difficult to avoid or negotiate, such as stones, tree limbs, wet surfaces, or blind corners. Objects or hazards on the road (not including vehicles) contribute to the risk of injury in one quarter of the injury cases.[1,29] Loss of balance, with no objects or vehicles involved, was the most commonly cited reason for sustaining an in-line skating injury.[1,8,10,48] Vehicles and equipment failure each contributed to injury less than 5% of the time. The prevalence of inexperience among injured in-line skaters was noted in a number of studies.[2,10,13,28] In one study, 46% of injured in-line skaters were first-time skaters who lost control and fell.[13] In summary, the inexperienced skater and the skater still mastering balance, control, and stopping are at risk for injury.

A skater's ability to deal with unexpected hazards also depends on the skater's skill level. In-line skating is a skilled activity that requires a learning phase and an appreciation for the potential hazards while in-line skating. For the novice skater, controlling speed going down hills can be especially challenging. During this initial period, precautions need to be taken while mastering the skills of balance, falling, and stopping. Practicing these skills on level ground in an area protected from obstacles and vehicles is recommended. Formal lessons from a certified instructor may also be beneficial during this stage.

Protective Equipment

Using protective equipment such as a helmet, knee pads, elbow pads, and wrist guards makes intuitive sense. However, in unobtrusive observational studies of in-line skaters and in injured populations, protective equipment was under-utilized. Helmet use ranged from 2.6% to 18.6%.[8,10,17,47] Of patients presenting to the emergency department with an in-line skating injury, no protective equipment was worn by 45.8% of patients in a study with a mean age 23.8 years,[10] whereas in a group of predominantly male children, 88% did not wear equipment.[8] Thirty-two percent of in-line skaters skating in a park in an observational study were not wearing protective equipment.[47] Wrist guards are the most popular piece of protective gear worn, with 45.7% to 65.2% of in-line skaters wearing them.[10,17,47] Adolescent males, children, and advanced skaters are the least likely to be seen wearing protective equipment.[47] Reasons given for not wearing protective equipment are that the gear is felt to be unnecessary, too hot, too uncomfortable, too expensive, and unattractive in appearance.[48]

The most comprehensive study done on protective equipment use was a case-control study of 161 patients obtained through the NEISS in the United States.[37] The odds ratio for wrist injury for those who did not wear wrist guards as compared to those who did, adjusted for age and sex, was 10.4 (95% confidence interval, 2.9 to 36.9). For elbow injury, the odds ratio was 9.5 (95% confidence interval, 2.6 to 34.4) for those who did not wear elbow pads, adjusted for number of lessons taken and whether or not they performed trick skating.[37] The evidence supporting the use of wrist guards is of considerable importance since wrist and forearm fractures account for 37% to 68.8% of the total injuries.[2,10,17,23,36] On the other hand, there is some concern that wrist splints may change the pattern of injury to a more complicated proximal forearm fracture. Four cases of open forearm fractures in in-line skaters wearing wrist splints have been reported to have occurred adjacent to the proximal border of the wrist splints.[7] The balance of evidence supports the use of wrist guards and ultimately standards need to be set similar to the Snell and ANSI standards in place for bicycle helmets.

The efficacy of helmet use in in-line skating is not known. The risk of injury to an in-line skater is comparable to the risk for a bicyclist with respect to speeds obtainable, exposure to motor vehicles, and road surfaces used. Bicycle helmets are typically used by in-line skaters but they are not designed to protect the occiput from a backward fall. This type of fall would be rare from a bicycle but not uncommon in in-line skating. A hockey-style helmet may provide some protection from this type of fall. No studies have determined the type of helmet best suited for in-line skating. Until such information is available, helmet use in in-line skating is recommended on the basis of experience with bicycling[41] and hockey.

Comparisons to Other Sports

Although there are many similarities between cycling and in-line skating, there have been no studies done that have compared the two. In-line skating has been compared to roller skating and skateboarding. For every in-line skating injury, there are an estimated 3.3 roller skating and 1.2 skateboarding injuries.[36] In-line skating injuries have been compared to other sport-related injuries in children that have presented to the emergency department through data obtained from the Canadian Hospitals Injury Reporting and Prevention Program database.[8] In-line skating had significantly greater number of fractures (55% versus 21% in other sporting activities) and of upper extremity injuries. In-line skaters also required more extensive treatment than children injured in other sports. Finally, the differences in injury patterns between ice hockey and hockey on in-line skates has been studied. In ice hockey there are more lacerations and an increased risk of head and neck injuries. In hockey using in-line skates, there were increased number of injuries due to checking and a decrease in number of injuries as a result of skate equipment.[16]

Concluding Remarks

In-line skating is a relatively new sport that has grown in popularity because of its broad appeal. It is an aerobic activity that carries a risk for traumatic injury. Although contusions and abrasions are the most common injuries, the most significant injury requiring emergent care is fracture of the wrist. Wrist splints and elbow pads have been shown to reduce injury and should be worn. Although there are no in-line skating studies to support the protective effect of helmets and knee pads, the prudent in-line skater should wear them as well, especially helmets, given what is known about the protective effect of helmets in cycling. Injuries are most commonly caused by falls resulting from loss of balance or speed. Stopping and controlling speed should be learned initially by taking lessons and by practicing in a safe area free from vehicles.

References

1. Adams SL, Wyte CD, Paradise MS, del Castillo J: A prospective study of in-line skating: observational series and survey of active in-line skaters-injuries, protective equipment and training. Acad Emerg Med 3:304–11, 1996.
2. Banas MP, Dalldorf PG, Marquardt JD: Skateboard and in-line skate fractures: a report of one summer's experience. J Orthop Trauma 6:301–5, 1992.
3. Berto F: A pedal revolution. Bicycling 30(3):172, 1989.
4. Burke ER: Proper fit of the bicycle. Clin Sports Med 13(1):1–14, 1994.
5. Burke ER, Newsom MM: Medical and Scientific Aspects Of Cycling. Champaign, Ill, Human Kinetics Publishers, 1988.
6. Calle SC, Eaton RG: Wheels-in-line roller skating injuries. J Trauma 35:946–51, 1993.
7. Cheng SL, Rajaratnam K, Raskin KB, Hu RW: "Splint-top" fracture of the forearm: a description of an in-line skating injury associated with the use of protective wrist splints. J Trauma 39(6):1194–7, 1995.
8. Ellis JA, Kierulf JC, Klassen, TP: Injuries associated with in-line skating from the Canadian hospitals injury reporting and prevention program database. Can J Public Health 86(2): 133–6, 1995.
9. Ellis TH, Streight D, Mellion MB: Bicycle safety equipment. Clin Sports Med 13(1):75–98, 1994.
10. Frankovich RJ, Petrella RJ, Luttanzio CN: In-line skating injuries patterns and protective equipment use. Phys Sports Med 24(4):57–62,2001.
11. Gregor R J, Broker JP, Ryan MM: The biomechanics of cycling. Exerc Sports Sci Rev 19:127, 1991.
12. Hannaford DR, Moran GT, Hlavac HF: Video analysis and treatment of overuse knee injuries in cycling: a limited clinical study. Clin Podiatr Med Surg 3(4):671, 1988.
13. Heller D: Rollerblading injuries. Hazard, Victoria, Australia 10:11–6, 1993.
14. Holmes JC, Pruitt AL, Whalen NJ: Cycling injuries. In: Nicholas JA, Hershman EB (eds): The Lower Extremity and Spine in Sports Medicine, 2nd edition. St Louis, Mosby-Year Book, 1995, pp 1559–76.
15. Holmes JC, Pruitt AL, Whalen NJ: Lower extremity overuse in bicycling. Clin Sports Med 13(1):187–203, 1994.
16. Hutchinson MR, Milhouse C, Gapski M: Comparison of injury patterns in elite hockey players using ice versus in-line skates. Med Sci Sports Exerc 30(9):1371–3, 1998.
17. Jacques LB, Grzesiak E: Personal protective equipment use by in-line roller skaters. J Fam Pract 38:486–8, 1994.
18. Kronisch RL: Mountain biking injuries. Phys Sportsmed 26(3):65–72, 1998.
19. Kronisch RL, Pfeiffer RP, Chow TK: Acute injuries in cross-country and downhill off-road bicycle racing. Med Sci Sports Exerc 28(11):1351–5, 1996.
20. Kronisch RL, Rubin AL: Traumatic injuries in off-road bicycling. Clin J Sport Med 4(4):240–4, 1994.
21. Li G, Baker SP: Exploring the male-female discrepancy in death rates from bicycling injury: The decomposition method. Accid Anal Prev 28(4):537–40, 1996.
22. Lofthouse GA: Traumatic injuries to the extremities and thorax. Clin Sports Med 13(1):113–35, 1994.
23. Malanga GA, Stuart MJ: In-line skating injuries. Mayo Clin Proc 70:752–4, 1995.
24. Melanson EL, Freedson PS, Jungbluth S: Changes in VO_2max and maximal treadmill time after 9 wk of running or in-line skate training. Med Sci Sports Exerc 28(11):1422–6, 1996.
25. Mellion MB: Neck and back pain in cycling. Clin Sports Med 13(1):137–64, 1994.
26. Menzies D: It's the wheel thing. Living Safety Spring:16–9, 1992.

27. Mitts KG, Hennrikus WL: In-line skating fractures in children. J Pediatr Orthop 16:640–3, 1996.

28. NEISS Estimates Reports: Estimates for the Calendar Year 1992. Washington, DC, National Injury Information Clearinghouse, US Consumer Product Safety Commission, 1992.

29. Orenstein JB: Injuries and small-wheel skates. Ann Emerg Med 27(2):204–9, 1996.

30. Pena N: The critical joint. Bicycling 32(5):74, 1991.

31. Powell EC, Tanz RR: In-line skate and rollerskate injuries in childhood. Pediatr Emerg Care 4:259–62, 1996.

32. Rappelfeld J: The Complete Blader. New York, St Martin's Press, 1992, pp ix-x.

33. Richmond DR: Handlebar problems in bicycling. Clin Sports Med 13(1):165–74, 1994.

34. Rodgers E: Working to beat the bans. Inline: The Skaters Magazine September:11, 1993.

35. Schieber RA, Branche-Dorsey CM: In-line skating injuries. Epidemiology and recommendations for prevention. Sports Med 19(6):427–32, 1995.

36. Schieber RA, Branche-Dorsey CM, Ryan GW: Comparison of in-line skating injuries with roller skating and skateboarding injuries. JAMA 271:1856–8, 1994.

37. Schieber RA, Branche-Dorsey CM, Ryan GW: Risk factors for injuries from in-line skating and the effectiveness of safety gear. N Engl J Med 335:1630–5, 1996.

38. Selbst SM, Alexander D, Ruddy R: Bicycle-related injuries. Am J Dis Child 141:140–4, 1987.

39. Thompson DC, Nunn ME, Thompson RS, et al: Effectiveness of bicycle safety helmets in preventing serious facial injury. JAMA 276(24):1974–5, 1996.

40. Thompson DC, Patterson MQ: Cycle helmets and the prevention of injuries. Sports Med 25(4):213–9, 1998.

41. Thompson DC, Rivara FP, Thompson RS: Effectiveness of bicycle safety helmets in preventing head injuries. JAMA 276(24):1968–73, 1996.

42. Thompson DC, Thompson RS, Rivara FP: Incidence of bicycle-related injuries in a defined population. Am J Public Health 80(11):1388–90, 1990.

43. Wallick ME, Porcari JP, Wallick SB, et al: Physiological responses to in-line skating compared to treadmill running. Med Sci Sports Exerc 27(2):242–8, 1995.

44. Weiss BD: Bicycle-related head injuries. Clin Sports Med 13(1):99–112, 1994.

45. Weiss BD: Clinical syndromes associated with bicycle seats. Clin Sports Med 13(1):175–86, 1994.

46. Wilber CA, Holland GJ, Madison RE, Loy SF: An epidemiological analysis of overuse injuries among recreational cyclists. Int J Sports Med 16(3):201–6, 1995.

47. Young CC, Mark DH: In-line skating. An observational study of protective equipment used by skaters. Arch Fam Med 4:19–23, 1995.

48. Young CC, Seth A, Mark DH: In-line skating: use of protective equipment, falling patterns, and injuries. Clin J Sport Med 8:111–4, 1998.

Chapter 51

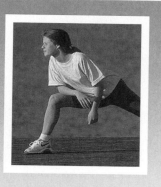

Dance

Carol C. Teitz, M.D.

Few injuries are unique to dance, although many injuries have unique dance-related causes. In order to understand dancers' injuries, we must consider the milieu in which the dancer lives and works. Dancers require flexibility, strength, coordination, rhythm, balance, and timing. Aesthetics are a major issue for performing dancers. Because many dance disciplines demand a thin body habitus, nutritional problems are rampant and lead to menstrual abnormalities, decreased bone mineral density, stress fractures, and scoliosis.[1,3,4,11,33,35] In addition, aesthetic demands also prevent dancers from using knee or ankle braces during performance.

DANCE TYPE

There are many dance disciplines, each of which has specific requirements and types of movements. Many dancers are multidisciplinary. Although no musculoskeletal injury occurs exclusively in a given dance form, to a certain extent different injuries are seen as a function of the specific dance discipline.

Aerobic Dance

Aerobic dance began as a high-impact form of dance. The injuries seen are similar to those seen in runners and include stress fractures, shin splints, and posterior tibial tendonitis.[2,6,9] These injuries can be prevented to a certain extent by a sensible training schedule, wearing shoes designed for aerobic dance, and by dancing on resilient floors.

A low-impact variation of aerobic dance was introduced to decrease the incidence of impact injuries. Low-impact aerobic dance involves keeping at least one foot in contact with the floor at all times. Upper extremity use above the head is encouraged to keep cardiac output high. Although there are fewer impact injuries, low-impact aerobic dance includes many lunges, which leads to patellofemoral problems. The overhead arm use also leads to symptoms of shoulder impingement.

Bench aerobics is designed to use big muscles such as hip flexors and gluteals. One can do high- or low-impact moves on the bench, with or without overhead arm motion. In this form of aerobic dance, the dancer steps on and off of a step/bench, which can range in height from 6 to 18 inches. Bench aerobics allows the dancer an opportunity to adapt her program to protect previously injured body parts.

Ballet

Ballet is a classical lyrical dance form with very specific named steps and movements that have been handed down without much change over the last 2 centuries.[32] In a typical ballet class, dancers begin with a routine of movements at the barre (railing) designed to stretch and strengthen muscles and joints, as well as to work on the fine points of technique. They then move to "center floor," where they work on movement across the room, turns, jumps, and combinations thereof.

A critical fundamental movement in ballet is the plié. A plié is a squat, although the feet are not "in parallel" as they are in typical athletics squats. Instead, they are in of 5 positions, all of which require "turnout" (Fig. 51-1). Ideally, turnout should reflect external rotation of the hip. During plié an imaginary plumb line dropped from the knee should pass through the center of the knee and ankle and land over the second toe.[28] Minor aberrations in plié technique, repeated over time, may produce clinical problems such as medial knee strain, patellofemoral pain, quadriceps tendonitis, medial ankle pain, and bunions.

Ballroom Dance

Ballroom dance includes dances such as the waltz, tango, rumba, and jitterbug. Although

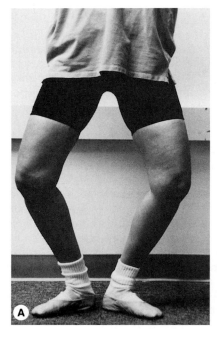
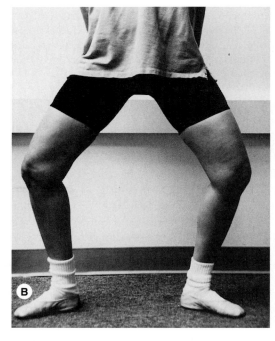
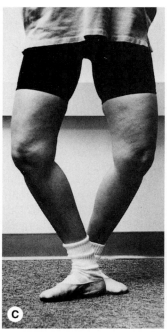
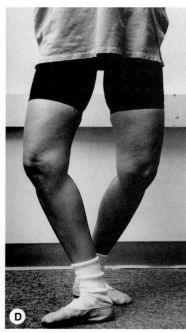
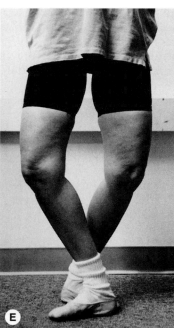

Figure 51-1. Demi-plié (half squat) in the 5 basic positions. **A**, first position; **B**, second position; **C**, third position; **D**, fourth position; **E**, fifth position. Notice that the knees are centered over the feet.

recreational ballroom dancers rarely push their physical limits, competitive ballroom dancers develop quite elaborate routines. These dancers usually wear high (3-inch) heels and have problems with ankle sprains, shin splints, and patellofemoral pain as well as being at risk for tearing menisci.

Folk Dance

Folk dances are ethnic dances specific to a certain culture or part of the world. Some are lyrical, whereas others, such as Eastern European dances, are vigorous and involve percussive movements. In the highland dances, much of the work is done on a flexed knee and on the ball of the foot. This often leads to patellofemoral complaints, metatarsal pain, Morton's neuromata, Achilles tendonitis, and ankle sprains. Stress fractures are also common in female folk dancers.

Jazz Dance

Jazz dancing is what most of us associate with Broadway dancing and is often a ballistic dance form. It incorporates many dance disciplines. Shoes can range from soft jazz slippers (like a laced-up ballet shoe) to heels or even tennis shoes depending on the theme of the piece. Traumatic injuries are more common than overuse injuries. These include patellar dislocations from rapid turns, hamstring tears from high kicks and splits, and miscellaneous contusions and fractures from falls and lifts.[34]

Modern Dance

Modern dance began as a purposeful move away from the rigid structure of classical ballet. Modern dancers contract, release, and fold the torso, flexing and extending, and their movements are more angular. Many of the movements are spiral rather than planar. The head and neck are more likely to move out of phase with the lower torso. Modern dance requires movements while sitting, lying, or kneeling on the floor as well as movements up and down to and from various levels. There are specific forms of modern dance and injuries in these dancers differ as a function of the particular technique.[25] Cervical and upper back strains are roughly twice as common in modern dancers as in ballet dancers.[20] In addition, patellar and meniscal injuries are common.

Tap Dance

Tap dance is a percussive form of dance involving rapid movements of the foot in an anterior and posterior direction. The key is rhythm. The gastrocsoleus muscles are working constantly and Achilles tendonitis can result. Most weight is borne on the ball of the foot, so metatarsalgia and Morton's neuromata are frequent problems. Strong trunk muscles, particularly the rectus abdominis, are required. The knees are almost always flexed; therefore good quadriceps control is required. Despite this, patellofemoral symptoms are rare because the knee is flexed only 15° to 20°.

ETIOLOGY OF INJURY

Most dancers' injuries are overuse injuries and few require surgery.[6,19,20,25,34] Associated risk factors include training errors (intensity, duration, or frequency), poor technique (positioning and muscle use), musculoskeletal imbalance (flexibility and strength), anatomic malalignment of the lower extremity (including leg-length discrepancy, abnormal rotation, angular deformity, and flat feet), and inappropriate equipment (shoe wear and floor surface).[2,17,24,25] Some of these problems can be avoided by selecting a dance discipline that compliments the dancer's lower extremity anatomic structure.

Training Schedule

First and foremost, overuse injuries are caused by too many repetitions of the same movement. Dancers, with the exception of aerobic dancers, typically do not engage in adjunctive training. Finding a time during which to rehabilitate an injury is difficult because dancers, like other athletes, do not want to stop dancing, and dance is not a seasonal "sport." Recreational dancers often are dependent on activity for psychological well being; professionals must dance for financial survival. In addition, most professional dancers are not on fixed salaries and are not covered by either health or industrial insurance.

Flexibility

Few dancers are truly hypermobile.[14] The need for flexibility is greatest in the spine, hips, and ankles. Most dancers have greater-than-average hamstring muscle flexibility but typically have tight iliotibial bands, gastrocsoleus muscles, and hip flexors.

Strength

Generally dancers tend to be more supple than strong.[12] Many dancers consider weight-lifting taboo, and fear development of defined musculature. Trunk strength is particularly important for centering body weight, especially during various maneuvers in which the dancer balances on one leg. Trunk strength is also required for lifting, and for various gymnastic-like maneuvers seen in modern and jazz dance. For balancing on the ball of the foot, peroneal, posterior tibial, and intrinsic foot muscle strengthening are critical. Cybex-testing quadriceps and hamstring muscles for strength and power is useful for pointing out deficiencies, setting goals, and assessing progress during the rehabilitation period.

Equipment

Equipment also can play an etiologic role in injuries. A dance floor should be resilient, yet firm. A sprung wood floor that absorbs some of the shock of jumping or percussive foot work can decrease the incidence of injuries such as stress fractures.[23] Shoes are important as well. Other than shoes for aerobic dance, most dance shoes have no shock absorbancy and no room for standard orthoses. Modern dancers often dance barefooted, making protective padding or adjustments for anatomic variations extremely difficult.

SPECIFIC INJURIES

This section describes musculoskeletal problems seen in various forms of dance. Those injuries common to other female athletes will be mentioned. However, the reader is referred elsewhere in this text for details on their presentation and treatment. Unless otherwise noted, these injuries are treated as in other athletes. Unique dance etiologic factors will be noted. Injuries that are seen almost exclusively in dancers will be discussed in detail.

Hip Injuries

Snapping Hip

The snapping hip is associated with ballet. It most commonly is due to the iliopsoas tendon snapping over the iliopectineal eminence and is usually due to imbalance between the rectus femoris and iliopsoas muscles. Because of its anatomic position, the iliopsoas is critical for centering body weight through the pelvis without excessively increasing or decreasing lumbar lordosis.[31] It also allows greater and more controlled flexion of the hip.

Snapping hip presents as an audible, low-pitched "clunk" in the groin during flexion, abduction, and external rotation of the hip (Fig. 51-2). Gradually, this movement will become associated with pain in the groin. The symptoms are typically unilateral and more common in the non-weight-bearing leg (the gesture leg). On examination, one may find pain with resisted use of iliopsoas. The dancer can usually readily reproduce the "clunk" for the examiner who cannot produce it by passive range of motion.

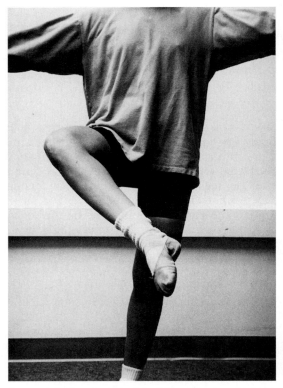

Figure 51-2. A typical hip "clunk" occurs when the hip is simultaneously flexed, abducted and externally rotated.

This problem is best treated by sending the dancer to a movement analyst, Pilates therapist, or physical therapist versed in dance. The dancer will be taught correct biomechanics and repatterning of muscle use in addition to iliopsoas stretching. If the dancer has become fixated with repetition of the "clunk," an element of tendinosis may be present and will require additional treatment. This will include ice-friction massage, nonsteroidal anti-inflammatory drugs, and telling the dancer to stop intentional snapping. Rarely, operative lengthening of the tendon is required.[22]

Knee Injuries

Patellofemoral Problems

Patellofemoral problems are rampant in aerobic dancers as a result of jumping (traditional aerobics), lunges (low impact), use of the step (bench), and the prevalence of lower extremity malalignment in these recreational dancers. The most common form of lower extremity malalignment seen, a triad of excessive femoral anteversion, external tibial torsion, and pronated feet, can produce patellar problems in dancers as in other athletes.[5] Other contributing factors may include tight hamstrings, quadriceps, or iliotibial bands. When no alignment abnormalities or tight tendons are noted, one should counsel the patient to make sure her knees are over her feet during lunges. For dancers with anatomic abnormalities, over-strengthening the vastus medialis obliquus muscle and stretching of the iliotibial band, hamstrings, and quadriceps muscles are helpful.

When ballet students develop retropatellar pain, it is often due to improper use of the quadriceps muscles. Many students contract their quadriceps muscles tightly during an entire plié, producing constantly high patellofemoral compression forces. In addition, quadriceps strains will result from chronic eccentric use. Teaching the student to use hip external rotators to initiate plié and adductors to return to the starting position will often eliminate this problem.[5]

Hyperextension of the knee, secondary to frequent equinus positioning of the foot, can contribute to the tendency for patellar subluxation. Hamstrings strengthening and working on centering body weight, especially during demi-pointe and pointe, will decrease the tendency toward hyperextension of the knee.

Medial Knee Strain

Medial capsular knee strain is seen predominantly in poorly trained ballet dancers, either children or adult beginners.[29] It presents as pain along the medial side of the knee with no history of specific injury. Pain is usually worse after class and gradually decreases if there is a day or two hiatus between ballet classes. There is no history of swelling or locking. Physical examination often reveals tenderness along the medial aspect of the knee but not specifically over the joint line. No effusion is present. Meniscal signs are lacking. One can confirm the suspicion of medial knee strain by asking the dancer to do a plié. If the positioning is inappropriate (Fig. 51-3), technique is quite likely the cause of this minor problem, and technical training is the best treatment.

Torn Meniscus

Meniscal tears occur in ballroom dancers when they turn on a fixed foot. The workup and treatment of this problem is no different in the dancer than in other athletes. During rehabilitation, special care must be given to achieving full range of motion and quadriceps strength.

Patellar Subluxation and Dislocation

Patellar subluxation and dislocation occur when initiating a turn or a jump associated with a turn

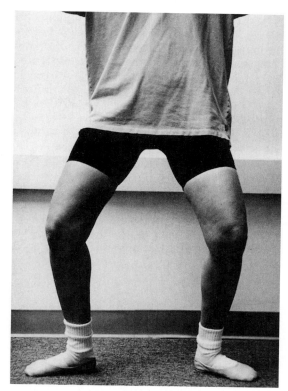

Figure 51-3. Inappropriate positioning, with the knees "inside" the feet, will cause strain on the medial capsule of the knee. Note that the feet face sideways while the knees face forward. Compare to the correct position shown in Figure 51–1B.

in midair. The torque necessary to start a turn comes from the foot pushing against the ground as the body begins to rotate.[15] Most dancers who have suffered a patellar dislocation will present as other athletes with this injury and should be evaluated for torn medial retinaculum, hemarthrosis, or osteochondral fractures, and treated accordingly. However, in dancers with marked ligamentous laxity, dislocation can occur without tearing the medial retinaculum. These dancers will report the knee "going out" but will not have much, if any, swelling or tenderness.

Proprioceptive training with tape is recommended to discourage hyperextension. Patellar restraining braces, though useful in providing additional support to the returning athlete, can be used by the dancer during class or rehearsal but usually cannot be worn in performance.

Anterior Cruciate Ligament Tears

Anterior cruciate ligaments (ACLs) are rarely injured in female dancers as a result of dance. However, special considerations pertain when treating ACL injuries in professional dancers. They cannot wear functional knee braces during performance. In addition, they require full extension of the knee both for stability and for aesthetic reasons. A loss of 5° to 10° of knee extension following ligament reconstruction procedures is incompatible with a career in dance. Dancers with a torn ACL have a difficult time turning as well as landing jumps. Furthermore, with regard to donor tendon, patellar tendon is not as good a choice as hamstring because of the increased incidence of patellofemoral problems afterward and the great demands on the patellofemoral joint in dancers. Despite muscular strengthening and reconstruction of a torn ACL, often the knee is perceived as less stable than before, perhaps because of the lack of proprioceptive input from the reconstructed ligament. For all these reasons, in a professional dancer, ACL injury may be the end of her career.

Foot and Ankle Injuries

Achilles Tendonitis

Achilles tendonitis is particularly common in all forms of aerobic dance. Failure to put the heel on the floor or bench, particularly when landing or stepping on and off the bench, overuses the Achilles tendon in both concentric and eccentric modes.

Anterior Ankle Impingement

Anterior ankle impingement presents as anterior pain during extreme ankle dorsiflexion, most commonly while landing a jump. The pain results from impingement of the anterior capsule and synovium. Occasionally these structures are pinched by an exostosis on the anterior talar neck, the tibial plafond, or both.[13] On physical examination one finds decreased and painful dorsiflexion of the ankle, and tenderness to palpation over the anterior joint line. Roentgenograms may reveal tibial or talar exostoses.

Treatment consists of temporary restriction of dorsiflexion, jumping, and deep pliés. A heel lift in street shoes is helpful. One can also use ice-friction massage and anti-inflammatory modalities. However, when an exostosis is present, symptoms will not usually resolve unless that exostosis is removed. This can be done through a small anterior approach medial to the tibialis anterior tendon. Arthroscopic excisions also have been described.[10]

Posterior Ankle Impingement

Posterior ankle impingement is a problem in ballet dancers. It presents as pain deep to the Achilles tendon during extreme ankle plantar flexion, particularly during relevé (heel raises) and especially en pointe (standing on the tips of one's toes). The pain results from impingement of the posterior capsule and synovium between the posterior lip of the tibia and the posterior tubercle of the talus or an os trigonum.[7] Physical examination will reveal decreased and painful plantar flexion, and tenderness posterolaterally deep to the Achilles tendon. A lateral roentgenograph of the foot taken with the ankle in maximal plantar flexion will often reveal a long posterior talar tubercle or os trigonum making contact with the posterior lip of the tibia. To decrease any swelling in the posterior synovium, one should restrict pointe and plantar flexion, use ice-friction massage and anti-inflammatory medication and modalities. In the professional dancer a surgical exostectomy may be required. Both medial and lateral surgical approaches have been described.[16]

Tendinitis About the Ankle

Peroneal and posterior tibial tendinitis are seen more often in the inexperienced student ballet dancer who, because of inadequate strength in both her trunk and lower extremities, is often poorly positioned in relevé.[8] Posterior tibial tendinitis also results from being en pointe on a short first toe. Treatment consists of anti-inflammatory medication and modalities, correcting inappropriate positioning, and using toe caps where necessary to equalize toe length. Tendinitis of the flexor hallucis longus can present as trigger toe. Tenosynovitis and nodules on the flexor hallucis longus tendon can produce catching of the interphalangeal joint of the flexed great toe such that it must be extended manually and does so with a sudden snap. Treatment consists of anti-inflammatory medication and modalities. Injection is not recommended. If conservative measures are not successful, surgical release of the tendon sheath is recommended.

Foot Problems

In ballet dancers, stress fractures commonly occur at the base of the metatarsal rather than in the metatarsal neck.[18] This may be related to the frequency of ballet dancers' positioning on the balls of their feet (demi-pointe) or on their toes (pointe) creating unusual stresses in the mid part of the foot.

Bunions and hallux rigidus are especially common in ballet dancers who have been en pointe.[21] Hallux rigidus is incompatible with dancing. These conditions, in part, may be related to shoe wear, toe lengths, and positioning of the trunk and feet.[30] For girls planning to dance in "pointe" shoes, the first 2 toes should be the same length. Toe caps or specially made orthoses can be placed in the box of the pointe shoe to even out toe lengths.

REHABILITATION PRINCIPLES

When rehabilitating the injured dancer, identifying and changing the factors that may have contributed to an overuse injury not only helps treat the problem, but also prevents recurrence. Dancers benefit from proprioceptive neuromuscular facilitation and visualization (ideokinesis) techniques that they learn easily.[26,27] When modifications to shoe wear are indicated, small felt pieces can be taped to the foot in place of orthoses. During the rehabilitation period, when possible, the dancer should be kept in class, restricting only those movements that may exacerbate the injury. This allows the dancer to stay conditioned, and to keep up with the choreography.

Ballet dancers can begin by practicing the usual sequence of barre exercises lying supine on the floor or by using a Pilates Reformer. The elimination of gravity allows concentration on appropriate muscle use. Once back in the dance studio, barre work only is begun. Movement to the center floor is gradual, without turns or jumps, with one at a time added when strength and range of motion are normal. For aerobic dancers, one can start with aqua aerobics, then step and finally low-impact or traditional aerobics. Ballroom, jazz, and folk dancers can initially "mark" steps (do them in place without any jumping or turning.)

CONCLUDING REMARKS

Dancers have many of the same injuries as other athletes. Understanding the dance-specific causes of these injuries as well as the requirements of the dance discipline allows the health care provider the best opportunity for success when treating an injured dancer.

References

1. Abraham SF, et al: Body weight, exercise and menstrual status among ballet dancers in training. Br J Obstet Gynaecol 89:507–10, 1982.
2. Belt C: Injuries associated with aerobic dance. Am Fam Physician 41:1769–72, 1990.
3. Benson JE, Geiger CJ, Eiserman PA, et al: Relationship between nutrient intake, body mass index, menstrual function, and ballet injuries. J Am Diet Assoc 89:58–63, 1989.
4. Brooks-Gunn J, Warren MP, Hamilton LH: The relation of eating problems and amenorrhea in ballet dancers. Med Sci Sports Exerc 19:41–4, 1987.
5. Clippinger-Robertson KS, Hutton RS, Miller DI, et al: Mechanical and anatomical factors relating to the incidence and etiology of patellofemoral pain in dancers. In: Shell CG (ed): The Dancer as Athlete. Olympic Scientific Congress Proceedings. Champaign, Ill, Human Kinetics Publishers, 1986, pp 53–72.
6. Garrick JG, Gillien DM, Whiteside P: The epidemiology of aerobic dance injuries. Am J Sports Med 14:67–72, 1986.
7. Hamilton WG: Stenosing tenosynovitis of the flexor hallucis longus tendon and posterior impingement upon the os trigonum in ballet dancers. Foot Ankle 3:74–81, 1982.
8. Hamilton WG: Tendinitis about the ankle joint in classical ballet dancers. Am J Sports Med 5:84–8, 1977.
9. Hickey M, Hager CA: Aerobic dance injuries. Orthop Nurs 13:9–12, 1994.
10. Jaivin JS, Ferkel RD: Arthroscopy of the foot and ankle. Clin Sports Med 3(4):761–81, 1994.
11. Kadel NJ, Teitz CC: Stress fractures in ballet dancers. Am J Sports Med 20:445–9, 1992.
12. Kirkendall DT, Calabrese LH: Physiological aspects of dance. Clin Sports Med 2:525–37, 1983.
13. Kleiger B: A tibiotalar impingement syndrome in dancers. Foot Ankle 3:69–73, 1982.
14. Klemp P, Stevens JE, Isaacs S: A hypermobility study in ballet dancers. J Rheumatol 11:692–6, 1984.
15. Laws K: The Physics of Dance. New York, Schirmer, 1984.
16. Marotta JJ, Micheli LJ: Os trigonum impingement in dancers. Am J Sports Med 20(5):533–6, 1992.
17. Micheli LJ: Overuse injuries in children's sports. Orthop Clin North Am 14:337, 1983.
18. Micheli LJ, Sohn RF, Solomon R: Stress fractures of the second metatarsal involving Lisfranc's joint in ballet dancers. J Bone Joint Surg 67A:1372–5, 1985.
19. Quirk R: Ballet injuries. The Australian experience. Clin Sports Med 2:507–14, 1983.
20. Rovere GD, Webb LX, Gristina AG, et al: Musculoskeletal injuries in theatrical dance students. Am J Sports Med 11:195–9, 1983.
21. Sammarco GJ, Miller EH: Forefoot conditions in dancers—part I. Foot Ankle 3:85–92, 1982.
22. Schaberg JE, Harper MC, Allan WC: The snapping hip syndrome. Am J Sports Med 12:361–5, 1984.
23. Seals JG: A study of dance surfaces. Clin Sports Med 2:557–61, 1983.
24. Solomon RL: In search of more efficient dance training. In: Solomon RL, Minton SC, Solomon J (eds): Preventing Dance Injuries, An Interdisciplinary Perspective. Reston, Va, American Alliance for Health, Physical Education, Recreation, and Dance, 1990, pp 191–222.
25. Solomon RL, Micheli LJ: Technique as a consideration in modern dance injuries. Physician Sportsmed 14:83–92, 1986.
26. Sweigard LE: Human Movement Potential: Its Ideokinetic Facilitation. New York, Harper & Row, 1974.
27. Teitz CC: Dance. In Griffin LY (ed): Rehabilitation of the Injured Knee. St Louis, CV Mosby, 1995, pp 274–82.

28. Teitz CC: Knee Problems in Dancers. In: Solomon RL, Minton SC, Solomon J (eds): Preventing Dance Injuries, An Interdisciplinary Perspective. Reston, Va, American Alliance for Health, Physical Education, Recreation, and Dance, 1990, pp 39–73.

29. Teitz CC: Sports medicine concerns in dance and gymnastics. Pediatr Clin North Am 29:1399–421, 1982.

30. Teitz CC, Harrington RM, Wiley H: Pressures on the foot in pointe shoes. Foot Ankle 5:216–21, 1985.

31. Trepman E, Walaszek A, Micheli LJ: Spinal problems in the dancer. In: Solomon RL, Minton SC, Solomon J (eds): Preventing Dance Injuries, An Interdisciplinary Perspective. Reston, Va, American Alliance for Health, Physical Education, Recreation, and Dance, 1990, 103–31.

32. Vaganova A: Basic Principles of Classical Ballet. New York, Dover, 1969.

33. Warren MP, Brooks-Gunn J, Hamilton LH, et al: Scoliosis and fractures in young ballet dancers: Relation to delayed menarche and secondary amenorrhea. N Engl J Med 314:1348–53, 1986.

34. Washington EL: Musculoskeletal injuries in theatrical dancers: site, frequency, and severity. Am J Sports Med 6:75–98, 1978.

35. Wolman RL, Clark P, McNally E, et al: Menstrual state and exercise as determinants of spinal trabecular bone density in female athletes. Br Med J 301:516–8, 1990.

Chapter 52

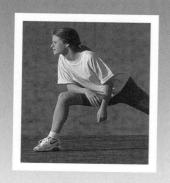

Equestrian

J. W. Thomas Byrd, M.D.

"If the world were a logical place, men would ride side saddle."

Rita Mae Brown
U.S. Polo Association Player

Equestrian competition is unique in the sports world. It is a team sport comprising of members from 2 different species (Fig. 52-1). Additionally, it is a sport in which men and women compete as equals. This is reflected by the fact that it is the only Olympic sport in which gender identity testing of the athletes is not mandatory.

The horse has been an integral part of America's heritage as well as mankind's climb through civilization. However, since the industrial revolution, the importance of the horse, once essential for military, industrial, and transportation purposes, has sharply declined. Still, the horse's role in recreational pursuits and the competitive arena has persisted and continues to occupy a prominent place in the modern-day sports world.

While historically, military and industrial purposes of the horse were strongly male dominated; currently, women maintain a majority role at almost every level of equestrian competition (Table 52-1).[35]

Probably nowhere are the challenges, contrasts, and paradoxes of both the female equestrian and sports injuries more clearly highlighted than in combined training. This includes dressage, cross-country, and stadium jumping (Fig. 52-2). In the discipline of dressage, the horse and rider perform a number of intricate maneuvers in an arena, challenging the horse's training and responsive skills; the performance, in some respects, is analogous to the compulsory phase

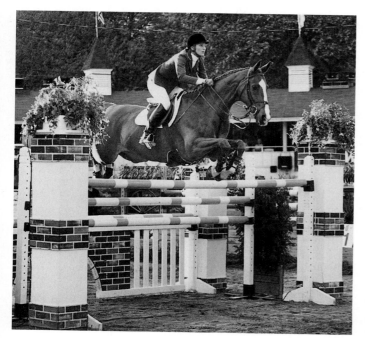

Figure 52-1. An equestrienne and her mount compete in Grand Prix Show Jumping. A team sport comprising members of 2 different species, they are intimately dependent upon one another for success as well as safety. (Courtesy of Pennington Galleries.)

Table 52-1. 1992–1993 Female Participation in Horse Organizations

	TOTAL MEMBERSHIP	TOTAL FEMALE	% FEMALE
Sanctioning Organizations			
American Horse Shows Association	58,000	47,560	82
American Quarter Horse Association	288,000	149,760	52
Breed Organizations			
American Morgan Horse Association	10,971	7131	65
American Paint Horse Association	35,108	17,905	51
American Saddlebred Horse Association	6182	4018	65
American Warmblood Society	268	214	80
Appaloosa Horse Club	24,375	12,188	50
International Arabian Horse Association	30,000	22,500	75
Palomino Horse Breeders of America	7618	4190	55
Other Organizations			
United States Dressage Federation	30,000	24,000	80
United States Combined Training Association	10,200	6630	65
Women's Pro Rodeo Association	1600	1600	100
American Vaulting Association	1256	678	54
International Hunter Futurity	1200	720	60
National Steeplechase & Hunt Association	1200	396	33
American Endurance Ride Conference	3870	2941	76
American Driving Society	2400	1200	50
The Carriage Association of America	3500	1400	40
International Side Saddle Organization	650	650	100
Youth Organizations/Division			
American Quarter Horse Association	26,000	20,540	79
American Morgan Horse Association	1668	1418	85
Appaloosa Horse Club	3211	1927	60
United States Pony Clubs	10,834	10,292	95
National 4-H	5,500,000	2,915,000	53
Intercollegiate Horse Show Association	4400	3740	85

From Racing Resource Group, Inc., P. O. Box 20069, Alexandria, Va, 22320, with permission.

in ice skating. The cross-country course requires the team to clear a number of challenging obstacles over variable terrain, testing both courage and strength. The final phase is stadium jumping, a more familiar sport because of its popular spectator format.

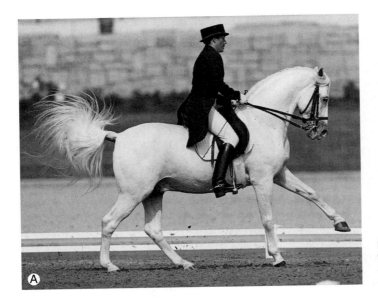

Figure 52-2. Combined training exemplifies the heterogenous nature of both the demands and the risks of equestrian disciplines. **A**, Dressage.

Illustration continued on following page

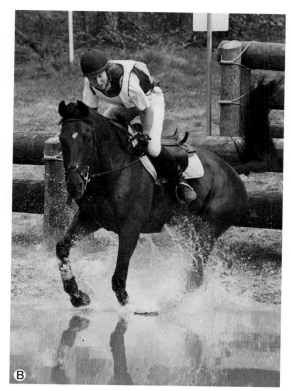

Figure 52-2 (*Continued*). **B,** Cross-country.

in this competition. Only then did women begin to establish their place in the sport, now representing a predominance of participants. As the Olympic sport in which gender is not an issue, both women and men alike are challenged by the spectrum of demands (and risks) ranging from the grace and charm of dressage, to the strength and courage of cross-country.

IMPLICATIONS OF GENDER-SPECIFIC ANATOMIC VARIATIONS

Historical teachings based on a male-dominated activity continue to influence current riding instruction where female participation prevails. This creates many potential sources for problems if not accounting for the musculoskeletal variations between men and women.[10]

Proper riding technique, as well as judging, during competition is often based on appearance, especially an upright, nonslouched posture. However, a properly balanced position for women can produce an entirely different outward appearance of posture because of the unique bony architecture of the female pelvis and lumbosacral spine. In this respect, based on outward appearances, form does not follow function.

Proportionate to the rest of her body, the female has a broader pelvis (Fig. 52-3). While this may superficially appear beneficial in straddling a horse, her unique pelvic construct influences the sitting position and, secondarily, the relationship of the torso. For example, the ischia, where weight is borne in the seated posi-

The origins of combined training are strongly seated in military heritage. Each of the disciplines tests a different necessary quality attributed to a good cavalry officer and his mount.

As cavalry units became obsolete, with an especially sharp decline following World War II, civilian participants began to recognize success

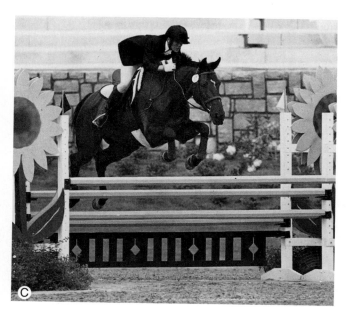

Figure 52-2 (*Continued*). **C,** Show jumping. (Courtesy of Pennington Galleries.)

MALE PELVIS

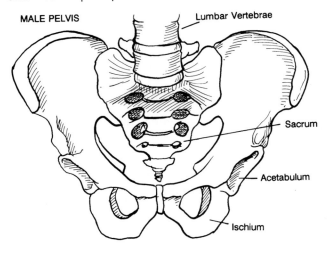

Lumbar Vertebrae

Sacrum

Acetabulum

Ischium

Figure 52-3. Front views of the bony pelvis highlight the distinguishing characteristics between the male and female architecture. These differences are prefaced on the need for a wide birth canal in the female to accommodate the passage of the head of the fetus, which is proportionately much larger than that of most mammals.

FEMALE PELVIS

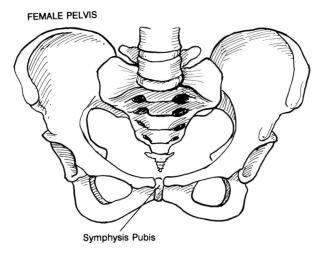

Symphysis Pubis

tion, are oriented more parallel in the male, allowing the ability to rock back and forth in the saddle more easily (Fig. 52-4). In the female pelvis, the ischia are oriented more obliquely and tend to cause the pelvis to rest with the pubis bone in a more downward position in what would be called an extended position of the pelvis (Fig. 52-4).

Pelvic extension inherently causes lumbar lordosis to maintain the center of gravity over the hips. Additionally, the relationship of the sacrum to the pelvis is oriented more horizontally and the lumbosacral articulation more obliquely in the female, further accentuating lumbar lordosis (Fig. 52-5).

These factors accentuate several differences in the outward appearance of the seated position between the male and female. First of all, the male can maintain a relatively flat back appearance, which is much more difficult for the female to achieve when the pelvis tends to rest in extension. Secondly, the female may tend to round the shoulders, flexing the upper thoracic

area to compensate for her increased lumbar lordosis. If this is misinterpreted as slouching, attempts to extend the spine will only accentuate the already excessive lumbar lordosis.

The lower center of gravity for the female does offer a modest advantage over her male counterpart, but there are many other interrelated variations of the female structure that will alter the outward appearance so often used in judging and instruction. For example, the wider pelvis necessitates a more valgus position at the knee to keep the mechanical axis centered under the body. These factors will have an effect on appearance when riding.

The significance of this is an awareness of the differences in riding technique between males and females. The dilemma has been heightened by a male-dominated influence in a sport that has recently become more female oriented.

Chronic low back pain is a frequent affliction of the equestrian. This is especially true for the female as a result of the position of the pelvis and lumbosacral spine assumed in horseback

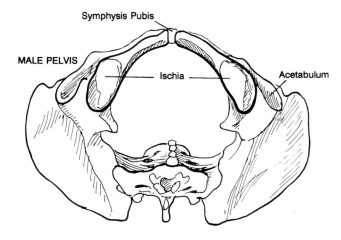

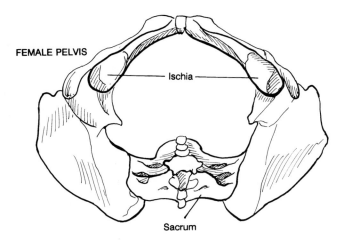

Figure 52-4. Viewed from below, the ischia are oriented more obliquely in the female, making it more difficult to rock back and forth in the seated position. In fact, this orientation causes the pelvis to rest with the pubis more downward in an extended position, necessitating a compensatory hyperlordosis of the lumbar spine.

riding. This condition may be readily accentuated when instructors try to apply male ideals of posturing to the female anatomy.

RIDING DURING PREGNANCY

There is very little scientific evidence to support the benefits of exercise during pregnancy or to define the physiologic risks to the mother and fetus.[7,21,29] Thus, any recommendations are made with a limited fund of knowledge and are usually based on empiric observation or a commonsense approach.

The decision to ride during pregnancy is to be made by the woman and her obstetrician. This requires that a proper examination be performed as well as routine follow-up to monitor any potential untoward effects of the exercise routine.[7] Any number of obstetric risk factors or other concerns may influence the decision not to ride.[2]

Novice or beginner riders should not ride during pregnancy. However, experienced riders

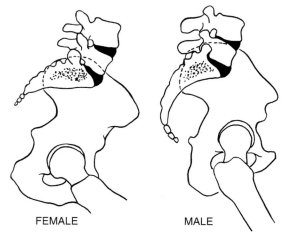

Figure 52-5. A line drawing from lateral roentgenograms of male and female pelves obtained with the subjects seated astride in a proper balanced seat position. In the female, the sacrum is foreshortened and oriented more horizontal relative to the rest of the pelvis, another accommodation to widen the birth canal. Consequently, the lumbosacral articulation has a more oblique angle, making it more susceptible to stresses on the lumbosacral joint. Additionally, the position of the female pelvis necessitates a greater degree of lumbar lordosis. (Courtesy of Deb Bennett, PhD., Equine Studies Institute, www.equinestudies.org.)

without other factors that represent a high-risk pregnancy may seek advice on how to continue a riding routine.

The biggest concern with riding during pregnancy is the risk of bodily injury, which is always a concern of any equestrian activity. Added to this is the risk of blunt or penetrating abdominal trauma to the uterus and fetus.[21] As enlargement occurs, this risk is heightened and thus riding should be discouraged or more significantly modified after the 16th week of pregnancy.

The enlarging uterus also accentuates lumbar lordosis, which is already problematic for the female equestrian.[2,29] Combined with breast enlargement, the center of gravity is altered and has an adverse effect on balance, which can further increase risk of injury because of a greater possibility of falling.

By the 8th week of gestation, the hormone relaxin has begun to induce softening of the connective tissues.[7,29] The effect is most apparent in the pelvis with increased mobility of the joints. The effect can result in increased pelvic discomfort as well as possibly a greater risk of ligamentous injury.

Pain and bleeding represent only a few of the recognized warning signs for immediate discontinuation of exercise, including horseback riding.[2] One of the greatest risks to the mother is musculoskeletal injury, while risks to the fetus include abruption of the placenta.[7]

If a woman chooses to ride during pregnancy, it is important to take all the normal precautions, including protective headgear and demonstrating modified intensity as gestation progresses. A commonsense approach is also important, not taking any unnecessary risks in either the activities that she chooses to participate in, or the mounts that she chooses to ride. Vigorous competition is probably contraindicated.[21]

OSTEOPOROSIS AND HORSEBACK RIDING

It is important to address the implications of osteoporosis in equestrian activities for several reasons. First of all, women are especially susceptible to the development of osteoporosis. Age is also a major variable in the development of osteoporosis. Since many women ride and riding is an activity that can be enjoyed through later years, osteoporosis needs to be given specific attention.

The biggest concern with osteoporosis is the increased risk of fracture as osteoporosis is implicated in approximately 1.5 million fractures each year.[1] Fractures also represent a sometimes serious type of equestrian injury, accounting for approximately 30% of injuries that require emergency department attention.[30] Consequently, the concern of this combination, osteoporosis and horseback riding, is further magnified.

Osteopenia refers to reduced bone density. Osteoporosis is but one form of osteopenia due to a reduced quantity of bone. The bone that is present is of normal quality, but it is simply present in reduced amounts.

A number of risk factors are known to be associated with the development of osteoporosis, including advanced age, female gender, estrogen deficiency, thin body habitus, heredity, and white and Asian races. Lifestyle risk factors include smoking, excessive alcohol intake, physical inactivity, excessive caffeine consumption, inadequate calcium intake, poor nutrition, and chronic illness. Osteoporosis has also been associated with certain disease states and drugs such as corticosteroids.

Although osteoporosis will occur in all people as they age, its rate of progression and effects can be modified with proper early diagnosis and treatment. The best form of management is prevention. Prevention and early management both require an awareness of the potential presence of osteoporosis. Unfortunately, osteoporosis is usually diagnosed only once a fracture has occurred. Although osteoporosis can be treated to reduce further bone loss, there are no proven methods of restoring lost bone. As quoted by my former Chief of Orthopaedics, James Harkess, "Bone density is much like virginity. Once it's lost, you never truly get it back."[27]

Thus, when significant risk factors are present, especially for the female with a recognized cause of estrogen deficiency, a physician should be consulted for an appropriate evaluation and recommendations. The implications of osteoporosis should be clearly recognized by those participating in equestrian activities, especially with regard to the risks of fracture, which can even occur spontaneously in association with severe osteoporosis.

However, awareness and prevention go beyond just those with recognized risk factors. Peak bone density occurs at the completion of longitudinal growth between the second and third decades. Small gains in bone mass may occur following completion of growth, but cease by age 30.[38] Attainment of peak density and subsequent maintenance of skeletal mass is most influenced by adequate dietary intake, exercise and a lifestyle emphasizing minimal alcohol and caffeine intake and avoidance of smoking.

HORSEBACK RIDING INJURIES

Interpreting injury data in horseback riding is difficult. Equestrian competition encompasses a very heterogenous population of activities. For example, falling from a horse, which may be a prelude to injury, is not an infrequent occurrence in steeplechasing, but ranges from uncommon in dressage, to unavoidable in rodeo. While it is therefore difficult to accurately ascribe risks in these defined areas, these do not even represent the environment where the majority of injuries occur. Most injuries, and perhaps the greatest risk of injury per exposure, occur in leisure riding or working activities. In these settings, while the numerator may be defined by injuries that occur requiring medical attention, the denominator of the number of people and hours of exposure in these activities is much less clear. Estimates of the number of participants in horseback riding activities in the United States range from 27,000,000 to 82,000,000, a greater than 3-fold discrepancy.[23,26]

Horseback riding ranks 13th in activities causing injury that require emergency room attention in the United States.[30] However, if an accident occurs, it is more likely to be severe, possibly leaving permanent injury or causing death.[8,20,28,31,37]

The possibility of injury cannot be completely eliminated. However, recently, studies of these accidents have suggested that prevention or reduction in the severity of injury is possible.[12–14,32]

Risk Factors

Some risk of injury will always exist in equestrian activities. The horse and rider are intimately dependent upon one another for safety as well as performance.

The horse typically outweighs the human by a thousand pounds or more. This is an animal that is powerfully influenced by the basic instincts of fright and flight. He exhibits a good memory, but poor reasoning. There is no such thing as a safe horse. Even a seemingly quiet animal can be spooked.

The rider is delicately balanced in unstable equilibrium over the horse's center of gravity. This balance is tenuously maintained by grip from the knees and thighs and using the stirrups as outriggers.

Horses are capable of reaching speeds of 35 to 40 miles/hour. The rider's head is typically carried approximately 9 feet off the ground. This combination of height and speed results in considerable forces that can be generated during a fall, potentially resulting in injury. Added to this are the variable surfaces that can be struck, including rocks, rails, and tree limbs.

Becker's principle states that the risk of head and neck injury in a sport is proportionate to the degree of head-forward stance adopted.[18] Although this is not unique to equestrian pursuits, perhaps nowhere is this more clearly exemplified than in many equestrian activities (Fig. 52-6).

As the jockey falls with the arms outstretched, she keeps her hands turned in. This forces the elbows to remain slightly flexed, softening the impact (Fig. 52-7). If the hands are turned outward, the elbows can lock in extension with more violent impact, resulting in a much greater risk of supracondylar fracture of the elbow or other fractures of the forearm, humerus, or shoulder. As the fall progresses, the jockey tends to duck, curl, and roll (Fig. 52-8). This serves 2 purposes. It dissipates the energy of the impact and makes the rider a smaller target for the hooves of following horses (Fig. 52-9).

As a consequence of this duck, curl, and roll mechanism, axial loading of the cervical spine is rarely a mechanism of injury. More common is the risk of flexion injury (Fig. 52-10), which carries with it a significant risk of neurologic deficit.

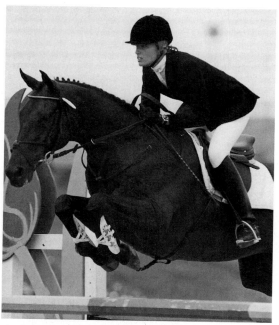

Figure 52-6. Becker's principle states that "the risk of head and neck injury in a sport is proportionate to the degree of head-forward stance adopted." This is frequently demonstrated in horseback riding. (Courtesy of Pennington Galleries.)

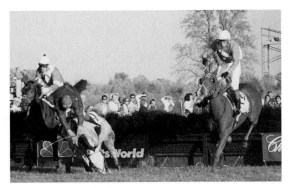

Figure 52-7. Photograph of a fall demonstrating that, as the jockey's arms are outstretched in front of her, the hands are turned inward, which keeps the elbows slightly flexed, lessening the impact. (Courtesy of Catherine French.)

Hyperextension injuries are much less common (Fig. 52-11), but tend to be more stable.

Another potentially devastating injury is the flexion injury to the thoracolumbar junction,

which carries with it a significant associated risk of neurologic injury, especially paraplegia (Fig. 52-12). This occurs from a fall, landing in the seated position with the torso forcibly flexed forward. Women may be more susceptible to this type of injury because of their lower center of gravity, while men are more susceptible to cervical and upper extremity injuries.

Working around horses introduces some potential for injury, especially if not respecting routine precautions. Firth has calculated that the kick from a horse's hoof can generate greater than 10 kilonewtons (1 ton) of force, representing considerable destructive power (Fig. 52-13).[24] Being butted by the head of a horse is also a potential source of facial trauma.

Brooks reviewed 83 horse-related central nervous system injuries, including 72 cranial and 11 spinal injuries.[18] Amongst this group, there were 7 fatalities. Twenty-two (26.5%) of the injuries occurred while the rider was

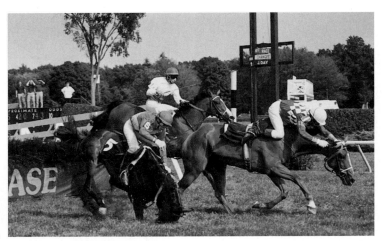

A

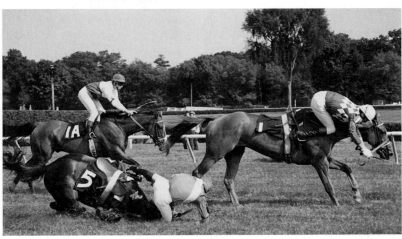

B

Figure 52-8. A & **B**, Serial photographs demonstrate the duck, curl, and roll maneuver adopted by jockeys. This serves 2 purposes: it dissipates the energy of the impact and makes the rider a smaller target for the hooves of following horses. (Courtesy of Catherine French.)

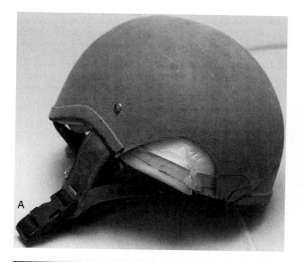

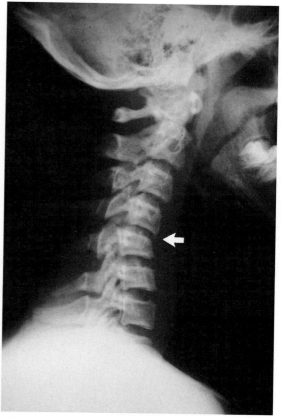

Figure 52-10. A forced flexion mechanism to the cervical spine in a horseback riding accident caused this C4/5 injury (arrow), which resulted in quadriplegia.

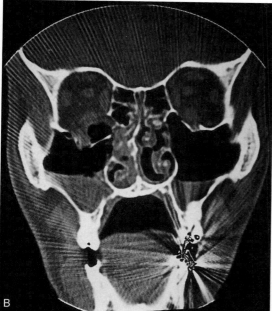

Figure 52-9. A, A helmet that meets the ASTM standards worn by a jockey trampled after a fall. The missing section of the helmet corresponds to the horse's hoof over the right brow and reflects that, while these types of helmets can lessen the severity of injuries, they will not prevent them. **B,** Facial CT scan reveals the bilateral orbital blowout and zygomatic arch fractures suffered from the blow.

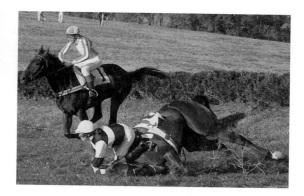

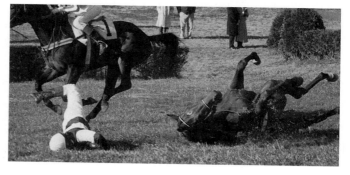

Figure 52-11. Serial photographs demonstrating a jockey's fall. The hands are late releasing from the reins and, thus, the arms never get out in front to initiate the duck, curl, and roll mechanism. Landing face first, the cervical spine is forced into hyperextension, but no major injury occurred. (Courtesy of Catherine French.)

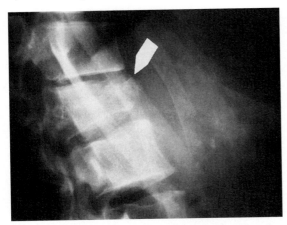

Figure 52-12. Fracture at the thoracolumbar junction (*arrow*) occurred when a rider was thrown, landing forcibly in the seated position. Paraplegia resulted.

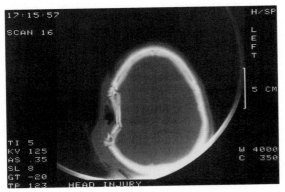

Figure 52-13. CT scan of the skull following a kick from a horse. No protective headgear was worn, and the blow was fatal.

unmounted (all cranial). Among the 61 injuries that occurred with the rider mounted, only 22 (36.0%) were wearing helmets. All spinal injuries occurred from a fall. Twenty-three (27.7%) of the 83 cases were legally intoxicated with a blood ethanol level greater than 0.1. Also of the 83, only 20 (24.1%) occurred during some form of organized competition.

With regard to risk factors, these data emphasize that: (1) a significant number of injuries (approximately 25%) occur unmounted; (2) of those that were mounted, most (approximately 33%) were not wearing helmets; (3) alcohol was a significant factor in over 25% of the injuries; and (4) less than 25% occurred during some form of organized competition.

Epidemiology

Mechanism of Injury

Approximately 84% of horse-related injuries occur in mounted situations, with the remaining

Table 52-2. Common Injuries in Equestrian Competition

BODY PART INJURED (1993–1994)		
Lower trunk	20,210	14.46%
Head	15,844	11.34%
Upper trunk	13,733	9.83%
Wrist	10,668	7.63%
Shoulder	10,228	7.32%
Ankle	7848	5.62%
Finger	7113	5.09%
Face	7070	5.06%
Lower arm	6742	4.82%
Lower leg	6412	4.59%
Foot	5901	4.22%
Knee	4893	3.50%
Hand	3781	2.71%
Elbow	3569	2.55%
Neck	3484	2.49%
Upper leg	3247	2.32%
Upper arm	2495	1.79%
25% to 50% body	1803	1.29%
Toe	1369	0.98%
Mouth	923	0.66%
Pubic region	904	0.65%
All parts body	733	0.52%
Eyeball	327	0.23%
Unknown	248	0.18%
Ear	219	0.16%
Total	139,764	100.00%

TYPE OF INJURY (1993–1994)		
Contusion/abrasion	42,382	30.95%
Fracture	40,131	29.30%
Strain/sprain	23,207	16.95%
Laceration	11,636	8.50%
Other	4983	3.64%
Concussion	4908	3.58%
Internal injury	2824	2.06%
Hematoma	1838	1.34%
Dislocation	1614	1.18%
Foreign body	914	0.67%
Unknown	694	0.51%
Amputation	379	0.28%
Puncture	356	0.26%
Avulsion	313	0.23%
Nerve damage	224	0.16%
Dental	224	0.16%
Crushing	149	0.11%
Derma/conjunct	115	0.08%
Burn	59	0.04%
Hemorrhage	0	0.00%
Submersion	0	0.00%
Radiation	0	0.00%
Poisoning	0	0.00%
Total	136,950	100.00%

Data from the National Electronic Injury Surveillance System (NEISS), US Consumer Product Safety Commission, National Injury Information Clearing House, Washington, DC.

16% occurring in horse management (loading, saddling, grooming, feeding, cleaning the stall, veterinary care, hoof care, and shoeing).[14] Most mounted accidents result from a fall from the horse. Injuries on the ground usually occur from being kicked by the horse, although trampling and crushing are also causative factors.

Type of Injury

In order of decreasing frequency, the most common injuries are bruises or abrasions, fractures, strains/sprains, lacerations, and concussions (Table 52-2).[30]

Body Part

The most common area of the body to be injured is collectively the upper extremity, followed by the trunk, lower extremity, and head/face (Table 52-2).[30] However, the most common cause of death is head injury (60% to 78%), followed by chest and abdominal injuries.[17,22]

Gender

According to several studies, females have proportionately more injuries than males.[11,14,15,20,37] It is possible that the greater strength of the male is an advantage in lessening the likelihood of injury. However, more deaths occur in the male population, which may suggest the risks that this group is willing to take compared to their female counterparts.[7,28,34] Interestingly, head injury as a cause of death is more prevalent in the female group.[17,22]

Age

Approximately 53% of injuries occur to riders less than 25 years of age.[30] Injuries to older riders tend to be more severe and more likely to cause death.

Location

Up to 98% of accidents have been reported to occur in leisure riding.[33] In Gleave's study, hacking is the activity implicated in 80% of injuries, while according to Whitlock's work, only 25% of injuries occurred during some type of organized competition.[25,39]

Treatment

The majority of injuries that require treatment are evaluated in emergency departments. In a survey of riders who sought medical treatment, treatment was administered in an emergency room (48%), in hospital with admission (29%), in a doctor's office (20%), and in a first-aid station (3%).[3]

Disability

Reflecting the severity of horse-related injuries, approximately 15% of riders reported permanent disability from horse-related accidents.[4] *Concussion* is defined as a momentary loss of memory, confusion or disorientation, as well as loss of consciousness. However, we now know that the results of repeated head injuries with concussion are cumulative, resulting in personality changes, decreased speed in problem-solving, loss of memory, impaired judgment, and distractibility.[36]

Death

The most common cause of death is head injury (60% to 78%), followed by multiple injuries (15%) frequently caused by catching the foot in the stirrup and being dragged by the horse.[17,22]

Protective Equipment

Protective Headgear

Proper protective headgear is an essential piece of equipment in all equestrian activities. There is no such thing as a safe horse, a safe environment, or a safe activity where headgear is not necessary.

Studies have shown that head injuries can be prevented or their severity reduced by wearing a properly constructed, fitted, and secured helmet.[14]

The current standards for equestrian protective headgear have been established by the American Society of Testing and Materials (ASTM) (Fig. 52-14).[5] Headgear that meets these standards is certified by the Safety Equipment Institute (SEI). The SEI seal is prominently displayed in all equipment that meets their certification.

The design of the helmet must incorporate several different parameters. It must be lightweight and comfortable, but also must be cosmetic in appearance to satisfy the traditional aspects of the equestrian world. Its outer shell must protect against penetrating blows and be round in shape to turn direct blows into glancing blows. The contour needs to protect the vulnerable areas of the skull without hindering mobility or obstructing vision. The liner serves to cushion the brain and there must be a harness assembly sufficient to prevent the helmet from being dislodged during a fall.

In addition to the design criteria, the helmet must be properly fitted to the rider.

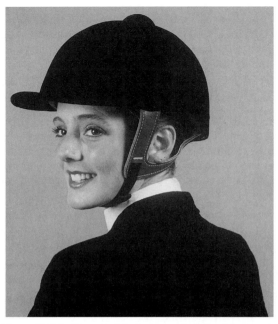

Figure 52-14. Characteristic features of a helmet that meets the standards established by the ASTM: lightweight and comfortable; cosmetic in appearance; outer shell to protect against penetrating blows; round shape to turn direct blows into glancing blows; contoured to protect the vulnerable areas of the skull; does not hinder mobility or obstruct vision; cushions the brain; harness assembly to prevent the helmet from being dislodged during a fall. (Courtesy of Lexington Safety Products.)

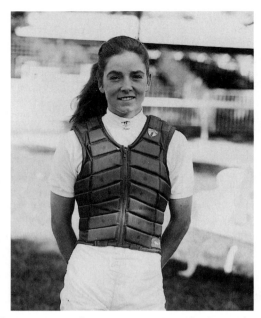

Figure 52-15. Body protectors are exceedingly popular in racing and jumping sports and are often mandatory, although little is known about their efficacy. (Courtesy of Cohen & Associates/Tipperary Sport Products.)

Protective Vests

Protective vests or "body protectors" are very popular, especially in equestrian disciplines where falls occur with some frequency, such as flat-track racing, steeplechasing, and combined training (Fig. 52-15). Despite their popularity, there is very little scientific evidence to accurately define how much protection is afforded by these vests.

There are currently no American standards for protective vests and no American manufacturers. Therefore, all vests presently being used are imported. The only standard currently in existence is that of the British Equestrian Trade Association (BETA) with guidance from Michael Whitlock, FRCS, one of Britain's most experienced jockey–physicians.[16] The materials from which these vests are constructed are tested in a laboratory by dropping a weighted object from a fixed height and measuring the dissipation of the impact by the material. There are currently 2 minimum standards, the BETA 5 (Blue Label) and the more recent BETA 7 (Red Label) which yields a higher level of protection. These standards test only the materials and not the construction of the vest other than to say that it must cover the torso and be properly fitted.

It appears that a properly constructed vest may offer some protection against direct blows and the type of injuries that a rider may expect from a contusion or possibly even a cracked rib.

Protective vests offer no protection against major spinal injuries, the most feared scenario because of permanent disability and paralysis. In fact, a poorly constructed vest might potentially heighten the likelihood of spinal injury. Also, placing excessive confidence in a vest could encourage a rider to take undue risks.

Prevention

In a national survey of riders, the order of most significant factors in rider safety were the experience of the rider; knowledge of the rider; training of the horse; and nature of the horse.[3] However, in a study of young riders, experience without knowledge increased the incidence of horse-related injuries. Experience may cause riders to attempt activities for which they are not qualified.

Horseback riders need appropriate training and education and must have guidance in the selection of their mounts. They then must demonstrate proficiency in these skills. This requires an instructor who emphasizes safety and should be certified through a nationally recognized organization such as the Horsemanship Safety Association, the American Riding Instructor Certification Program, the

Association for Horsemanship Safety and Education, or the United States Dressage Federation (Table 52-3).

Proper headgear is essential to all mounted situations. It must meet ASTM standards and be SEI certified. Additionally, it must be properly fitted to the rider and properly secured at all times. Observation of routine precautions in unmounted situations with horses is also important.

Riding equipment should be inspected regularly and replaced if worn. Saddles must fit snugly and the girth checked frequently to ensure that the saddle will not slip while riding. All riders should wear heeled, smooth-soled footwear with adequate ankle support and avoid loose fitting clothes that may catch on tree limbs or other objects while riding.

Injury Management

The key to any management opportunity is to emphasize injury prevention. However, injury occurrence cannot be avoided completely and appropriate preparations must be made for their assessment.

Most injuries occur not in the competitive arena, but in leisure, recreational, and working environments. This is difficult to regulate or prepare for, but certain steps can be taken.

A first-aid kit should be available in any barn, stable, or other area where horseback-riding activities occur. It should be equipped to handle the common types of injuries that may be seen. Additionally, a phone should be available. Affixed in a very visible location next to the phone should be a list of instructions. This should include where to call for emergency services and directions to your location so that whoever uses the phone can give this information.

For organized competitive events, injury management can be more comprehensive. This usually includes on-site physician and ambulance coverage with a plan to provide the most immediate assessment of injuries and adequate backup systems. Protocols have been developed by the American Medical Equestrian Association (AMEA) specifically for these purposes.[19]

Table 52-3. Rider Instructor Certification Programs

The Association for Horseman Safety and Education

American Riding Instructor Certification Program

Horsemanship Safety Association

United States Pony Clubs, Inc.

United States Dressage Federation

CONCLUDING REMARKS

The horse is an integral part of our heritage. We are witnessing the completion of a transition from its once important military and industrial uses to increasing popularity in recreational and competitive arenas. Accompanying this transition is its change from a male-dominated activity to one in which female involvement is predominant.

This shift in demographics has not come without some hardship for the female participant. The equestrian world is one steeped in tradition. We must be careful not to relearn Mark Twain's observation that "tradition is the logic of fools." Riding instruction is often based on historical concepts, and for women this may mean learning to ride like a man. This is accentuated in competition, where judging is often highly subjective, based on the qualities of proper posture of the rider.

The female body habitus is significantly different from that of the male. We are still learning how these variations may affect the optimal functional alignment when sitting astride a horse, which may produce a significantly different outward appearance of posture. A position that works best for a man, tried and true through centuries of evolution on horseback, may not necessarily apply to a woman. We know that the differences in body build influence both the acute and chronic injury patterns that occur.

Other unique female health issues that bear special attention in horseback riding include pregnancy and osteoporosis. Conversely, alcohol, a recognized factor in a significant number of severe injuries, knows no gender.

As has been stated, equestrian competition is unique in the sports world. It is a rare sport in which men and women compete as equals, and the only such Olympic sport. Additionally, it is a team sport comprising members from 2 different species. They are intimately dependent upon one another, both for success as well as safety.

Injury in this sport cannot be completely prevented. However, the risks can be minimized and the severity of injury lessened. This requires proper schooling in horsemanship skills, matching of the horse with the rider's ability, and use of proper equipment that is in good working order and properly fitted.

Most injuries do not occur during organized competition, but occur in leisure riding. Thus, mandates and regulatory activities are often ineffectual. Therefore, education and understanding and awareness of injuries and injury prevention are the most effective means of reducing risks. This has been a main focus of the

American Medical Equestrian Association (P.O. Box 130848, Birmingham, AL 35213), a non-profit organization of health-care professionals and other organizational representatives with an interest in safety.

We also know that with the heterogenous nature of various equestrian organizations, and the vaguely defined demographics of many of the populations that are involved, it is often difficult to accurately define risks. The sparsity of data emphasizes the importance of further properly constructed research.

References

1. American Academy of Orthopaedic Surgeons: Live It Safe, AAOS Committee on Public Education. Rosemont, Ill, American Academy of Orthopaedic Surgeons, 1992.
2. American College of Obstetricians and Gynecologists: Exercise during pregnancy and the postnatal period, ACOG Technical Bulletin 189. Washington, DC, ACOG, 1994.
3. American Medical Equestrian Association: 1990 rider survey. AMEA News 1(1), 1991.
4. American Medical Equestrian Association: Vest survey. AMEA News 3(3):6–7, 1993.
5. American Society for Testing and Materials: Standards of 1995 (F-1163,90A), Volume 15. Philadelphia, American Society for Testing and Materials, 1995.
6. Aronson H, Tough SC: Horse-related fatalities in the province of Alberta, 1975–1990. Am J Forensic Med Pathol 14(1):28–30, 1993.
7. Artal R, Wiswell RA, Drinkwater BL, St. John-Repovich W: Exercise guidelines for pregnancy. In: Artal R, Wiswell RA, Drinkwater BL (eds): Exercise in Pregnancy. Baltimore, Williams & Wilkins, 1991, pp 299–312.
8. Barone GW, Rogers BM: Pediatric equestrian injuries: a 14 year review. J Trauma 29(2):245–7, 1989.
9. Becker T: Das stumpfe Schadel trauma als sportunfall. Mschr Unfallheilkd 62:179, 1959.
10. Bennett D: Who's built best to ride? Equus 140:58–64, 1994.
11. Bernhang AM, Winslett G: Equestrian injuries. Physician Sportsmed 11(1):90–7, 1983.
12. Bixby-Hammett DM, Brooks WH: Neurologic injuries in equestrian sports. In: Jordan BD, Tsairis P, Warren RF (eds): Sports Neurology. Philadelphia, 1989, pp 229–34.
13. Bixby-Hammett DM, Brooks WH: Head and spinal injuries associated with equestrian sports. In Torg JS (ed): Athletic Injuries to the Head, Neck and Face, 2nd edition. St Louis, CV Mosby, 1991, pp 133–41.
14. Bixby-Hammett DM: USPC completes ten-year accident study. USPC News 51, 1992.
15. Bixby-Hammett DM: Pediatric equestrian injuries. Pediatrics 89(6):1173–6, 1992.
16. British Equestrian Trade Association Body and Shoulder Protector Standard, 1995.
17. Brooks WH, Bixby-Hammett D: Prevention of neurologic injuries in equestrian sports. Physician Sportsmed 16(11):84–95, 1988.
18. Byrd JWT: Risk factors of head and neck injuries in equestrian activities. In: Hoerner E (ed): Head and Neck Injuries in Sports, ASTP STP 1229. Philadelphia, American Society for Testing and Materials, 1994.
19. Byrd JWT: Planning event coverage: equestrian emergency medical protocols. Waynesville, NC, American Medical Equestrian Association, 1993.
20. Christey GI, Nelson DE, Rivera FP, et al: Horseback riding injuries among children and young adults, J Fam Pract 39(2):148–52, 1994.
21. Clapp JF: A clinical approach to exercise during pregnancy, Clin Sports Med 13(2):443–58, 1994.
22. Common injuries in horseback riding: a review. Sports Med 9(1):36–47:1990.
23. DeBenedette V: People and horses: the risks of riding, Physician Sportsmed 17(3):251–4, 1989.
24. Firth JL: Equestrian injuries. In: Schneider RD, Kennedy JC (eds): Sports Injuries. Baltimore, Williams & Wilkins, 1985, pp 431–49.
25. Gleave JRW: The impact of sports on a neurosurgical unit. Read before Britain Institute of Sports Medicine Symposium, Cambridge, England, 1975.
26. Grossman JAI, Kulund D, Miller C, et al: Equestrian injuries, results of a prospective study. JAMA 240(17):1881–2, 1978.
27. Harkess Society 1995 Annual Meeting, Nashville, Tenn.
28. Ingemarson H, Grevsten S, Thorsen L: Lethal horse-riding injuries, J Trauma 29(1):25–30,1989.
29. Mullinax KM, Dale E: Some considerations of exercise during pregnancy. Clin Sports Med 5(3):559–63, 1986.
30. National Electronic Injury Surveillance System. Washington DC, US Consumer Product Safety Commission, National Injury Information Clearing House, 1993.
31. Nelson DE, Rivara FR, Condie C, Smith SM: Injuries in equestrian sports. Physician Sportsmed 22(10):53–60, 1994.
32. Nelson DE, Rivera FP, Condie C: Helmets and horseback riders. Am J Prev Med 10(1):15–9, 1994.
33. Phillips GH, Stucky WE: Accidents to rural Ohio people occurring during recreational activities. Cooperative Extension Service, Ohio State University, Extension Bulletin MM295, Circular 166, 1969.
34. Pounder DJ: The grave yawns for the horseman, equestrian deaths in South Australia 1973–1983. Med J Austral 141:632–5, 1984.
35. Racing Resource Group, Inc: 1992–93 female participation in horse organizations. Alexandria, Va, Equestrian Resources.
36. Rimel RW, Giordani B, Barth JT, Boll TJ and Jane JA: Disability caused by minor head injury Neurosurgery 9(3):221–8, 1981.
37. Sherry K: In: Horse Related Injuries, 7th edition. Hazard, Victorian Injury Surveillance System. Royal Children's Hospital, Parkville, Victoria, Australia, 1991.
38. Snow-Harter CM: Bone health and prevention of osteoporosis in active and athletic women. Clin Sports Med 13(2):389–404, 1994.
39. Whitlock M: Equestrian injuries in England. Presented at Second International Conference on Emergency Medicine, Barnet General Hospital, Hertfordshire, England, 1988.

Chapter 53

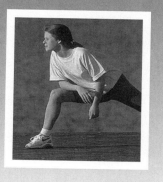

Fencing

Julie Moyer Knowles, Ed.D., A.T.C., P.T.

Fencing, one of the original sports of the Olympic Games, involves 2 opponents trying to score points against one another by having one's weapon touch an opponent's valid target area, while staying within a designated area on a 2- by 14-meter playing strip.

The actions of fencing are so fast that they are scored electrically. A green light comes on when a fencer makes a valid hit, a red light illuminates when the opponent makes a valid hit, and a white light indicates a touch made outside of the valid target area. Each time a fencer touches the opponent in a valid manner and on a valid target, a point is awarded. The first fencer to score 15 points (in direct elimination rounds) or 5 points (in double elimination rounds) wins that particular game, called a *bout*. Fencing combines athleticism with mental sharpness.

HISTORY OF THE SPORT

Fencing has a history that extends back to the time of primitive man, when hand weapons were used in battle against men and for hunting against animals. The Chinese, around 2000 BC, began to develop these weapons into more useful tools. In approximately 1200 BC, these hand-held weapons, along with hand shields and face masks, were used in sport by the Egyptian Pharaoh Ramses III; hence, the use of fencing as a sport began. However, it was not until the 15th century, when the Spanish Maitres d' Armes began teaching the art of fencing, that modern-day fencing truly originated.[1]

Most of the rules governing fencing were first adopted in 1914 by the Federation Internationale de Escrima (FIE). This international fencing association, which is the governing body for the technical rules in the sport of fencing, was first developed because of differences in fencing rules between countries during the Olympic Games (Shaw, USFA Historian, unpublished correspondence, 1995).

In the United States the sport of modern fencing is governed by the United States Fencing Association (USFA). Since 1914, when most of the rules governing fencing were adopted, there have been some rule changes, primarily concerning the electronic scoring apparatus, protective equipment, safety, expansion of the role of the female, and drug testing.

PARTICIPATION, UNIQUENESS, AND COMPARISONS TO OTHER SPORTS

Participation

The sport of fencing involves 3 types of blunted weapons: the foil, the epee, and the saber (Fig. 53-1). While all weapons are composed of a flexible steel blade, the 3 are different in that they have their own rules of play and unique design. In particular, the blade and the guard, a hand protector near where the hand grips the weapon, are different.[9]

In foil competition, the only touches that are considered valid are those confined to the trunk. The limbs and the head are excluded. Since the limbs are excluded there is a smaller guard, or protective device, around the hand. In contrast, the guard diameter of the epee is up to 1.5 cm wider. During epee competition the whole body of the fencer is the target, including her clothing, equipment, and hand. Therefore, this larger guard helps protect the hand from trauma.

In contrast to the foil and epee, which are thrusting weapons only utilizing the end of the weapon, the saber combines both thrusting and cutting moves with the edge and the back edge of the weapon. Many hits made to the guard are considered invalid and the fencer is penalized. A valid point in saber competition is awarded when the target is touched by the opponent's

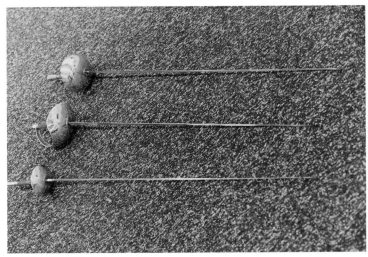

Figure 53-1. The three weapons of fencing. Top to Bottom: Epee, saber, and foil. (From Moyer JA, Jaffe R, Adrian M: Fencing. In: Fu F, Stone D (eds): Sports Injuries. Philadelphia: Williams & Wilkins, 1994, pp 333–48, with permission.)

weapon at any part of the body above a horizontal line formed at the top of the thighs.

Unique Medical Rules

The USFA has implemented a program that helps monitor and improve the health care of fencers involved with the organization. The USFA Athletic Training Sports Medicine Committee was established to provide medical health care professionals (qualified physician or athletic trainer) at every open national competition and national championships overseen by the USFA. The primary purpose of the Athletic Training Committee is to provide emergency management, stabilization, and treatment of injuries that occur during the fencing competition. In addition, monitoring of the medical status of elite, world-class fencers is also done. Physicians and trainers who volunteer are put on the USFA Medical Volunteer Corps list. Every year the USFA may submit the name of a physician or a trainer from the USFA Medical Volunteer Corps to the United States Olympic Sports Medicine Committee National Governing Body for consideration for the United States Olympic Sports Medicine Volunteer Program (Table 53-1).

It is important that health care providers be familiar with the sport and restrictions placed on the sport when providing care. For example, if any type of taping must be done, one must take care not to interfere with the electrical current needed for proper scoring during the competition. In addition, if electric devices, such as a transcutaneous electrical nerve stimulation unit, are used to help relieve pain between bouts, care

must be taken that these wires are removed prior to competition. It is advisable that any time tape is used on the weapon hand or around the target area, or if any type of electric device is used, preapproval be obtained from the Director of the Rules Committee prior to the start of competition.

Injury Comparisons to Other Sports

Comparatively speaking, the injuries that occur during fencing are less severe than those of other contact sports. There are, however, certain specific injuries that historically have resulted in significant and even life-threatening situations. In particular, severe puncture wounds resulting from a broken blade penetrating an opponent have occurred.[4,12,13] There have been at least 2 immediate deaths associated with a weapon penetrating a face mask.[4] There has also been a case where brain penetration has occurred and the athlete survived with permanent amnesia.[13] Therefore, it is important for the health care provider to be well versed in the management of medical emergencies, including stabilizing nonextractable foreign objects and managing cardiorespiratory distress. The health care provider should also be well trained in control of hemorrhage, management of foreign bodies, such as slivers of metal, especially in the eye, and management of a punctured lung.

In order to treat injuries, the health care provider should have appropriate supplies available at the competition site. Some supplies may be provided by the USFA or the local organizing committee. Table 53-1 includes a list of supplies. Other supplies and equipment that may

Table 53-1. Responsibilities of Local Organizing Committee and Medical Personnel at USFA Events

The duties of the **local organizing committee** shall include the following:
1. Coordinate medical coverage through the assistance of the USFA's Medical Commission.
2. Notify the area hospital when and where the fencing event is going to be held.
3. Provide food, housing, and transportation reimbursement for the trainer and physician. If a local athletic trainer and/or physician cannot be obtained or if the USFA/local organizing committee chooses to bring in a trainer/physician from outside the area, the trainer/physician must also be supplied with a vehicle for local transportation and medical purposes.
4. Mail the completed treatment report forms and initial evaluation forms to both the USFA Headquarters and the Medical Commission.
5. If the trainer or physician engaged is not familiar with fencing, the local organizing committee along with a fencing official shall instruct the medical personnel as to their duties.
6. Events with a higher number of entrants require additional staffing. Each event should have at least one physician and one trainer present at all times (Nationals, 3 trainers, 2 physicians, minimal).
7. Notify USFA headquarters of all serious injuries or injuries requiring hospital transport.
8. Notify the trainer and physician of the ambulance response time and transportation time, and give the medical staff a map of the area, including competition site, hotel, and hospital.
9. Find a suitable training room area in close proximity to the actual competition. Communication devices between the training room, physician, and committee are recommended.
10. Medical personnel should be provided with adequate medical supplies. An example of supplies used for a 4-day tournament follows:

   - 80 rolls (2 cases) $1\frac{1}{2}$-inch white tape
   - 8-oz can tape spray
   - 4 Ace wraps (4-inch)
   - 8 oz hydrogen peroxide
   - Box 100 knuckle Band-Aids
   - Pack 100 sterile 3×3-inch gauze
   - 1 bottle (100) aspirin
   - 1 bottle (100) acetominophen
   - 4-oz tube bacitracin
   - Rubber gloves
   - Eye wash
   - Crutches
   - 5 rolls prewrap
   - Pack (minimum 100) mid-size supermarket plastic bags and biohazard bags
   - 400 Cups
   - 2 1-gallon water coolers
   - Ice
   - 20 treatment report forms
   - 20 initial evaluation forms

11. Contact the local medical groups and licensure committee to confirm temporary medical practice of out-of-state medical personnel.

The duties of the **athletic trainer** shall include the following:
1. Provide prevention and immediate care of injuries to athletes and supportive staff.
2. Arrange for transportation of injured persons to the hospital.
3. Make necessary referrals to the physician.
4. Bring his/her own standard trainer's kit.
5. Maintain treatment reports and initial evaluation forms.
6. Notify the local organizing committee of all serious injuries or injuries requiring hospital transport.
7. All medical personnel (including physicians) are responsible for their own malpractice insurance; however, because the services are of a volunteer nature, in some states the Good Samaritan Law may cover emergency care of injuries.

The duties of the **physician** shall include the following:
1. Fulfill the role as described in the rules and regulations involving the determinations if an injury is a result of trauma (ie, rule out cramps).
2. Determine and make a record of all interruptions of combat granted.
3. If a 10-minute request is denied, the physician must issue a warning and subsequently notify the bout committee as a repetition of the offence will result in exclusion.
4. In addition to the above requirements in the rules of fencing, the physician must provide emergency treatment of injuries as necessary or as requested by the athletic trainer.

From Moyer JA, Jaffe R, Adrian M: Fencing. In: Fu F, Stone D, (eds): Sports Injuries. Philadelphia, Williams & Wilkins, 1994, pp. 333–48, with permission.

be helpful are a sterile suturing kit, electric cautery, intravenous fluids, an eye kit with fluorescein/blue light, and a vacuum splint kit.[9]

GENDER DIFFERENCES, PHYSIOLOGIC DEMANDS, AND INJURY TRENDS

Gender Differences

Women were first permitted to participate in fencing long before many other sports, especially contact sports. One reason women were excluded from other sports was because those sports caused the female to become flushed and red in the face. It was thought that this sweating and redness could possibly arouse men and could be a hindrance to the physical well-being of women. Governing personnel felt that at least the women in fencing were covered with attire so that men could not see such physiologic responses (Shaw, USFA Historian, unpublished correspondence, 1995).

Women first became involved in the sport of fencing in the United States around 1888 after a Viennese traveling corps of fencers demonstrated fencing by women at the New York Fencers Club. After that, fencing lessons for women began throughout the United States. In 1924 during the Paris Olympics, women were first allowed to participate in fencing competition using the foil only. The other weapons were considered too strenuous for women. Of the 3 weapons, the foil was believed to be the most basic, had the smallest target area, and was believed to be a training weapon; therefore, it was thought to be manageable by the female.

Women also had a different target area. To score a point in foil, a vital organ (trunk) had to be struck in a stabbing manner. A vital organ hit (a death blow) was always considered a good hit. The groin was not considered a valid touch (point) in the female fencer. In men, however, the groin area was considered a vital organ and consequently a valid touch. It wasn't until the 1960 Olympics in Rome that the target area of the female fencer was changed to be the same as that of the male.

Today, women compete in all 3 weapons internationally, with all target areas being the same as men's, although not all competitions have female participants in all weapons. Gender discrepancies still exist in the sport of fencing. While foil competition for women is standard, it was not until 1989 that a second weapon, the epee, was added to the World Championships,

and not until 1996 that epee was added to the Olympic Games.

Physiologic and Biomechanical Considerations

The development of proper strength, flexibility, coordination, balance, cardiovascular status, and proprioception is important for the elite fencer. Musculoskeletal endurance is also very important since most competitions require the fencer to compete in multiple bouts in a day, several days in a row.

The arm that holds the weapon, and the lead leg (the forward lunging leg) especially, require special evaluation and exercise in order to ensure proper technique, proper physiology, and injury avoidance. The weapon hand and forward leg have been shown to be significantly stronger than the contralateral limb because of the mechanics of the sport.[11] Because of their usage, these dominant limbs tend to be more prone to overuse injuries.

Since the pattern of movement promotes muscular asymmetry, it is also important for the nondominant side to be well conditioned outside of the sports arena. Many acute lower extremity injuries occur to the trial limb. Since females in general have about one half the upper body strength of men of comparable weight and size, it is essential to emphasize a bilateral upper extremity program for female fencers.[7] The mechanics of the sport also reveal that core stability exercises of the trunk may be very beneficial. Lastly, in addition to physical training, mental training is also a very large component to sports conditioning in fencing.[6]

Injury Trends: Chronic Disorders

Over the past 10 years, as fencing has gained popularity in the United States, participants are starting the sport at a much earlier age. The most significant injury trend has therefore involved chronic and overuse injuries. Impingement syndrome of the dominant shoulder has increased, especially with epee fencers, who internally rotate the dominant arm and perform long and frequent lunges with a thrusting upper extremity movement. Plantar fasciitis is also very common and is often associated with poor fencing footwear. Patellofemoral disorders are increasing, especially as the number of female adolescent participants rises. Also, recurring groin strains of the trail leg and lower back strains continue to occur.

PROTECTIVE EQUIPMENT, ENVIRONMENT, AND INJURIES

Protective Equipment

Proper equipment and technique play an extremely important role in the safety of the sport. The need to enforce this evolved after the development of electric fencing, when the blades became stiffer and heavier, and the sport became more athletic. Once the Directors (officials) no longer had to actually see a touch in electric fencing, the opponents were allowed to stand much closer to one another, and the competition began to last longer.[2]

Through time and usage, the blades of the fencing weapons develop small cracks, which, until recently, often went undetected. Under stress of competition, these cracks can cause breaks in the blade and could possibly lead to a penetration injury to an opponent. In order to prevent this type of injury a nondestructive evaluation (NDE) of fencing blades is being investigated. In this procedure, prior to competition, an athlete's blade is passed through an electromagnetic probe that can detect imperfections in the blade.[2]

While weapons as well as other equipment, such as the mask, must be presented by the fencer to the weapons inspection officer prior to any official event, the NDE form of testing is not mandatory at all events even though it has proven itself effective in the detection of blade defects.[14]

Another means under investigation to help prevent fencing injuries is replacing steel blades with blades made of a composite material. As has been shown in other sports, such as tennis and golf, composites tend to be extremely strong, yet lightweight and flexible. With stronger and more durable weapons, it is believed that the incidence of serious injuries as well as minor bruising could be lowered.[2]

Face masks, clothing, gloves, vests, and chest protectors are other forms of protective equipment used by fencers. Certain clothing requirements are specific to the weapon being used, since the target area is different from weapon to weapon. For example, the clothing in epee is more protective, since the entire body is a target. The jacket must cover the whole front of the trunk and must be made of a lining of double thickness on the weapon arm from the sleeve down to the elbow, and covering the flank in the region of the axilla.[14] Also, in order to prevent hand or upper extremity injuries, a glove on the weapon hand is worn with the cuff of the glove fully covering approximately one half of the dominant forearm in epee.[14]

Other forms of protective clothing include breast protectors made of a rigid material. Breast protectors are mandatory for all female participants; however, protection for the female or male genitals is optional. Although these and other FIE standards have reduced the risk of serious penetration injuries, bruising injuries are still a problem. Therefore, research regarding modification of clothing to minimize forces absorbed by the body are being investigated.

Footwear is becoming more of a concern in fencing as the incidence of lower chain disorders increases.[9] The 2 current problems with fencing footwear are lack of support and lack of proper sizing. Fencing shoes are primarily made in men's sizes, forcing most women, who generally have narrower feet, to wear wider shoes than what would be indicated.[2]

Environment

The field of play in fencing is known as the strip, or *piste*. It is 14 meters long and 1.8 to 2 meters wide.[14] The USFA Safety Committee is working with the USFA/American Society for Testing and Materials (ASTM) to investigate evaluation methods in determining strip safety. This includes determining adequate friction ratios between the strip and the floor, and establishing impact absorption criteria in order to minimize overuse injuries.[2]

Other environmental concerns include spectator injuries, many of which occur in other fencers. Frequently fencers who are watching a competition in between their own bouts become injured by competing fencers because of the close and often constrained resting space between strips.

Also, proper air conditioning is necessary in the fencing environment. The requirements and necessity of protective clothing decrease the athlete's ability to expel heat and thus increase the chance of acquiring heat-related disorders.[9]

Injuries

Two different studies have been conducted by the USFA that examine the distribution and types of fencing injuries. In the first study, the USFA's Athletic Training Committee analyzed injury data obtained at major fencing competitions. Since these were major competitions, the study primarily involved the more elite fencers. During major competitions over a 2-year period, 586 injuries (323 acute) were reported by fencers to medical personnel. Approximately 30% of all injuries reported were in female fencers, while 70% were from male fencers. Some of the gender differences were associated with fewer female participants. Also, there were more injuries with the epee than with any other weapon, most likely because of the epee fencer's larger target area.[9,10]

The types and locations of fencing injuries reported are listed in Tables 53-2 and 53-3. The most commonly reported injuries were sprains, at 33%. Strains were second at 24%, heat disorders were third at 18%, and contusions were fourth at 6%.[9,10]

When examining just the female competitors, the ankle, hand, and fingers had the highest incidence of injury. Sprains and heat disorders, including cramps, were the most common types of acute injury.[9,10]

The USFA has regulations regarding withdrawal of a competitor for medical reasons, including cramping and nonacute injuries. One rule allows for a 10-minute maximum break for an injury incurred during the bout and confirmed by an FIE medical representative, or by the physician or athletic trainer on duty. The break is timed by the official overseeing the bout. If prior to the end of the 10 minutes the qualified medical professional feels that the fencer is incapable of continuing, he or she will notify the official that the fencer should be withdrawn if in an individual event, or replaced if in a team event. At any other time during that day if the fencer does return to competition he or she may not withdraw from a bout because of the same injury without completely forfeiting the bout. In team events, a fencer who is withdrawn by a designated medical official may, if approved by that medical official, fence later that same day in other matches. It should also be noted that heat cramps are not considered injuries and therefore the 10-minute injury time-outs are not given for this disorder.[14]

The second USFA-supported study was much more inclusive in that both the recreational as well as the competitive fencer was surveyed, regardless of age or acuteness of injury. In this study, 1603 fencers (19% of the USFA membership) responded to a 25-question survey emphasizing training and competitive injuries that occurred within the previous one-year period, as well as the fencer's most serious injury. Twenty-eight percent of the respondents were female, and 72% were male. Many of the respondents were not at the competitive level found in the previous study; 36% reported less than 3 years experience and only 23% had more than 12 years experience fencing.[3]

The injury types and factors contributing to fencing injuries reported in this study are given in Tables 53-4 and 53-5. Strains (27%) and sprains (24%) were the most commonly reported injuries; however, it should be noted that these "diagnoses" were not always made by qualified medical personnel. Lacerations and puncture wounds accounted for 6% of the worst injuries within the previous year. Seventeen percent of the reported injuries were to the knee, while 14.5% were to the ankle. The survey also found that one third of all reported injuries were of gradual onset.[3]

Both studies found ankle sprain in particular to be an extremely common injury.[3,9] This is not surprising since, as previously mentioned, there is relatively poor footwear in the sport, and the biomechanical positioning (flexed, externally rotated, and valgus stress) of the trail leg promotes excessive eversion. The knee was the second most commonly injured body part when looking at acute, high-level competitive injuries. Again, the biomechanical positioning of the trail leg promotes not only acute knee injuries such as medial collateral ligament sprains and meniscal tears, but also various recurring and chronic injuries such as patellofemoral dysfunction.[5] Other biomechanical and postural-related disorders, some of which can be helped with specialized orthotic inserts, include plantar fasciitis, iliotibial band syndrome, and low back pain.

When fencing injuries are adjusted for exposure time, men and women incur about the same number of fencing injuries.[4] As can be seen in the previously mentioned survey by Carter and Heil of the 455 female fencers who responded to the survey, 46% did not have any injuries in the previous year, as compared to 48% of the men.[3] Similar results finding no gender difference were also reported in a collegiate fencing study.[8]

CONCLUDING REMARKS

Although not as frequent as other comparable contact sports, severe injuries in fencing do occur, especially penetration wounds. Although the USFA and FIE have established protective equipment and technique regulations to help prevent these serious injuries, they still occur and therefore require that trained medical personnel be present during all sanctioned competitions.

Because of the unique biomechanics of fencing (the position of the trail leg and weapon arm in particular) sprains, strains, and overuse injuries are quite common. Many of these injuries can be minimized by total-body conditioning to

Table 53-2. Types of Acute Fencing Injuries (%)

WEAPON	CONTUSIONS	FRACTURES/ RUPTURES	HEAT-RELATED DISORDERS	MISCELLANEOUS SYSTEMIC DISORDERS	OPEN WOUNDS/ LACERATIONS	SPRAINS	STRAINS	ROW % (NUMBER)
Women's foil	2.5	0.3	2.8	—	2.8	4.0	2.8	15.2(49)
Women's epee	0.3	0.3	2.5	—	0.9	1.9	0.9	6.8(22)
Women's saber	0.3	—	0.6	—	—	—	—	0.9(3)
Men's foil	0.3	—	1.2	—	1.9	3.4	3.7	10.5(34)
Men's epee	2.5	0.6	6.8	0.3	9.3	18.0	8.4	45.8(148)
Men's saber	0.3	—	4.0	—	2.5	5.9	8.0	20.7(67)
TOTAL	6.2	1.2	17.9	0.3	17.4	33.2	23.8	100

From Moyer JA, Jaffe R, Adrian M. Fencing. In: Fu F, Stone D, (eds): Sports Injuries. Philadelphia: Williams & Wilkins, 1994; 333–348, with permission.

Table 53-3. Location of Fencing Injuries (%)

WEAPON	ANKLE	CLAVICLE	FINGER	FOOT	FOREARM	GROIN	HAND	HEAD	HEEL	HIP	KNEE	LOWER BACK	NECK	SHIN	SHOULDER	THIGH	THUMB	TOE	UPPER BACK	UPPER ARM	WRIST	ROW % (NUMBER)
Women's foil	3.7	—	1.2	1.5	0.3	—	—	0.6	0.6	0.3	0.9	0.3	—	—	—	1.5	0.6	2.5	0.6	0.3	0.6	15.2(49)
Women's epee	1.5	0.6	0.3	0.3	0.9	—	—	1.5	—	—	—	—	—	—	0.3	0.3	—	0.3	—	—	0.3	6.8(22)
Women's saber	0.3	—	—	—	—	—	—	0.3	—	—	—	—	—	0.3	—	—	—	—	—	—	—	0.9(3)
Men's foil	1.2	—	0.6	0.9	0.6	—	0.3	0.6	0.3	0.3	0.9	0.6	0.3	—	0.6	0.6	0.3	—	0.3	0.3	0.9	10.5(34)
Men's epee	9.0	—	0.3	2.5	2.8	0.3	1.9	3.7	—	1.9	3.7	2.2	0.9	0.6	4.6	4.6	0.3	—	0.3	0.3	2.2	45.8(148)
Men's saber	3.7	—	0.3	0.6	0.6	0.3	0.3	1.9	0.3	1.9	2.5	1.9	0.6	0.3	1.9	1.9	0.3	—	0.6	1.2	0.6	20.7(67)
TOTAL	15.8	0.6	2.8	5.9	5.3	1.2	2.5	8.4	1.2	5.9	8.0	5.0	2.2	0.9	5.6	10.5	1.5	2.5	2.2	2.2	4.6	100

From Moyer JA, Jaffe R, Adrian M: Fencing. In: Fu F, Stone D, (eds): Sports Injuries. Philadelphia: Williams & Wilkins, 1994, pp. 333–48, with permission.

Table 53-4. Worst Injury in Past Year and Worst Injury in Fencing Career

TYPE OF INJURY	WORST IN LAST YEAR (%)	WORST IN CAREER (%)
Strain (muscle)	26.0	22.0
Sprain (ligament)	23.9	21.8
Tendinitis	14.5	14.4
Cartilage tear	5.3	7.5
Puncture	3.3	4.9
Torn tendon	2.4	3.8
Fracture	2.1	3.6
Laceration	3.0	3.5
Other	18.9	18.5

From Moyer JA, Jaffe R, Adrian M: Fencing. In: Fu F, Stone D, (eds): Sports Injuries. Philadelphia, Williams & Wilkins, 1994, pp 333–48, with permission.

Table 53-5. Factors Contributing to Worst Injury in Past Year and Worst Injury During Fencing Career

	WORST IN LAST YEAR (%)	WORST IN CAREER (%)
Personal factors	48.3	46.2
Poor technique	12.2	14.7
Inadequate warm-up	13.2	11.2
Fatigue	11.0	10.0
Dangerous tactics	2.4	2.5
Other	9.5	7.8
Behavior of others	12.7	13.7
Dangerous tactics by opponent	8.5	9.0
Poor coaching	1.0	1.6
Poor officiating	1.6	1.4
Other	1.6	1.6
Equipment and facilities	27.9	27.8
Strip	9.6	9.7
Shoes	9.5	8.3
Weapon	4.5	4.6
Jacket	0.8	1.3
Mask	0.4	0.5
Lighting	0.4	0.5
Other	2.7	2.9
No identifiable contributing factors	11.1	12.4

From Moyer JA, Jaffe R, Adrian M: Fencing. In: Fu F, Stone D, (eds): Sports Injuries. Philadelphia, Williams & Wilkins, 1994, pp 333–48, with permission.

decrease asymmetry, as well as by good coaching.

When injuries are adjusted for exposure time, no real gender difference can be seen between male and female fencers. However, through history and even to today, although to a lesser degree, women do not have the same international fencing competition privileges as men and the rules of their competitions are gender biased.

References

1. Campos J: The Art of Fencing. New York, Vantage Press, 1988.
2. Carter C, Heil J: Safer fencing for everyone. Am Fencing 42(3):13–4, 1992.
3. Carter C, Heil J, Zemper E: What hurts and why. Am Fencing 43(3):16–29, 1993.
4. Crawford AR: Death of a fencer. Br J Sports Med 18(3):220–2, 1984.
5. Gray WJ, Bassett FH: Ostechondritis dissecans of the patella in a competitive fencer. Orthop Rev 19(1):96–8, 1990.
6. Heil J, Zemper E, Carter C: Behavioral factors in fencing injuries. Presented at the VIIth World Congress of Sports Psychology. Lisbon, 1993.
7. Klafs CE, Arnheim DD: Modern Principles of Athletic Training. St Louis, CV Mosby, 1977.
8. Lanese R, Strauss R, Lerman D, et al: Injury and disability in matched men's and women's intercollegiate sports. Am J Public Health 80(12):1459–62, 1990.
9. Moyer JA, Jaffe R, Adrian M: Fencing. In: Fu F, Stone D (eds): Sports Injuries. Philadelphia, Williams & Wilkins, 1994, pp 333-48.
10. Moyer JA, Konin JG: An overview of fencing injuries. Am Fencing 42(4):25, 1992.
11. Nystrom J, Lindwall O, Ceci R, et al: Physiological and morphological characteristics of world class fencers. Int J Sports Med 11(2):136-9, 1990.

12. Roi GS, Fasc A: Survey of requests for medical assistance during fencing matches. Ital J Sports Trauma 10(1):55–62, 1988.
13. Squire LR, Amaral DG, Zola-Morgars S, et al: Description of brain injury in the amnesic patient N.A. based on magnetic resonance imaging. Exp Neurol 105(1):23–35, 1989.
14. US Fencing Association: USFA Rules. Colorado Springs, Colo, USFA, 1990.

Chapter 54

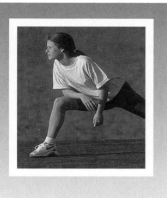

Women's Field Hockey and Lacrosse

Jean A. Miles, P.T., A.T.C., C.S.C.S.

Field hockey and lacrosse both came to the United States from Great Britain in the early 1900s. While their origins stem from different parts of the world, they both strongly appealed to women at a time when few athletic endeavors were available to them. Their popularity continues today, with participation in field hockey and lacrosse beginning in middle school and carrying over to the postcollegiate club organizations found in many urban areas.

This chapter will individually address each sport, beginning with the basics of the game and concluding with injury trends. Possible recommendations regarding injury reduction will be made when plausible.

FIELD HOCKEY

Field hockey was introduced to English women in the mid-19th century, although it hails from India. It quickly became the dominant women's sport. Constance M. K. Applebee, a British woman, is credited with bringing field hockey to a sports symposium at Harvard University in 1901. She was subsequently invited to introduce the game to several northeastern colleges, eventually ending up at Bryn Mawr. Her love of the game continued as she organized clubs, and she was ultimately instrumental in the development of the governing body of the sport, the United States Field Hockey Association (USFHA), in 1922.

Today the USFHA is the national governing body of both men's and women's field hockey. Women's field hockey is played extensively internationally and has been an Olympic sport since 1980.[1]

Sport Specifics

Field hockey is played with 11 members on each team. The field measures 100 yards long and 60 yards wide. Game length is dependent upon level of competition: collegiate, 35-minute halves: high school, 30-minute halves; and middle school, 25-minute halves.

Equipment is minimal. Shin guards, made of plastic or fiberglass, and mouth guards are the only required elements (except for the better-protected goalie). Shoes generally have cleats of rubber or plastic, and turf shoes are used if warranted.

The field hockey stick is like no other in sport, as it has one flat side and one curved side. This ensures that the stick is turned when changing direction, dictating a right-to-left style of game. It is made of wood, and runs from 35 to 38 inches in length.

The goalie is by far the best protected from the $5\frac{1}{2}$ ounce, dense plastic ball. She wears a wire basket mask, neck protector, chest protector, padded apron for the thighs and pelvis, leg pads, and square toe protectors.

Injury Trends

Unfortunately, field hockey does not have a complete injury reporting system at every level of competition. The most complete study of injury has been done by the division of Sports Science of the National Collegiate Athletic Association (NCAA). The NCAA Injury Surveillance Survey (ISS) has compiled injury data on all levels of collegiate field hockey from 1986 to 2000. In their reports, an *injury* is defined as an event that "(1) occurs as a result of participation in an organized intercollegiate event, (2) requires medical attention by an athletic trainer or team physician, and (3) results in restriction of the student-athlete's participation for one or more days beyond the day of injury."[3] An *athletic exposure* is defined as "one athlete participation in one practice or game where he or she is exposed to the possibility of athletic injury."[3] The injury rate is then determined to be "a ratio of the number of injuries in a particular category to the number of athlete exposures in that category."[3]

Figure 54-1 depicts data from the past 10 years, relating injury rates to pre-, regular-, and postseason play. Preseason activity consistently yields the most number of injuries.

This is not really surprising, given that athletes come in after a summer away from a school setting with questionable levels of fitness to begin several sessions of practice a day. Postseason injury rates are routinely lower given better fitness, a season of game experience, and fewer athletes on the whole participating in this part of the season.

There is often much made about the connection of playing on artificial turf and increasing number of athletic injuries,[5] so we examine that aspect specific to field hockey in Figure 54-2. Over the last 6 years, injury trends seem to indicate that the number of natural-turf injuries has stayed the same, while playing on artificial turf has increased the number of days missed because of injury. Interestingly enough, the number of exposures to artificial surfaces still dwarfs natural turf by approximately 50%.[3]

Figure 54-3 illustrates above-the-neck, head, and concussion injuries. Clearly, above-the-neck injuries dominate the game of field hockey. In the 1999 to 2000 season, injuries were tallied by the NCAA as follows: head,[4] eye,[2] face,[3] and teeth.[2]

While these are not the most prevalent injuries found in this study, the statistics substantiate concerns by researchers abroad. A group of British researchers have found the number of dental and facial injuries in international field hockey to be approximately 54%.[2] They believe the use of a mouth protector would greatly cut down on injuries necessitating a visit to a physician and/or dentist.

Figure 54-4 illustrates injury rates of 16 sports and gives an overall picture of how field hockey injury rates compare to others tracked by the NCAA. Field hockey rates in the lower third of sports that produce injuries, with 7.6/1000 athletic game exposures.

LACROSSE

Lacrosse is deeply embedded in Canadian culture. It was developed by the North American Indians as a violent training exercise to simulate battle. It was adopted and named by the French settlers of Canada. The men's game was first introduced into the United States in the 1870s, while the women's game came from Great Britain in the early 1900s.[6]

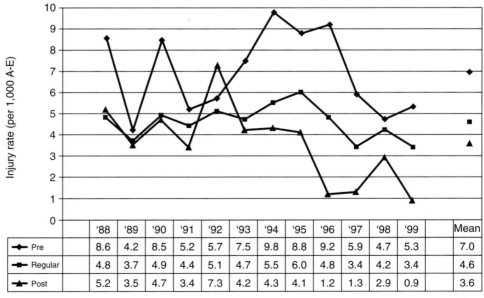

	'88	'89	'90	'91	'92	'93	'94	'95	'96	'97	'98	'99		Mean
Pre	8.6	4.2	8.5	5.2	5.7	7.5	9.8	8.8	9.2	5.9	4.7	5.3		7.0
Regular	4.8	3.7	4.9	4.4	5.1	4.7	5.5	6.0	4.8	3.4	4.2	3.4		4.6
Post	5.2	3.5	4.7	3.4	7.3	4.2	4.3	4.1	1.2	1.3	2.9	0.9		3.6

Figure 54-1. Field hockey: pre-, regular-, and postseason injury rates, total (practice and game). Preseason: prior to first regular season game; postseason: following regular season games. A-E, athletic exposure. (Data from NCAA Injury Surveillance System, 2000.)

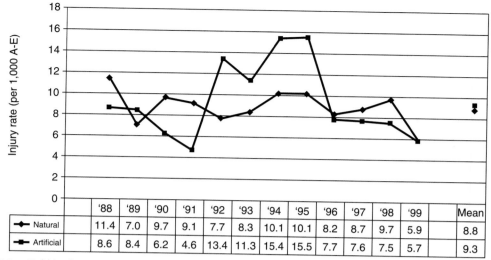

Figure 54-2. Field hockey: game surface injury rates. A-E, athletic exposure. (Data from NCAA Injury Surveillance System, 2000.)

	'88	'89	'90	'91	'92	'93	'94	'95	'96	'97	'98	'99	Mean
Natural	11.4	7.0	9.7	9.1	7.7	8.3	10.1	10.1	8.2	8.7	9.7	5.9	8.8
Artificial	8.6	8.4	6.2	4.6	13.4	11.3	15.4	15.5	7.7	7.6	7.5	5.7	9.3

Today lacrosse is enjoying a large growth spurt, with 69 schools adding programs from 1995 to 2000. This is an increase in collegiate teams of 48.25%.[4] The former United States Women's Lacrosse Association, now known as United States Lacrosse, has separate divisions for men's and women's programs, and is located in Baltimore, Maryland.

Sport Specifics

Women's lacrosse is a noncontact game of skill, speed, and stamina. It is played on a field with no official boundaries. Goals are 100 yards apart, and only dangerous obstacles, such as trees or immovable objects, qualify as out of play.

Women's lacrosse is a game known for its speed of passing to advance the ball up the field.

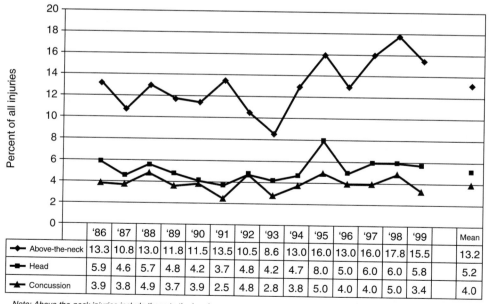

	'86	'87	'88	'89	'90	'91	'92	'93	'94	'95	'96	'97	'98	'99	Mean
Above-the-neck	13.3	10.8	13.0	11.8	11.5	13.5	10.5	8.6	13.0	16.0	13.0	16.0	17.8	15.5	13.2
Head	5.9	4.6	5.7	4.8	4.2	3.7	4.8	4.2	4.7	8.0	5.0	6.0	6.0	5.8	5.2
Concussion	3.9	3.8	4.9	3.7	3.9	2.5	4.8	2.8	3.8	5.0	4.0	4.0	5.0	3.4	4.0

Note: Above-the-neck injuries include those to the head, eyes, ears, nose, face, chin, jaw, mouth, teeth and tongue. Injuries to the head are a subset of these injuries and primarily consist of concussions.

Figure 54-3. Field hockey: above-the-neck and head injury and concussion percentages, total (practice and game). (Data from NCAA Injury Surveillance System, 2000.)

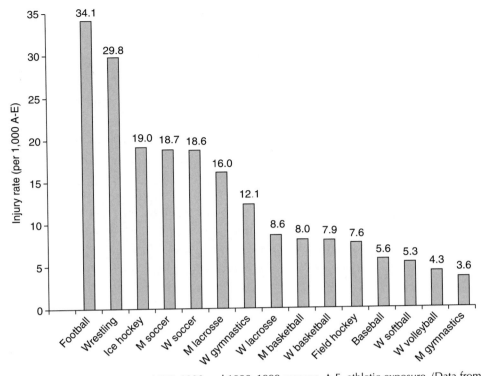

Figure 54-4. Game injury rate summary, 1997–1998 and 1998–1999 seasons. A-E, athletic exposure. (Data from NCAA Injury Surveillance System, 2000.)

There are 12 players on each team. Although 4 players must be behind the 50-yard line at all times, any player may run anywhere on the field. Women play two 30-minute halves.

Women's lacrosse, unlike the men's game, allows checking to the stick only when the ball is in it. There is a "protective sphere" around a player's head that can not be crossed by a stick at any time without penalty. No shots at the goalie's head are allowed.

Equipment requirements are few. Currently, in college lacrosse, only mouth guards are mandatory. High-school players are required to wear goggles and, in some states, a helmet. Gloves, while optional, are a popular choice because they cut down on the number of hand lacerations and exposures to blood.[9] Sticks, once traditionally wooden, may now be of molded plastic.

Once again, the goalie is the most protected player, wearing a helmet, throat and chest protectors, and leg pads.

Injury Trends

Although this sport spans a population from middle school past the collegiate years, the NCAA is the only source of consistent injury information. Definitions of injuries and injury rates are consistent with those previously used in this chapter.[4]

To give a sense of injury trends, Figure 54-5 depicts injury rates of pre-, regular-, and post-season activity. As with field hockey, preseason exposures resulted in more injuries, and postseason play was the least injury-producing time of the season.

The influence of artificial surfaces on injuries is illustrated in Figure 54-6. Of the 40 schools reporting to the NCAA for the academic year 1999 to 2000, only approximately 32% of collegiate contests were played on an artificial surface.[4] The data support the belief that more injuries occur on artificial surfaces.

Figure 54-7 displays the injury trends of above-the-neck and head injury rates.

Statistics furnished by the NCAA for the academic year 1999 to 2000 documented injuries above the head as follows: teeth,[1] nose,[6] eyes,[5] and head.[5] The top injury mechanisms for the past 5 years have been collisions with the ball and/or stick.[4]

Eye injuries have been cited twice in the literature as a concern with women's lacrosse.[7,8] Researchers in both Canada and Philadelphia were concerned with cases of ocular trauma, resulting from lack of protective eyewear. Both groups concluded protective eyewear should be mandated.

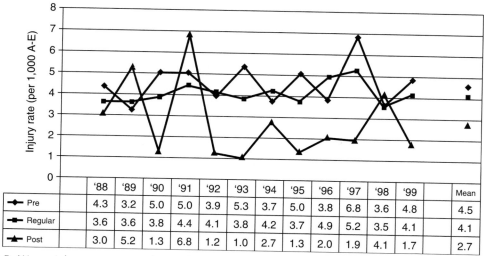

Figure 54-5. Women's lacrosse: pre-, regular-, and postseason injury rates, total (practice and game). Preseason: prior to first regular season game; postseason: following regular season game. A-E, athletic exposure. (Data from NCAA Injury Surveillance System, 2000.)

	'88	'89	'90	'91	'92	'93	'94	'95	'96	'97	'98	'99		Mean
Pre	4.3	3.2	5.0	5.0	3.9	5.3	3.7	5.0	3.8	6.8	3.6	4.8		4.5
Regular	3.6	3.6	3.8	4.4	4.1	3.8	4.2	3.7	4.9	5.2	3.5	4.1		4.1
Post	3.0	5.2	1.3	6.8	1.2	1.0	2.7	1.3	2.0	1.9	4.1	1.7		2.7

Tables 54-1 and 54-2 list the most common injuries by body part and injury classification. The ankle, upper leg, and knee have been consistently involved in the majority of women's lacrosse injuries in the past 10 years.[4]

Strains and sprains account for most of these injuries. Surprisingly, the third most prevalent type of injury in 1997 to 1998 was first-degree concussion; this may be due to the more athletic and aggressive nature of women's lacrosse being played currently.

Hand injuries, although small in number, have been documented as being primarily preventable with the use of gloves.[9]

When compared to other sports tracked by the NCAA (Fig. 54-8), women's lacrosse falls in the lower half of surveyed sports in regard to injuries, at 8.6/1000 athletic game exposures.[4]

CONCLUDING REMARKS AND RECOMMENDATIONS

While both field hockey and lacrosse require very little protective equipment, they enjoy a relatively small ratio of injuries per athletic exposure. Incidence of injury statistics primarily relate to the lower extremity, however, any evidence of above-the-neck and head injuries should be addressed by each individual sport.

Field hockey requires the use of shin and mouth guards to protect its players.

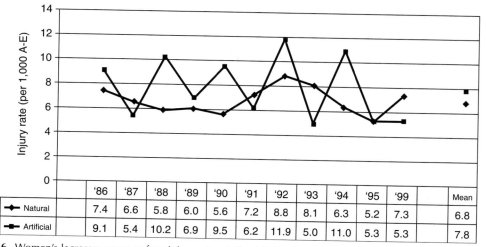

	'86	'87	'88	'89	'90	'91	'92	'93	'94	'95	'99		Mean
Natural	7.4	6.6	5.8	6.0	5.6	7.2	8.8	8.1	6.3	5.2	7.3		6.8
Artificial	9.1	5.4	10.2	6.9	9.5	6.2	11.9	5.0	11.0	5.3	5.3		7.8

Figure 54-6. Women's lacrosse: game surface injury rates. A-E, athletic exposure. (Data from NCAA Injury Surveillance System, 2000.)

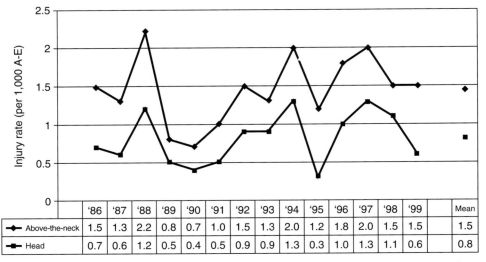

Figure 54-7. Women's lacrosse: above-the-neck and head injury rates, game. Note: head injuries are primarily concussions. A-E, athletic exposure. (Data from NCAA Injury Surveillance System, 2000.)

The prevalence of lower body strains and sprains is support for further emphasis on good off-season and year-round strength and fitness training.

Lacrosse, requiring only a mouth guard, has greater potential for possible injury prevention. The prevalence of first-degree concussions is alarming to health professionals. While many

Table 54-1. Top Three Body Parts Injured in Women's Lacrosse

PRACTICE									
YEAR	NO. TEAMS	NO. INJURIES	1ST	% TOTAL INJURIES	2ND	% TOTAL INJURIES	3RD	% TOTAL INJURIES	
1999–2000	40	152	Ankle	18%	Lower leg	13%	Foot	13%	
1998–1999	31	85	Knee	19%	Ankle	14%	Upper leg	12%	
1997–1998	41	157	Upper leg	18%	Lower leg	17%	Ankle	14%	
GAME									
		NO. INJURIES	1ST	% TOTAL INJURIES	2ND	% TOTAL INJURIES	3RD	% TOTAL INJURIES	
		57	Knee	28%	Upper leg	16%	Head	9%	
		52	Ankle	21%	Head	15%	Knee	15%	
		74	Knee	22%	Ankle	20%	Head	15%	
TOTAL (PRACTICE AND GAME)[a]									
YEAR	NO. TEAMS	NO. INJURIES	1ST	% TOTAL INJURIES	2ND	% TOTAL INJURIES	3RD	% TOTAL INJURIES	
1996–1997	51	259	Ankle	17%	Upper leg	16%	Lower leg	12%	
1995–1996	43	206	Ankle	16%	Upper leg	16%	Knee	13%	
1994–1995	36	154	Ankle	22%	Knee	12%	Upper leg	11%	
1993–1994	32	188	Ankle	19%	Upper leg	18%	Knee	11%	
1992–1993	31	138	Ankle	22%	Upper leg	15%	Knee	14%	
1991–1992	30	156	Ankle	17%	Upper leg	14%	Lower leg	14%	
1990–1991	32	167	Ankle	23%	Upper leg	18%	Knee	15%	
1989–1990	18	83	Ankle	22%	Knee	15%	Upper leg	10%	
1988–1989	27	153	Ankle	19%	Upper leg	17%	Knee	15%	
1987–1988	25	146	Ankle	21%	Upper leg	19%	Knee	13%	
1986–1987	26	166	Knee	19%	Ankle	14%	Upper leg	13%	

[a]Data collected from 1986–1987 to 1996–1997 show combined injury rates for practice and game.
Data from NCAA Injury Surveillance System, 2000.

Table 54-2. Top Three Types of Injuries in Women's Lacrosse

				PRACTICE					
YEAR	NO. TEAMS	NO. INJURIES	1ST	% TOTAL INJURIES	2ND	% TOTAL INJURIES	3RD	% TOTAL INJURIES	
1999–2000	40	151	Strain	28%	Sprain	24%	Stress Fracture	10%	
1998–1999	31	85	Sprain	28%	Strain	28%	Contusion	7%	
1997–1998	41	157	Strain	31%	Sprain	19%	Concussion	9%	

				GAME				
YEAR	NO. INJURIES	1ST	% TOTAL INJURIES	2ND	% TOTAL INJURIES	3RD	% TOTAL INJURIES	
	57	Sprain	30%	Strain	25%	Contusion	16%	
	52	Sprain	38%	Strain	17%	Contusion	17%	
	74	Sprain	36%	Strain	20%	Concussion	15%	

				TOTAL (PRACTICE AND GAME)[a]				
YEAR	NO. TEAMS	NO. INJURIES	1ST	% TOTAL INJURIES	2ND	% TOTAL INJURIES	3RD	% TOTAL INJURIES
1996–1997	51	259	Strain	34%	Sprain	26%	Contusion	7%
1995–1996	43	206	Strain	37%	Sprain	18%	Contusion	8%
1994–1995	36	154	Strain	22%	Sprain	22%	Contusion	8%
1993–1994	32	188	Strain	26%	Sprain	20%	Contusion	10%
1992–1993	31	138	Strain	25%	Sprain	22%	Contusion	10%
1991–1992	30	156	Strain	39%	Sprain	23%	Inflammation	7%
1990–1991	32	167	Strain	32%	Sprain	24%	Contusion	9%
1989–1990	18	83	Strain	27%	Sprain	22%	Tendinitis	8%
1988–1989	27	153	Strain	30%	Sprain	22%	Fracture	11%
1987–1988	25	146	Strain	28%	Sprain	26%	Contusion	9%
1986–1987	26	166	Strain	28%	Sprain	21%	Tendinitis	9%

[a]Data collected from 1986–1987 to 1996–1997 show combined injury rates for practice and game.
Data from NCAA Injury Surveillance System, 2000.

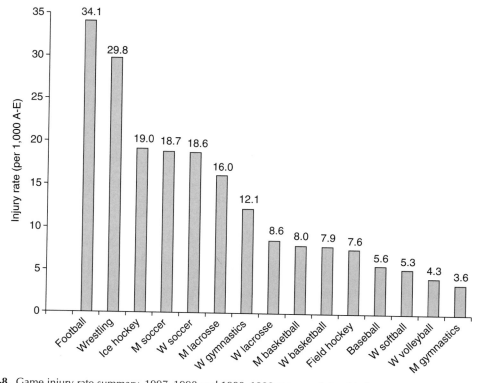

Figure 54-8. Game injury rate summary, 1997–1998 and 1998–1999 seasons. A-E, athletic exposure. (Data from NCAA Injury Surveillance System, 2000.)

debate that the use of helmets or goggles will only serve to increase the aggressiveness of women's lacrosse, some believe the sphere around the head is not adequate protection given that the ball and stick are constantly above shoulder level.

The data clearly demonstrate that the lower body is at greatest risk for injury.

Conditioning programs are most important in this sport, as teams often start training in cold, snowy weather, only to travel to warm, humid conditions. This may be partly responsible for the increase in the preseason injury rate.

All athletes, but especially women, need to have their fundamental nutritional needs evaluated throughout the season. Preseason training may require a higher calorie count for increased energy demands, while injury healing can definitely be enhanced with a balanced nutritional program.

Acknowledgments

Conclusions drawn from or recommendations based on the data provided by the NCAA are those of the author based on analyses/evaluations of the authors and do not represent the views of the officers, staff or membership of the NCAA.[3,4]

References

1. Axton WF, Martin WL: Spaulding Field Hockey. Indianapolis, Ind, Masters Press, 1993.
2. Bolhuis JH, Leurs JM, Flogel GE: Dental and facial injuries in international field hockey. Br J Sports Med 21(4):174–7, 1987.
3. Dick R: Field Hockey. NCAA Injury Surveillance System, 2000.
4. Dick R: Women's Lacrosse. NCAA Injury Surveillance System, 2000.
5. Eggers-Stroder G, Hermann B: Injuries in field hockey. Sportverletz Sportschad 8(2):93–7, 1984.
6. Hanna M: Lacrosse for Men and Women. New York, Hawthorn/Dutton, 1980.
7. Lapidus CS, Nelson LB, Jeffers JB, et al: Eye injuries in lacrosse. J Trauma 32(5):555–6, 1992.
8. Livingson LA, Forbes SL: Eye injuries in women's lacrosse. J Trauma 40(1):144–5, 1996.
9. Mayer NE, Kenney JG, Edlich RC et al: Fractures in women lacrosse players. J Emerg Med 5(3):177–80, 1987.

Chapter 55

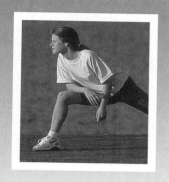

Figure Skating

Leisure Yu, M.D., Ph.D.
Angela D. Smith, M.D.

Figure skating combines speed with the athleticism and grace of ballet. The strength required to achieve such perfection depends on technical skills and physical stamina. In the last decade, the number of competitive figure skaters has grown 65 to 68% per year, with over 90% of the increase occurring in the last 5 years. This increase is due to the tremendous publicity from the Winter Olympic Games and to the commercialization of this sport in skating arenas, theater performances, and television programs.

The total number of registered skaters in North America in 1997 to 1998 was over 340,000 (data obtained from registered skaters of all ages from Canadian Figure Skating Association, United States Figure Skating Association, and Ice Skating Institute of America, 1997). The United States Figure Skating Association (USFSA) and the Canadian Figure Skating Association (CFSA) members are eligible for International Skating Union-sponsored Olympic competition. Female competitive figure skaters outnumber male skaters by 15:1 at lower levels of competition and that ratio decreases to 4:1 at the senior levels. More adult skaters are joining the competitive ranks. This trend is certain to continue as more competitions for adults are made available. The first Adult National Figure Skating Championships were held in 1995.

Serious young competitive skaters often modify their school attendance or switch to private tutoring or correspondence courses around the age of 8. Depending on the specific discipline—singles, pairs, or dance—the on-ice training time ranges from 15 to 30 hours per week, spread over 5 to 7 days. Competitive skaters spend additional time (5 to 15 hours per week) on off-ice activities, including strength training programs, music selection, and costume development. A skater's coach may often engage a choreographer, a ballet instructor, and a trainer to complete the training staff. The physical, mental, and financial costs associated with this challenging but beautiful sport can be burdensome. Parents who encourage their children to skate should review their goals with objectivity. Many figure skaters of all ages participate for the exercise, creativity, and speed possible on the ice. Additional benefits also include development of self-confidence, expression, and discipline. Only an elite few become millionaire performers, but competitive skaters turn to coaching or rink management, or volunteer their time so others can discover the lifelong joys of skating.

HISTORY AND CURRENT COMPETITIVE TRENDS IN FIGURE SKATING

The first Figure Skating World Championships were held in St Petersburg (Leningrad) in 1896 and the first Olympic figure skating events were during the London Games of 1908. Until 1979, competitive figure skating involved jumps in which only 1 or 2 revolutions were performed. However, triple jumps are now required for top competitors. Dick Button introduced the double axle in 1948 and the triple loop at the 1952 Olympics.[10] Twenty-six years later, Vern Taylor successfully executed a triple axle, completing $3\frac{1}{2}$ revolutions in the 1978 World Championships in Ottawa, Ontario. In 1988, Kurt Browning completed a quadruple toe-loop for the first time in World Championships. At the 1992 Olympic Games in Albertville, France, 13 skaters performed a triple axle, while 4 skaters attempted quadruple toe-loops.[22]

Now, champion female figure skaters perform 6 to 8 triple jumps or combinations of triples and doubles in their competitive routine. In the 1998 Olympic Games in Nagano, Japan, Tara

Lapinski at the age of 14 performed a triple loop-triple loop combination in her long program to become the youngest figure skating gold-medal Olympian. It is now common for juvenile girls as young as age 8 or 9 to perform double-revolution jumps. Prepubertal girls at the United States Junior Olympic level perform triple jumps routinely.

Artistic talent plays a very significant role in addition to technical skills. Michelle Kwan was the first figure skater ever to receive 8 perfect (6.0) scores for the artistic component of her long program during the 1998 US National competition. She accomplished this by completing 8 triple and triple combination jumps in a lyrical, flowing performance. To achieve a high level of proficiency, the training season for competitive skaters has become year round with little cross-training in other sports. The emotional and physical stresses are particularly exaggerated during the fall and winter months, when both nonqualifying and qualifying (national and international levels) competitions take place. Figure skaters participate in singles and pairs in competitions.

The status of synchronized or team skating continues to evolve. There are usually 14 to 24 members on a team. In the United States, participants are 98% female, whereas the Russian teams are typically made up of equal numbers of male and female skaters. Synchronized skating currently has no Olympic status. Its first World Championship event was held in the year 2000 in Minneapolis.

SPECIFIC PHYSICAL DEMANDS AND PROBLEMS OF FIGURE SKATING

The physical demands of figure skating are noteworthy. Skaters' programs, both long (4 minutes for senior females, 4.5 minutes for senior males) and short (2 minutes), are conducted at intensities requiring maximal aerobic and anaerobic conditioning.

Supramaximal Effort

When an athlete begins to exercise, oxygen consumption increases linearly with increasing physical intensity. After a while oxygen consumption and heart rates level off despite an increasing exercise load. The oxygen consumption, when it no longer responds to physical demand, is called maximum oxygen consumption, or VO_2max ($mL/min^{-1}/kg^{-1}$). Lactic acid, a by-product of anaerobic metabolism, begins to accumulate when a skater reaches 50% to 90% of VO_2max.[46]

This anaerobic state occurs when near maximal heart rate (190 to 200 beats/min), and VO_2max are held for the duration of the program. Several studies of skaters performing their long programs showed that the average heart rate leveled near 195 beats/min, serum lactate averaged 7 to 8 mM, and VO_2max at 40 to 50 $mL/min^{-1}/kg^{-1}$.[1,12] Thus, having a high VO_2max and being able to produce and tolerate high levels of lactic acid are competitive necessities in order for skaters to succeed.

National Championship junior-level female skaters monitored during actual competition[1,46] already had heart rates of 200 beats/min within the first 1 to 2 minutes of their long programs. Their average serum lactate value was 15 mM (the highest value was just under 20 mM). These young skaters were able to sustain very high heart rates and produced elevated levels of lactic acid, indicating that even young competitive skaters perform at near-maximum aerobic and anaerobic capacity. These VO_2max and lactate levels and heart rates are seen in trained athletes performing supramaximal effort to exhaustion.[14] It is no wonder that figure skaters sometimes complain of fatigue at the end of their long program. In order to be able to mount a physiologic response of this magnitude, skaters are encouraged to understand the need to train properly. The statement, "a great skater is a better athlete," forms the basis of this conditioning program.

Conditioning Program

The systematic approach to prioritizing both off-ice and on-ice training allows skaters to physically peak at the appropriate time for competitions. This is known as "periodization." Periodization reduces the potential for injury and maximizes a skater's performance. McMaster and colleagues[27] were the first to evaluate interval off-ice training programs that led to a 9% increase in oxygen utilization capacity and a 10-second average reduction in timed effort at a half-mile skate. Objectively, these skaters were able to complete the freestyle routine (3 minutes duration) with greater speed after a 3-month training program. Subjectively, skaters were less fatigued during the final minute of the programs. A figure skater, therefore, optimally trains with 2 parallel programs: one off-ice and the other on-ice. Both programs are monitored and progressively changed to achieve maximum performance outcome. The off-ice training program is important in reducing on-ice injury. This is especially true in pairs. Yu[48] showed that in skaters who trained with a cumulative daily off-ice program of 60 minutes or more significantly reduced their on-ice injury rate. This off-ice program amounts to core body development involving flexibility, strength training, and plyometrics. Other off-ice training programs include aerobic endurance exercises such as running, biking, or slideboarding as well as ballet for grace, posture, and expression.

Figure skating jumps and spins require significant energy. Skaters utilize strength and speed to produce angular momentum for jump rotation. During spin, skaters rotate rapidly, averaging 3 to 6 revolutions per second and generating up to 200 to 300 pounds of centrifugal force.[30] Upper and lower body strength are required to keep arms and legs in a closed "tight" position to counteract centrifugal force.[27,36] A kinematic study showed that male skaters generated higher angular momentum and faster maximal rotational velocity at take-off in performing triple axels than in single or double axels.[20] Jump height determines the length of time in the air and remains relatively unchanged between single, double, and triple axels. However, horizontal velocity and flight distance is decreased in the triple axel. Thus, in a triple axel, angular momentum is achieved at the expense of horizontal velocity and flight distance. Knoll and Hildebrand[22] emphasized the importance of developing a fast approach, an explosive take-off, and an ability to quickly attain the rotating position. Podolsky and coworkers[35] showed that higher jumps of both female and male figure skaters were highly correlated with the strength of their knee extension and flexion, hip extension and flexion, and shoulder abduction and adduction muscles. These were correlated with jump height in both single-axel and double-axel jumps.

Exercise-Induced Bronchospasm

Competitive figure skaters perform supramaximal exercise in cold, dry air, an environment that often precipitates exercise-induced asthma or bronchospasm (EIB).[7] The incidence of EIB (female and male) ranges from 30% to 50% in previously undiagnosed healthy figure skaters.[9,46] A similar incidence of EIB was also observed in a cold, humid ice arena.[5] Farber and coworkers[9] and McKenzie[26] showed that 15 minutes of continuous exercise at an intensity equivalent to 60% VO_2max provided a significant protective effect in athletes with EIB. This probably relates to the theory that high-intensity exercise resulted in the depletion of a bronchospasm mediator from the mast cell, leading to a refractory period before the mediator can be replenished. Generally, inhalation or oral medication is recommended for the symptomatic asthmatic skater. A skater who chronically experiences fatigue or shortness of breath during skating may not be "out of shape" and should be evaluated for possible EIB by a sports medicine physician knowledgeable in the field.

GENDER-SPECIFIC DEMANDS IN FIGURE SKATING

Female figure skaters often commit to the sport beginning at age 3 or 4, some 3 years before male skaters. The distribution by age from USFSA shows 50% of registered female members versus only 25% for male members occurs between ages 6 and 18. The competitive edge, therefore, goes to the female skater, who can optimize performance and avoid injury at a young age. Female skaters, however, have specific demands that are almost unique to the sport of figure skating.

Physiologic Changes at Puberty

Female skaters undergo a dramatic change in hormone levels, body habitus, emotional makeup, and physiologic events on reaching puberty. The onset of menses itself is delayed by a year (average age of onset 13.7 years) in competitive figure skaters compared with nonskater females (average age 12.6 years).[40] Forty percent of female skaters had menstrual irregularities: oligomenorrhea (20%) and amenorrhea (20%).[40] Athletic amenorrhea does not appear to have a direct association with the body fat.[28,39] On the other hand, intense physical activity and daily high energy expenditure with insufficient caloric intake are associated with oligomenorrhea and amenorrhea.[24]

The need to be a thin skater for biomechanical reasons (such as pairs and dance lifts, rotational speed in jumps and spins, and for aesthetic desires) is thwarted by weight gain. The distribution of weight to the breast, buttock, and thigh areas alters the mechanics of jumps and spins. Female skaters often are frustrated by their inability to maintain prepubertal levels of multirevolution jumps. To reflect such change and the change in the body's center of mass, coaches and skaters often comment that their "timing is off." Loss of flexibility is another physiologic change that may affect a skater's ability to perform Bielmann spins or full splits after puberty. Adolescence is a very difficult time for the female skater. Coaches, family, and other support team members should be especially sensitive to the needs of the female skater at puberty. Female skaters should be encouraged with patience and understanding. It is not unheard of for skaters to leave figure skating at this time to try to "recapture their childhood," spend more time with school friends, or reorient their sports activities.

Body Composition

The increased energy imbalance between high-intensity activities and diminished dietary intake has raised concern that skaters may be shorter in stature compared with less-active young women. However, Slemenda and Johnson[40] showed that there were no differences in height between 22 competitive skaters (25 to 40 hours on-ice per week of training) and nonathletic controls. The skaters were thinner than their nonskating controls (18.7% versus 24.3% body fat). Olympic-level female skaters' caloric intake is similar to female gymnasts and ballet dancers. However, skaters and ballet dancers have the lowest percentage of body fat (13%) compared to gymnasts (17%)[46] and their age-matched control peers (25% to 28%).[40,46]

The bone mineral density (BMD) in skaters is of significant interest as menstrual irregularity adversely affects it.[16,24] Among the 22 competitive female figure skaters Slemenda and Johnson[40] studied, the BMD in the arms, ribs, and spine was not statistically significant from that of the control group. However, the BMD of the trunk, legs, pelvis, and total body was significantly higher among skaters than among control subjects. These findings suggest that intense weight-bearing and impact-loading activities may diminish the negative effects of hormonal irregularities on bone mass. In the smaller group of skaters with menstrual irregularities, an insignificant 2% BMD deficit was observed.

Dietary Habits

During this adolescent time of dramatic biologic changes, a female skater's perception of body image and related dietary habits is important for long-term health and fitness. Female skaters not only develop dietary habits different from male skaters, it also appears that these dietary changes become more prominent with age. Olympic-level female skaters' total energy intake is approximately 55% to 76%[40,46] of the recommended daily allowances (RDA) for moderately active nonskating females. A skater's energy imbalance may be inadequate for performing prolonged, strenuous physical activity. Diminished caloric intake is of major concern as the female skaters are young, and the decreased food intake predisposes female skaters to menstrual irregularities.

Rucinski[38] showed the diminished dietary intake of vitamins, iron, and calcium in female skaters. In contrast, male skaters met the RDA for caloric intake. Using the Eating Attitude Test (EAT), a rating scale used to evaluate behaviors and attitudes found in anorexia nervosa, Rucinski[38] showed that there was a negative linear relationship between the EAT score and dietary intake for energy, iron, and thiamine in the female skater. Though not statistically significant, a negative trend was observed for other nutrients. Analysis of similar data for male skaters showed no significant correlation between EAT and dietary intake, but positive trends were observed. Rucinski's[38] study showed that the pressure on competitive male skaters for thinness did not compare with the pressure indicated by female skaters. The diminished caloric intake, with its inverse relationship to EAT scores seen in older groups of female skaters with the mean age of 17.6 years and 5.2 years postpuberty,[38] was not observed in a younger group of female skaters with the mean age of 13.7 years and 1.3 years postpuberty.[49] This preoccupation with thinness appears to be exaggerated in the female competitive figure skaters and may increase with age. It is not clear whether the risk factors also include performance standings. Nutrition counselors, therefore, should be familiar with adolescent skaters' goals and assist them in establishing nutritional practices that optimize the necessary lean body mass and provide adequate energy and essential nutrients, but maintain body weight within the range determined to be optimal for the individual skater. No optimal weight or body fat percentage applicable to all competitive female skaters has been determined.

EPIDEMIOLOGY OF FIGURE SKATING INJURIES

There are no published longitudinal prospective studies of figure skating injuries among females alone. It is logical to assume that more female than male skaters are likely to be injured since they predominate in this sport by a ratio of 15:1 during the competitive ages of 6 to 25 years. Meta-analysis of injury data is limited because the published reports use different injury severity criteria. In cross sport comparisons it is fairly accurate to say that figure skaters are less likely to sustain catastrophic injuries than elite female gymnasts or male football players of similar ages.

Surprisingly, the elimination of compulsory figures following the 1990 competitive season may have actually contributed to decrease in skating-related injuries. It is the impression of Paul Comper[8] that the decrease in on-ice injuries between the periods immediately before and after the elimination of the figure skating competition may be related to the skaters' tendency to use time previously spent in figures in more off-ice conditioning activities.

Injury Rates for Skaters

The earliest available English language retrospective study of figure skating injuries was conducted by Smith and Micheli[44] on 19 young skaters, a few of whom competed at the national level. The skaters completed a history and a physical examination. The mean age of the skaters was 13.8 years, ranging from 11 to 19 years. The average duration of skating was 4.5 years. Fourteen skated in ladies, 3 in men's, and 2 in pairs events. All skaters trained 4 to 6 hours a day, 6 days a week, 48 to 51 weeks a year. Serious injury was defined as disabling a skater from all practice for more than 72 hours. Fifteen girls were able to recall a total of 33 injuries, while 4 boys recalled a total of 19 injuries. Of the 52 total injuries reported by the skaters, 16 were the result of acute injuries and 36 resulted from overuse or stress. The authors calculated an incidence of 0.12 serious injuries per competitive year per skater. Using Chambers'[6] method to examine the incidence of acute orthopaedic injuries among school-age athletes, Smith and Micheli obtained the following indices: 0.05 for skating, 0 for swimming, 0.14 for baseball, 0.85 for gymnastics, and 1.72 for football.

The longest prospective study was performed by Smith and Ludington[43] on pair skaters and ice dancers over a 4-year period. The number of males and females were equal each year of the study. At least 85% of the skaters competed at national or international levels. The average age for female subjects was 18 ± 3.6 years and for male subjects was 21.9 ± 3.7 years. The average weight for female subjects was 46 ± 5 kg and for male subjects was 66 ± 8 kg. Skaters were examined and encouraged to report all injuries. A serious injury was defined as an injury requiring the skater to either alter training significantly or to cease training completely for at least 7 consecutive days. During the first competitive season of that study, 48 skaters sustained 33 serious injuries. Within this group, an average of 1.4% serious injuries was found for senior pair females (versus 0.4 for males); 1.2 for senior dance females (versus 1.0 for males); 0.5 for junior pair females (versus 0.8 for males); and 0.5 for junior dance females (versus 0.0 for junior dance males and novice skaters). There was no correlation between injury incidence and age, height, weight, or national ranking. There was an apparent correlation between injury rate and the difficulty of moves performed only in the pair skater group. Lifting maneuvers caused 11 of the serious injuries. Few of the serious injuries were thought to be preventable. However, the subsequent 3 years of the study showed a reduction in both the serious and less serious injuries as flexibility, strength training, and other interventions were introduced.[42]

Kjaer and Larsson[21] prospectively followed 8 elite Danish single figure skaters (3 men, 5 women) for a period of 1 year. An injury was recorded if it led to time lost from practice or competition. All injured skaters were examined by a physician. Skaters trained 29 ± 4 hours per week with 80% of the time on ice and 20% of the time off ice. The injury incidence was recorded as 1.4 injuries per 1,000 hours of training, with 56% of the injuries acute and 44% chronic injuries. Six of the skaters sustained 18 injuries, with 8 of the injuries due to overuse injuries and 7 involving the lower extremity. The injuries resulted in a mean of 4 days lost from training or competition. The authors noted only 83% of the registered injuries were recalled by skaters when a retrospective questionnaire was administered at the end of the observation period.

Garrick[13] surveyed all the competitors in the 1981 US National Championships, and 70 of the skaters responded to a written questionnaire. The skaters reported a total of 150 injuries sustained during their careers. Brock and Striowski[3] surveyed 64 Canadian National Team skaters by a mailed questionnaire with a follow-up phone call and input from the skaters' coaches. Sixty competitors responded, including 32 women and 28 men. There were 29 single skaters, 18 ice dancers, and 13 paired skaters. The skaters trained an average of 27.2 hours per week on ice, and spent 5.6 hours per week on conditioning off ice and 12 minutes per week on preskating warm-up and stretching exercises. Twenty-eight skaters sustained an injury that caused loss of training or competition time or a decrease in performance rating. Fourteen skaters had acute injuries and 12 reported overuse injuries. Two reported injuries were unrelated to skating. Four of the 12 overuse injuries were caused by skating boots. There were no differences between the training patterns, skating level, boot type, height, weight, and body fat percent of the injured and uninjured skaters. The authors calculated injury rates (dividing the number of injuries by the number of participants per year) for the ice skaters at 47%, compared with 138% for elite female gymnasts and 81% for boys in football. The gymnasts spent a similar amount of time training as the skaters, whereas football players spent fewer hours per week in football practice.

Fortin and Roberts[11] surveyed 53 skaters who sought medical treatment at the 1987 US National Championships, from a total of 200 competitors. Seventeen of the skaters had sustained an injury during that competition and others sought treatment for previous injuries. One third of the injured skaters were pair skaters, and one fourth were ice dancers. These results differed slightly from the findings of Garrick,[13] who showed that single skaters were at greater risk of injury when he surveyed a group of all competitors 5 years earlier.

Brown and McKeag[4] studied 7 pair skating teams in a single training center by a written questionnaire. They evaluated injury patterns during pairs' and singles' events. Only 11 of the 14 skaters responded. The average age for the females (14.0 years) was 4 years younger than their male counterparts (18.1 years). The girls started skating at an average of 6.5 years of age, more than 3 years earlier than the boys. The pairs skated an average of 18.9 hours per week. Thirty-nine injuries from singles skating and 9 injuries from pair skating caused them to miss at least 1 day of training. The study showed that even with an average loss of 10.3 successive days of training during each injury, only 22% of the injuries were treated by a physician. Single female skaters were less likely to report injuries than single male skaters, 38% and 72%, respectively. Of the 9 pair skating injuries, 3 were concussions and 3 were fractures or dislocations. The predominant injuries from single skating were hip injuries in females and knee injuries in males.

Injury Rates for Recreational Skaters

The female recreational skater, unlike her elite sister, presents with different injury rates. Williamson and Lowden[47] evaluated ice skating injuries after the opening of a new ice rink, which provided many people with the chance to skate for the first time. They evaluated all patients coming to a nearby hospital for 2 months after the opening of the ice rink. There were 203 ice skating injuries, 113 in females and

90 in males, with a mean age of 21 years. The prevalence of skating injuries was far in excess of those from roller skating (100 in 3 months) and skateboarding (75 in 3 months) at hospitals with a similar drawing population. It was interesting to note, however, that the weekly incidence of injuries per thousand visits to the ice rink declined over the first 10-week period, with a correlation coefficient of -0.88. Serious injury rate declined from 0.14% initially to 0.03% of participants.[37] Further analysis of their data showed that the hospital's workload represented 1% of all emergency department visits. This represented an injury rate of 0.31% of all who skated at the rink during the study period.

Newton[31] also evaluated emergency department visits by ice skaters for 3 months following the opening of a new ice rink. Skating injuries accounted for 2.2% of the patients seen in the emergency department, with a risk-of-sustaining-an-injury rate of 0.037%. The overall injury rate (including first-aid records) was 0.1%, which was similar to that of the study reported by Radford and colleagues.[37] This study did not evaluate the injury patterns by gender. However, 67% described themselves as first-time skaters or novices. The majority of the group sustaining injury was aged 16 to 20 years. Bernard and coworkers[2] evaluated a total of 169 injured recreational skaters over one calendar year (1984). Fifty-nine percent of the patients were female and 41% were male. The average age at the time of injury was 16.4 years. Fifteen percent required hospital admission, primarily due to fractures.

Injury Severity of Figure Skating

Definitions of injury severity differ from publication to publication. In Brock and Striowski's[3] study of acute figure skating injuries, the average time before returning to practice was 12 days. However, the average time for skaters to achieve full recovery was 11 weeks, which was skewed by 2 skaters with meniscal injuries. The average time of return to practice for tendinitis and patellofemoral pain was 18 days, and the average time for full recovery was 9 weeks. The Smith and Ludington[43] study defined significant alteration of the training program for at least 7 consecutive days as the criterion for serious or significant injury. There were 33 serious injuries among 48 skaters within the first year of study. Smith's prospective study of 305 consecutive, competitive season injuries of National and World team members found only 6 injuries that required greater than 28 days for full recovery. These included a concussion, herniated lumbar disk, severe lumbar strain, tibial stress fracture, a painful multipartite patella that required partial resection, and a comminuted patellar fracture sustained in an auto accident (unpublished data).

Injury Type and Location

Competitive Figure Skater Injuries

In most of the studies, competitive figure skaters' injuries (serious and minor) have been evenly divided between acute and overuse injuries. Overuse injuries occur more frequently among females and acute injuries among males. Serious injuries, however, were more likely to be acute.[6,43,44] Injuries of single skaters tend to involve, in order of decreasing frequency, the lower extremity, low back, upper extremity, and head and neck.[11,13] Overuse injuries of the knee (patellofemoral syndrome, jumper's knee, etc) and hip (bursitis, tendinitis, muscle strain, etc) were no different from those seen in other sports and responded well to known standard treatment regimens of muscle rehabilitation. Lower extremity injuries occurred most commonly around the knee. Female skaters had a higher incidence and level of pain in hips and feet than male skaters. Recently, the authors have noticed an increased incidence (4 cases in 2001 versus 1 case in 2000) of low-back pain associated with lumbar-5 pars fracture in competitive skaters performing triple-triple jumps.

Among 11 pair skaters questioned in one training center, the leading injury was muscle pull (31%), followed by fractures (21%).[4] Fractures accounted for 48% of lost training days. Other studies reported markedly lower fracture rates. Pair skaters sustained additional injuries to the shoulder girdle, wrist, and low back from the lifting maneuvers. Female pair skaters had the highest risk of sustaining injury (Smith and Ludington[43]). Most of the serious pair skater injuries were caused by throw jumps. In a throw jump, the female skater is hurled into the air and across the ice, at the same time performing a 1- to 3-revolution jump and then landing on one foot. Serious injuries are rarely seen in lower-level pair skaters, presumably due to less difficult technical jumps, slower speed, and lower body center of gravity. Upper extremity injuries in pair skaters were more likely to occur in the wrist and shoulder and less likely in the elbow and hand (Brown and McKeag,[4] Smith, unpublished data). Female ice-dancers had higher risk for injury than their male partners.[43]

Acute Knee Injuries. Meniscus injuries are infrequent among competitive figure skaters and career-threatening knee injuries are extremely rare. Anterior cruciate ligament (ACL) injuries, interestingly, have not been reported until recently.[32] The relative paucity of internal derangement of the knee may be inherent in the sport of figure skating. Almost all of the jumps are landed skating backward, where cocontraction of quadriceps and hamstring muscles are essential for control. Furthermore, the leg lands in an open kinetic position on a slippery gliding surface. A recent report of ACL injuries[32] seen in one female single skater and one male skater occurred during incompletely performed triple jumps. The incomplete rotation resulted in a forward landing position with momentary fixation (closed kinetic position) of the blade on the ice and overactive quadriceps reflex. Following their ACL reconstructions, the female skater returned to competitive skating, but the male skater quit the sport at age 19.

Acute Ankle Injuries and Stress Fractures. Smith's unpublished data on 305 injuries of competitive skaters at one training center showed that 12 of 305 injuries were ankle sprains. Of the 12 ankle sprains, 2 occurred off the ice, 3 were recurrent (related to a previous injury), and 2 were caused by throw jumps. Therefore, only 5 of the 305 injuries were first-time on-ice ankle sprains sustained by single skaters. Her findings contrasted with those of Kjaer and Larsson,[21] whose study group of 8 skaters sustained 6 on-ice ankle sprains during the 1-year study period.

Pecina and coworkers[34] evaluated the frequency of stress fractures among 42 world-class figure skaters through a retrospective questionnaire study. Nine skaters, 5 female and 4 male, had sustained stress fractures. The time span from onset of symptoms to definite diagnosis ranged from 2 to 10 weeks. Four of the stress fractures occurred during preseason off-ice training associated with increased running mileage. Five stress fractures occurred during the season. In all situations, the fracture involved the take-off leg. Two skaters had a tarsal navicular stress fracture, 2 had a Jones fracture of the fifth metatarsal, and one fractured the anterior cortex of the middle third of the tibia. Of the 9 injured skaters, 8 were treated nonoperatively. One skater with a Jones fracture was treated surgically. All skaters were able to resume a preinjury level of activity 3 to 7 months after treatment began. Stress fractures, therefore, should be included in the differential diagnosis of the skaters' lower extremity pain as they occur relatively often among all athletes comprising about 5% of all sports injuries,[17,25] although they have been reported less frequently among competitive skaters. The present authors are not aware of any case of death or permanent paralysis during competitive figure skating. There are no studies to suggest long-term disability resulting from injuries sustained in competitive figure skating.

Avulsion injuries, muscle strains, and stress fractures that cause pain during walking should be put to complete rest, possibly requiring crutches or even a cast for 2 to 3 weeks, until pain free. Recent advances in early stress fracture healing may include the use of low intensity pulsed ultrasound[23] in skeletally mature skaters.

In synchronized team skating, lacerations about the legs, elbows, and hands, as well as shoulder strain, appear to be the most common injuries. Overuse injuries involving feet of synchronized ice skaters have been reported by Kennedy and coworkers[19] in 31 skaters (28 female, 3 males). Most of these injuries were presumably related to boot wear.

Recreational Figure Skater Injuries

Ice skating injury in the general population is quite different from that of competitive single skaters. Upper extremity injuries, especially fractures, predominate over lower extremity injuries. Williamson and Lowden's study[47] found 48 upper extremity fractures compared with 13 lower extremity fractures in a total of 203 skaters who presented to the emergency department. Forty-seven percent of the fractures were seen in patients over 25 years and only 26% of the fractures were seen in patients under 25 years. Lacerations were sustained mainly on the hands or fingers, followed by the face and the lower extremity. Bruises and sprains were most common in the knee, followed by the wrist, the ankle, and then the elbow. The majority of the mechanisms of injury in recreational skaters were due to falling. The rest were collisions with another skater.[2,31,37] Oakland's[33] study found 77 fractures and 8 dislocations seen in 467 patients over a 1-year period following the opening of a local ice rink. Alcohol consumption was mentioned as a contributing factor in 25 of the 77 fractures. Twenty-three patients required admission as the result of head injuries, although there were no skull fractures. Thirty-three skaters required an operative procedure under anesthesia.

Figure Skating Injury Prevention and Treatment

The first step to injury prevention in any sport, including figure skating, is fitness. This involves a daily routine of warm-up and cool-down,

stretching for flexibility, strengthening for core body development, and plyometric exercises for jumping. Appropriate periodization of strength training, plyometric exercises, and cardiovascular interval drills may optimize the skater's performance at key events during the season.

Figure skating has inherent risks because of speed and technical flexibility demands. Smith and coworkers[45] investigated the relationship between thigh muscle flexibility and anterior knee pain in 46 adolescent elite junior skaters over an 18-month period. Anterior knee pain, including jumper's knee, Osgood-Schlatter disease, and patellofemoral disorders, was observed in 30% of the skaters. Female skaters (38%) had more complaints than males (20%). Poor flexibility of the quadriceps muscles was associated with all types of anterior knee pain, and poor flexibility of the hamstrings was associated with patellofemoral pain. Three fourths of the skaters who improved their quadriceps flexibility eliminated their knee pain. However, at the US Olympic Training Center, Katz and colleagues[18] tested 8 figure skaters and found no relationship between the quadriceps/hamstring isokinetic torque power ratio and the incidence of knee injury, which was reported in 50% of the skaters tested.

In the skeletally immature skater, sites of muscle attachment should be evaluated for apophysitis or epiphyseal avulsion. A relatively common injury is iliac crest apophyseal avulsion. This injury often requires 2 to 3 months for healing. Skaters with this injury often have pain in the flank (abdominal transversalis), lumbar, and gluteal muscles, with tenderness in the iliac crest area. Frequently skaters will also have pain or tightness in the iliopsoas and quadriceps muscles. Roentgenograms show increased distance from the epiphysis and the bone. Magnetic resonance image (MRI) studies will show edema around the epiphysis and in muscle groups that attach there. The iliac crest avulsion injury often occurs on the side contralateral to the landing leg, where rotational torque pull is the greatest.

Bursitis of the foot is a common complaint in figure skaters. This is because of the stiffness of skating boots. New skating boots should be worked over and loosened up to the same "softness" of the old boot before skating in them. The offending area of the boot should be punched out and silicone gel pads used. Bursal aspiration with an injection of steroid and using coban wrap may rarely be considered. Finally, surgical bursectomy is occasionally needed for recalcitrant cases. The best way to treat bursitis is to never let it begin to be a chronic problem. It is better to operate on the boot than on the skater. Stress fracture and fracture healing time may be shortened by the use of low-intensity pulsed ultrasound.[15]

Equipment

As early as 1979 Ferstle[10] recommended a return to more flexible skating boots. Still, most advanced skaters prefer very rigid boots. These boots allow minimal inversion or eversion and very little plantar flexion of the ankle. The skater wearing stiff boots dorsiflexes the ankle by pushing the tibia against the tongue and laces of the boot, often causing anterior tibial bursitis. The authors strongly advocate flexible boots and have presented a functional pair actually worn by a competitive skater.[41] However, manufacturers have not found a large market share for such a boot. Younger skaters may be advised to begin wearing boots that are more flexible than the extremely rigid boots favored by competitors currently. More flexible boots allow the muscles of the foot and leg to develop appropriately so that when the skater is ready to attempt more difficult jumps, they can rely on their muscles to provide both jumping height and landing strength.[29]

CONCLUDING REMARKS

Competitive figure skating increasingly demands physical stamina, technical skills, and artistry. The female skater commits herself to full-time skating at a very young age. Owing to the nature of the sport and preoccupation with thinness, many female skaters consume an inadequate amount of calories. This diminished intake in the face of increased energy consumption places her at high risk of endocrinopathy associated with menstrual cycle irregularity. However, the high-impact nature of the sport seems to protect her from the injurious effects of hormonal imbalances on bone mineral density.

Evidence suggests that off-ice programs diminish the incidence of overuse injuries when combined with flexibility programs. Competitive figure skating requires the female skater to perform at supramaximal levels in both the long and the short programs. The periodization of her off-ice and on-ice training not only allows her to be able to achieve these supramaximal efforts, but also optimizes her performance during competitions.

The female pair skater is more likely to be injured than any other skater in singles or in pairs. Overall, the injury rate for figure skaters is much lower than that of elite gymnasts.

Competitive skaters' injuries are rarely career or life threatening. As our understanding of the biomechanical, physiologic, and psychological demands of ice skating grows, we anticipate an improved multidisciplinary approach to training and injury prevention for competitive skaters.

References

1. Aleshinsky SY, Podolsky A, McQueen C, et al: Strength and conditioning program for figure skating [roundtable discussion]. Natl Strength Condit Assoc J 10:26–30, 1988.
2. Bernard AA, Corlett S, Thomsen E, et al: Ice skating accidents and injuries. Injury 19:191–2, 1988.
3. Brock RM, Striowski CC: Injuries in elite figure skaters. Physician Sportsmed 14:111–5, 1986.
4. Brown EW, McKeag DB: Training, experience, and medical history of pair skaters. Physician Sportsmed 15:101–13, 1987.
5. Buch B, Smith A, Padman R: Incidence of exercise-induced bronchospasm in elite figure skaters. Presented at the American College of Sports Medicine Annual Meeting, Baltimore, 1989.
6. Chambers RB: Orthopaedic injuries in athletes (ages 6–17), comparison of injuries occurring in six sports. Am J Sports Med 7:195–7, 1987.
7. Chen WY, Horton DJ: Heat and water loss from the airways and exercise-induced asthma. Respiration 34:305–13, 1977.
8. Comper P: The Impact of Removing Compulsory Figures from Figure Skating: The Sports Medicine and Sports Science of Skating. San Jose, Calif, January 1996.
9. Farber MO, Mannix ET, Palange P, et al: Exercise-induced asthma in elite figure skaters. Clin Res 39:754, 1991.
10. Ferstle J: Figure skating: in search of the winning edge. Physician Sportsmed 7:129–33, 1979.
11. Fortin JD, Roberts D: Competitive figure skating injuries. Arch Phys Med Rehabil 68:642, 1987.
12. Gaisl G, Wiesspeiner G: Training prescriptions for 9 to 17-year-old figure skaters based on lactate assessment in the laboratory and on ice. In: Rutenfranz J, Rolf M, Ferdinand K (eds): Champaign, Ill, Human Kinetics Publishers, 1985, pp 59–65.
13. Garrick JG: Figure skating injuries. Med Sci Sports Exerc 14:141, 1982.
14. Gastin PB, Costill DL, Lawson DL, et al: Accumulated oxygen deficit during supramaximal all-out and constant intensity exercise. Med Sci Sports Exerc 27:255–63, 1995.
15. Heckman J, Ryaby J, McCabe J, et al: Acceleration of tibial fracture-healing by non-invasive, low-intensity pulsed ultrasound. J Bone Joint Surg 76A:26–34, 1994.
16. Howat P, Carbo M, Mills G, Wozniak P:. The influence of diet, body fat, menstrual cycling, and activity upon the bone density of females. J Am Diet Assoc 89:1305–7, 1989.
17. Hukko A, Orava S: Stress fractures in athletes. Int J Sports Med 8:221–6, 1987.
18. Katz AL, Stone J, Van Handel P: Injury status and isokinetic torque and power of quadriceps and hamstrings muscles: normative data on elite athlete groups. In: Tenenbaum G, Eiger D (eds): Life Sciences. Proceedings of the Maccabiah-Wingate International Congress. The Emmanuel Gill Publishing House, Israel Wingate Institute for the Physical Education and Sports 1989, pp 264–78.

19. Kennedy D, Klupp N, Wirth J, Periman PR: Overuse injuries of precision ice skating. Sports Med News September:12, 1992.

20. King DL, Arnold AS, Smith SL: A kinematic comparison of single, double, and triple axels. J Appl Biomech 10:51–60, 1994.

21. Kjaer M, Larsson B: Physiological profile and incidence of injuries among elite figure skaters. J Sports Sci 10:29–36, 1992.

22. Knoll K, Hildebrand F: Entwicklungsstand der drei-und vier-factisprunge im eiskunstlauf (Developmental standing of triple and quadruple jump in figure skating). Trainingslehre December 15:11–4, 1992.

23. Kristiansen T, Ryaby J, McCabe J, et al: Accelerated healing of distal radial fractures with the use of specific, low-intensity ultrasound. J Bone Joint Surg 79A:961–73, 1997.

24. Loucks AB: Effects of exercise training on the menstrual cycle: existence and mechanism. Med Sci Sports Exerc 22:275–80, 1990.

25. Matheson GO, Clement DB, McKenzie DC, et al: Stress fractures in athletes. A study of 320 cases. Am J Sports Med 15:46–58, 1987.

26. McKenzie DC, McLuckie SL, Stirling DR: The protective effects of continuous and interval exercise in athletes with exercise-induced asthma. Med Sci Sports Exerc 26:951–6, 1994.

27. McMaster WC, Liddle S, Walsh J: Conditioning program for competitive figure skating. Am J Sports Med 7:43–7, 1979.

28. Mickelsfield LK, Lambert EV, Fataar AB, et al: Bone mineral density in mature, premenopausal ultramarathon runners. Med Sci Sports Exerc 27:688–96, 1995.

29. Montag WD: The figure skating boot. In: Segesser B, Pforringer W (eds): The Shoe in Sport. St Louis, Year Book Medical Publishers, 1987, pp 175–80.

30. Nash HL: U. S. Olympic figure skaters: honing their performances. Phys Sport Med 6:181–5, 1988.

31. Newton AP: Ice skating injuries: a survey of cases seen in an accident and emergency department. J Roy Nav Med Serv 77:71–4, 1991.

32. Nichols A, Yu L, Garrick J, Raqua R: Anterior cruciate ligament injury in two international figure skaters. Mechanism of injury. The Third Congress on the Sports Medicine and Sports Science of Skating. Philadelphia, January 1998.

33. Oakland CDH: Ice skating injuries: can they be reduced or prevented? Arch Emerg Med 7:95–9, 1990.

34. Pecina M, Bojanic I, Dubravcic S: Stress fractures in figure skaters. Am J Sports Med 18:277–9, 1990.

35. Podolsky A, Kaufman KR Cahalan TD, et al: The relationship of strength and jump height in figure skaters. Am J Sports Med 18:400–5, 1990.

36. Poe CM, O'Bryant HS, Laws DE: Off-ice resistance and polymetric training for singles figure skaters. Strength Condition 68–76, 1988.

37. Radford PJ, Williamson DM, Lowdon IMR: The risks of injury in public ice skating. Br J Sports Med 22:78–80, 1988.

38. Rucinski A: Relationship of body image and dietary intake of competitive ice skaters. J Am Diet Assoc 89:98–100, 1989.

39. Sanborn CF, Albrecht BH, Wagner WN: Athletic amenorrhea: lack of association with body fat. Med Sci Sports Exerc 19:207–11, 1987.

40. Slemenda CW, Johnson CC: High intensity activities in young women: site-specific mass effects among female figure skaters. Bone Miner Res 20:125–32, 1993.

41. Smith A: An articulated skate boot. International Congress on the Sports Medicine and Sports Science of Skating. San Jose, Calif, January 1996.

42. Smith A: Reduction of injuries among elite figure skaters. A 4-year longitudinal study. Med Sci Sports Exerc 23(Suppl 4):151, 1991.

43. Smith AD, Ludington R: Injuries in elite pair skaters and ice dancers. Am J Sports Med 17:482–8, 1989.

44. Smith AD, Micheli LJ: Injuries in competitive figure skaters. Physician Sportsmed 19:36–47, 1982.

45. Smith AD, Stroud L, McQueen C: Flexibility and anterior knee pain in adolescent elite figure skaters. J Pediatr Orthop 11:77–82, 1991.

46. USFSA/USOC Sports Science and Medicine Camp Report. Colorado Springs, Colo, 1995.

47. Williamson DM, Lowden IMR: Ice skating injuries. Injury 17:205–7, 1986.

48. Yu L: Injuries of national and international competitive skaters. International Congress on the Sports Medicine and Sports Science of Skating. San Jose, Calif, January 1996.

49. Ziegler P, Heusley S, Roepke JB et al: Eating attitudes and energy intakes of female skaters. Sports Sci Med Exerc 30:583–6, 1998.

Chapter 56

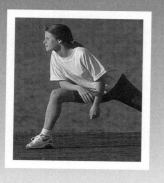

Golf

John R. McCarroll, M.D.

Golf is one of the most popular sports in the world. In every community in the United States there are more golf courses being built, and more people of all ages and gender becoming involved in golf. Until recently very little was written about the frequency and treatment of golf injuries, especially in women. Only 3 articles have looked at men and women separately.[14–16] Dr. William J. Mallon[11] has authored a column in *Golf Digest*, and between 1985 and 1991 he received over 1400 letters concerning golf injuries and illness. Although not scientific, these letters constitute a fairly large body of data concerning injury patterns in the recreational female golfer (Table 56-1). Mallon[11] found that the lower back was the most commonly injured body part in the female golfer (45%), followed by the left elbow (27%), the left wrist (14%), and the left shoulder (4%).

McCarroll and Gioe[14] found the left wrist was injured in 31.3% of golfers, followed by the lower back in 22.4%, and the left hand in 9%. The left shoulder, elbow, and knee injuries were very similar in frequency (Table 56-2). McCarroll[12] also looked at injuries in the female amateur golfer (Table 56-3). In the amateur golfer the left elbow was most commonly injured (35.4%), followed

by the lower back in 27%, left shoulder in 16%, and hand and wrist in 14.5% of players.

Most of these injuries are caused by frequent player practice, resulting in overuse syndromes. Other causes, such as poor swing mechanics, hitting an object other than the ball, and poor warm up, are summarized in Table 56-4.

GOLF SWING BIOMECHANICS

To evaluate, treat, and prevent golf injuries it is important to understand the biomechanics of the golf swing. For the purpose of this chapter the golf swing will be broken down into 3 stages: take-away, impact, and follow-through. The golf swing occurs in 2 planes: the plane of the backswing and the plane of the downswing. The swing evolves in 3 dimensions: vertical, lateral, and rotatory.[10]

Take-Away

Take-away consists of the setup and movement to the top of the backswing (Fig. 56-1). This

Table 56-1. Injury Complaints from *Golf Digest*

INJURY SITE	NO. INJURIES IN FEMALES (*N* = 311)
Lower back	111 (45%)
Left elbow	68 (27%)
Lateral elbow	49 (20%)
Medial elbow	19 (8%)
Left wrist	35 (14%)
Left shoulder	10 (4%)
Left ankle	7 (3%)
Right hip	4 (2%)
Left hip	4 (2%)
Right knee	3 (1%)
Left knee	1 (<1%)

Adapted from JR McCarroll: The frequency of golf injuries. Clin Sports Med 15(1): 1–7, 1996, with permission.

Table 56-2. Professional Golf Injuries (LPGA)

INJURY SITE	NO. INJURIES REPORTED (*N* = 201)
Left wrist	63 (31.1%)
Lower back	45 (22.4%)
Left hand	18 (9%)
Left knee	12 (6%)
Left elbow	9 (4.5%)
Foot	9 (4.5%)
Right wrist	9 (4.5%)
Right shoulder	9 (4.5%)
Left shoulder	6 (3%)
Ribs	6 (3%)
Ankle	6 (3%)
Cervical spine	3 (1.5%)
Right elbow	3 (1.5%)
Groin	3 (1.5%)

Adapted from JR McCarroll: The frequency of golf injuries. Clin Sports Med 15(1): 1–7, 1996, with permission.

Table 56-3. Golf Injuries in the Amateur Female

INJURY SITE	NO. INJURIES REPORTED (N = 124)
Elbow	44 (35.4%)
Lateral	34 (27.4%)
Medial	10 (8.1%)
Lower back	34 (27.4%)
Shoulder	20 (16.1%)
Hand and wrist	18 (14.5%)
Knee	14 (11.3%)
Ankle	10 (8.1%)
Ribs	6 (4.8%)
Hip	4 (3.2%)
Neck	2 (1.6%)
Forearm	2 (1.6%)

Adapted from JR McCarroll: The frequency of golf injuries. Clin Sports Med 15(1): 1–7, 1996, with permission.

stage starts when the golfer addresses the ball. The golfer rotates the knees, hips, and lumbar and cervical spine while the head remains relatively stationary. The weight shifts to the right side. As the backswing continues, the left arm (in the right-handed golfer) is raised and swings across the trunk. Electromyelographic studies have shown that the only muscle activity in the upper extremities during the take-away stage is that of the suprascapularis of the left arm.[7] There is hyperabduction of the left thumb, radial deviation of the left wrist, and dorsiflexion of the right wrist. However, less than 25% of golf injuries occur during this stage of the swing.

Impact

The impact stage consists of the downswing and impact of the club with the ball (Fig. 56-2). There are more than twice as many injuries during the impact stage as there are during the take-away stage. During the downswing the club covers the same range of motion (ROM) as in the take-away, but moves about 3 times as fast.

As the downswing begins the golfer shifts weight to the left side by moving the hip toward the target. Good golfers actually begin this hip movement about 0.1 second before the downswing starts.[1,4] To develop maximum acceleration in the downswing stage, a golfer applies the stretch reflex principle. When the whole muscle is stretched, the muscle spindles produce a reflex contraction of their host muscles. As a result, the contractile force of the muscle increases and facilitates a recoil of elastic tissues. Increasing the flexibility of the major muscle groups can further develop this principle. The farther the golfer can rotate the shoulders away from the target, the greater club head speed that can be generated—thus increasing distance.

This counterclockwise torque in the upper body is generated by the buttocks, quadriceps, hamstrings, and lower back muscles. The torque causes moderate levels of activity in the pectoralis major, latissimus dorsi, and rotator cuff muscles in both shoulders.[7] During the downswing, the wrist applies a negative torque by remaining cocked. At this time, the right wrist is in maximum dorsiflexion; the left thumb is hyperabducted, and the left ulnar nerve, elbow, and forearm muscles are under tension. When the club is approximately horizontal to the ground, both wrists uncock, which accelerates the club into the ball. The pectoralis major, subscapularis, and latissimus dorsi of both arms power these movements.[7]

The impact stage of the golf swing begins the instant before contact when the club head has obtained its maximum velocity, and ends the instant the ball has completely left the club. From a performance aspect, the purpose of impact is to hit the ball as far as possible in the proper direction. From a safety aspect, the purpose of the impact stage is to have a smooth transition from acceleration to deceleration.

Table 56-4. Mechanisms of Injury

INJURY	PROFESSIONAL GOLFER	AMATEUR GOLFER
Overuse from play/practice	270	204
Poor swing mechanics	0	150
Hit ground—divot	40	171
Over swing	0	85
Poor warm-up	0	60
Twist during swing	18	22
Grip or swing change	0	26
Fall	2	24
Bending over putt	5	8
Injury caused by cart	0	18
Hit by ball	3	36

Adapted from JR McCarroll: The frequency of golf injuries. Clin Sports Med 15(1): 1–7, 1996, with permission.

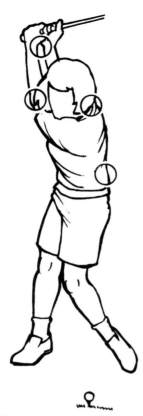

Figure 56-1. The golfer has moved the club to the top of the backswing. The circles indicate areas of stress.

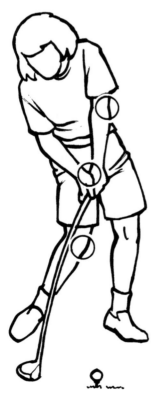

Figure 56-2. The impact stage. The circles show areas of stress.

At impact 80% to 95% of the weight has been transferred to the left side.[18] This is true of low- and high-handicap golfers. Skilled golfers, however, generally have their weight supported toward the heel of the foot, whereas, lesser skilled golfers tend to support themselves on the middle of the foot.[4] This implies that skilled golfers probably get more counterclockwise rotation during the swing.

During impact, valgus stress occurs on the right knee, both wrists are under compression, and the extension muscles of the left elbow contracts. The left wrist, hand, and elbow are often hurt during the compression of impact.

Follow-Through

About 25% of all golf swing injuries occur during follow-through (Fig. 56-3). After impact, the left forearm supinates, the right forearm pronates, and the lumbar and cervical spines rotate and hyperextend in the right-handed golfer. Hip rotation is also completed. The subscapularis (along with reduced levels of the latissimus dorsi and pectoralis muscles of both arms) continues to be active, decelerating the swing.[7] Both knees rotate, the right knee flexes, and the left knee everts. At this point all the weight should be transferred to the left side. As the club decelerates, the golfer extends the back into a reverse-C position (Fig. 56-4A). This position was once

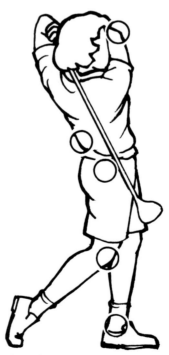

Figure 56-3. Once the golfer has impacted the ball, the follow-through stage begins and ends with completion of the golf swing. The circles show areas of stress.

thought to be essential to playing golf—this is not necessarily true of the more modern golf swing. Most injuries in this stage occur in the back, secondary to the reverse-C position.

The golf swing is the cause of many injuries. However, to avoid these injuries, the golfer must correct the faulty swing mechanics. Professional golf instructors, using years of experience, and equipped with video recorders, can correct the mechanics of the golf swing to prevent injuries and change abnormal stresses applied to various body parts. Also, there are many different types of clubs, shafts, and other equipment. A golf instructor should be consulted before making a final decision on what equipment to use.

INJURIES AND TREATMENT

Hand and Wrist

Hand and wrist injuries account for nearly 18% of all golf injuries.[15] Tendinitis is the most commonly seen problem in the wrist and forearm of the golfer. This is the result of the repetitive motions of the wrist and forearm during the swing and stress at impact. Tendinitis may involve any of the tendons about the wrist. The pain is usually aching or burning in nature.

On physical examination, there may be tenderness over the tendon, especially with resisted motions of the wrist. There may be crepitus felt along the tendons associated with motion.

Tendinitis is treated with rest and/or modification of activities, anti-inflammatory medication, and ice. Other modalities, such as phonophoresis with 10% hydrocortisone cream and ultrasound, or electrogalvanic stimulation (EGS), as described by Standish and coworkers,[19] are also helpful. The golfer is started on a functional progression golf program before returning to full activity (Table 56-5).

De Quervain's disease is tenosynovitis of the first dorsal compartment of the wrist and is a common condition. The author has seen many professional golfers who have developed this disease as a result of repetitive practice. A positive Finkelstein's test is diagnostic. The thumb and hand are forcibly deviated toward the ulnar side of the wrist, producing exquisite pain over the radial styloid process and the common sheath of the first compartment. This test is similar to the mechanisms used in hitting a golf ball, especially at preimpact and impact. Conservative treatment of de Quervain's involves splinting, ice, and medication. Injection or operative treatment is considered only in resistant cases.

The hook of the hamate is a long, thin bone that is subject to injury as it projects toward the palmar surface of the hand.[20] In golfers, fractures occur when the grip of the club strikes the hook of the hamate. Clinically, the golfer has tenderness over the hook of the hamate. Roentgenograms should include anteroposterior, lateral, oblique, and carpal tunnel views of the wrist. If these views are negative, but a fracture is still suspected, a bone scan or computed tomography (CT) scan may be helpful. In the acute, nondisplaced fracture treatment is a short-arm cast and rest for 6 weeks. The incidence of nonunion of this fracture is high. A badly displaced fracture, or a nonunion of the fracture, requires surgical excision.

The golfer may suffer from other miscellaneous hand and wrist conditions, including ligamentous sprains, carpal tunnel syndrome, Guyon's canal syndrome, or impaction/impingement syndromes.[3,9,17] Occult or overt ganglia, ulnar compression syndromes, and distal radial ulnar joint syndrome, may result from the golf swing and must be considered when treating hand and wrist injuries.

Elbow

Golfers may suffer 2 common elbow injuries: medial and lateral epicondylitis.[21] These may be caused by faulty swing mechanics or overuse from repetitive swinging throughout the season. Tennis and golfer's elbow develop simultaneously with essentially the same symptoms, treatment, and prognosis. They differ only in site of inflammation. In the author's experience, medial epicondylitis occurs more often in golf than in tennis, but lateral epicondylitis is the most common injury in both.

Occurring in varying degrees of disability, epicondylitis may be mild, with pain felt only when the golfer swings the club. In more severe cases, sufferers may find themselves unable to perform even simple activities of daily living. The diagnosis of epicondylitis can usually be determined by a series of simple tests. Tenderness to palpation over either epicondyle, or pain with resisted dorsi or volar flexion of the wrist, is diagnostic. Tendinitis is by far the most common of all elbow injuries, but radial tunnel syndrome and ulnar nerve entrapment must also be considered. Furthermore, radiating pain may be caused by degenerative changes in the region of C5 and C6.

Treatment is divided into 4 stages:

1. Relief of acute or chronic inflammation is accomplished with rest, ice, anti-inflammatory medications, and splinting.[2]

Table 56-5. Interval Golf Rehabilitation Program[a]

WEEK	MONDAY	WEDNESDAY	FRIDAY
1	5 min chip and putt 5 min rest 5 min chip and putt	5 min chip and putt 5 min rest 5 min chip and putt 5 min rest 5 min chip and putt	5 min chip and putt 5 min rest 5 min chip and putt 5 min rest 5 min chip and putt
2	10 min chip and putt 10 min rest 10 min short iron	10 min chip and putt 10 min rest 10 min short iron 10 min rest 10 min short iron	10 min chip and putt 10 min rest 10 min short iron 10 min rest 10 min short iron
3	15 min short iron 10 min rest 15 min long iron 10 min rest 15 min long iron	15 min short iron 10 min rest 15 min long iron 10 min rest 15 min long iron	15 min short iron 10 min rest 15 min long iron 10 min rest 15 min long iron
4	Repeat Friday of week 3	Play 9 holes	Play 18 holes

[a]Do flexibility exercises before hitting and use ice after hitting.
From JR McCarroll: Golf. In: Fu FH, Stone DA (eds): Sports Injuries: Mechanisms, Prevention, Treatment. Baltimore, Williams & Wilkins, 1994, pp. 375–81, with permission.

2. Increased forearm strength, flexibility and endurance is needed. This is accomplished through eccentric exercises and cross-friction massage that stresses flexibility of the muscles and increased strengthening.

3. One must correct poor technique in order to ensure the injury will not recur. The author decreases movement of force at the wrist by altering the swing mechanics. Equipment changes also may be necessary to correct the force that is placed on the forearm muscles. Few equipment changes are available to golfers to alleviate symptoms of tendinitis in the elbow, however, a larger grip size has been helpful to some golfers. Graphite shaft clubs cause less torque and may relieve some stress in the epicondyle area. Elbow supports provide a reactive force against the contractile muscles, and either spread the force over a wider area or decrease the contractile pull of the epicondyle, and thus, can be helpful.

4. Steroid injections are used when other treatments have not relieved the pain. If injections do not help, and all other conservative treatment has failed, surgery may be considered.

Shoulder

Repetitive overuse syndromes are the most common cause of shoulder pathology in golfers. However, previous insults, incomplete recovery from those insults, degeneration of general body strength, and lack of conditioning by nonuse or extended time of play must also be considered as precipitating factors. Inflammation of the rotator cuff musculotendinous units is initially reversible. With continued repetitive insults, soft-tissue structures microscopically tear, articular cartilage degenerates, osseous tissue produces osteophytes, and the labral rim erodes. At this stage, spontaneous reversibility is doubtful. When scarring, decreased ROM, instability, and impingement occur, surgical intervention and rehabilitation are necessary for recovery. Total-body conditioning before playing golf is advisable, however, special attention should be given to the shoulder joint. Strengthening and proper swing mechanics must be stressed in order to prevent overuse injuries.

Back

Injuries to the back, especially the lumbar spine, are some of the most common injuries in both professional and amateur golfers (see Tables 56-1 to 56-3). The repetitive, compression, and increased rotational forces placed on the back during the golf swing affect the bony structures, intervertebral discs, ligaments, and muscles of the lower back. The reverse-C position (Fig. 56-4A) was once thought to be essential. By holding this position through impact, the golfer promotes correct ball trajectory, better body leverage, and solid impact. Many players exaggerate this position in an effort to hit the ball farther, and through repetitive practice such golfers have paid the penalty of severe back problems. It is now thought that a more upright finish (Fig. 56-4B) puts less stress on the lower back.

Hosea and coworkers[5,6] studied the kinematic and myoelectric analysis of the golfer's back. They found that the period from initiation of the backswing to the end of the follow-through

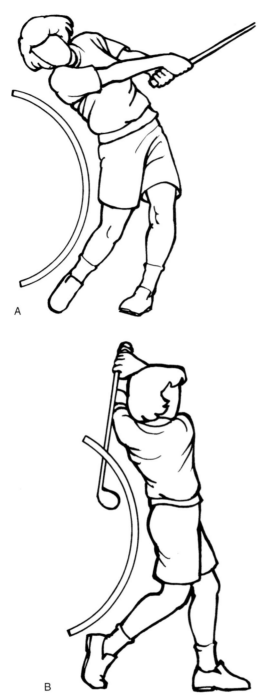

the backswing to ball impact, while amateurs covered the same portion of the swing in 0.37 seconds. Yet both groups achieved nearly the same club head velocity at impact (2.317 + 3.52 m/sec for pros versus 20.02 + 1.84 m/sec for amateurs). The professional group generated more than 34% greater peak club head acceleration, which occurred just before impact.

The golf swing produced a complex loading pattern, involving large shear, lateral bending, compression, and axial torsional loads with rapid changes in directional forces. The amateurs generated an average of 596.74 + 514.01 N in peak shear load at the L3 to L4 segment after impact, yet the large standard deviation indicated a wide variation in mechanics present in this group. The professionals averaged 329.36 + 141.27 N or 80% less peak shear load. Furthermore, the amateurs generated 81% greater peak lateral bending force than the professionals. This is well-demonstrated by the professional golfer's classic weight shift from right to left side when changing direction from take-away to follow-through; whereas the amateur golfer reveals a common problem of swinging from the top or reverse pivoting causing the upper torso actually to lean from the ball at impact.

Although the professionals generated a greater peak compression load than amateurs, both groups generated more than 8 times their body weight at the peak in the lower back. There were 2 peaks of compression forces, at the top of the backswing and during follow-through (see Figs. 56-1 to 56-3). The amateur golfers generated a peak torsion load of 85.4 + 34.21 N, while the load of professionals was 50% less. Yet despite the lower torque force, the professionals generated 34% greater club head acceleration at impact, indicating that they use the arms and wrists instead of the trunk, unlike most amateurs. Myoelectric analysis revealed that the left external, and to a lesser degree, the left rectus abdominis, and left L3 paraspinal initiate the take-away. The right-sided muscles lead from the top of the backswing through impact. It is during this period that the peak muscle forces occur. Anterior muscles continue to fire during the follow-through, while the paraspinals are essentially inactive. The right-sided external oblique and abdominal rectus muscles developed a higher peak activity than the left, while the paraspinals are nearly symmetrical. The amateurs, who demonstrated higher shear, lateral bending, and torsional loads, also generated a higher peak total overall activity of the tested muscles.

Hosea and colleagues[5,6] demonstrated that the magnitude of force on the lumbar spine dur-

Figure 56-4. **A**, The golfer is in the reverse-C position. This golfer experiences more torque and increased risk of spinal injury. **B**, This golfer is in a more erect position, producing less stress to the lower back.

averaged 1.55 seconds for professional golfers compared with 1.86 seconds for amateur golfers. The backswing averaged 49% of the total swing (0.76 seconds) for pros compared with 53% (nearly 1 second) in amateurs. Professionals took 0.23 seconds from the top of ing the golf swing is sufficient enough to produce pathologic changes over time. These changes most likely occur at the intervertebral disc, pars interarticularis, and/or facet joints.

To evaluate lower back problems, the physician should consider the use of routine roentgenography, CT, bone scanning, and magnetic resonance imaging (MRI) in addition to the physical examination. Treatment of lower back problems includes anti-inflammatory medications and physical therapy. It is also important that the golfer's swing be analyzed to identify faulty swing mechanics. The presence of rapid and intense loading of the lumbar spine (in what was previously considered a nonstrenuous sport) indicates the need for preparticipation conditioning, reasonable practice patterns, and thorough warm-up before play.

Lower Extremities

The lower extremities are the foundation for the swing. Proper leg action promotes good rhythm, balance, and tempo. Injuries to the lower extremities, although not as frequent as upper extremity injuries in golf, can be bothersome. McCarroll and Mallon[15] found the knee was injured in 6.6% of professional golfers and 9.3% of the amateur golfers.

The most common hip problem seen in golfers, especially females, is trochanteric bursitis. This is an inflammatory condition of the bursa overlying the greater trochanter and is usually caused by rotation of the hip during practice, overuse in the frequent golfer, combined with walking on uneven terrain. Treatment includes rest, ice, anti-inflammatory medication, and physical therapy, which may include cross-friction massage, ultrasound, and stretching of the usually tight tensor fascia latae or iliotibial band.

The author has treated 5 young golfers (between 35 to 40 years old) who have arthritic changes of both hips. These golfers complained of decreased hip motion, especially with abduction and internal rotation. Each experienced aching associated with playing. None of these golfers had past medical indications for arthritis. Roentgenograms showed early arthritic changes about the hip, with narrowing of the joint space. Four of the 5 responded to anti-inflammatory medication and physical therapy. One of the gentlemen, however, continued to have joint deterioration, and eventually underwent total hip arthroplasty. He has returned to golf, but the opposite hip has developed similar symptoms.

Other common injuries of the lower extremities are meniscus tears (usually degenerative), patellofemoral syndrome, calf strains, Achilles tendinitis, and plantar fasciitis.[13]

CONDITIONING

Golf demands a high degree of refined motor skills. There are many frustrated golfers lacking physical conditioning. The weekend golfer, and even the professional golfer, must condition her body before going to the course or assume the risks of injury. Injuries, sore muscles, and frustrating days on the golf course can be eliminated with year-round conditioning.

There are 4 types of exercises that will help female golfers prevent injuries. Stretching exercises are used to maintain complete ROM of the hamstrings, back, and shoulders. Without complete ROM and flexibility, the golf swing will put abnormal stress on various body parts.

Golf is not a strength game like other sports. Strength in itself will not enable the individual to hit a ball farther and longer. However, it will allow the skilled player to strike shots with a more consistent, explosive power over extended periods. Any golfer with a weak muscle area, especially in the shoulder or back, is at risk for a golf injury. One can use equipment such as Nautilus, Universal gym, or home devices such as free weights or weighted clubs to increase strength.

These workout programs also developed the endurance needed to walk long distances, climb hills, and repeat the swing over and over during a game. There are various muscles that must be strengthened to improve basic golf skills. Table 56-6 reviews a workout program for golfers. For the golfer who does not have access to specialized exercise equipment, an excellent reference book of home exercises is available.[8]

Cardiovascular exercise for endurance is another essential part of conditioning. Climbing hills and walking 18 holes is impossible without a cardiovascular system that will respond to strenuous exercise. The golfer should follow a preseason conditioning program that includes jogging, cycling, walking, and/or stair-stepping machines to reach ideal cardiovascular condition for the sport.

In many sports such as football, basketball, and baseball, injured athletes are put through a functional progression and rehabilitation program before returning to their sport. Table 56-5 is an example of an interval golf rehabilitation program to return the injured golfer safely to play.

Golfers are athletes, because golf is a sport. To play it well one must have athletic ability,

Table 56-6. Nautilus Workout Program for Golfers

EXERCISE[a]	MUSCLES	SKILLS
Hip, back	Buttocks, lower back	Driving power, walking endurance
Leg extension	Quadriceps	Driving power, walking endurance
Leg curl	Hamstrings	Hip turn, driving power
Double shoulder (lateral press)	Deltoids	Club control, impact velocity
Double shoulder (seated press)	Deltoids, triceps	Shoulder turn, club extension
Pull over	Latissimus dorsi	Shoulder turn, club extension
Wrist curl	Forearm flexors	Club head control, impact power, acceleration
Reverse wrist curl	Forearm extensors	Club head control, acceleration

From Peterson J: Conditioning for a Purpose—the West Point Way. West Point, NY, Leisure Press, 1977, with permission.
[a]Perform one set of 8 to 12 repetitions of each exercise. Take no more than 60 seconds to perform each set. Rest no more than 30 seconds between each set.

strength, agility, coordination, and endurance. The golf swing is physically demanding and can contribute to various types of injuries. The wrist, back, and shoulder are the most frequently injured body parts. These injuries can be prevented or reduced by a combination of proper conditioning, correct swing mechanics, and prompt and appropriate treatment of injuries when they occur.

Suggested Readings

Gluten G (ed): Golf injuries. Clin Sports Med 15(1), 1996.
Stover CN, McCarroll JR, Mallon W (eds): Feeling Up to Par: Medicine from Tee to Green. Philadelphia, FA Davis, 1994.

References

1. Cochran A, Stobbs J: The Search for the Perfect Swing. Portsmouth, NH, Heinemann Educational, 1968.
2. Curwin S, Standish WD: Tendinitis: Its Etiology and Treatment. Lexington, Mass, DC Heath, 1986.
3. Dobyns JH, Sim FH, Linscheid RL: Sports stress syndromes of the hand and wrist. Am J Sports Med 6:236–53, 1978.
4. Hay JG: The Biomechanics of Sports Techniques. Englewood Cliffs, NJ, Prentice-Hall, 1973.
5. Hosea TM, Gatt CJ, Calli KM, et al: The golfer's back: a kinematic and myoelectric analysis. Presented at the American Orthopaedic Society for Sports Medicine Meeting and the First Scientific Meeting of Golf Science. Edinburgh, Scotland, 1991.
6. Hosea TM: Mechanical Analysis of the golfer's back. In: Stover CN, McCarroll JR, Mallon W (eds): Feeling Up to Par: Medicine from Tee to Green. Philadelphia, FA Davis, 1994.
7. Jobe FW, Moynes DR, Antonelli DJ: Rotator cuff function during a golf swing. Am J Sports Med 14:388–92, 1986.
8. Jobe FW, Moynes DR, Antonelli DJ: 30 Exercises for Better Golf. Inglewood, Cal, Champion Press, 1986.
9. Linscheid RL, Dobyns JH: Athletic injuries in the wrist. Clin Orthop 198:141–51, 1985.
10. Maddalozzo GF: Anatomical and biomechanical analysis of the full golf swing. Nat Strength Coaches Assoc J 9:4–6, 1990.
11. Mallon WJ: Ask the doctor {semimonthly column}. Golf Digest 1986–1991.
12. McCarroll JR: The frequency of golf injuries. Clin Sports Med 15(1):1–7, 1996.
13. McCarroll JR: The lower extremity. In: Stover CN, McCarroll JR, Mallon WJ (eds): Feeling Up to Par: Medicine from Tee to Green. Philadelphia, FA Davis, 1994, pp 165–9.
14. McCarroll JR, Gioe TJ: Professional golfers and the price they pay. Physician Sportsmed 10:64–8, 1982.
15. McCarroll JR, Mallon WJ: Epidemiology of golf injuries. In: Stover CN, McCarroll JR, Mallon WJ (eds): Feeling Up to Par: Medicine from Tee to Green. Philadelphia, FA Davis, 1994, pp 9–13.
16. McCarroll JR, Rettig AC, Shelbourne KD: Injuries in the amateur golfer. Physician Sportsmed 18:122–6, 1990.
17. Rettig AC: The wrist and hand. In: Stover CN, McCarroll JR, Mallon WJ (eds): Feeling Up to Par: Medicine from Tee to Green. Philadelphia, FA Davis, 1994, pp 151–62.
18. Richards J, Farrell M, Kent J, et al: Weight transfer patterns during the golf swing. Res Q Exerc Sport 56: 361–5, 1985.
19. Standish WD, Rubinovich RM, Arwin S: Eccentric exercise in chronic tendinitis. Clin Orthop 208:65–8, 1986.
20. Torisu T: Fracture of the hook of the hamate by a golf swing. Clin Orthop 83:91–4, 1972.
21. Weston PA: Injury from a disrupted golf ball. Lancet 1(8007):375, 1977.

Chapter 57

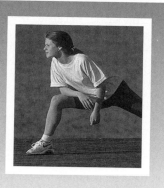

Gymnastics

Susan M. Ott, D.O.

The sport of women's artistic gymnastics has changed dramatically over the last 20 years. The participation and popularity of the sport has increased significantly and will most likely continue to grow. Gymnastics is unique among sports in that as the athlete advances toward the elite level of the sport, she must continually learn new skills. In most sports the same basic skills are performed at every level of participation; it is only the proficiency with which those skills are performed which changes. This is a sport in which early participation is the norm, with the trend toward starting at even younger ages. It is not uncommon for children to begin gymnastics training at 2 to 3 years of age. The average age of the United States national team has declined from the 1960s through the 1990s, but this trend is now changing since an Olympic team member now must turn 16 during the Olympic year in order to participate in the games.

It is important for the health care provider to understand the equipment, training techniques, and conditioning programs used in gymnastics as well as gymnasts' health care needs when treating these athletes. Because of the nature of the sport of gymnastics it is usually possible for training to continue on some level despite injury. It is also important for the health care provider to account for the skill level of the patient when formulating a treatment plan.

HISTORY

Gymnastics began as a competitive sport during the 1800s, but it has existed for over 2000 years as an activity. The Sokols and the Turnvereins established the first gymnastics clubs and exhibitions. Gymnastics was first introduced to the United States in the 1830s. In 1881 the European Gymnastics Federation (now the International Gymnastics Federation, FIG) was established, and in 1883 the Amateur Athletic Union (AAU) took control of gymnas-

tics in the United States. Gymnastics first appeared in the Olympics during the 1896 games. Male athletes from 5 countries competed in the events of horizontal bar, parallel bars, pommel horse, rings, and vault. The first world championships were held in 1903, and during the 1904 Olympic games the men's team combined competition was added. Track and field events were held during the world gymnastics championships until 1954. Women's gymnastics became an Olympic event during the 1928 games and the United States sent its first women's Olympic team to the 1936 games. The current governing body for gymnastics in the United States is USA Gymnastics, formerly known as the United States Gymnastics Federation, which was established in 1970. The sports of rhythmic gymnastics, trampoline, and tumbling are also governed by USA Gymnastics.

USA Gymnastics provides coaches, athletes, and parents with information on coaching and safety, as well as conditioning and nutrition. An athlete wellness program has been established which provides information on health care issues for gymnasts, and has established a health care referral network of professionals with experience in treating gymnasts. This network consists of physicians, psychologists, nutritionists, athletic trainers, and physical therapists available as a resource for coaches, athletes, and parents. USA Gymnastics has made a position statement regarding eating disorders and the female athlete triad. This information is available on the USA Gymnastics website (http://www.usa-gymnastics.org) and through its publications.[21,39]

LEVEL OF COMPETITION AND PARTICIPATION

The image that most of the public has of a female gymnast is that of the elite or Olympic gymnast. While these are the most visible athletes in the sport, they also make up the smallest percentage of thousands of athletes. USA Gymnastics estimates there are approximately 55,000 athletes in the competitive women's program. Of those, only 190 are elite gymnasts.[39] Competitive club gymnastics begins at level 4 and goes to level 10 followed by the elite level.[39] Table 57-1 summarizes the number of participants at each level.[39] When treating gymnasts it is important to know what level they compete at. By asking the simple question, "What level are you?" the health care professional can garner a fairly good idea of the amount of training the athlete is doing and how intense that training is. In general the higher the competitive level, the more hours trained per week and the higher the risk of injury.

There are several other levels of participation in gymnastics. There are recreational programs, noncompetitive classes, and precompetitive classes. Some areas of the country have high school gymnastics programs. The skill level of high school gymnasts varies greatly. Many colleges and universities have gymnastics teams. As in any NCAA sport there are divisions I, II, and III for the sport of gymnastics. Most collegiate gymnasts are at least level 8 and most are level 9 or above.

OTHER USA GYMNASTICS— SANCTIONED SPORTS

The sports of rhythmic gymnastics, trampoline, and tumbling are also governed by USA Gymnastics. Trampoline made its Olympic debut during the 2000 games. Rhythmic gymnastics became an Olympic sport in 1984 and a medal sport in 1996. Rhythmic gymnasts compete in the events of rope, hoop, ball, clubs, and ribbon. There is also a group event consisting of 5 athletes working as a unit. The routines are performed to music on a 13- × 13-meter floor with the various apparatus. The sport of rhythmic gymnastics requires extreme flexibility and stresses leanness in the athletes. Leaping ability

is also important in this sport.[25,28] The injuries sustained by rhythmic gymnasts are similar to those sustained by dancers. Because of the repetitive nature of their sport and the extreme flexibility it requires, rhythmic gymnasts are at risk for overuse injuries. Low back pain is the most common complaint.[24] As in artistic gymnastics, rhythmic gymnasts are at risk for eating disorders and disordered eating.

INJURY RATES

Numerous studies have examined injury rates among gymnasts.[5,12,17,19,22,29,31,32,34,38,40,46–49] There have been studies that have looked at injury rates among college, high school, club, and noncompetitive gymnasts. Only one study has attempted to asses the long-term effects of injuries sustained during the athlete's competitive career.[22] Each of these studies has concluded that gymnastics is a sport that carries a high risk of injury and that risk increases with the increasing ability of the athlete. National Collegiate Athletic Association (NCAA) data indicate that gymnastics carries the highest incidence of injury among all women's intercollegiate sports.[26] Most studies agree that floor exercise and tumbling carry the highest risk of injury and vault the lowest.[5,17,40,46] A study by Sands and colleagues[46] of NCAA division I athletes documented that 71% of the time the gymnast was training with an injury, and that a new injury occurred 9% of the time. That study also documented an increased risk of injury during competition and just prior to competition. Thirty-eight percent of the injuries sustained during the study period were overuse injuries.[46] Caine and coworkers[5] surveyed 50 club gymnasts. Six of the 50 athletes were injured at the onset of the study. Of the remaining 44 athletes, 38 had trained with pain in the 2 weeks prior to the study. The Caine study documented a reinjury rate of 32%.[5] These studies document that training with an injury and/or pain is common in gymnastics and that overuse injuries are common as well.

EQUIPMENT AND EVENTS

There are 4 events in women's gymnastics: vault, uneven parallel bars, balance beam, and floor exercise. Dance and tumbling are traineds as part of the events of floor and beam. Other equipment used in training gymnasts includes mats, tumble tramps, trampolines, spotting belts, foam-filled pits, and spring boards. There are certain injuries that are specific to each event.

Table 57-1. Number of Female Gymnasts per Training Level in the United States

TRAINING LEVEL	NUMBER OF ATHLETES
Level 4	11,247
Level 5	18,446
Level 6	9012
Level 7	5890
Level 8	4956
Level 9	3104
Level 10	1767
Elite	190

Vault

In the vault event in women's gymnastics, the gymnast is required to propel herself over the vaulting horse. This is accomplished by running down a carpeted runway, jumping onto the springboard, and perfoming the vault over the horse. Some vaulting horses are spring-loaded to absorb forces and to give the athlete additional push off the apparatus. In 2001 a new vaulting table was approved for use at the senior level. The new apparatus was designed to reduce injuries associated with the standard vaulting table. It was first used at the 2001 World Gymnastics Championships.

Several studies have documented that the event of vault is responsible for the lowest percentage of injuries in women's gymnastics.[16,17,46] Overuse injuries such as shin splints can be attributed to this event. Acute injuries are usually due to falls onto or off of the horse or badly landed vaults. Yerchenko vaults or round-off entry vaults are allowed only at the highest level of competition because of the high risk of injury associated with this type of vault.[32] Twisting vaults account for a large number of knee injuries.[12,22,32] If the gymnast does not have enough height to complete the twisting component in the air, her foot can plant on the mat as her body continues to twist, resulting in injury. This is a common mechanism for anterior cruciate ligament (ACL), medial collateral ligament (MCL), and meniscal injury.[2]

Uneven Parallel Bars

The event of uneven parallel bars, or bars, is the women's event that has changed the most over the last 2 decades. The bars have become smaller and more rounded, and the gymnasts now compete with bars much further apart. How high the bars are and the distance between them varies with the age, size, and ability of the gymnast. Injury during uneven bars work is often due to a fall off of or onto the equipment or a poorly landed dismount.[23,33] Priest and Wiese in a study of elbow injuries in gymnastics found that uneven bars is the event with the highest incidence of elbow injuries.[41,42]

Women's uneven bars has become more similar to the event of men's high bar and many of the release moves now done by the women originated in the men's event. With the increase in the number and difficulty of release moves done on bars, the risk of injury has also increased. The number of giant swings done by the women has increased as well. This move places tremendous stress across the upper extremity.[3,6] When an athlete begins L-grip giants, a movement that is performed with the forearms in a hypersupinated position with a forward grip on the bar, wrist pain can become a complaint or a chronic problem worsened.

An injury specific to uneven bars and men's high bar and unique to the sport of gymnastics is called *grip lock*. Most gymnasts use doweled grips for bars. The grips serve to protect the hands from friction injury, to increase the athlete's grip on the bar, and to maintain the fingers in a flexed position. Grip lock occurs when the doweled grip becomes locked on the bar, but the gymnast's momentum continues to carry her through the skill. The forces propelling the gymnast around the bar are transmitted to the wrist and forearm and can result in fracture. Forces transmitted to the distal radius from routine use of doweled grips are a potential cause of chronic wrist pain in gymnasts.[45]

Balance Beam

The balance beam is 4 feet high, 4 inches wide and 16.5 feet long. It is leather covered and padded, and some are spring-loaded. Injuries on balance beam are usually due to falls onto or off of the equipment or a poorly landed dismount. The springboard is frequently used for mounting the beam. When learning new skills on beam a low beam, only a few inches off the ground, is used first and the height gradually increased. Finger and toe injuries frequently occur if the athlete lands on a flexed digit, or catches a finger or toe on the edge of the beam. Figure 57-1

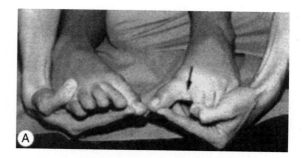

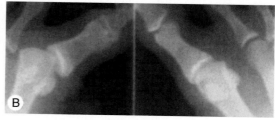

Figure 57-1. A, This collegiate gymnast sustained multiple dislocations of the first metatarsal phalangeal joint, one of which was open, due to repetitive injuries on the balance beam. **B,** Preoperative stress roentgenograms of the same athlete. (Courtesy of M.L. Ireland, MD)

demonstrates stress testing of an intercollegiate gymnast who sustained recurrent injuries to the great toe when landing on the beam, resulting in medial dislocations, one of which was open.

Floor Exercise and Tumbling

The event of floor exercise is competed to music on a 40- × 40-foot carpeted mat. Most gymnasts practice and compete on a spring-loaded floor. The springs under the mat give the athlete additional push off as well as provide a more cushioned landing surface. Floor exercise has dance and tumbling elements. Tumbling and floor are responsible for the highest percentage of injuries in women's gymnastics.[5,17,32,38,46,49] Overuse injuries such as shin splints and wrist pain can occur. Tumbling passes that are landed short or twisting elements that are landed poorly account for most acute injuries.[32,47]

COMMON GYMNASTICS INJURIES

Back Injuries

Back pain is a common complaint among gymnasts.[17,46] High-impact landings and repetitive hyperextension of the lumbar spine contribute to back pain in this group of athletes.[20] Roentgenograms should be obtained in athletes who present to the physician's office, or with a history of back pain of more than 2 weeks' duration. If roentgenograms are negative, single-photon emission computed tomography (SPECT) scanning should be done to rule out spondylolysis, which is fairly common in the female gymnast.[1,8,14,27] Spina bifida can be associated with spondylolysis. Vertebral end plate fractures have been reported in gymnasts as well.[35] Fractures should be treated with bracing and rest.[8] Other potential causes of back pain that should be ruled out include discogenic pain, tumor, diskitis, and infection.[18,33,35]

Once fracture has been ruled out, back strains in gymnasts can be treated conservatively with physical therapy, nonsteroidal anti-inflammatory drugs (NSAIDs), and activity modification.[18,24] Training modifications should include limiting the number of high-impact landings and repetitive hyperextension. Landings can be cushioned by increasing matting, using sting mats, and tumbling on tumble tramps or into a pit. Physical therapy that focuses on upper and lower back strengthening, abdominal strengthening proprioception, and core stability should be emphasized.[37]

Wrist Injuries

A study by Difiori and coworkers[13] indicates that approximately 80% of gymnasts will experience wrist pain at some point in their career. Wrist pain is so common in this population it is almost considered the norm. Wrist injuries and wrist pain are common in gymnastics owing to the fact that the upper extremities become weight bearing.[9] Young gymnasts have been reported to have stress changes of the distal radial epiphysis. Repetitive axial compression forces on the distal radius can cause epiphyseal reactions or fracture. Radial growth arrest with subsequent ulnar overgrowth can occur.[4,7,10,11,15,44] In a study of nonelite gymnasts Difiori and colleagues[11] found that 25% of the athletes in the study had radiographic findings consistent with stress injury of the distal radius and a more positive ulnar variance than age-predicted norms. Scaphoid fractures and injury to the triangular fibrocartilage complex can also occur.[9,15] Roentgenographic examination should be done on any gymnast presenting to the physician's office with wrist pain. Many gymnasts use wrist braces with a hyperextension block to decrease wrist pain and theoretically prevent injury. There are several commercially available types of braces, but there are no outcome studies evaluating their efficacy.

Elbow Injuries

Elbow injuries are fairly common in gymnasts and are probably underdiagnosed. Elbow dislocations can occur and are usually due to a fall off a piece of equipment onto an outstretched hand.[41,42] The injury is confirmed with roentgenograms. Care should be taken to rule out vascular injury. Postreduction films should be obtained to be sure no fracture is present. Figure 57-2 demonstrates a right elbow dislocation with a left elbow fracture dislocation. This injury occurred in a level 10 athlete who fell from the uneven bars during practice.

Osteochondritis dessicans of the capitellum can occur and is probably underrecognized. Because of the fact that the upper extremities are weight bearing and tremendous stresses are placed across the elbow, gymnasts are at increased risk for this injury. Loose bodies can occur and result in locking symptoms. Figure 57-3 demonstrates osteochondritis dessicans of the capitellum with loose body formation in this gymnast turned cheerleader. The loose bodies were removed arthroscopically. A careful ligamentous examination should be done in the face of osteochondritis in order to rule out medial elbow instability.

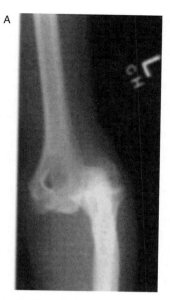

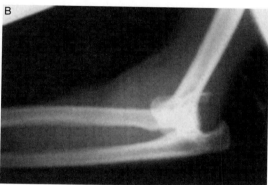

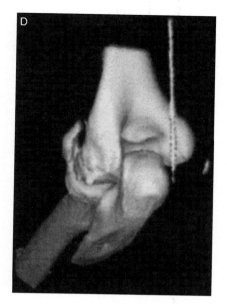

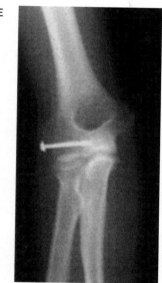

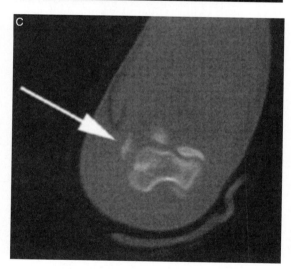

Figure 57-2. This level 10 gymnast sustained a right elbow dislocation and a left elbow fracture dislocation after a fall from the uneven bars. The medial epicondyle fracture was treated with open reduction and internal fixation. **A & B,** Preoperative radiographs. **C,** CT scan. **D,** Three-dimensional view. **E,** Postoperative roentgenogram. (Courtesy of M.L. Ireland, MD)

Shoulder Injuries

Shoulder injuries are becoming more common in the sport of gymnastics, and many athletes are having problems with chronic instability. In most injury surveys done in gymnastics populations indicate that while shoulder injuries are common, they are not the most or least frequent complaint. Superior labrum anterior posterior (SLAP) lesions have been reported in gymnasts and should be in the differential of shoulder pain in a gymnast not responding to conservative care.[6] Rotator cuff tears are rare in young athletes, and instability is the more likely diagnosis. An assessment of the scapulothoracic musculature should be done as part of the shoulder examination. Athletes with weak scapulothoracic musculature and a weak upper

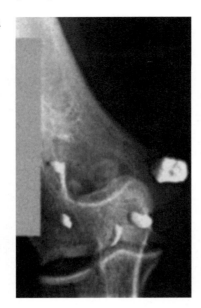

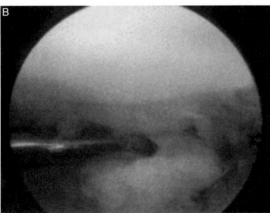

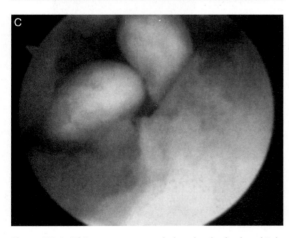

Figure 57-3. This gymnast turned cheerleader had multiple loose bodies and osteochondritis dessicans of the capitellum. **A,** Preoperative roentgenogram. **B & C,** Intraoperative arthroscopic views. (Courtesy of M.L. Ireland, MD)

back are at increased risk for shoulder injury. Physical therapy should focus on rotator cuff strengthening and scapulothoracic stabilization.

Chronic instability or shoulder pain not responding to conservative care may need operative intervention.

Knee Injuries

Knee injuries in gymnastics fall into the categories of overuse injuries and acute injuries. Overuse injuries include patellofemoral stress syndrome, Osgood–Schlatter disease, symptomatic medial plica, and tendinopathies.[2,26] Errors in technique, underconditioning, and overconditioning may be the cause of overuse injuries in the gymnast. Most overuse injuries can be treated conservatively with physical therapy, NSAIDs, and activity modification. Care should be taken to rule out tumor, infection, discoid meniscus, and osteochondritis dessicans.[2]

Acute knee injuries frequently occur when landing twisting elements on any of the events.[22,32] As the gymnast lands the skill, if she is not high enough the foot plants and the body continues to twist. This is a common mechanism of injury for ACL, MCL, and meniscal injury. Hyperextension injuries can occur on any of the events and, while less common than twisting injuries, can also result in ACL injury. Most MCL injuries can be treated conservatively. ACL and meniscal injuries should be addressed operatively in active individuals. Roentgenograms should be taken to evaluate the skeletal maturity and to rule out fracture. Mechanisms of injury that may cause a ligamentous injury in an adult may cause fracture in a skeletally immature individual. In young athletes with ACL injuries, surgical decisions may need to be changed if the athlete is skeletally immature. This is especially important in gymnasts, as they tend to lag behind the norm in attaining maturity.[30]

Leg, Foot, and Ankle Injuries

As in most other sports, the ankle is frequently injured in gymnastics as well. Inversion ankle sprains are common. Oftentimes a short landing will add a dorsiflexion component to the injury, resulting in a high ankle sprain. Subluxing peroneal tendons are another potential source of lateral ankle pain. Other causes include talar dome fracture, lateral ankle impingement syndrome, osteochondritis dessicans of the talus, and stress fracture of the lateral malleolus. Ankle sprains not responding to conservative care should be evaluated for these possible problems.[26]

Foot injuries are common in gymnastics as well. Gymnastics is one of the few sports in which no shoes are worn. Some athletes wear socks or gymnastics slippers, but it is essentially a no-shoe sport. Posterior tibialis tendonitis is not uncommon. The mechanism is frequently repetitive landings on the beam with the arch of the foot straddling the beam, forcing the foot into pronation and external rotation. Toes can be injured on the beam as a result of bad landings or landing on a flexed toe. Toes also can be jammed into the bar during uneven bars work. Stress fractures of the metatarsals are less common as are injuries to Lisfranc's joint. Young gymnasts often suffer from Sever's disease, which can be treated conservatively. Achilles tendonitis and Achilles tendon rupture are other potential foot injuries that can occur in gymnastics.

In the leg, shin splints, or medial tibial stress syndrome, commonly occurs in gymnasts. Running for vault and tumbling, dance elements, and high impact landings contribute to this overuse injury. Care should be taken to rule out exertional compartment syndrome. Stress fracture is another potential source of anterior tibial pain. Shin pain not responsive to conservative care should be evaluated for stress fracture with roentgenograms and a bone scan.[26] In athletes with documented stress fracture a careful nutritional and menstrual history should be obtained in order to rule out athletic amenorrhea and the female athlete triad.[16,26]

Disordered Eating and the Female Athlete Triad

Disordered eating is often underdiagnosed in female athletes, including young female gymnasts. Although studies assessing eating disorders in female gymnasts compared to their nonathletic peers have not uniformly demonstrated an increased prevalence of eating disorders in this population, most of the studies have assessed gymnasts in the college setting, with few studies assessing the younger (more common) club gymnast. In addition, there is a lack of well-controlled studies assessing disordered eating in this population, and an urgent need for studies defining the prevalence of disordered eating in the sport, as well as optimal strategies for prevention and treatment. Both artistic and rhythmic gymnasts, however, are *at risk* for disordered patterns of eating, including restrictive eating, as well as binge–purge behaviors.[21,36,50] Coaches, athletes, and parents need to be aware of the increased risk of disordered eating and have mechanisms in place for prevention.[21,26,36,50] According to the American Psychiatric Association definitions, eating disorders are gross disturbances in eating behavior

that typically begin during adolescence or early adult life. Athletes with bulimia participate in recurrent episodes of binge eating followed by purging or other compensatory behavior to prevent weight gain.[16] These athletes are often normal in weight. Athletes with anorexia nervosa refuse to maintain body weight over the minimal norms for height, and have an intense fear of gaining weight, a distorted body image, and amenorrhea. Some athletes will have a combination of anorexia and bulimia. More commonly, the female athlete may exhibit disordered patterns of eating, less severe than frank anorexia or bulimia nervosa. However, there are still significant medical, psychological, and orthopaedic health risks associated with disordered eating. The athlete, coach, parents, and medical practitioner should be aware of not only the risk of disordered eating in these athletes, but also the common misconceptions among female athletes in order to counsel them regarding their nutritional and hormonal health and well-being.[16,21,26,36,50]

In addition to disordered eating, the other components of the female athlete triad include amenorrhea and osteoporosis. The health care provider should fully evaluate a female athlete with amenorrhea to exclude other causes of amenorrhea. Gymnasts have a later onset of menses than age-matched controls.[30] Fortunately, gymnasts have been found to have increased bone mineral density in most instances, despite the possible presence of menstrual dysfunction and/or disordered eating.[43] This increased bone density is likely due to the high-impact forces on bone, in addition to other factors. Attention to nutrition and hormonal status remains important to optimize bone health.[21,36] The female athlete triad is a multifactorial problem best treated by a team of health care professionals. While the best treatment is prevention, if the triad is present, it should be treated by a team consisting of a physician, nutritionist, and psychologist or psychiatrist, ideally with expertise or significant knowledge of the triad problems. USA Gymnastics developed a task force in response to the female athlete triad in 1995,[50] and has a referral system in place of specialists in these areas throughout the country.

TREATING THE INJURED FEMALE GYMNAST

Gymnasts are a unique group of athletes. Understanding the basics of their sport and the level at which they compete and train will help the health care professional when treating an injured gymnast. Knowledge of common overuse and acute injuries sustained in gymnastics is also helpful in caring for these athletes. Owing to the uniqueness of the sport, some degree of training can usually continue despite injury. If the lower extremity has been injured, bars can still be trained, with the exception of dismounts. If the upper extremity has been injured, lower extremity conditioning can still be done and dance for floor and beam can be trained. A high index of suspicion for disordered eating and the female athlete triad should be maintained for all gymnasts and additional care should be taken in athletes who have risk factors, whose weight is low for height, or who are amenorrheic or oligomenorrheic, and for those who have sustained stress fractures.

References

1. Anderson K, Sarwark JF, Longue ES, Shafer MF: Quantitative assessment with SPECT imaging of stress injuries of the pars interarticularis and response to bracing. J Pediatr Orthop 20(1):28–33, 2000.
2. Andrish JT: Knee injuries in gymnastics. Clin Sports Med 4(1):11–21, 1985.
3. Aronen JG: Problems of the upper extremity in gymnasts. Clin Sports Med 4(1):61–8, 1985.
4. Beunen G, Galina RM, Claessens AL, et al: Ulnar variance and skeletal maturity of the radius and ulna in female gymnasts. Med Sci Sports Exerc 31(5):653–7, 1999.
5. Caine JV, Jackson DW: An epidemiologic investigation of injuries affecting young competitive female gymnasts. Am J Sports Med 17(6):811–20, 1989.
6. Caraffa A, Cerulli G, Buompadre V, Appoggetti S: An arthroscopic and electromyographic study of painful shoulders in elite gymnasts. Knee Surg Sports Traumatol Arthros 4(1):39–42, 1996.
7. Chang CY, Shih C, Penn IW, et al: Wrist injuries in adolescent gymnasts of a Chinese opera school: radiographic survey. Radiology 195(3):861–4, 1995.
8. Cuillo JV, Jackson DW: Pars interarticularis stress reaction, spondylolysis and spondylolisthesis in gymnasts. Clin Sports Med 4(1):95–110, 1985.
9. De Smet L, Claessens A, Fabry G: Wrist pain in gymnasts. Acta Orthop Belg 59(4):377–80, 1993.
10. Difiori JP, Mandelbaum BR: Wrist pain in a young gymnast: Unusual radiographic findings and MRI evidence of growth plate injury. Med Sci Sports Exerc 28(12):1453–8, 1996.
11. Difiori JP, Puffer JC, Mandelbaum BR, Dorey F: Distal radial growth plate injury and positive ulnar variance in nonelite gymnasts. Am J Sports Med 25(6):763–8, 1997.
12. Difiori JP, Puffer JC, Mandelbaum BR: Factors associated with wrist pain in the young gymnast. Am J Sports Med 24(1):9–14, 1996.
13. Dixon M, Fricker P: Injury to elite gymnasts over 10 years. Med Sci Sports Exerc 25(12):1322–9, 1993.
14. Dutton JA, Hughes SP, Peteres AM: SPECT in the management of patients with back pain and spondylolysis. Clin Nucl Med 25(2):93–6, 2000.
15. Gabel GT: Wrist pain in gymnasts. Clin Sports Med 17(3):611–21, 1998.
16. Gadpaille WJ, Feicht-Sandborn C, Wagner WW: Athletic amenorrhea major affective disorders and eating disorders. Am J Psychol 144(7):939–42, 1987.
17. Garrick JG, Requa RK: Epidemiology of women's gymnastics injuries. Am J Sports Med 8(4):261–4, 1980.
18. Garry JP, McShane J: Lumbar back pain in adolescent athletes. J Fam Pract 47(2):145–9, 1998.
19. Goldberg MJ: Gymnastics injuries. Orthop Clin North Am 11(4):717–26, 1980.
20. Hall SJ: Mechanical contribution to lumbar stress injuries in female gymnasts. Med Sci Sports Exerc 18(6):599–602, 1986.
21. Hecht S, Nattiv A, Balagne G, Marshall NT: Gymnastics and the female athlete triad. In: Marshall NT (ed): The Athlete Wellness Book. Indianapolis, Ind, USA Gymnastics Publications, 1999.
22. Hudash-Wadley G, Albright J: Women's intercollegiate gymnastics: injury patterns and "permanent" medical disability. Am J Sports Med 21(2):314–20, 1993.
23. Hunter LY, Torgan C: Dismounts in gymnastics: should scoring be reevaluated? Am J Sports Med 11(2):208–10, 1983.
24. Hutchinson MR: Low back pain in elite rhythmic gymnasts. Med Sci Sports Exerc 30 (11):1686–8, 1998.
25. Hutchinson MR, Tremain L, Christiansen J, Beitzel J: Improving leaping ability in elite rhythmic gymnasts. Med Sci Sports Exerc 30(10):1543–7, 1998.
26. Ireland ML: Special concerns of the female athlete. In: Fu F (ed): Sports Injuries: Mechanisms, Prevention and Treatment, Baltimore, Williams & Wilkins, 1994, pp 153–87.
27. Jackson DW, White LL, Crinicione RJ: Spondylolysis in the female gymnast. Clin Orthop Rel Res 117:68–73, 1976.
28. Kirby RL, Simme FC, Symington VI, Garner JB: Flexibility and musculoskeletal symptomatology in female gymnasts and age matched controls. Am J Sports Med 9(3):160–4, 1981.
29. Kolt GS, Kirkby RJ: Epidemiology of injury in elite and subelite female gymnasts: a comparison of retrospective and prospective findings. Br J Sports Med 33(5):312–8, 1999.
30. Lindholm C, Hagenfeldt K, Ringertz BM: Pubertal development in elite juvenile gymnasts. Effects of physical training. Acta Obset Gynecol Scand 73(3):269–73, 1994.
31. Lowry CB, Leveau BF: A retrospective study of gymnastics injuries to competitors and noncompetitors in private clubs. Am J Sports Med 19(4):237–9, 1982.
32. McAuley E, et al: Injuries in women's gymnastics. The state of the art. Am J Sports Med 15(6):558–65, 1987.
33. McCormack RG, Athwal G: Isolated fracture of the vertebral articular facet in a gymnast. A spondylolysis mimic. Am J Sports Med 27(1):104–6, 1999.
34. McLuckie G: The agony of victory. How gymnasts lose by winning. OSU Quest Winter:12–3, 1987.
35. Micheli LJ: Back injuries in gymnastics. Clin Sports Med 4(1):85–93, 1984.
36. Nattiv A, Mandelbaum BR: Injuries and special concerns in female gymnasts: Detecting, treating, and preventing common problems. Phys Sports Med 21:66–82, 1993.
37. O'Sullivan PB, Phyt GD, Twomey LT, Allison GT: Evaluation of specific stabilizing exercise in the treatment of chronic low back pain with radiologic diagnosis of spondylolysis or spondylolisthesis. Spine 15(22):2959–67, 1997.
38. Ott SM, Krahe DH, Sefcik R: Injury patterns and incidence in club gymnasts: a one year survey. J Am Osteopath Acad Assoc 36(1):61–5, 1999.

39. Pesic L: Fast facts. USA Gymnastics 29(2):32, 2000.
40. Pettrone FA, Ricciardeli E: Gymnastics injuries: The Virginia experience 1982–1983. Am J Sports Med 15(1):59–62, 1987.
41. Priest JD: Elbow injuries in gymnastics. Clin Sports Med 4(1):73–83, 1985.
42. Priest JD, Weise DJ: Elbow injuries in women's gymnastics. Am J Sports Med 9(5):288–95, 1981.
43. Robinson TL, Snow-Harter C, Taafe DR, et al: Gymnasts exhibit higher bone mass than runners despite similar prevalence of amenorrhea and oligomenorrhea. J Bone Miner Res 10:26–35, 1995.
44. Ruggles DL, Peterson HA, Scott SG: Radial growth plate injury in a female gymnast. Med Sci Sports Exerc 23(4):393–6, 1991.
45. Samuelson M, Reider B, Weiss D: Grip lock injuries to the forearm in male gymnasts. Am J Sports Med 24(1):15–8, 1996.
46. Sands WA, Schultz BB, Newman AP: Women's gymnastics injuries a 5-year study. Am J Sports Med 21(2):271–6, 1993.
47. Snook GA: Injuries in women's gymnastics a 5-year study. Am J Sports Med 7(4):242–4, 1979.
48. Snook GA: A review of women's collegiate gymnastics. Clin Sports Med 4(1):31–7, 1985.
49. Wieker GG: Injuries in club gymnasts. Phys Sports Med 13(4):63–6, 1983.
50. USA Gymnastics Task Force: USA Gymnastics response to the female athlete triad. Technique 15:16–22, 1995.

Chapter 58

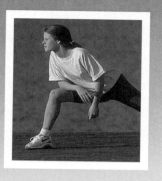

Judo and Taekwondo

Jennifer A. Stone, B.A., M.S.

Judo and taekwondo are martial arts that are part of the Olympic Summer Games. Men's judo became a medal sport in 1964, and women's judo in 1992. Taekwondo for both men and women was a demonstration sport in 1988 and 1992 and became an official Olympic sport in 2000.

Judo is a Japanese martial art that uses throws, pins, and submission holds (arm bars and chokes). Judo matches are won by submission holds or throwing or pinning an opponent for points. Women's matches are 4 minutes long. Competitors compete in 8 weight classes, with women competing in the under-48-kg through the over-78-kg classes plus the open category. The open category, not included in the Olympic Summer Games, is open to all competitors irrespective of body weight. The judo uniform, known as the *gi*, consists of white cotton pants and a jacket with reinforced sleeves and shoulders. Rules detail the gi fit to prevent competitors from gaining an advantage by tightly tailoring the gi. Women wear a plain white T-shirt under the gi. The jacket is fastened by a colored belt indicating the athlete's skill level. Everyone starts at a white belt and may progress to a black belt, which itself has 10 levels. Females do not wear any special protective equipment.

Taekwondo is a Korean kicking and punching martial art. Points are scored by kicking or punching the opponent "accurately and powerfully." The scoring area is the trunk for punches and kicks and the face for kicks only. Matches are three 3-minute rounds, with 1 minute of rest between rounds. The Olympic Games have different weight classes from other international competitions. For all international competitions other than the Olympic Games, women compete in 8 weight classes, from under 47 kg to over 72 kg. The Olympic Games have only 4 weight classes, from under 49 kg to over 67 kg. The competitive uniform is a *dobok*, white pants and a white V-neck top. The top is secured by a belt indicating the athlete's skill level, ranging from white through black, which has 10 levels itself. Female competitors must wear the following protective equipment: chest protector, head protector, breast protector, groin protector, and forearm and shin guards. All protective equipment but the chest protector and head protector are worn under the dobok.

In both martial arts, belt advancement is by tests, also called forms, in which throws (in judo) and kicks and punches (in taekwondo) are performed in a prescribed sequence and judged on technical proficiency. There are forms competitions in both judo and taekwondo, but Olympic competition involves fighting, not forms.

Both martial arts use mats called *tatamis*, straw mats with a nonsticky covering. The mat area for judo is 12 × 12 meters, with a competitive area of 8 × 8 meters. For taekwondo, a canvas "ring," covers the tatami and has the same dimensions as the judo tatami. In both, referees control the match and award penalties. Judo uses 2 mat judges and a referee to score a match. With manual scoring, taekwondo uses 4 mat judges to score; the referee only breaks ties. With electronic scoring, taekwondo uses 3 mat judges; the referee does not score.

Because of the combative nature of martial arts, injuries do occur. Little information about injuries and injury rates is published in the medical literature. Much information is anecdotal and published in sport magazines. Most articles report total injuries rather than differentiating male from female injuries.

A major concern of women in martial arts is competition during pregnancy. Authors writing for 2 different karate publications stated that forms competition is permissible within the comfort level of the athlete, although they thought fighting during pregnancy was not prudent because of the possibility of abdominal trauma.[1,2] Until recently, the international federations for both judo and taekwondo required a negative pregnancy test within 4 weeks of major competitions for all female athletes.

JUDO INJURIES

The only published study on judo injuries is that by Ransom and Ransom[7] who surveyed brown- and black-belt competitors at 3 judo competitions, the 1986 and 1987 Ladder tournaments and the 1988 Missouri state judo championships. They asked competitors about previous practice or competition injuries. These judo players reported 485 injuries, with the most commonly injured body parts being the foot and toes (18.5%) followed by the shoulder (16%), hand (10.7%), knee (9.1%), ankle (7.4%), wrist (6.2%), clavicle (4.9%), nose (4.5%), ribs (3.7%), teeth (7.9%), ears (2.5%), legs (1.6%), groin (1.6%), arms (1.2%), eyes (0.8%), and jaw (0.4%); internal injuries occurred in 0.4%. They did not separate injuries by sex nor indicate injury severity and/or time lost from participation.

Various authors[3, 4, 6] state, without providing data, that judo athletes tend to suffer upper extremity (especially elbow) injuries. They speculate that these injuries are caused by improper falling and stress the importance of learning break falls. Soft mats are mentioned as a cause of both upper and lower extremity injuries since they do not permit the extremity to slide on the mat.

Judo tatamis are put together in 1- × 1-meter sections, and while they fit together tightly, it is possible to get a foot or toe caught in a crack between mats. Vigilance in mat inspection prior to practice or competition minimizes this risk. Also, it is possible that the foot can become fixed to the mat, much as a cleat gets stuck in the grass or turf. This stops the foot from sliding and causes forces to be transmitted higher up the extremity. Depending on position and type of throw, injuries occur to any joint and range in severity from mild sprains to total dislocations. Ensuring the tatamis are of high quality and are properly maintained reduces, but does not eliminate, this problem.

Since judo is a throwing sport, injuries to the upper extremity occur as the athlete tries to stop a throw or reduce the quality of the throw by putting a hand on the mat. When the hand is planted on the mat, injuries occur all along the upper extremity, from the hand and fingers up to and including the shoulder. As with lower extremity injuries, most are minor sprains and strains, but dislocations are not uncommon.

Another potential injury situation results from the arm bar. This hold is an elbow joint lock applied with an extension/valgus force. The opponent is allowed time to submit; however, he or she does not always do so in a timely fashion. While a posterior elbow dislocation can occur, the more common injury is an elbow ulnar collateral ligament sprain.

Closed head injuries from hitting the head on the mat are a possibility. However, a more real danger is from a choke hold, which puts pressure on the carotid arteries, temporarily depriving the brain of blood and causing the athlete to "go out." Usually, the competitor gives up prior to going out; however, potential cerebrovascular problems are possible, especially in participants with pre-existing vascular disease.

TAEKWONDO INJURIES

Injuries in regional and international taekwondo competitions have been described by several authors. Sherrill[8] surveyed injuries at the 1987 and 1988 Midwest Taekwondo Championships, involving 722 competitors, and reported that numbers of injuries increased with increasing skill level. Black-belt competitors were the most likely injured, suffering 12 of 34 reported injuries, and white-belt competitors the least, only 1 of 34 injuries. A majority of the injuries, 23 of 34, occurred during fighting as opposed to forms (1) or breaking (10). All injuries resulted in less than 7 days of disability. Sherrill did not report injuries by sex.

Siana and coworkers[9] documented injuries requiring hospitalization at the 1983 Taekwondo World Championships. Of 346 competitors, not reported by sex, 15 were hospitalized, 11 with head/neck injuries and 4 with limb injuries. Head and neck injuries consisted of 6 fractures, mostly facial bones, 1 concussion, 2 contusions/lacerations, 1 dental fracture, and 1 epistaxis. All competitors with facial fractures were wearing mouth protection at the time of injury. Limb injuries included 1 ulnar fracture and 3 contusions, 1 of the upper extremity and 2 of the lower extremity. They did not report injuries not requiring hospitalization as these were treated at the competition site.

Zemper and Pieter[10] collected data at the 1988 US Olympic Taekwondo Trials using a standardized form and on-site medical providers as data collectors. Most injuries were contusions, occurring in 17 of 27 (64%) male competitors and in 15 of 20 (75%) female competitors. One athlete of each sex suffered a concussion. No females suffered fractures, but 4 males did. Males were injured most frequently by receiving a blow (63%), but female injuries were evenly divided between those occurring while receiving and delivering blows (35% each). The foot was the most commonly injured body part (5 of 27 injuries to males and 8 of 20 injuries to females). Statistics indicated a time-loss injury rate of 23.58/1000 athlete/exposures for males, similar to that in soccer and football, and of 13.51/1000 athlete/exposures for females, similar to that in gymnastics and soccer.

Pieter and Lufting[5] reported injuries at the 1991 Taekwondo World Championships. These championships had 433 competitors, 160 females and 273 males. They enlisted ringside physicians and team physicians as data collectors, using the same form Zemper and Pieter used. Twenty-two serious injuries, more than 1 day time loss, occurred, 4 to females and 18 to males. There were 10 fractures, 2 in females and 1 in a male, and 9 concussions, 1 in a female and 8 in males. Most injuries occurred while receiving a blow, 2 in females and 14 in males, and only 1 each while delivering a blow. They could not discern any injury pattern among weight classes. According to exposure data, taekwondo competitors at the international level have higher rates of concussion and fracture than American football players.

While other injuries do occur, the vast majority of taekwondo injuries are contusions, especially to the feet and arms. Feet are injured delivering blows, and arms while defending blows. Better protective equipment could reduce the severity of many of these contusions. Foot padding must take into account protection for the athlete delivering the blow but not increase the risk of injury to the opponent from a rigid device.

Closed head injuries can and do occur, as the head is a target for kicks. Present protective headgear is constructed of vinyl foam. As with foot protection, headgear is a compromise between protecting the wearer and keeping the opponent safe.

CONCLUDING REMARKS

The martial arts of judo and taekwondo as practiced at the national and international levels are combative sports with one athlete fighting another. Competitors are matched by weight. Little information exists in the medical literature about injuries in judo, and no source differentiates injuries suffered by females from those of males. More definitive information is available for taekwondo, indicating that females are injured with a lower frequency than males, and injuries suffered by females are equally distributed between those occurring while delivering and while receiving a blow. Injury rates may be decreased by attention to personal equipment and mats as well as through conditioning and technique instruction. Proper conditioning includes flexibility, strength training, and cardiovascular conditioning. Proper technique requires a skilled instructor who provides correct instruction in offensive and defensive techniques.

References

1. Birrer RB, Birrer C: An official medical report: the female athlete in the martial arts. Official Karate 13:28–30, 57–8, 1981.
2. Birrer RB, Birrer CD: Safety for women: a doctor's notes on treatment and prevention of injuries. Karate Illustr 15:53–7, 1984.
3. Kurland HL: Mat dangers—aikido and judo injuries compared. Black Belt 18:41–5, 62, 1980.
4. McLatchie GR: Injuries in combat sports. In Reilly T (ed): Sports Fitness and Sports Injuries. Boston, Faber & Faber, 1981, pp 168–74.
5. Pieter W, Lufting R: Injuries at the 1991 taekwondo world championships. J Sports Traumatol 16:49–56, 1994.
6. Purcell M: Judo. In Adams S, Adrian M, Bayless MA (eds): Catastrophic Injuries in Sports. Indianapolis, Ind, Benchmark Press, 1987, pp 179–83.
7. Ransom SB, Ransom ER: The epidemiology of judo injuries. J Osteopath Sports Med 3:12–4, 1989.
8. Sherrill PM: Martial art injuries at a major midwest tournament: results of a cumulative 2 year study and a comparison with other recent studies. J Osteopath Sports Med 3:8–11, 1989.
9. Siana JE, Borum P, Kryger H: Injuries in taekwondo. Br J Sports Med 20:165–6, 1986.
10. Zemper ED, Pieter W: Injury rates during the 1988 U.S. Olympic team trials. Br J Sports Med 23:161–4, 1989.

Chapter 59

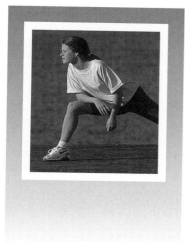

Racquet Sports

Beven P. Livingston, M.S., P.T., A.T.C.
T. Jeff Chandler, Ed.D., C.S.C.S.*D., FACSM
W. Ben Kibler, M.D.
Marc R. Safran, M.D.

Racquet sports require a combination of physical agility, tactical analysis, eye-to-hand (racquet-to-ball) coordination, as well as mental toughness. Over the past several years, more women have been competing in racquet sports, including badminton, squash, racquetball, and tennis, in order to develop and maintain physical fitness and health. Maylack[33] estimated that by 1980, there were more than 28 million racquet sports participants, but only recently have concerted efforts been made to study and understand the sport science of racquet sports. There are few studies of female-related factors associated with participation in racquet sports.

The purpose of this chapter is to present the most current information on the female in racquet sports as it relates to the required musculoskeletal and physiologic demands, performance parameters, and injury risks.

MUSCULOSKELETAL AND PHYSIOLOGIC DEMANDS

Racquet-sport participants of all ages and abilities enter their respective sport with different levels of fitness. As these individuals participate in a particular sport, their musculoskeletal and physiologic systems adapt to its demands. With the accurate measurement of these adaptations, individuals can compare their profiles with an ideal profile, with the goal of improved performance and decreased injury risk in the sport. This framework can be represented by the "critical point interaction" (Fig. 59-1). Each sport places inherent demands on each individual musculoskeletal base. Out of this critical point interaction comes performance and injury risk.

Performance parameters in racquet sports are generally less for female athletes compared to their male counterparts of the same age and ability level. This would be expected in racquet sports, as in other sports, because of such variables as increased body fat, decreased muscle strength, and decreased speed and agility. In this section, we will discuss the musculoskeletal demands of racquet sports on strength and range of motion, as well as physiologic demands on the cardiovascular system, metabolism, and energy expenditure, and the relationship of these variables to performance.

Racquetball

There are few studies on females and the musculoskeletal and physiologic demands of racquetball. Most researchers have studied only male racquetball players.[18,35,39]

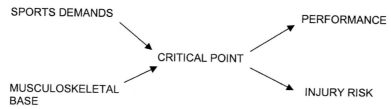

Figure 59-1. The critical point interaction.

One study[44] reported on comparisons of the physiologic demands of racquetball between males and females. Cardiovascular data were collected by heart rate measurement every 5 seconds during a match (Fig. 59-2). All participants (9 males and 7 females; mean age 27 years) were matched with a playing partner according to skill level. Both men and women played with a mean relative heart rate of 92% of their maximum. Blood lactate measures were taken at the beginning of each match, and 2 to 2.5 minutes after the completion of each game. The females' prematch mean lactate measure was 14% of maximum and the postgame levels were 22% of maximum. In absolute terms, lactate measurements ranged from 4.5 to 9.0 mM/L. The mean oxygen consumption (VO_2max) for the females determined by treadmill testing was 40.6 mL/kg/min, a rather low value compared to those seen in other sports. It was concluded that the physiologic demands of racquetball were similar in males and females, and with a relatively low VO_2max requirement, suggesting that aerobic demands are relatively low in racquetball.

Squash

Squash is a physiologically demanding sport that is popular worldwide and played in all seasons, yet there are few good studies on the musculoskeletal or physiologic demands on the female athlete. Todd and Mahoney[47] reported on the musculoskeletal and physiologic characteristics of elite male squash players by measuring strength of the abdominal muscles through sit-ups in 1 minute at 43.3 ± 2.0, grip strength at 507.4 ± 16.7 N, and flexibility of the hamstrings and low back through a sit and reach test at 28.0 ± 1.6 cm. Montpetit and colleagues[36,37] reported heart rates ranging from 150 to 172 beats/minute or from 80% to 95% of maximum, yet most of these data were collected on male participants (Table 59-1).

Owing to some reports of sudden death in squash players,[38] there has been an interest in blood pressure changes during the game of squash. Brigden and coworkers[7] reported that although there was an 18% rise in systolic blood pressure early in the game, there was no prolonged pressor response. Numerous investigators have reported low levels of lactate (2 to 4 mmol/L) as a result of squash games lasting 25 to 90 minutes.[2,4,20,34] Montpetit[36] reported the average percent VO_2max was 57%, slightly higher in squash players as compared to 51% for racquetball players.

In the studies of female squash players, there are few data on the physiologic demands; however, assuming similar responses as males, the research demonstrates that squash is a moderate-to high-intensity, intermittent exercise. Sport-specific performance enhancement for squash

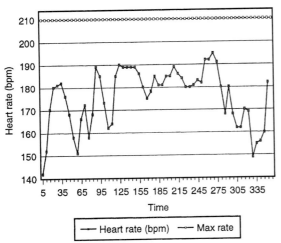

Figure 59-2. Heart rate responses (5-second samples) for a female during a racquetball game. (Adapted from Salmoni AW, Sidney K, Michel R, et al: A descriptive analysis of elite-level racquetball. Res Q Exerc Sport 62(1), 109–114, 1991, with permission.)

Table 59-1. Mean Heart Rate and Percent of Maximum Heart Rate During a Game of Squash

REFERENCE	GRADE AND TYPE OF PLAYERS	MEAN HEART RATE	% HRMAX
Blanksby et al (1973)[6a]	Middle-aged inactive	172	95
	Middle-aged active	150	94
	A grade	160	82
Montgomery et al (1981)[35a]	Young recreational	167 ±11	86
Northcote et al (1983)[37a]	Recreational	149 ±18	80 +/- 10
Mercier et al (1987)[34]	Medium-skill	157 ±13	85
	High-skill	153 ± 9	84
Montpetit et al (1987)[36]	Medium-skill	147 ± 18	80
Visser et al (1987)[48a]	Recreational	164 ± 22	89

Adapted from Montpetit R. Applied physiology of squash. Sports Med 10(1):36, 1990, with permission.

would involve interval training at high intensities with sport-specific work–rest intervals.

Badminton

Badminton is one of the most popular sports in the world and is played from youth to old age at both recreational and competitive levels. There are, however, very few studies on the musculoskeletal and physiologic demands of this sport. Coad and colleagues[12] and Docherty[15] found the average rally to last around 5 seconds followed by an average recovery of 5 to 10 seconds, and high-class matches may last 1 hour. Given this combination of power and endurance, Hughes[24] set out to study these demands on 13 senior national squad members, both males and females, during several situations. He determined that during various training routines and competition, the heart rate was 80% of maximum 85% of the time. He also noted that mean VO_2max was 51.5 mL/kg/min, and the blood lactate measures for both the males and females were 4.0 mM/L, the exception being during the shadow drills, when blood lactate measures reached 7.2 mM/L. Dias and Ghosh[14] looked at similar parameters in a group of 5 female badminton players ages 13 to 14, both before and after a 3-week training schedule. They found similar results: heart rate between 78% and 90% of maximum, and blood lactate measures of 3.9 mM/L, again except for the shadow drills, where it was recorded as an average of 6.2 mM/L. Improvement of the VO_2max was an average of 6% and the range of $_{Tvent}$ values was reported at 7% to 12% after training. In summary, badminton is similar in its physiologic demands to squash and racquetball.

Tennis

In the athletic population, it is well known that males are generally stronger than females and females are generally more flexible than males.[28] Flexibility deficits at the shoulder in internal rotation[9] as well as muscle strength deficits in external rotation[8] have been presented in the literature in both male and female tennis players. In a cross-sectional study, Kibler and coworkers[30] demonstrated that both males and females adapt equally to lose flexibility in glenohumeral shoulder internal rotation. Thirty-nine members of the US National Team were tested in shoulder internal and external rotation. Both males and females were found to have decreased internal rotation with increasing age and years of tournament play. Females demonstrated the

same degree of deficits as males. These findings were confirmed in a longitudinal study.[42] They followed tennis players over 4 years and showed significant decrease in internal rotation in both males and females to the same extent.

The role of musculoskeletal inflexibility has been identified in male and female tennis players compared to athletes competing in other sports.[9] Eighty-six male and female junior elite tennis players were compared to 139 nontennis athletes on certain range-of-motion measurements. Tennis players were significantly more flexible in both dominant and nondominant shoulder external rotation and were significantly less flexible in the sit and reach, dominant shoulder internal rotation, and nondominant shoulder internal rotation.

Specific areas of muscle weakness and/or strength imbalances have been identified in tennis players.[8] Twenty-four male and female college tennis players were tested on a Cybex 340 isokinetic dynamometer on bilateral shoulder internal/external rotation. Subjects produced significantly more torque in internal rotation at both 60° and 300°/sec in the dominant arm compared to the nondominant arm. By increasing the strength of the internal rotators without subsequent strengthening of the external rotators, a muscle imbalance is created that may increase the athlete's risk of injury. The external rotator muscles also have been shown to be more prone to fatigue than the internal rotators.[16] It is apparent that female tennis players acquire musculoskeletal adaptations with intense play, including a decrease in range of motion at the shoulder and other areas, and muscle strength and endurance imbalance at the shoulder. These findings may have important implications for both performance and injury prevention.

Kraemer and colleagues[32] have looked at several performance variables in female tennis players. Generally, there was a low correlation of strength with ball velocity, indicating that skill plays a large role in force production. The isokinetic and isometric measurements of knee flexion and knee extension were the most highly correlated variables with ball speed. Training these muscles would be of importance in improving ball velocity in tennis. Flexibility and joint laxity measurements correlated highly with ball velocity. This is important, as females have been shown to be more flexible than their male counterparts.[28]

The metabolic aspects of tennis have been studied in male tennis players[5] and female tennis players.[40] Male elite tennis players attained a VO_2max on treadmill testing of approximately

58.5 mL/kg/min. In a study of 10 female junior players, ranking 15 or above in their state, VO_2max was measured at 48 mL/kg/min.[40] Female athletes in this study demonstrated significantly greater grip strength in the preferred hand, and no difference in skinfold measurements between the preferred and nonpreferred sides. Circumference measures of the preferred forearm were significantly greater than those of the nonpreferred side. Circumference measures of the upper arm tended to be bigger in the preferred arm, but the difference was insignificant. It was concluded that female elite tennis players differed from young untrained females, demonstrating a higher VO_2max, increased grip strength in the preferred hand, increased forearm girth, and an increased ventilatory capacity.

Fox[19] estimated the metabolic demands in the sport of tennis at 70% anaerobic alactic, 20% lactic anaerobic, and 10% aerobic. Tennis involves intermittent bouts with variable intensity and duration, followed by a brief rest period. The dominant energy pathway is the anaerobic alactic system during play. The alactic anaerobic system is recharged by the aerobic system between points. The anaerobic lactic system is less involved in tennis owing to the length of the points.

Work–rest intervals in the sport of tennis have been studied at the professional and recreational levels. In the 1988 US Open, the average point in the women's finals (Graf vs Sabatini) was 10.8 seconds with an average rest of 16.2 seconds on points within a game.[10] In the men's finals (Lendl vs Wilander), the average point was 12.2 seconds with a rest period of 28.3 seconds within a game. The overall work:rest ratio including rest between games and court changes was 1:2.7 in the women's finals and 1:3.4 in the men's finals. For the female players, 62% of the points were less than 10 seconds, 25% were 10 to 20 seconds, and only 13% were over 20 seconds. For recreational tennis players, work–rest intervals have been reported on clay at a ratio of 16.7:29.2 seconds in males and 15.8:33.6 seconds in females.[29] On hard courts, the average work:rest ratio was 12.7:28.4 in males and 14.2:32.5 in females. These data suggest that the primary energy system used during the tennis point is the alactic anaerobic system, with the aerobic system engaged primarily during recovery.

Elliott[17] examined the physical variables related to performance in 11-, 13-, and 15-year-old tennis players. In females, height and mass were not discriminating factors related to performance. Body composition was significantly lower in 11- to 15-year-old female tennis players compared to an age-matched control group. These results were similar to the results in male players in each age classification.

To meet the inherent sports demands in tennis, muscle activation is organized into patterns to generate force, accept loads, and stabilize joints. These patterns involve sequential activation of muscles to link and harmonize movement of several joints to create kinetic chains. These chains should develop the appropriate forces and motions to achieve the high velocities needed without putting excessive stress on any one segment. In general, the large muscles of the legs, hips, and trunk should generate force and rotational momentum, and the smaller muscles of the upper back and arm should control joint motions and regulate forces. This pattern uses ground reaction forces and can be considered to be a "push-through" type of method of generating force and arm speed. It is known from many studies that females do not activate the hip and leg muscles to the same degree as males in running and jumping activities. Preliminary studies from our lab show that females do not activate hip and trunk muscles in tennis strokes in the same pattern that would create the "push-through" sequence. They use their trunk abductor muscles rather than their hip abductors in the service motion, creating a "pull-through" sequencing for arm motion that may create overload conditions by developing increased stresses in the arm and shoulder in order to maintain high performance levels.

INJURIES IN RACQUET SPORTS

Few good epidemiologic studies exist that accurately demonstrate the incidence and type of injuries that occur in racquet sports. Most reports are either anecdotal or based on individual questionnaires. However, in order to give a better representation of injuries that occur in racquet sports, data must be categorized into 2 types: traumatic injuries and overload injuries. Traumatic injuries are those that occur as a result of a single incident or force, such as a sprained ankle or getting hit in the eye by a racquetball. Overload injuries are the result of a series of repetitive forces that overwhelm the tissue's ability to repair itself, such as "tennis elbow" or Achilles tendinitis.

Squash and Racquetball

An 8-year retrospective study by Chard and Lachmann[11] at their sports injury clinic revealed 631 injuries due to racquet sports, 59% of which were in squash participants. The ratio of male to female injuries was 2:1. It appears from this study that squash players were 3 times more likely than other racquet sport participants to present with an injury. The injuries affected the knee, lumbar region, ankle, and various muscles (especially the calf) (Fig 59-3). Eighty percent were acute traumatic-versus overload-type injuries. There was, however, a larger percentage of females than males with rotator cuff tendinitis.

Sonderstrom and Doxanas[46] in a retrospective review of racquetball injuries showed 75% occurring in males and 25% in females. Fifty-seven percent of the injuries were acute facial injuries and occurred more commonly in novice players. Of the nonfacial type injuries, the highest occurrence was that of ankle sprains. Rose and Morse,[43] Berson,[6] and Barrell[3] all reported on the high incidence of ocular trauma in squash and racquetball, including hyphemas, retinal detachment, retinal hemorrhage, cataracts, and increased risk of future glaucoma. The most effective treatment, of course, is prevention, and there are various protective eyeguards now available.

In summary, it would appear that women are less likely to suffer injuries in squash and racquetball than men. Furthermore, most of the injuries are traumatic, with a high incidence of eye injuries, calf muscle injuries, and ankle sprains. These observations are consistent with the high level of stress and risk of physical contact involved in these 2 racquet sports.

Badminton

Badminton, the world's fastest racquet sport and one of the most widely played sports in the world, has received little sports medicine interest. An article by Jorgensen and Winge[26] reported that it is a relatively low-risk sport dominated by overload injuries. The single most frequent injury is Achilles tendinitis, followed by "tennis elbow." Men have a higher risk than women when time of exposures is considered. Chard and Lachmann[11] also supported the findings of higher incidence of lower limb injuries (59%) and an increased frequency of lateral epicondylitis (9.4%) similar to tennis. Their study demonstrated a high incidence of knee injuries in badminton (65.5%), primarily collateral ligament, cruciate ligament, and meniscal injuries.

In contrast to squash and racquetball, injuries seen in badminton are more often overload-type injuries to the lower extremity, with males being at a greater risk than females.

Tennis

Tennis, more than any of the other racquet sports, has received considerable epidemiologic attention. Analysis of injuries sustained in tennis competition reveals that (1) they are very common; (2) they occur throughout the body; (3) they cause relatively mild disability; (4) they occur frequently as a result of microtrauma and infrequently from macrotrauma; and (5) very few studies have looked at gender differences in injuries.

Most studies of injury patterns have been done on elite or competitive athletes. Table 59-2 summarizes injury incidence reports from several studies: an international study,[31] a United States Tennis Association (USTA) study,[29] a Belgian study,[48] and a Danish study.[49] Table 59-3 shows injury sites from these plus an American study.[25] Table 59-4 breaks these injuries into types, either macrotrauma (sprains and fractures) or microtrauma (overload). Table 59-5 shows the types of injuries for each anatomic site. These studies, although limited owing to the population studied, population size, and lack of a common definition of injury, are similar in their findings and probably do represent injury profiles in competitive tennis players.

Injury occurrence in both male and female competitive tennis players is quite high. Fifty to ninety percent of players reported an injury in the 12 months prior to the questionnaire (Table

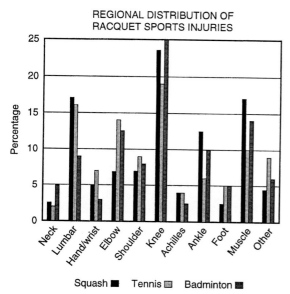

Figure 59-3. Regional distribution of racquet sports injuries. (Adapted from Chard MD, Lachmann SM: Racquet sports–patterns of injury presenting to a sports injury clinic. Br J Sports Med 21(4):150–3, 1987, with permission.)

Table 59-2. Injury Incidence

STUDY	TOTAL PLAYERS	PLAYERS WITH INJURY (%)	TOTAL NUMBER OF INJURIES
International			
English	17	11 (64.7)	14
Swedish	13	12 (92.3)	18
American	33	18 (54.5)	27
Total	63	41 (65.1)	59
USTA	34	22 (64.7)	26
Belgian	127	110 (87)	167
Danish	88	68 (77.2)	81

Table 59-3. Injury Site

	INTERNATIONAL (%)	USTA (%)	BELGIAN (%)	AMERICAN (%)
Shoulder	7 (22)	4 (15)	21 (13)	(14.1)
Elbow	2 (6)	1 (4)	10 (9)	(10.4)
Back	4 (12.5)	2 (8)	31 (18.5)	(22.3)
Knee	4 (12.5)	5 (19)	33 (20)	(18)
Ankle and foot	6 (18)	7 (27)	26 (15.5)	(18)

Table 59-4. Injury Type

	MACROTRAUMA (%)	MICROTRAUMA (%)
Overall (USTA and American)	33	67
Overall (International)	31	69
Overall (Belgian)	24	76
Overall (Danish)	29	71
Individual—Shoulder	6	94
Individual—Back	25	75
Individual—Knee	42	58
Individual—Foot and ankle	48	52

59-4). These injuries were spread throughout the entire body, reflecting the stresses applied to all parts of the body during tennis (Table 59-5). In general, the injuries tended to cause mild disabilities. The only study that closely followed "down time" showed that the mean time away from sport was 3.1 weeks, and no player had to give up tennis directly because of the injury.

In Chard and Lachmann's[11] retrospective study, they reported fewer injuries in tennis than in squash and badminton. Lower limb injuries predominated (45%), yet upper limb injuries (35%) were more common than in the other racquet sports. Injuries to the knee, patellofemoral type, occurred commonly, followed by back injuries, of which 43% were due to disc prolapse.

Table 59-5. Tennis Injury Type by Anatomic Site

	TOTAL	MALE	O/S + F	FEMALE	O/S + F
Shoulder	20	7	7/0	13	13/0
Elbow	7	4	4/0	3	3/0
Wrist	8	3	2/1	5	4/1
Back	9	6	5/1	3	1/2
Hamstrings	5	4	4/0	1	1/0
Knee	16	10	4/6	6	3/3
Achilles	5	2	2/0	3	3/0
Ankle	12	6	0/6	6	0/6
Foot	8	5	4/1	3	1/2
			32/15		29/14

O, Overload; S, sprain; F, fracture.
From Kibler WB, McQueen C, Uhl TL: Fitness evaluations and fitness findings in competitive junior tennis players. Clin Sports Med 7:2, 1988, with permission.

Further studies include one by Kibler and colleagues[28] in which they surveyed elite international and American junior tennis players. He found 100 total injuries had occurred in 63 of 97 junior tennis players over an 18-month period prior to the study. The most common anatomic areas affected were the shoulder, the knee, and the ankle (Fig. 59-3). It was also noted that overload injuries represented 63% of the cases.

Allman[1] estimated that one-half of all tennis players will suffer at some time in their playing career from an affliction commonly known as "tennis elbow." The nature and pathology of this condition is still debated. Gardner, cited by Colt,[13] identified age as a factor and stated that women were more affected than men. Other studies have implicated such factors as inexperience, equipment, and improper technique.[21,23]

Safran has used a validated injury questionnaire to examine injury prevalence and incidence among male and female junior tennis players over several years in national tournaments. Sixteen- and 18-year-old boys sustained more new injuries during the USTA National Hardcourt Championships compared to girls at the USTA Girls' 16's National Championships over the 3 years studied (Table 59-6). However, there was no significant difference in the overall rate of injury (new and recurrent) between boys and girls. Boys and girls had a similar rate of lower extremity injury, both in incidence and prevalence, however, the amount of lower extremity injuries was disproportionately greater in girls as compared with boys. Injuries to the abdomen, back, and groin were significantly fewer in females as compared with males. Both boys and girls have a high rate of injury to the back and shoulder, while girls have more injury to the feet, leg/calf, and wrist. Boys sustain more injuries to the ankle, groin, and hand. For both boys and girls, strains predominated, followed by inflammation, then sprains. Boys have a greater incidence of contusion, abrasions, and lacerations.

Using the questionnaire data of the Girls' 16's USTA National Championships participants over the last 4 years, and the Boys' USTA National Championships more recently, those who are injured during the national championships play and practice more, per year, than those who were not injured during the same tournaments. Females injured during the 1998 tournament played and practiced 11% more per year than those who were not injured, and males injured during their 1998 nationals played and practiced twice as much per year as those who were not injured. Ninety-nine percent of injured females jogged and 77% weight-lifted as part of their training program as compared to uninjured females, of whom 82% jogged on the average 10% less mileage than the injured females and only 50% weight-lifted. There was no difference between injured and uninjured males for running or weight-lifting.

1998 was the first year in which the validated tennis questionnaire was applied to both the boys and girls nationals to assess the prevalence of injury in these elite junior players (Table 59-7). For 1998, only 23% of girls and 45% of boys noted no injury that kept them from playing for one week or more, while 53% of females and only 29% of males noted more than one tennis injury in the past. Low back pain was the most common ailment that has kept elite junior boys and girls from play. Pain in the front of the shoulder was the next most prevalent injury in girls, followed by dominant wrist injury, nondominant wrist injury, and elbow pain. Boys noted similar rates of injury to the elbow, dominant wrist, and pain in the front and back of the shoulder.

The questionnaire revealed that at the 1998 USTA Girls' 16's National Championships, 35%

Table 59-6. Prevalence of Injury or Pain

	MALES	FEMALES
Low back pain	31%	47%
Pain—front of shoulder	17%	31%
Pain—back of shoulder	15%	15%
Elbow	22%	25%
Dominant wrist	19%	29%
Nondominant wrist	6%	25%

Self-reported, closed-ended questionnaire administered at the 1998 USTA Girls' 16's National Tennis Championships and the 1998 USTA Boys' National Hardcourt Championships about injury or pain that prevented the player from playing, practicing, or competing in tennis for at least 7 days.

Table 59-7. Incidence (New Injuries Only) and Prevalence (New and Recurrent Injuries) of Injury During the 1996–1998 USTA National Championships

	MALES	FEMALES
New injuries—incidence (per 100 athletes)	13.2	8.9
New injuries—incidence (per 1000 athletic exposures)	2.9	1.6
New or Recurrent Injury—Prevalence (per 100 athletes)	19.0	17.8

Injuries reported to the medical staff during the 1996–1998 USTA Girls' 16's National Tennis Championships and the 1996–1998 USTA Boys' National Hardcourt Championships.

noted shoulder pain currently or in the past (56% of these were anterior shoulder pain, 15% posterior shoulder pain, and 31% both anterior and posterior shoulder pain). For the 16- and 18-year-old participants at the 1998 USTA Boys' National Championships, 25% noted previous or current shoulder pain (38% anterior shoulder pain, 30% posterior shoulder pain, and 32% noted both anterior and posterior shoulder pain).

At the 1998 USTA Girls' National Championships, 25% noted elbow pain currently or in the past, while 22% of participants at the 1998 USTA Boys' National Championships reported previous or current elbow pain.

At the 1998 USTA Girls' 16's National Championships, 29% noted dominant wrist pain and 25% noted nondominant wrist pain currently or in the past. For the male participants at the 1998 USTA Boys' National Championships, 19% noted previous or current dominant wrist pain and 6% noted nondominant wrist pain.

In summary, most injuries that occur in tennis represent the overload type, such as rotator cuff tendinitis and "tennis elbow" in the upper extremity and patellofemoral-type problems in the lower extremity. Young females may have a slightly higher incidence of lower extremity injuries, as well as an equally high incidence of upper extremity injuries, compared to males, but it appears injuries are due more to the demands of the game and musculoskeletal adaptations than they are to gender.

INTERVENTIONAL STRATEGIES FOR INJURY PREVENTION

It is an enticing thought that since many of these injuries proceed through a rather long process of gradual damage before producing clinical symptoms, recognition of athletes in the preclinical stages could be accomplished and adequate steps could be undertaken to prevent further progression. It is also enticing to think that if all the sports-specific demands could be identified, then skill training programs could be designed to stay within certain limits, or "doses," and conditioning programs could be designed to optimize the musculoskeletal base for a particular sport. Research along these lines is proceeding, and early evidence points to support for these thoughts. Most of the research concerning tennis has already been presented. Reviews of the role of subclinical adaptations in injury causation and the role of strengthening in injury prevention point to positive results from improvement

of these important parameters. Because of these findings, interventional strategies should be actively pursued in tennis injury work.

Identification of muscle weaknesses and inflexibilities can best be approached through a sports-specific preparticipation examination. By testing specific anatomic areas with tests relatively specific for the sport or activity, a profile of musculoskeletal "readiness" for play can be identified. Conditioning programs based on correcting deficits and strengthening areas of high demand can then be constructed. These have shown promise in decreasing injury. "Fine tuning" of both the examination process and the conditioning programs will allow better results in the future.

This process of "prehabilitation," or prospective conditioning, is also important in young elite athletes who have the prospect of more intensive play as they get older. Studies have shown that adaptive changes occur as a result of playing sports in tennis players as young as 12 to 13 years of age. Injuries are not prevalent in this age group, but are seen with high incidence in the 15- to 18-year-old group. It is surmised that the younger athlete's adaptive changes may be creating biomechanical deficits that predispose the athlete to injury with continued, increased use. The areas of injury in the players (the shoulder, back, and knee) correspond with the areas of demonstrated inflexibility and weakness. In the young athlete, much work is now being directed toward defining the proper exercise dose to prevent such adaptations and defining the most appropriate conditioning programs, given the age and physical limitations in these athletes.

CONDITIONING FOR TENNIS

Owing to factors such as the length of the season, the musculoskeletal maladaptations that occur with the sport, and the sport-specific injury patterns, it is necessary to discuss the sport-specific aspects of conditioning for tennis. A conditioning program for tennis can be divided into the following areas: prehabilitation (the correction of musculoskeletal maladaptations that may predispose the tennis player to injury), resistive training, and, finally, sprint/interval, footwork, and speed training.

Prehabilitation

Prehabilitation exercises would consist of exercises to correct musculoskeletal deficits found in a preparticipation evaluation of the tennis player. At the elite level, such exercises are important both to prevent injury and to improve performance. At the recreational level, these exercises are important to prevent injury and to allow the player to continue to enjoy and benefit from the sport of tennis. Typical goals of a prehabilitation program might be:

1. To improve internal rotation range of motion on the dominant arm;
2. To improve external rotation strength and endurance;
3. To improve the strength of the scapular stabilizing musculature;
4. To improve low back and hamstring flexibility; and
5. To correct any individual weaknesses in terms of strength and range of motion.

Resistive Training

Resistive training for the tennis player is an important goal if the player is interested in preventing injuries and improving performance. Resistive training includes not only weight training, but also drills for abdominal strength, medicine ball drills for total-body strength, and calisthenic exercises. By improving strength, power is increased, which is becoming an increasingly important component of tennis. Also, short-term endurance is increased, which is of tremendous importance to the tennis player. Conditioning with medicine balls has the advantage of conditioning the entire kinetic chain in a way that promotes improved power in the tennis stroke.

Sprint/Interval, Footwork, and Speed Training

As previously mentioned, the sport of tennis is generally played in short bursts of activity. Interval training in the off-season progressing to shorter bursts of activity as the tennis season approaches is likely the best way to train for tennis. Interval training can provide an aerobic base that can be maintained by sprint training during the season. It is possible that extensive aerobic training during the season would interfere with the production of strength and power. Particularly for competitive tennis players, training in 10- to 20-second bursts is more specific to tennis performance than running long distances. By training in shorter bursts for long periods of time, the aerobic energy system will be utilized during the recovery process between exercise bouts, which is the same way it is used in a tennis match (ie, recovery between points).

One problem that often arises with competitive tennis players is that there is no off-season in which to condition. The best answer is found in the concept of periodization. By carefully planning the competitive year and by choosing the times of the year when the player wants to be at his or her best, a schedule of conditioning can be incorporated into this plan. Typically, there will be an off-season, a preseason, and an in-season leading to a peak. After a peak, there should be some time of active rest, where the athlete is allowed time to recover from intense competition. An athlete who would like to peak twice in a period of 4 to 6 weeks will not likely have the opportunity for active rest or for going into an off-season phase.

FEMALE ATHLETE TRIAD

A final issue of consideration for the female athlete in racquet sports is the female athlete triad. This refers to the inter-relatedness of eating disorders, amenorrhea, and osteoporosis, which may lead to morbidity or mortality. Sports that pose a risk are those in which low body weight or a lean physique is advantageous. Fortunately, this is not true in most cases with racquet sports as they lend themselves to being more anaerobic, power sports. Of further consideration is the effect of exercise on bone mass. A study by Kannus and coworkers[27] comparing tennis and squash players' dominant and nondominant arms for bone mineral content as affected by starting age and age of menarche found that the benefit of playing is 2 times greater if females start playing at or before menarche. Although bone mineral density in specific sites may increase as a result of stresses placed on the site, specific increases have been shown to occur even in an amenorrheic and oligomenorrheic athlete.[41,45] Although female racquet sport athletes do not appear to be a high-risk population, health-care professionals need to continue to work closely with the athletes and offer appropriate prevention and treatment measures as early as possible, while continuing to promote safe and healthy exercise.

Racquet sports have a wide appeal to the population, including women of all ages. Future research will enhance our knowledge of the physiologic and metabolic demands of the sports as they relate specifically to women, and the findings will continue to educate participants in order to reduce the number and severity of injuries that may result.

References

1. Allman FL: Tennis elbow: etiology, prevention and treatment. Clin Orthop 3:308, 1975.
2. Ayling JH, Bennett S, Davidson I, Major P: The influence of squash play on plasma glucose and lactate. J Sports Sci 2:165, 1984.
3. Barrell GV, Cooper PJ, Elkington AR, Macfadyen JM: Squash ball to eye ball: the likelihood of squash players incurring an eye injury. Br Med J (Clin Res Ed) 283:893–5, 1981.
4. Beauchamp L, Montpetit R: The oxygen consumption during racquet-ball and squash matches. Can J Appl Sports Sci 5:273A, 1980.
5. Bergeron MF, Maresh CM, Kraemer WJ, et al: Tennis: a physiological profile during match play. Int J Sports Med 12:474–9, 1991.
6. Berson BL, Rolnick AM, Ramos CG, et al: An epidemiologic study of squash injuries. Am J Sports Med 6:34, 1981.
6a. Blanksby BA, Elliott BC, Bloomfield J. Telemetered heart rate responses of middle-aged sedentary males, middle-aged active males and 'A' grade male squash players. Med J Australia 2: 477–481, 1973
7. Brigden GS, Hughes LO, Broadhurst P, Raftery EB: Blood pressure changes during the game of squash. Eur Heart J 13:1084–7, 1992.
8. Chandler TJ, Kibler WB, Stracener EC, et al: Shoulder strength, power, and endurance in college tennis players. Am J Sports Med 20(4):155–8, 1992.
9. Chandler TJ, Kibler WB, Uhl TL, et al: Flexibility comparisons of junior elite tennis players to other athletes. Am J Sports Med 18(2):134–6. 1990.
10. Chandler TJ: Work/rest intervals in world class tennis. Tennis Pro January/February:4, 1991.
11. Chard MD, Lachmann SM: Racquet sports-patterns of injury presenting to a sports injury clinic. Br J Sports Med 21(4):150–3, 1987.
12. Coad D, Rasmussen B, Mikkelson F: Physical demands of recreational badminton. In: Terauds J (ed): Science in Racquet Sports. Del Mar, Cal, Academic Publishers, 1979, pp 43–54.
13. Colt E: Tennis elbow. Br Med J 4:679, 1970.
14. Dias R, Ghosh AK: Physiological evaluation of specific training in badminton. In: Reilly T, Hughes M, Lee A (eds): Science and Racket Sports. London, E & FN Spon, 1994, pp 38–43.
15. Docherty D: A comparison of heart rate response in racquet games. Br J Sports Med 16:96–100, 1982.
16. Ellenbecker TS, Roetert EP: Testing isokinetic muscular fatigue of shoulder internal and external rotation in elite junior tennis players. J Orthop Sports Phys Ther 29:275–81, 1999.
17. Elliott BC, Ackland TR, Blanksby BA, Bloomfield J: A prospective study of physiological and kinanthropometric indicators of junior tennis performance. Austral J Sci Med Sport December:87–92, 1990.
18. Faria IE, Lewis F: Metabolic response to playing racquetball. Med Sci Sports Exerc 15:147, 1982.
19. Fox EL, Matthews DK: Interval Training. Philadelphia, WB Saunders, 1974.
20. Garden G, Hale PJ, Horrocks PM, et al: Metabolic and hormonal responses during squash. Eur J Appl Physiol 55:445–9, 1986.
21. Gerberich SG, Priest JD: Treatment for lateral epicondylitis: variables related to recovery. Br J Sports Med 19:224, 1985.
22. Gruchow HW, Pelletier D: An epidemiologic study of tennis elbow. Am J Sports Med 7:234, 1979.
23. Hang Y, Peng S: An epidemiologic study of upper extremity injury in tennis players. J Formosan Med Assoc 83:307, 1984.
24. Hughes MG: Physiological demands of training in elite badminton players. In: Reilly T, Hughes M, Lee A (eds): Science and Racket Sports. London, E & FN Spon, 1994, pp 32–7.
25. Hutchinson MR, Laprade RF, Burnett QM: Injury surveillance at the USTA Boys' Tennis Championships: a 6-year study. Med Sci Sports Exerc 28:826–30, 1995.
26. Jorgenson U, Winge S: Injuries in badminton. Sports Med 10(1):59–64, 1990.
27. Kannus P, Haapasalo H, Sankelo M, et al: Effect of starting age of physical activity on bone mass in the dominant arm of tennis and squash players. Ann Intern Med 123:27–31, 1995.
28. Kibler WB, Chandler TJ, Uhl TL, et al: A musculoskeletal approach to the preparticipation physical evaluation. Am J Sports Med 17:525–31, 1989.
29. Kibler WB, Chandler TJ: Racquet sports. In: Fu FH, Stone DA (eds): Sports Injuries, Mechanisms, Prevention, Treatment. Baltimore, Williams & Wilkins, 1994.
30. Kibler WB, Chandler TJ, Livingston BP, Roetert EP: Shoulder range of motion in elite tennis players. Effect of age and years of tournament play. Am J Sports Med 24(3):279–85, 1996.
31. Kibler WB, McQueen C, Uhl TL: Fitness evaluations and fitness findings in competitive junior tennis players. Clin Sports Med 7:403–16, 1988.
32. Kraemer WJ, Triplett NT, Fry AC, et al: An in depth sports medicine profile of women college tennis players. J Sports Rehab 4:79–98, 1995.
33. Maylack FH: Epidemiology of tennis, squash, and racquetball injuries. Clin Sports Med: Injury Treatment and Prevention 7(2):233–52, 1988.
34. Mercier M, Beillot J, Gratas A, et al: Adaptation to work load in squash players: laboratory tests and on-court recordings. J Sports Med 27:98–104, 1987.
35. Montgomery DL: Heart rate response to racquetball. Physician Sportsmed 9(10):59–62, 1981.
35a. Montgomery DL. Malcolm V, McDonnell E. A comparison of the intensity of play in squash and running. Physician Sportsmed 9:116–119, 1981.
36. Montpetit RR, Beauchamp L, Leger L: Energy requirements of squash and racquetball Physician Sportsmed 15:106–12, 1987.
37. Montpetit RR: Applied physiology of squash. Sports Med 10(1):31–41, 1990.
37a. Northcote RJ, MacFarlane P, Ballantyne D. Ambulatory electrocardiography in squash players. Br Heart J 50:372–377, 1983.
38. Northcote RJ, Evans ADB, Ballantyne D: Sudden death in squash players. Lancet 1: 148, 1984.
39. Pipes TV: The racquetball pro: A physiological profile. Physician Sportsmed 7(10):91–4, 1979.
40. Powers SK, Walker R: Physiological and anatomical characteristics of outstanding female junior tennis players. Res Q Exerc Sport 53(2):172–5, 1982.
41. Robinson T, Snow-Harter C, Gillis D, et al: Bone mineral density and menstrual cycle status in competitive female runners and gymnasts. Med Sci Sports Exerc (Suppl) 25:S49, 1993.
42. Roetert EP, Ellenbecker TS, Brown SW: Shoulder internal and external range of motion in nationally ranked tennis players: a longitudinal analysis. J Strength Cond Res 14:140–3, 2000.
43. Rose CP, Morse JO: Racquetball injuries. Physician Sportsmed 7:73, 1979.

44. Salmoni AW, Sidney K, Michel R, et al: A descriptive analysis of elite-level racquetball. Res Q Exerc Sport 62(1):109–14, 1990.

45. Snow-Harter C, Bouxsein M, Lewis B, et al: Effects of resistance and endurance exercise on bone mineral status of young women: a randomized exercise intervention trial J. Bone Miner Res 7:761, 1992.

46. Soderstrom CA, Doxanas MT: Racquetball: a game with preventable injuries. Am J Sports Med 10:180, 1982.

47. Todd MK, Mahoney CA: Determination of pre-season physiological characteristics of elite male squash players. In: Reilly T, Hughes M, Lee A (eds): Science and Racquet Sports. London, E&FN Spon, 1995, pp 81–6.

48. Verspeelt P: A review of tennis-related injuries in Flemish high level players. In: Krahl H, Pieper H-G, Kibler WB, Renstrom P (eds): Tennis: Sports Medicine and Science. Dusseldorf, Rau, 1995, pp 47–51.

48a. Visser FC, Mihciokur M, Van Duk CN, den Engelsman J, Roos JP. Arrhythmias in athletes: comparison of stress test. 24h Holter and Holter monitoring during the game in squash players. Eur Heart J 8: 29–32, 1987

49. Winge S, Jorgenson U, Nielson L: Epidemiology of injuries in Danish championship tennis. Int J Sports Med 10:368–71, 1989.

Chapter 60

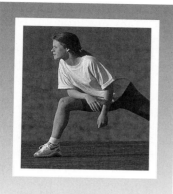

Rowing

Timothy M. Hosea, M.D.
Jo A. Hannafin, M.D., Ph.D.

HISTORY OF ROWING

With the enactment of Title IX, there has been nearly a doubling of the number of intercollegiate rowing programs for women in the United States (Fig. 60-1). These opportunities have rekindled interest and enthusiasm for a sport that was once the greatest spectator sport in the United States.[14]

The rowing stroke originated sometime after 1000 BC when it was discovered that an oar working against a fulcrum was mechanically more efficient than a paddle. Eventually the seated position with a sliding seat was found to allow an even greater force be exerted against the oar, thus generating greater boat speed. In the United States, boatmen were able to help support themselves professionally with rowing. In 1716, Thomas Dogget, a British actor, endowed annual races in England for apprentice boatmen. By the time of the Civil War, the Biglen and Ward brothers and James Hanlon had gained a national reputation in the United States racing for $350 to $3000 a race. These

individuals provided the sporting public with their first heroes and they were promoted by various companies, including Hops Bitters, a medicine that called itself the "Invalids Friend and Hope." Murad cigarettes originated a trading card series of 25 collegiate rowers in 1911.[14]

In 1896, rowing was one of the inaugural events of the modern Olympic games, although the event was canceled because of poor weather conditions. The first Olympic regatta for heavyweight men occurred in the 1900 Olympics, and women began participating in 1976. With the 1996 Olympic games in Atlanta, the rowing competition was expanded to include lightweight men and women for the first time.[14]

With the rapid growth and interest in rowing in the United States, a great deal of attention has been focused in the injury patterns occurring in this sport. Generally speaking, the majority of rowing injuries are overuse injuries. Any abrupt changes in training level, alterations in technique or the type of boat rowed, and rapid increases in training volume contribute to their occurrence. In order to better understand, evalu-

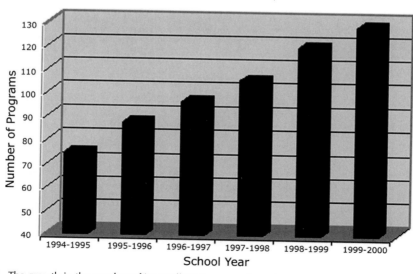

Figure 60-1. The growth in the number of intercollegiate women's rowing programs since the passage of Title IX.

ate, and treat the rowing injuries, a thorough understanding of the sport is essential. The type of boat they row can characterize rowers. Sweep rowing involves the use of a single oar (Fig. 60-2A); the shells are composed of 2, 4, or 8 rowers. Sculling utilizes 2 oars working together (Fig. 60-2B), and may include a single individual or 2 or 4. At the intercollegiate and international levels, a team of rowers may participate in the open or lightweight classifications. Special attention must be provided to all rowing athletes to encourage proper nutrition and appropriate evaluation to realistically determine which athletes participate in the open or lightweight categories.

Rowing is an unusual sport in that the athletes sit facing the stern of the boat with their feet anchored in sneakers attached to a foot stretcher. At the finish and release of the rowing stroke, the knees are fully extended, and the elbows are flexed to the body at waist height (Fig. 60-3A,B). The recovery phase begins with the movement of the hands away from the body toward the stern of the boat followed by the forward flexion at the hip (Fig. 60-3C,D). When the body and shoulders are forward of the hips and the hands past the knees, the legs slowly begin to flex until the catch position, where the knees are flexed approximately 110° to 120°, the hips are maximally flexed and the shoulders are fully extended (Fig. 60-3E). At this compressed position, there is a great deal of potential energy stored in the legs, back, and arms in preparation for the drive phase of the stroke. At the catch, the oar is placed in the water followed by the legs driving the body back toward the bow of the boat, pulling the boat past the anchored oar (Fig. 60-3F,G). The back, shoulders, and arms act as connections so that the force generated by the legs can be applied to the oar and not

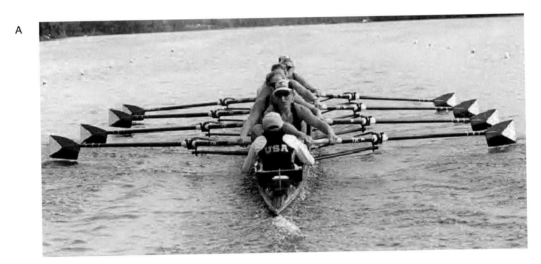

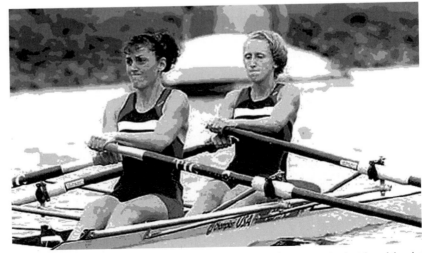

Figure 60-2. **(A)** In sweep rowing, each rower has one oar, with equal number of rowers on both sides of the shell. The shells are composed of 2, 4, or 8 rowers. **(B)** In sculling, each rower has an oar in each hand. The shells hold 1, 2, or 4 rowers.

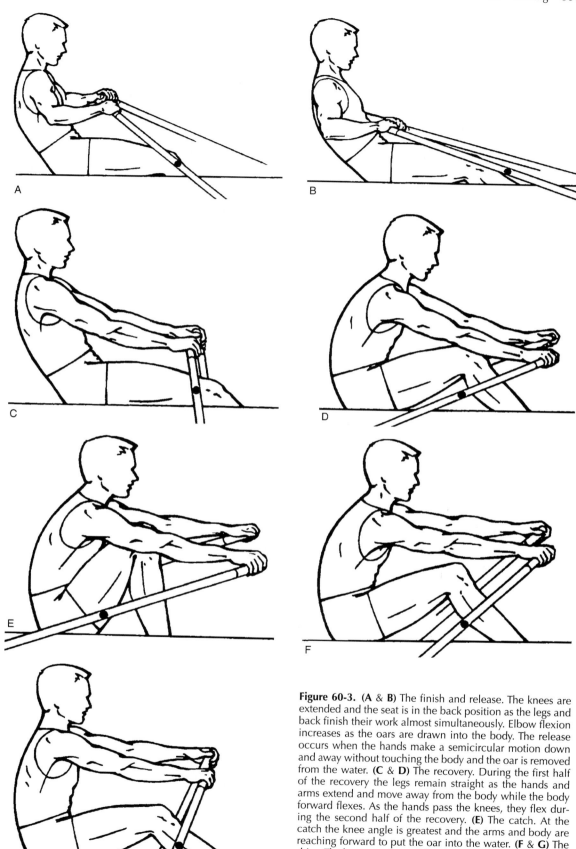

Figure 60-3. (A & B) The finish and release. The knees are extended and the seat is in the back position as the legs and back finish their work almost simultaneously. Elbow flexion increases as the oars are drawn into the body. The release occurs when the hands make a semicircular motion down and away without touching the body and the oar is removed from the water. **(C & D)** The recovery. During the first half of the recovery the legs remain straight as the hands and arms extend and move away from the body while the body forward flexes. As the hands pass the knees, they flex during the second half of the recovery. **(E)** The catch. At the catch the knee angle is greatest and the arms and body are reaching forward to put the oar into the water. **(F & G)** The drive. The legs extend, providing the power of the stroke at the beginning of the drive, without any change in the body angle or arm extension. The body angle increases, the elbows flex, and the knees fully extend during the last portion of the drive.

dissipated. The drive phase ends at the finish and the same cycle is repeated over and over for the length of the race or practice.

Myoelectric analysis of a female Olympian demonstrates the firing of the rectus femoris and thoracic paraspinal muscles initiating the drive phase of the rowing stroke. The rectus femoris provides the power and the thoracic and lumbar paraspinal muscles stabilize the spine to enable the transfer of power to the oar. As the knees and hips extend during the drive the gluteus maximus and hamstrings fire, controlling the drive and stabilizing the pelvis. The back acts as a braced cantilever and provides an additional source of power by extending from 30° of flexion to approximately 30° of extension. Again, the L3 paraspinal activity during this phase of the stroke reflects the corresponding increase in the lumbar shear loads (Fig. 60-4A,B).[7]

The force generated by the legs and back is then transmitted to the oar through the shoulders, which are stabilized by the latissimus dorsi and serratus anterior. Peak acceleration at mid drive causes these muscles to fire maximally and in unison. During the later part of the drive the rectus femoris continues to fire, keeping the knees extended as the arms pull the oar into the body. At the finish, the previously mentioned major muscle groups generate minimal activity while the rectus and external oblique muscle fire,

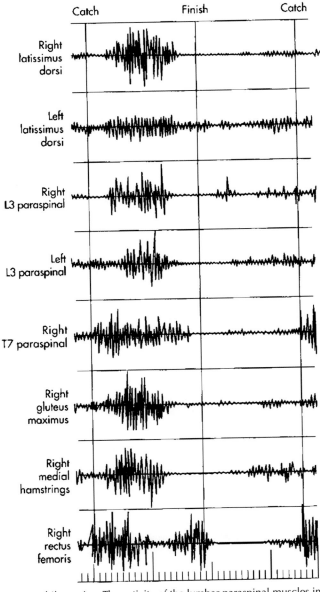

A

Figure 60-4. (A) Myoelectric activity while rowing. The activity of the lumbar paraspinal muscles increases as the shear load affecting the lumbar spine increases, thus enabling the transfer of the power generated by the legs to the oar.

Illustration continued on following page

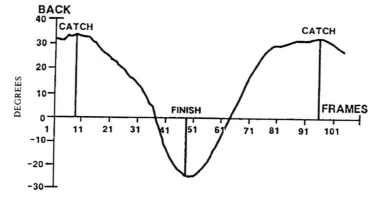

Figure 60-4*(Continued)*. **(B)** A typical example of the trunk motion during a rowing stroke, with approximately 30° of flexion at the catch and a smooth transition to extension at the finish.

stabilizing the trunk, which is in an extended position. During the recovery phase with the body in a forward position and the knees and hips flexing and compressing there is little or no activity of the paraspinal muscles, reflecting the minimal load in the lumbar disc. The hamstrings then fire submaximally to flex the knee and initiate movement back up the slide to the catch position to begin the next stroke.[10]

ROWING INJURIES

The injuries affecting rowers are primarily overuse injuries. Review of the injury patterns at rowing programs of Harvard and Rutgers universities revealed 180 injuries to oarsmen and -women over a 3-year period (Fig. 60-5).[7] At these institutions the knee was the most com-

mon site of complaint, followed by the back, upper extremity, and ribcage. The high incidence of foot and ankle injuries was related to accidents occurring while running to and from the boathouse and will not be included in this discussion.

Rowing involves a continuous, repetitive motion during which the stresses are continually increased or decreased depending on the stroke phase. Off-water training for rowing also involves similar activities, such as weight-lifting, running, stair-running, cross-country skiing, rowing in tanks, and the use of the rowing ergometer. Such activities predispose individuals to stress fractures, which in our rowing population primarily affect the ribs. The rowing stress pattern is also thought to be responsible for the high incidence of back problems and will be discussed further in this chapter. The majority of

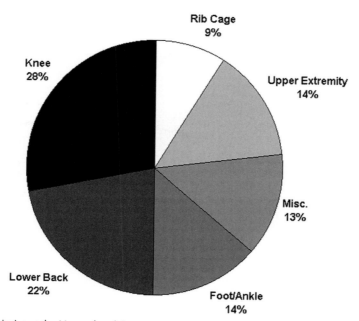

Figure 60-5. Rowing injuries at the Harvard and Rutgers programs.

the knee injuries involve chondromalacia patella, and iliotibial band friction syndrome, reflecting the constant flexion and extension of the knee under load. The necessity to feather the oar in and out of the water results in the high incidence of extensor tenosynovitis and wrist injuries seen in this group. In this chapter, we will discuss extensor tenosynovitis, rib stress fractures, chondromalacia patella, iliotibial band friction syndrome, and low back pain in the rowing athlete.

Extensor Tenosynovitis of the Wrist

During the rowing stroke, the oar blade is removed from the water at the finish. It is then feathered parallel to the water and rerotated back perpendicular at the catch just prior to its placement into the water. When feathering, the following muscles are utilized: the abductor pollices longus, extensor pollices brevis, the extensor carpi radialis longus and the extensor carpi radialis brevis. Surgical exploration has revealed that extensor tenosynovitis of the wrist in rowers is caused by compression of the radial extensor tendons beneath the swollen hypertrophied abductor pollices longus and extensor pollices brevis (Fig. 60-6).

Extensor tenosynovitis is a common overuse injury in rowers and generally manifests itself in early spring when there is a return to high-intensity rowing in the water and relatively cold weather. This is associated with pain, swelling, and crepitus with motion of the involved tendons. It is a cause of considerable functional disability not only with rowing, but occasionally with activities of daily living.

Conventional treatment involves rest with the use of a cock-up wrist splint, anti-inflammatory medications, and physical therapy modalities such as ultrasound and whirlpool. Local corticosteroid injections may be helpful.

In the authors' experience, conservative management has generally provided relief in 2 to 3 weeks. The key to prevention is keeping the hand and wrist as warm as possible, thus the rower should make sure to wear long sleeves. Also helpful are commercially available fleece covers, that cover the hand, wrist and oar while rowing.

Although the authors have no experience with operative treatment, excellent results with surgical decompression of the abductor longus and extensor brevis have been reported by Williams.[18]

Chondromalacia Patellae and Iliotibial Band Friction Syndrome

Not only does rowing involve loading the patellofemoral joint, but the training activities designed to increase the strength of the quadriceps mechanism include running upstairs, squats, and squat jumps. In the authors' survey of rowing injuries, the knee was the most commonly affected site. Chondromalacia patellae and iliotibial band (ITB) friction syndrome were the most common diagnosis present in the rowing population.

Rowing requires the forceful extension of the knee from nearly full flexion to full extension under a tremendous load, thus giving rise to the significant number of knee injuries found in the rowing population. At the catch, the knee flexion angle ranges up to 120° and the legs then extend during the drive phase of the stroke to full extension at the finish.

If the rower has either genu valgum or genu varum, rowing will cause either chondromalacia,

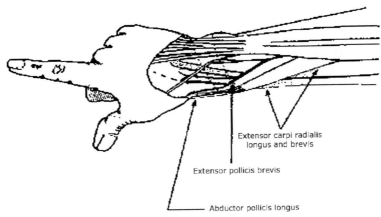

Extensor carpi radialis longus and brevis

Extensor pollicis brevis

Abductor pollicis longus

Figure 60-6. Diagram of the extensor aspect of the distal forearm with the abductor pollicis longus and extensor pollicis brevis overlying the radial extensors of the wrist proximal to the extensor retinaculum (From Williams J: Surgical management of traumatic non-infective tenosynovitis of the wrist extensors. J Bone Joint Surg 59B:408, 1977, with permission.)

in the case of genu valgum, or ITB friction, in the case of genu varum. Patellofemoral pain is commonly found in those with genu valgum or the "malicious malalignment" syndrome. Malicious malalignment occurs in the presence of increased femoral anteversion of the femoral neck and corresponding secondary external rotation of the tibia. Chondromalacia patellae presents with complaints of anterior knee pain with rowing and other training activities. Pain with ascending and descending stairs, swelling, crepitus, and/or a clicking sensation during the rowing stroke may be present. Examination of the knee generally reveals lateral patella facet tenderness and tracking. Of particular note in the rowing population is the presence of a tight quadriceps and ITB. Rarely does a rower have a negative Ober test, or the ability to touch her heel to her buttock with the hip extended. The authors' treatment for individuals with chondromalacia of the patella consists of nonsteroidal anti-inflammatory drugs (NSAIDs) and an aggressive stretching program of the anterior hip, quadriceps, and ITB. In addition, strengthening the vastus medialis obliquus with progressive ankle resistance is an important component of the rehabilitation program. On occasion, McConnell taping techniques have been helpful. In the markedly symptomatic rower, the authors recommend ceasing all rowing and squatting activities until pain relief can be obtained. Surgical management of this problem has rarely been necessary in the rowing population. However, a novice rower with significant pre-existing chondromalacia patellae associated with pain and crepitus should be very cautious with initiating participation in this particular activity.

The ITB friction syndrome is also fairly common in the rowing population. This condition occurs secondary to pressure from the ITB against the lateral femoral condyle as it moves from a position anterior to the lateral femoral condyle in extension to one posterior with knee flexion (Fig. 60-7). The ITB rises as the tendinous extension of the fascia covering the gluteus maximus and tensor fascia lata muscles proximally and attaches to the Gerdes tubercle on the proximal aspect of the lateral tibia metaphysis. While sending fibers to the lateral intermuscular septum and the lateral aspect of the patella over the lateral femoral condyle, the ITB is free to glide anteriorly and posteriorly. Either motion produces inflammation over the lateral femoral condyle, resulting in pain localized over the lateral femoral condyle. ITB friction syndrome may also present with crepitus and swelling over the lateral aspect of the knee.

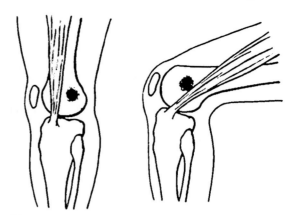

Figure 60-7. With motion of the knee, the ITB passes over the prominent lateral femoral condyle, and can result in inflammation and pain. (From Boland AL, Hurlstyn MJ: Soft tissue injuries of the knee. In: Nicholas JA, Hershman EB (eds): Spine and Lower Extremities in Sports Medicine. St Louis, CV Mosby, 1995, p 928, with permission.)

The Ober test is universally positive and the ITB friction syndrome generally occurs in individuals with a slight genu varum. Joint effusion, lateral joint line tenderness, and evidence of meniscal derangement or ligamentous instability are not present. Treatment for the ITB friction syndrome consists of active rest, ice, anti-inflammatory medications, ultrasound, and occasional local steroid injection to reduce the inflammatory reaction. In addition, comprehensive stretching exercises are used to correct the static contracture (Fig. 60-8). We eliminate stair-running and squatting activities. These individuals can usually continue rowing except in the most severe cases.

Low Back Pain

Low back pain is a common complaint in the rowing population. Howell's studies of elite lightweight female rowers revealed an 82.2% incidence of low back compared to an age and sex match incidence in the general population of 20% to 30%.[8] Stallard stated that "a back ache is suffered by almost all those in serious rowing training."[16] The authors' review of 2 intercollegiate programs revealed that the lower back is the second most common area injured. Kinetic and myoelectric analysis of the lower lumbar spine reveals significant loading with each stroke. The back functions as a braced cantilever during the rowing stroke and is the major connection in the transfer of power from the legs to the oar. These forces are similar with sculling and ergometer rowing. Sweep rowing adds a torsional and lateral bending stress to the already-existing sheer and compression components of the sculling stroke. At the catch, there is a rapid

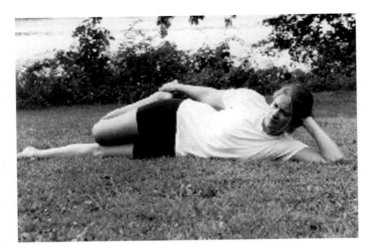

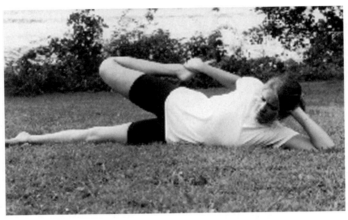

Figure 60-8. (**A** & **B**) Quadriceps-stretching exercise.

Illustration continued on following page

generation of force at the oar. This force accelerates to a peak at mid drive and tapers to a finish. The pattern is similar for both men and women. The anterior shear load at the L3-4 motion segment mirrors the resistance applied to the oar (Fig. 60-9). The peak of the anterior shear load affecting the L3-4 motion segment averages 848 N for the men and 717 N for the women. These are essentially the same for both sexes when normalized for body weight. The trunk moves from approximately 30° of flexion at the catch to 28° of extension at the finish. While both sexes finish the rowing stroke with essentially the same amount of extension, the men demonstrated a greater flexion angle at the trunk at the catch (see Fig. 60-4B). Compression forces at the L3-4 motion segment averaged 3919 N for the men and 3330 N for the women. The peak compression load occurs during the latter portion of the drive phase as the upper dorsal thorax passes over the pelvis into the extended position. At this point the peak compression load averages 6066 N for the men and 5031 N for the women, or when normalized for body weight, 7 times body weight for the men and 6.85 times body weight for the women.[7]

The mechanics of the rowing stroke with its repetitive cyclic and intense loading of the lumbar spine explains the increased incidence of lumbar spine injuries in rowing population. The forces generated with the rowing stroke are similar to those that have been shown to produce pathologic changes in cadaveric specimens.[1,2] While the spinal motion segment is well suited to resist compression, as the disc degenerates and loses its shock-absorbing capability, it becomes susceptible to injury and also transmits a significant load to the facets and posterior structures. The facets are well oriented to resist sheer forces, and when combined with compression, resist 33% to 50% of the corresponding sheer force, with the intervertebral disc resisting the balance. Thus, the rowing stroke puts considerable pressure in the posterior elements of the spine, which may result in bony injury of the lumbar spine.[15]

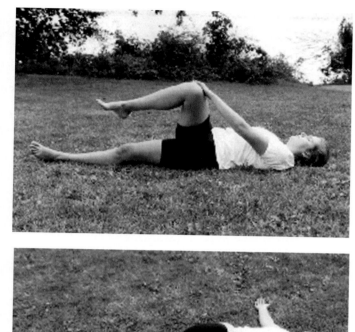

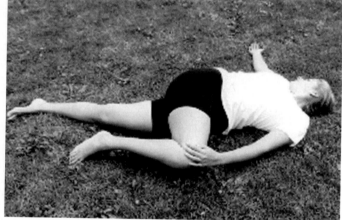

Figure 60-8 *(Continued).* **(C & D)** ITB-stretching exercise.

Illustration continued on following page

Also of interest is the occurrence of central disc herniation related to the use of the ergometer and sculling. In the adolescent and young adult, this may present with an absence of neurologic findings, only persistent lower lumbar back pain without radiation into the legs.[13] Although the rowing stroke subjects the lumbar spine to significant mechanical loads, it is important to consider all causes of low back pain in the differential diagnosis (Table 60-1). Back pain in the rowing population can be described as mechanical, discogenic, spondylolytic, or, in the masters rower, facet arthropathy related. Mechanical lower back pain is generally localized to the lumbar area. It is associated with significant muscle spasm and may begin gradually with episodic exacerbation. Quite often in the adolescent or intercollegiate rower, this ill-defined low back pain without radicular symptoms signals early disc degeneration or central herniation. The pain is generally exacerbated with activity and relieved with rest and NSAIDs. Prevention must include a comprehensive

trunk-strengthening program, proper use of rowing technique, and a thorough warm-up with stretching prior to rowing. *Discogenic lower back pain* refers to disorders of the intervertebral disc that result in nerve root irritation sciatica. However, in the older rower, facet arthropathy may also cause sciatica. The herniated nucleus pulposus commonly occurs in a third decade. However, in the rowing population disc herniation is common in all age groups. They generally are associated with a specific event where a "snap" or "pop" may be felt in the lower spine with associated lower back pain. Within 24 to 48 hours the leg pain develops accompanied by dermatomal-specific physical findings (Table 60-2). A herniated disc typically occurs in a lower lumbar motion segment. An L3-4 herniation produces an L4 radiculopathy with pain radiating from the posterior lateral thigh across the patella and the anterior medial leg. Weakness of the quadriceps and, in chronic cases, atrophy are present. The knee deep tendon reflex may be diminished with

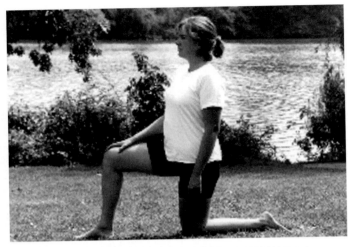

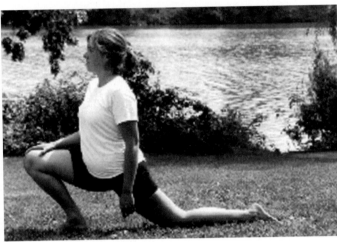

Figure 60-8 *(Continued)*. **(E & F)** Anterior hip-stretching exercise.

decreased sensation over the anterior medial thigh. The L4-5 motion segment affects the L5 nerve root, with associated pain radiating down the posterior lateral thigh and anterior lateral leg. Weakness of the extensor hallucis longus and anterior tibialis may be present. An L5-S1 herniation affects the S1 nerve root, resulting in pain radiating down the posterior lateral aspect of the thigh and leg. There may be decreased sensation along the lateral aspect of the heel and foot, weakness of plantar flexion with associated atrophy of the soleus and gastrocnemius, and absence of the ankle deep tendon reflexes. Treatment for discogenic lower back pain includes cessation of rowing, active rest as tolerated, local modalities, NSAIDs, and, on occasion, antispasmodic medications. The patient with a documented neurologic deficit should be followed very closely. If there is no resolution or improvement of the deficit or if radicular pain persists after 14 days of treatment, further workup is indicated.

Lumbar spine roentgenograms are obtained to rule out other pathologies such as spondylolysis, infection, tumors, segmental instability, and fracture. In addition, magnetic resonance imaging (MRI) is an excellent means of imaging disc pathology. If necessary, metrizamide may be added to this study to enhance its specificity.

In general, individuals with disc herniation do well with conservative management. When most of the acute symptoms have subsided and the pain has largely resolved, a comprehensive rehabilitation program begins starting with hamstring and lumbosacral stretching exercises associated with the instruction of body mechanics and progressing to Williams flexion and abdominal strengthening exercises. McKenzie lumbar extension exercises are an essential component of the rehabilitation of a disc herniation. In those individuals with a persistent symptomatic radiculopathy, epidural corticosteroid injections may be warranted. However, if the neurologic deficit persists or progresses despite

Table 60-1. Etiologic Factors in Low Back Pain

I. Congenital disorders
  A. Facet tropism (asymmetry)
  B. Transitional vertebra
    1. Sacralization of lumbar vertebra
    2. Lumbarization of sacral vertebra
II. Tumors
  A. Benign
    1. Tumors involving nerve roots or meninges (eg, neurinoma, hemangioma, meningioma)
    2. Tumors involving vertebrae (eg, osteoid osteoma, Paget's disease, osteoblastoma)
  B. Malignant
    1. Primary bone tumors (eg, multiple myeloma)
    2. Primary neural tumors
    3. Secondary tumors (eg, metastases from breast, prostate, kidney, lung, thyroid)
III. Trauma
  A. Lumbar strain
    1. Acute
    2. Chronic
  B. Compression fracture
    1. Fracture of vertebral body
    2. Fracture of transverse process
  C. Subluxated facet joint (facet syndrome)
  D. Spondylolysis and spondylolisthesis
IV. Toxicity
  A. Heavy metal poisoning (eg, radium)
V. Metabolic disorders (eg, osteoporosis)
VI. Inflammatory diseases (eg, rheumatoid arthritis, ankylosing spondylitis)
VII. Degenerative disorders (eg, spondylosis, osteoarthritis, herniated disc, herniated nucleus pulposus, spinal stenosis—nerve root entrapment syndrome)
VIII. Infections
  A. Acute (eg, pyogenic disc space infections)
  B. Chronic (eg, tuberculosis, chronic osteomyelitis, fungal infection)
IX. Circulatory disorders (eg, abdominal aortic aneurysm)
X. Mechanical causes
  A. Intrinsic (eg, poor muscle tone, chronic postural strain, myofascial pain, unstable vertebrae)
  B. Extrinsic (eg, uterine fibroids, pelvic tumors or infections, hip diseases, prostate disease, sacroiliac joint infections and sprains, untreated lumbar scoliosis)
XI. Psychoneurotic problems (eg, hysteria, malingering, compensatory low back pain—"green poultice" syndrome)

From Keim HA, Kirkaldy-Willis WH: Low back pain. Clin Symp 32(6):8, 1980. Copyright © 1980 CIBA-GEIGY Corporation, all rights reserved; with permission.

conservative management, and if it correlates with objective findings on physical examination as well as diagnostic studies, surgical intervention may be indicated. For individuals with persistent radicular and lower symptoms, no clearly defined neurologic deficits, and negative diagnostic studies, conservative management is indicated. Surgical intervention is never indicated in the absence of a clear-cut anatomic lesion.

Spondylolysis is a defect of the pars interarticularis and in most cases represents a stress-type injury caused by repetitive loading of the lumbar spine. The rower usually presents complaining of lower back pain, generally without sciatica. The pain is localized over the pars lateral to the midline and exacerbated with hyperextension of the spine. There are no neurologic deficits. Roentgenograms should include lumbar posterior oblique views, which optimize identification of the pars defect. Often when roentgenograms are inconclusive, a single-photon emission computed tomography (SPECT) bone scan will provide visualization of the defect.[3] Symptomatic individuals should follow a comprehensive back program with emphasis in lower extremity and trunk stretching as well as strengthening. While the person is symptomatic, rowing should be avoided. For individuals with persistent symptoms and a positive bone scan, bracing may be helpful.

Facet joint arthropathy is a result of aging and minor trauma. Rowers with degenerative facet changes generally complain of a vague back pain without radicular symptoms. As this process develops the pain is described as deep, dull, and aching and may be referred to the lumbosacral area, buttocks, and upper thighs. It is generally exacerbated by ambulation and relieved by sitting.

Physical examination may reveal loss of normal lumbar lordosis with a decreased lumbar range of motion. Significant paraspinal spasm may be present, and the pain is elicited by palpation over the affected facet joints. The neurologic examination reflects the level of the motion segment involved with associated nerve root compression. However, when the facet hypertrophy is extensive the nerve root exiting one level below may be compressed, presenting a complex clinical picture. Imaging studies, including roentgenography, MRI, and metrizamide-enhanced MRI, will be helpful in defining the pathology. Limitation of activity, NSAIDs, and lumbar support will generally provide relief. With cessation of symptoms, a trunk and hamstring stretching and strengthening program should be instituted.

Low back pain in the rowing population is common and directly related to the loads placed on the lumbar spine during participation in this activity. Proper management requires an accurate diagnosis. In addition, the management must emphasize maintaining aerobic performance of the rower while rehabilitating the lower back injury.

Ribs and Thorax

Pain associated with the ribcage is a common complaint in the rowing population. The vast majority of these injuries are rib stress fractures.

Table 60-2. Clinical Features of Herniated Lumbar Discs

L3–4 DISC; L4 NERVE ROOT	
Pain	Lower back, hip, posterolateral thigh, across patella, anteromedial aspect of leg
Numbness	Anteromedial thigh and knee
Weakness	Knee extension
Atrophy	Quadriceps
Reflexes	Knee jerk diminished
L4–5 DISC; L5 NERVE ROOT	
Pain	Sacroiliac region, hip, posterolateral thigh, anterolateral leg
Numbness	Lateral leg, first webspace
Weakness	Dorsiflexion of great toe and foot
Atrophy	Minimal anterior calf
Reflexes	None, or absent posterior tibial tendon reflex
L5–S1 DISC; S1 NERVE ROOT	
Pain	Sacroiliac region, hip, posterolateral thigh/leg
Numbness	Back of calf; lateral heel, foot, and toe
Weakness	Plantarflexion of foot and great toe
Atrophy	Gastrocnemius and soleus
Reflexes	Ankle jerk diminished or absent

From Boden SD, Wiesel SW, Laws ER, et al: The Aging Spine. Philadelphia, WB Saunders, 1991, with permission.

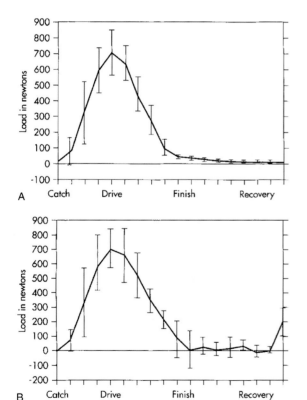

Figure 60-9. **(A)** The force at the oar measured with a strain gauge shows the rapid acceleration in the first half of the drive phase, peaking at mid-drive and tapering to the finish. **(B)** The shear load on the lower back mirrors the load applied to the oar. With the acceleration of the knees and back, the lumbar shear load peaks at mid-drive and tapers to the finish. There is minimal shear force affecting the lumbar spine during the recovery phase.

Studies of collegiate rowing programs and the Canadian National Rowing Team revealed that rib stress fractures make up about 10% of the rowing injuries (Bachus R: Personal communication, 1996).[6,7] Stress fractures of the ribs have been associated with throwing, golfing, rowing, canoeing, and swimming.[4,5,11,12,17] While the vast majority of rib stress fractures reported in literature involve the first rib, the ribs primarily affected in rowers are the fifth through ninth ribs. Biomechanical analysis of the ribs in rowing reveals the greatest bending moment occurs at the junction of the middle third of the rib and the posterior lateral segment. This is the site of the majority of the fractures in the rowing population. It has been proposed that the opposing actions of the serratus anterior and external oblique muscles are the major contributor to development of the stress fracture.[9] The serratus anterior muscle originates at the medial border of the scapula and inserts into the anterior lateral aspect of the first through ninth ribs and interdigitates with the origin of the external oblique muscle on the fifth through ninth ribs (Fig. 60-10). Utilizing wire electromyography electrodes, the serratus anterior muscle was found to fire maximally at the catch phase of the rowing stroke. This activity continues through the drive phase and turns off at the finish (Fig. 60-11). The activity of this muscle stabilizes the scapula, maintaining the connection allowing transfer of the power generated by the legs to the oar.[7]

The external oblique muscle has been found to increase the lateral segment bend of the rib

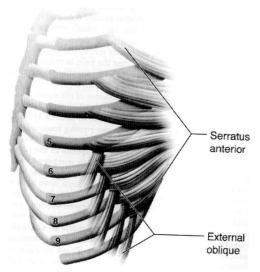

Serratus
anterior

External
oblique

Figure 60-10. Diagram of the anatomy of the serratus anterior and external oblique muscles showing the interdigitation of these muscles on the fifth to ninth rib. (From Karlson KA: Rib stress fractures in elite rowers. Am J Sports Med 26:516, 1998, with permission.)

rowers train with long aerobic workouts on the water and spend a significant length of time on the rowing ergometer. As with stress fractures in other locations, the rib stress fracture generally presents with a vague, ill-defined thoracic discomfort before progressing to an obviously painful stress fracture. Recognizing the insidious onset and changing the rib stress patterns at that time may prevent the onset of an acute fracture. The stress fracture presents with a sharp stabbing pain that is exacerbated by coughing, deep breathing, and changing position. It has been accompanied on occasion by winging of the scapula. The pain is generally discretely localized by the affected rib in the posterior lateral corner and radiates into the anterior axillary line. The pain is also produced with thoracic compression as well as stressing the serratus anterior muscle on the affected side. Diagnosis confirmed by a bone scan, which identifies the increased uptake in the rib (Fig. 60-12). Occasionally the acute stress fracture may be seen on routine roentgenography but generally the roentgenograms become positive late in the healing process when the fracture callus becomes visible. The authors have seen one case of a hypertrophic nonunion following an unrecognized stress fracture (Fig. 60-13). Rib stress fractures generally heal within 6 to 8 weeks. With the onset of symptoms, the rower should cease all activities until activities of daily living can be performed comfortably. At this point, the rowers continue to avoid rowing activities but begin cross training to maintain fitness, utilizing devices such as a bicycle ergometer and StairMaster. Running and impact-loading activities tend to exacerbate the discomfort and are to be avoided during the early healing phase. As a fracture heals and the

by pulling it inward and downward. It is assumed to fire maximally at the finish of the rowing stroke when the shoulders are behind the hips and the scapulae are fully retracted. With the serratus anterior muscle firing eccentrically, the opposing actions of these 2 muscles result in a repetitive bending force in the middle segment of the rib. With intense training and increasing loads this off-and-on firing pattern results in a fatigue mode of stress loading, which may result in a rib stress fracture.[9]

Rib stress fractures generally occur during periods of intense training, with a relatively low stroke rate and high load per stroke. This occurs during the fall and winter training, when the

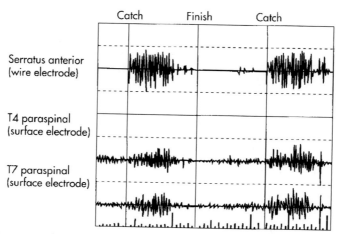

Figure 60-11. Myoelectric activity of the serratus anterior and thoracic musculature during the rowing stroke. The activity of the serratus anterior is maximal during the drive phase, corresponding to the stabilization of the scapula allowing for the transfer of power to the oar.

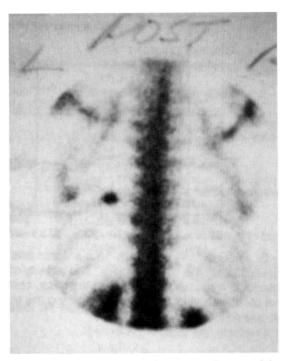

Figure 60-12. Bone scan revealing a stress fracture of the left posterior seventh rib.

rower becomes less symptomatic, training on the rower ergometer is allowed, with minimal resistance at a relatively high stroke rate. The rower then progresses slowly, increasing the resistance and lowering the stroke rate as tolerated until normal activities can be resumed. Symptomatic relief is provided with analgesics and NSAIDs. The use of a transcutaneous elec-trical nerve stimulation unit has been helpful on occasion, while in the authors' experience rib belts have not been helpful. It is recommended that serratus stabilization exercises such as push-ups plus, upper extremity step-ups, and serratus rhythmic stabilization be used as part of the rower's regular training program to prevent this injury from occurring (Fig. 60-14). The key to minimizing the disability associated with a rib stress fracture is early identification during the ill-defined aching phase, at which point cessation of rowing may prevent the progression to full-blown stress fracture symptoms.

CONCLUDING REMARKS

Rowing provides an excellent aerobic and anaerobic form of exercise. The injury pattern in the sport is related to overuse. Inappropriate training patterns and poor technique will predispose the rower to injuries. However, with proper coaching, cross training, and a comprehensive stretching program, a large number of these injuries may be prevented.

For those individuals wishing to begin serious rowing participation but with a pre-existing condition such as significant patellofemoral chondromalacia or a pre-existing serious lower back diagnosis such as disc herniation, spondylolisthesis, and spondylolysis, careful guidance is imperative. This may include discouraging participation altogether.

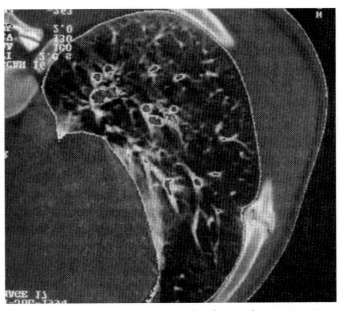

Figure 60-13. CT scan of a hypertrophic nonunion of a rib stress fracture in a 20-year-old rower.

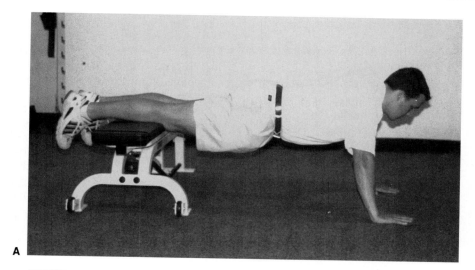

A

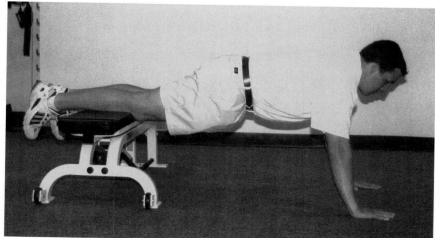

B

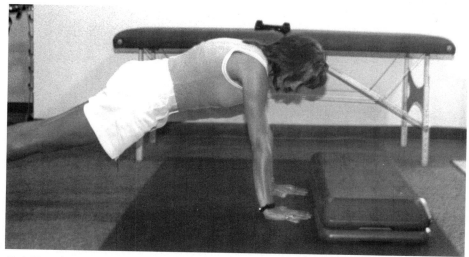

C

Figure 60-14. (**A** & **B**) Push-up plus. The rower is in the prone position with the legs on the floor or a straight bench (**A**). With the arms straight and the shoulders and back in a level position, the rower pushes upward, causing the thoracic region to become rounded (**B**). (**C** & **D**) Upper extremity step-ups. Body position begins with a kneeling position to a full push up position (**C**) to a leg-elevated position. In proper form the rower's arms are straight, shoulders level, and back straight.

Illustration continued on following page

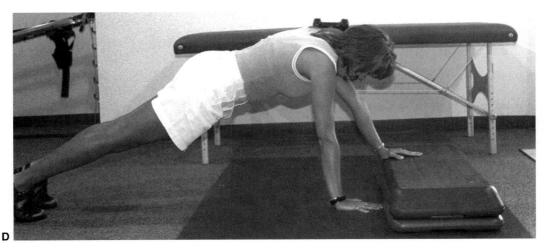

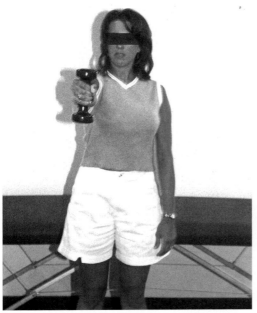
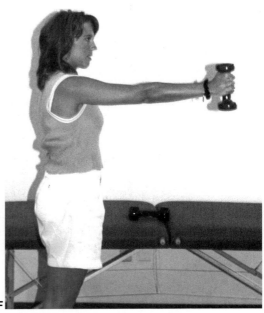

Figure 60-14. (*Continued*). The rower's weight shifts onto one arm while stepping on the plate (**D**). The opposite arm follows, so both arms are placed on the plate. The rower then steps down, alternating the arms. (**E** & **F**) Serratus rhythmic stabilization. The rower sits or stands with good posture. Beginning with the arm at a 90° angle of forward elevation, the athlete presses/pushes the weight forward. While holding the weight forward, the athlete spells the alphabet or makes a star shape with the arm, keeping the elbow locked in full extension.

References

1. Adams, MA, Hutton, WC: The effect of fatigue on the lumbar intervertebral disc. J Bone Joint Surg 65B:199, 1983.
2. Adams MA, Hutton WC: Gradual disc prolapse. Spine 10:524, 1985.
3. Collier BD, Johnson RF, et al: Painful spondylosis or spondylolisthesis studies by radiography and single-photon emission computerized tomography. Radiology 154:277, 1985.
4. Curran DB, Kelly DA: Stress fractures of the first rib. Am J Orthop 8:16, 1966.
5. Gurtler R, Pavlov H, Torg JS: Stress fracture of the ipsi-lateral rib in a pitcher. Am J Sports Med 13:277, 1985.
6. Holden D, Jackson D: Stress fractures of the ribs in female rowers. Am J Sports Med 13:342, 1985.
7. Hosea T, Boland A, et al: Rowing injuries. Postgrad Adv Sports Med 3:1,1989.
8. Howell D: Musculoskeletal profile and incidence of musculoskeletal injuries in lightweight female rowers. Am J Sports Med 12:278, 1984.
9. Karlson K: Rib stress fractures in elite rowers: a case series

10. Korzeniowski K: Basic Rowing Technique in U.S.: Rowing Instructor Manual Level I. Indianapolis, Ind, 1993, pp 15–37.
11. Lord MJ, Ha K: Stress fractures of the ribs in golfers. Am J Sports Med 24:118, 1996.
12. Maffuuli N, Pintore E: Stress fracture of the sixth rib in a canoeist. Br J Sports Med 24:247, 1990.
13. McClean M, Hosea TM: Central disc herniation in the intercollegiate rowing population. Am J Sports Med, 2002 (submitted for publication).
14. Mendenhall TC: A Short History of American Rowing. Boston, Charles River Books, 1980.
15. Schultz AB, Andersson GBJ: Analysis of loads on the lumbar spine. Spine 6:76, 1981.
16. Stallard MC: Backache in oarsman. Br J Sports Med 14:105, 1980.
17. Taimela S, Kajala UM, et al: Two consecutive rib stress fractures in a female competitive swimmer. Clin J Sports Med 6:204, 1995.
18. Williams J: Surgical management of traumatic non-infective tenosynovitis of the wrist extensors. J Bone Joint Surg 59B:408, 1977.

Chapter 61

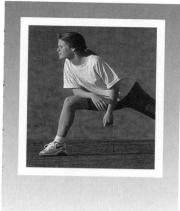

Soccer

Margot Putukian, M.D.
Bert R. Mandelbaum, M.D.
Douglas W. Brown, M.D.

In recent years, interest in playing soccer has exploded, with 200,000,000 players worldwide. The female soccer player is now very popular, but historically she was not. In 1921, the European Football Association banned female participation in soccer. In 1971, this ban was lifted, furthering participation of athletes. In 1972, Title IX was enacted within the National Collegiate Athletic Association (NCAA) in an attempt to equalize the number of men's and women's athletic teams in the United States collegiate environment. This had a dramatic effect on the creation of female soccer programs. In 1986, there were only 230 programs in the NCAA[83]; by 1997, there were 696. The 1991 World Cup in China allowed female soccer players to be showcased on an international front. The United States women's team won the World Cup. The evolution in the United States has continued to be rapid, with significant developments and increased participation of youth and females. In the United States, 43% of active players are female; whereas, worldwide, female players only account for 22% of active players. The future appears to be extremely exciting. The Women's World Cup hosted by the United States in 1999 laid the groundwork for increased participation and enhanced spectator interest. The purpose of this chapter is to focus on the gender-specific characteristics of the female soccer player with respect to performance, injury care, and injury prevention.

PERFORMANCE AND GENDER DIFFERENCES

Soccer demands a combination of endurance running and discontinuous sprinting. The sport-specific skills used in soccer include quick turns, pivots, jumps in the air, and both forward and backward running. All surfaces of the body are utilized with the exception of the arms and hands, though these are used frequently during throw-ins and in goalkeeping. There is a reliance on lower extremity and trunk strength, but also balance and proprioception. It has been documented that the female athlete runs approximately 8471 meters in a game. The average sprint is 14.9 meters long with an average of 100 sprints per game. The average percent body fat is between 19% and 22%. The average maximum oxygen consumption (VO_2max) ranges between 47 and 56 mL/kg/min.[27] Compared to female runners, female soccer players have a higher percent body fat and a lower VO_2max. These European data from 1986 may not reflect the current-day soccer player.[27] One might expect that the level of fitness of the female soccer player in the United States would reflect a lower percent body fat and a higher VO_2max. The benefits of athletic participation by females are significant. Overall lifestyle improvements include a lower teen pregnancy rate, less drug and alcohol use and abuse, higher graduation rates, improved self-esteem and body image, less depression, and improved teamwork, cooperation, goal-setting, and acceptance of others.[90] Despite these outstanding benefits, there are significant risks associated with female athletic participation.

The physiologic demands of soccer require proper nutrition and hydration. This is especially true when the ambient temperature is high or the playing situation demands multiple games be played with little time for restoration of energy and fluids. The female athlete has special nutritional needs that may play a role in performance.[14] An understanding of the special needs of the female player is important in the education of athletes as well as in the organization of their training.

Iron deficiency is the most common nutritional deficiency in the female athlete. The most common cause of iron deficiency in women is poor dietary intake in combination with the blood loss of menstruation. A nutritional survey at the beginning of the season can help determine if an athlete is obtaining sufficient iron intake. A screening assessment of hemoglobin and/or ferritin can be useful in further assessing for iron deficiency or low iron stores.

Fluid ingestion during soccer activity is important to provide an energy source to supplement the body's limited stores and to replace the water and electrolytes lost through sweating. The optimal fluid content and timing of replacement should be individualized to meet the demands of the intensity and duration of exercise, the ambient temperature and humidity, and the individual preferences of the athlete.

The primary cause of fatigue in soccer play is the depletion of carbohydrate reserves. Most athletes will not drink enough on their own to replace losses; thirst does not stimulate drinking enough replacement fluid. Studies have demonstrated that when an individual is dehydrated by as little as 2%, exercise performance is impaired. If 5% of body weight is lost, work capacity can diminish by approximately 30%.[101]

The most serious side effect of dehydration is the inability to dissipate heat, which can result in heat exhaustion and heat illness. This was well demonstrated in a youth soccer tournament in Minnesota, where modifications made decreased the incidence of heat-related illness.[36] Risk factors for heat-related illness include preexisting medical disease (diabetes, cardiovascular disease, alcoholism, hyperthyroidism), prepubertal or older age, poor conditioning, inadequate acclimatization, dehydration, obesity, fatigue, prior heat injury, and current or recent febrile illness. Certain drugs can also increase the risk for heat injury.

Adding carbohydrate to fluids ingested during soccer activity can delay muscle glycogen depletion and maintain hydration.[23] Depletion of muscle glycogen can occur with either 90 to 180 minutes of continuous exercise at 60% to 80% of VO_2max, or 15 to 30 minutes of exercise at 90% to 130% VO_2max performed in 1- to 5-minute intervals.[19,58] The benefits of ingesting carbohydrate are sparing of muscle glycogen stores, enhanced performance and work output, and increased time to exhaustion.[22,49,56,81] It has also been demonstrated that the timing of carbohydrate ingestion after exercise is important in replenishing depleted glycogen stores. Ingesting carbohydrate as soon after exercise as possible will maximize the replacement of muscle glycogen energy stores in preparation for the next game or practice.

The use of carbohydrate and fluid ingestion in soccer performance has been examined prospectively using muscle biopsies obtained before and after a game. Glucose polymer ingestion before and during a soccer match resulted in a glycogen content in the vastus lateralis musculature 31% higher than that in muscles of players given a placebo solution.[64] Foster and coworkers performed a similar study assessing the effects of glucose polymer solution ingested between 2 successive indoor games. This study was a single-blind, crossover study in which each player served as his own control. The amount of time spent running, cruising, or sprinting was measured in both the first and second halves of both games. There was no difference in the amount of time spent walking in the first or second halves, and no difference in the amount of time spent cruising or sprinting in the first half. However, in the second half, the athletes given glucose polymer solution spent 40% more time sprinting and cruising and overall covered 20% more distance than when they did not have glucose polymer.[41]

These studies emphasize the need for proper energy and fluid replacement during soccer, not only to prevent dehydration and heat-related illness, but also to optimize performance. The American College of Sports Medicine (ACSM) recommendations are very useful for the exercising athlete.[4] Their recommended amount of carbohydrate to maintain glucose levels and spare muscle glycogen is 30 to 60 g/hr; the amount of fluid replacement may vary depending on the environmental conditions. Because athletes can be dehydrated and not feel thirsty, they may need to be reminded to drink early and at regular intervals during exercise. Fluid replacement should take precedence over substrate when exercising in the heat. Adding sodium may be useful in maintaining the osmotic drive to drink and enabling the kidneys to hold on to sodium, and in making fluids more palatable.[4]

INJURY CARE

It has been documented in several studies that in a comparison to age-matched male controls, females sustained an increased number of injuries.[38,102] We know that male and female athletes under the age of 10 experience minimal to no injuries.[7,53,59] The incidence of injury increases with age, and is up to 10-fold higher in high school athletes than in those under 10 years.[53,113] The overall injury incidence in soccer is favorable, with fewer injuries than in

American football. Studies are often difficult to compare because they often use different definitions for injury. However, most studies consistently show that in the younger age group girls have a higher injury incidence than boys for outdoor soccer. Injury rate and distribution data were recorded from 1988 to 1997 for the USA Cup Soccer competition, a 6-day event with 800 teams from 23 countries participating in age groups from under 12 to under 19.[35] Injury rates were reported in detail as per 1000 player hours, and comparisons of age groups under 12, under 14, under 16, and under 19, and gender were provided. The injury rates for both genders declined over the 10-year span of the Cup study. There was a slightly higher aggregate injury rate for females, but the difference became less significant as the tournament matured. Females were 1.6 times more likely to sustain heat illness than males. Engstrom and colleagues reported an incidence per 1000 player hours of 12 for girls versus 5 for boys,[38] and Schmidt-Olson and coworkers reported an incidence per 1000 player hours of 17.6 for girls versus 7.4 for boys.[102]

Injury patterns, risk factors, and prevention strategies are summarized in dissertations focusing on the female soccer player.[15,108] In a prospective study over one outdoor soccer season, adolescent females were compared to males in European football. The overall injury incidence was 6.8 per 1000 hours (games and practice); 9.1 and 1.5 injuries per 1000 player hours occurred in games and practices, respectively. Ankle sprain was the most frequent type of injury. Fifty-six percent of the ankle sprains were reinjuries.[108]

At the collegiate level the incidence of injury between men and women appears to equalize. The National Collegiate Athletic Association (NCAA) utilizes a well-established Injury Surveillance System (ISS) to track men's and women's sports injuries, using time lost from play because of injury as their definition of injury.[82]

Soccer injury rates reported by the NCAA ISS for the years 1999 to 2000 list the rate numbers per 1000 athletic exposures in practices and games. There are 3 categorizations (Table 61-1). The first is by diagnosis: sprain, incomplete or complete; strain, incomplete or complete; dislocation, partial or complete; fracture; stress fracture; and concussion.[82] These injury types apply to any and all body parts. The second categorization is by body part involved. Lower extremity injuries are most common. The third categorization is by field surface. Concussions were 4.3:1 more common in women than men.

Complete tears were more common in female athletes in practice (2.67:1) and in games (5.23:1). Stress fractures were more common in females, in a ratio of 3.5:1. The female:male ACL injury ratios were 1.8 in practices and 5.78 in games.

The types of injury that occur in indoor and outdoor soccer are similar in both body part affected and severity. Studies of the injury incidence in indoor soccer are limited to only a few studies, and only 2 studies have included women. Lindenfeld demonstrated an equal incidence of injuries in men and women in a 7-week indoor soccer league play, with 5.04 and 5.03 injuries per 100 player hours, respectively.[69] Their injury definition included any injury in which the player left the game or requested medical attention, or for which play was stopped. They did demonstrate a higher incidence of ACL injuries in women compared to men in this study. Putukian and colleagues demonstrated a similar overall injury incidence in men and women during a 3-day indoor tournament, with 5.79 and 4.74 injuries per 100 player hours, respectively.[94] In this study, there was no significant difference in ACL injuries, although the number of ACL injuries that occurred was small.

In games played on natural grass, overall injury rates were 6 times higher in males and 4.3 times higher in females. On artificial grass, overall injury rates were the same in men and lower in women, with injuries in games 5 times more common in men and 4 times more common in women.[82] Hormonal influences have been linked to injury. The menstrual cycle and its relation to soccer injuries was prospectively studied by Moller-Nielsen.[80] The study showed that women soccer players were more susceptible to traumatic injuries during the premenstrual and menstrual periods compared to the rest of the menstrual cycle ($P < 0.05$), especially among players with premenstrual symptoms such as irritability, swelling/discomfort in the breasts, and swelling/congestion in the abdomen. It was also found that women using oral contraceptive pills had a lower rate of injury ($P < 0.05$) compared to women who were not on the pill. The results can be explained by the fact that oral contraceptives ameliorate some symptoms of the premenstrual and menstrual periods, which might also affect coordination and hence the risk of injury.[80] Further research is needed. There is no suggestion to change the female athlete's schedule based on the time of her menstrual cycle.[45]

Lindenfeld and coworkers demonstrated that female players suffered a significantly higher rate

Table 61-1. Soccer Injury Rates, 1999–2000: Injury Rates Per 1000 Athletic Exposures

	PRACTICES			GAMES		
DIAGNOSIS	Males	Females	Ratio F/M	Males	Females	Ratio F/M
Laceration	0.01	0.01	1.00	0.78	0.37	0.47
Ligament sprain (incomplete tear)	1.15	1.01	0.88	6.09	4.64	0.76
Ligament sprain (complete tear)	0.06	0.16	2.67	0.31	1.62	5.23
Muscle-tendon strain (incomplete tear)	1.37	1.97	1.44	3.74	2.72	0.73
Muscle-tendon strain (complete tear)	0.01	0.05	5.00	0.00	0.04	—
Dislocation (partial)	0.04	0.04	1.00	0.31	0.40	1.29
Dislocation (complete)	0.04	0.01	0.25	0.20	0.04	0.20
Fracture	0.16	0.13	0.81	1.09	1.10	1.01
Stress fracture	0.02	0.07	3.50	0.08	0.07	0.88
Concussion	0.03	0.13	4.33	1.37	1.95	1.42
BODY PARTS INVOLVED						
Lower back	0.08	0.15	1.88	0.43	0.44	1.02
Pelvis, groin, hip	0.47	0.53	1.13	1.21	0.52	0.43
Upper leg	0.72	1.20	1.67	2.77	1.77	0.64
Knee	0.55	0.68	1.24	3.24	3.98	1.23
ACL	0.05	0.09	1.80	0.23	1.33	5.78
Patella	0.07	0.06	0.86	0.16	0.15	0.94
Lower leg	0.32	0.34	1.06	1.21	1.33	1.10
Ankle	0.92	0.98	1.07	4.37	3.57	0.82
Heel/Achilles	0.11	0.13	1.18	0.12	0.29	2.42
Foot	0.28	0.19	0.68	1.05	0.77	0.73
Neck	0.01	0.02	2.00	0.12	0.29	2.42
Shoulder	0.09	0.09	1.00	0.66	0.40	0.61
Clavicle	0.04	0.01	0.25	0.12	0.11	0.92
AC separation	0.01	0.00	0.00	0.20	0.07	0.35
Elbow	0.01	0.02	2.00	0.16	0.15	0.94
Forearm	0.01	0.00	0.00	0.16	0.07	0.44
Wrist	0.04	0.02	0.50	0.20	0.26	1.30
Hand	0.02	0.01	0.50	0.04	0.11	2.75
Finger(s)	0.04	0.02	0.50	0.04	0.18	4.50
Thumb(s)	0.05	0.05	1.00	0.20	0.00	0.00
Head	0.04	0.15	3.75	1.95	2.13	1.09
Eye	0.01	0.02	2.00	0.12	0.15	1.25
FIELD SURFACE						
Natural grass	4.00	4.90	1.23	24.20	21.00	0.87
Artificial grass	4.90	4.40	0.90	24.70	17.60	0.71
Nongrass (gym floor, etc.)	7.40	2.90	0.39	0.00	0.00	—

From NCAA: 1999–2000 NCAA Injury Surveillance System, Indianapolis, Ind, 2000, with permission.

of knee ligament injuries compared to males in a study of indoor soccer.[69] The reason for the difference between males and females remains unclear, but some investigators have discussed a relative lack of physical fitness in female athletes compared to males as one possible cause. This may to some extent be due to factors such as training background. The differences may also be due to intensity during training sessions and/or the amount of training. The training time for female elite players was approximately half of that of male elite players. The training habits have changed rapidly since the late 1980s, so this important question requires further investigation. Although there are similarities in the incidence and the type of injuries, there are also

significant differences in comparison to male soccer players. Knapik and colleagues demonstrated in a prospective study of female collegiate athletes that flexibility and lower extremity strength imbalances of more than 15% were associated with a 2.6 times increased injury rate.[61]

Additional risks include amenorrhea, disordered eating, premature osteoporosis, and a higher level of stress fractures.[90] Overall, in evaluating the medical and orthopaedic issues within a women's teams program, there are 4 major areas that need to be addressed. These include ACL injuries, stress fractures, ankle sprains with ankle impingement syndromes, and head injuries. There has been significant research addressing both knee and ankle injuries in soccer, as well as programs to prevent these injuries in the soccer player.[29,31,36,37,39,40,42, 46,52,96,104, 105,114] Focus on each of these issues follows in detail.

Knee Injuries

In soccer the rate of ACL tears per 1000 athletic exposures in the female is 0.31 as compared to 0.13 in the male, a 40% greater incidence. Female soccer players show a higher rate of knee and ACL injuries compared to their male counterparts.[2,5]

Noncontact ACL injuries in men compared to women over a 10-year period are shown in Figure 61-1. This increased incidence in ACL injuries for women compared to men is of significant concern and has not fallen from 1989 to 1999.[2,5] From NCAA statistics of universities surveyed, for each year there was a statistically significant difference in ACL injury rates by gender. The average female : male ratio was 2.75 from 1989 through 1999.[82]

The youth injury incidence is between 11.7% and 19%.[7,60,102] In an NCAA study on knee injury, Arendt and Dick in 1995 found a female rate of 1.6 per 1000 exposures as compared to 1.3 in age-matched males.[5]

Noyes in 1983 indicated that 78% of ACL injuries occurred as a result of a noncontact mechanism.[88] Arendt and Dick found that noncontact injuries were significantly more common in the female athlete ($P < 0.01$), but that noncontact and contact mechanisms were equal in the male athlete.[5] The contact mechanisms, as demonstrated by Ekstrand in 1983, include charge or block tackling and foul play, especially tackles from behind.[32] Boden and Garrett have further articulated the mechanism of injury by evaluating 85 athletes with ACL tears and found that 72% involved noncontact deceleration occurring at an average knee flexion of 23°. The exact mechanisms include pivot in 23%, a varus moment in 19%, hyperextension in 13%, valgus in 6%, and contact varus in 2%.[12] Shoemaker found that the anterior tibial force was maximum with knee at 25° of flexion, internal torque, and a varus moment.[106] Noonan and Woo concluded that ACL rupture occurs at 2000 N, this being the critical threshold.

The risk factors for injury to the ACL are divided into intrinsic and extrinsic factors. As

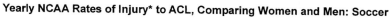

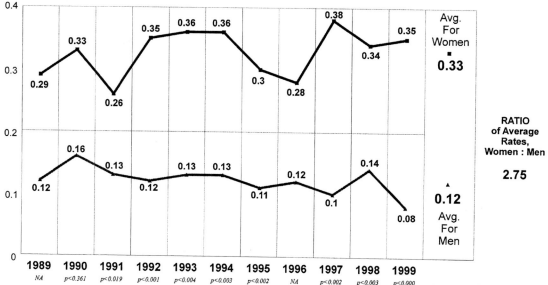

Figure 61-1. The NCAA Injury Surveillance System from the 1989–1990 through the 1999–2000 seasons shows statistically significant higher rates of ACL injuries in women compared to men for all years. These rates were significant for each year as noted under the years on bottom of the graph. The average ratio was 0.33 in women compared to 0.12 in men. On average, women were 2.7 times more likely than men to have an ACL tear. Rates are given per 1000 athlete exposures. (Figure design copyright 2001, Mary Lloyd Ireland, MD. Statistical data from NCAA Injury Surveillance System 1999–2000, NCAA, PO Box 6222, Indianapolis, Indiana.)

an intrinsic factor the quadriceps is the major antagonist of the ACL, and the hamstring is an agonist. During gait and heel strike, the quadriceps becomes activated, creating an eccentric contraction that limits flexion, facilitating extension and resulting in greater forces on the ACL.[6,11] With respect to the female athlete, Wojtys demonstrated that, overall, there is less quadriceps and hamstring isokinetic strength in the female athlete. In addition, in the female the quadriceps is recruited first, which is in contradistinction to the male, who recruits the hamstring first. Furthermore, the maximal hamstring torque and recruitment of that torque takes longer to attain in males.[118] Level of aerobic and anaerobic fitness is a possible risk factor and cause for ACL injury. It has been proposed that females have a higher incidence of ACL injuries because of poor fitness, although more research is needed in this area. Wojtys and coworkers demonstrated that female players were significantly weaker.[118] Limb alignment is another intrinsic factor that may be related to ACL injury. Gray and colleagues demonstrated that there is no correlation between Q angle, femorotibial alignment, and ACL injury.[44] Dynamic, not static anatomic differences, are the most important factors in the increase of ACL injuries. In the flexed hip and knee position without limb rotation ("get down"), the hamstrings and hip external rotators and abductors can fire quickly and reduce ACL tear likelihood.[55]

The dimensions of the intercondylar notch as defined by a smaller notch width index correlates significantly with ACL tears. Souryal and Laprade also concluded that there were no male–female differences in this association.[112] It is well known that the ACL deficiency, and hence instability, has a greater potential for further injury and degenerative osteoarthritis.[63,112]

Identification of the athlete with anterolateral rotatory instability is essential to limit participation in high school, collegiate, and professional soccer. Anterolateral rotatory instability is not to be confused with hyperlaxity or hypermobility, which is present commonly in the female athlete and has not been correlated with a greater risk of knee injury.[43] In contradistinction, Nicholas thought that there was a strong correlation with injury.[85] Most recently, a physiologic explanation has been offered by Liu that the increased elasticity may come from a direct estrogen–relaxin response, as estrogen and progesterone inhibit fibroblast proliferation. The question that remains is, what is the relationship between normal cyclic hormonal changes and the connective tissue's normal and pathologic responses to adaptive changes of sports participation.[70]

During the athletic participation, the athlete depends on neuromuscular balance, proprioception, reflexes, and reaction time for good performance. Proprioception has 3 components: (1) sensory modality of the joint, (2) kinesia or movement of the joint, and (3) position of the joint. Proprioception of the knee can be measured with a Fastex (Cybex Brand), which can measure balance, coordination, reaction time, and single-stance stability. Perhaps proprioception may be central to the etiology of ACL injuries. Caraffa and colleagues found that ACL injury occurred after landing.[18] In the female high school basketball athlete, Henning and colleagues showed that, with training proprioceptive strategies, the incidence of ACL injuries may be influenced.[50,51] Proprioception must be discussed with respect to 3 distinct populations: (1) the normal athlete who is at risk for injuring the ACL, (2) the athlete whose ACL has been partially or completely torn, and (3) the athlete whose ligament has been torn and reconstructed and who has been rehabilitated back to sport. The question in each of these athletic groups is how optimally to restore proprioceptive function. Barrack and Skinner declared that, with ACL injury, there was a "partial differentiation" of the knee.[9] This theory corroborated Solomonow's theory that a diminished hamstring reflex results in less stabilization.[109] Clearly, the function of the ACL is to protect from anterolateral subluxation of the tibia with ground reactive forces. This is most optimally measured in physical examination utilizing the Lachman, anterior drawer, and pivot-shift tests, videotape analysis of an athlete with an ACL deficiency, and observation of body position and kinetics that are significantly different in comparison to that of the non-ACL-injured athlete. It is well accepted that ACL reconstruction, followed by an accelerated and a comprehensive rehabilitation program, will restore proprioceptive function.[65]

Extrinsic risk factors include the field, synthetic or otherwise, and grass turf where there may be holes or uneven surfaces.[33] There are some who believe that even a dry hard surface may be causative.[33] Shoes have also been theorized to have a role in ACL tears. Lambson demonstrated that football cleats with an edge design have a significant correlation to ACL tears.[62] Lastly, it is well known that foul-play rule violations result in a greater potential for knee injury.[28,30]

Meniscal injuries are common in soccer players, especially in older players. The mechanism of injury is no different than in other sports, though the sport-specific rotational activity during kicking may contribute to the occurrence of this injury. Meniscal injuries are further complicated in the setting of ACL injury. Neyret performed a retrospective study of 77 soccer players with both ACL and meniscal injuries. Five years after having a rim-preserving meniscectomy, those individuals who were ACL deficient were less likely to still be playing soccer (52% versus 75%), less happy with their knees (74% versus 97%), and more likely to have roentgenographic evidence of osteoarthritis (77% versus 24%).[84]

With the explosive growth of female soccer participation has come a greater number of knees and a greater possibility of ACL injuries.[5] The mechanism of ACL injury is multifactorial, with both intrinsic and extrinsic variables. Since all these factors work in concert, that can be an important variable at one time or another. It is imperative from the perspective of the design of a prevention program to identify risks by evaluating epidemiologic patterns of incidence and prevalence and then communicating them back to athletes, parents, coaches, athletic trainers, and physicians. Specific prevention programs have been designed for snow skiing and soccer.[45] The PEP (Prevent Injury and Enhance Performance) program is being introduced in Southern California.[45] (Refer to the American Academy of Orthopaedic Surgeons website: www.aclprevent.com.)

Stress Fractures

Stress fractures remain one of the most common problems in all sports, as well as women's soccer.[75,77] Why are they so common? Theories include the following:

1. Soccer fields are too hard, with impact overload occurring over time.
2. A functional shoe design deficit involving the cleats causes force to be concentrated to the fifth metatarsal.
3. The training parameters of duration, intensity, and frequency have been increased in a very steep progression.
4. The level of fitness is insufficient to adapt to the level of training and competition.
5. Abnormalities in nutrition, and disordered eating and hormonal deficiencies, are prevalent.

In recent years, the concept of the "female athlete triad" has been commonly upheld.[90] This theory relates to the association of stress fractures with disordered eating and amenorrhea. Drinkwater and colleagues demonstrated that past and present menstrual patterns have a relationship to bone mineral density and stress fractures.[25] It has also been shown that athletes with stress fractures have a low bone mineral density, a low calcium intake, a negative calcium balance, menstrual irregularities, and lower oral contraceptive use.[71] Lindburg and coworkers found that in amenorrheic athletes, there was a lower bone mineral density in 49% who had a stress fracture history.[68] It appears that the menstrual dysfunction occurs at the hypothalamic–pituitary level. Gonadotropin-releasing hormone plays the most important role in stimulation of luteinizing hormone (LH) and follicle-stimulating hormone (FSH), as these central changes are most impactful. It has been demonstrated that menstrual dysfunction is associated with low bone mineral density.[18a,24,42a,68,71] Thus it is concluded that a relationship exists between exercise and sports and the central physiologic neuroendocrine response that results in a decrease in bone density and the predilection for stress injury to bone.

Eating disorders are quite common in athletes. In a survey study in 182 collegiate athletes, 32% demonstrated at least one type of pathologic eating behavior, including bingeing (20%), purging (20%), use of diet pills or diuretics (25%), and use of laxatives (16%).[85] The negative consequences of disordered eating include infertility, thermoregulatory disturbances, depression, poor performance, immune dysfunction, poor healing, low bone mineral density, and stress fractures.[90]

The etiology of stress fractures is multifactorial. Activity accounting for exercise duration, intensity, and frequency as a dose-response curve has been proposed by Mandelbaum.[73] Normal connective tissue and bone adaptation occurs in a cyclic progression. Bone/tissue adaptation is negative with non-weight-bearing and immobilization and positive with low-, mid-, and high-level exercise. As athletes continue to practice a cyclic progression, they stay on the performance side of the curve. A significant breach in the training pattern or a disordered eating problem coupled with oligomenorrhea or amenorrhea can result in immediate shifting from the cyclic progression curve to the injury zone with resultant stress fractures. This particular practice is an excellent means of reviewing the multifactorial etiology in a dynamic fashion and learning how to train an athlete optimally to prevent these problems over time.[54]

Ankle Sprains

Ankle sprain is the most common injury in soccer and occurs most commonly as the athlete inverts the ankle.[34,36] The spectrum and severity of injury to the ankle includes injury to the lateral ligaments, articular cartilage, and even bone. The athlete by history only will describe a momentary twist as the mechanism of injury. The physical examination reveals swelling, tenderness and a decreased range of motion. Swelling must be controlled immediately with elevation, compression, and ice. Gradual weight-bearing, strength, proprioceptive training, and rehabilitation exercises are essential for the rapid return to training and competition. Prevention strategies include taping, bracing, and proprioceptive training.

If there is persistent pain after sprain, repeat roentgenography with talar views should be done. The soccer athlete depicted in Figure 61-2 sustained an inversion injury and had pain over the lateral talar dome. Initial roentgenograms showed radiolucency at the anterolateral talus (Fig. 61-2A). A magnetic resonance imaging (MRI) scan confirmed acute fracture with bony edema and fracture fragment (Fig. 61-2B,C). The fracture was treated with non-weight-bearing and immobilization. Foot and ankle injuries must be diagnosed early and treated until completely healed. The foot in a soccer shoe and the demands placed on it require normal function. Ankle impingement syndromes with osteophytes anteriorly on the talus and tibia are commonly seen but often are asymptomatic. MRI is necessary if there is persistent pain and swelling. Arthroscopy may be necessary if the talus fracture

is displaced or diagnosed late.[72] Knowledge of these syndromes is necessary.[72] The soccer athlete depicted in Figure 61–3 had fallen with the foot plantarflexed and had posterior ankle pain. Roentgenograms confirmed an os trigonum fracture. The fracture healed uneventfully and the athlete returned to soccer at 3 months.

Head Injuries

Heading the ball in soccer is one of the sport-specific skills that makes soccer unique. In a typical male professional soccer player's career, it has been estimated that approximately 300 games are played and 200 blows to the head are sus-

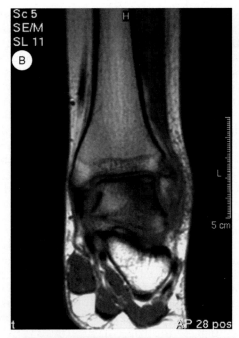

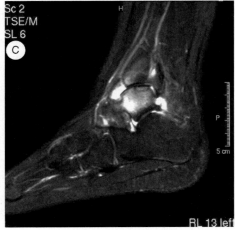

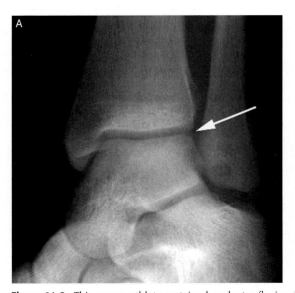

Figure 61-2. This soccer athlete sustained a plantar flexion inversion injury to her ankle. She reported soreness over the anterolateral aspect (*arrow*) of the talus. The roentgenogram (**A**) suggested a radiolucency, which was confirmed with anteroposterior (**B**) and lateral (**C**) MRI scans. At the 8-week follow-up continued radiolucency but no evidence of displacement and progressive healing without displacement of the fragment was seen. (Copyright 2001, Mary Lloyd Ireland, MD.)

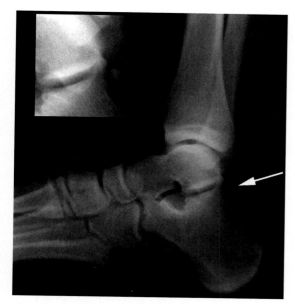

Figure 61-3. This player slid with the foot plantar flexed while playing soccer. Lateral view shows an os trigonum fracture (*arrow*). (Copyright 2001, Mary Lloyd Ireland, MD.)

tained.[117] The head is used to clear the ball defensively, pass to a teammate, and strike the ball toward the goal. The kicked ball travels at an approximate average speed of 114 km/hr, and from 10 meters away strikes with an impact of 116 kpm.[103,107] The ball stays in contact with the head from 1/63 to 1/128 seconds.

Heading technique is complex and varies for different game situations. It has been compared to a catapult, where both the upper and lower body go into extension prior to impact, then contract forcefully such that the head strikes through the ball as the trunk goes into flexion. Skilled players maintain their neck rigidly as the head impacts the ball, which acts to decrease the angular acceleration of the head and ultimately protect the athlete from head and neck injury.[16,115] There has been speculation that the greatest risk for head and neck injury from heading may occur in the younger player, who has not yet mastered proper technique.

There has been concern that cumulative traumatic encephalopathy, or the "punch-drunk" syndrome, described in boxers[47,74] can occur in soccer players. It has been assumed that this syndrome is due to the repetitive minor impacts that occur from heading. The assumption that heading in and of itself can cause damage is not well founded, and it may be that significant or cumulative concussions may be more important considerations.

Central cerebral atrophy on CT in Norwegian professional soccer players has been reported and is more likely to be present if a player was a "typical header" (ie, likely to head the ball).

Electroencephalographic changes and neuropsychological changes have also been reported in former soccer players.[110,115,117] A more recent cross-sectional study compared neuropsychological tests in amateur soccer players to those in swimmers and track athletes and found that soccer players scored significantly lower on some of these tests.[76] Although they provide useful information, these studies have been faulted because of methodological problems, including lack of good control groups, and lack of screening for acute head injuries, previous motor vehicle accidents, or alcohol use. A recent well-controlled study of US National players found no statistical differences between soccer players and track athletes on MRI assessment.[57]

Neuropsychological testing is an exciting new area of sports medicine research that has recently gained more attention in the assessment of head injury and cognitive function in athletes. There is good evidence that neuropsychological testing provides a reliable assessment and quantification of brain functioning by examining brain–behavior relationships.[67] Specifically, the tests can be used to assess speed of information processing, reaction time, attention and concentration, scanning and visual tracking ability, memory recall, and problem-solving abilities. The tests have been useful in detecting mild head injuries.[1,20,26,66,78,98,99] Neuropsychological testing can be used to detect acute and chronic head injury, and may be more sensitive in assessing cognitive function[3,91] than classic medical testing. Neuropsychological testing has been investigated in relationship with MRI and CT in head-injured patients, and has been shown to correlate with the location, severity, and resolution of injury demonstrated by MRI.[66]

Tysvaer used neuropsychological testing in former professional soccer players and found mild to severe deficits in attention, concentration, memory, and judgment in 81% of former players, compared to 40% with only a mild degree of impairment in controls.[116] No baseline tests had been performed in these athletes prior to their soccer activities. Matser recently published a cross-sectional study using neuropsychological testing and found that soccer players scored significantly lower in tests of planning and memory compared to control athletes (swimming and track).[76] This study also found that soccer players had a higher use of alcohol and had more sport-related concussions. They also found that the number of concussions was inversely related to their performance on several neuropsychological tests. They did not explain how they obtained some of their data or how severe the concussions were, and also did not report on the performance when these sport-related concussions were excluded. Yet, they concluded that repetitive heading in soccer might explain the poor performance in cognitive function.

All of these studies have not gained recognition because they have significant flaws in methodology, including lack of proper control groups, no control for acute head injuries, and lack of screening for other problems (motor vehicle accidents) and alcohol use. Very few well-controlled, prospective studies have been performed. In addition, modifications in the game, such as a ball that is less likely to absorb water, may affect some of the injury patterns seen in more recent times.

There have been no long-term prospective studies to assess the long-term effects of head injury and concussions in soccer, nor are there any that assess the long-term effects of heading, an integral part of the sport. The effect of severe and/or multiple concussions on cognitive function may be more important than that of repetitive heading, and in the studies to date, concussions and repetitive heading have not been separated.

The first prospective study to assess the effects of heading on cognitive function was a pilot study in collegiate soccer players.[92] This prospective cross-over study of male and female players demonstrated no differences in cognitive function as assessed by a battery of neuropsychological tests performed before and after a single practice session. Participants served as their own controls on 2 separate practice days when they either did or did not participate in heading the ball for 20 minutes out of a 90-minute session.

A larger battery of neuropsychological tests have been performed on these same collegiate athletes on a yearly basis. These athletes have had neuropsychological testing performed as part of their participation in the Penn State Concussion Program.[26] This is a longitudinal study using neuropsychological tests to assess the effects of concussion in several sports at the college level. For the soccer players at Penn State University, neuropsychological testing is performed yearly and preliminary results have demonstrated that heading has no effect on cognitive function over the course of one season of play.[93] These 2 prospective studies demonstrate that heading in and of itself does not appear to adversely affect cognitive function as assessed by neuropsychological tests. Ongoing research is addressing whether changes in cognitive function occur in soccer players over the course of their college career. Whether significant or repetitive concussions may be the source of the

deficits found in the earlier European studies of soccer players remains a question that further research will need to address.[93]

Head injuries do occur in soccer, accounting for 1.2% to 8% of all injuries, depending on the study. The head injuries that occur most commonly are concussions, which generally occur as a result of impact with another player, the ground, or the goal posts. From 1996 to 1997, head injuries occurred at an incidence of 0.46 injuries per 1000 athlete exposures in women's NCAA soccer, accounting for 4.4% of the total injuries seen.

At the high school level, recent data have demonstrated that mild traumatic brain injury occurs at a rate of 1.14 and 0.92 per 100 player-seasons in girls and boys, respectively, accounting for 4.3% and 3.9% of the total injuries reported for those sports.[89] Generally, the acute head injuries seen in soccer occur from impact of the head with another player, the ground, or the goal posts. In fact, in the study by Boden, none of the concussions occurred from purposeful heading of the ball.

The concussion incidence in elite female US college soccer players has recently been reported to be slightly lower than that reported in the NCAA as a whole at 0.4 per 1000 athlete exposures compared to 0.6 for men.[13] Over a 2-year period in the Atlantic Coast Conference, 26 athletes sustained concussions: 17 (59%) were men and 12 (41%) were women. Twenty concussions (69%) occurred in games. None of the concussions resulted from intentional heading of the ball. The incidence was 0.96 concussions per team per season and the overall incidence was 0.6 per 1000 athlete exposures for men and 0.04 per 1000 athlete exposures for women. By grades of concussion, 21 (72%) were grade I and 8 (22%) grade II; none were grade III. The most common mechanism was contact with an opponent's head, 8 (28%), or the ball, 7 (24%).[13]

US Olympics Sports Festival female and male soccer players from 1993 were asked about previous head injury frequency and sequelae. There were 74 concussions in 39 male players and 28 concussions in 23 female players. Being dazed and dizziness were the most common symptoms reported. The odds were 50% that a man and 22% that a woman would sustain a concussion in a 10-year period.[8]

As mentioned previously, neuropsychological testing is becoming a more useful tool in the assessment of head injury in several sports, including soccer. If obtained as part of a preseason assessment, these tests can also be used to determine if a concussive injury has occurred and whether an athlete has returned to baseline function or remains impaired. These data have been used in college athletes and aid in making return-to-play decisions.[26] In prospective research, neuropsychological testing has been performed as part of the Penn State Concussion Program with athletes who participate in football, soccer, basketball, ice hockey, lacrosse, and wrestling. These tests demonstrate that neuropsychological testing is sensitive in detecting deficits when an athlete has sustained a concussion and that the more severe the injury, the more significant the deficits are. Other conclusions from this research thus far are as follows: (1) Athletes self-report a significant number of mTBI (mild traumatic brain injury) during high school. (2) Marked individual variability exists on neuropsychological tests, making baseline testing critical. (3) Marked variability exists between sports and sexes on neuropsychological tests. (4) Neuropsychological tests are sensitive to detection of cognitive impairment following mTBI. (5) Neurologic symptoms do not correspond perfectly to neuropsychological data; at 48 hours postinjury, symptoms do not differentiate injured from noninjured players, whereas neuropsychological tests do.[7] Most athletes return to baseline function within one week of mTBI, some with continuing cognitive deficits and postconcussive symptoms.[9] Athletes sustaining mTBI show greater variability in test scores than controls.[10] Although verbal learning and memory tests appear to be very sensitive to the effects of concussion, several measures differentiated groups at different times. Thus, no one test adequately assesses the complexity of cognitive problems postinjury.

The data also suggest that when a concussion is more severe, a higher percentage of neuropsychological tests are abnormal and stay below the baseline for a longer time. In addition, because individuals have different strengths and weaknesses in cognitive function, a baseline is necessary, and likely a battery of tests instead of a few selected tests. With more severe injuries, more of the neuropsychological tests reveal abnormalities, and the length of time that these deficits persist also increases.

Postural sway, in conjunction with neuropsychological testing, has also been used to assess head-injured athletes. Guskiewicz used both cognitive tests (Trail Making Test, Digit Span Test, Stroop Test, and Hopkins Verbal Learning Test) and a test measuring postural sway (NeuroCom Smart Balance Master) to assess athletes with and without head injury.[48] They found that in injured individuals, postural sway testing was abnormal one day after injury,

whereas cognitive tests remained the same. Three to 5 days later these differences persisted, though the differences in postural sway were no longer statistically significant. A Balance Error Scoring System (BESS) has also been developed as a measure of postural sway and can be used in the absence of force platform equipment to assess the effect of concussion in the athlete.[97]

These new tools for assessing concussion in athletes may change the way that athletes are evaluated in the future. Preseason physical examinations that include tests of cognitive function or postural sway may help the physician and athletic training staff in making return-to-play decisions based on more objective data. As more prospective long-term research is completed, we will know more about the natural history of concussion in sport as well as the differential effects of heading and concussion as they relate to cumulative cognitive function. This research will undoubtedly aid health care providers in providing optimal care to the soccer player.

The management and assessment of the head-injured soccer player remains difficult and controversial. Athletes should be closely assessed for abnormalities in cognitive function, evidence for underlying intracranial abnormalities, and cervical spine injury, and not allowed to return to play if they are symptomatic. Several concussion classification systems and return-to-play guidelines exist in the literature and are not discussed further here.[17,21,95] This is an area where exciting new research is ongoing.

PREVENTION

In soccer, Ekstrand has demonstrated that implementation of a multilevel approach to soccer in the male athlete can diminish injuries by 75%.[30] The elements of a prevention program for the female athlete should consist of the following:

1. Correction of training problems. In the female it is essential to recognize that *more is not better*, and that *quality should be considered over quantity* at all times.
2. Provision of optimum equipment, including shin guards and shoes, and maintenance of good-quality fields.
3. Prophylactic ankle taping or bracing with proprioceptive ankle taping.
4. Controlled rehabilitation and identification of those athletes who have not healed adequately or have been rehabilitated.
5. Exclusion of players with marked knee ligament instability and optimal conditioning

and rehabilitation for those athletes who have normal knees and those who have undergone reconstruction.

6. Education about the importance of disciplined play and the significantly increased risk of injury from foul play.
7. Supervision of games by health care professional(s) and athletic trainer(s).
8. Identification and treatment of those athletes with eating disorders, and provision of supplementation with calcium, iron, calories, and other components when appropriate.
9. Identification and treatment of menstrual abnormalities.

CONCLUDING REMARKS

Comparing genders, there are specificities and complexities with respect to performance and injury that make care of the female soccer athlete special. With the rapid expansion of female participation in soccer in the United States and worldwide, a heightened level of awareness of these unique aspects is required. Physiologically, the female performs with less power, strength, and agility and lower levels of aerobic and anaerobic fitness. The incidence and type of ankle injuries are similar in male and female soccer athletes. There are significant differences with respect to ACL injuries and stress fractures. Preventive strategies can have a significant impact on injury patterns and rates. The health care provider should continue to educate athletes, coaches, and parents.

FUTURE

The World United Soccer Association (WUSA) launched its first season in April 2001. It comprises 8 teams from the United States and other countries. The inaugural game was held April 14, 2001, featuring the Washington Freedom, starring Mia Hamm, and San Jose CyberRays, starring Brandi Chastain. The game was won by the Washington Freedom, 1–0, in front of 35,000 fans at RF Kennedy Stadium in Washington, DC.

Young female soccer players with role models like these women playing professional soccer will further enhance the benefits of participation in soccer. The WUSA players are very happy and humble, and they love to interact with the fans, particularly the young soccer players. The medical staff is very interested in following these elite professional soccer athletes to evaluate their past and present injuries and medical conditions. An exiting future awaits female soccer players.

Acknowledgment

Thanks to Mary Lloyd Ireland, MD, for her assistance in the preparation of this chapter.

References

1. Abreau F, Templer DI, Schuyler BA, et al: Neuropsychological assessment of soccer players. Neuropsychology 4:175–81, 1990.
2. Aendt EA, Agel J, Dick R. Anterior cruciate ligament injury patterns among collegiate men and women. J Athlet Train 34(2):86–92, 1999.
3. Alves WM, Rimel RW, Nelson WE: University of Virginia prospective study of football induced minor head injury: status report. Clin Sports Med 6(1):211–8, 1987.
4. American College of Sports Medicine: Position stand on exercise and fluid replacement. Med Sci Sports Exerc 28(1)i—vii, 1996.
5. Arendt E, Dick R: Knee injury patterns among men and women in collegiate Basketball and Soccer. Am J Sports Med 23:694–701, 1995.
6. Arms S, Pope M, Johnson, RJ, et al: The biomechanics of anterior cruciate ligament rehabilitation and reconstruction. Am J Sports Med 12:8–18, 1984.
7. Backous DD, Friedl KE, Smith NJ, et al: Soccer injuries and their relation to physical maturity. Am J Dis Child 142:839–42, 1988.
8. Barnes BC, Cooper L, Kirkendall DT, et al: Concussion history in elite male and female soccer players. Am J Sports Med 26(3):433–8, 1998.
9. Barrack RL, Skinner HB, Buckley SL: Proprioception in the anterior cruciate deficient knee. Am J Sports Med 17:1–6, 1989.
10. Barth JT, Alves WM, Ryan TV, et al: Mild head injury in sports: Neuropsychological sequelae and recovery of function. In: Levin HS, Eisenberg HM, Benton AL (eds): Mild Head Injury. New York, Oxford, 1989, pp 257–75.
11. Berchuck M, Andriacchi T, Bach B, et al: Gait adaptations by patients who have deficient anterior cruciate ligaments. J Bone Joint Surg 72A:871–7, 1990.
12. Boden BP, Dean GS, Feagin JA, et al: Mechanisms of anterior cruciate ligament injury. Orthopaedics 23(6): 573–8, 2000.
13. Boden BP, Kirkendall DT, Garrett WE: concussion incidence in elite college soccer players. Am J Sports Med 26(2):238–41, 1998.
14. Brewer J: Nutritional aspects of women's soccer. J Sports Sci 12:S35–8, 1994.
15. Brynhildsen J, Ekstrand J, Jeppsson A, et al: Previous injuries and persisting symptoms in female soccer players. Int J Sports Med 11:489–92, 1990.
16. Burslem L, Lees A: Quantification of impact accelerations of the head during the heading of a football. In: Reilly T, Lees A, Davids K, et al (eds): Science and Football: Proceedings of the First World Congress of Science and Football. London, E&FN Spon Ltd, 1987, pp 243–8.
17. Cantu RC: Return to play guidelines after a head injury. Clin Sports Med 17(1):45, 1998.

18. Caraffa A, Cerulli G, Projetti M, et al: Prevention of anterior cruciate ligament injuries in soccer. A prospective controlled study of proprioceptive training. Knee Surg Sports Traumatol Arthrosc 4:19–21, 1996.

18a. Chan CE, Martin MC, Genant HK et al: Decreased spinal content in amenorrheic women. JAMA 251:626–9, 1984.

19. Coggan AR, Coyle EF: Carbohydrate ingestion during prolonged exercise: effects on metabolism and performance. Exerc Sport Sci Rev 19:1–40, 1991.

20. Collins MW, Grindel SH, Lovell MR, et al: Relationship between concussion and neuropsychological performance in college football players. JAMA 282:964–70, 1999.

21. Colorado Medical Society: Guidelines for the Management of Concussion in Sports. Colorado Medical Society, Sports Medicine Committee, May 1990 (revised May 1991).

22. Coyle EF, Coggan AR, Hemmert MK, Ivy J: Muscle glycogen utilisation during prolonged strenuous exercise when fed carbohydrates. J Appl Phys 61:165–72, 1986.

23. Coyle EF, Montain SJ: Carbohydrate and fluid ingestion during exercise: are there trade-offs? Med Sci Sports Exerc 24(6):671–8, 1992

24. Drinkwater BL, Bruemmer B, Chestnut CH III: Menstrual history as a determinant of current bone mineral density in young athletes. JAMA 263:545, 1990.

25. Drinkwater, BL, Nilson, K, Chesnut, CH, et al: Bone mineral content of amenorrheic and eumenorrheic athletes, N Engl J Med 311:277–81, 1984.

26. Echemendia RJ, Putukian M, Mackin RS, et al: Neuropsychological test performance prior to and following sports-related mild traumatic brain injury. Clin J Sport Med 11(1):23–31, 2001.

27. Ekblom B (ed): Football (Soccer). An IOC Medical Commission Publication. Oxford, Blackwell Scientific Publications, 1994.

28. Ekstrand J, Gillquist J: The avoidability of soccer injuries. Int J Sports Med 4:124–8, 1983.

29. Ekstrand J, Giliquist J: The frequency of muscle tightness and injuries in soccer players. Am J Sports Med 10:75–8, 1982.

30. Ekstrand J, Gillquist J: Soccer injuries and their mechanisms: a prospective study. Med Sci Sports Exerc 15:267–70, 1983.

31. Ekstrand J, Gillquist J, Liljedahl SO: Prevention of soccer injuries. Supervision by doctor and physiotherapist. Am J Sports Med 11:116–20, 1983.

32. Ekstrand J, Gillquist J, Moller M, et al: Incidence of soccer injuries and their relation to training and team success. Am J Sports Med 11:63–7, 1983.

33. Ekstrand J, Nigg BM: Surface-related injuries in soccer. Sports Med 8:56–62, 1989.

34. Ekstrand J, Tropp H: The incidence of ankle sprains in soccer. Foot Ankle 11:41–4, 1990.

35. Elias SR. 10-year trend in USA Cup soccer injuries: 1988–1997. Med Sci Sports Exerc 33(3):359–67, 2001.

36. Elias SR, Roberst WO, Thorson DC: Team sports in hot weather: Guidelines for modifying youth soccer. Physician Sportsmed 19(5):67–78, 1991.

37. Engstrom B, Forssblad M, Johansson C, et al: Does a major knee injury definitely sideline an elite soccer player? Am J Sports Med 18:101–5, 1990.

38. Engstrom B, Johansson C, Tornkvist H: Soccer injuries among elite female players. Am J Sports Med 19:372–75, 1991.

39. Ettlinger C, Johnson F, Shealy J: A method to help reduce the risk of serious knee sprains incurred in alpine skiing. Am J Sports Med 23:531–7, 1995.

40. Feagin J, Lambert K: Mechanism of injury and pathology of anterior cruciate ligament injuries. Orthop Clin North Am 16:41–5, 1985.

41. Foster C, Thompson NN, Dean J, Kirkendall DT: Carbohydrate supplementation and performance in soccer players. Med Sci Sport Exerc 18:8–12, 1986.

42. Friden T, Erlandsson T, Zatterstrom R, et al: Compression or distraction of the anterior cruciate injured knee: Variations in injury pattern in contact sports and downhill skiing. Knee Surg Sports Traumatol Arthrosc 3:14–147, 1995.

42a. Georgiou E, Ntalles K, Papageorgiou A et al: Bone mineral related to menstrual history. Acta Orthop Scand 60:192–194, 1989.

43. Goodshall RW: The predictability of athletic injuries: A eight-year study. J Sports Med 3:50–4, 1975.

44. Gray J, Taunton JE, McDenzie DC, et al: A survey of injuries to the ACL of the knee in female basketball players. Int J Sports Med 6:314–6, 1985.

45. Griffin LY. Prevention of Noncontact ACL Injuries. Rosemont, Ill, American Academy of Orthopaedic Surgeons, American Orthopaedic Society for Sports Medicine, 2001.

46. Grood E, Suntay W, Noyes F, et al: Biomechanics of the knee-extension exercise. Effect of cutting the anterior cruciate ligament. J Bone Joint Surg 66A:725–34, 1984.

47. Haglund Y, Eriksson E. Does amateur boxing lead to chronic brain damage? A review of some recent investigations. Am J Sports Med 21:97–109, 1993.

48. Guskiewicz KM, Riemann BL, Perrin DH, Nashner LM: Alternative approaches to the assessment of mild head injury in athletes. Med Sci Sports Exerc 29(7):S213–21, 1997.

49. Hargreaves M, Costill DL, Coggan A, Nishibata I: Effect of carbohydrate feedings on muscle glycogen utilization and exercise performance. Med Sci Sports Exerc 16(3):219–22, 1984.

50. Henning CE: Injury prevention of the anterior cruciate ligament. An Update on Sports Medicine. Proceedings from the Second Scandinavian Conference in Sports Medicine, Soria Moria, Norway, 1986, pp 222–9.

51. Henning CE, Griffis ND, Vequist SW, et al: Sport-specific knee injuries. In: Renstrom PAFH (ed): Sports Injury Prevention and Care. Encyclopaedia of Sports Medicine: An IOC Medical Commission Publication: I(A–178), 1994.

52. Hirowaka S, Solomonow M, Lu Y, et al: Anterior-posterior and rotational displacement of the tibia elicited by quadriceps contraction. Am J Sports Med 20:299–306, 1992.

53. Hoff GI, Martin TA: Outdoor and indoor soccer: injuries among youth players. Am J Sports Med 14:231–3, 1986.

54. Ireland ML, Wall C: Epidemiology and comparison of knee injuries in elite male and female United States basketball athletes. Med Sci Sports Exerc 22:S82, 1980.

55. Ireland ML: Anterior cruciate ligament injury in female athletes: Epidemiology. J Athlet Train 34(2):150–4, 1999.

56. Ivy JL, Miller W, Dover V, et al: Endurance improved by ingestion of a glucose polymer supplement. Med Sci Sports Exerc 15(6):466–71, 1983.

57. Jordan SH, Green GA, Galanty HL, et al: Acute and Chronic Brain Injury in United States National Team Soccer Players. Am J Sports Med 24(2):205–10, 1996.

58. Keizer HA, Kulpers H, van Kranenburg, Geurten P: Influence of lipid and solid meals on muscle glycogen and resynthesis, plasma fuel hormone response, and maximal physical working capacity. Int J Sports Med 8(2):99–104, 1987.

59. Keller CS, Noyes FR, Buncher CR: The medical aspects of soccer injury epidemiology. Am J Sports Med 15:230–7, 1987.
60. Kibler WB: Injuries in adolescent and preadolescent soccer players. Med Sci Sports Exerc 25:1330–2, 1993.
61. Knapik JJ, Baumn CL, Jones BH, et al: Pre-season strength and flexibility imbalances associated with athletic injuries in female collegiate athletes. Am J Sports Med 19(l):76–81, 1991.
62. Lambson RB, Barnhill BS, Higgins RW: Football cleat design and its effect on anterior cruciate ligament injuries. A three-year prospective study (see comments). Am J Sports Med 24:155–9, 1996.
63. LaPrade RF, Burnett QM: Femoral intercondylar notch stenosis and correlation to anterior cruciate ligament injury. A prospective study. Am J Sports Med 22:198–202, 1994.
64. Leatt PB, Jacobs I: Effect of glucose polymer on glycogen depletion during a soccer match. Can J Sport Sci 14(2):112–6, 1989.
65. Lephart SM, Pincivero DM, Giraldo JL, Fu M: The role of proprioception in the management and rehabilitation of athletic injuries. Am J Sports Med 25:130–7, 1997.
66. Levin HS, Amparo E, Eisenberg JM, et al: Magnetic resonance imaging and computerized tomography in relation to the neurobehavioral sequelae of mild and moderate head injuries. J Neurosurg 66:706–13, 1987.
67. Lezak M: Neuropsychological Assessment, 3rd edition. New York, Oxford University Press, 1995.
68. Lindberg JS, Fears YvB, Hunt MM, et al.: Exercise induced amenorrhea and bone density. Ann Intern Med 101:647–8, 1984.
69. Lindenfeld TN, Schmitt DJ, Hendy MP, et al: Incidence of injury in indoor soccer. Am J Sports Med 22:364–71, 1994.
70. Liu SH, Yu WD, Panossian V, et al: Female sex hormones influence the cellular metabolism of the female human anterior cruciate ligament. Cabaud Memorial Award. Presented at the American Society of Sports Medicine Annual Meeting, Sun Valley, Idaho, June 23, 1997.
71. Myburgh KH, Badrach LK, Lewis B, et al: Bone mineral density at axial and appendicular sites in amenorrheic athletes. Med Sci Sports Exerc 25:1197–1202, 1993.
72. Mandelbaum, BR, Knapp, TP: Ankle impingement syndromes in soccer. In: Garrett WE (ed): The U.S. Soccer Sports Medicine Book. Baltimore, Williams & Wilkins, 1996.
73. Mandelbaum, BR, Knapp, TP: Stress fractures. In: Garrett WE (ed): The U.S. Soccer Sports Medicine Book. Baltimore, Williams & Wilkins, 1996.
74. Martland HS: Punch drunk. JAMA 91:1103–7, 1928.
75. Matheson GO, Clement DB, McKenzie DC, et al: Stress fracture in athletes. Am J Sports Med 15:46–58, 1987.
76. Matser EJT, Kessels AG, Lezak MID, et al: Neuropsychological impairment in amateur soccer players. JAMA 282:971–3, 1999.
77. McBryde AM: Stress fractures in athletes. J Sports Med 3:212–7, 1975.
78. McLatchie G, Brooks N, Galbraith S, et al: Clinical neurological examination, neuropsychology, electroencephalography and computed tomographic head scanning in active amateur boxers. J Neurol Neurosurg Psych 50:96–9, 1987.
79. McNair P, Marshall R, Matheson J: Important features associated with acute anterior cruciate ligament injury. NZ Med J 103:537–9, 1990.
80. Moller-Nielsen J, Hammar M: Women's soccer injuries in relation to the menstrual cycle and oral contraceptive use. Med Sci Sports Exerc 21:126–9, 1989.
81. Murray I, Eddy DE, Murray TW, et al: The effect of fluid and carbohydrate feedings during intermittent cycling exercise. Med Sci Sports Exerc 19(6):597–604, 1987.
82. National Collegiate Athletic Association: NCAA Injury Surveillance System. Indianapolis, Ind, NCAA, 2000.
83. National Collegiate Athletic Association. NCAA Injury Surveillance System, 1986–1996. Indianapolis, Ind, NCAA.
84. Neyret P, Donell ST, DeJour D, DeJour H: Partial meniscectomy and anterior cruciate ligament rupture in soccer players. A study with a minimum of 20 years follow up. Am J Sports Med 21(3):455–60, 1993.
85. Rosen LW, McKeey DB, Hough DO, et al: Pathogenic weight control behaviors in female athletes. Physician Sports Med 14:79–86, 1986.
86. Nisel IR: Mechanics of the knee joint: A study of joint and muscle load with clinical applications. Acta Orthop Scand 216(Sl56):142, 1985.
87. Norwood L, Cross M: The intercondylar shelf and the anterior cruciate ligament. Am J Sports Med 5(4):171–6, 1977.
88. Noyes F, Mooar P, Matthews D, et al: The symptomatic ACL-deficient knee. J Bone Joint Surg 65A:154–74, 1983.
89. Powell JW, Parber-Foss KD: Traumatic brain injury in high school athletes. JAMA 282:958–63, 1999.
90. Putukian M: The female athlete triad. Clin Sports Med 17:675–96, 1998.
91. Putukian M, Echemendia RJ: Managing successive minor head injuries: Which tests guide return to play? Physician Sportsmed 24(11):25–38, 1996.
92. Putukian M, Echemendia RJ, Mackin S: Acute effects of heading in soccer: A prospective neuropsychological evaluation. Clin J Sports Med 10:104–9, 2000.
93. Putukian M, Echemendia RJ, Evans TA, Bruce J. Effects of heading contacts in collegiate soccer players on cognitive function: Prospective neuropsychological assessment over a season. Presented at American Medical Society for Sports Medicine Annual Meeting, San Antonio, Texas, April 9, 2001.
94. Putukian M, Knowles WK, Swere S, Castle NG: Injuries in Indoor Soccer. The Lake Placid Dawn to Dark Soccer Tournament. Am J Sports Med 24(3):317–322, 1996.
95. Quality Standards Subcommittee, American Academy of Neurology, Practice Parameter; The management of concussion in sports (sun-miary statement) Neurology 48:581–585, 1997.
96. Renstrom P, Arms S, Stanwyck T, et al.: Strain within the anterior cruciate ligament during hamstring and quadriceps activity. Am J Sports Med 14:83–87, 1986.
97. Riemann BL, Guskiewicz KM: Effects of mild head injury on postural stability as measured through clinical balance testing. J Athlet Train 35(1):19–25, 2000.
98. Rimel RW, Giordam B, Barth JT, et al: Disability caused by minor head injury. Neurosurgery 9(3):221–228, 1981.
99. Rimel RW, Giordani B, Barth JT, et al: Moderate head injury: Completing the clinical spectrum of brain trauma. Neurosurgery 11(3):344–51, 1982.
100. Roos H, Ornell M, Gdrdsell P, et al: Soccer after anterior cruciate ligament injury—an incompatible combination? A national survey of incidence and risk factors and a 7-year follow-up of 310 players: see comments. Acta Orthop Scand 66:107–12, 1995.
101. Saltin B, Costill DL: Fluid and electrolyte balance during prolonged exercise. In Horton ES, Terjung RL (eds): Exercise, Nutrition and Metabolism. New York, Macmillan, 1998, pp 150–8.
102. Schmidt-Olsen S, Jorgensen U, Kaalund S, Sorenson J: Injuries among young soccer players. Am J Sports Med 19:273–5, 1991.

103. Schneider PG, Lichte H: Untersuchungen zur Groesse der Kraileinwirkung beim Kopfballspiel des Fussballers. Sportarz Sportmed 26:10, 1975.

104. Shelbourne K, Nitz P: The O'Donoghue triad revisited. Am J Sports Med 19:474–7, 1991.

105. Sherman MF, Warren RF, Marshall JL, Savatsky GJ: A clinical and radiographic analysis of 127 anterior cruciate insufficient knees. Clin Orthop 227:229–37, 1988.

106. Shoemaker S, Adams D, Daniel D, et al: Quadriceps/anterior cruciate graft interaction: An in vitro study of joint kinematics and anterior cruciate graft tension. Clin Orthop 294:379–90, 1993.

107. Smodlaka VN: Medical aspects of heading the ball in soccer. Physician Sportsmed 12(2):127–31, 1984.

108. Soderman K: The Female Soccer Player: Injury Pattern: Risk Factors, and Intervention. Umea, Sweden, Kerstin Soderman, 2001.

109. Solomonow M, Baratta R, Zhou BH, et al: The synergistic action of the anterior cruciate ligament and thigh muscles in maintaining joint stability. Am J Sports Med 15:207–13, 1987.

110. Sortland 0, Tysvaer AT: Brain damage in former association football players. Neuroradiology 31:44–8, 1989.

111. Sortland 0, Tysvaer AT, Storli OV: Changes in the cervical spine in Association football players. Br J Sports Med 16:80–4, 1982.

112. Souryal TO, Freeman TR: Intercondylar notch size and anterior cruciate ligament injury in athletes. A prospective study. Am J Sports Med 21:535–9, 1993.

113. Sullivan JA, Gross RH, Grana WA, et al: Evaluation of injuries in youth soccer. Am J Sports Med 8:325–7, 1980.

114. Torzilli P, Deng X, Warren R: The effect of joint-compressive load and quadriceps muscle force on knee motion in the intact and anterior cruciate ligament sectioned knee. Am J Sports Med 22:105–12, 1994.

115. Tysvaer AT: Head and neck injuries in soccer. Impact of minor trauma. Sports Med 14(3):200–13, 1992.

116. Tysvaer AT, Lochen EA: Soccer injuries to the brain: a neuropsychologic study of former soccer players. Am J Sports Med 19(1):56–60, 1991.

117. Tysvaer AT, Storli OV, Bachen NI: Soccer injuries to the brain: a neurologic and electroencephalographic study of former players. Acta Neurol Scand 80:151–6, 1989.

118. Wojtys EM, Wylie BB, Huston LJ: The effects of muscular fatigue on neuromuscular function and anterior tibial translation in healthy knees. Am J Sports Med 24:615–21, 1996.

Chapter 62

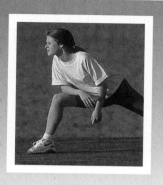

Softball

Robert G. Hosey, M.D.
John P. DiFiori, M.D.

1996 marked the inaugural year for women's softball as an Olympic sport. The gold medal winning performance of the United States team thrust a relatively unknown group of athletes into the national spotlight while providing international exposure for their sport. Currently, millions of women participate in softball on a recreational or competitive basis and the increased exposure provided by the Olympic Games can be expected to translate into higher participation rates in the future. As with all sports, there are specific medical issues that are commonly encountered in softball. This chapter will deal with those that pertain particularly to the sport of women's fast-pitch softball. Specifically, the physical demands of softball, the epidemiology and etiology of softball injuries, and injury-prevention strategies will be addressed. In addition, we will examine the rules of softball and make a comparison to the game of baseball.

HISTORY

Games played with the tools of a bat and a ball can be traced back through civilization to the prehistoric era. In fact, there is no known culture in the world that does not have some form of a bat and ball game. The game of softball is a relative newcomer, having evolved over the last 120 years. Softball, like baseball, can trace its roots back to a 16th-century game played in England called rounders. In the United States, by the 19th century the game had undergone many rule revisions and numerous variations existed. At this time the game became known as townball because nearly every town had a different set of rules for the game.[34]

Modern-day baseball originated from a version of the game as it was played in Cooperstown, NY, the location of the Baseball Hall of Fame. As the game of baseball was taking shape in upstate New York, softball would find its origin elsewhere. One story suggests that the game was inspired by a group of Ivy League alumni from Harvard and Yale who played the first softball game using a boxing glove and a stick. Another historical report places the birthplace of softball in Chicago in the 1880s, where the game formed from an indoor version of baseball. In either case, the first official rules for an outdoor version of the game were developed in 1895. In the late 1890s the game was adopted by a group of firemen in Minnesota and played in the lots behind the fire station. The team was named the Kittens and for many years the game was known as kitten ball. It also was known as mush ball, big ball, and later diamond ball.[21] It wasn't until 1933 that softball was given its official name. Softball spread worldwide as US servicemen introduced the game to several other countries during World War II. Since that time the sport has continued to gain in popularity. Today many versions of the game still exist, including fast-pitch softball, which is the type played by the majority of women softballers. Today, women's fast-pitch softball is played at the competitive level in youth leagues, high schools, all divisions of the National Collegiate Athletic Association (NCAA), on the international level, and in professional leagues.

UNIQUE ASPECTS OF SOFTBALL

While many variations exist in the game of softball, this chapter will concentrate on fast-pitch softball. It is difficult to view a softball game without drawing comparisons to the game of baseball. The 2 sports require similar skills, play by similar rules, have a common origin, and incur similar risks. With the exception of the pitching position, the techniques used in throwing, hitting, fielding, and running the bases are nearly identical for baseball and softball. However, there are several aspects of the game that make it clearly distinct from baseball. Perhaps the most noticeable difference is in equipment. The balls used in softball are much larger than regulation baseballs. They are not, as the name implies, soft, however. The bats used in softball possess a somewhat thinner barrel than their baseball counterparts but are routinely constructed of the same material, aluminum. Because batted softballs do not travel nearly as far as baseballs struck with the same velocities, softball field dimensions are accordingly smaller. Base paths register 60 feet in distance compared to 90 feet in baseball. Outfield dimensions commonly are set at a radius of 200 feet from home plate in softball, while outfield fences in baseball typically run 1.5 to 2 times that distance. Even more distinct is the landscape surrounding the pitching area. On softball fields this area is flat and only designated by a circle of chalk. Baseball fields have mounds for the pitchers to throw from, which commonly rise 2 to 3 feet from the level playing surface. Another major difference is the distance from the pitcher to home plate, a distance of 40 feet in softball, compared to 60 feet, 6 inches in baseball. Uniforms worn by players may also differ. Many collegiate softball teams wear shorts instead of long pants as part of their attire.

The rules governing fast-pitch softball are generally similar to those of baseball but some significant differences are noteworthy. For instance, base runners in softball are not allowed to take a lead from a base prior to the pitching of the ball. As a result, "pick-off" attempts by the pitcher are not part of the game and pitchers use the wind-up motion with runners on base. There are also several rules regarding the act of pitching that differ between the sports which can go into great detail and are beyond the scope of this chapter.

Also seen in many collegiate and scholastic softball games is the institution of a "mercy rule," which states that if a team is ahead by a certain number of runs (usually 10) after completion of the 5th inning, then the game is terminated at that point. The mercy rule is designed to limit the overall time of games in which one team has built an "insurmountable" lead. In addition, all starting players in softball are allowed to re-enter the game one time after they have been removed. They must, however, return to their original spot in the batting order.

While these differences exist, the flow of the 2 games remains remarkably similar and easy to follow.

THE WINDMILL THROWING MOTION

Perhaps the most striking feature of fast-pitch softball is the pitching. It quickly distinguishes fast-pitch softball from all other bat and ball sports. Ball speeds generated by these windmill-style pitchers often reach 50 to 70 miles/hr. When considering the fact that the pitcher's mound is a mere 40 feet away, this would be equivalent to an 80- to 100-miles/hr fastball in baseball. The force needed to generate these ball speeds is produced by a windmill-type windup and underhand delivery of the ball. This pitching motion has been analyzed by Maffet and colleagues using intramuscular EMG, high-speed cinematography, and motion analysis.[16] From this study the windmill pitching technique has been divided into phases corresponding to positions of the clock (Fig. 62-1). The initial motion starts with the wind-up, which varies from pitcher to pitcher.

From the 6 o'clock position at the end of the wind-up phase the ball is brought sequentially counterclockwise going from the 6 o'clock to the 3 o'clock position in phase 2, 3 o'clock to 12 o'clock in phase 3, 12 o'clock to 9 o'clock in phase 4 and finally, 9 o'clock to ball release and

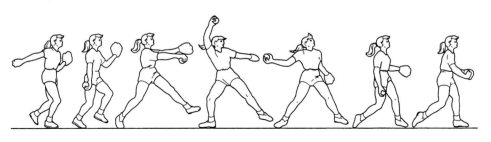

Wind-up	6 O'clock	3 O'clock	12 O'clock	9 O'clock	Ball release	Follow-through

Figure 62-1. The windmill pitching technique. (Adapted from Atwater A: Biomechanics of overarm throwing movements and of throwing injuries. Exerc Sport Sci Rev 7:43–85, 1979, with permission.)

follow-through. During the pitching motion the arm initially elevates in an internally rotated position to 180°. From this point at the top of the pitch the arm is adducted as the body rotates, transferring momentum to the pitching arm. Nearly simultaneously with the release of the ball, the pitching arm contacts the lateral hip and thigh, which stops forward progression of the humerus. The player's weight begins on the ipsilateral side, is transferred forward in phases 2 and 3, then lands on the contralateral foot at the end of phase 4, producing momentum that is transferred to the pitch as the body rotates back to the forward position. Electromyographic analysis in this study revealed several interesting findings. The pectoralis major muscle was primarily responsible for adducting the arm across the body in phases 4 and 5, which contributed to the power of the pitch. The pectoralis major along with the subscapularis provided stabilization against anterior forces. The serratus anterior worked in synchrony with the pectoralis major in an attempt to stabilize the scapula, which acts as a platform for transferring forces to the ball. Lastly, muscle action following release of the ball was minimal. This suggests that much of the momentum is stopped when the arm contacts the hip and thigh.

Overall, the windmill motion allows the pitcher to generate significant arm velocity, which is transferred to the pitched softball. Because of the underhand motion used, typical injuries seen in repetitive overhand-throwing athletes are likely to be avoided. Other problems, however, may arise and will be discussed later in the chapter.

INJURY RISKS IN SOFTBALL

As with other sports certain inherit risks are involved in playing softball. The field dimensions of the softball diamond place players in close proximity to the batter and to each other. This creates the risk of being struck by the ball or by another player. Pitchers appear to have the greatest disadvantage, standing only 40 feet from home plate and in many instances ending up in a vulnerable position following a pitch. Fixed objects around the playing field, including the dugout, backstop, and outfield fences, all have injury-causing potential for the unsuspecting player that collides with them. Much of the danger can be lessened by adequately padding these structures.

The use of standard bases has been cited as a major source of injuries in softball.[5–7,29] Standard bases are "fixed" by means of a post into the ground and do not give way with contact. As a result, standard bases pose a risk for injuries, especially during sliding. (see discussion under Etiology of Injuries). Less obvious sources of potential risk include prolonged sun exposure. Collegiate softball double headers (which are a routine part of collegiate softball schedules) can last up to 6 hours, requiring players to spend extended amounts of time exposed to harmful ultraviolet rays.

Softball players are susceptible to a number of musculoskeletal overuse injuries. In particular, the motion of overhand throwing places the shoulder and elbow at risk for repetitive microtrauma, which may lead to injury of muscles, tendons, nerves, and bones. Although pitchers use a different mechanism of propelling the ball, they too are vulnerable to overuse injuries.

PARTICIPATION INFORMATION

Softball is recognized as the most popular team sport in the nation, boasting over 40 million male and female players at all levels of play.[6] In the United States an estimated 5.9 million girls ages 6 to 17 play softball. More than 350,000 play scholastically at the high school level, representing over 15,000 high schools. At the collegiate level there are more than 1300 softball programs encompassing all divisions of the NCAA.[37] In 1997, a professional league, the Women's Pro Fast Pitch (WPF) was established. Currently the WPF consists of 6 teams with approximately 100 total players in the league.

It has been estimated that 1 in 6 women in the United States plays softball and that greater than 60% of all softball players are between the ages of 18 and 44.[21,37] These numbers may rise in the future. The inauguration of women's fast-pitch softball into the modern Olympics as a medal sport in 1996 is likely to bolster interest in the sport and increase participation numbers.

EPIDEMIOLOGY OF SOFTBALL INJURIES

The sports medicine literature is quite limited in regard to injury data for women's fast-pitch softball. However, the NCAA has compiled injury statistics on sanctioned sports for the past few decades. Injury incidence rates expressed as the number of injuries per 1000 exposures (an exposure consists of one practice or game) are calculated on an annual basis for most sports. This allows comparison within and between sports. As of the 1995 to 1996 season, the injury rate for women's softball was 15% higher than that of baseball. For injuries that resulted in more than 7 days of lost participation, the rate for women's softball was identical to that of baseball. The percentage of injuries that resulted in the need for subsequent surgery was 0.3 % higher for softball compared to baseball (Table 62-1).[19]

Data looking at younger age groups are sparse. A study performed in Ontario, Canada, investigated injury rates among several amateur softball and baseball teams for one season in 1989.[23] The study looked at participants of varying ages (from 8 to 19 and above), level of play, and gender. Injury rates were recorded per 1000 games. The softball teams were either fast-pitch or slow-pitch. The injury rate for female softball players was 6.6 per 1000 games, while that for males was 4.6 per 1000 games. When the data were stratified by age, differences in injury rates were limited to players older than 13 years of age. The authors noted that the older age groups tended to be involved in leagues playing fast-pitch softball. Other data, gathered from Australian softball players, indicates that females ages 10 to 19 are the most commonly injured group.[20]

These data suggest that female softball players are at a slightly increased risk of injury compared to their male counterparts (playing baseball or softball) for the above-mentioned age groups. The reasons for such differences are unclear; more research in this area is needed.

PHYSICAL DEMANDS OF SOFTBALL

Softball may be viewed as both a power sport and a finesse sport. Power is needed to be successful in running, throwing, and hitting. Agility and finesse are crucial to fielding the ball.

Short bursts of activity followed by longer periods of rest are common in softball. Long periods of aerobic activity are not required during game situations.

Some of the literature suggests that as nonendurance athletes, women softball players

do not reap the physiologic benefits of sustained physical activity. Rivera and coworkers studied 12 female softball players from the Puerto Rican National team and found these athletes to demonstrate below-optimal levels of cardiorespiratory endurance, muscular strength, and flexibility. This study also found them to have high levels of body fat.[25] Comparing elite softball players with field hockey and netball players in South Australia, Withers and coworkers noted softballers to have the lowest maximum anaerobic power and intermediate maximum aerobic power among the groups. No significant difference in body fat was noted. The authors concluded that differences in power likely reflected the different demands of these sports.[36] However, echocardiographic and maximum oxygen consumption (VO_2max) assessments of women softball players reach different conclusions. Rubal and coworkers reported a mean VO_2max of 55.3 mL O_2/kg*min in a group of women collegiate softball champions compared to 40.3 mL O_2/kg*min for a group of sedentary controls. Further analysis found that softball players demonstrated a resting bradycardia and echocardiographic evidence of eccentric hypertrophy, findings representative of beneficial physiologic adaptation.[26,27] At this time there are no large studies describing the physiologic profiles of women softball players. Because of the small sample sizes used in these studies, the conclusions may not be generalizeable to all populations. And the more recent emphasis of year-round strength training and conditioning further limits the applicability of these data to the contemporary softball player.

ETIOLOGY OF INJURY

As previously noted, softball players encounter significant risk of injury during the course of participation. Softball injuries may be categorized based upon the mechanism of injury, including throwing injuries, running injuries, collision injuries, and sliding injuries.

Table 62-1. Injury Statistics for Collegiate Softball and Baseball

	SOFTBALL	BASEBALL
Injuries per 1000 exposures	3.9	3.4
Injuries per 1000 exposures with > 7 days lost participation	1.2	1.2
Percentage of injuries requiring surgery	5.9	5.6

[a]Data from NCAA injury statistics through the 1995–1996 year.[20]

Table 62-2. Biomechanics of Overhand Throwing

MUSCLE	ACTION OF MUSCLE	PHASE OF THROWING[a]	
Deltoid Rotator cuff	Hold arm elevated at 90° Movement of shoulder from flexion to extension	Early cocking	(drawing A)
Subscapularis Serratus anterior	Decelerates shoulder's external rotation Controls scapulothoracic joint	Late cocking	(drawing B)
Serratus anterior Triceps Pectoralis major Latissimus dorsi	Provides stable glenoid for humeral rotation Rapid extension of the elbow Provide thrust to forward moving throwing arm	Acceleration	(drawing C)
Biceps Supraspinatus Subscapularis	Deceleration of elbow Deceleration of arm in space Internal rotation of the shoulder	Follow-through	(drawing D)

[a]See Figure 62-2.
Adapted from Jobe FW, Moynes DR, Tibone JE, et al: An EMG analysis of the shoulder in pitching. A second report. Am J Sports Med 12(3): 218–20, 1984, and Jobe FW, Tibone JE, Perry J, et al: An EMG analysis of the shoulder in pitching. A preliminary report. Am J Sports Med 11(1): 3–5, 1983.

Throwing Injuries

The biomechanics of overhand throwing have been well studied. Jobe and coworkers used EMG to identify muscle firing patterns of the shoulder throughout the stages of the throwing motion (Table 62-2; Fig. 62-2).[8,9] Differences and similarities between the windmill softball pitch and baseball pitch have also been identified (Table 62-3).[16] Atwater further looked at the biomechanics of overhand throwing in both men and women in a kinematic study. She noted that skilled women and men moved through nearly the same joint range of motion while throwing, but the women moved somewhat more slowly.[1]

Since softball players perform the overhand throwing motion thousands of times in a season, it is not unexpected that some will develop shoulder or elbow pain. Abrupt changes in intensity of throwing, duration of throwing, poor technique, abnormal throwing mechanics, or joint laxity may predispose to throwing-related injuries. Injuries to the shoulder and elbow and surrounding soft tissue structures are numerous. Some of the more common problems are listed in Table 62-4. Their diagnosis and management is discussed in detail elsewhere in this text.

Injuries to Softball Pitchers

Despite the underhand throwing motion, softball pitchers are not immune to upper extremity injury. In a study of 24 NCAA Division I softball pitchers, Loosli and coworkers found that 20 had been injured during the course of the softball season, experiencing a total of 26 injuries. Seventeen of the injuries involved the upper extremity, with 50% of all injuries affecting the shoulder or elbow. Furthermore, 21 of the 26 injuries were classified as overuse injuries, with the most common diagnosis being tendonitis.[15] The windmill motion employed may also lead to rather unique injuries. Jowett and Brukner reported an unusual case of a fifth metacarpal stress fracture in a softball pitcher.[10] They postulated that the fracture resulted from repetitive abduction forces involved in the grip and release of the ball in conjunction with the muscle forces exerted by the extensor carpi ulnaris. The patient recovered after 6 weeks of rest and modification of her ball grip.

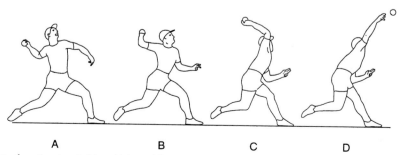

Figure 62-2. Range of motion in pitching. (Adapted from Atwater A: Biomechanics of overarm throwing movements and of throwing injuries. Exerc Sport Sci Rev 7:43–85, 1979, with permission.)

Table 62-3. Comparison of the Baseball and Softball Pitch

	BASEBALL	SOFTBALL
Position of the humerus	Abducted	In the plane of the body
Power generation	Pectoralis major	Pectoralis major
	Internal rotation of humerus	Adduction of humerus across the body
Deceleration of pitching arm	Eccentric muscle contraction	Contact of arm with hip
Provides stabilization against anterior forces	Anterior wall muscles	Anterior wall muscles
Provides scapulohumeral synchronization	Serratus anterior	Serratus anterior

Adapted from Maffet MW, Jobe FW, Pink MM, et al: Shoulder muscle firing patterns during the windmill softball pitch. Am J Sports Med 25(3): 369–74, 1997, with permission.

Stress fractures of the middle one third of the shaft of the ulna have also been reported.[33] Computed tomography sections of the forearms of 6 windmill-style softball pitchers with this injury revealed smaller cross-sectional areas of the middle third of the ulna than at other sites. Based on this information, the injuries were thought to be a result of excessive torsional stress on the bone. The torsional stress appears to be due to excessive pronation of the forearm during the follow-through phase of the pitch. Deceleration of the arm mainly occurs as the forearm strikes the hip, with the release of the ball as previously noted.[16] This repetitive loading of the medial aspect of the forearm may contribute to fatigue fracture of the ulna.

Injury to nerve structures of the upper extremity, including the radial and ulnar nerves, have likewise been documented.[15,30] Radial neuropathy was reported in 2 cases by Sinson and coworkers in which the radial nerve was entrapped proximally. As the radial nerve passes under the fibrous arch of the lateral head of the triceps, it may be tethered. In conjunction with the traction forces applied to the radial nerve by windmill motion, this may prove to be sufficient to result in a neuropathy. This may be similar to the injury to the ulnar nerve seen in baseball pitchers that results from excessive valgus overload.

Another neurologic injury that may be encountered in softball players is thoracic outlet syndrome (TOS). In general, TOS occurs when the great vessels and nerves of the upper extremity become entrapped or compressed as they exit the region surrounding the axilla. TOS is characterized by a constellation of symptoms, which may include any or all of the following: pain localized to the shoulder, neck, upper extremity, or face, parasthesias, numbness, swelling, weakness, or skin color changes of the proximal and or distal aspect of the upper extremity. Specific symptom patterns may be identified according to the primary neurovascular structures being compressed. Four symptom patterns have been described.[11] The lower trunk pattern is the most common, with symptoms including pain and paresthesias of the neck and shoulder that may radiate to medial forearm and fourth and fifth fingers. Grasp weakness may also be present. The upper trunk pattern consists of paresthesias and pain in the face, neck, and shoulders that may radiate to the lateral forearm. The patient with the rare vascular pattern may present with either venous (edema, cyanotic discoloration of arm) or arterial (numbness, exertional fatigue, and temperature change of the arm) symptoms. A mixed pattern of neurologic and vascular symptoms is also possible. TOS occurs twice as often in women compared with men[22] and has been reported in baseball pitchers.[31] While there are no epidemiologic data in female softball players, it is our experience that TOS does occur in this population.

Multiple anatomic variants that may predispose to developing TOS have been identified, including the presence of a cervical rib, exuberant callus formation following a clavicular fracture, fibromuscular bands within the scalene muscles, and pectoralis minor hypertrophy.[31] In throwing athletes symptoms are often aggravated by a particular aspect of throwing (eg, cocking phase) and may be reproducible by having the patient repeat the maneuver. Classic provocative maneuvers include the Adson test, the Wright test, and the costoclavicular compression test.

Table 62-4. Common Elbow and Shoulder Problems in Softball Players

ELBOW	SHOULDER
Medial epicondylitis	Rotator cuff injuries
Ulnar collateral ligament injury	Bicipital tendonitis
Loose body formation	Glenoid labral lesions
Posterior impingement	(or tears)
Osteochondritis dissecans	Glenohumeral instability
Osteochondroses	

The Adson test involves having the patient extend her neck and turn her head to the affected side while taking a deep breath. The examiner feels for diminishing presence of the radial pulse with the arm abducted and externally rotated.[32] The Wright test is performed by having the patient take a deep breath and turn her head to the unaffected side while the examiner passively abducts and externally rotates the affected arm. A test is considered positive if the radial pulse disappears or the symptoms are reproduced. The costoclavicular compression test has the patient assume an exaggerated military posture with shoulders being drawn back and downward while the examiner again measures the quality of the radial pulse in the affected arm.

Although many patients with TOS will have a positive provocative test, the tests have rather high false-positive and false-negative rates and they should not be relied on to make the diagnosis.[12,24]

Ancillary tests that may prove helpful in the diagnosis of TOS include plain roentgenography, electromyography (EMG), sensory evoked potentials, venography/arteriography, magnetic resonance imaging (MRI), and magnetic resonance arteriography (MRA). Plain roentgenography can detect bony abnormalities such as a cervical rib, degenerative disease of the cervical spine, and hypertrophic callus from an old clavicular fracture.

EMG can help in excluding a cervical radiculopathy, brachial plexus injury, or other nerve entrapment. Arteriography and venography are indicated if vascular symptoms or signs are present. More recently, MRI and MRA have been employed in diagnosing TOS.

MRI used in conjunction with MRA is able to provide quality images of the brachial plexus and determine the presence of any vascular occlusion or compression.[4]

Treatment of TOS includes symptomatic relief through the use of rest, icing, and non-steroidal anti-inflammatory drugs. Physical therapy is aimed at posture correction and strengthening of the scapular stabilizers and shoulder girdle. Surgical treatment may be necessary for those individuals with symptoms that do not improve with conservative measures.

Running-Related Injuries

Running from base to base, chasing down a fly ball, and moving quickly to field a ground ball necessitate the use of bursts of speed. Fast, forceful muscle contractions of the large muscle groups of the lower extremities are needed to produce these efforts. Consequently, acute injuries such as muscle strains or tears and ligamentous sprains of the lower extremities may occur during the course of a contest. Many other conditions may develop secondary to overuse or a combination of acute and chronic injury. Some of the more common problems that are encountered are included in Table 62-5.

Collision Injuries

Collision in softball can transpire in one of 3 ways: player versus player, player versus ball, and player versus field obstacle. Poor communication between players on the same team can result in collisions, often at high rates of speed. Base runners may purposefully run or slide into a defender. Perhaps the best example of this occurs when the catcher is awaiting a throw from the field and blocks home plate to prevent the runner from scoring. The runner, in an attempt to beat the throw or jar the ball loose, may collide with the catcher at full speed. These scenarios have the potential to produce serious injury.

Likewise, lack of familiarity with the playing field could mean colliding with a wall, fence, tarp, or other stationary object. For this reason players should be aware of the ground rules specific for each field and take time before a game to survey the field and note any potential hazards (eg, the field tarp that is commonly along side the playing field should be out of play).

Perhaps the most prevalent collision danger is that of the ball, thrown or batted, striking a player. Injuries caused by blunt softball trauma can range from minor injuries such as contusions to more serious, even fatal, injuries. Pitched softballs can reach a velocity of up to 70 miles/hr and batted balls can reach higher velocities. Since players may be as close as 40 feet from the batter, it is thus easy to understand that batted balls, which take unanticipated hops off the playing surface, can cause significant injuries. Specific injuries resulting from collisions with a softball include contusions and fractures. The facial region seems to be particularly

Table 62-5. Injuries Associated with Running in Softball

Muscle strain (quadriceps, hamstrings, gastrocnemius-soleus, etc)
Ankle sprain
Medial tibial stress syndrome
Stress fractures
Achilles tendinitis
Patellofemoral pain
Plantar fasciitis

prone to such injuries. Mandible, nasal, and orbital fractures are not uncommon in bat and ball sports. Injuries to the hands are also frequently observed. Included among these are mallet injury to the distal interphalangeal joints, volar plate injuries, metacarpal fractures, and collateral ligament injuries. Degroot and Mass reviewed 119 hand injuries in 108 softball players and found that injuries to the distal and proximal interphalangeal joints were common, with mallet injuries and volar plate injuries accounting for the majority of visits.[3]

More rarely, life-threatening injury may occur. Internal carotid artery dissection has been reported following blunt trauma from a softball. Schievink and coworkers described 2 cases of softball players who were struck in the anterolateral aspect of the neck and subsequently developed traumatic dissection of the carotid artery.[28] One patient suffered a resultant Horner syndrome and the other had transient cerebral ischemic symptoms. Both patients were also noted to have a low carotid bifurcation during evaluation, which the authors considered a possible risk factor for traumatic dissection.

A particularly serious injury caused by blunt trauma is commotio cordis. *Commotio cordis* is defined as sudden death from cardiac arrest after a blunt blow to the chest in the absence of structural cardiovascular disease.[17] Commotio cordis may occur in softball athletes who are struck in the precordial area with the ball or during a collision. It occurs predominately in young athletes, males more often than females, with the most reported cases in baseball and softball.[17] The underlying cause is thought to be the development of ventricular fibrillation following the chest wall impact.[14,17]

In a recent case study Link and coworkers reported a case of commotio cordis in a 14-year-old boy and documented ventricular fibrillation 6 minutes after the boy had collapsed.[13]

In a swine animal model of commotio cordis, Link and coworkers demonstrated that there appears to be a critical window of the cardiac cycle during which the heart is susceptible to commotio cordis.

This study found that if a chest wall blow was delivered within 30 to 15 msec before the peak of the T wave on the electrocardiogram, ventricular fibrillation resulted 9 of 10 times.[14]

Sudden death is far too frequently the end result of commotio cordis. In a series of 25 patients suffering commotio cordis, all 25 died despite resuscitative measures.[17] Recently, however, a small number of survivors have been reported.[13,18]

Early recognition is the key to management of commotio cordis. In one case series nearly half of the victims collapsed instantaneously, while in the others cardiac arrest was not immediate. Some individuals were able to speak, cry out, or perform brief physical activity prior to collapsing.[17] Cardiopulmonary resuscitation (CPR) should be initiated immediately following determination of a pulseless, apneic patient. Of the survival cases reported all had CPR started within 3 minutes.[13,18] Underlying cardiac structural and conduction abnormalities should be investigated in cases of survival.

Sliding Injuries

Sliding is a tactic typically employed by base runners to avoid being tagged out by a defender. Historically, sliding was performed using a feet-first technique. Currently, many players use a head-first technique at least on an occasional basis. The mechanisms of these 2 types of sliding have been examined in professional baseball players.[2] Using high-speed cinematography the sliding act was broken down into 4 distinct phases: sprint, attainment of sliding position, airborne, and landing. Initial impact with the ground following the airborne phase was determined to be a likely source of injury. For feet-first slides, the leading foot struck the ground first, followed by the tucked foot and knee. Head-first slides placed the hands and knees at risk of injury because these slides involved landing on the hands and knees prior to the chest and thighs contacting the ground. While it seems logical that head-first slides would result in proportionally more injuries to the upper extremities and feet-first slides in lower extremity injuries, there are no epidemiologic data at this time to support this theory.

Sliding injuries account for up to 71% of recreational softball injuries.[5] Other studies have indicated that the use of standard bases is the major underlying cause of sliding injuries and that by using break-away or impact bases up to 98% of sliding injuries could be prevented.[5–7,29] Despite these findings the transition to the use of break-away bases has been slow, with the majority of games continuing to be played using standard bases.[4a]

Injuries sustained from sliding predominantly involve sprains and fractures of the ankle and hand/wrist.[6,35] The rapid deceleration associated with sliding combined with striking an immobile base is the likely mechanism for the majority of injuries. Until recently, softball sliding injury data had mainly been collected using recreationally active subjects and have not differentiated between sliding technique. Prospective data from NCAA Division I women's collegiate softball teams show an injury rate of 12.13 per 1000 sliding attempts. Head-first slides had an injury rate of 19.46 compared to 10.04 for feet-first slides (per 1000 slides).[4a] These preliminary data indicate an important difference between the 2 different sliding techniques and does suggest that the incidence of sliding injuries in women's collegiate softball is significant.

INJURY PREVENTION

While not all softball injuries can be avoided, preventive measures should be maximized to ensure the safest environment for all athletes. Equipment plays an enormous role in injury prevention. Over the past 50, years tremendous strides have been made to improve softball equipment. Similarly, rules have changed to enforce the use of safety gear. Batting helmets are required at all levels of competitive softball and provide protection from batted and thrown balls. Catchers must use extensive protective gear, including chest protectors, shin guards, throat guards, and masks. Plastic molded cleats have replaced metal spikes at most levels. Gloves are better designed to absorb and distribute impact. The revolutionary new aluminum bat designs, however, may be a step in the opposite direction. Because aluminum bats are lighter, hitters are able to increase bat velocity, which in turn increases the velocity of the batted ball. This coupled with the relatively short distance between batter and fielder may increase the risk of injury from a batted ball. This may necessitate modification of aluminum bats in the future. Measures to this effect have already been undertaken in baseball. The NCAA recently recommended aluminum bats not exceed 2 5/8 inches in diameter and a length-to-weight unit differential of no more than 3. (A 34-inch bat must weigh at least 31 ounces).

The use of break-away or impact bases, as previously noted, can substantially decrease the number of injuries from sliding. Playing recreational softball games on fields using break-away bases resulted in significantly fewer sliding injuries than playing on fields with stationary bases (0.3% per game versus 7.2%).[7] Similar results were observed by Sendre and coworkers in their study using impact bases. A sliding injury occurred in 2.6% of games using standard bases compared to 0.08% of games using impact bases.[29]

The grounds crew also plays a large role in assuring a safe playing environment. Well-manicured fields reduce the likelihood of bad bounces or twisted ankles or knees on uneven surfaces. Padding of outfield walls, backstops, and dugouts can further diminish serious injury from collisions. Protective fencing around the dugout area may lessen the chance of a player being struck by a batted or thrown ball. Learning proper technique for fielding, base running, sliding, throwing, and pitching at early ages with proper supervision may also be helpful in reducing injuries. Coaches can help by ensuring player compliance with all rules and safety regulations of the game, and by implementing appropriate flexibility and warm up sessions prior to practice and games.

In-season and off-season conditioning programs should be employed by competitive softball players in order to both help prevent injury and improve performance. (Specific conditioning and flexibility programs are discussed elsewhere in the book.)

Future preventive efforts may include the mandatory use of break-away bases. Equipment modifications may also be instituted. The use of mouthguards may decrease the number of dental injuries. The use of softer materials in the manufacturing of balls and the return to the use of wooden bats have also been a topic of discussion. A study looking at the etiology of commotio cordis found a decreased rate of inciting ventricular fibrillation following chest-wall impact with softer "safety balls" compared to regulation baseballs.[20]

Finally, field dimensions could be altered to reduce the potential for batted-ball injuries. While all these changes are possible, any significant change that might alter the character or flow of the game should be well thought out prior to suggesting implementation.

References

1. Atwater A: Biomechanics of overarm throwing movements and of throwing injuries. Exerc Sport Sci Rev 7:43–85, 1979.
2. Corzatt RD, Groppel JL, Pfautsch E, et al: The biomechanics of head-first versus feet-first sliding. Am J Sports Med 12(3):229–32, 1984.
3. Degroot H, Mass DP: Hand injury patterns in softball players using a 16 inch ball. Am J Sports Med 16(3):260–5, 1988.
4. Esposito MD, Arrington JA, Blackshear MN, et al: Thoracic outlet syndrome in a throwing athlete diagnosed with MRI and MRA. J Magnet Reson Imag 17:598–9, 1997.
4a. Hosey RG, Puffer JC: Baseball and softball sliding injuries: Incidence and the effect of technique in

collegiate baseball and softball players. AJSM 28(3):360–363, 2000.

5. Janda DH, Hankin FM, Wojtys EM: Softball injuries: Cost, cause and prevention. Am Fam Phys 33(6):143–4, 1986.

6. Janda DH, Wild DE, Hensinger RN: Softball injuries: Aetiology and prevention. Sports Med 13(4):285–91, 1992.

7. Janda DH, Wojtys EM, Hankin FM, et al: Softball sliding injuries: A prospective study comparing standard and modified bases. JAMA 259(12):1848–50, 1988.

8. Jobe FW, Moynes RD, Tibone JE, et al: An EMG analysis of the shoulder in pitching. A second report. Am J Sports Med 12(3):218–20, 1984.

9. Jobe FW, Tibone JE, Perry J, et al: An EMG analysis of the shoulder in throwing and pitching. A preliminary report. Am J Sports Med 11(1):3–5, 1983.

10. Jowett AD, Brukner PD: Fifth metacarpal stress fracture in a female softball pitcher. Clin J Sport Med 7(3):220–1, 1997.

11. Karas SE: Thoracic outlet syndrome. Clin Sports Med 9:297–310, 1990.

12. Leffert RD: Thoracic outlet syndrome and the shoulder. Clin J Sport Med 2:439–52, 1983.

13. Link MS, Ginsburg SH, Wang PJ, et al: Commotio cordis. Cardiovascular manifestations of a rare survivor. Chest 114(1):326–8, 1998.

14. Link MS, Wang PJ, Pandian NG, et al: An experimental model of sudden death due to low-energy chest-wall impact (commotio cordis). N Engl J Med 338(25): 1805–11, 1998.

15. Loosli AR, Requa RK, Garrick JG, et al: Injuries to pitchers in women's collegiate fast-pitch softball. Am J Sports Med 20(1):35–7, 1992.

16. Maffet MW, Jobe FW, Pink MM, et al: Shoulder muscle firing patterns during the windmill softball pitch. Am J Sports Med 25(3):369–74, 1997.

17. Maron BJ, Poliac LC, Kaplan JA, et al: Blunt impact to the chest leading to sudden death from cardiac arrest during sports activities. N Engl J Med 333(6):337–42, 1995.

18. Maron BJ, Strasburger JF, Kugler JD, et al: Survival following blunt chest impact-induced cardiac arrest during sports activities in young athletes. Am J Cardiol 79(6):840–1, 1997.

19. National Collegiate Athletic Association: Injury Surveillance System, 1997–1998. Overland Park, Kan, National Collegiate Athletic Association,1998.

20. National Sport Information Centre Australian Sports Commission: Softball at the Australian Institute of Sport. Belconnen ACT, Australia, 1996. Website http://www.ausport.gov.au/aissof.html.

21. National Broadcasting Company: Softball: Did you know. 1996. Website http://www.olympic.nbc.com /sports/softball/did.html.

22. Nichols AW: The thoracic outlet syndrome in athletes. J Am Board Fam Pract 9(5):346–55, 1996.

23. Ontario Amateur Baseball and Softball Injuries Study–1989. Published by the Ministry of Tourism and Recreation. Province of Ontario, Toronto, Canada, 1990.

24. Rayan GM, Jensen C: Thoracic outlet syndrome: provocative examination maneuvers in a typical population. J Shoulder Elbow Surg 4:113–7, 1995.

25. Rivera MA, Ramirez-Marrero FA, Rivas CA, et al: Anthropometric and physiologic profile of Puerto Rican athletes: female softball. P R Health Sci J 13(4): 255–60, 1994.

26. Rubal BJ, Al-Muhailani, Rosentswieg J: Effects of physical conditioning on the heart size and wall thickness of college women. Med Sci Sports Exerc 19(5):423–9, 1987.

27. Rubal BJ, Rosentswieg J, Hamerly B: Echocardiographic examination of women collegiate softball champions. Med Sci Sports Exerc 13(3):176–9, 1981.

28. Schievink WI, Atkinson JL, Bartleson JD, et al: Traumatic internal carotid artery dissections caused by blunt softball injuries. Am J Emerg Med 16(2):179–82 1998.

29. Sendre RA, Keating TM, Hornak JE, et al: Use of the hollywood impact base and standard stationary base to reduce sliding and base-running injuries in baseball and softball. Am J Sports Med 22(4):450–453, 1994.

30. Sinson G, Zager EL, Kline DG: Windmill pitcher's radial neuropathy. Neurosurgery 34(6):1087–9, 1994.

31. Strukel RJ, Garrick JG: Thoracic outlet compression in athletes: a report of four cases. Am J Sports Med 6:35–9, 1978.

32. The classic. Surgical treatment for symptoms produced by cervical ribs and the scalenus anticus muscle. By Alfred Washington Adson. 1947. Clin Orthop 207:3–12, 1986.

33. Tanabe S, Nakahira J, Bando E, et al: Fatigue fracture of the ulna occurring in pitchers of fast-pitch softball. Am J Sports Med 19(3):317–21, 1991.

34. Townball: Description and rules. 1998. Website http://www.sirius.com/~cmonser/Townball.html.

35. Wheeler BR: Slow-pitch softball injuries. Am J Sports Med 12(3):237–40, 1984.

36. Withers RT, Roberts RG: Physiologic profiles of representative women softball, hockey and netball players. Ergonomics 24(8):583–91, 1981.

37. Women's Pro Fastpitch: Facts. Website http:// www.womensprofastpitch.com/facts.htm.

Chapter 63

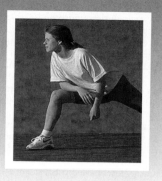

Swimming and Diving

William C. McMaster, M.D.

Swimming is enjoyed by a larger number of participants of all ages and skill levels than any other sport activity. Swimming and diving competitions for men were included from the beginning of the modern Olympiad movement, 1896, and for women since the 1912 Games at Stockholm. The advent of Masters' competitive programs, for men and women, and the inclusion of women in triathlon activities has encouraged athletic participation for women beyond the school-age years.

SWIMMING INJURIES

Biomechanics and Injury Patterns

Epidemiologic studies have demonstrated that aquatic sport activities have a low injury potential.[3,9,10,17] While serious injuries are not a major concern, repetitive microtrauma can have a significant impact on the swimmer's capacity to train and compete to his or her potential. Kennedy and Hawkins reported a study of 2496 swimmers, 261 (10.46%) of whom had orthopaedic complaints.[22] Ninety percent of these involved the shoulder, calf, or foot. There were 85 calf and foot problems divided equally among the 4 competitive strokes. All 70 knee problems were caused by the whip kick during breaststroke.

Understanding the phases of swimming strokes is necessary to treat swimmers. The 4 strokes are freestyle (front or crawl), butterfly, backstroke, and breaststroke. The components of the competitive strokes are reach or entry, catch, pull, and recovery.[11,16]

In 1968, "Doc" Counsilman published a textbook, *The Science of Swimming*.[11] This is a classic textbook still used by coaches and beneficial for the practitioner to understand the mechanical principles involved in swimming for each stroke. To treat swimmers and make the correct diagnosis, one must understand the nor-

mal biomechanics and consequent stresses on the musculoskeletal system. The degree of knee flexion varies, depending on the stroke (Fig. 63-1).[49] The phases of strokes and demands on shoulder and knee should be understood.[43] The biomechanical demands involved in propelling the body through the water create unique traumatic injury patterns. The rehabilitation of injured joints must focus on stabilization of hypermobile joints, strengthening, and correction of posture.[21]

The unique aspects of the kick in breaststroke make it the stroke most likely to cause knee pain

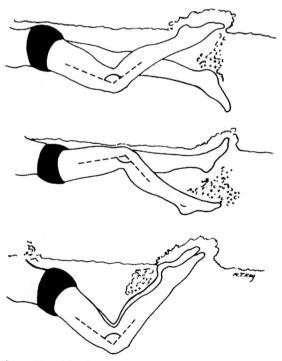

Figure 63-1. The degree of knee flexion varies depending on the stroke. Shown are flexion angles in (top to bottom) the freestyle, backstroke, and butterfly. (From Rodeo SA: Knee pain in competitive swimming. Clin Sports Med 18(2): 383, 1999, with permission.)

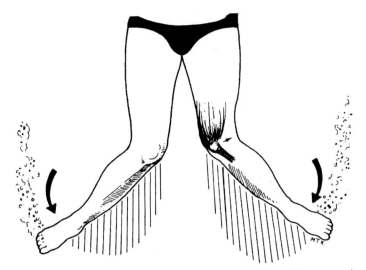

Figure 63-2. The breaststroke kick involves extension of the knees and the "catch" of the water (shaded area). (From Rodeo SA: Knee pain in competitive swimming. Clin Sports Med 18(2): 381, 1999, with permission.)

(Fig. 63-2).[47] The narrow whip kick puts distraction forces on the medial aspect of the knee. With more intense and longer workouts for the breaststroker, knee problems are common. The leg action is divided into 4 phases, the "catch," downsweep, insweep, and recovery. During the catch (Fig. 63-3A), the knees are fully bent greater than 90° and the feet are above the buttocks and close to each other.[48] The feet change inward in the whip part of the kick. The propulsion-generating movement occurs here. The hip is turned externally so the feet face backward and upward with toes lateral during the downsweep (Fig. 63-3B).[48] In the insweep, the feet continue to turn in and the legs finish with extension and are brought together and held in an extended position for a fraction of a second. At recovery at the end of the propulsive part of

the kick, the feet are together and then the feet are brought up to the buttocks by flexing of the knees. In the breaststroke, new techniques of holding the head high make the shoulder more vulnerable. The muscle actions involved in the phases of catch, downsweep, insweep, upsweep, and recovery are shown in Figure 63-4.

Butterflyers have the most shoulder injuries. The stroke is divided into catch, downsweep, insweep, and recovery (Fig. 63-5). During the catch, the arm is maximally extended (Fig. 63-5A). In entry, the hands are pitched in internal rotation at 45° to slice the water. The elbows are extended and the hands enter the water in line with the shoulder. During the downsweep, the hands pass outside shoulder width and move downward and outward in a circular path, the elbows bend, and the hands reach their deepest

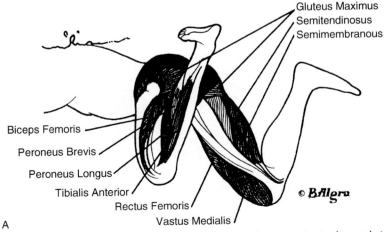

A

Figure 63-3.A. In the breaststroke, activity of muscles varies. The musles that are active in the catch (**A**) and downsweep

Illustration continued on following page

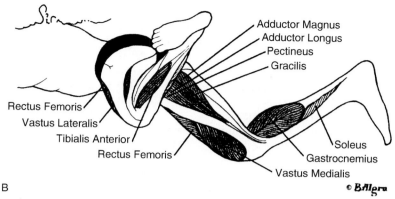

B

Figure 63-3 *(Continued).* **(B)** are shown. (From Rodeo S: Swimming the breaststroke—a kinesiological analysis and considerations for strength training. Natl Strength Condition Assoc J Sept.-Oct: 6, 1984, with permission.)

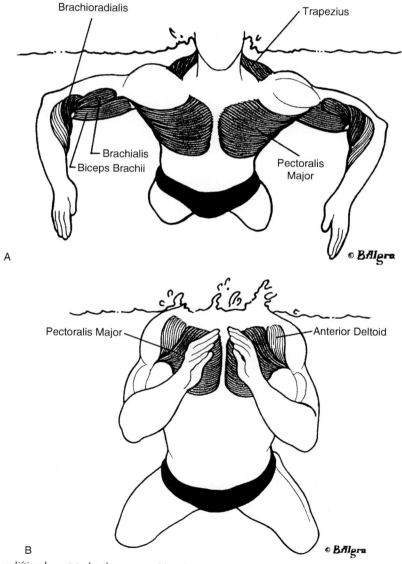

Figure 63-4. In the uplifting breaststroke the arm position is very important. Those muscles active during downsweep and insweep **(A)** and recovery **(B)** are shown. (From Rodeo S: Swimming the breaststroke—a kinesiological analysis and considerations for strength training. Natl Strength Condition Assoc J Sept.-Oct: 5, 1984, with permission.)

point.[48] During insweep (Fig. 63-5B), the arms and hands travel inward toward the midline and the hands pass beneath the elbows, somewhat like a sculling action. The recovery occurs as the hands turn inward and release their pressure on the water and the elbows break the surface of the water first, followed by the hands.[48]

In swimming programs, resistive weight training began 3 decades ago. In the past, weight training was identified as increasing the potential for injury in swimmers.[19] Rehabilitation programs are implemented for prevention of injury. These focus on stabilization for lax joints, postural correction, strengthening, and knee flexibility. Proper techniques and timing of the strengthening program are important for injury prevention.

Neck Injuries and Referred Pain

Neck and shoulder problems can plague swimmers. Fortunately, no catastrophic head and neck injuries have been reported in organized competitive swimming.[9] When age-related degenerative cervical disc disease and/or osteoarthritic degeneration of the facet joints of the cervical spine occurs, neck-related complaints might result. Nerve root impingement, from a herniated nucleus pulposus or from degenerative osteophytes projecting into the neuroforamina, may be responsible for neck and/or arm pain radiating into the fingers. As the C5 and C6 nerve roots supply the motor and sensory investment about the shoulder, root dysfunction from this level could result in shoulder complaints. Patients with arthritis and limited range of neck motion may find correct breathing techniques difficult and painful.

Although unusual, a vascular cause for shoulder pain is subclavian vein thrombosis.[64] Damage to the axillary vein by stretching or impacting against the first rib may result in local thrombosis.[18,39] The symptoms include arm pain with exertion and inability to swim effectively. The signs are swelling of the arm and distention of the distal veins without change when the arm is elevated. This precludes swimming training and has led to retirement from competition. In the author's personal clinical experience with this entity in swimmers, vein thrombosis is related to heavy-resistance weight training.

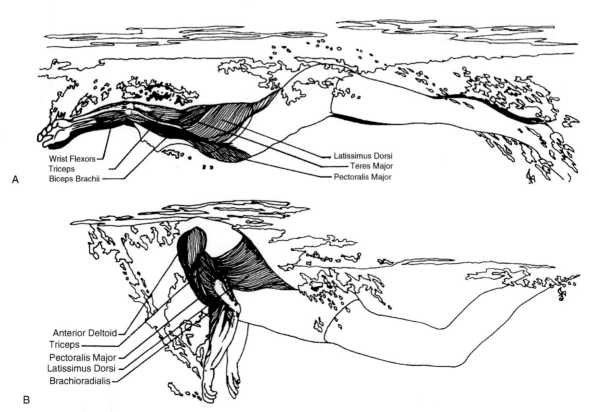

Wrist Flexors
Triceps
Biceps Brachii

Latissimus Dorsi
Teres Major
Pectoralis Major

A

Anterior Deltoid
Triceps
Pectoralis Major
Latissimus Dorsi
Brachioradialis

B

Figure 63-5. In the butterfly stroke muscle activity is highest during the catch and downsweep **(A)**, then insweep and upsweep **(B)**. The active muscles are shown. (From Rodeo S: The butterfly—a kinesiological analysis and strength training program. Natl Strength Condition Assoc J Aug-Sept: 4, 1985, with permission.)

Thoracic outlet syndrome may be important in any overhead athlete.[14] The upper extremity vascular supply and the brachial plexus exit the neck and upper thorax over the first rib and between the scalene muscles. Impingement of the brachial plexus and/or artery on these structures may cause arm problems during exertion. The result is undue fatigue, aching, and inability to perform repetitive or prolonged activities requiring overhead position of the arms. Often the problem is noted also during sleep. Operative removal of the first rib or scalene muscle release may be required to relieve symptoms if physical therapy exercise programs fail. Following surgery, return to the same level of swimming is not predictable or common.

Shoulder Injuries

The term "swimmer's shoulder" was first used by Kennedy and Hawkins in 1974 to refer to tendinitis of the supraspinatus and/or biceps tendon.[23] Swimmer's shoulder occurs in 3% to 50% of swimmers. The multiple factors involved in development of swimmer's shoulder are training patterns, intensity and distance, biomechanics, physiologic laxity, shoulder strength and balances, compressive subacromial space forces, distraction, glenohumeral forces, core strength and amount of shoulder roll, and the biomechanics of the stroke.

Compared to recreational swimmers, elite swimmers have greater multidirectional laxity.[66] Females have increased generalized joint laxity relative to males, but generalized joint laxity does not correlate with shoulder laxity. There are conflicting reports on shoulder laxity and gender. In a review of multidirectional instability in patients who were treated operatively, the numbers were greater in females, 94 (55%), compared with males, 77 (45%). The number or gender of patients who were treated nonoperatively was not reported.[6] In female athletes at the college level, the overall injury rate for exposure was less than in other collegiate athletic populations. Cross-training injuries predominantly involved the lower extremity, and swimming injuries involved the shoulder. The overall injury rate per 1000 exposures was 2.12, with 45% due to swimming, 44% to cross training, and 11% unrelated to athletics. The ratio of upper to lower extremity injuries due to swimming was 3:1, whereas the ratio for cross training was 1:4.[28] This is thought to be both genetic and acquired. Generalized joint laxity was also more common in elite swimmers.

A survey comparing 100 collegiate and Masters' teams has been published. Although there were similar percentages of swimmer's shoulder in the collegiate and Masters' groups—47 and 48%, respectively–, problems occurred at lesser distances and intensities in the Masters' group. Therefore, fatigue may be associated with the development of swimmer's shoulder and a strengthening program should be implemented prior to development of symptoms.

Shoulder joint arthritis, unusual in the young, may be more common in the Masters' group. Rotator cuff arthropathy, associated with chronic massive rotator cuff tear, is unusual in the swimmer. A common sequela of years of inflammatory tendinitis and bursitis in the overhead athlete, disruption of the supraspinatus portion of the rotator cuff may occur with a surprisingly functional shoulder in some individuals. Most, however, will be impaired and unable to train or compete. In older individuals, glenohumeral arthritis with a normal rotator cuff is rarely seen in swimmers who swam with their age group and beyond.

Biomechanics

The shoulder is an intrinsically unstable joint consisting of a large humeral head resting against a flat glenoid surface enlarged and deepened by a fibrocartilaginous labrum. The shoulder capsule generates negative pressure relative to the atmosphere and results in a small suction stabilizing effect for the joint. The glenohumeral ligaments have been identified as the primary joint stabilizers in both the anterior and, recently, the posterior capsule.[59,63] The rotator cuff musculature functions as a secondary line of stability whose primary responsibility is glenohumeral motion and centering of the humeral head against the glenoid. The more superficial shoulder muscular layer functions to provide motion and precise positioning. However, no amount of strength of the muscular investment seems able to prevent subluxation or dislocation of the glenohumeral joint if the primary capsular restraints are incompetent.

In swimming, most of the propulsive force is generated by the arms with the legs providing stabilization as well as propulsive force.[43,57] The shoulder joint of any overhead athlete is subject to a variety of repetitive microtrauma or overuse syndromes.[13,33,34,44,45] It is interesting, however, that not all swimmers training under similar load conditions, will develop significant interfering shoulder complaints. Most will escape any problems at all. The reasons for this are likely multifactorial. As a consequence, there probably is no truly definable entity of "swimmer's shoulder."

Significant torque and shear forces occur in the glenohumeral joint during the propulsive phase of swimming enhanced by the length of the lever arm extending from the propeller hand to the shoulder joint axis.[57,58] Fine-wire electromyography studies have demonstrated the proportionate contribution of shoulder muscle groups to the various phases of the swimming stroke pattern. In particular, infraspinatus and teres minor seem to have a minor role during the swimming stroke.[3,40,41,42] The serratus anterior functions near maximal during each stroke and may fatigue with training at the subscapularis and the serratus anterior.[40] The pectoralis major and latissimus dorsi propel the body and the infraspinatus is active only to externally rotate the arm during midrecovery. Placement of the hand in the water is by the deltoid and supraspinatus and the scapula is positioned before the arm by the rhomboids and upper trapezius. During the breaststroke, the serratus anterior and teres minor muscles in normal shoulders fire 15% above manual maximal test throughout the cycle. Specific programs to avoid injury must include endurance training of the serratus anterior and teres minor, as well as balancing internal and external rotation musculature of the shoulder.[56]

These muscles are overshadowed by the more powerful swimming muscles, the adductors and internal rotators.[15] A series of studies was conducted in swimmers and demonstrated, in both males and females, shifts in rotator cuff force couples previously noted in nonaquatic overhead athletes.[1,20,65] There is an adaptive shift in the torque ratios of adduction:abduction and external:internal rotation to favor adduction and internal rotation in male swimmers and water polo players.[29,30] Similar changes were also noted in female swimmers (Table 63-1). In a stable shoulder, these adaptations seem to be well tolerated. In the individual with an unstable shoulder, the external rotators will work to restrain the humeral head against anterior translation during the press and insweep phases of the freestyle stroke.[57] This may lead to fatigue and inflammation and may account for the paradoxical posterior pain in the shoulder with anterior subluxation or dislocation.

Specific rehabilitation programs have been designed for injury prevention. In the shoulder, the primary diagnosis must be made in order to implement the appropriate treatment. A primary diagnosis of instability could involve a capsular glenohumeral ligament injury, a capsular labral problem, or a rotator cuff tear (articular side, bursal side). In the freestyle stroke, "impingement syndrome" is common and the rehabilitation program must promote equilibrium of shoulder complex and proper stroke mechanics.[2] Rehabilitation programs should be implemented prior to injury, particularly about the shoulder.[21]

To moderate these adaptive changes, a remedial exercise protocol was developed and tested.[31] Refer to the referenced article for a full description of exercises and protocol. While the results of this study did not demonstrate statistically significant differences, a trend toward normalization of the rotator cuff shifts was noted. Table 63-2 presents the study's training protocol. The suggested weights are for college-age athletes and appropriate adjustments should be made for the younger or older athlete. A safe starting weight resistance for any exercise should allow the athlete to complete a 20 reps/3 sets protocol from the onset. The protocol should be done every other day.

Table 63-1. Rotator Cuff Force Couple Ratios (Cybex at 30°/sec)

FEMALE SWIMMERS VERSUS CONTROLS			
RATIO	CONTROL	SWIMMERS	P
External:Internal			
R arm	.74±.10	.63±.10[a]	.024
L arm	.74±.13	.65±.13	.144
Adduction:Abduction			
R arm	1.65±.21	2.13±.42 [a]	.004
L arm	1.57±.12	1.99±.24[a]	.000

[a]p<.05.

Table 63-2. Guidelines for Rotator Cuff Exercise Protocol (College-Age Female Swimmers)

EXERCISE	START WEIGHT[a]	REPS	NO. SETS	WEIGHT CHANGE	GOAL WEIGHT
1	3	20	3	1 lb/2 wks	10
2	2	20	3	1 lb/2 wks	7
3	2	20	3	2 lb/2 wks	12
4	5	20	3	2 lb/2 wks	15
5		10	1	add 4 /2 wks	30 reps

[a]Note: The starting weights are only suggestions. Use a starting weight that allows the athlete to complete the full 20 rep/3 sets from the onset.

The specific exercises are described as follows:

Lateral Abduction. This is done in the standing position. The weight is held in the hand with the thumb positioned forward with the elbow straight. The weight is raised 70° and then returned to the starting position.

Supraspinatus. This is done in the standing position. The weight is held in the hand with the thumb rotated downward toward the floor. Maintaining this position of the thumb, and with the elbow straight, the arm is raised 70° in a plane 45° from the nose.

External Rotators. This is done lying on the side. The body is maintained in a straight alignment. With the arm at the side, the hand grasps the weight straight forward, the elbow is bent to 90°, and the arm is rotated 90° outward keeping the elbow in contact with the side. The side of exercise should be alternated between sets.

Shoulder Instability

Instability is the primary diagnosis in most shoulder conditions. Other diagnoses include glenoid labrum tear, subacromial bursitis, and rotator cuff tendinitis associated with impingement syndrome.[32,36,37] Anterior instability has been long recognized. It is now well understood that instability in other directions is also important and must be carefully assessed for.[4, 38] The multidirectionally lax shoulder joint may be subluxing or dislocating, anterior, inferior, posterior, and, to some extent, superior. This may potentiate the impingement of the rotator cuff between the rising humeral head and the acromion and may be magnified in the individual who has an extended type II or III acromion or a convex shape to the subacromial profile.[7,37] Impingement results in abrasion damage to the rotator cuff and secondary tendinitis.

In the young athlete, rotator cuff avulsions are unusual. Partial thickness tears, particularly on the articular surface at the attachment site to the greater tuberosity, are more common. Arthroscopic, mini-open, or open repairs of the rotator cuff in athletes are required if the cuff is torn through and through.[46, 52, 62] Although masters level swimmers may have true compressive impingement and failure of the rotator cuff, in young swimmers, an underlying instability, often multidirectional, must be suspected as the primary cause of rotator cuff pathology. Thus, treating the tendinitis symptoms may improve but not completely cure the athlete whose shoulder is unstable. We have confirmed our clinical impressions that excess laxity of the shoulder joint in aquatic athletes does correlate to the report of disabling pain. A statistically significant correlation between a shoulder laxity score and the presence of significant interfering shoulder pain was demonstrated in a group of elite-level swimmers.[35] There appears to be a range of physiologic shoulder laxity that is compatible with painless performance and probably is necessary to be biomechanically efficient. Indeed, such a factor may be operating to select individuals who are most successful in swimming. The threshold from physiologic laxity to pathologic instability is narrow. Once the shoulder is unstable, there is an increased potential to damage intra-articular structures and stretch the capsule even further.

The treatment for disabling instability of the shoulder is surgical. With arthroscopic or open techniques, the labrum is reattached and/or the capsule tightened. After surgery, return to swimming competition depends on operative findings and the procedure done, not level of pain or whether the procedure was done open or arthroscopic. Care must be taken not to overconstrain the shoulder. Loss of external rotation may limit a swimmer's return to efficient and successful swimming.

Knee Injuries

Breaststroker's Knee

Knee pain occurs commonly in swimming but breaststrokers are the most common group with knee complaints. Most knee pain is related to the breaststroke. The differential diagnosis for "breaststroker's knee" includes medial collateral ligament (MCL) sprain, patellofemoral stress syndrome, symptomatic plica, patellar subluxation, and rarely medial meniscus tear. Kennedy and Fowler described breaststroker's knee MCL sprain.[24,61] Stulberg and Shulman described breaststroker's knee by site of regional tenderness on physical examination. Of 23 swimmers with knee pain, 18 had tenderness over the medial patellar facet and 5 over the MCL.[61] Keskinen reported the findings in breaststroker's knee as tenderness over the medial plica and synovitis of the medial compartment.[25] Rovere and Nichols found that a significant number of breaststrokers had a thickened medial synovial plica.[51] It is difficult to document the exact cause of breaststroker's knee, as these medial structures are all under tension. Early recognition of knee pain and repeated examination to make the correct diagnosis is necessary.

Assessment of biomechanics of the stroke should be done. Modifications to the stroke include keeping legs together during the recovery and thrush phases of the whip kick. Hip stretching to increase hip internal rotation and quadriceps and hip strengthening also have been suggested.[49]

The position of the knee center relative to the hip during the breaststroke kick has a direct relationship to the stress in the MCL and capsule of the knee joint.[60] The optimum initiating position for the breaststroke kick is with the hip and knee centers aligned. If the knee center position is wider or narrower, increased tensile force on the medial joint structures will result. When high forces are created with the leg in external rotation, sprains of the MCL can occur. The more severe sprains occur in water polo players using the egg beater kick or exploding to throw or get to the play.

Patellar Instability

Variations in development of the patellofemoral joint and in the nature of swimming repetitive and open chain motions combine to create disorders. The depth of the trochlear groove and the length and attachment of the patellar tendon are genetically determined. If the patellar tendon attachment to the tibial tubercle is in an externally rotated position and the patellar tendon is long, the patella is potentially unstable and rotated in the trochlear groove. Rehabilitation, not surgery, is the treatment. Quadriceps and core strengthening is necessary. Additional measures include McConnell taping and exercises designed to decrease the lateral thrusting of the patella and re-coordinate the firing of the vastus medialis.[27]

Patellar Tendinitis

Inflammation of the patellar tendon can occur proximal ("jumper's knee") or distal to the tibial tubercle attachment site (Osgood–Schlatter's disease, or tibial tubercle apophysitis). High tensile loads generated in running, jumping, plyometric exercise, hard kicking, forceful extensions, and squats in weight training result in damage to the tendon–bone attachment site. The mechanism is repetitive tensile overload of the tendon attachment site. Training for swimming requires both open and closed chain exercises. Treatment includes reduction in painful activities such as plyometric training, strengthening of the core and quadriceps, and stretching.

Muscle Strain

Muscle strains most common in breaststrokers occur during an eccentric muscular contraction with large internal stresses. Quadriceps or adductor strains are serious, with recurrent problems common. A careful, slow rehabilitation process with stretching and strengthening is required.

Meniscus Injury

The fibrocartilaginous meniscus of the knee may be injured during flexion, twisting, and extension movements of the knee. As the knee bends under load, the meniscus may get trapped between the joint surfaces, producing a tear that may cause pain, snapping or popping, and possible locking of the knee. The breaststroke kick can be compared to performing a medial McMurray test again and again. Owing to the peripheral and limited blood supply, meniscal tears will usually not heal. Treatment of symptomatic meniscus tears is arthroscopic surgery. In the Masters age group, tearing of a meniscus as part of the arthritic process is not uncommon. Arthroscopic results of meniscectomy are predictably positive, but in the arthritic knee, medial plicae may recur.

DIVING INJURIES

Epidemiology

Fortunately, no fatalities or catastrophic or serious injuries have been reported to the National Center for Catastrophic Sports Injuries from 1982 to 1997.[9] Two cases of fatal head injuries have occurred in competitive diving. Both divers were attempting a reverse $3\frac{1}{2}$ tuck somersault from the 10-meter platform.[8,26] No cases of cervical spine injuries or paralysis have occurred according to reports from the National Collegiate Athletic Association (NCAA) or the Federation Internationale de Natation Amateur (FINA).[12] Fortunately, the serious catastrophic and fatal injuries have not occurred in organized competitive diving.[53]

Competitive diving injuries are related to the biomechanics of diving. The dive is divided into 3 phases: take-off, flight, and entry. The position of the upper extremities just before flat-handed entry and at the moment of impact with the water surface is shown in Figure 63-6.[55] The scapula becomes more upwardly rotated and protracted and the elbows are extended. The forces that are transmitted to the wrist,

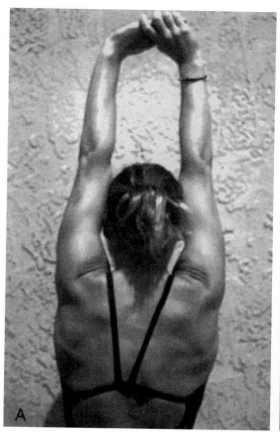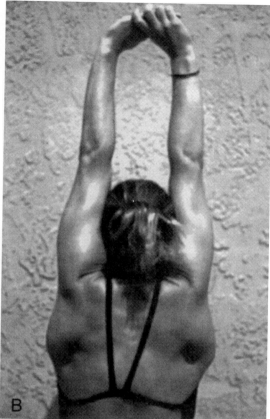

Figure 63-6. Position of the diver's upper extremities just before entry in the flat-handed entry technique **(A)** and at the moment of impact with the water surface **(B)**. Note the change in the position of the scapulae. (From Rubin BD: The basics of competitive diving and its injuries. Clin Sports Med 18(2):297, 1999, with permission.)

elbow, and shoulder are great, resulting in compression of the wrist and elbow and potential instability of the shoulder. Speeds of as high as 35 miles/hr at entry in a 10-mm dive have been measured. As the height increases, the speed and forces at water entry are magnified and acceleration increases in a function of time squared.

The exact incidence of injury in divers is difficult to track. No large series with exposures per diving hour or participants have tracked this. The design of studies has been case reports. A summary of these series is shown in Table 63-3.[54] There were no gender differences in these studies. There are certain trends toward increasing numbers of injuries with increasing training, competition, pool training over dry land training, platform over springboard training, and practice over competition. The most common injury involves the low back (Rubin B, personal communication). Diving has the highest incidence of spondylolisthesis (with true isthmic pars interarticularis lesions). The

Table 63-3. Incidence of Injury in Diving by Anatomic Location

LOCATION	RUBIN AND RICHARDSON (1981) (N = 37)	MUTOCH (1988) (N = 10)
Spine/trunk		
Neck	40%	10%
Back	61%	28%
Upper extremity		
Shoulder	32%	21%
Hand/wrist	29%	24%
Lower extremity		
Knee	27%	
Ankle	19%	

From Rubin BD, Anderson SJ: Diving. In: Cain DJ, Caine CG, Lindner KJ (eds): Champaign, Ill, Human Kinetics Publishers, 1996, p178, with permission.

incidence was 83.3% in diving, 44.8% in weight lifting, 32.3% in wrestling, 37.9% in gymnastics, and 24.5% in track and field.[50] Knee injuries do occur and are most commonly patellofemoral. Back injuries far outweigh the other injury patterns seen.[50]

Neck and Spine Injuries

Neck injury is associated with poor head position with sudden flexion or extension of the neck at water impact. Acute problems such as herniated nucleus pulposus may result. In the long term changes of degenerative disc disease and secondary spondylosis may be seen. The lumbosacral spine may also be injured in divers and the injuries may be in common with those of other sports that load the lumbosacral spine, including weight lifting, gymnastics, and acrobatics. Musculoligamentous strains are most common but herniation of the nucleus pulposus with classic sciatica can result. Stress fractures of the pars interarticularis from high shear stresses may cause pain and spasm. Young individuals may develop secondary vertebral slippage or spondylolisthesis. While rest will resolve most complaints, surgery for unresolved sciatica or high-grade vertebral slip may be necessary. Significant spinal pathology from any cause will likely preclude participation in diving competition.

Shoulder Injuries

Shoulder injuries are more common in divers, particularly women. Multidirectional laxity with subsequent rotator cuff weakness and scapular stabilizer dysfunction are common. This results from a combination of distraction forces on the capsule and rotator cuff and compression forces in the subacromial space. Triceps strain is also seen as a result of failure to lock the elbows out and is more frequent in younger divers and platform divers.

In diving, the shoulder is often involved in the older platform diver. The physiologic laxity progresses to frank anterior inferior instability. Treatment is surgical stabilization from an anterior approach and restoration of the anterior glenohumeral ligament, capsular integrity, and closure of the rotator cuff.

Hand and Wrist Injuries

Hand injuries are usually caused by impact with the surface and attempts to "save" dives by forcefully changing wrist position during entry. These forces may result in wrist injuries such as carpal subluxation and, if ligaments are torn, can result in wrist bone instability that will require surgical repair or reconstruction. Repeated high stresses may produce dorsal impaction syndrome, stress fractures of the distal epiphysis or scaphoid and avascular necrosis of the lunate. These problems are not treated simply and can result in secondary arthritic changes of the wrist joint that will be significantly disabling.

CONCLUDING REMARKS

Knowledge of the biomechanics of swimming and diving allows improvement of precise diagnosis and specific treatment programs. Although injuries are not always catastrophic, they can be frustrating for the athlete. To minimize the time away from the sport, early diagnosis must be made and treatment and training modifications implemented early.

Acknowledgments

Special thanks to Mary Lloyd Ireland, M.D., for assistance in reviewing the manuscript.

References

1. Aldernick GJ, Kuck DJ: Isokinetic shoulder strength of high school and college-aged pitchers. J Orthop Sports Phys Ther 7:163–72, 1986.
2. Allegrucci M, Whitney SL, Irrgang JJ: Clinical implications of secondary impingement of the shoulder in freestyle swimmers. J Orthop Sports Phup Ther 20(6):307–18, 1994.
3. Backx, FJ, Erich WB, Kemper AB, VerBeek, AL: Sports injuries in school-aged children. Am J Sports Med 17:234–40, 1989.
4. Bigliani LU, Pollock RG, McIlveen SJ, et al: Shift of the posterior inferior aspect of the capsule for recurrent posterior glenohumeral instability. J Bone Joint Surg 77A:1101–20, 1995.
5. Birrer P: The shoulder, EMG, and the swimming stroke. J Swim Res 2:20–3, 1986.
6. Brown GA, Tan JL, Kirkley A: The lax shoulder in females. Clin Orthop Rel Res 372:110–22, 2000.
7. Burkhart SS: Congenital subacromial stenosis. Arthroscopy 11:63–8, 1995.
8. Caine DJ, Caine CG, Lindner KJ: Epidemiology of Sports Injuries. Champaign, Ill, Human Kinetics Publishers, 1996.
9. Cantu RC, Mueller RC: Fatalities and catastrophic injuries in high school and college sports, 1982–1997. Physician Sportsmed 27(8):35–48, 1999.
10. Clark KS, Buckley WE: Women's injuries in collegiate sports. Am J Sports Med 8:187–91, 1980.
11. Counsilman JE: The Science of Swimming. Englewood Cliffs, NJ, Prentice–Hall, 1968.
12. DeMers G: Competitive diving and swimming. In: Adams SH, et al (eds): Catastrophic Injuries in Sports: Avoidance Strategies. Salinas, Cal, Coyote Press, 1984, pp 22–37.
13. Dominguez RH: Shoulder pain in age group swimmers. In: Erickson B, Furberg B (eds): Swimming Medicine IV. Baltimore, University Park Press, 1978, pp 105–9.

14. Fechter JD, Kuschnerfkenal SH: The thoracic outlet syndrome. Orthopedics 16:1243–51, 1993.
15. Fowler PJ: Shoulder injuries in the mature athlete. Adv Sports Med Fitness 1:225–38, 1988.
16. Fowler PJ: Swimming. In: Fu FH, Stone DA (eds): Sports Injuries: Mechanisms, Prevention, Treatment. Battimore, Williams & Wilkins, 1994, pp 633–48.
17. Garrick J, Requa R: Injuries in school-aged children. Pediatrics 61:465–9, 1978.
18. Gloviczki P, Kazmier FJ, Hollier LH: Axillary–sub clavian venous occlusion: The morbidity of a nonlethal disease. J Vasc Surg 4:333–7, 1986.
19. Greipp JF: Swimmer's shoulder: The influence of flexibility and weight training. Physician Sportsmed 13:92–105, 1985.
20. Hinton RY: Isokinetic evaluation of the shoulder rotational strength in high school baseball pitchers. Am Sports Med 16:274–9, 1986.
21. Kenal KAF, Knapp LD: Rehabilitation of injuries in competitive swimmers. Sports Med 22(5):337–47, 1996.
22. Kennedy JC, Hawkins RJ: Breaststroker's knee. Physician Sportsmed 2:33, 1974.
23. Kennedy JC, Hawkins RJ: Swimmer's shoulder. Physician Sportsmed 2(4):35, 1974.
24. Kennedy J, Hawkins R, Krissof W: Orthopaedic manifestations of swimming. Am J Sports Med 6:309–22, 1978.
25. Keskinen K, Eriksson E, Limo P: Breaststroke swimmer's knee: A biomechanical and arthroscopic study. Am J Sports Med 8:228–31, 1980.
26. Kimball RJ, Carter RL, Schneider RC. Competitive diving injuries. In: Schneider RC (ed.): Sports Injuries: Mechanisms, Prevention, and Treatment. Baltimore, Williams & Wilkins, 1985, pp 192–211.
27. McConnell J: The management of chondromalacia patella: a long term solution. Austral J Physiother 32:215–23, 1986.
28. McFarland EG, Wasik M: Injuries in female collegieate swimmers due to swimming and cross training. Clin J Sport Med 6(3):178–82, 1996.
29. McMaster WC, Long S, Caiozzo V: Isokinetic torque imbalances in the rotator cuff of the elite water polo player. Am J Sports Med 19:72–5, 1990.
30. McMaster WC, Long S, Caiozzo V: Shoulder torque changes in the swimming athletes.
31. McMaster WC: Assessment of the rotator cuff and a remedial exercise program for the aquatic athlete. In: Miyashita J, Mutoh M, Richardson AB (eds): Medicine and Science in Aquatic Sports, Vol 39. Basel, S. Karge, 1994, pp 213–217.
32. McMaster WC: Glenoid labrum tears in swimmers: a cause of shoulder pain. Am J Sports Med 14:383–7, 1986.
33. McMaster WC: Painful shoulder in swimmers: a diagnostic challenge. Physician Sports med 14:108–22, 1986.
34. McMaster WC, Troup J: A survey of interfering shoulder pain in United States competitive swimmers. Am J Sports Med 21:67–70, 1993.
35. McMaster WC, Roberts A, Stoddard T: A correlation between shoulder laxity and interfering pain in competitive swimmers. Am J Sports Med 26:83–6, 1998.
36. Meyers JF: Arthroscopic management of impingement syndrome and rotator cuff tears. Adv Sports Med Fitness 2:243–60, 1989.
37. Neer CS: Impingement lesions. Clin Orthop Rel Res 173:70–7, 1983.
38. Neer CS, Foster CR: Inferior capsular shift for involuntary and multidirectional instability of the shoulder. J Bone Joint Surg 62A:897–908, 1980.
39. Nermers DW, Thorpe PE, Knibble MA, Beard DW: Upper extremity venous thrombosis. Orthop Rev 19:164–72, 1990.
40. Nuber GW, Jobe FW, Perry J, et al: Fine wire electromyography analysis of muscles of the shoulder during swimming. Am J Sports Med 14(1):7–11, 1986.
41. Pease DC, Cappaert JM, McDonald K, et al: Biomechanical and electromyographical differences between swimmers with injured and non-injured shoulders. Med Sci Sports Exerc 24:S173, 1993.
42. Pink M, Perry J, Browne A, et al: The normal shoulder during freestyle swimming: An electromyographic and cinematographic analysis of twelve muscles. Am J Sports Med 19(6):569–79, 1991.
43. Richardson AB: The biomechanics of swimming: the knee and shoulder. Clin Sports Med 5:103–13, 1986.
44. Richardson AB: Overuse syndrome in baseball, tennis, gymnastics, swimming. Clin Sports Med 2:379–90, 1983.
45. Richardson AB, Jobe FW, Collins WR: The shoulder in competitive swimming. Am J Sports Med 8:159–63, 1980.
46. Rockwood CA, Willows GR, Burkhead WZ: Debridement of degenerative, irreparable lesions of the rotator cuff. J Bone Joint Surg 77A:857–66, 1995.
47. Rodeo S: The butterfly: A kinesiology analysis and strength training program. Natl Strength Condition Assoc J 7(4):4–10;74, 1985.
48. Rodeo S. Swimming the breaststroke—a kinesiological analysis and considerations for strength training. Natl Strength Condition Assoc J 6(4):4–6, 74–76,80, 1984.
49. Rodeo SA: Knee pain in competitive swimming. Clin Sports Med 18(2):379–87, 1999.
50. Rossi F: Spondylolysis, spondylolisthesis and sports. J Sports Med Phys Fitness 18(4):317–40, 1978.
51. Rovere G, Nichols A: Frequency, associated factors, and treatment of breaststroker's knee in competitive swimmers. Am J Sports Med 13:99–104, 1985.
52. Roye RP, Grana WA, Yates CK: Arthroscopic subacromial decompression: two to seven year follow-up. Arthroscopy 11:301–6, 1995.
53. Rubin BD: Injuries in competitive diving. Sports Med Dig 9:1–3, 1987.
54. Rubin BD, Anderson SJ. Diving. In: Cain DJ, Caine CG, Lindner KJ: Champaign, Ill, Human Kinetics Publishers, 1996, pp. 176–85.
55. Rubin BD: The basics of competitive diving and its injuries. Clin Sports Med 18(2):293–303, 1999.
56. Ruwe PA, Pink M, Jobe FW, et al: The normal and the painful shoulder during the breaststroke. Electromyographic and cinematographic analysis of twelve mucles. Am J Sports Med 22(6):789–96, 1994.
57. Schleihouf RE, Grey L, De Rose J: Three dimensional analysis of hand propulsion in the front crawl stroke. In: Hollander AP, Huijung, PA, de Groot, G (eds.): Biomechanics and Medicine in swimming, Vol 14. Champaign, Ill, Human Kinetics Publishers, pp. 173–83.
58. Schleihauf R: Swimming skill: a review of basic theory. J Swim Res 2:11–20, 1986.
59. Schwartz RE, O'Brien SJ, Warren RF: Capsular restraints to anterior-posterior motion of the shoulder. Orthop Trans 12:277, 1988.
60. Stalberg SD, Schulman K, Stuart S, Culp P: Breastroker's knee: pathology, etiology, and treatment. Am J Sports Med 8:164–71, 1980.
61. Stulberg S, Shulman K, Stuart S, et al. Breaststroke's knee: Pathology, etiology, and treatment. Am J Sports Med 8:164–71, 1980.
62. Tibone JE Elrod B, Jobe FW, et al: Surgical treatment of tears of the rotator cuff in athletes. J Bone Joint Surg 68A:887–91, 1986.

63. Turkel SJ, Panio MW, Marshall JL: Stabilizing mechanisms preventing anterior dislocation of the glenohumeral joint. J Bone Joint Surg 63A:1208–17, 1981.

64. Vogel CM, Jensen JE: Thrombosis of the subclavian vein in a competitive swimmer. Am J Sports Med 13–299–72, 1985.

65. Wilk KE, Andrews JR, Arrigo CA: The abductor and adductor strength characteristics of professional baseball pitchers. Am J Sports Med 23:307–11, 1995.

66. Zemak MJ, Magee DJ: Comparison of glenohumeral joint laxity in elite and recreational swimmers. Clin J Sport Med 6(1):40–7, 1996.

Chapter 64

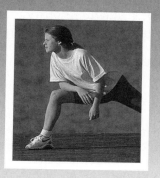

Track and Field

Susan L. Snouse, A.T.C.

The sport of track and field consists of over 20 different events. Track and field is also known as "athletics" to the majority of the world. While each event has its differences, all the track and field events have a running, jumping, or throwing component involved. In comparison to many other sports, most events in track and field require very little additional equipment for competition to take place.

Track or running events are split into different categories: sprints (100-meter, 200-meter, 400-meter), middle distance (800-meter, 1500-meter), distance (3000-meter and longer), hurdles (110-meter, 400-meter), relays (4 × 100-meter, 4 × 400-meter), and race walking (10-km and 20-km for females, 20-km and 50-km for males). Field events involve 2 categories: jumping events (high jump, long jump, triple jump, pole vault) and throwing events (discus, hammer throw, javelin, shot put).

Track events take place on a 400-meter oval track (except for distances greater than 10 km) in a counterclockwise direction. Field events take place in the infield of the track. Field events often take place prior to the running events to decrease the chance of injury by a throwing implement.

With the large number of participants and the simultaneous but diverse events, the sport of track and field can be a challenge for the sports medicine professional to cover. Track and field athletes present with a wide range of injuries and illnesses.

HISTORY OF TRACK AND FIELD

Track and field is one of the oldest sports known to civilization.[20] Track and field is also one of the original and most popular of Olympic sports. The Greeks introduced the sport of track and field as a method to train their soldiers by turning physical training into sport competi-

tions.[6] Track and field consists of elements needed for military maneuvers: running, jumping, and throwing.[1] These movements are among the most fundamental and natural activities known to humans.

Dominated by males for centuries, it wasn't until 1891 that the first female running event was recorded.[7] In the 1896 Olympic Games, a female entered the marathon under the pseudonym of Melpomene and finished the then 24-mile event in 4 hours and 30 minutes.[7,12]

Females made their official Olympic track and field debut in the 1928 Olympic Games.[7,12] Five events were held: 100-meter, 800-meter, 4 × 100-meter relay, high jump, and discus throw. Several females collapsed at the end of the 800-meter race, although whether this was due to heat or lack of fitness is debated.[7,12] Regardless, the International Olympic Committee (IOC) felt it was dangerous for females to run long distances and events longer than 200 meters were prohibited for females until the 1960 Olympic Games.[12] It was not until the 1972 Olympic Games that a track event over 800 meters was added.

The women's marathon was added to the Olympic Games in 1984. That race is notable for Joan Benoit's outstanding winning performance. However, many individuals remember that race because of the slow, stumbling finish of Gabriel Anderson-Scheiss and her subsequent collapse at the finish line. Her collapse was due to heat exhaustion, but it prompted many in the general public to question the ability of women to participate in long-distance running. Fortunately, this athlete suffered no permanent injury from her heat illness, and she joined the medical and scientific community in educating the general public about the hazards of heat illnesses and the techniques that can be used to prevent such problems.

In the past, there was a significant gender gap in the number of track and field events held at the Olympics. This gap narrowed during the 1990s, and by 1996, males competed in 24 Olympic track and field events and females in 20 events. With the addition of the hammer throw and pole vault for females in the 2000 Olympic Games, the gender gap has neared equality in Olympic track and field.

SPORT INFORMATION FOR TRACK AND FIELD

There is a great deal of repetitious movement in all the events of track and field. The runners, jumpers, and throwers all train by constantly practicing the demanding skills of their event in the quest of perfect technique. This repetition contributes to the great number of overuse injuries seen in track and field athletes.

Except for 3 throwing events (discus, hammer, shot put), running or race walking is involved in some aspect of each track and field event. The running gait is a sequence of stance, swing, and float phases that occur 800 to 1500 times per mile.[15,22] A force of 2 to 5 times body weight is experienced by the foot and that force is transferred up the kinetic chain.[5,14-16,22] As the speed of gait increases, the stance phase decreases in length while the swing phase and float phase increase. The float phase occurs in fast running when neither foot is in contact with the ground.[22]

The stance phase consists of foot strike, mid support, and take-off.[22] Foot strike usually occurs at the posterolateral aspect of the heel.[14] At this point, the foot is a rigid lever and the tibia is externally rotated. As the foot makes contact, the calcaneus everts and the transverse tarsal joints unlock, causing the foot to become more flexible and to pronate for shock absorption.[16,22]

The swing phase involves follow-through, forward swing, and foot descent.[22] On the forward swing, as the swing leg passes the stance leg, external rotation of the stance pelvis occurs. This external rotation causes inversion on the calcaneus, which locks the transverse tarsal joint. The rigid lever of the foot is necessary for propulsion.

Running speed is a function of stride length and stride frequency. Stride length is determined by the athlete's leg length, muscle strength, and running mechanics. Stride frequency is a function of the athlete's leg length, genetic factors, and training.[8] Running styles differ with the different events. Foot strike occurs for sprinters at their toes, while distance runners have foot strike at their heel or mid-foot.

Jump events all have an approach, take-off, flight, and landing phase. In the approach, the athlete sprints down a runway to provide the velocity needed for a powerful take-off. With jumps, the athlete continuously moves her body with muscular effort while striving for greatest distance or height.[9] It is often in the landing phase that the athlete is at risk for serious injury.

The throwing events have 2 phases, launch and flight. The launch phase involves moving the body with the purpose of a forceful release of the implement. The airborne trajectory of the implement is the flight phase.[9] No matter what implement is being thrown, an athlete must contend with gravity on every throw.[9]

The running surface of a track can also affect performance. A variety of different surfaces are found in track facilities, including synthetic material, cinders, gravel, and even asphalt. The synthetic surfaces are mandatory for elite competitions. Sprinters prefer that surfaces be hard to achieve faster times. Distance runners prefer a softer track that provides more shock absorption. One concern with synthetic tracks is the amount of heat they absorb. This additional heat can contribute to heat illnesses suffered by athletes and officials.

Several environmental factors can affect track and field performances. These include wind speed (a tailwind improves running times, whereas a headwind hinders running times) and air density (increased altitude can improve sprint times and distances for jumps).[21] Sprinters and jumpers like to compete in warm temperatures because the heat gives them the feeling of being extra "loose" and warmed-up prior to their event. For comfort and avoidance of heat illnesses, distance runners prefer cooler temperatures.

The sprint events (100- to 400-meter) require fast reactions, explosive starts, and sustained top speed through the entire race. Anaerobic power and strong musculature are important for sprinters. The use of blocks, staying in the lane, and a crouched start are requirements for sprinting.[23] It is often in the sprint events that acute muscle strains occur, particularly strains of the hamstring muscles.

Not only must the middle-distance runners have a solid aerobic base, but they must also train their anaerobic system for the harsh pace. Many of the elite athletes competing in the 800-meter event now consider it a long sprint. Blocks are not used and lane restrictions are only in effect for the first lap of the race. With fewer lane restrictions, however, contact can occur between the runners. Injuries from this contact can include spike wounds in the lower leg or multiple contusions and/or abrasions from falls. Overuse injuries tend to be the most common injuries in middle-distance runners.

Distance runners train to improve their aerobic thresholds, as 75% to 90% of the energy used is produced aerobically.[8] The elite distance runner must also be able to sprint at any point, thus anaerobic training is necessary. Overuse injuries, including stress fractures, and environmental factors are concerns in these events.

The hurdle events combine sprinting with the clearing of 10 hurdles over 2 distances. Timing and flexibility are critical in this event.[20] The athletes often have to be able to switch lead legs. Hurdlers experience overuse injuries to the lower extremity, contusions from hitting the hurdle with their trail leg, and abrasions from falls.

Relays involve 4 runners handing off a baton over 2 distances. The shorter relay (4 × 100-meter) has a blind exchange of the baton, and this is where most mistakes happen. The 3 relay exchanges must occur in a passing zone that is 20 meters long or a disqualification occurs.[23] Hand injuries, including lacerations, contusions, and sprains, do occur with the exchanges.

The race-walking athlete must have foot contact with the ground at all times (heel of advancing foot must touch before the rear foot lifts) and the knee must be straightened. With this technique, the hip abductors and adductors are used, contributing to the event's unique form. Overuse injuries develop, particularly in the Achilles tendon and the posterior knee.

In the high jump, the athlete must take off from one foot but there are several acceptable forms for going over the bar. The best-known method, the Fosbery flop, has the athlete planting the foot, rotating the body, and going backward over the bar. Head and cervical spinal injuries can occur with improper landing or if the athlete misses the landing pads.

The long jump involves a sprint, a foot plant, and a forward leap as far as possible into a sand pit. In the long jump and triple jump, fouls are called if the athlete steps past a line on the take-off. A putty-like substance called plasticine is placed directly beyond this line to mark any fouls. One should be aware that the plasticine could provide a soft surface for the athlete's spike to get caught in and cause a lower leg injury.

The triple jump involves 3 interdependent jumps in one sequence. The athlete must be an excellent sprinter and have great rebound ability. As in the long jump, there is considerable

stress on the joints of the lower extremities and overuse injuries, such as patellar tendinitis and acute ankle sprains from awkward landings, occur.

The pole vault is a spectacular event that involves sprinting down a runway while carrying a fiberglass pole. This pole gets planted in a box at the base of the pit. The athlete is vaulted into the air and lands on a mat past the bar. Catastrophic injuries can occur if the pole breaks, the athlete errs on the pole plant, or in the landing.[20]

Discus involves approximately 2 body spins and then a powerful release of an aerodynamic disc. All throwing events involve the risk of serious injury for spectators and others if a throw is mishandled. Female throwing implements are lighter than those required for male participants. Discus athletes often suffer overuse injuries of the upper extremity.

Hammer is the most technically challenging of the throwing events. The weight is attached via a wire cable to a handle that the athlete releases after a repetitive rotary motion. A large wire cage is necessary for the protection of fellow athletes and spectators. The hammer event is often held at a different location than the rest of the track and field events because of the space needs as well as the problems that may occur on the infield on the impact of the hammer. Besides upper extremity overuse injuries, the rotary component of the hammer throw can cause lumbar and thoracic injuries.

In the javelin throw, a foul occurs if the athlete crosses the foul line or if any part of the javelin except the tip strikes the ground. The javelin athlete is allowed a run-up and performs a crossover maneuver prior to the throw. With the run-up and one-sided nature of the sport, upper and lower extremity injuries are possible.

With the shot put, the athlete may only use one hand to throw the implement. The athlete may use an explosive squat/thrust motion or a spin motion similar to what is used in the discus to propel a heavy metal ball. As with other throwing events, a foul is called if the athlete's foot touches the circle or falls outside of the circle. Technique errors and the explosiveness of the throw can cause trunk as well as upper or lower extremity injuries.

The multi-events are the decathlon (10 events) for males and the heptathlon (7 events) for females. These events are spread out over 2 days, rotating running, throwing, and jumping events. The athlete is scored in each event and the overall point leader wins. Because of the high volume of work needed for these events, overuse injuries are common. Traumatic injuries in the multi-events are similar to what one would see in individual events (eg, ankle sprains in the long jump take-off or landing).

PHYSIOLOGIC CHARACTERISTICS OF TRACK AND FIELD

While trained male runners have between 4% and 10% body fat, trained female runners have 12% to 18% body fat.[7,24] This additional body fat places a higher demand on the female's oxygen transportation system. Conversely, this additional body fat is thought to provide additional energy stores for females in road events such as the ultramarathon (races longer than 26 miles).

Maximum oxygen consumption (VO_2max) values in elite female athletes are 16% to 25% lower than those in elite males.[7,17] Male elite runners also have a greater heart volume than elite female runners.[7] Male and female runners have similar lower extremity strength when using lean body mass as the measure. However, male runners have significantly more upper body strength than female runners. Upper body strength is especially important in the sprint events[7] and throwing events.

Compared to males, females tend to have narrower shoulder girdles, a wider pelvis, shorter bones that are less dense, larger Q angles, a lower center of gravity, and greater genu valgus.[7,11,24] The female's wider pelvis, weaker thigh musculature, and greater Q angle is thought to place greater stress on the knee, lower leg, and ankle.[7]

ORTHOPAEDIC AND MEDICAL CONCERNS IN TRACK AND FIELD

Epidemiology of Injury

Knutzen and Hart reviewed the epidemiology of running injuries and found many of the studies were limited to a specific population (marathon and road runners), did not separate level of experience or gender, and frequently had weak data collection methods. In the few studies on running injuries in which Knutzen and Hart did find separate gender data, it appeared that males and females had similar annual injury incidence rates, with the rate for males ranging from 49% to 52% and that for females ranging from 46% to 49%.[15] Colliton reported that the overall incidence of injuries in female runners was no greater than that in male runners.[7]

In a review study on injuries in field events, Alexander did not find a study looking only at field events but did find studies that combined field with track injuries. Alexander summarized that 4 out of every 5 injuries occurred during a track event rather then a field event and that the pole vault was the field event with the highest risk of injury.[1]

Few studies focused on the elite track and field athlete. The author reviewed the USOC medical records for the 1992 Olympic Games. The 1992 US Olympic Track and Field team data were chosen because the author had been one of the assigned personnel for providing medical coverage to this team. At the 1992 Olympic Games, a total of 625 US athletes competed. One hundred and twenty-three members, or 19.7%, of this delegation were track and field athletes. Figure 64-1 shows the gender breakdown of this team.

A total of 930 injury and illness evaluations were recorded within the US delegation (580 injuries and 350 illnesses). The evaluations were classified as follows: 30% lower extremity injuries, 13% upper extremity injuries, 19% other injuries, and 38% illnesses (Fig. 64-2). The top 3 illnesses involved the upper respiratory tract, gastrointestinal tract, and skin. For the track and field athletes, a total of 106 injury and illness evaluations (or 11% of the total evaluations) were recorded. The track and field evaluations were classified as follows: 49% lower extremity injuries (male, 29; female, 23), 5% upper extremity injuries (male, 3; female, 2), 20% other injuries (male, 11; female, 10), and 26% illnesses (male, 10; female, 18). Figure 64-3 shows this breakdown. Considering the nature of track and field, it is not surprising that a higher percentage of lower extremity injuries occurred in these athletes compared to the rest of the delegation.

Finally, the 106 evaluations were broken down into gender-specific injuries and illnesses (male injuries, 43; male illnesses, 10; female injuries, 35; female illnesses, 18; Fig. 64-4). Despite being fewer in number, the female track and field athletes had a larger number of illnesses compared to the male track and field athletes. Future research is needed to assess gender differences in track and field athletes, as well as in athletes in other sports.

Footwear

There is no single shoe that fits all the needs of the sport of track and field. The different events require different shoes; a runner in a track and field meet would use a lightweight, flexible shoe with spikes, while a thrower might use a heavier, rigid hightop shoe with spikes.[14] Many world-

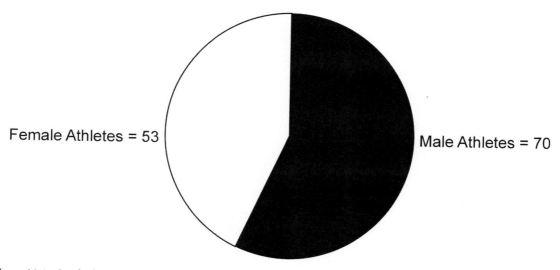

Figure 64-1. Gender breakdown of the 1992 US Olympic Track and Field Team — (123 athletes).

class sprinters have their shoes molded to their individual foot and will wear these custom-built spikes for only one or two races. Spikes are designed to provide additional grip or traction on the track and are for short-term use only. Spikes do not give the support or shock absorption needed for heavy training. Spikes that do not fit properly or that are worn too long increase the risk of lower extremity injury. Training flats or traditional running shoes are used for daily training of a track and field athlete. Athletes and the general public need to be aware that these shoes quickly lose their shock

absorption and, regardless of external appearance, should be replaced every 250 to 500 miles.[14,22]

As important as picking the appropriate model for their event, each athlete needs to pick shoes that meet their anatomic needs. An athlete with pes planus (Fig. 64-5) overpronates. Pronators should pick shoes that have a straight or combination last for the control and stability it can provide.[14] An athlete with pes cavus (Fig. 64-6) has a high arch and an inflexible foot, and supinates. Supinators should choose a shoe with a curved or semicurved last for its shock absorp-

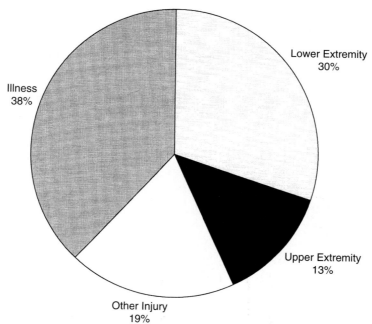

Figure 64-2. Injury or illness percentage breakdown for the 1992 US Olympic Team, total delegation—(625 athletes).

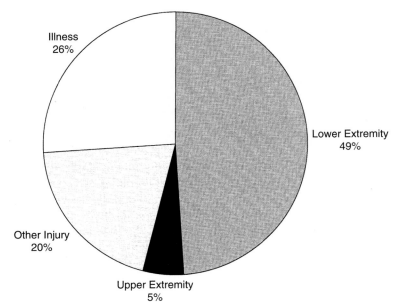

Figure 64-3. Injury or illness percentage breakdown for the 1992 US Olympic Team, track and field delegation—(123 athletes).

tion and flexibility.[14] Orthotics are often extolled as a runner's savior from injuries. An orthotic is defined by Hunter, Dolan, and Davis as "a device that is placed in a person's shoe to reduce or eliminate pathological stresses to the foot or other portions of the lower kinetic chain."[10] If an individual has anatomic abnormalities, orthotics should be used only if the individual has accompanying symptoms of pain.

There are 3 types of orthotics available: rigid, semirigid, and soft. The rigid orthotics are made of a hard plastic material and are designed to provide complete motion control. The rigidity frequently makes athletic participation difficult.

Semirigid orthotics use a combination of materials such as plastics, foams, and cork. Semirigid orthotics are commonly used in athletic participation because they provide moderate motion control with shock absorption. Soft orthotics are made of a viscoelastic material called Sorbothane, felt, or foam. They are designed for providing shock absorption, protection of soft tissue, and minor motion control.[10,22]

Illness and Injury

Illnesses affecting track and field athletes can include upper respiratory tract infections, asthma,

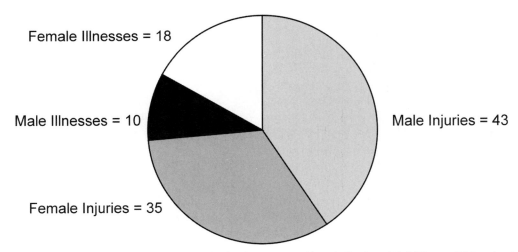

Figure 64-4. Injury and illness breakdown by gender for the 1992 US Olympic Track and Field Team—(106 evaluations).

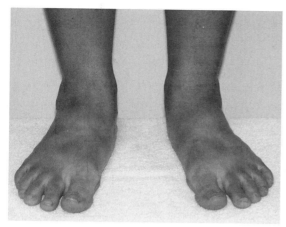

Figure 64-5. Athlete with pes planus.

gastrointestinal illnesses, and diarrhea.[20] Because track and field athletes are exposed to the environment, they are subject to cold or heat illnesses. Fluid replacement should be strongly encouraged in these athletes.

Many female track and field athletes, particularly distance runners, will attempt to decrease their body weight in the hope of improving performance.[13] Resulting disordered eating patterns and the athlete's intense training may contribute to an energy-deficit state and the development of the female athlete triad. As many as 50% of competitive athletes may be amenorrheic.[7] In addition to the potential hazard of menstrual dysfunction on the skeleton, female athletes should be informed that the absence of menstruation is not an effective form of contraception.

In elite track and field events, there has been a great deal of media attention about the positive drug tests that have occurred since 1988. Anabolic steroids have been the pharmaceutical class most often abused. Anabolic steroids and certain other medications have been banned

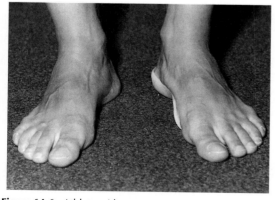

Figure 64-6. Athlete with pes cavus.

by the IOC, the US Olympic Committee (USOC), and the National Collegiate Athletic Association. The status of any medication can be checked by calling the USOC Drug Education Hotline at (800) 233-0393.

The personnel providing medical coverage of a track and field meet should "think prevention." Heat illnesses may be prevented by ensuring adequate supplies of fluids are present and easily accessible to the athletes and officials. In addition, holding practices and competitions during times of day during lowest heat and humidity is imperative. Having sponges or ice towels available for distance runners is helpful. Injuries from throwing implements can be avoided by using safe cages and a large, open throwing field, and announcing when field events are taking place over the public address system. Delay in provision of medical attention to stricken athletes is prevented by having a central medical tent and also dispersing medical staff members at specific sites on the track. The most common treatments that the athletes will request are assistance with stretching, massage, and ice.

As stated previously, overuse injuries are common in track and field because of the repetitive motions. Acute injuries can also occur either from maximal muscle contraction[1] or mishaps in the field events, such as sprained ankle in a long jump take-off or cervical spine trauma in a pole vault landing.

Training errors are the frequent culprit in track and field injuries. A common rule for training, especially in running, is never to increase the workload by more than 10% a week. Training errors can include any of the following: increasing mileage, abrupt increase frequency and/or intensity training on a hard or different surface, consistently running in one direction or on a banked surface, excessive hill training, or training in worn-out or improper shoes. Runners are often extremely inflexible. A proper warm-up and cool-down should be encouraged, as well as a quality stretching program.

The majority of running and jumping injuries involve the lower extremities, while throwers' injuries often involve the upper extremities and trunk.[1] Knutzen and Hart found that the most frequent injury (12.7% to 29.5%) in runners was to the knee.[15] Female runners report more complaints of patellofemoral pain, and appear to have a higher incidence of stress fractures and medial tibial stress syndrome than male runners,[15,22] although the increased incidence of stress fractures in females is more evident in military studies than has been demonstrated in the athletic population.[4,18]

Specific types of injuries seen in the lower extremity include blisters, callosities, sesamoiditis, Morton's neuroma, plantar fascitis, Achilles tendinitis, medial tibial stress syndrome (shin splints), stress fractures, muscle strains, patellofemoral stress syndrome, popliteal tendinitis and iliotibial band syndrome.[2,3,18]

Stress fractures are of particular importance to females. Contributing risk factors to stress fractures include low bone density, menstrual dysfunction, disordered eating, faulty biomechanics, prior fracture history, and training errors.[3,18,19] For females, common sites of stress fractures include the tibia, metatarsals, fibula, navicular, femoral tarsal neck, and, less commonly, the sacrum and the pubic bone.

Trunk injuries can include sprains, strains, spondylolysis, sacroiliac dysfunction, and fractures from improper landing in the jump events. Upper extremity injuries include shoulder impingement, rotator cuff strains, bicipital tendinitis, medial epicondylitis, and wrist and finger strains or tendinitis.

CONCLUDING REMARKS

Track and field involves a wide assortment of activities that often take place concurrently. While many injuries seen in track and field are related to overuse, acute injuries do occur. Of concern in the field events are inadvertent contact with a throwing implement and, in the jumping events, a fall. The medical staff must be aware of the potentially catastrophic results of an implement striking or spearing an athlete, official, or spectator. Other factors causing injuries include environmental concerns, anatomic structure, and training errors. Female track athletes are at risk for patellofemoral stress syndrome, stress fractures, and other overuse injuries. Special attention to nutritional and hormonal factors and bone health concerns is imperative. Further study is needed to assess medical and orthopaedic concerns in female athletes participating in track and field, as well as outcome studies to assess prevention and treatment strategies for common problems in this population.

References

1. Alexander MJL. Injuries in field events. In Caine D, Caine C, Lindner KJ (eds): Epidemiology of Sports Injuries. Champaign, Ill, Human Kinetics, 1996.
2. Bennell KL, Bruckner PD: Epidemiology and site specificity of stress fractures. Clin Sports Med 16:179-96, 1997.
3. Bennell KL, Malcolm SA, Thomas SA, et al: Risk factors for stress fractures in female track and field athletes: A retrospective analysis. Clin J Sports Med 5:229–35, 1995.
4. Bennell KL, Malcolm SA, Thomas SA, et al: The incidence and distribution of stress fractures in competitive track and field athletes: A twelve month prospective study. Am J Sports Med 24(2):211–7, 1996.
5. Caborn DNM, Grollman LJ, Nyland JA, Brosky T: Running. In Fu FH, Stone DA (eds): Sports Injuries: Mechanisms, Prevention, Treatment. Baltimore, Williams & Wilkins, 1994, pp 565–89.
6. Ciullo JV, Shapiro JD. Track and field. In Fu FH, Stone DA (eds): Sports Injuries: Mechanisms, Prevention, Treatment. Baltimore, Williams & Wilkins, 1994, pp 649–77.
7. Colliton JW: Running. In: Agostini R, Titus S (eds): Medical and Orthopedic Issues of Active and Athletic Women. Philadelphia, Hanley & Belfus, 1994, pp 406–18.
8. Derse E, Stolley S (eds): AAF/CIF Cross Country Coaching Manual. Los Angeles, Health For Life Publishers, 1994, pp 59–88.
9. Hubbard M: The throwing events in track and field. In: Vaughan CL (ed): Biomechanics of Sport. Boca Raton, Fla: CRC Press, 1989, pp 214–37.
10. Hunter S, Dolan MG, Davis JM: Foot Orthotics in Therapy and Sport. Champaign, Ill, Human Kinetics, 1995, pp 1–9.
11. Hutchinson MR, Ireland ML: Knee injuries in female athletes. Sports Med 19(4):288–302, 1995.
12. Jaffe R: History of women in sports. In: Agostini R, Titus S (eds): Medical and Orthopedic Issues of Active and Athletic Women. Philadelphia, Hanley & Belfus, 1994, pp 1–5.
13. Johnson MD: Disordered eating. In: In: Agostini R, Titus S (eds): Medical and Orthopedic Issues of Active and Athletic Women. Philadelphia, Hanley & Belfus, 1994, pp 141–51.
14. Kelly PJ: Athletic footwear. In: Street SA, Runkle D (eds): Athletic Protective Equipment: Care, Selection and Fitting. Boston, McGraw Hill, 2000, pp 59–76.
15. Knutzen K, Hart L: Epidemiology of running injuries. In Caine D, Caine C, Lindner KJ (eds): Epidemiology of Sports Injuries. Champaign, Ill, Human Kinetics, 1996.
16. Mann RA: Biomechanics of running. In: D'Ambrosia RD, Drez D Jr (eds): Prevention and Treatment of Running Injuries, 2nd edition. Thorofare, NJ, Slack, 1989, pp 1–20.
17. Micheli L: Female runners. In: D'Ambrosia RD, Drez D Jr (eds): Prevention and Treatment of Running Injuries, 2nd edition. Thorofare, NJ, Slack, 1989, pp 199–208.
18. Nattiv A: Stress fractures and bone health in track and field athletes. J Sci Med Sport 3(3):267–78, 2000.
19. Otis CL: Stress fractures in athletes. In: Agostini R, Titus S (eds): Medical and Orthopedic Issues of Active and Athletic Women. Philadelphia, Hanley & Belfus, 1994, pp 325–32.
20. Otis CL: Track and field. In: Agostini R, Titus S (eds): Medical and Orthopedic Issues of Active and Athletic Women. Philadelphia, Hanley & Belfus, 1994, pp 455–8.
21. Putnam CA, Kozey JW: Substantive issues in running. In Vaughan CL (ed): Biomechanics of Sport. Boca Raton, Fla: CRC Press, 1989, pp 1–33.
22. Reid DC: Sports Injury Assessment and Rehabilitation. New York, Churchill Livingstone, 1992, pp 1131–58.
23. Track & Field News: Big Red Book. Mountain View, Calif, T&FN Press, 1995, pp 84–96.
24. Wells CL: Women, Sport & Performance: A Physiological Perspective. Champaign, Ill, Human Kinetics, 1985, pp 3–18.

Chapter 65

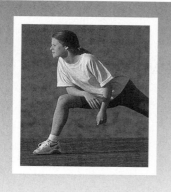

Volleyball

William W. Briner, M.D., FACSM
Holly J. Benjamin, M.D., FAAP

In recent decades, the sport of volleyball has become truly international. In fact, according to the Federation Internationale de Volleyball (FIVB), volleyball's international federation, there are 800 million players worldwide, which would make it the world's most popular participation sport. Perhaps the basis of this popularity is that it can be played and enjoyed by individuals of all ages and skill levels. As many as 130 countries play volleyball, but only 50 countries acknowledge the sport as a major one. In the United States, the vast majority of competitive players, especially at the younger age levels, are female.

HISTORY

Volleyball was invented in 1895 by William G. Morgan, the physical education director for the YMCA in Massachusetts. His goal was to create a game that would be less stressful than basketball on the bodies of young men, yet still be enjoyable and competitive, and keep them fit. Originally, the game was called *mintonette*, but it was renamed *volleyball* several years later by Alfred T. Halstead of Springfield College in Massachusetts. Although it was invented in the United States, some of the best volleyball teams at the world level currently are European, Asian, and South American. At this elite level, volleyball is a highly competitive, explosive sport where a spiked ball may travel at up to 90 mph.

Volleyball has a long Olympic history. It has been contested since 1964 in Tokyo on indoor hard-court surfaces. The 1996 Olympics in Atlanta marked the first time that there were 2 different volleyball competitions. Both men and women competed indoors on 6-player teams and outdoors on 2-player teams on the sand. Sand volleyball originated on the beaches of Southern

California. This 2-person game was first played competitively in the 1960s. Since this sport grew in popularity in the United States and internationally throughout the 1990s, sand volleyball was introduced into the Olympics as a full medal sport in Atlanta without having previously been a demonstration sport.

OVERVIEW

Sport-Specific Skills

In general, all of the players on a volleyball court engage in each of the various sport-specific skills during the course of a game. These skills have varying risks of injury. Play is always initiated with the serve, during which the player usually tosses the ball into the air, then strikes it with the hand overhead (Fig. 65-1). Until recently, most players served with both feet on the ground. However, the jump serve gives teams an advantage to score points and has become more popular. Recreational players may be more likely to utilize an underhand serve. After the serve, the opposing team attempts to bump or "pass" the ball (Fig. 65-2). This skill is almost always performed with the elbows extended and the hands below the waist. Next, the ball is typically "set." In setting, the ball is played with the fingertips of both hands simultaneously and directed toward the net, where it can be hit or spiked by a teammate. In volleyball injury surveys, the skills of serving, passing, and setting have not been associated with high numbers of injuries.[7,8,15,27,28,33,34]

The act of "spiking" or attacking the ball is quite similar to an overhead throwing motion (Fig. 65-3). When spiking, the player jumps high into the air and contacts the ball at the highest point of her jump. There is a cocking period just prior to the point of contact when

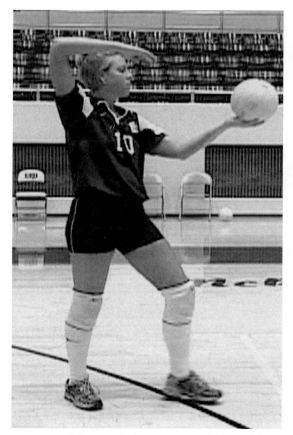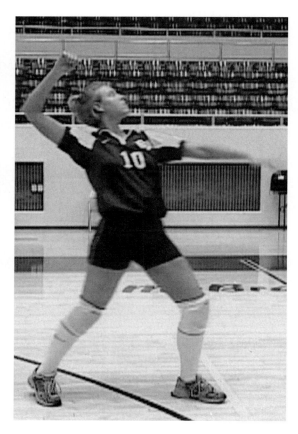

Figure 65-1. The serve initiates play. Arm, body, and foot position for the early part of the serve.

the shoulder is abducted and externally rotated with the elbow flexed. Then, as the ball is contacted, there is a forceful forward flexion and internal rotation of the shoulder with concurrent elbow extension. This skill has been associated with a fairly high incidence of injury.[8,15,27,33,34]

Players on the opposing team will attempt to block a spike by reaching over the net with their hands overhead while their shoulders are maximally forward flexed. Blockers attempt to force the ball back onto the hitter's side within the boundaries of the court. Blocking has been associated with the highest rate of injury in volleyball injury surveys.[7,8,15,27,33]

If the ball is spiked past the block, the blocking team must bump or "dig" the ball. The object is to keep it from touching the ground. Often the player is required to move quickly. Sometimes it is even necessary to dive to play the ball up into the air (Fig. 65-4). Defense has been associated with a small number of volleyball injuries.[8,15,28,34]

Divisions Within the Sport of Volleyball (Levels of Play)

Most volleyball players are involved in the game occasionally at a recreational level, or they may play more frequently in leagues that are sanctioned locally. Players who are more serious may wish to join USA Volleyball, which is the national governing body for the sport in this country. Leagues and tournaments are sanctioned by USA Volleyball on indoor hard courts and outdoors on grass and sand. Young players who wish to play competitively often join volleyball clubs and play in amateur junior tournaments. Interscholastic competition usually starts at the level of high school. Almost all high schools field volleyball teams for girls. Historically, boys' high school volleyball has been more popular on the West Coast, but recently, it has begun to be offered at the varsity level in high schools across the United States. Players who excel in high school may have the option of playing intercollegiate volleyball. Beyond this level, there is the United States National Team for men and

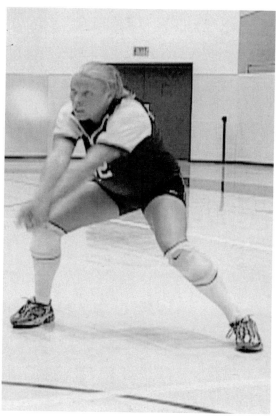

Figure 65-2. The receiving team bumps or "passes" the shot. The pass is performed with elbows extended and hands below the waist.

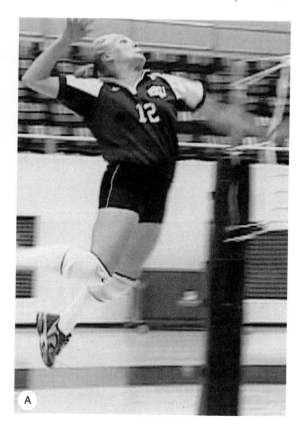

A

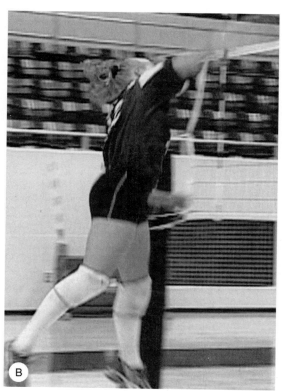

B

Figure 65-3A,B. When spiking the ball, a player jumps high into the air and contacts the ball at the highest point of her jump playing at the net.

women. There have also been professional indoor leagues for elite women players in some European countries, Japan, and the United States.

Professional beach volleyball began to flourish in the early and mid-1990s. There have been professional tours during the summer for men and women in the United States with tournaments in cities across the country. The Association of Volleyball Professionals (AVP) has been the governing body for men at this level in the United States. The Women's Professional Volleyball Association (WPVA) has been the national governing body for women's professional beach volleyball. At this high level 2 players cover a sand court that is the same size as an indoor court on which 6 players play. Since this is the division of the sport that offers the most prize money, most players feel that this is the highest level of competition in volleyball. The FIVB also sanctions professional 2-on-2 beach tournaments for men and women. There has been a professional 4-on-4 sand volleyball tournament for men and women as well.

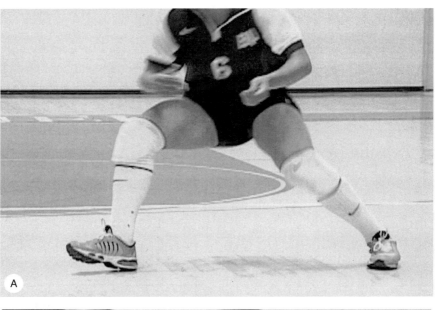

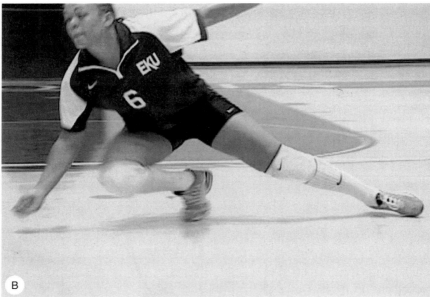

Figure 65-4A,B. Defense or "digging" may involve rapid lateral movements.

Comparisons With Other Sports

Comparing injury data between sports (and even among different studies of the same sport) is often difficult because different definitions of injury are utilized in different studies. However, it seems that the frequent jumping inherent in the sport of volleyball may be particularly risky.[7,8,15] A Dutch study of school children who participated in athletics found that those who played sports with a high "jump rate" were much more likely to be injured. Volleyball also had the highest injury rate of all sports analyzed in this population during practice.[1] Another study reviewed the rehabilitation records of 106 patients who were treated for volleyball injuries. Jumping and landing were associated with a significant majority (63%) of those injuries.[15]

Overuse injury to the dominant shoulder of volleyball players is quite common. It may be that volleyball players are particularly at risk for the forces that cause impingement since they strike the ball at a position of maximal shoulder abduction. This action is somewhat similar to a tennis serve, however, hitters in volleyball perform huge numbers of repetitions of this skill, and the ball is much heavier than a tennis ball.

Unlike most sports, volleyball is contested on several different surfaces. There is some evidence that injury is less likely on softer surfaces. An analysis of patellar tendinitis found this condition to be less common among players who played on wood surfaces than among those who played on harder concrete or linoleum.[12] Elite college players also reported 5-fold fewer injuries per hour on sand than on wood surfaces.[8] There is little data available with respect to volleyball injuries on grass surfaces.

Unique Risks of Volleyball

Injuries that are common and specific to this sport are discussed elsewhere in the chapter, as are gender-specific implications for injury. If there is one aspect of volleyball that makes players particularly susceptible to injury, it is probably the frequent jumping that occurs with competing and practicing. The most common injuries in the acute setting are the ankle sprain, which typically occurs when landing from a jump, and patellar tendinitis, or "jumper's knee," from overuse.

Volleyball players as a group are particularly committed to jump training. This training may involve a variety of techniques, including plyometrics or "drop jumps" from a platform above the landing surface followed by an immediate springing upward. This type of training has been demonstrated to increase vertical jump height.[5] When performed correctly in a setting with adequate instruction, plyometrics probably do not increase the risk of patellar tendinitis.[10,12] However, many players report that their tendinitis becomes symptomatic with jump training,[7,8] and it may be possible to identify players at particular risk for this injury. Patellar tendinitis has been found to be more common in those who play or train more than 4 times weekly, those in the age range of 20 to 25, and those who have been involved in volleyball from 2 to 5 years.[12]

Participants

As noted above, there may be as many as 800 million volleyball players worldwide. According to USA Volleyball, there were 34.1 million players in this country in 1998, of whom 122,968 players were registered with USA Volleyball, and 65% of these were junior players less than age 18. With respect to interscholastic competition, in 1998 there were 12,896 high schools that offered varsity girls volleyball to 370,957 participants. In 1998, volleyball was the third most popular sport for girls behind basketball and track and field. For this same year there were 1441 high schools offering boys' varsity volleyball to 32,375 participants. Volleyball was the 11th most popular sport for high school boys in 1998.

At the intercollegiate level, 920 schools offered volleyball for women, while only 68 colleges and universities played men's varsity volleyball in 1998, according to the NCAA. At the NCAA division I level, women's programs may offer 12 scholarships to varsity volleyball players, and men's programs may offer 4.5 scholarships to varsity players. There were 294 schools offering 3528 scholarships for women and 22 schools offering 99 scholarships for men in 1998. It is readily apparent that the vast majority of scholarship volleyball players are female.

Rules Considerations

The rule in volleyball that has the most direct impact on injuries is the center line rule (Fig. 65-5). The center line is a line immediately beneath the net in indoor volleyball that separates the 2 sides of the court. Players from one side may not cross this line during play. However, a player is judged to have violated the center line only if her foot is entirely across the line. If any portion of the foot makes contact with the line, then no violation has occurred, and play continues. The majority of ankle sprains are inversion injuries that occur in this attack zone. Most often, a blocker lands on the foot of a spiker from the opposing team whose foot has come partially under the net.[3]

A study was undertaken in Norway to analyze the effect of a change in the center line rule in the interest of decreasing ankle sprains. Basically, the rule was changed such that any portion of the foot coming in contact with the line would be judged as a violation (Fig. 65-6). Unfortunately, when the rule change was tested in exhibition tournament play, it was felt that there was an unacceptably high number of game interruptions because of the change[2] and the study was stopped before it could be implemented on a wider scale. However, these investigators were able to demonstrate a significant decrease in ankle sprains by utilizing the "new rule" during practice.[2] This would almost certainly be a reasonable recommendation during practice for all indoor teams.

GENDER-SPECIFIC IMPLICATIONS FOR INJURY

Volleyball players are not immune to the risk factors for injury that affect all female athletes.

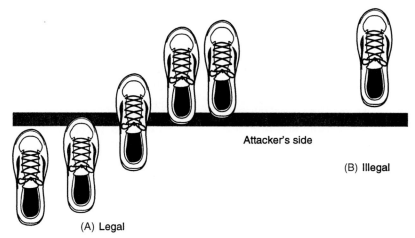

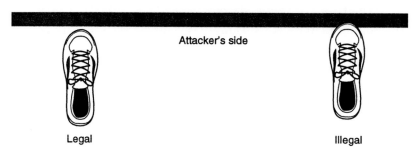

Figure 65-5. Current center line rule. **(A)** A player's foot landing in contact with the center line in any of the positions shown is legal, according to volleyball rules. **(B)** The foot must be entirely across the line to be judged illegal.

Figure 65-6. New center line rule. If a player's foot makes any contact with the center line, this is a violation of the rule.

While the female athlete triad has not been seen frequently among volleyball players, thin, osteoporotic women may place themselves at increased risk for lower extremity stress fractures because of the high frequency of jumping in volleyball. Stress fractures in volleyball players are almost always season-ending injuries. Team physicians who care for volleyball athletes should keep the female athlete triad in mind when performing preparticipation physical examinations.

There is some suspicion that anterior cruciate ligament (ACL) injury is more common among female than male volleyball players. This has certainly been suspected by coaches, and has been reported on in the lay volleyball literature.[22] The only large series of ACL injuries in volleyball players in the sports medicine literature reported on 52 injuries among higher-level Italian players.[11] Some of these injuries also involved the menisci, and all of these injuries were season ending. The vast majority of injuries in this series occurred with landing from a jump in the attack zone. The demographics of the population from which this series was recorded were not well defined. However, it is interesting to note that there are more male volleyball players in Italy than there are female players. Prospective data on ACL injury per exposure to volleyball competition and practice for men and women might help to better define the scope of this problem.

Several theories have been advanced to explain why women may be more susceptible to ACL injury than men. These include a narrower intercondylar notch in women, wider Q-angles that may increase valgus forces at the knee, and greater laxity of female joints. Since almost all of these injuries in volleyball occur when landing from a jump, and knee hyperextension is a fairly common mechanism of injury to the ACL in this situation, it may be reasonable to recommend that female volleyball players practice landing from jumping with their knees in slight flexion. This would probably be a reasonable suggestion to make to coaches during jump training to possibly decrease the chance of ACL injury. That team physician might also consider this advice for players in whom knee recurvatum is identified during the preparticipation examination.

Specific Physiologic Demands

Volleyball is almost entirely an anaerobic sport. Training to enhance maximal anaerobic power and vertical jump height will likely enhance the chances of success in volleyball. Aerobic conditioning may be beneficial for longer matches and in situations where multiple matches must be contested on the same day. There is evidence that plyometric training increases an athlete's vertical jump.[5] This type of training typically involves "depth jumps," where the athlete jumps from a height then bounds upward again immediately upon landing. The result is a very forceful concentric and eccentric contraction of the muscles involved in jumping. For this reason, it is best to do plyometric training near the beginning of practice before the muscles have become fatigued to minimize injury risk.[5] When this training is performed in a supervised setting with an experienced coach, it does not seem to increase the chance of injury.[10,12] In general, plyometrics should not be done daily.

Injury Trends by Level of Participation

There is not much definitive data on injury trends with respect to level of play. Two studies that used a similar definition of injury may allow for some comparisons on this topic. The definition of injury in both of these was "any condition that resulted in the athlete presenting to the medical staff at the tournament." At the 1995 US Olympic Festival, there was an injury rate of 1 per 25 hours training and competing in volleyball.[8] The injured were elite collegiate players with a mean age of 20.2 years. During the 1987 National Amateur Volleyball Tournament in the United States, an injury rate of 1 per 50 hours was found during competition.[28] The athletes in this population represented various ages and levels of play. It seems that more elite players may be at greater risk of injury. Perhaps these athletes placed greater cumulative stresses on their bodies by playing more frequently and with greater intensity than players at lower levels.

COMMON INJURIES IN VOLLEYBALL

Injuries in volleyball have been examined in different settings. The rate of injury varies between studies depending on the population and the definition of injury utilized. In the 2 studies that documented injury rates during tournament competition, most of the injuries were minor and did not result in any time lost from play.

Injuries during the course of 1 year have also been examined retrospectively. Among 86 Scottish National League players an injury rate of 53% was found. The definition of injury was "any condition resulting in 2 or more days missed from play." Most of these injuries were of mild severity, and only 26% resulted in more than 2 weeks missed from play.[34] The injury rate among 93 elite college-age volleyball players in the United States was 81.7% over 1 year. In this study, the definition of injury utilized was "any condition resulting in at least 1 day missed from play." The majority of these injuries resulted in less than 4 days missed from play.[8]

Patellar tendinitis is the most common overuse injury in volleyball.[8,10,28] Ankle sprains are the most common acute injury, representing 15% to 60% of injuries recorded.[3,8,28,34] The shoulder is involved in 8% to 20% of volleyball injuries. The most common shoulder injury is tendinitis of the biceps and rotator cuff tendons.[8,28,34] Suprascapular neuropathy has been reported to be fairly common in elite players[9,18] and more specific to the sport of volleyball. Hand injuries due to blocking are also fairly frequent in volleyball. Acute knee ligamentous injuries are rare but may result in significant "down time" from sport. Back injuries may account for up to 14% of volleyball injuries.[8,15,34]

Patellar Tendinitis

Etiology and Diagnosis

Patellar tendinitis is common in volleyball because of the frequent jumping that is inherent in competition and training. Pain occurs most frequently at the lower pole of the patella, with less frequent involvement of the upper pole and tibial tuberosity.[10] These are the areas where tenderness is palpable on examination. Pathologic studies have demonstrated inflammation localized to the bone–tendon junction.[10] More recent data have demonstrated that these are not truly inflammatory cells and that this process may be more appropriately referred to as a chronic "tendinosis."[24] While diagnostic ultrasonography may be useful when evaluating some types of tendon pathology, it does not seem to be particularly helpful in patellar tendinitis.[24]

Mechanism

This condition is more common among the players who can generate the greatest power during a rebound jump.[24] These are usually also the players who have the quickest and highest jumps.[24] Those with deeper knee flexion angles on jumping and landing seem to be at risk as well.[26] It is probably the rapid eccentric contraction of the quadriceps muscle that occurs with landing from a jump that results in pain and pathologic changes in the tendons of these players.[10,24]

Management, Rehabilitation, and Return to Play

Medical treatment for volleyball players is similar to that for other athletes with this condition. Anti-inflammatory agents may be helpful for short periods (2 to 3 weeks) when there is an acute flare-up of pain. Ice after activity seems to be beneficial. Modalities such as electrical stimulation may also be helpful in the acute period. All athletes with patellar tendinitis should be evaluated for tight hamstrings. If the hamstrings are functionally tight, the knee extensor mechanism is under constant stress, which probably contributes to overuse. For those with recurrent episodes of symptoms, a recommendation should probably be made to the coach to evaluate jumping form, with particular attention to knee flexion angles at takeoff and landing from jumping. This angle should probably not exceed 90°.[26] Patellar tendinitis is a condition that rarely results in a volleyball player missing time from practice or competition. However, symptoms that limit a player's ability to perform may indicate that an alteration in the training regimen should be considered.

Prevention

As we have noted, the athletes who are most likely to be afflicted with this condition are, in fact, the ones who are likely to be the most proficient jumpers on the team.[24] This is probably the group of players who stand to benefit the least from jump training. Athletes who already have a high vertical jump and have had symptomatic patellar tendinitis might best be advised to spend time working on other skills relevant to volleyball while their teammates are jump training.

Ankle Sprains

Etiology, Mechanism, and Diagnosis

Ankle sprains in volleyball occur most frequently when a blocker lands on the foot of a spiker from the opposing team that has come underneath the net on a hard-court indoor surface.[3] There is really nothing about this inversion injury or its management that is unique to volleyball. Tenderness is most frequently palpable in the area of the anterior talofibular ligament. Edema may occur inferior and anterior to the lateral malleolus.

Management

Acute treatment should include rest, ice, compression, and elevation until the initial edema and inflammation has begun to subside. Anti-inflammatory agents may be beneficial during the first 2 to 3 weeks following injury.

Rehabilitation and Return to Play

Functional exercise of the musculotendinous support structures of the ankle, particularly the peroneal muscles, seems to be helpful. Closed-chain balancing exercises may help to facilitate proprioception.[31] A progressive program that gradually approximates volleyball-specific weight-bearing activities is felt to be helpful in returning the athletes to play as expeditiously as possible.[2,7,31] When the player is able to jump and land without pain, and rapid side-to-side cutting maneuvers do not cause pain or a feeling of instability, return to play may be contemplated. Protective bracing or taping should be considered.

Protective Bracing and Prevention

Ankle taping has been shown to restrict inversion motion.[19,23] High-top shoes also may be beneficial.[14] Semirigid ankle supports have been demonstrated to decrease inversion range of motion during athletic activities.[14,16] There is some evidence that these supports may be superior to ankle taping because they do not lose their ability to restrict inversion as tape does after several repeated cycles of vertical jumping.[16,23] A prospective study of air-stirrup ankle supports demonstrated them to be effective for secondary prevention of ankle sprains. Among ankles that had suffered a previous sprain, there was a 5-fold decrease in ankle sprains during a soccer season with this support device. There was not a significant difference in number of sprains with the use of the air-stirrup in ankles that had not suffered a previous sprain.[29]

In the Norwegian study that was mentioned previously, a rule change during practice helped to decrease the incidence of sprains. Basically, during practice, players were not allowed to let their foot come into contact with the center line at all.[2] A second component of this study was proprioceptive balance training, which was taught to all of the teams in the study and continued for 10 weeks. These 2 concurrent interventions resulted in a 2-fold decrease in ankle sprain incidence over the course of a season.[2]

Shoulder Tendinitis

Etiology, Mechanism, and Diagnosis

Overuse of the biceps and rotator cuff tendons may result in tendinosis of these structures. This probably occurs secondary to repeated cycles of abduction and external rotation followed by forceful extension and internal rotation of the shoulder at the point of contact with the ball during spiking and overhead serving. This condition is common among athletes who play frequently, but it rarely results in down time from competition or training. Diagnosis of this condition is typically clinical and is similar to that for shoulder tendinitis in any other setting. Impingement maneuvers and tests aimed at isolating the involved tendons aid in establishing the diagnosis. Some centers find diagnostic ultrasonography to be a helpful tool.[6,25]

Management, Rehabilitation, and Return to Play

If scapulothoracic instability can be demonstrated on examination, then this should be addressed first in a rehabilitation program. Rotator cuff strengthening exercises would follow after that. Volleyball players may develop an altered arc of rotation similar to that seen in other athletes who perform frequent overhead activities.[7] There is usually increased external and decreased internal rotation, especially with shoulder abduction. If this is identified in a symptomatic shoulder, it should be addressed with a stretching program. If there is evidence on examination of a full-thickness rotator cuff tear, then that possibility should be evaluated and treated prior to the athlete's return to play.

Suprascapular Nerve Entrapment: A Volleyball-Specific Injury?

Suprascapular neuropathy is a fairly rare condition that is surprisingly common among elite volleyball players. At the 1985 European Championships, 13% of 96 athletes evaluated were found to have this problem.[9] A similar study of top-level German players found an incidence of 32% among 66 athletes.[18] When this nerve becomes entrapped in volleyball players, it is almost always compressed at the spinoglenoid notch such that the terminal branch, which supplies motor fibers to the infraspinatus muscle, is involved. The majority of players in both of these series were asymptomatic.

Mechanism, Diagnosis, and Treatment

A likely mechanism that has been advanced by one group that has studied this condition extensively is that the "floater" serve that is frequently used in indoor volleyball may be implicated.[9] To execute this serve, players use an overhand motion similar to throwing a ball, however, just after making contact, the arm swing is halted in order to impart as little spin as possible to the ball. When the ball is served without spin, air currents cause it to move erratically, making it difficult to pass. When the overhand motion is stopped prior to follow-through, a forceful deceleration of the upper extremity occurs secondary to strong eccentric contraction of the shoulder external rotators, principally the infraspinatus. This may result in stretching of the nerve between the myoneural junctions and the spinoglenoid notch. Compression of the suprascapular nerve at this site is rare in athletes who are not volleyball players. A more common site is at the suprascapular notch, resulting in supraspinal and infraspinatus weakness.

Another mechanism for this condition may be compression of the terminal branch of the suprascapular nerve by a ganglion cyst. Such a case has been described in a volleyball player.[32] One series of 6 patients with isolated paralysis of the infraspinatus muscle found 4 patients to have ganglion cysts causing nerve compression. These cysts were identified by magnetic resonance imaging (MRI) and ultrasonography.[30] Another series of 27 patients with a space-occupying lesions compressing the suprascapular nerve has been reported. Twenty-one of these lesions were ganglion cysts and all were identifiable by MRI.[13] If suprascapular neuropathy is identified in a symptomatic patient, ancillary studies should include electromyography/noncontrast ultrasonography and MRI.

The usual finding on physical examination is isolated infraspinatus weakness in the dominant shoulder. A 22% loss of strength in external rotation has been reported.[9,18] Some athletes may be symptomatic with shoulder pain when they present with weakness in shoulder external rotation. Surgical decompression of the suprascapular nerve with or without restoration of symmetrical strength in external rotation is necessary prior to return to play.

Hand Injuries

While hand injuries in volleyball are fairly common, they are rarely a presenting complaint to the medical staff. This may be because players perceive them as minor injuries and continue to play in spite of them. Only a small number of hand injuries have been recorded in the volleyball injury surveys.[4] However, a series of 226 hand injuries in volleyball players in the Netherlands has been described. These injuries occurred over a 5-year period and were analyzed retrospectively. Sprains and strains were the most common types of injuries (39%), followed by fractures (25%) and contusions (16%). Injuries were more common among the lower-level recreational players. Thirty-seven percent of injuries occurred playing defense, 36% occurred during blocking, and 18% occurred with falls. The thumb metacarpophalangeal joint was the most frequent location of ligamentous injury.[4] The radial collateral ligament of this joint is particularly vulnerable to injury during blocking.

Most finger sprains and closed fractures can be managed with appropriate splinting and taping. Collateral ligament injuries to the interphalangeal joints must be "buddy taped" to the adjacent finger to provide adequate support. Volleyball players frequently tape fingers individually, which offers little biomechanical support.

One player was wearing a ring that got tangled in the net, resulting in a near-amputation of the ring finger. This case demonstrates that it is important to advise volleyball players not to wear jewelry while playing. These investigators also cautioned that many hand injuries resulted in late sequelae. They advised that early medical attention for hand injuries may be beneficial in decreasing the chance of long-term complications.[4]

Other unusual hand injuries that have been described in indoor volleyball players include 2 cases of possible fatigue fracture of the pisiform bone. This may have been secondary to contact with the ball or the floor.[20] Three cases of antebrachial-palmar hammer syndrome were reported in one series.[21] This condition is caused by blunt trauma to the radial and ulnar arteries and may result in vasospasm of these arteries. Pain, pulselessness, and distal cyanosis may occur. It may be possible that the "pancake" maneuver is implicated in all of these injuries. This is a defensive maneuver in which the player slides her hand under the ball with the palm on the floor and the fingers extended. When this is done correctly, the ball bounces up off of the hand and remains in play. However, the hand is between a hard-driven ball and the floor, which may leave it vulnerable to injury.

Acute Knee Injuries

In volleyball injury surveys, the acute knee injuries are, fortunately, quite rare.[8,15,28,34]

A series of 52 serious knee ligament injuries in volleyball players has been described. These injuries occurred over several years, and all required surgery. The most frequent mechanism of injury was landing from a jump in the attack zone. All of the athletes in this series had ACL injuries. Many also injured the meniscus cartilage.[11] There were more women than men in this series.

Other Injuries

Low back injuries may account for up to 14% of volleyball injuries.[4,28,34] This is usually mechanical back pain that frequently occurs secondary to landing from jumping. Fortunately, herniated lumbar discs are rare among volleyball players.[7,8,28,34] Decreasing the number of repetitions of jumping activity, and jumping on a softer surface (such as sand), may help to decrease low back symptoms among volleyball players. An appropriate rehabilitation exercise program may also be beneficial in preventing recurrences.

Finally, there has been one reported case of a traumatic myocardial infarction during volleyball competition. A 41-year-old male was hit in the chest by a spiked volleyball. He was thought to have sustained a traumatic coronary artery thrombosis resulting in an acute apical myocardial infarction.[17] This patient had pre-existing coronary artery disease and it may have been that contact of the ball against his chest caused a proximal plaque to dislodge, resulting in distal artery obstruction.

CONCLUDING REMARKS

Volleyball is a very popular participation sport that is enjoyed all over the world. There are many more females than males who play this sport competitively in the United States, especially in interscholastic competition. The overwhelming majority of volleyball injuries are related to landing from a jump. The frequent jumping inherent in the sport may be the most significant risk factor in volleyball. The most common acute injury in volleyball is the inversion ankle sprain and the most common overuse injury is patellar tendinitis. Suprascapular neuropathy is a fairly prevalent condition among elite volleyball players and is caused by unique overhead maneuvers involved in the game. Many athletes who have this condition are asymptomatic but have shoulder external rotation weakness. Though ACL injury is rare in volleyball, there is significant suspicion that it may be more frequent in female players than in males. Lower extremity injury can be prevented to some extent by taking specific measures to avoid ankle sprains, close supervision of jump training, and training on softer surfaces such as sand.

References

1. Backx FJG, Beijer HJM, Erich WBM: Injuries in high-risk persons and high-risk sports. Am J Sports Med 19(2):124–30, 1991.
2. Bahr R, Bahr IA, Lian O, et al: A two-fold reduction in the incidence of ankle sprains in volleyball after introduction of a prevention program (abstr). Med Sci Sports Exerc 28(5) Suppl 55:29, 1996.
3. Bahr R, Karlsen R, Lian O, et al: Incidence and mechanisms of acute ankle inversion injuries in volleyball. Am J Sports Med 22(5):595–600, 1994.
4. Bhairo NH, Nijsten MWN, van Dalen KC, et al: Hand injuries in volleyball. Int J Sports Med 13:351–4, 1992.
5. Bobbert MF: Drop jumping as a training method for jumping ability. Sports Med 9(1):7–22, 1990.
6. Brenneke SL, Morgan CJ: Evaluation of ultrasonography as a diagnostic technique in the assessment of rotator cuff tendon tears. Am J Sports Med 20(3):287–9, 1992.
7. Briner WW, Kacmar L: Common injuries in volleyball: mechanisms of injury, prevention and rehabilitation. Sports Med 24(1):65–71, 1997.
8. Briner WW, Pera CE: Volleyball injuries at the 1995 U.S. Olympic Festival. Int J Volleyball Res 1(1):7–11, 1999.
9. Ferretti A, Cerullo G, Russo G: Suprascapular neuropathy in volleyball players. J Bone Joint Surg 69A(2):260–3, 1987.
10. Ferretti A, Ippolito E, Mariani P, et al: Jumper's knee. Am J Sports Med 11(2):58–62, 1983.
11. Ferretti A, Papapndrea P, Conteduca F, et al: Knee ligament injuries in volleyball players. Am J Sports Med 20(2):203–7, 1992.
12. Ferretti A, Puddu G, Mariani PP, et al: Jumper's knee: an epidemiological study of volleyball players. Physician Sportsmed 12(10):97–103, 1984.
13. Fritz RC, Helms CA, Steinbach LS, et al: Suprascapular nerve entrapment: evaluation with MR imaging. Radiology 182:437–44, 1992.
14. Garrick JG, Requa RK: Role of external support in the prevention of ankle sprains. Med Sci Sports Exerc 5(3):200–3, 1973.
15. Goodwin-Gerberich SG, Luhmann S, Finke C, et al: Analysis of severe injuries associated with volleyball activities. Physician Sportsmed 15(8):75–9, 1987.
16. Greene TA, Hillman SK: Comparison of support provided by a semirigid orthosis and adhesive ankle taping before, during, and after exercise. Am J Sports Med 18(5):498–506, 1990.
17. Grossfield PD, Friedman DB, Levine BD: Traumatic myocardial infarction during competitive volleyball: a case report. Med Sci Sports Exerc 25(8):901–3, 1993.
18. Holzgraefe M, Kukowski B, Eggert S: Prevalence of latent and manifest suprascapular neuropathy in high-performance volleyball players. Br J Sports Med 28(3):177–9, 1994.
19. Hughes LY, Stetts DM: A comparison of ankle taping and a semirigid support. Physician Sportsmed 11(4):99–103, 1983.
20. Israeli A, Engel J, Ganel A: Possible fatigue fracture of the pisiform bone in volleyball players. Int J Sports Med 3: 56–7, 1982.
21. Kostianen S, Orava S: Blunt injury of the radial and ulnar arteries in volleyball players: a report of three cases of the antebrachial-palmar hammer syndrome. Br J Sports Med 17(3):172–6, 1983.
22. Kraft D: On a tear. Volleyball Dec:64–9, 1995.
23. Laughman RK, Carr TA, Chao EY, et al: Three-dimensional kinematics of the taped ankle before and after exercise. Am J Sports Med 8(6):425–31, 1980.
24. Lian O, Engebretsen L, Ovrebo RV, et al: Characteristics of the leg extensors in male volleyball players with jumper's knee. Am J Sports Med 24(3):380–4, 1996.
25. Olive RJ Jr, Marsh HO: Ultrasonography of rotator cuff tears. Clin Orthop 282:110–3, 1992.
26. Richards DP, Ajemian SV, Wiley JP, et al: Knee joint dynamics predict patellar tendinitis in elite volleyball players. Am J Sports Med 24(5):676–83, 1996.
27. Schafle MD: Common injuries in volleyball. Sports Med 16(2):126–9, 1993.
28. Schafle MD, Requa RK, Patton WL, et al: Injuries in the 1987 National Amateur Volleyball Tournament. Am J Sports Med 18(6):624–31, 1992.
29. Surve I, Schwellnus MP, Noakes T, et al: A five-fold reduction in the incidence of recurrent ankle sprains in soccer players using the sport stirrup orthosis. Am J Sports Med 2(5):601–6, 1994.
30. Takagishi K, Saitoh A, Tonegawa M, et al: Isolated paralysis of the infraspinatus muscle. J Bone Joint Surg 76B:584–7, 1994.
31. Tropp H, Askling C, Gillquist J: Prevention of ankle sprains. Am J Sports Med 13(4):259–62, 1985.
32. Wang DH, Koehler SM: Isolated infraspinatus atrophy in a collegiate volleyball player. Clin J Sports Med 6(4):255–8, 1996.
33. Watkins J: Injuries in volleyball. In: Renstrom PAFH (ed): Clinical Practice of Sports Injury Prevention and Care. Oxford, Blackwell Scientific Publications, 1994, pp 360–74.
34. Watkins J, Green BN: Volleyball injuries: a survey of injuries of Scottish National League male players. Br J Sports Med 26(2):135–7, 1992.

Chapter 66

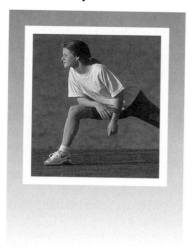

Winter Sports

SKIING, SPEED SKATING, ICE HOCKEY

David M. Joyner, M.D.
Susan L. Snouse, A.T.C.

SKIING

Skiing is an extremely exciting winter sport. An elite skier must not only have adequate aerobic capacity, muscular strength, and agility, but must also have excellent reaction time and eyesight. Defined simply, skiing is gravity or self-propulsion on snow by means of elongated runners.[12] Modern skiing can be divided into 2 major categories: Alpine (downhill skiing) and Nordic (cross-country skiing). Ski jumping and Nordic combined skiing have evolved into separate winter sports. Freestyle skiing (aerials and moguls) and snowboarding are 2 recent popular additions to the skiing family.

History of Skiing

The origins of skiing can be traced back almost 4000 years to the region that is now Norway and Sweden.[1] The first skis were probably made from bone and were used as a means of transportation across frozen land. In the mid 1800s, Norwegians developed bindings, which increased one's command over the skis. Skiing evolved from a form of transportation to a competitive activity. As skiing spread through Europe and Asia, the emphasis changed from flat skiing to traversing mountainous slopes. The speeds obtained in downhill skiing propagated the sport of Alpine skiing.

Skiing came to the United States with Norwegian immigrants in the 1850s. The focus of skiing at that time was Nordic skiing and its use for transportation. It was many years before the sporting aspect of Alpine and Nordic skiing became popular in the United States. It was not until 1934 that the first tow rope was installed, in Woodstock, Vermont.[1]

While freestyle skiing and snowboarding evolved in the 1970s, it wasn't until the 1990s that both emerged as popular sports for competitors and spectators alike. Snowboarding has gone from an activity banned at most ski resorts to the fastest-growing winter sport.

Sport Information for Skiing

The basic equipment for each category of skiing is similar: the skis, a binding system, and possibly poles. Alpine and freestyle accessories are designed for speed and control. The Alpine and freestyle binding is designed to fix both the heel and the toe of the boot to the ski, and to release when the stress becomes too high. The snowboard is a single board with a binding system designed to affix both heel and toe to the board. Nordic equipment is lighter and allows the skier to stride without stress. The Nordic binding is designed to hold the tip of the boot in place, while allowing the heel to rise up off the ski. Nordic boots are less stiff than their Alpine equivalents. The binding may be considered the most important part of the boot-binding–ski unit because it connects the leg of the skier with the lever of the ski.[16]

Skiing became an Olympic sport in 1924, at the first separately held Olympic Winter Games. Alpine skiing for females was introduced at the 1936 Olympic Winter Games. Events in Alpine skiing involve skiers following a premarked course. Five different Alpine skiing events are contested at the Olympic Winter Games. The downhill event occurs on a mile-long course where the skiers obtain speeds greater than 145 km/hr. Slalom tests the ability of the racer to turn quickly and accurately through gates that are positioned close to one another. Giant slalom combines the technique of both downhill and slalom. The 2 newest events, super G and the combined (one downhill and one slalom run combined for the best time) also combine the techniques and courses of the downhill and slalom.

Nordic, or cross-country, events take place over various distances on a premarked course. The course combines both flat and hilly terrain. The female events are the 5-, 10-, 20-, and 4 × 5-km relays. The distances for males are longer. The Nordic combined (males only) and biathlon combine ski jumping and shooting, respectively, with cross-country skiing.

Freestyle skiing has 3 disciplines that both males and females compete in: acro (ballet), aerials, and moguls. Only aerials and moguls are contested at the Olympic Winter Games. Moguls made their medal debut in the 1992 Olympic Winter Games and aerials became a medal sport in the 1994 Olympic Winter Games. Snowboarding, a recent addition to the Olympic Winter Games, made its debut in the 1998 games. Both males and females compete in the disciplines of slalom and half-pipe.

In the 1998 Olympic Winter Games in Nagano, Japan, there were 7 skiing categories: biathlon, Nordic combined, Alpine skiing, cross-country skiing, freestyle, ski jumping, and snowboarding. Females competed in all but Nordic combined and ski jumping.

Etiology of Injury and Medical Considerations for Skiing

Statistical data dividing ski injuries into male and female categories are rare. Injury patterns have been reported separately for Nordic and Alpine skiers. The Nordic injury rate is from 0.2 to 0.5/1000 skier days.[32] Nordic skiing injuries are relatively rare, and are usually the result of training errors. A similar injury pattern between Nordic skiers and distance runners has been suspected, because the 2 share similar biomechanical movements, at least in the lower extremities. Tendinitis of multiple upper extremity groups, in addition to the hip extensors and adductors, is not uncommon. The ankle ligaments and the Achilles tendon are also susceptible. Skin injuries secondary to ill-fitting boots do occur. Back pain can also be a Nordic skier complaint. This may result from fatigue fractures of the pars intra-articularis or muscle inflammation.[15] All such injuries are treated with rest, ice for the initial 48 hours, and maintenance of fitness level by cross-training until the sport can be slowly reintroduced.

The Alpine injury rate seems to vary between the 3/1000 skier day ratio reported by Johnson and coworkers[13] and the 4.2/1000 skier day ratio found in the general inquiry study by Scherer, Ascher, and Lecher.[25] The majority of injuries sustained in Alpine skiing are to the lower extremity, with knee sprains the most common, although the second most common overall injury is to the thumb.

Despite the obvious trauma-related injuries one would imagine from falling and hitting frozen earth, there are other causes of injury to consider. The very nature of skiing as a winter sport leaves the skier at the mercy of the environment. Skiers are vulnerable to altitude and exposure to the wind and sun. Frostbite and hypothermia in the skier are always risks. Data on these injuries are sparse.

Alpine skiing offers many more avenues for traumatic injury. Falls can result in head trauma or cervical spine injuries. The part of the body most commonly injured during Alpine skiing is the knee joint. With the advent of the stiffer, higher ski boot, it is thought that the transmission of stress is now located in the knee.[14,16] Rather than ending at the distal ankle, the higher boot now traverses the tibia at a stronger point, less likely to fracture. The resultant load on the knee can result in medial cruciate ligament stretch or tear or a more catastrophic anterior cruciate ligament (ACL) sprain or rupture. Meniscal tears are much less common.[21] The tibia is not immune to fracture, however, a bending injury, where the tibia is forced over the top of the stiff boot, can still result in this bone injury. Femur fractures also occur in both Alpine and freestyle competitions.

Skier's or gamekeeper's thumb is the most common upper extremity injury. Disruption of the ulnar collateral ligament results from the thumb planting in the snow while the force of the skier's body or the ski pole itself causes abduction and hyperextension. If unstable, this injury may require surgical intervention. After a fall, the skier may experience bony or soft-tissue shoulder injuries. Humeral fractures, glenohumeral dislocation, acromioclavicular joint separation, and rotator cuff tears are all possible.

SPEED SKATING

Speed skating consists of 2 disciplines: long-track speed skating (LTSS) and short-track speed skating (STSS). The sports are similar in that both involve skating on 14- to 18-inch blades at high velocities in a counterclockwise direction. LTSS utilizes a 400-meter oval course with 2 skaters competing on separate tracks. The skaters race the clock and have only one opportunity to produce a winning time. Contact between the skaters is prohibited. The recent invention of "clap" skates has increased not only the skaters' speeds (velocities greater than 56 km/hr[15]) but also the possibility of acute injuries from falls.

STSS takes place on a 30- × 60-meter ice sheet with a pack of 4 to 6 skaters on a 111-meter course. A STSS race has heats, quarterfinals, semifinals, and finals. The skater must finish first or second in 3 races to advance to the finals. STSS also offers a team relay event. With speeds over 40 km/hr, a small track, and potential contact from other skaters, STSS has a greater risk of acute injury.

History of Speed Skating

Archaeological findings date skating back 3000 years.[20,31] It has been suggested that a piece of bone was first used to slide across ice, whether this be by accident[20,31] or design.[11] It has also been suggested that skating could have evolved from skiing.[20] Whatever its origin, skating's original function was transportation and was often done by hunters.

Wooden skates were the next advancement and were cultivated in the Netherlands.[11] Hybrid skates using both wood and iron appeared in the mid 1200s.[11] These skates consisted of a wood platform and iron blades. All-iron skates were the next development, appearing in 1572.[11] The advantage of all-iron skates was that the blade was directly attached to the boot, which was an improvement over the ill-fitting wood platforms. Lighter steel blades were first manufactured in 1850.[11] This advancement revolutionized skating and increased its accessibility to the public. The all-iron skate remains the basis for today's skate.

In the Netherlands, skating evolved from a form of transportation to a sport in the late 1600s. The first competitions involved packs of skaters who skated on canals between cities in long-distance races. Unlike modern speed skating courses, these courses were often linear.

Sport Information for Speed Skating

LTSS international competition began in 1885 and the first World Championships were held in 1891.[20,31] In 1892 the International Skating Union (ISU) was formed and the rules and regulations of speed skating were developed. The ISU continues to organize world championships and govern international speed skating. In the United States, both disciplines are governed by an organization called US Speedskating.

LTSS was first included in the Olympic Winter Games in 1924. At that time, the Olympic Winter Games speed skating events were only open to males. Female speed skating was a demonstration sport in the 1932 Olympic Winter Games,[4] but it did not make its official debut until the 1960 Olympic Winter Games. Both sexes compete in 5 distances. For females these are the 500-, 1000-, 1500-, 3000-, and 5000-meter events.

With the invention of artificial ice in the 1800s, pack-style skating, or STSS, moved indoors. While national competitions have been held since the early 1900s, international competition did not begin until 1976 and the first STSS World Championships were held in 1980 (Susan Polakoff-Shaw, former USS Media Relations Director, personal communication). STSS was a demonstration sport in the 1988 Olympic Winter Games. The sport achieved full medal status in the 1992 Olympic Winter Games. Included in the Olympic Winter Games of 1992, 1994, and 1998 were a limited number of events (the 500-, 1000-, and 3000-meter relays for females, and the 5000-meter relay for males).

Biomechanical studies of speed skaters have shown that skating efficiency is affected most by the skater's pre-extension knee angle, stroke frequency, and the air and ice friction.[7,10,31] In studies comparing males to females, female speed skaters often exhibit larger pre-extension knee angles than male skaters.[10,31] In physiologic studies, the maximum oxygen consumption (VO_2max) of male and female elite long-track speed skaters was average when compared to other athletes.[7,8] When correlated to fat-free body weight, there were no significant differences in VO_2max between the sexes. The percentage of body fat for male skaters averaged 7.4% and for females averaged 16.5%.[4] The investigators suggested that in LTSS, female skaters could especially benefit from increased conditioning and decreased body fat.[7,30]

Etiology of Injury and Medical Considerations for Speed Skating

A review of literature did not find any epidemiological studies of injuries for either LTSS or STSS. Table 66-1 lists the medical information collected at the 1994 and 1998 Olympic Winter Games by the United States Olympic Committee (USOC) Sports Medicine Division. Injury and illness occurrence rates for LTSS and STSS were comparable to those of other sports. However, both long- and

Table 66-1. Statistics from the Olympic Winter Games, 1994–1998

	1994	1998
Total athletes	155	195
Long-track speed skaters	16 (10% of athletes)	16 (8% of athletes)
Short-track speed skaters	10 (6% of athletes)	12 (6% of athletes)
Total injury evaluations	123	145
Long-track speed skaters	13 (11% of evaluations)	11 (8% of evaluations)
Short-track speed skaters	9 (7% of evaluations)	6 (4% of evaluations)
Total illness evaluations	104	153
Long-track speed skaters	13 (13% of evaluations)	11 (7% of evaluations)
Short-track speed skaters	8 (8% of evaluations)	8 (5% of evaluations)
Total prescriptions filled	243	310
Long-track speed skaters	23 (9% of total)	18 (5% of total)
Short-track speed skaters	13 (5% of total)	12 (4% of total)
Total treatments	1671	2896
Long-track speed skaters	301 (18% of total)	376 (13% of total)
Short-track speed skaters	250 (15% of total)	262 (9% of total)

Medical data collected from the 1994 and 1998 Olympic Winter Games by the United States Olympic Committee (USOC) Sports Medicine Division.

short-track speed skaters received a larger percentage of medical treatments than their delegation size might suggest. In 1994 and 1998, speed skating athletes comprised 17% and 14% of the total athlete delegation but received 33% and 21% of the total medical treatments. Unlike several other winter sports teams, speed skating teams travel with a certified athletic trainer and the athletes are accustomed to receiving sports medicine treatment. Both disciplines receive high amounts of manual therapy (massage, mobilization techniques, etc) similar to athletes competing in track and swimming.

Injury and illness occurrence rates for members of the United States Olympic STSS Team were tracked by the USOC during the 1993–1994 season. Nine athletes (5 males and 4 females) were followed for a 30-week period; 308.5 hours of on-ice training and 279 hours of off-ice training (cycling, running, pliometrics, weights) were recorded. On-ice injuries occurred every 10.6 hours during training, while off-ice injuries occurred every 9.3 hours during training. Significant gender differences emerged: female athletes sustained 72% of the on-ice injuries, 57% of the off-ice injuries, and 81% of non-sport-related injuries and illnesses.

The new "clap" skates in LTSS are designed so that the skater's toe remains affixed to the blade while the heel can lift up. This allows the skater to create more power with each stroke. While the "clap" skate has increased the skater's times, there has also been a decrease in the stability of the skater. Contact with the rink's outer pads is a greater hazard than in the past. There are a variety of risk factors in STSS. Falls onto the ice or into rink walls and collisions with

opponents can cause contusions, lacerations, sprains/strains, and fractures.

Specific injuries often seen include callosities, corns, and hammertoes caused by ill-fitting boots. As many skaters do not wear socks, tinea pedis can become a problem. Tibialis anterior, extensor hallucis longus, or extensor digitorum longus tendinitis secondary to "lace bite" from improperly tied laces is common. Lacerations are of significant concern, particularly in STSS. In the USOC's experience, 3 severe medial shin lacerations occurred to US skaters between November 1993 and November 1994, 2 of which also involved tibial fractures. The junior author witnessed an Australian skater receive a severe femoral artery laceration in international competition in October 1994. Lacerations can also occur in LTSS, particularly at the start if the athlete falls onto his or her own blade. Such an occurrence produced a testicular laceration in one athlete (USOC data).

Overuse injuries such as patellar tendinitis, patellofemoral disorders, and iliotibial band syndrome occur and are often due to the constant repetitive motions in one direction. Mechanical low back pain due to the extreme flexion necessary in competitive speed skating is a frequent occurrence. Both disciplines involve an explosive start that can cause muscle strains, especially in the hip flexors and adductor muscles. Fractures can occur in speed skating secondary to falls. A femoral fracture and a tibial fracture have been documented in the past year at USOC training centers. While catastrophic injuries are uncommon, because of the velocities obtained, the risk does exist. In December 1993, a Dutch skater sustained an axial-loaded cervical spine fracture after colliding into unpadded boards. There was neurologic involvement and the athlete remains quadriplegic.

During outdoor skating, LTSS skaters can face subzero temperatures and experience the full range of cold-induced injuries. Speed skaters, like many elite athletes, are susceptible to colds, upper respiratory tract infections, and viral syndromes.[33] Treatment of these respiratory illnesses is symptomatic.[6,33]

ICE HOCKEY

Ice hockey is an extremely fast, high-contact skating team sport, played on ice in rinks of varying size. Ice hockey has experienced a surge in participation over the last 15 years. Registered ice hockey teams in the United States jumped from 10,490 to 14,347 in 8 years,[5] a 73% increase. Registration of individual female ice hockey players has skyrocketed from 6336 in 1990 to 27,273 in 1997 (Kristine Pleiman, former USA Hockey Media Director, personal communication).

The object of an ice hockey game is simple: to place a puck (a hard 3-inch rubber disc) in the opponent's goal, using "sticks" to propel the puck. Teams consist of one goalie, 2 defense persons, and 3 forwards. An ice hockey game is played in three 20-minute periods. In international tournaments, the game is played on a 30×60-meter rink. The larger size of the international rink is advantageous for a team that relies on speed skills and play-making abilities.

Ice Hockey History

Ice hockey started as a combination of ice skating and field hockey. The word *hockey* most likely derived from the french word *hoquet*, or shepherd's staff.[18,19] While games have been reported as early as the mid 1850s, formal organization began in Canada in the 1880s.[18,19,28] Professional leagues were started soon after the inception of the game and ice hockey for males made its debut in the 1920 Olympic Games in Antwerp.[18]

Females were involved with ice hockey as early as 1892 in Canada.[28] Leagues were formed in Canada and the United States in the 1920s and 1930s. As with other female sports (baseball) after World War II, there was decreased interest in female hockey. It wasn't until the 1960s that interest returned and leagues formed in Canada and the United States. Today, the NCAA recognizes female ice hockey as an emerging sport. In the United States, USA Hockey governs amateur ice hockey for both male and female athletes.

In 1992, the IOC and the International Ice Hockey Federation (IIHF) voted to include ice hockey as a medal sport for females in the 1998 Olympic Winter Games. The IIHF coordinated world championship tournaments in 1990, 1992, 1994, and 1997. The order of finish has been the same for all 4 championships: Canada first, United States second, and Finland third. Women participated in their first Olympic Winter Games in 1998. The order of finish was the United States first, Canada second, and Finland third.

Sport Information for Ice Hockey

Ice hockey makes great anaerobic demands, although aerobic conditioning is also necessary. While players generally play 30 to 80 seconds in a shift,[9] the player may skate a total of 2 to 4 miles in a single game.[23] Forward skating speeds have been recorded at 56 km/hr and backward skating at 27 km/hr.[19] In looking at elite male ice hockey players, it was found that the athletes worked at approximately 70% to 80% of their maximal aerobic power.[9] Elite male ice hockey players averaged 10% body fat.[26] No studies were found that compared male to female ice hockey players.

Many US rinks are smaller than international-sized rinks and thus many US players rely on checking (the practice of blocking or ramming an opponent into the boards) to control the games.[19] At this time in international play, female players are limited to modified body checking and any legal contact must take place near the puck. This rule was implemented to decrease injuries and to promote equal play,[28] however, many females play in men's leagues that do allow checking and several females have played goalie in professional minor leagues.

Because of the nature of the sport, use of equipment is mandatory for the athlete's safety. According to IIHF and USA Hockey rules, helmets are mandatory and females are required to wear a full face mask. The helmet should fit snugly and utilize a 4-point fit (like a football helmet). Mouthguards are not mandatory in international play, but their use is highly encouraged. The use of custom-fitted mouthguards has greatly increased compliance in the US Women's Ice Hockey Team. Kevlar throat protectors are requirements in many leagues and countries.

Ice hockey athletes wear shoulder and elbow pads. Shoulder pads can vary in size and the amount of protection they offer. A previous problem for the female ice hockey player was finding equipment that fit properly. Several manufacturers now design equipment specifically for females. Gloves are a universal requirement. A recent trend of wearing shorter-cuff gloves for more wrist motion may increase the risk of injury.

Similar to their male counterparts, female ice hockey players wear a protective cup. Padded hockey pants provide protection from the hips to the top of the knees. Shin pads should cover from the top of the knees to the ankles. Like speed skaters, ice hockey players look for snug-fitting skates and often do not wear socks to improve their ability to "feel" the ice. Many ice hockey players prefer leather skates that have plastic shields on the outside for ankle support and protection.[9] A 10- to 12-inch blade unit is riveted into the base of the boot.

Etiology of Injury and Medical Considerations for Ice Hockey

There are numerous epidemiologic studies of male ice hockey injuries.[3,18,26] Bahr cites data that show approximately 80 injuries per 1000 player hours.[3] A large difference seems to exist in the amount of injuries occurring in training versus those occurring in competition (1.5 incidents per 1000 hours versus 38.0 incidents per 1000 hours).[17]

Injury and illness occurrence rates for members of the US Women's Ice Hockey Team were tracked during the 1995 season. Two international tournaments and practice sessions were followed for a 4-week period. Forty-four hours of practice and 16 hours of games were recorded. Thirty-nine injuries occurred in practice sessions (one incident every 0.89 hour). Eighteen injuries occurred in the games (one incident every 1.12 hours). Twenty-five illnesses were recorded (USOC data).

Ice hockey presents many opportunities for injury: hard ice surface, unpadded rink walls, and contact with equipment and other players. Pucks often travel at speeds of greater than 100 miles/hr.[18,19] Prevention of injuries through the use of proper and well-fitting equipment is vital. Rules to keep sticks lower, prohibition of back checking, and stringent equipment requirements have been instituted in an attempt to decrease injury occurrence.[19]

Common injuries in ice hockey include contusions, lacerations, sprains/strains, and fractures. Facial lacerations and eye injuries occur frequently in male ice hockey players.[3,18,22]

Facial injuries are fewer in females because of the face mask requirement. In a review of USOC data and female ice hockey players, no females in USOC data were found to have received facial lacerations and only one female player was found to have sustained a facial fracture.[27] Lacerations from the skate blades can occur between pads on the forearms or shins.[3]

Head and cervical spine injuries result from contact with the boards. A rising trend in axial-loaded cervical spine injuries has been noted with the advent of mandatory helmet use,[24,29] possibly because helmets give the athlete a feeling of "invincibility." In any event, ice hockey players are going into the boards with catastrophic results.[24,29] Lumbar strains are common with the athlete's flexed skating position and constant rotation. The lack of lumbar and hamstring flexibility in many ice hockey players may precipitate lumbar strains.[2] Spondylosis and spinal stress fractures have been reported as well.[3]

Shoulder injuries, including acromioclavicular joint and clavicle fractures, are frequent in ice hockey.[3,18] These are often caused by high-velocity contact with the boards or other players. Groin strains are common (from the explosive starts and rapid changes in direction). Knee injuries can range from traumatic bursitis to torn cruciate and collateral ligaments. The lack of foot fixation often aids the athlete with instabilities.[18] "Lace bite" may explain a nagging foot or ankle problem.

Illnesses tend to be of the respiratory tract. Transmission of rhinoviruses and other infections is frequently the result of inhaling infected droplets or touching a mucus membrane after contact. Frequent hand washing, eliminating sharing water bottles and towels, and the proper use of tissues must be stressed to minimize contamination.[6]

CONCLUDING REMARKS

Skiing, speed skating, and ice hockey are all technically challenging, action sports. Injuries can be expected while participating in any of these sports. Injury factors include environmental concerns, contact with objects, or self-induced muscle strains. Further study is necessary to investigate increased safety and female participation in these sports. For athletes subjected to drug testing, medication use should be checked with the applicable sport body.

References

1. The Academic American Encyclopedia. On-line edition. Danbury, Conn, Groiler Electronic Publishing, 1993.
2. Agre JC, Baxter TL, Casal DC, et al: Musculoskeletal characteristics of professional ice-hockey players. Can J Sport Sci 12(4):202–6, 1987.
3. Bahr R, Bendiksen F, Engebretsen L: 'Tis the season: diagnosing and managing ice hockey injuries. J Musculoskel Med 12(2):48–56, 1995.
4. Bland JH, Casey MJ: Women in winter sports. In: Casey MJ, Foster C, Hixson EG (eds): Winter Sports Medicine. Philadelphia, FA Davis, 1990, pp 42–55.
5. Blase K: USA hockey: a vision for the 1990s. In: Grana WA, Lombardo JA, Sharkey BJ, Stone, JA (eds): Advances in Sports Medicine and Fitness, Vol 3. Chicago, Year Book, 1990, 245–56.
6. Casey MJ, Dick EC: Acute respiratory infections. In: Casey MJ, Foster C, Hixson EG (eds): Winter Sports Medicine. Philadelphia, FA Davis, 1990, pp 112–28.
7. De Groot G, Hollander AP, Sargeant AJ, et al: Applied physiology of speed skating. J Sport Sci 5(3):249–59, 1987.
8. Foster C, Thompson NN: The physiology of speed skating. In: Casey MJ, Foster C, Hixson EG (eds): Winter Sports Medicine. Philadelphia, FA Davis, 1990, pp 221–40.
9. Green H, Bishop P, Houston M, et al: Time-motion and physiological assessments of ice hockey performance. J Appl Physiol 40(2):159–63, 1976.
10. Greer NL: Biomechanics of skating. In: Casey MJ, Foster C, Hixson EG (eds): Winter Sports Medicine. Philadelphia, FA Davis, 1990, pp 240–47.
11. Holum D: The Complete Handbook of Speed Skating. Hillside, IL, Enslow, 1984, pp 5–16.
12. The Hutchinson Encyclopedia. On-line edition. Oxford, UK, Helicon, 1995.
13. Johnson RJ, Ettlinger CF, Cambell RJ, Pope MH: Trends in skiing injuries: analysis of a six year study (1972–1978). Am J Sports Med 8:106–13, 1980.
14. Johnson RJ: Epidemiology of Alpine ski injuries and ski injury research. Presented at the Winter Sport and Common Sports Injury Conference, Vail, Colo, 1990.
15. Johnson RJ, Incavo SJ: Cross-country ski injuries. In: Casey MJ, Foster C, Hixson EG (eds): Winter Sports Medicine. Philadelphia, FA Davis, 1990, pp 302.
16. Johnson RJ, Incavo SJ: Alpine skiing injuries. In: Casey MJ, Foster C, Hixson EG (eds): Winter Sports Medicine. Philadelphia, FA Davis, 1990, pp 352–5.
17. Jorgensen U, Schmidt-Olsen S: The epidemiology of ice hockey injuries. Br J Sports Med 20(1):7–9, 1986.
18. Minkoff J, Varlotta GP, Simonson BG: Ice hockey. In: Fu FH, Stone DA (eds): Sports Injuries: Mechanisms-Prevention-Treatment. Baltimore, Williams & Wilkins, 1994, pp 397–444.
19. Morgan JV: Ice hockey injuries. In: Casey MJ, Foster C, Hixson EG (eds): Winter Sports Medicine. Philadelphia, FA Davis, 1990, pp 269–74.
20. Muller DL, Renstrom PAFH, Pyne JIB: Ice skating: figure, speed, long distance, and in-line. In: Fu FH, Stone DA (eds): Sports Injuries: Mechanisms-Prevention-Treatment. Baltimore, Williams & Wilkins, 1994, pp 445–54.
21. Paletta GA Jr, Levine DS, O'Brien SJ, et al: Patterns of meniscal injury associated with anterior cruciate ligament injuries in skiers. Am J Sports Med 20(5):542–7, 1992.
22. Pashby T: Epidemiology of eye injuries in hockey. In: Castaldi CR, Hoerner ET (eds): Safety in Ice Hockey, Vol 1. Phildelphia, American Society for Testing and Materials, 1989, pp 29–31.
23. Percival L: The Hockey Handbook, revised edition. Toronto, McClelland & Stewart, 1992.
24. Reynen PD, Clancy WG: Cervical spine injury, hocicey helmets and face masks. Am J Sports Med 22(2):167–70, 1994.
25. Scherer MA, Ascherl R, Lechner RF: The value of epidemiologic studies of ski injuries. Sportverletzung Sportschaden 6(4):150–5, 1992.
26. Sim FH, Simonet WT, Melton LJ, Lehn TA: Ice hickey injuries. Am J Sports Med 15(1):30–40, 1987.
27. Snouse SL, Casterline MA, Stephens BA: Zygomatic arch fracture in women's ice hockey. Athlet Ther Today 3(6):13–4, 1998.
28. Stewart B: She shoots . . . she scores! Toronto, Doubleday Canada, 1993, pp 23–33, 41–4.
29. Tator CH, Edmonds VE, Lapczak L: Spinal injuries in ice hockey: review of 182 North American cases and analysis of etiologic factors. In Castaldi CR, Bishop PJ, Hoerner ET (eds): Safety in Ice Hockey, Vol 2. Phildelphia, American Society for Testing and Materials, 1993, pp 11–20.
30. van Ingen Schenau GJ, de Groot G: On the origin of differences in performance level between elite male and female speed skaters. Hum Movement Sci 2:151–9, 1983.
31. van Ingen Schenau GJ, de Boer RW, de Groot G: Biomechanics of speed skating. In: Vaughan CL (ed): Biomechanics of Sport. Boca Raton, Fla, CRC Press, 1989, pp 121–67.
32. Westten N: Injuries in long distance cross-country and downhill skiing. Orthop Clin North Am 7:1–2, 1976.
33. Woods MP: Medical aspects of speed skating. In: Casey MJ, Foster C, Hixson EG (eds): Winter Sports Medicine. Philadelphia, FA Davis, 1990, pp 248–53.

Chapter 67

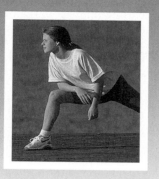

Olympic Sports

David M. Joyner, M.D.

Participation in Olympic sports has undergone dramatic evolution in the 12 centuries since the first competitions. From a one-event, one-day foot race held to honor Zeus in 776 BC to the 296-medal event, $2\frac{1}{2}$-week gathering that comprised the 2000 Olympic Games in Sydney, growth and change have been key to the existence of the Olympic Games. When the ancient Olympics came to an end in 394 AD over religious concerns (or lack of them), women did not participate in the Olympics; however, the number of events and participants had increased significantly. The idea of the Olympic Games arose as a salute to the gods, and in the ancient forum contained both athleticism and aestheticism. Theater and music were an integral part of the celebrations. Somewhere along the time line, the focus shifted to a more professional athletic participation, honoring the athlete in addition to, or instead of, the gods. This shift was a major factor in the demise of the ancient games. The Games were revived in 1896 under the guidance of Pierre de Coubertin. Considered by many to be the father of the modern Games, he espoused a creed, "The important thing in the Olympic Games is not winning, but taking part."

Taking part may not always be good enough for the athletes, though. Winning is often the ultimate goal. To that end, problems have arisen of both a biologic and philosophical nature. At the Games of the XXIX Olympiad in Sydney in 2000, more athletes than ever before entered more events than ever before. Females, especially, have grown in their access and ability to compete. In Sydney, 118 events were specific to females, with an additional 12 mixed events.

DRUG TESTING

"Whereas the International Olympic Committee (IOC) has established rules prohibiting the use of certain substances and methods intended to enhance and/or having the effect of enhancing athletic performance, such practices being contrary to medical ethics, and which are referred to generally as 'doping'."[5]

Man has always strived to succeed. The forum of sport, with the Olympic Games as its highlight, is no exception. The personal desire to be the best, to become a legend, in addition to increasing financial and celebrity status, pushes the boundaries of human performance. With the advent of synthetic agents to enhance that performance, it seems a way to improve on nature has been found. In an effort to retain the "natural" in a natural athlete, and to protect the athlete from potentially harmful and irreversible side effects, a number of international governing bodies realized the necessity of banning certain substances and methods from competition. The IOC Medical Code is standard for the Olympic Games. Although substances such as cocoa leaves and poppy plants were used to alter performance for hundreds of years, it was not until the 1960s that the athletic world realized the intensity of the problem. A Danish cyclist at the 1960 Games in Rome and a British cyclist in the Tour de France both died during their events from the effects of amphetamines. These incidents spurred the beginning of standardized drug testing.[2] Much of the early work in developing the actual tests was done by Beckett. He used gas chromatography to check urine samples primarily for stimulants (personal communication, Don Catlin, MD, Director, UCLA Olympic Analytical Laboratory, Los Angeles, Calif.)

The evolution of drug testing has continued since the early days. The initial focus on screening for performance enhancing substances, such as amphetamines, has expanded to include performance-impairing agents, such as narcotics, and chemically manipulative agents, such as probenecid. Table 67-1 lists classes of substances,

Table 67-1. Classes of Substances, Drugs, and Methods Prohibited or Restricted by the IOC

PROHIBITED CLASSES OF SUBSTANCES

Stimulants
Narcotics
Anabolic agents
Diuretics
Peptide and glycoprotein hormones and analogues

CLASSES OF DRUGS SUBJECT TO CERTAIN RESTRICTIONS

Alcohol
Marijuana
Local anesthetics
Corticosteroids
Beta-blockers

PROHIBITED METHODS

Blood doping
Pharmacologic, chemical, and physical manipulation

drugs, and methods prohibited or restricted by the IOC.[5] The IOC provides both a definition of doping and a categorical breakdown of prohibitive substances and methods: "Doping consists of the administration of substances belonging to prohibited classes of pharmacological agents and/or the use of various prohibited methods."[5]

The development of drug testing for Olympic athletes has not been without controversy. Medications from diuretics to beta-blockers are used to treat hypertension. Testosterone is used to treat males with hypogonadism. Where the medical indications and legislated infractions blur is a source of continuing discussion. The end result should always ensure the safety and health of the athletes.

GENDER VERIFICATION

"All competitors taking part in women's events . . . or as the female competitor of a mixed team in which one or more of the competitors must be female shall be subject to gender verification."[5]

The exact origin of the need for gender verification is unclear. At least in the 1930s, the media fostered a notion that some female athletic competitors were indeed male.[6] The whispering continued and grew louder with increasing public support of athletics in the 1950s and 1960s. Physical inspection of the female athlete began. Subsequent embarrassment over the visual and sometimes manual examinations necessitated a change.

At the 1968 Games in Mexico City, buccal smear (or sex chromatin testing) was first used. This measures the X chromatin mass of the individual. Problems with this testing have been debated by physicians and geneticists from the beginning. Because it looks at genetic markers and not the appearance of the individual, the buccal smear does not distinguish between genetic and anatomic sex. Individuals with 45X (Turner) syndrome would demonstrate a male sex chromatin pattern though appear phenotypically female.[4] Research and data collected by Ferguson-Smith and Ferris show the rate of ineligible females determined by this method to be 1 in 504.[3]

Polymerase chain reaction (PCR) testing is an alternative to the buccal smear. This tests for the presence of Y-specific DNA, rather than for X chromatin mass. Again, debate continued for the reasons stated above. The PCR test is a strictly genetic measure. Thus, individuals with the XY androgen insensitivity syndrome would be classified as males, even though they have a female phenotype and the condition gives them no athletic advantage.[1] At the Nagano Games, buccal cytology brush sampling applying PCR was used.

The International Amateur Athletics Federation (IAAF) convened regarding the issue of laboratory-based gender verification and reached a different conclusion than the IOC. In 1991, the IAAF abolished the laboratory-based gender verification testing and replaced it with a screening health examination for both males and females. In 1992, regular screening proved difficult, and screening the gender of a participant at IAAF events became optional.[7]

During the 1996 IOC World Conference on Women and Health, the IOC passed a resolution to "discontinue the current process of gender verification during the Olympic Games." The IOC Athletes' Commission in 1999 recommended to the IOC Executive Board that gender verification testing be discontinued. At the 109th IOC session in Seoul, South Korea, in June 1999, the decision was made to abolish testing, which became effective at the 2000 Olympic games in Sydney, Australia.[7]

ILLNESS AND INJURIES

"Whereas the IOC medical code is essentially intended to safeguard the health of athletes, and to ensure respect for the ethical concepts implicit in fair play, the Olympic Spirit and medical practice."[5]

A traveling event such as the Olympics presents a wide variety of medical concerns.

Attention must not be focused only on athletic injuries such as fractures and muscle pulls; illness can strike an athlete as well.

Travel to different parts of the world can result in "jet lag" or altered sleep patterns. Although an athlete's diet is closely monitored, a change in fresh fruits, vegetables, or water can cause gastrointestinal problems. Obviously, the weather conditions necessary to promote winter and summer sports can leave the athlete vulnerable to the elements. Frostbite, windburn, sunburn, heat exhaustion, and dehydration can all affect the athlete's performance and health. A breakdown of injury patterns for females at the 1994 Olympic Winter Games in Lillehammer, Norway, showed 59 total injuries. Of these, muscle strains were most prevalent at 15, followed by contusions, sprains, and bursitis. There were no fractures recorded. Total illnesses numbered 51. Upper respiratory tract infection was the leading culprit, followed by sinusitis, gastritis, and pharyngitis (unpublished data, correspondence with the United States Olympic Committee Sports Medicine Division).

CONCLUDING REMARKS

The evolution of female participation in the Olympic Games, from its 2-event beginning in the 1900 Games to its 130 events in the millennial 2000 Games in Sydney, has been remarkable. New or modified events for women at the Sydney Games included trampoline, water polo, modern pentathlon, hammer, pole vault, weightlifting, tae kwon do, triathlon, sailing 49er class, trap and skeet shooting, and synchronized swimming duet (personal communication, Steve Saye, Associate Director, International Games Preparation Division, USOC). At the 2002 Olympic Winter Games in Salt Lake City, women's bobsleigh, skeleton, and cross-country ski sprints were added to the Games, thus leaving only nordic combined and ski jumping without female events. Female participation in Olympic sports will continue to expand over time. It is hoped that research and advances in sports medicine for females will follow the same course.

References

1. Anderson C: Olympic row over sex testing. Nature 353:784, 1991.
2. Dugal R, Bertrand M: The technological deterrent to doping at the Montreal Olympics. Canadian Research, May–June 1976.
3. Ferguson-Smith M, Ferris E: Gender verification in sport: The need for change? Br J Sports Med 25:17–21, 1991.
4. Ljungqvist A, Simpson JL: Medical examination for the health of all athletes replacing the need for gender verification in international sports. JAMA 267:850–2, 1992.
5. Medical Code, International Olympic Committee. Lausanne, Switzerland, International Olympic Committee, 1995, pp 2–11.
6. Simpson JL, Ljungqvist A, de la Chapelle A, et al: Gender verification in competitive sports. Sports Med 16:305–15, 1993.
7. Simpson JL, Ljungqvist A, Ferguson-Smith MA, et al: Gender verification in the Olympics. JAMA 284:1568–9, 2000.

Final Thoughts

Athletic competition has never been more important to women. Thanks to new laws and new attitudes, doors of opportunity have swung open in every school and on every playground in America.

In professional sports, women are excelling across the board. From Wimbledon to Madison Square Garden, female athletes are making their marks, setting new records and making themselves legends and role models for young girls everywhere. This extraordinary social development compares to the great civil rights movement in its breadth and depth and in its meaning to millions of young women, not only in the United States but also throughout most of the world.

Women can play the game! And furthermore, we can play it with a grace and style that is uniquely our own. As physicians who have devoted their careers to sports medicine, we can honestly say that in the last 20 years we have witnessed the dawning of a new day for female athletes. A new era that is not just filled with new laws and new opportunity, but with the sound we love the most: the wonderful cacophony of young girls on the playground, running, jumping, kicking, swinging, and having fun, just like all of the other kids.

We reject the notion that women in professional sports must ultimately be judged on whether or not they can compete either physically or economically with men. To begin with, there is no question that most women are not physically equipped to participate in full contact sports, such as football and boxing and let's face it, that is where the real money is. We can see no change in this situation anywhere on the current horizon.

Women versus men competitions, even well meaning contests in tennis and golf, are cheap theatrics and ultimately demean the participants. In the final analysis, only the vast American market, with its impersonal forces and its immutable laws of survival, will determine what sports and what athletes the public will pay to see perform, not legislation or philosophical debate. Let women be women, and everything else will sort itself out as the sports themselves, as well as the athletes and our society evolve over time.

Women can play the game! And now they must be encouraged at every level to get involved and to learn at an early age the importance of physical fitness and its vital connection to enjoying life to the fullest. Obese young girls often turn into obese adults, with accompanying physical and psychological problems, and every school in the nation must now target obesity with the same intensity of purpose that accompanied historic national efforts to eradicate childhood diseases.

At the opposite end of the food abuse scale are the widespread pandemics of eating disorders, now reaching unprecedented levels of affliction. Coaches and trainers in relevant sports, such as gymnastics and track and field, must become proactive in screening their teams for problems related to anorexia and bulimia. They must work with parents and primary care physicians and orthopaedic surgeons to intervene early in the development of the problem to prevent the real danger of life threatening situations.

These problems and many others are covered in depth in *The Female Athlete*. And of course, we want to thank all of the contributors to this volume for their hard work and their insights into the problems facing the female athlete today. We and the contributors share a common goal: to support and encourage the development of women in sports. We may disagree from time to time about the medicine or the politics, but we must all stand aside as this great movement continues to swell and gather speed and moves across the country, sweeping aside all the doubts, the derision, and the ideological demagoguery that leaves the air crystal clear and singing. Women can play the game!

Mary Lloyd Ireland, M.D.
Aurelia Nattiv, M.D.

781

Index

Note: Page numbers followed by f indicate figures; those followed by t indicate tables.